1. Loyalty
2. Helping others
3. determination / hope

everything that's
meant to be will
be

happens for
a reason

484
752
3702

The Professional Medical Assistant

An Integrative, Teamwork-Based Approach

The Professional Medical Assistant

An Integrative, Teamwork-Based Approach

Sharon Eagle, RN, MSN
Former Director, Medical Assisting Program
Wenatchee Valley College
Wenatchee, WA

Cindi Brassington, MS, CMA (AAMA)
Professor of Allied Health
Quinebaug Valley Community College
Danielson, CT

Candy Dailey, RN, MSN, CMA (AAMA)
Instructor, Medical Assistant Program Director, Health Occupations Instructor
Nicolet Area Community College
Rhinelander, WI

Cheri Goretti, MA, MT (ASCP), CMA (AAMA)
Professor and Medical Assisting Program Director
Quinebaug Valley Community College
Danielson, CT

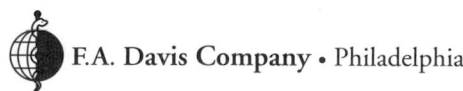

F.A. Davis Company • Philadelphia

F. A. Davis Company
1915 Arch Street
Philadelphia, PA 19103
www.fadavis.com

Printed in the United States of America

Last digit indicates print number: 10 9 8 7 6 5 4 3 2 1

Senior Acquisitions Editor: Andy McPhee
Manager of Content Development: George W. Lang
Developmental Editor: Brenna H. Mayer
Art and Design Manager: Carolyn O'Brien

As new scientific information becomes available through basic and clinical research, recommended treatments and drug therapies undergo changes. The author(s) and publisher have done everything possible to make this book accurate, up-to-date, and in accord with accepted standards at the time of publication. The author(s), editors, and publisher are not responsible for errors or omissions or for consequences from application of the book, and make no warranty, expressed or implied, in regard to the contents of the book. Any practice described in this book should be applied by the reader in accordance with professional standards of care used in regard to the unique circumstances that may apply in each situation. The reader is advised always to check product information (package inserts) for changes and new information regarding dose and contraindications before administering any drug. Caution is especially urged when using new or infrequently ordered drugs.

Library of Congress Cataloging-in-Publication Data
The professional medical assistant: an integrative, teamwork-based approach / Sharon Eagle ... [et al.].
    p. ; cm.
  Includes index.
  ISBN-13: 978-0-8036-1668-4
  ISBN-10: 0-8036-1668-6
  1. Physicians' assistants. I. Eagle, Sharon.
  [DNLM: 1. Physician Assistants. 2. Clinical Competence. 3. Patient Care Team. W 21.5 P9635 2009]
  R697.P45P76 2009
  610.73'72069—dc22

                                                                              2009002947

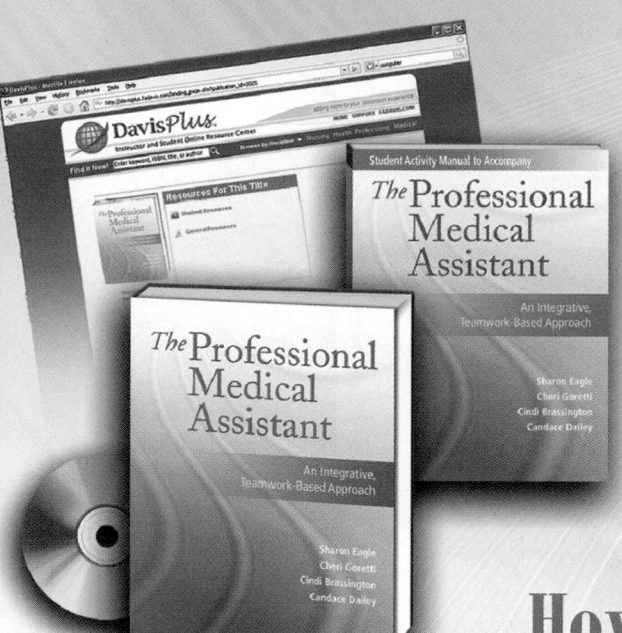

Success from Front to Back!

From front to back, **The Professional Medical Assistant** meets every need with a **unique approach** to administrative and clinical skills that truly reflects the real world in which MAs practice.

How it Works...

The Complete MA Package –

Text, Activity Manual, CD-ROM, and Online Resources!

✓ **Promotes critical thinking and problem solving.**

✓ **Features a step-by-step, chapter-by-chapter, body systems approach.**

✓ **Addresses structure and function and medical terminology.**

✓ **Includes lifespan coverage with chapters on pediatrics and geriatrics.**

✓ **Offers full chapters covering bioethics, legal issues, HIPAA, and patient rights.**

✓ **Highlights the importance of accurate documentation.**

✓ **Provides ICD-9 codes for quick reference.**

❶ Integrated Approach

Prepares students for all aspects of the front and back office.

❸ Multiple Learning Styles

Reflects all the various ways students learn and instructors teach.

❷ Teamwork Building

Provides problem-solving and team-building activities for a variety of scenarios.

Front office–Back office connection

Caring for stroke victims

Patients who suffer from stroke and other neurological injuries receive their early care in the hospital. However, those who recover will return to the medical office for follow-up care. Many of them may be struggling with some residual neurological deficit that impacts their ability to move, process information, respond, and speak. Therefore, medical assistants must remember to be patient, speak clearly, and allow such patients ample time to respond.

Team Work Exercises

1. Teams will select or be assigned one of the following assignments.

   ● Research about the Mini Mental State Examination. Return to class with the following information prepared:

   a. purpose of the tool

   b. type of clients most commonly evaluated with this tool

   c. how the results are scored

   d. implications of low scores

   e. a role-play scenario in which the medical assistant evaluates the patient using the tool.

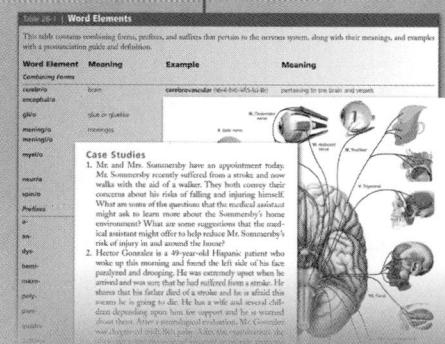

Designed for Success

The Professional Medical Assistant

An Integrative, Teamwork-Based Approach

Sharon Eagle
Cheri Goretti
Cindi Brassington
Candace Dailey

CHAPTER 26

Neurology

An easy-to-read writing style directly addresses what **MAs** need to know.

Learning Objectives
Upon completion of this chapter, the student will be able to:
- identify key structures of the neurological system
- discuss the roles played by the neurological system
- define and spell terms related to neurology
- describe the role of the medical assistant in the neurologist's office
- identify common neurological diseases and disorders
- list commonly used word elements related to the neurological system
- give at least 10 examples of how new neurological related terms may be created by combining prefixes, suffixes, and combining forms
- describe the medical assistant's role in assisting with neurological procedures
- describe physical examination techniques used to evaluate the neurological system.

CAAHEP Competencies
Clinical Competencies
Patient Care
Prepare patients for and assist with routine and specialty examination
Prepare patients for and assist with procedures, treatments, and minor office surgery
General Competencies
Legal Concepts
Document appropriately

Patient Instruction
Instruct individuals according to their needs

ABHES Competencies
Communication
Use appropriate medical terminology
Administrative Duties
Perform diagnostic coding
Clinical Duties
Prepare patients for procedures
Prepare patient for and assist physician with routine and specialty examinations and treatments and minor office surgeries
Collect and process specimens
Perform immunology testing
Instruction
Teach patients methods of health promotion and disease prevention
Procedures
Assisting with a neurological examination
Assisting with lumbar puncture

Chapter Outline
Structures and Functions of the Nervous System
Structures of the Nervous System
Neuron
Central nervous system
Peripheral nervous system

and Disorders
Disorders of the Central Nervous System
Stroke
Transient ischemic attack
Migraine headache
Epilepsy
Encephalitis
Meningitis
Traumatic brain injury
Spinal cord injury
Parkinson disease
Multiple sclerosis
Brain tumor
Amyotrophic lateral sclerosis
Bell palsy
Peripheral neuropathy
Carpal tunnel syndrome
Spinal stenosis
Neurology Procedures
Assisting with Examination
Nervous System Tests
Electroencephalography
Lumbar puncture
Computed tomography
Magnetic resonance imaging
Chapter Summary
Team Work Exercises
Case Studies
Resources

Learning Objectives and **CAAHEP** and **ABHES Competencies** clearly define the knowledge, skills, and procedures to be mastered upon completion of the chapter.

Key Terms with definitions are cited at the beginning of each chapter.

Key Terms
affect
Emotional state or mood
aura
Subjective sensation that occurs prior to and signals the onset of a migraine headache or a seizure
bradykinesia
Extreme slowness in movement
Brudzinski sign
Patient response in which neck flexion causes flexion of the hips when the patient is lying in a supine position
central nervous system
Nerve tissue that comprises the brain and spinal cord
cerebral concussion
Brief loss of consciousness or brief episode of disorientation or confusion following

fibrillation
Spontaneous muscle contraction or quivering
homeostasis
State of equilibrium in the body
Kernig sign
Reflexive hamstring contraction and pain when attempting to extend the leg after flexing the hip
motor nerves
Nerves involved in movement
myelin
Layer of phospholipids and protein that forms the myelin sheath of neurons and acts as electrical insulation
neuron
Nerve cell
neurotransmitter
Chemical that plays an important role in nerve impulse transmission
nuchal rigidity
Condition that involves pain and stiffness of the neck and a resulting reluctance to flex the head forward
paresthesia
Abnormal sensation
peripheral nervous system
Portion of the nervous system outside the central nervous system that conveys sensory and motor impulses
sensory nerves
Nerves that convey sensory information
spinal fusion
Surgical immobilization of adjacent vertebrae
thrombotic
Caused by a blood clot
transection
Cutting

Structures and Functions of the Nervous System

The nervous system
ostasis, the
ronment of
computer,
amounts of
messages th

Structure
An understanding of the nervous system m
most essential element, the neuron. While th
functions as an integrated system, it is more e
when divided into its two major parts: the
system (CNS) and the peripheral nervous sys

Neuron
A neuron includes a cell body, dendrites, and axon. The cell
body houses the nucleus and organelles, which are a variety
of specialized structures within the cell. Dendrites resemble
branches coming off of the cell body, much like the branches
of a tree. The axons of a neuron are as short as a few millimeters or as long as a meter. They are cordlike projections
that are sometimes covered in a myelin sheath made up of a
specialized layer of cells. (See Figure 26-1.) Neuron cell
bodies grouped together form gray matter. Axons bundled
together form white matter, named for the whitish hue of
the myelin sheaths. Within the PNS, bundles of axons are
called *nerves*.

Crystal-clear, full-color illustrations make basic and advanced concepts easy to understand and easy to follow.

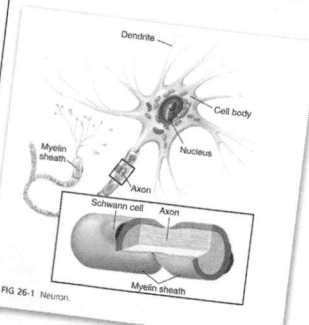

FIG 26-1 Neuron.

Neurology Procedures

Neurology is a medical specialty that focuses on the study and treatment of diseases and disorders of the nervous system. A physician who specializes in this area of medicine is a neurologist.

Assisting with Examination
The medical assistant must prepare the patient for neurological evaluation by first checking vital signs and updating
health history, including data regarding medications, allergies, family history, and recent symptoms of concern to the
patient. In addition, the medical assistant should pay special
attention to subtle clues about neurological functioning and
possible deficits. While it is the neurologist's role to conduct
a thorough neurological evaluation, any significant observations made by the medical assistant might help the physician
identify issues of special concern. Thus, the medical assistant
should note the patient's general appearance, hygiene, dress,
and **affect**, which is the emotional reaction, associated with
an experience (also called *mood*). She should note whether
the patient understands and responds appropriately to questions and commands, as well as any difficulty with short-
term memory and disturbances in gait, movement, strength,
coordination, or speech. She should then assist the patient as
needed with undressing and positioning and also assist the
neurologist as needed with the examination and any procedures. (See *Procedure 26-1: Assisting with a neurological
examination*, page xxx.)

Nervous System Tests
The medical assistant working in the neurology department
may help with patient evaluations by conducting or assisting
with a variety of diagnostic procedures. Each of these procedures helps to evaluate the patient's condition and to gather
data necessary for the diagnosing and treatment of neurological disorders.

Electroencephalography
Electroencephalography is the process of amplifying,
recording, and analyzing the electrical activity of the brain.
The printed record obtained is called an electroencephalogram (EEG). A variety of electrodes are placed at specific
sites on the patient's scalp. (See Figure 26-13.) The

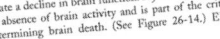

FIG 26-13 Patient undergoing EEG testing.

causes waveform changes. For example, *delta waves* are slow,
irregular waves normally found only in infants, small children, and sleeping adults. They are an abnormal finding in
wakeful adults. *Theta waves* are slow, regular waves that indicate a decline in brain function. A *flatline* EEG indicates
an absence of brain activity and is part of the criteria for
determining brain death. (See Figure 26-14.) EEG has

Alpha: Relaxed
Beta: Alert
Theta: Drowsy
Delta: Sleeping

1 sec

FIG 26-14 EEG wave patterns.

Migraine Headache
ICD-9-CM code: 346.9 (unspecified)
Migraine headaches are a familial disorder marked by
episodes of severe throbbing headache that is commonly
unilateral and sometimes disabling. They affect more than
28 million Americans and are three times more common in
women than in men.

The cause of migraine headaches is not fully understood,
although they tend to run in families, are worse early in life,
and generally improve in later years. Current theories about
causes include involvement of the trigeminal nerve, imbalances in such chemicals as serotonin, and vascular dilation
and inflammation. Many risk factors and potential triggers
have also been identified, including hormonal changes and

Diseases and disorders include **ICD-9 Codes** for quick reference and emphasize integration of the front and back office.

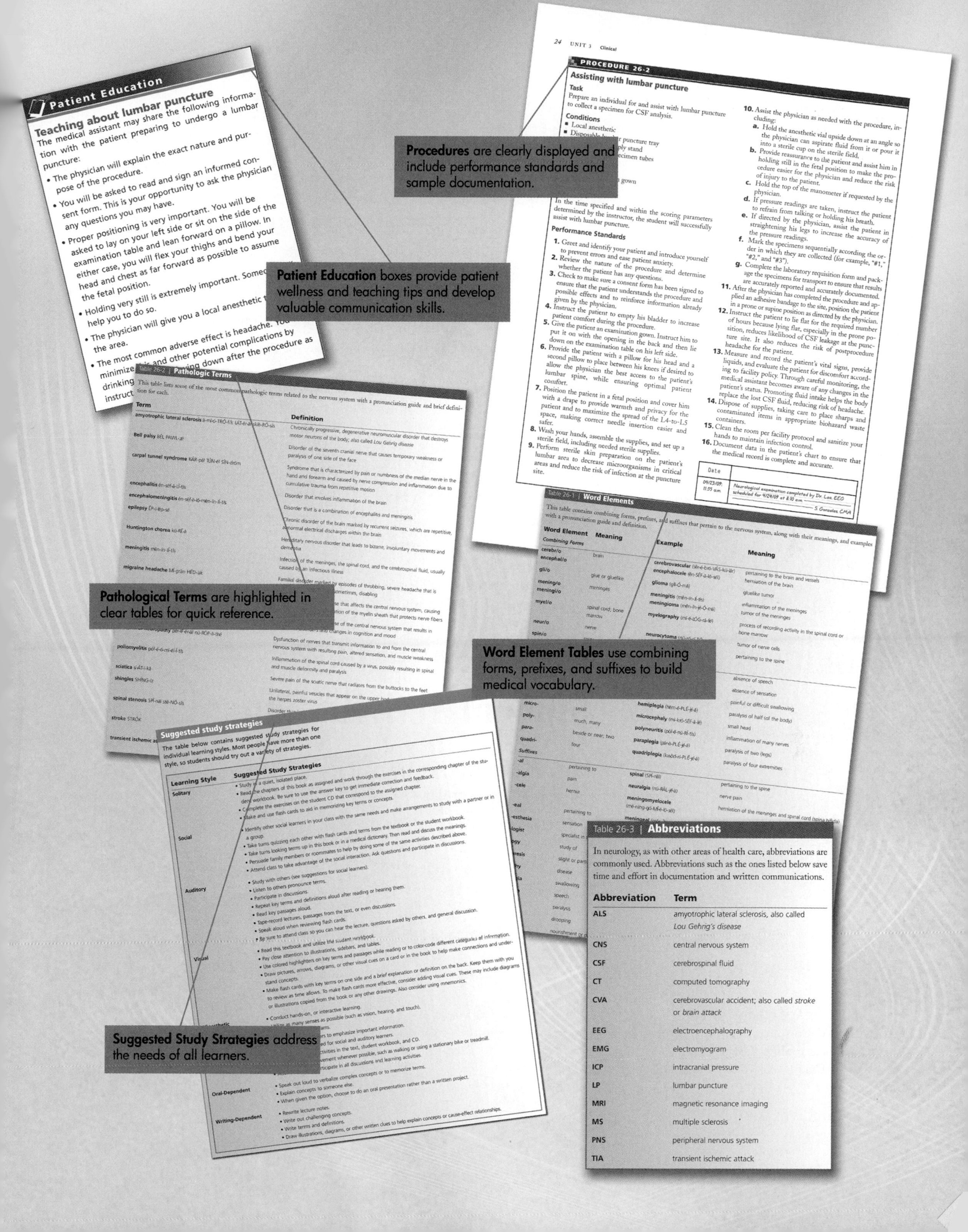

Patient Education

Teaching about lumbar puncture

The medical assistant may share the following information with the patient preparing to undergo a lumbar puncture:

- The physician will explain the exact nature and purpose of the procedure.
- You will be asked to read and sign an informed consent form. This is your opportunity to ask the physician any questions you may have.
- Proper positioning is very important. You will be asked to lay on your left side or sit on the side of the examination table and lean forward on a pillow. In either case, you will flex your thighs and bend your head and chest as far forward as possible to assume the fetal position.
- Holding very still is extremely important. Someone help you to do so.
- The physician will give you a local anesthetic the area.
- The most common adverse effect is headache. You minimize this and other potential complications by drinking after the procedure as instruct

Procedures are clearly displayed and include performance standards and sample documentation.

Patient Education boxes provide patient wellness and teaching tips and develop valuable communication skills.

Pathological Terms are highlighted in clear tables for quick reference.

Word Element Tables use combining forms, prefixes, and suffixes to build medical vocabulary.

Suggested Study Strategies address the needs of all learners.

---

24   UNIT 3   Clinical

PROCEDURE 26-2

Assisting with lumbar puncture

Task
Prepare an individual for and assist with lumbar puncture to collect a specimen for CSF analysis.

Conditions
- Local anesthetic
- Disposable lumbar puncture tray
- ply stand
- specimen tubes
- gown

In the time specified and within the scoring parameters determined by the instructor, the student will successfully assist with lumbar puncture.

Performance Standards

1. Greet and identify your patient and introduce yourself to prevent errors and ease patient anxiety.
2. Review the nature of the procedure and determine whether the patient has any questions.
3. Check to make sure a consent form has been signed to ensure that the patient understands the procedure and possible effects and to reinforce information already given by the physician.
4. Instruct the patient to empty his bladder to increase patient comfort during the procedure.
5. Give the patient an examination gown. Instruct him to put it on with the opening in the back and then lie down on the examination table on his left side.
6. Provide the patient with a pillow for his head and a second pillow to place between his knees if desired to allow the physician the best access to the patient's lumbar spine, while ensuring optimal patient comfort.
7. Position the patient in a fetal position and cover him with a drape to provide warmth and privacy for the patient and to maximize the spread of the L4-to-L5 space, making correct needle insertion easier and safer.
8. Wash your hands, assemble the supplies, and set up a sterile field, including needed sterile supplies.
9. Perform sterile skin preparation on the patient's lumbar area to decrease microorganisms in critical areas and reduce the risk of infection at the puncture site.

10. Assist the physician as needed with the procedure, including:
    a. Hold the anesthetic vial upside down at an angle so the physician can aspirate fluid from it or pour it into a sterile cup on the sterile field.
    b. Provide reassurance to the patient and assist him in holding still in the fetal position to make the procedure easier for the physician and reduce the risk of injury to the patient.
    c. Hold the top of the manometer if requested by the physician.
    d. If pressure readings are taken, instruct the patient to refrain from talking or holding his breath.
    e. If directed by the physician, assist the patient in straightening his legs to increase the accuracy of the pressure readings.
    f. Mark the specimens sequentially according the order in which they are collected (for example, "#1," "#2," and "#3").
    g. Complete the laboratory requisition form and package the specimens for transport to ensure that results are accurately reported and accurately documented.
11. After the physician has completed the procedure and applied an adhesive bandage to the site, position the patient in a prone or supine position as directed by the physician.
12. Instruct the patient to lie flat for the required number of hours because lying flat, especially in the prone position, reduces likelihood of CSF leakage at the puncture site. It also reduces the risk of postprocedure headache for the patient.
13. Measure and record the patient's vital signs, provide liquids, and evaluate the patient for discomfort according to facility policy. Through careful monitoring, the medical assistant becomes aware of any changes in the patient's status. Promoting fluid intake helps the body replace the lost CSF fluid, reducing risk of headache.
14. Dispose of supplies, taking care to place sharps and contaminated items in appropriate biohazard waste containers.
15. Clean the room per facility protocol and sanitize your hands to maintain infection control.
16. Document data in the patient's chart to ensure that the medical record is complete and accurate.

Date	
09/23/09 11:55 a.m.	Neurological examination completed by Dr. Lee. EEG scheduled for 9/24/09 at 8:30 a.m. ———————— S. Gonzales, CMA

Table 26-2 | **Pathologic Terms**

This table lists some of the most common pathologic terms related to the nervous system with a pronunciation guide and brief definition for each.

Term	Definition
amyotrophic lateral sclerosis a-mīo-TRŌ-fĭk LAT-ĕr-ăl-sklĕ-RŌ-sĭs	Chronically progressive, degenerative neuromuscular disorder that destroys motor neurons of the body; also called Lou Gehrig disease
Bell palsy BĔL PAWL-zē	Disorder of the seventh cranial nerve that causes temporary weakness or paralysis of one side of the face
carpal tunnel syndrome KAR-păl TŬN-ĕl SĬN-drōm	Syndrome that is characterized by pain or numbness of the median nerve in the hand and forearm and caused by nerve compression and inflammation due to cumulative trauma from repetitive motion
encephalitis ĕn-sĕf-ă-LĪ-tĭs	Disorder that involves inflammation of the brain
encephalomeningitis ĕn-sĕf-ă-lō-mĕn-ĭn-JĪ-tĭs	Disorder that is a combination of encephalitis and meningitis
epilepsy ĔP-ĭ-lĕp-sē	Chronic disorder of the brain marked by recurrent seizures, which are repetitive, abnormal electrical discharges within the brain
Huntington chorea kō-RĒ-ă	Hereditary nervous disorder that leads to bizarre, involuntary movements and dementia
meningitis mĕn-ĭn-JĪ-tĭs	Infection of the meninges, the spinal cord, and the cerebrospinal fluid, usually caused by an infectious illness
migraine headache MĪ-grān HĔD-āk	Familial disorder marked by episodes of throbbing, severe headache that is sometimes, disabling
	se that affects the central nervous system, causing tion of the myelin sheath that protects nerve fibers
neuropathy pŏ-ik-ē-ăl nŏ-ROP-ă-thē	se of the central nervous system that results in and changes in cognition and mood
poliomyelitis pŏl-ē-ŏ-mī-ĕl-Ī-tĭs	Dysfunction of nerves that transmit information to and from the central nervous system with resulting pain, altered sensation, and muscle weakness
sciatica sī-AT-ĭ-kă	Inflammation of the spinal cord caused by a virus, possibly resulting in spinal and muscle deformity and paralysis
shingles SHĬNG-lz	Severe pain of the sciatic nerve that radiates from the buttocks to the feet
spinal stenosis SPĪ-năl stĕ-NŌ-sĭs	Unilateral, painful vesicles that appear on the upper body herpes zoster virus
stroke STRŌK	Disorder in
transient ischemic a	

Table 26-1 | **Word Elements**

This table contains combining forms, prefixes, and suffixes that pertain to the nervous system, along with their meanings, and examples with a pronunciation guide and definition.

Word Element Combining Forms	Meaning	Example	Meaning
cerebr/o	brain	cerebrovascular (sĕr-ē-brō-VĂS-kū-lĕr)	pertaining to the brain and vessels
encephal/o		encephalocele (ĕn-SĔF-ă-lō-sēl)	herniation of the brain
gli/o	glue or gluelike	glioma (glĭ-Ō-mă)	gluelike tumor
mening/o	meninges	meningitis (mĕn-ĭn-JĪ-tĭs)	inflammation of the meninges
meningi/o		meningioma (mĕn-ĭn-jē-Ō-mă)	tumor of the meninges
myel/o	spinal cord; bone marrow	myelography (mī-ĕ-lŎG-ră-fē)	process of recording activity in the spinal cord or bone marrow
neur/o	nerve	neurocytoma (nū	tumor of nerve cells
spin/o			pertaining to the spine
micro-	small	hemiplegia (hem-ē-PLE-jē-ă)	absence of speech
poly-	much, many	microcephaly (mī-krō-SĔF-ă-lē)	absence of sensation
para-	beside or near; two	polyneuritis (pŏl-ē-nū-RĪ-tĭs)	painful or difficult swallowing
quadri-	four	paraplegia (păr-ă-PLĒ-jē-ă)	paralysis of half (of the body)
Suffixes		quadriplegia (kwŏd-rĭ-PLĒ-jē-ă)	small head
-al	pertaining to	spinal (SPĪ-năl)	inflammation of many nerves
-algia	pain		paralysis of two (legs)
-cele		neuralgia (nū-RĂL-jē-ă)	paralysis of four extremities
	hernia	meningomyelocele (mē-nĭng-gō-MĪ-ĕ-lō-sēl)	pertaining to the spine
-eal	pertaining to	meningeal	nerve pain
-esthesia	sensation		herniation of the meninges and spinal cord
-logist	specialist in		
-opy	study of		
-sis	slight or part		
	disease		
	swallowing		
	speech		
	paralysis		
	drooping		
	nourishment		

Suggested study strategies

The table below contains suggested study strategies for individual learning styles. Most people have more than one style, so students should try out a variety of strategies.

Learning Style	Suggested Study Strategies
Solitary	• Study in a quiet, isolated place. • Read the chapters of this book as assigned and work through the exercises in the corresponding chapter of the student workbook. Be sure to use the answer key to get immediate correction and feedback. • Complete the exercises on the student CD that correspond to the assigned chapter. • Make and use flash cards to aid in memorizing key terms or concepts.
Social	• Identify other social learners in your class with flash cards and terms from the textbook or the student workbook. Make arrangements to study with a partner or in a group. • Take turns quizzing each other with flash cards and terms in a medical dictionary. Then read and discuss the meanings. • Persuade family members or roommates to help by doing some of the same activities described above. • Attend class to take advantage of the social interaction. Ask questions and participate in discussions.
Auditory	• Study with others (see suggestions for social learners). • Listen to others pronounce terms. • Participate in discussions. • Repeat key terms and definitions aloud after reading or hearing them. • Read key passages aloud. • Tape-record lectures, passages from the text, or even discussions. • Speak aloud when reviewing flash cards. • Be sure to attend class so you can hear the lecture, questions asked by others, and general discussion.
Visual	• Read this textbook and utilize the student workbook. • Pay close attention to illustrations, sidebars, and tables. • Use colored highlighters while reading or to color-code different categories of information. • Draw pictures, arrows, diagrams, or other visual cues on a card or in the book to help make connections and understand concepts. • Make flash cards with key terms on one side and a brief explanation or definition on the back. Keep them with you to review as time allows. To make flash cards more effective, consider adding visual cues. These may include diagrams or illustrations copied from the book or any other drawings. Also consider using mnemonics.
Kinesthetic	• Conduct hands-on, or interactive learning. • utilize as many senses as possible (such as vision, hearing, and touch). • ams. • ed to emphasize important information. • ed for social and auditory learners, and CD. • activities in the text, student workbook, and CD. • movement whenever possible, such as walking or using a stationary bike or treadmill. • participate in all discussions and learning activities.
Oral-Dependent	• Speak out loud to verbalize complex concepts or to memorize terms. • Explain concepts to someone else. • When given the option, choose to do an oral presentation rather than a written project.
Writing-Dependent	• Rewrite lecture notes. • Write out challenging concepts. • Write terms and definitions. • Draw illustrations, diagrams, or other written clues to help explain concepts or cause-effect relationships.

Table 26-3 | **Abbreviations**

In neurology, as with other areas of health care, abbreviations are commonly used. Abbreviations such as the ones listed below save time and effort in documentation and written communications.

Abbreviation	Term
ALS	amyotrophic lateral sclerosis, also called Lou Gehrig's disease
CNS	central nervous system
CSF	cerebrospinal fluid
CT	computed tomography
CVA	cerebrovascular accident; also called stroke or brain attack
EEG	electroencephalography
EMG	electromyogram
ICP	intracranial pressure
LP	lumbar puncture
MRI	magnetic resonance imaging
MS	multiple sclerosis
PNS	peripheral nervous system
TIA	transient ischemic attack

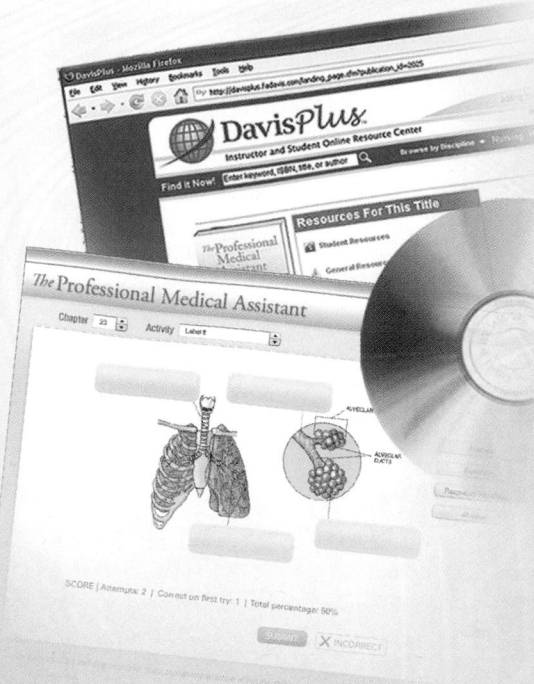
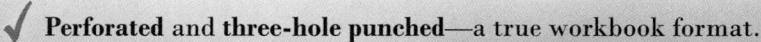
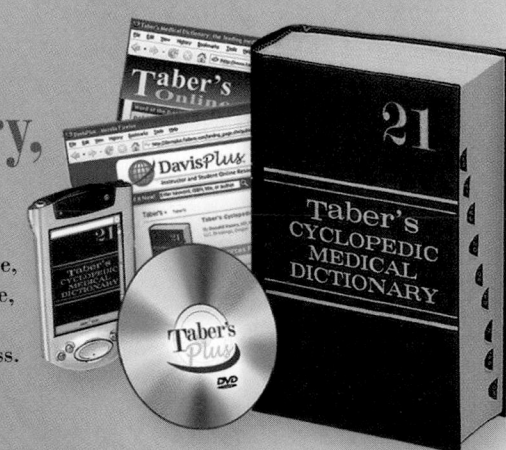

Dedication

Thanks to my children Brad, Brian, and Nicole for your love and encouragement; to my daughters-in-law and son-in-law, Melissa, Sayo, and Adam for loving my children and for your patience with their mother; to my grandsons Gabe, Seth, and Isaac for enriching our family in such an amazing way; to my siblings, Rob, Steph, Rick, Roger, and Troy, though some of us are miles apart, we are always close in spirit; to my mother Durmma, for your unfailing love and support; and to my cowriters, Cindi, Cheri, and Candy, your support, commitment, work ethic, warmth, humor, and friendship have made this an awesome journey.—SE

Thanks to my husband Gary for your help with orthopedics, acupuncture, and "does this sound right?" Sadie and Hannah, my ever-understanding daughters for cooking, cleaning, doing laundry, and taking care of Mom through this project, I love you all.—CB

Thank you to my loving, supportive parents, Bill and Mary Jane Schultz, who taught me the importance of hard work and education; my husband, Bucky, who inspires me every day; my children, Bill, Deuce, Matthew, and Elizabeth, and siblings, Kirby, Brian, and Stephanie, for strength in family; my incredible repertoire of colleagues and friends who encourage and rejuvenate me with every conversation—Becki, Dr. Nick, Ann, Connie, Shelly, Julie, Deb, Nancy, Holly, Tracey, the Wisconsin Medical Assistant Educators Group, the Dream Team, and my Lake Lucerne family.—CD

Thanks to Dean Huard and President Williams for the support you gave me throughout this project as well as all of the students who have touched my life and have, in their own way, contributed to this book. To the Dream Team, I enjoyed sharing this journey with a group of fabulous individuals and I value your friendship immensely. Lastly, to my family, John, Lynn, and Jill, for your understanding, patience, and help while I spent countless hours working on the book. This is for you, and I love you all!—CG

Preface

The profession of medical assisting has evolved dramatically since its inception more than 50 years ago. Expectations placed on medical assistants continue to increase. Individuals entering and working in this dynamic field are challenged more than ever before to meet the demands of the profession and evolve with it. Developing a sound knowledge base is mandatory. Maintaining currency in knowledge and skills is crucial. Demonstrating flexibility on the job is critical. Working effectively and efficiently as team members is of the utmost importance. Those characteristics, so essential to the profession and so highly valued by employers, are the pervasive themes of this text.

Our Approach

By integrating the content, focusing on building teamwork skills, and providing opportunities for students of all learning styles, *The Professional Medical Assistant: An Integrative, Teamwork-Based Approach* helps learners move from novice students to competent professionals.

Integrated Content

We have chosen to present this text as a unified whole to allow students to learn within the full context of medical assisting practice. Other comprehensive textbooks present sterile divisions between general, administrative, and clinical units. To divide the content in such a manner emphasizes the disconnect that already exists between the front and back office. In truth, neither can survive without the other, and both areas thrive when all individuals make the same commitment to work together as a team.

Keeping the text unified has allowed us to present content the way most instructors present it in class—by making full use of teachable moments, the times when an individual is particularly responsive to learning something new. Rather than presenting, say, medical coding content solely in the administrative section of the book, we also present it at opportune moments in the clinical section, listing pertinent ICD-9-CM codes, for instance, at the beginning of each discussion of a disease. Rather than covering patient education solely in the clinical section, we also present it at appropriate times in the administrative section. We chose this integrated approach because

that's the way faculty teach, students learn, and medical assistants practice.

Teamwork

Health care employers highly prize medical assistants who demonstrate the ability to work well with others as effective members of the health care team. The importance of teamwork is emphasized throughout this book in the written text, sidebars, and activities. Special recurring sidebars clarify the connections between the front and back office by pointing out how team members from different areas of the medical office can work together in a cooperative, efficient manner.

Activities in the text and workbook provide opportunities for students to practice and develop the skills necessary for good teamwork, especially communication and active problem-solving. These activities help students adopt and maintain a flexible attitude, demonstrated by a willingness to help meet the needs of patients, coworkers, and supervisors. By emphasizing skill maintenance and flexibility, this text encourages students to avoid restricting themselves to one narrow area of comfort. Rather, it urges them to become diverse and proficient in all areas of knowledge and skill and carry this commitment beyond graduation into the workplace for the duration of their careers. By committing themselves to lifelong learning and skill maintenance, they will find themselves among the most valued and respected members of the health care team, regardless of where they choose to work.

Multiple Learning Styles

We have embedded within the textbook, workbook, and student and instructor ancillaries a wide variety of exercises and activities to help meet the learning needs of all students. The first chapter introduces learning styles and helps students choose the most effective study techniques for them, such as study groups vs. solitary study or tape recording lectures. By addressing learning styles clearly and uniformly, we aim to enhance the entire learning experience for students and teaching experience for faculty.

Competency Development

This comprehensive text covers a wide range of topics in medical assisting theory and clinical competency, or skill. It supports competency acquisition by providing clear, thorough explanations within the text, detailed step-by-step procedures, and full-color photos and illustrations that show how to perform the necessary competencies. Procedures within this text are written in a student-friendly, step-by-step format so that students can easily refer to them as they learn and practice. Rationales are also included within the procedures to help students understand the reason for certain steps to help them become more than mere technicians and begin to function as knowledgeable professionals.

The Instructor's Resource Disk (IRD) contains in-depth procedure checklists, and the student disk offers fun animations and interactive activities, also available on the DavisPlus website (www.davisplus.fadavis.com). All activities support learning, review, repetition, and competency in all requirements.

Demonstration of competency is an important part of the learning process and is the gold standard for verifying a student's ability. It also provides critical data for program evaluation and maintenance of accreditation. To address the need for such verification, the text clearly identifies competencies specifically required by the Commission on Accreditation of Allied Health Programs (CAAHEP) and the Accrediting Bureau of Health Education Schools (ABHES). It also includes additional competencies common to the health care setting. Competencies are addressed in most of chapters of this text as appropriate to the subject matter. The instructor can easily locate each competency by referring to the Index of Competencies in Appendix C. In addition, the IRD contains information to help instructors evaluate student competence.

Gender References

We recognize and welcome the increasing number of men entering the profession of medical assisting. We desire to treat all individuals referenced in this text with the courtesy and respect they deserve but find it awkward and cumbersome to consistently use gender-neutral references. Therefore, because the vast majority of individuals within this profession are female, this text refers to students and medical assistants as female. It refers to physicians alternately as male or female because recent data indicate that nearly one-half of those currently graduating from medical school are female. It also alternates references to patients as male or female, with preference shown only when discussing disorders or situations that overwhelmingly apply to one sex more than the other.

Features

Content within this text is organized according to general, administrative, and clinical subject areas. The user-friendly writing style engages the learner and explains the subject matter in a manner that is clear and simple, but sufficiently detailed to inform without overwhelming. Numerous features of the text are designed to enhance student learning.

Reference Lists

Each chapter includes several reference lists that indicate the information addressed in the chapter, including:

- clear learning objectives that indicate what the student should learn from reading the chapter
- key competencies addressed in the chapter for the Committee on Accreditation of Allied Health Programs (CAAHEP) and the Accrediting Bureau of Health Education Schools (ABHES)
- list of procedures included in the chapter
- chapter outline
- table of key terms from the chapter along with brief definitions with the corresponding term in the text set in boldface to emphasize its importance.
- bulleted chapter summary located at the end of each chapter for a quick review of the chapter highlights
- resource list at the end of each chapter that provides students with sources of current information, including books, journals, and Internet sites and encourages students to expand their learning by conducting their own information search.

Body Systems and Specialties

Several chapters in the clinical unit address body system and specialty information. Key features of these chapters include:

- consistent organization of all body system chapters to clearly identify information on anatomy and physiology, medical terminology, and pathology, testing, and treatment
- information on structure and function for each body system to help students understand anatomy and physiology
- medical terminology related to body systems with an emphasis on relevant combining forms, abbreviations, and pathologic terms
- most common diseases and disorders seen by medical assistants for each body system along with the appropriate ICD-9-CM code used for each disorder
- discussion of the role of the medical assistant in each specialty, along with commentary about specialized diagnostic tests, procedures, and treatments.

Other Critical Information

In addition to comprehensive body system and specialty reviews, other chapters highlight critical information, including:

- *Chapter 1*, "Succeeding as a Student," sets the stage for success by helping students develop strategies for test-taking, anxiety reduction, and self-care.
- *Chapter 3*, "Professionalism," stresses issues so important to prospective employers, including dependability, flexibility, positive attitude, tact, appropriate appearance, and ability to function as a team player.

- *Chapter 7*, "HIPAA and a Patient's Rights," is devoted to information about a patient's rights and the role and responsibilities of the medical assistant in maintaining protected health and personal information without unnecessarily preventing patients from access to their medical records. In addition, it reviews the responsibilities of a HIPAA compliance officer.
- *Chapter 8*, "Bioethics," introduces students to ethical principles and philosophies and helps them better understand how they can identify and respond to ethical issues in the workplace.
- *Chapter 14*, "Medical Records Management," discusses electronic medical records and how personnel in the medical office can transition from paper-based medical records to electronic medical records.
- *Chapter 16*, "Coding and Insurance," introduces students to ICD-9-CM and CPT-4 coding. Examples and activities included help students gain competency. ICD-10 coding is also introduced.
- *Chapter 23*, "Essentials of Medical Terminology," introduces students to basic medical terminology, including key categories of medical word elements and the steps to medical term translation. A comprehensive list of prefixes and suffixes is provided. Organization of medical terminology content in this text introduces terminology to the novice or serves as a review for those who have already completed a medical terminology course.
- *Chapter 34*, "Geriatrics," describes the physiological changes caused by the aging process in each body system as well as diseases and disorders associated with aging. It also explores special needs of the geriatric population related to communication, safety, mobility, pain management, and end-of-life care.
- *Chapter 42*, "Hematology and Coagulation Procedures," *Chapter 43*, "Clinical Chemistry and Serological Procedures," and *Chapter 44*, "Urinalysis," include normal values for common laboratory tests.
- *Chapter 46*, "Bioemergency Response and Preparedness," addresses the medical assistant's role in responding to biological emergencies and pandemics.

Sidebars, Tables, and Procedures

In addition to the individual chapter features, all chapters include numerous sidebars, tables, and procedures that highlight important information or provide additional information on an important subject. These elements include:

- procedures written in a clear, step-by-step format with rationales provided in a different color to help students quickly grasp and understand *why* a step should be performed
- charting examples included for procedures that require documentation to help students begin to learn how to document care

- informational sidebars that highlight specific information and provide additional detail
- recurring *Front Office–Back Office Connection* sidebars that emphasize the critical nature of teamwork that must occur on an ongoing basis between administrative and clinical medical assistants as well as other members of the health care team
- recurring *Patient Education* sidebars strategically placed throughout the text that capitalize on the "teachable moments" that occur in relation to specific topics and address patient education in a way that is more specific and, therefore, more useful than a list of generic teaching tips placed at the end of a chapter
- numerous tables and colorful illustrations located throughout the text that clarify and emphasize specific information

Learning Activities

Two groups of learning activities at the end of each chapter challenge students to think critically and apply the information they have learned from the chapter. These activities include:

- team work exercises that allow students to work cooperatively as members of a group
- case studies that provide real-life scenarios, which require the student to problem-solve using the information supplied and the knowledge gleaned from the chapter.

Appendices

Also included are several key appendices that provide helpful information for using the book and enhancing student learning. Appendices include:

- complete glossary of key terms from the text
- key abbreviations from the text listed in table format
- index of all competencies included in the chapters as well as an indication of work product requirements for those competencies
- outlines of the content on the CAAHEP and ABHES certification examinations
- list of over 200 of the most commonly prescribed drugs, including generic and trade names.

Support Materials

Several additional resources are available that will enhance the instructor's and student's use of the textbook.

- **Instructor's Resource Disk** (IRD) helps instructors to administer examinations, design course content, provide student activities, and track student performance. Features include:
  - test bank with more than 1,500 multiple-choice test questions that require critical thinking as well as memory

recall, with each question categorized as *general, administrative,* or *clinical*

- function that enables the instructor to select questions from the test bank to create tests, including tests similar in format and subject matter to the certification examination
- chapter outlines to aid instructors in developing lecture notes
- sample syllabi for semester-based courses as well as module-based courses
- additional classroom activities not included in the text or student workbook
- detailed PowerPoint presentations for each chapter, including photos and illustrations from the text
- competency checklists in Microsoft Word format for each procedure included in the text so that instructors can print and use the checklists as they are designed or modify them as desired to meet individual program needs.

- **Student workbook** includes a variety of learning activities that incorporate various student learning styles. Activities include:

  - key term review
  - medical terminology review
  - chapter review
  - anatomy identification
  - disease or condition identification
  - competency checklists that correspond to each procedure within the text
  - office projects that require students to apply knowledge and skills learned from a chapter to the performance of specific activities for those chapters that do not contain formal procedures, including creating educational or informational bulletin boards, sponsoring blood pressure clinics within the community, and hosting guest speakers for the benefit of the class and entire student body
  - critical thinking exercises that require students to use the reasoning process, to apply what they have learned, and to work cooperatively together to solve problems, including case studies, research activities, and team work exercises.

- **Student Activity Disk** includes interactive, fun learning activities, including:

  - Match It Up
  - Categorize This!
  - Don't Tip the Scale!
  - What Is It?

  - Label It
  - Wheel of Terminology
  - Flash Cards
  - Multiple Choice
  - Fill It In.

- **DavisPlus website** includes additional learning activities and colorful animations designed specifically for medical assistant students as well as many others designed for all allied health students.

The complete *Professional Medical Assistant* package provides learners and educators with an exciting, comprehensive suite of information and activities. It provides learners with foundational information to launch their careers and guide them on their journey to becoming health care professionals. We have enjoyed the challenge and privilege of creating this comprehensive learning package. It is our hope that educators and students alike will find it equally enjoyable to use.

—Sharon Eagle
Cindi Brassington
Candy Dailey
Cheri Goretti

Contributors

The authors would like to acknowledge two individuals whose contributions to the text have ensured its quality and accuracy:

Wilbert S. Ching, BSMT, CPT (NPA)
Phlebotomy Instructor
Quinebaug Valley Community College
Program Coordinator and Instructor (Health Services)
American Red Cross of Central Massachusetts

Linda Howrey, EJD, CCS-P
Managing Partner, Howrey and Associates
Member, AHIMA President's Council in Physician Practice

Reviewers

Darlene Kaye Acton, CMA (AAMA)
Director
Medical Assisting Department
Alamance Community College
Graham, NC

Carole Berube, MA, MSN, BSN, RN
Professor Emerita in Nursing, Instructor in Health Sciences
Bristol Community College
Health Sciences
Fall River, MA

Kay E. Biggs, BS, CMA (AAMA)
Coordinator/Advisor Medical Assisting
Columbus State Community College
Medical Assisting
Gahanna, OH

Beth Anne Buchholz, CMA (AAMA)
Medical Assistant Program Director
Wichita Area Technical College
Health Sciences
Wichita, KS

Carmen Carpenter, RN, MS, CMA (AAMA)
Chair
Allied Health and Medical Assisting
South University
West Palm Beach, FL

Mary Ann Crandall, RN, BS, MS
Instructor
Extended Campus Programs
Southern Oregon University
Ashland, OR

Michael Lewis Decker, RMA
Instructor
Vatterott College
Medical Assistant Program
Omaha, NE

Linda Demain, LPN, BS in BQM & HRD
Medical Externship Advisor
Wichita Technique Institute
Mulvane, KS

Peter Doolin, MEd, MT (ASCP), RMA
Instructor, Medical Program
McFatter Technical Center
Davie, FL

Theresa Errante-Parrino, CMA (AAMA), EMTP, BMO, MEd
Medical Assisting Program Director
Indian River Community College
Fort Pierce, FL

Tracie Fuqua, B.S., CMA (AAMA)
Program Director, Medical Assisting
Wallace State Community College
Athens, AL

Anne D. Gailey, CMA (AAMA)
Certified Medical Assistant
Medical Assisting Instructor
Ogeechee Technical College
Medical Assisting Program
Allied Health Department
Statesboro, GA

Marcie C. Jones, CMA (AAMA), CLC
Medical Assisting Program Director
Gwinnett Technical College
Health Sciences and Personal Services
Lawrenceville, GA

V. Maloof, MD
Phlebotomy Program Director, Educator
Griffin Technical College
Medical and Public Services Department
Morrow, GA

Maureen Elizabeth Russell Messier, AS, BA, RMA, CMA (AAMA)
Instructor
Branford Hall Career Institute
Medical Assisting Department
Unionville, CT

Pat G. Moeck, PhD, MBA, BA, CMA (AAMA)
Director, Medical Assisting Program
El Centro College
Health and Legal Studies
Dallas, TX

Lisa Nagle, CMA (AAMA), BSEd
Program Director/Instructor, Medical Assisting Program
Augusta Technical College
Augusta, GA

Tracy Thomas, RMA
Instructor
St. Louis College of Health Careers
Medical Assistant Program
St. Louis, MO

Marilyn M. Turner, RN, CMA (AAMA)
Director
Medical Assisting Program
Ogeechee Technical College
Allied Health Department
Statesboro, GA

Karon G. Walton, CMA (AAMA)
Clinical Coordinator/Instructor
Augusta Technical College
Medical Assisting Program
Augusta, GA

Deborah L White, CMA (AAMA), MS
Program Coordinator
Trident Technical College
Medical Assisting Program
Charleston, SC

Danielle Schortzmann Wilken, MS, MT (ASCP)
Health Sciences Department Chair
Goodwin College
Avon, CT

Kari Williams, BS, DC
Program Director
Medical Office Technology
Front Range Community College
Longmont, CO

Acknowledgments

The authors would like to thank the F.A. Davis editorial and production team for their contribution to this project:

- Andy McPhee, *Acquisitions Editor,* who provided the perfect balance of guidance and support
- Margaret Biblis, *Publisher,* Health Professions and Medicine, whose "behind-the-scenes" support we have continually felt and appreciated
- Brenna Mayer, *Developmental Editor,* whose attention to detail, consistency, and quality have made this the high-quality text that it is.

In addition, we wish to acknowledge and thank these dedicated individuals who also helped in this publication:

- George W. Lang, *Manager of Content Development*
- Karen Carter, *Developmental Editor*
- Yvonne N. Gillam, *Associate Developmental Editor*
- Elizabeth Y. Stepchin, *Developmental Associate*
- Kimberly Harris, *Administrative Assistant*
- Stephanie A. Casey, *Administrative Assistant*
- Kirk Pedrick, *Electronic Product Development Manager, Electronic Publishing*
- Frank J. Musick, *Developmental Editor, Electronic Publishing*
- Carolyn O'Brien, *Design Manager*
- Kate Margeson, *Illustrations Coordinator*
- Robert Butler, *Production Manager*
- David Orzechowski, *Managing Editor*
- Virgil Lloyd, *Promotions Manager.*

Contents at a Glance

Contents

UNIT I

General-Transdisciplinary

Succeeding as a Student

Learning Objectives

Upon completion of this chapter, the student will be able to:

- define the key terms
- identify their learning style
- describe study strategies relevant to their learning style
- differentiate between visual, auditory, kinesthetic, solitary, and social learners
- describe symptoms of burnout
- discuss factors that contribute to burnout
- design and describe a self-care plan that will help prevent burnout.

CAAHEP Competencies

General Competencies

Patient Instruction

Instruct individuals according to their needs

ABHES Competencies

Instruction

Instruct patients with special needs

Teach patients methods of health promotion and disease prevention

Chapter Outline

The Journey Begins

Learning Styles

Solitary Learners

Social Learners

Auditory Learners

Visual Learners

Kinesthetic Learners

Oral-Dependent Learners

Writing-Dependent Learners

Test-Taking Strategies

Anxiety Reduction

Preparing for the examination

Just before the examination

During the examination

Practical Strategies

Self-Care

Body Mechanics

Safe Lifting

Chapter Summary

Team Work Exercises

Case Studies

Resources

Key Terms

body mechanics
The conscious coordination of the nervous and musculoskeletal systems to preserve and protect posture, balance, and body alignment while bending, lifting, and performing activities of daily living (ADLs)

burnout
Decreased physical, emotional, or mental energy secondary to ongoing intensive demands without sufficient physical or emotional rest

learning style
Manner in which a person most effectively learns

mnemonic
Technique used to enhance memory, such as creating a word from the first letters of a series of words

self-care
Activity that supports and nurtures an individual's physical, mental, spiritual, or emotional health and well-being

The Journey Begins

Medical assisting is an exciting and rewarding career. However, the journey for each individual really begins when she steps into the role of the student. Programs of medical assisting are designed to provide students with foundational knowledge in two general ways. The first building block of this foundation is through theory (lecture) classes, which provide information about everything from medical terminology, body structure and function, and pharmacology to medical office procedures, coding, and many other content areas. The second building block is through laboratory and clinical courses, which provide students with the opportunity to acquire skills though hands-on practice. Both areas provide students with a sound knowledge base and the administrative and clinical skills necessary for a successful career as a medical assistant.

Learning Styles

Embarking on this program of study requires a serious commitment of time, money, energy, and other resources. Therefore, students naturally wish to be as successful as possible in their endeavors. An important way a student can ensure her chance of success is by taking the time to determine her **learning style**. This information will then help her identify learning activities that will be most effective. All people have learning styles, but no two people are exactly alike. Understanding more about learning styles will aid students in choosing the most effective study techniques for them, such as study groups versus solitary study or tape recording lectures versus creating **mnemonics**, which are words created from the first letters of a series of words to help remember a concept. Most people are actually a combination of styles, but one tends to be dominant. The most common learning styles are:

- solitary
- social
- auditory
- visual
- kinesthetic. (See *Learning in practice.*)

Solitary Learners
Solitary learners usually prefer to study alone because they find the conversation of others to be distracting rather than helpful. They should spend the majority of their study time alone in a quiet place and may wish to avoid study groups.

Social Learners
Social learners are the opposite of solitary learners. They are easily distracted when trying to study alone and prefer to

Learning in Practice

As a student moves on to become a professional medical assistant, she must remember that her patients will each have their own learning styles, too. As she teaches them about medications, lifestyle modifications, or other health practices, she must utilize strategies that best help them learn, understand, and remember what she has taught. Because she will likely not have time to conduct an intensive evaluation of each patient's learning style, she must develop a teaching routine that appeals to as many styles as possible.

have company when studying. They find that discussion with others helps them to "think out loud," or process information to gain a deeper understanding. The exchange of ideas and hearing others verbalize concepts is very helpful to them.

Auditory Learners

Auditory learners need to hear the spoken word. When they try to read or study silently, their minds wander. Auditory input, even by means of talking to themselves, helps them process information and gain deeper understanding. Few people are strong auditory learners, yet nearly everyone has an auditory component to their learning style. Therefore, most individuals benefit from combining auditory activities with their other study strategies.

Visual Learners

Visual learners may find their minds wandering when listening to a speaker without the benefit of interesting visual aids. They may often wonder why they have such a hard time paying attention and why they struggle so hard to remember what was said. Individuals with this learning style must see the information with their own eyes. Doing so helps them take in new information, process it, and understand it. They will sometimes say that after being exposed to information in a strongly visual manner, they can later "see" it in their mind's eye and remember it long after.

Kinesthetic Learners

Kinesthetic learners need hands-on interaction to learn. Sitting still for long periods of time is difficult for these people. They benefit far more from hands-on activities than from observation. While most adults are predominantly visual-kinesthetic learners, most people possess some of the traits of all of the styles described. Therefore, any of the suggested strategies may help students learn.

Oral-Dependent Learners

Oral-dependent learners can enhance their learning by verbalizing concepts and thinking aloud even if they are talking only to themselves. Describing and explaining concepts to a partner who can ask questions and give feedback is especially helpful.

Writing-Dependent Learners

Writing-dependent learners can enhance their learning by taking notes during lecture, writing out challenging concepts, or creating tables and diagrams or other written illustrations. These people may find that recopying their lecture notes is immensely helpful. (See *Suggested study strategies*, page 6.)

Test-Taking Strategies

Throughout their course of study, all students take many written examinations. Once they have completed their programs, most will take the CMA or RMA certification examination. Needless to say, test taking is commonly an anxiety-producing event for many people. For some students, anxiety may be so severe that it hinders their ability to be successful. It is a frustrating experience for students to study hard, feel prepared, and then test poorly because of severe anxiety. Many test-taking strategies, then, address reducing anxiety levels before and during the examination. Other strategies address more practical actions to take during the examination to aid memory and avoid common pitfalls.

Anxiety Reduction

A mild level of anxiety can be useful if students learn to channel their nervous energy in positive ways, such as devoting time to study and prepare for tests. During the test, a mild level of anxiety can actually help students stay awake and alert. However, excessive anxiety becomes a hindrance and can impair a student's ability to focus and problem solve. Therefore, students serve themselves well to identify, learn, and practice strategies that help keep their anxiety under control before and during a test.

There are many techniques that can be employed to reduce feelings of anxiety and help students focus on the task at hand. Not all techniques work equally well for everyone. Therefore, students should take time to try different strategies to find what best suits their individual needs. Some strategies address actions to take just before the examination or during the examination. Others address actions to take in preparing for the examination and require more time or practice to be effective.

Students who suffer extreme anxiety should meet with a counselor. Most colleges have counselors on campus who

Suggested study strategies

The table below contains suggested study strategies for individual learning styles. Most people have more than one style, so students should try out a variety of strategies.

Learning Style	Suggested Study Strategies
Solitary	• Study in a quiet, isolated place. • Read the chapters of this book as assigned and work through the exercises in the corresponding chapter of the student workbook. Be sure to use the answer key to get immediate correction and feedback. • Complete the exercises on the student CD that correspond to the assigned chapter. • Make and use flash cards to aid in memorizing key terms or concepts.
Social	• Identify other social learners in your class with the same needs and make arrangements to study with a partner or in a group. • Take turns quizzing each other with flash cards and terms from the textbook or the student workbook. • Take turns looking terms up in this book or in a medical dictionary. Then read and discuss the meanings. • Persuade family members or roommates to help by doing some of the same activities described above. • Attend class to take advantage of the social interaction. Ask questions and participate in discussions.
Auditory	• Study with others (see suggestions for social learners). • Listen to others pronounce terms. • Participate in discussions. • Repeat key terms and definitions aloud after reading or hearing them. • Read key passages aloud. • Tape-record lectures, passages from the text, or even discussions. • Speak aloud when reviewing flash cards. • Be sure to attend class so you can hear the lecture, questions asked by others, and general discussion.
Visual	• Read this textbook and utilize the student workbook. • Pay close attention to illustrations, sidebars, and tables. • Use colored highlighters on key terms and passages while reading or to color-code different categories of information. • Draw pictures, arrows, diagrams, or other visual cues on a card or in the book to help make connections and understand concepts. • Make flash cards with key terms on one side and a *brief* explanation or definition on the back. Keep them with you to review as time allows. To make flash cards more effective, consider adding visual cues. These may include diagrams or illustrations copied from the book or any other drawings. Also consider using mnemonics.
Kinesthetic	• Conduct hands-on, or interactive learning. • Utilize as many senses as possible (such as vision, hearing, and touch). • Draw pictures or diagrams. • Use colored highlighters to emphasize important information. • Try strategies suggested for social and auditory learners. • Complete learning activities in the text, student workbook, and CD. • Incorporate body movement whenever possible, such as walking or using a stationary bike or treadmill. • Attend class and participate in all discussions and learning activities.
Oral-Dependent	• Speak out loud to verbalize complex concepts or to memorize terms. • Explain concepts to someone else. • When given the option, choose to do an oral presentation rather than a written project.
Writing-Dependent	• Rewrite lecture notes. • Write out challenging concepts. • Write terms and definitions. • Draw illustrations, diagrams, or other written clues to help explain concepts or cause-effect relationships.

provide free services to students. They have expertise in such areas and can provide specific guidance and instruction. They can also provide referrals to a private therapist if appropriate.

Preparing for the Examination

Examples of anxiety management strategies that students can learn to use in preparing to take an examination include biofeedback and meditation and relaxation.

Biofeedback

Biofeedback is a type of therapy that teaches a person to control her autonomic (involuntary) nervous system. Techniques include the use of a variety of technologies that provide feedback about physiologic functions. Such technologies include:

- electromyography (EMG), which provides feedback about muscle tension
- skin sensors, which provide feedback about skin temperature
- electroencephalography (EEG), which provides feedback about brain wave activity
- electrodermal response (EDR), which provides feedback about sweat gland activity.

The person undergoing biofeedback receives feedback by way of sounds through headphones or blinking lights when changes in her pulse, blood pressure, brain waves, or muscle contractions occur. This biological feedback helps her develop increased awareness of her body. With this increased awareness, she learns to recognize relationships between sensations and actual levels of function. Once her skills are developed, she can then use learned techniques, such as muscle relaxation and breathing, to create the changes she desires without the assistance of technology. Through this process, a person can learn how to exercise voluntary control over bodily functions that were previously involuntary or unconscious. People usually master the skill after 10 to 12 sessions and are able to use it when needed. Many people with a number of conditions, including anxiety, hypertension, migraine and tension headaches, attention deficit hyperactivity disorder (ADHD), and attention deficit disorder (ADD), have found biofeedback useful.

Meditation and Relaxation

Many kinds of meditative and relaxation techniques are useful in relieving anxiety, easing depression, reducing pain, and promoting healing. Many forms exist and all work by inducing a deep state of relaxation. Some of the most common techniques include slow, rhythmic breathing; progressive relaxation of muscle groups; calming of the mind; and imagery or visualization. When using imagery, the person usually imagines himself in an environment that is safe, pleasant, soothing, and relaxing. These techniques promote physical and emotional relaxation and promote the production of endorphins and enkephalins (a natural morphine-like substance produced in the body). These techniques are most effective when practiced regularly. Conditions that respond to meditation include anxiety, headache, hypertension, insomnia, and backache.

Just Before the Examination

For most students, keeping test anxiety at bay begins before the examination. Taking care to avoid other highly anxious students just before the examination and relaxing in a quiet, calm environment can be helpful. Some possibilities include quiet study in the library, listening to soothing music with headphones, or performing relaxation exercises while sitting in the car. Other test preparation activities include getting enough sleep the night before and eating a nutritious meal before the examination so that energy levels do not drop during the examination. Some students benefit by drinking a cup of coffee or tea prior to the test, because a small amount of caffeine helps them remain awake and alert. However, drinking too many caffeinated beverages will lead to increased anxiety. Caffeine also has a diuretic effect, so too much may result in the need for frequent bathroom breaks. In addition, adequate hydration helps students feel and think their best. However, consuming large volumes of liquids should be avoided because doing so will also increase the need for trips to the bathroom.

During the Examination

Students can employ specific strategies during the examination to keep their anxiety levels low. For example, those who find themselves distracted by others should try to sit near the front of the room or in a corner where they are less likely to notice what others are doing. They can ask permission to wear ear plugs or headphones to reduce distractions from room noise.

Practical Strategies

As soon as the examinations are distributed, the student should do an information "dump" by writing memorized facts in the margins of the examination. Doing so will avoid the danger of forgetting such information and will free the student to concentrate on the examination. Examples of such data include formulas, laboratory values, and normal vital signs for various age groups. Other strategies can help students effectively read questions on the examination and select answers. Some suggestions include:

- covering potential answers until the questions have been read twice
- carefully reading potential answers one at a time (while keeping others covered)
- going back and reading the question one more time before selecting the answer

- avoiding overanalyzing questions by selecting the best answer from the choices available based on the data at hand and then moving on
- resisting the temptation to go back and change answers without an *extremely* good reason for doing so
- double-checking to make sure all questions have been answered before turning in the examination.

Self-Care

Most people are drawn to the health care professions because of a combined interest in medicine and a desire to help others and to make a difference in the world. This desire will serve them well in their careers but can also be their undoing because caregivers sometimes have a tendency to take good care of everyone but themselves. Ignoring their needs can eventually put them at great risk of **burnout**, a syndrome in which an individual feels physical, emotional, or mental exhaustion caused by ongoing intensive demands without sufficient physical or emotional rest. New medical assistants are usually so enthusiastic about their careers that they find it difficult to imagine themselves ever feeling burned out. However, no one is immune. Furthermore, burnout rarely occurs suddenly. Rather, it usually develops slowly over a period of time and may become profound before an individual is fully aware. Therefore, all new medical assistants should develop a plan now to avoid burnout later. (See *Symptoms of burnout*.)

Many factors contribute to burnout but a key factor is the neglect of **self-care**. Self-care is any activity that supports and nurtures an individual's physical, mental, spiritual, or emotional health and well-being. Providing effective self-care entails taking full responsibility for nurturing and keeping oneself physically, emotionally, and mentally healthy. Some people have a hard time doing this and feel guilty when they spend time on themselves. Yet they may find themselves feeling needy and resentful when their needs go unmet and may even begin to feel resentful of others for failing to meet their needs. This has a negative impact on their relationships. Such individuals are at high risk for eventual burnout. To avoid this risk, they must learn to grant themselves permission to provide self-care, understanding that caring for oneself is a critical first step in being able to effectively care for others. A key principle in self-care is finding ways to create balance among work, play, rest, family obligations, and self-care needs. Medical assistants who develop and consistently use a plan of self-care find their effectiveness in their professional and personal lives is enhanced. (See *Self-care strategies to avoid burnout*.)

Body Mechanics

Body mechanics can be defined as the conscious coordination of the nervous and musculoskeletal systems to preserve and protect posture, balance, and body alignment while bending, lifting, and performing activities of daily living (ADLs). An important part of self-care involves the practice of good body mechanics, which protects the medical assistant and others with whom she works from injury. Making the effort to learn and develop good body mechanics should be viewed as an investment that produces real rewards. Preventing injury saves the medical assistant untold pain, suffering, lost work, and lost income and may even prevent permanent disability. In addition, it saves the employer costs in terms of insurance and staffing issues. Furthermore, it might save patients from injury as well, which benefits everyone. In fact, it really takes no more time to develop good habits and to do things correctly than to develop bad habits and do things improperly.

Back injuries are among the most common type of workplace injury and usually occur as a result of improper lifting. Typical injury involves the strain of lumbar muscles. More severe injuries involve intervertebral disk herniation or rupture. Such injuries can put the medical assistant out of work for weeks or even months. Surprisingly, not all back injuries occur while moving or lifting heavy objects. Many individuals suffering from back pain recite stories of feeling a "pop," "twinge," or some other sensation followed by severe pain when doing something as seemingly innocent as bending over to retrieve a dropped pen. Therefore, good body mechanics and a safe lifting technique should be employed for any lifting or transferring demands, regardless of the weight involved.

Safe Lifting

Before lifting any item, the medical assistant should evaluate the size and weight of the object to determine whether help is needed. The extra few minutes required to get help is well worth the benefit of avoiding injury and lost work time. If the item is too heavy to be safely lifted by one person, the

---

Symptoms of burnout

A practicing medical assistant should watch out for these common symptoms of caregiver burnout:

- fatigue
- depression
- loss of interest in or enthusiasm for the job
- insomnia
- excessive need for sleep
- loss of empathy for clients
- feelings of anger or frustration.

Self-care strategies to avoid burnout

The table below lists some of the most common factors that contribute to burnout as well as self-care strategies that can help avoid them.

Burnout Factor	Self-Care Strategy
Stressful work environment	Utilize stress reduction strategies (meditation, exercise, relaxation, etc.)
Feeling unsupported by boss/manager	Set and adhere to healthy, effective boundaries in work and personal relationships
Conflict among coworkers	Create positive, nurturing relationships; participate in meaningful spiritual activities
Long work hours; inability or unwillingness to take time off	Make time for fun and recreational activities
Insufficient or poor quality sleep	Get an adequate amount of quality sleep each night (7 to 8 hours for most adults)
Substance abuse (self or family members); dysfunctional or stressful relationships; pent-up anger or frustration over unresolved issues	Seek professional counseling for major unresolved issues or dysfunctional relationships
Poor nutrition	Follow a commonsense balanced nutritional plan (avoid fad diets)
Lack of quality physical exercise	Participate in regular physical exercise (minimum of 3 days/week)
Medical illness	Practice good body mechanics; achieve and maintain optimal body weight
Financial stress	Develop and follow a budget; get advice from a credit counselor if necessary

medical assistant should get the help of a second person or use an approved lifting device. When lifting and moving numerous items, it is always better to make more frequent trips carrying fewer items than try to save time by carrying too much. (See Chapter 35, "Orthopedics," for more information on safely assisting and transferring patients.) When lifting an object, the medical assistant should adhere to the following guidelines:

- Stand as close to the item as possible.
- Tighten the stomach muscles and tuck the pelvis.
- Bend the knees rather than the back, keeping feet shoulder-width apart.
- Firmly grasp the item and hug it as close to the body as possible.
- Keeping the back as straight as possible, lift by straightening the knees.
- Consciously use the leg muscles, rather than back muscles, to do the work of lifting.
- Move the feet in the direction of the lift but do not twist. (See Figure 1-1.)

For most busy professionals, finding time for self-care activities is challenging. Yet, when one weighs the many benefits of self-care against the risks of burnout or injury, the choice becomes easier. For most individuals, it is helpful to view the time spent in self-care activities as an investment in their career and relationships that will reap benefits for years to come.

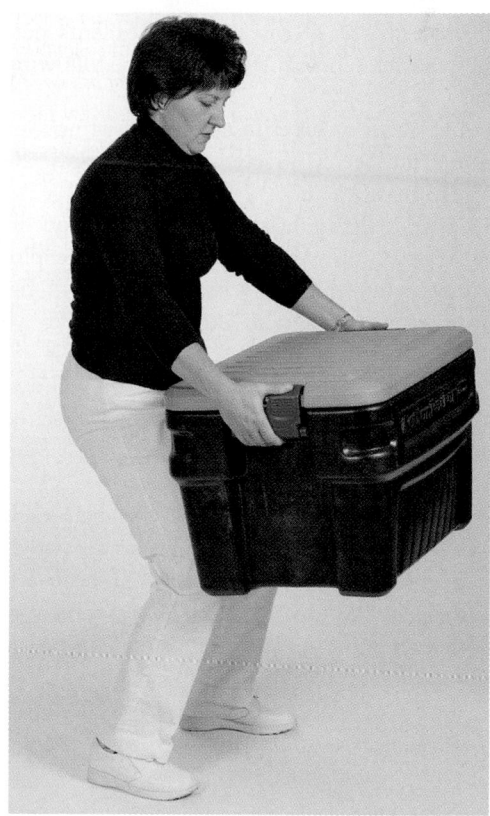

FIG 1-1 Proper lifting technique.

Chapter Summary

- All people have learning styles, but no two people are exactly alike. Most people are a combination of solitary, social, auditory, visual, kinesthetic, oral-dependent, and writing-dependent learners, with one or two areas being dominant. Different study strategies are effective for different types of learners.
- Students should try out a variety of test-taking strategies to find what works for them. Many such strategies can reduce anxiety prior to and during an examination, help with concentration and focus, and help the student be more successful.
- Numerous factors, such as long work hours and a stressful work environment, contribute to feelings of burnout. The development of good self-care habits is important to help prevent burnout and keep job satisfaction high. Each person should develop a good self-care plan that addresses such issues as exercise, rest, and nutrition.
- Development of good body mechanics is critical to workplace safety and self-care. An important example is learning to lift safely to avoid injury to the back.

Team Work Exercises

1. Divide into groups of three to five students per group. Within your team take turns sharing the following information:
   a. why you chose a career in medical assisting
   b. where you see yourself in 5, 10, and 20 years (professionally)
   c. what type of learning style you believe you have and what type of study strategies you want to explore
   d. what activities you enjoy in your nonwork time that reduce your feelings of stress and make you feel nurtured, rested, or energized
   e. at least two different activities that you will do at least once per week for the remainder of the school term that will contribute to your physical, emotional, psychological, or spiritual well-being.
2. Divide into teams of three to five members each. Each team will select one of the learning styles listed below. Over the next week (or time frame indicated by your instructor), your team will gather information about your assigned learning style and then return to present your information to the class. Design your presentation with the learning needs of all styles in mind. Your presentation should include descriptive information about the learning style and study strategies that might work for individuals with this style.
   a. Visual
   b. Auditory
   c. Kinesthetic
   d. Social
   e. Solitary

Case Studies

1. Mary Franklin is a coworker who comes to you for advice. She is a CMA who has worked in the family medical clinic for the past 5 years. She states that she is feeling unhappy and just isn't enjoying her work like she used to. She notices that she has less patience with clients and finds herself feeling overwhelmed and exhausted most of the time. She states that she would like to quit work for a while, but being a single mother of two teenagers she cannot afford to do this. You suspect that Mary may be experiencing burnout.
   a. What potential symptoms of burnout is Mary exhibiting?
   b. What questions might you ask her to further determine whether she might be experiencing burnout?
   c. Since Mary cannot afford to quit working, what advice might you offer to help her experience more job satisfaction?
2. Hilda Velasquez has just graduated from an accredited program of medical assisting and will be starting her new job soon. She is very excited about her new career and the work that she will be doing to help people with their health care needs. She has heard that some medical assistants burn out after a few years on the job and doesn't want that to happen to her. Describe a plan of self-care that Hilda might follow that will help her continue to enjoy her job for many years to come.

Resources

- Applied Psychophysiology and Biofeedback: *www.aapb.org*
- Free learning styles inventory test: *www.learning-styles-online.com*
- Help Guide: *www.helpguide.org/mental/burnout_signs_symptoms.htm*

The Profession of Medical Assisting

accredit
To certify as having met specific standards set by regional or national organizations

administrative medical assistant
Person who works in a medical office primarily in the front office areas, performing clerical, reception, or medical records duties

certification
Issuance of a certificate by a professional organization to an individual who has met a specified standard of education or training and has, therefore, earned the right to exercise certain skills

clinical medical assistant
Person who works in a medical office primarily in the back office areas, assisting the physician with patient care, procedures, and diagnostic testing

delegation
Act of assigning tasks to another person who then legally acts as the assigner's representative

float
Ability to fulfill a temporary assignment to work in a different area from the one in which an individual usually works

scope of practice
Legal description of professional responsibilities and duties that may be performed by a licensed or certified individual

Role Description

Medical assistants can work in various settings within health care; however, most medical assistants work in ambulatory settings, such as clinics and medical offices. Medical assistants work as part of the health care team performing clinical and administrative procedures. Because they are multiskilled professionals, they are commonly described as the most versatile members of the health care team. On any given day, a medical assistant might aid a physician in the examination of elderly patients, assist in the care of prenatal clients, give immunization injections to infants, administer medications, perform electrocardiograms (ECGs), draw blood for laboratory tests, file medical records, schedule appointments, enter data into a computer, and any number of other duties. Some medical assistants work primarily as **clinical medical assistants**, sometimes called *back office medical assistants*, helping with such hands-on duties as examinations and treatments. Others work primarily as **administrative medical assistants**, sometimes called *front office medical assistants*, where they perform a variety of clerical duties, such as reception, scheduling, billing, and coding. Others work in offices where they serve in both areas. Because of their versatility, medical assistants are sometimes **floated**, which means they are temporarily moved from one area to another within a facility in order to help where they are most needed. (See *Maintaining versatility*.)

Medical assistants perform clinical and administrative tasks as **delegated**, or assigned, by the physician, supervisor,

Front office–Back office connection

Maintaining Versatility

Medical assistants are educated and trained to work in virtually any area of the medical office. This versatility is a key reason they are so highly valued by employers. Yet, after beginning their careers, most medical assistants find jobs working in areas of preference. Over time, these medical assistants feel more and more reluctant to venture out of the area that has become their comfort zone. Sadly, this results in a loss of the very flexibility and versatility that initially made them so attractive to their employers. Medical assistants should remember that maintaining versatility not only enhances their value to their employers but also opens more doors of opportunity for future role enhancement and promotion. With this in mind, medical assistant students are encouraged to develop a career plan that will help them maintain and further develop their knowledge and skills in all areas. Such a plan might include these strategies:

• attending continuing education conferences and workshops that offer administrative and clinical content

Historically, most medical assistants were trained on the job. Many such individuals have attained a commendable level of knowledge and skills in this manner. However, there is little consistency in the training that occurs on the job, and employers bear the burden of such training. Therefore, employers appreciate the opportunity to hire individuals who are already fully trained and qualified. Therefore, it is best for medical assistants to attend and graduate from **accredited** programs of medical assisting. These programs have been certified as having met specific standards set by regional or national organizations.

Students who enroll in accredited programs can rest assured that they will receive excellent education and training that meets the standards and expectations of future employers. They will be prepared to enter the profession and work in virtually any ambulatory health care setting. Furthermore, as graduates of accredited programs, they will be eligible to take an examination to earn their **certification** credentials, which are an indication that they have met specific requirements and earned the right to exercise certain skills.

or nurse. Duties that can be delegated include those within the medical assistant's legal scope and for which she has received appropriate training. Such tasks must also be within the delegator's **scope of practice**, which is the legal description of professional responsibilities and duties that may be performed by a licensed or certified individual. Scope of practice is determined primarily by a state practice act. Tasks must also be within the bounds of the medical assistant's education, training, and experience. The scope of practice for medical assistants varies from state to state, but in most states medical assistants work as agents of the physician and are under his or her supervision. (See *Common skills of the medical assistant*.)

Career Opportunities for Medical Assistants

Medical assistants are commonly employed in primary care settings, such as family practice clinics where patients of all ages are seen for wellness checks as well as nonemergency care of injury and illness. Specialty offices also employ medical assistants in administrative and clinical roles, making it

Continued

Common skills of the medical assistant—cont'd

- Assist as appropriate in first aid or cardiopulmonary resuscitation (CPR)
- Collect and prepare specimens for testing
- Perform basic laboratory testing
- Administer medications (in most states) under the supervision of the physician
- Authorize drug refills as directed
- Phone prescriptions to the pharmacy
- Obtain an electrocardiogram (ECG)
- Prepare and assist with x-rays
- Assist in minor surgical procedures

- Prepare sterile trays and equipment
- Sanitize equipment and supplies
- Sterilize equipment using autoclave, steam, or chemical methods
- Gather patients' medical histories
- Provide patient education
- Obtain and record vital signs
- Remove sutures
- Apply and change dressings
- Prepare examination rooms

possible for medical assistants to specialize in an area of interest. Other, less traditional sites known to employ medical assistants include laboratories and research clinics. (See *Health care specialties*.)

Credentialing

A medical assistant can earn one of two credentials. She can become a certified medical assistant (CMA) or a registered medical assistant (RMA). These credentials are not legally required for employment as a medical assistant. However, individuals with these credentials are highly sought after by employers who understand that such individuals have demonstrated a specific level of competence in educational knowledge as well as clinical and administrative skills in order to have earned the credential.

The CMA and RMA credentials are sometimes confused with certificates of attendance awarded for completion of

Health care specialties

The list below indicates many of the health care specialties that employ administrative and clinical medical assistants.

- Family practice
- Pediatrics
- Geriatrics
- Cardiology
- Neurology
- Pulmonology
- Obstetrics
- Gynecology and women's health
- Urology and men's health
- Orthopedics
- Endocrinology
- Gastroenterology
- Podiatry
- Dermatology
- Nephrology
- Eyes, ears, nose, and throat
- Urgent care

- Psychiatric–mental health
- Oncology–hematology
- Internal medicine
- Minor surgery
- Community health
- Public health
- Rehabilitation
- Rheumatology
- Infectious disease
- Occupational medicine
- Laboratory
- Diagnostic imaging and radiology
- Sport's medicine
- Physical therapy
- Chiropractic
- Naturopathy
- Work injury
- Pain management

individual classes or workshops. However, they are not the same thing. They represent a much more comprehensive level of education and skill than what might be provided by any single class or workshop. Only individuals who have earned the CMA and RMA certification credential are entitled to use the letters CMA or RMA (in capitals) after their names to designate their level of educational achievement. (See *Teaching patients about the medical assistant's role.*)

Whether a medical assistant elects to earn the CMA or RMA credential is a matter of personal preference. There is very little difference between the two as far as knowledge, skills, or scope of practice. Students interested in becoming credentialed should visit the websites listed at the end of this chapter, gather information about each, and make an informed choice.

Certified Medical Assistant

Medical assistants earn the CMA credential by passing an examination offered by the American Association of Medical Assistants. To be eligible to take the examination, a person must have graduated from a program of medical assisting that is accredited by the Commission on Accreditation of Allied Health Education Programs (CAAHEP) or by the Accreditation Bureau of Health Education Schools (ABHES). Students wishing to sit for the certification examination offered by the AAMA can take their exam within a 3-month period after applying for the examination.

Teaching patients about the medical assistant's role

Many people do not understand the professional role of medical assistants and commonly confuse them with nurses, nurses' aides, or physician assistants. Therefore, medical assistants should take advantage of opportunities to educate patients about their role. They can easily do this when they introduce themselves to patients by offering a brief explanation of their role and their educational training. Some points of clarification they might share include:

- Medical assistants are not the same as nurses, nurses' aides, or physician assistants.
- Medical assistants are not licensed but commonly do earn certification.
- Medical assistants are educated, trained, skilled professionals whose jobs usually involve helping the physician with patient care in the medical office.
- Medical assistants may be graduates of 1- or 2-year programs of medical assisting.

Upon successful completion of the examination, medical assistants earn the privilege of using the CMA (AAMA) title after their name on their name badge and on all official documents. Recertification occurs every 5 years by continuing education or by reexamination.

Registered Medical Assistant

Medical assistants earn the RMA credential by passing an examination offered by the American Medical Technologists (AMT), a national certifying organization for laboratory professionals. There are three ways that individuals may qualify for the examination. They must have:

1. Graduated from a medical assisting program accredited by the ABHES or an organization approved by the U.S. Department of Education

2. Graduated from a formal medical services program of the U.S. Armed Forces

3. Been employed in the profession of medical assisting for at least 5 years.

RMA examinations are offered at testing center locations throughout the country every week. Upon successful completion of the examination, medical assistants earn the privilege of using the RMA credential after their name on their name badge and on all official documents. (See Figure 2-1.)

Professional and Regulatory Organizations

There are several organizations that set the standards for the profession of medical assisting. These organizations and their role in the profession of medical assisting are described in the following sections.

American Association of Medical Assistants

The American Association of Medical Assistants (AAMA) was founded in 1956 to promote the profession of medical assisting. The AAMA has since promoted the CMA credential as the minimum standard for entry to practice and established the national CMA certification program. They administer the CMA examination to graduates of accredited programs and also publish the journal *CMA Today*.

American Medical Technologists

The American Medical Technologists (AMT) organization formed the RMA program and offers national RMA certification to eligible candidates who successfully pass the RMA examination. The AMT offers credentialing examinations for other health-care-related fields as well, including certified

A

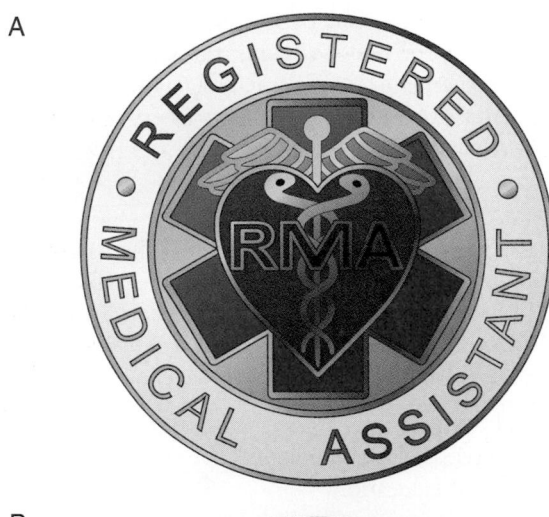

B

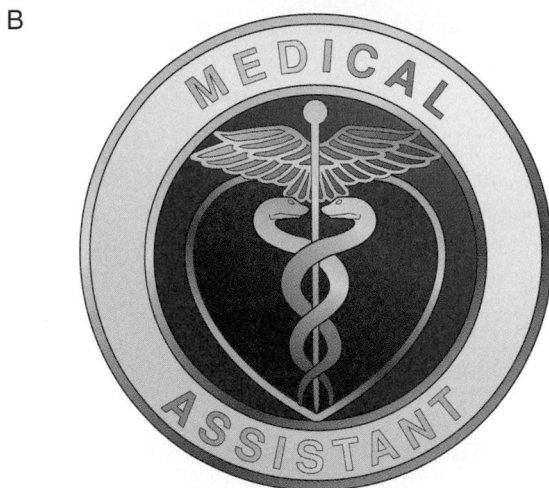

FIG 2-1 Certification pins. (A) RMA pin. (B) CMA pin.

office laboratory technicians (COLT), phlebotomy technicians (RPT), medical technologists (RMT), and medical laboratory technicians (RMLT). The AMT also publishes the journal *AMT Events.*

Accrediting Organizations

Students who are interested in attending a school of medical assisting should carefully consider their options. Consideration should be given to attending accredited programs that have met the accrediting organization's high standards for faculty qualifications, facilities, curriculum, clinical experience, and other factors. Students who attend accredited programs can feel assured that they will receive a good education. The two organizations that confer accreditation to medical assistant programs include the CAAHEP and the ABHES. Over 700 programs are currently accredited by these two organizations in the United States.

Chapter Summary

- Medical assistants work primarily in ambulatory settings, such as clinics and medical offices. Because they are multiskilled professionals, they are commonly described as the most versatile members of the health care team.
- Some medical assistants work primarily as clinical, or back office, medical assistants helping with such hands-on duties as examinations and treatments. Others work primarily as administrative, or front office, medical assistants, where they perform a variety of clerical duties, such as reception, scheduling, billing, and coding.
- Medical assistants perform clinical and administrative tasks as delegated by the physician, supervisor, or nurse.
- Students who enroll in accredited programs can rest assured that they will receive excellent education and training that meets the standards and expectations of future employers.
- Medical assistants are commonly employed in primary care settings, such as family practice clinics, but also may work in specialty areas.
- Individuals with the CMA or RMA credential are highly sought after by employers who value hiring well-educated and trained individuals.
- Medical assistants earn the CMA credential by passing an examination offered by the American Association of Medical Assistants (AAMA).
- Medical assistants earn the RMA credential by passing an examination offered by the American Medical Technologists (AMT), a national certifying organization for laboratory professionals.
- The AAMA was founded in 1956 to promote the profession of medical assisting and has since promoted the CMA credential as the minimum standard for entry to practice.
- The AMT organization formed the RMA program and offers national RMA certification to eligible candidates who successfully pass the RMA examination.
- Students who attend accredited programs of medical assisting can feel assured that they will receive a good education.

Team Work Exercises

1. Divide into four teams and complete these assignments as indicated by your instructor:
   a. Two teams will visit and review information available on the AAMA and AMT websites (see website addresses below). Each team will create a poster that summarizes the information available at their website and present it to the rest of the class.

b. One team will create a poster or multimedia presentation that illustrates the various pathways an individual might take to pursue a career in medical assisting. The presentation should include information about on-the-job training versus formal education and credentialing issues (such as national certification in the form of the CMA and RMA and "certification" by the state). The team must present the posters to the rest of the class.

c. One team will collect examples of professional medical assisting journals and create poster presentations that describe typical content in each of these journals.

2. Divide into two teams. Each team will research and present to the rest of the class how one earns:

a. RMA credential

b. CMA certification.

Include the steps involved and information about applying for and taking the national examinations.

Case Studies

1. Jon Alexander is a medical assistant who has worked in the urology department for the past 10 years since he graduated from a medical assisting program. He is good at his job and feels comfortable in this department. However, he is beginning to feel like his career has gone as far as it can in this area. Furthermore, he confesses that his interest in urology is lessening and he would like to try working in a different area. However, he is reluctant to venture out of his comfort zone. Help Jon develop a plan for making a change in his medical assistant career.

2. Isabella Rousseau is a newly graduated medical assistant working in a family practice clinic. She has noticed that many of her patients seem confused about her role. Sometimes they call her the "nurse" or the "physician assistant," which makes her feel uncomfortable. She does not wish to misrepresent herself, yet she does not want to embarrass her patients by correcting them. Describe some strategies she might employ to appropriately respond to her patients and clarify her role.

Resources

- Information regarding accredited programs of medical assisting or CMA examination: AAMA, 20 North Wacker Drive; Suite 1565; Chicago, IL 60606-2903 or *www.aama-ntl.org*

- Applications and further information about the RMA credential: Registrar's Office, American Medical Technologists, 710 Higgins Rd., Park Ridge, IL 60068-5765 or *www.amt1.com*

Professionalism

Learning Objectives

Upon completion of this chapter, the student will be able to:

- define key terms
- list and describe the characteristics of a professional
- discuss the medical assistant's responsibility as a positive role model
- describe a personal plan to avoid potential barriers to professionalism
- explain what is meant by the term *team player* and discuss the medical assistant's role as a member of the health care team.

CAAHEP Competencies

General Competencies

Professional Communications

Recognize and respond to verbal communications

Recognize and respond to nonverbal communications

ABHES Competencies

Professionalism

Project a positive attitude

Be a "team player"

Exhibit initiative

Adapt to change

Evidence a responsible attitude

Be courteous and diplomatic

Communication

Recognize and respond to verbal and nonverbal communication

Professional components

Allied health professions and credentialing

Chapter Outline

Characteristics of a Professional

Accuracy

Courteousness and Respectfulness

Dependability

Flexibility

Commitment to Lifelong Learning

Tactfulness

Accountability

Positive Attitude

Professional Appearance

Daily hygiene

Makeup

Jewelry

Tattoos

Hair

Attire

Medical Assistant as a Role Model

Qualities of a Good Role Model

Barriers to Professionalism

Bad Habits

Reactive versus Proactive

Personal Problems at Work

Rumors and Gossip

Becoming a Team Player

Chapter Summary

Team Work Exercises

Case Studies

Resources

Key Terms

accountable
Willingness to account for or be responsible for one's own actions

continuing education units
Credits awarded for attendance at classes, workshops, or seminars

courteous
Behavior that is polite, considerate, and helpful

dependable
Characteristic of being reliable and trustworthy

flexible
Adaptable to change; able to bend without breaking

reactive
Responding without considering the situation at hand

respectful
Behavior that treats a person or object with honor or esteem

tactful
Displaying sensitivity and courtesy in behavior and comments to avoid offending others

Characteristics of a Professional

Because many patients view medical assistants as representatives of the physician and health care facility, one of the unofficial duties of medical assistants is public relations. Keeping this in mind, medical assistants must consistently demonstrate professional behavior in all of their interactions with others. Not surprisingly, the qualities of professionalism that patients seek in their health care providers are the very same qualities that employers look for when hiring a medical assistant:

- accuracy
- courteousness and respectfulness
- dependability
- flexibility
- commitment to lifelong learning
- tactfulness
- accountability
- positive attitude
- professional appearance.

Accuracy

A medical assistant should strive for accuracy in everything she does. When a medical assistant performs accurately, she sends the message that she cares about safety and quality. Through her dedication to quality and efficiency, she will reap many rewards, including fewer errors, less need for damage control, and greater job satisfaction. In addition, patients will form a more positive impression of her, her coworkers, and her employers. Of even greater importance is the safety and well-being of patients who rely on health care providers to administer medications accurately and perform procedures safely. When dealing with human lives, it does not pay to take short cuts.

Courteousness and Respectfulness

Courteous behavior should be standard practice for a medical assistant as she interacts with patients and coworkers. This behavior is polite, considerate, and helpful. Even simple measures, such as making eye contact to acknowledge someone's presence, smiling, and saying "please," "thank you," and "you are welcome," go a long way in creating a pleasant, professional environment. **Respectful** behavior is similar to courteous behavior and involves treating others with honor, esteem, courteous regard, and thoughtful consideration.

Dependability

Dependability is critically important in winning the trust and respect of others. Being **dependable** means that a person is reliable and trustworthy. These qualities are important to everyone with whom the medical assistant interacts. Her employer depends on her to demonstrate consistent punctuality and performance. Coworkers depend on her to help out in a cooperative manner. Patients depend on the medical assistant to relay messages, return phone calls, and carry out other promised duties in a timely and professional manner.

Flexibility

Flexibility is the quality of being adaptable to change. One common analogy regarding flexibility is a tree branch, which is able to bend with the wind without breaking. In a fast-paced health care environment, unexpected events commonly occur. A medical assistant who is adaptable to change and able to "think on her feet" will thrive. A medical assistant who demonstrates the ability to recognize problems and move quickly toward a solution will earn the appreciation of her employer and coworkers. (See *Flexibility equals value.*)

Commitment to Lifelong Learning

Medical assistants are members of a profession in which things are continually changing. New medications enter the market frequently. Technology is becoming integrated into nearly every aspect of health care and technological changes continue to develop at a dizzying pace. It seems that new tests, treatments, and procedures enter the health care scene daily. Current understanding of the human body and the disease process also continues to deepen as a result of ongoing research. Keeping up with this fast-paced and ever-changing profession requires a commitment from all members of the health care team. Medical assistants are no exception. Anyone who enters a health care profession must be willing to commit herself to lifelong learning in order to stay current.

There are a number of ways medical assistants can pursue continuing education, including attending workshops, college classes, and reading professional journals. Most health care employers offer mandatory and optional continuing education courses. Medical assistants can benefit greatly from attending as many of these offerings as possible. A medical assistant should keep a personal folder or notebook in which she records all continuing education activities. In many cases, **continuing education units** (CEUs) are offered for these activities. CEUs are credits awarded for the attendance of classes, workshops, or seminars that are designed to keep individuals current in their field of expertise. They may be required for earning or renewing licensure or certification. The medical assistant may also categorize these units according to their general area, such as administrative or clinical and so forth. When it is time for medical assistants to renew certification, the needed data will be organized and close at hand. (See *Learning with a buddy.*)

Tactfulness

A **tactful** person is one who demonstrates the ability to respond to others with sensitivity and courtesy in their behavior and comments to avoid giving offense. Such persons are commonly described as *diplomatic*. Being tactful requires a medical assistant to think before she speaks, especially when tempers rise. She must resist the impulse to be so honest that her patient or coworker is offended. She must also strive to state things in a positive manner, using an even,

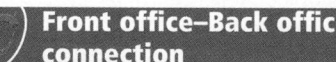

Front office–Back office connection

Flexibility Equals Value

When a coworker asks for help, the last thing she wants to hear is "that's not my job." Regardless of whether a medical assistant primarily works in the administrative or clinical setting, she can earn the respect and high regard of her coworkers and employer by demonstrating her willingness to help out when and where she is needed. For example, if the receptionist or administrative medical assistant is overwhelmed with ringing phones, the clinical medical assistant might step in to help answer phones. If the back office is short-staffed or overwhelmed with unexpected events, the administrative medical assistant might help out by weighing patients, escorting them to examination rooms, and checking their vital signs. Medical assistants will do well to remember the old saying, "What goes around, comes around." The person a medical assistant helps out today will feel more inclined to return the favor the next time she is in need.

Front office–Back office connection

Learning with a Buddy

To remain current and educated in all settings in her field, a medical assistant should consider teaming up with another medical assistant who works in an area different from hers. She can make an agreement to teach the other medical assistant something new about her area of expertise at least once each month in exchange for the same education from her learning "buddy." For example, an administrative medical assistant might review the latest changes in coding or data entry with her friend who is a clinical medical assistant. In return, the clinical medical assistant might teach her administrative medical assistant friend about the newest types of medications or diagnostic tests.

pleasant tone of voice. Because the medical assistant cannot take back words once they leave her mouth, it is always better to be discreet and say less, rather than more, when she is unsure of what to say. Language use should include proper grammar and be free of slang terms and vulgarity. In doing so, she creates a more professional impression and enhances effectiveness and accuracy when communicating with someone from another culture who speaks another language.

Accountability

The medical assistant who is **accountable** for her actions is someone who is willing to take responsibility for what she does. She must also admit her errors and work positively to take corrective measures if needed. In addition, a medical assistant who is accountable is empowered to create the positive work environment she wishes to experience, rather than feeling powerless to effect change or feeling victimized by others.

Positive Attitude

In most work environments, and especially in health care, attitude is everything. The saying "Hire the attitude, and train the skill" is common among health care employers. While doing so is not realistic in many cases, the statement points out how highly most employers value having employees with positive, professional attitudes. It also points out how difficult it can be to work with, not to mention change, someone with a bad attitude.

Attitudes *can* be changed, but the motivation for change must come from the individual. Therefore, it is up to each person to notice her responses, thoughts, feelings, habits—all of the things that go into her attitude—and then make the effort toward needed change. It takes work, but the results are well worth it. However, many people find it challenging to view themselves objectively.

Therefore, even though it feels risky, it may be enormously helpful for a medical assistant to solicit feedback from friends and coworkers. A safe way to begin might be to approach a trusted friend by saying, "I am setting some goals for myself in the area of professionalism. I would appreciate some honest feedback based on your observations. Regarding my general attitude and communication with others, what do you think are my greatest strengths? And what are some areas you believe I need to strengthen?" The next step is to set simple, measurable goals, such as getting though one work day without discussing personal problems, complaining about work conditions, or watching the clock. On a more positive note, one could make a mental (or actual) list of the things about the job that are enjoyable, positive, or interesting and then review the list at the start and end of each day. Focusing on the positive can have a significant impact on a person's outlook. Since attitudes seem to be contagious, medical assistants should commit themselves to spreading positives ones.

Professional Appearance

Appearance is a critical part of the professional role. Generally, the more conservative a person's appearance on the job, the better. Working on the job as a medical assistant is not the time to express individuality in a flamboyant or radical manner.

Daily Hygiene

Daily hygiene for the medical assistant should include a shower, use of a deodorant, and good oral hygiene. She should pay special attention to her hands, because keeping her skin clean and intact will protect the medical assistant and her patients from microorganisms. She should avoid fragrances, because not everyone appreciates them. More importantly, many patients and even other health care workers suffer from allergies and respiratory disorders, and some fragrances could exacerbate their symptoms.

Makeup

The medical assistant should be conservative with the application of makeup, keeping it to a minimum. She must keep her fingernails clean, smooth, and no longer than the tip of her finger. She should avoid long nails and artificial nails, because they tend to harbor microorganisms which can then be passed from person to person.

Jewelry

Jewelry should be conservative and minimal. Acceptable jewelry might include an engagement ring and/or wedding band, a wristwatch, and a single pair of small earrings. Jewelry related to body piercing is not appropriate in the health care setting.

Tattoos

A medical assistant should think carefully before making the decision to get a tattoo, because tattoos are deemed unprofessional by many people. Any tattoos the medical assistant already has should be covered if possible.

Hair

Men and women alike should keep their hair clean, neatly styled, out of the face, and pulled back when assisting with sterile procedures so that the sterile field and patient are not compromised. While many people enjoy expressing themselves through their hairstyles, medical assistants should resist the urge to wear wild hairstyles to work. A conservative appearance is always perceived as more professional.

Attire

Clothing should be clean and wrinkle-free and conform to the standards designated by the employer. In most cases, a medical assistant wears a uniform, good-quality scrubs, or professional-looking clothes, such as slacks and a shirt or a

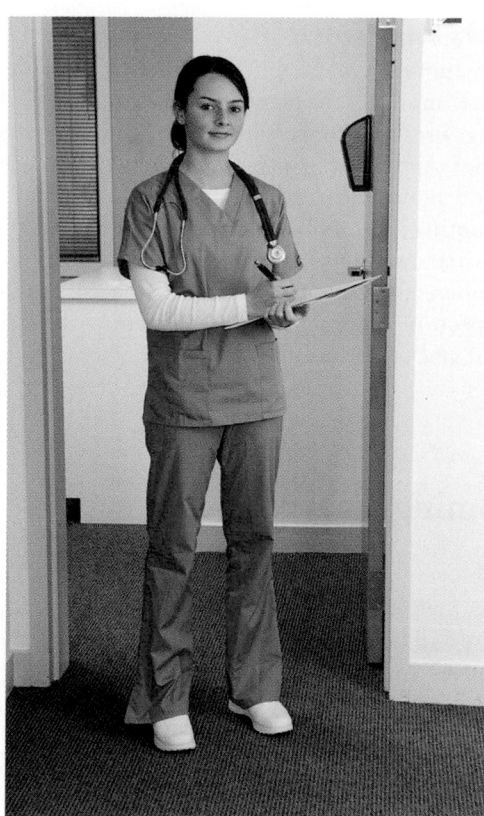

FIG 3-1 Professional attire for a medical assistant.

dress with a white laboratory coat and a name badge (see Figure 3-1). The medical assistant must be sure to button a laboratory coat when performing invasive procedures, such as injections and drawing blood. Because a medical assistant is exposed to ill patients continually, daily laundering of professional clothing is a must. She must wear undergarments, which should be flesh- or neutral-colored and free of designs or lettering so that they do not show through the uniform.

A medical assistant commonly spends a great deal of time on her feet. Therefore, comfortable, good-fitting shoes are of utmost importance. Shoes should conform to the dress code of the facility, and the medical assistant must keep them clean and in good repair. Many health care providers (male and female) who spend long hours on their feet make it a habit to wear support hose, which are available in knee-high length in a variety of colors. They come in various compression strengths and help reduce leg fatigue and aching and minimize the development of varicose veins.

Medical Assistant as a Role Model

Everyone is a role model in some respect. Everyone has some degree of influence on those with whom they come into contact. Some people welcome this responsibility, while others do not. When a person takes on a professional role, especially in a service-oriented profession such as medical assisting, this kind of responsibility takes on special meaning. Patients look to health care providers for help, information, and guidance. Furthermore, they observe and take note of such characteristics as lifestyle, attitude, behaviors, and habits—healthy and unhealthy. They may be inspired by good examples of healthful living and may be negatively influenced by unhealthful ones. With this power of influence in mind, the medical assistant must carefully consider the type of role model she wishes to be.

Qualities of a Good Role Model

Good role models practice what they preach. While no one leads the perfect life, health care professionals are viewed by others as examples of how one ought to live. At the very least, health care workers should avoid flaunting bad habits in front of patients (such as smoking in front of the medical building). Better yet, they should strive to develop the same healthful habits that they encourage in their patients. (See *Teaching by example*.)

Patient Education

Teaching by Example

Patients sometimes learn more from the medical assistant by her actions than from her words. Because she is a role model, the information that she gives patients about lifestyle modification will have a greater impact if the patients see her practicing what she preaches. If she teaches them about weight loss or smoking cessation, yet is significantly overweight herself or smells of tobacco smoke, her message loses impact.

On the other hand, if patients see a medical assistant who practices healthy behaviors, it makes a positive impression. They are then more likely to heed her words of advice. Although this may not seem fair, it is true. So the medical assistant should take every opportunity to lead others by example. Healthy behaviors for the medical assistant that have an impact on patients and patient education include:

- getting regular exercise, such as going to the gym, walking the dog, and riding a bike
- eating a nutritious diet
- finding a balance between work and play
- getting regular health checkups
- maintaining optimal weight
- avoiding tobacco or illicit drug use.

Barriers to Professionalism

In addition to qualities of professionalism that a medical assistant should look to acquire, there are some barriers to professionalism that she should try to avoid, including:

- indulging in unhealthy or impolite habits
- being reactive
- bringing personal problems to work
- engaging in rumors and gossip.

Bad Habits

The medical assistant should carefully consider eliminating behaviors that are unhealthful as well as those deemed ill-mannered or unprofessional. At the very least, she should refrain from such habits while performing her job. Examples of such behaviors include tobacco use, gum chewing, and vulgar language.

Reactive Versus Proactive

The hallmark of a true professional is the ability to maintain a professional demeanor under trying circumstances. Because the fast-paced environment of the medical office can be stressful, a medical assistant may, at times, find her energy and enthusiasm diminishing. When her energy lags and her patience runs low, her temper may easily flair. As a result, the medical assistant may be **reactive**, or respond without considering the situation at hand, resulting in words and actions that she regrets later. To avoid such situations, the medical assistant should strive to develop good organizational strategies to minimize the risk of such events and effective coping skills to better deal with them if they occur. She will expend less energy striving to behave professionally in a stressful situation than she would trying to apologize or make amends to upset patients or coworkers if she loses her temper.

Personal Problems at Work

If a medical assistant is not careful, problems and stresses from her personal life may threaten to intrude into the workplace and impact her attitude, energy level, and ability to focus. In these times especially, it is important for her to remember that each patient deserves the same measure of caring, attention, and respect, regardless of the medical assistant's personal issues. Therefore, she must learn how to place such personal problems aside when she goes to work each day, so she can give her full attention to the job at hand. Learning to focus on her immediate situation will assist the medical assistant in making this transition each day. Furthermore, if she discusses personal problems repeatedly in the workplace, she may eventually alienate her coworkers and have a negative impact on patients.

Rumors and Gossip

Because rumors and gossip have a negative impact on employee morale, the medical assistant should avoid engaging in such conversations at all costs. She must remember that the "grapevine" generally distorts the truth more and more with each retelling of a story. It is also worth noting that nobody is immune to the pain and damage that gossip inflicts. Professional medical assistants must understand that the best way to earn the goodwill and respect of coworkers is to treat them with respect and goodwill and to assume the best of others, rather than the worst.

Becoming a Team Player

All employers agree that one of the qualities they most desire in their employees is the ability to be a team player. With an individual sport, such as running a marathon, a person sets individual goals, plans independently, and develops a strategy based on personal strengths and weaknesses. The person relies only on herself to accomplish the task, arrives at the finish line alone, and takes personal credit for the accomplishment. With a team sport such as soccer, goals are shared by the entire team, and the game plan is communicated and agreed upon between players. On the field, players pass the ball to each other and lend support when and where it is needed. Everyone contributes to the process, and nobody performs alone. Personal sacrifices are made for the good of the team with the goal of achieving a team victory. Credit for the results, regardless of the final score, is shared by everyone on the team. Even players who may not particularly like one another understand that the welfare of the team comes before personal issues. They learn to work together effectively—putting personal feelings aside—and as a result develop a measure of respect for one another.

Similarly in the health care setting, such goals as providing top-quality patient care and creating a profitable medical practice are shared by the entire team. Effective communication is critical to the process and members of the team lend one another support when it is needed. Nobody performs in isolation. Everyone's contribution and cooperation is essential. On occasion, personal sacrifices are made for the good of the team so that the goals can be achieved. Although it is preferable, it is not mandatory for all employees to like one another. Even so, they must develop the ability to work together in a cooperative and respectful manner. Medical assistants who develop the ability to be true team players will be highly appreciated and valued by everyone.

Chapter Summary

- Medical assistants are viewed as representatives of the physician and the health care organization. Therefore, they must consistently demonstrate professional behavior in all of their interactions with others.
- Medical assistants should strive for accuracy in everything they do. When a medical assistant performs accurately, she indicates that she adheres to the standard of care and takes care in all that she does to avoid errors. Through her dedication to quality and efficiency, she will reap many rewards, including fewer errors, less need for damage control, and greater job satisfaction.
- Courteous behavior that is polite, considerate, and helpful should be standard practice for medical assistants as they interact with patients and coworkers.
- Being dependable means being reliable and trustworthy. These qualities are important to everyone with whom medical assistants interact.
- Medical assistants who are adaptable and flexible will quickly earn the appreciation of their employers and coworkers.
- Medical assistants are members of a profession in which things are continually changing. They must be willing to commit themselves to lifelong learning in order to keep up. Some ways they can do this is by attending workshops and college classes and reading professional journals.
- A tactful person is one who demonstrates the ability to respond to others with sensitivity and courtesy to avoid causing offense. Because the medical assistant cannot take back words once they leave her mouth, it is always better to be discreet and say less, rather than more, when she is unsure of what to say.
- Accountability refers to a willingness to be responsible for and answer for one's actions, own up to any errors, and work positively to take any corrective measures if needed.
- In most work environments, and especially in health care, attitude is everything. The saying "Hire the attitude, and train the skill" is common among health care employers. Attitudes *can* be changed, but the motivation for change must come from within the individual.
- Appearance is a critical part of the professional role. Generally, the more conservative a person's appearance is on the job, the better. Paying careful attention to appearance includes taking care with hygiene, wearing minimal makeup and jewelry, avoiding displaying tattoos, and keeping hair out of the face and eyes. Clothing should be neat and clean and conform to standards designated by the employer. Because medical assistants commonly spend long days on their feet, they should carefully select footwear and hosiery.
- Patients look to health care providers for help, information, and guidance. Furthermore, they observe and take note of such things as lifestyle, attitude, behaviors, and habits—healthy and unhealthy. Medical assistants must be aware that they are role models and strive to be positive ones.
- Potential barriers to professionalism include such bad habits as tobacco use, gum chewing, and vulgar language. Other barriers include being reactive rather than proactive when responding to others, bringing personal problems to work, and participating in gossip.
- All employers agree that one of the qualities they most desire in their employees is the ability to be a team player. Professional medical assistants should recognize that the welfare of the team sometimes must take priority over personal issues, and everyone's contribution and cooperation is essential. Medical assistants who develop the ability to be true team players will be highly appreciated and valued by everyone.

Team Work Exercises

1. Gather into teams of three to four students each. Each team will select one of the following assignments:
   a. Each team member must interview someone who works in a managerial or supervisory capacity (in any profession) and ask them to identify what qualities they look for in prospective employees. Each person should report her findings back to the team. The team must then prepare a poster presentation based on the compiled results.
   b. Each team member should contact the nearest local AAMA chapter and find out what types of continuing education unit (CEU) offerings or meetings are planned during the next 3 months. The team should report its findings to the class.
   c. Contact the national AAMA and find out what types of CEU offerings or meetings are planned during the next year. Report your findings back to the class.
2. Gather into teams of three to four students each. Read the scenario below together. Brainstorm with your team members and come up with a plan for addressing the issue in a positive and professional manner.
   A coworker in your medical office has good skills as a CMA but has poor personal hygiene. On several occasions, you and others have noticed that she has bad breath and occasional body odor. You like her and respect her knowledge and skills. However, you are concerned about the impact that this problem has on others, especially patients.

Case Studies

1. Olivia Bianchi works as an administrative CMA in a sports medicine clinic. She tells you she is feeling frustrated with her job and her coworkers, and cannot understand why they do not seem to like her. She states that she gets paid on an hourly basis to work from 9:00 a.m. to 5:00 p.m., 4 days a week. She says she thinks that others in the office resent her because she doesn't have to work 5 days a week like they do and she has an active personal life. She has seen some roll their eyes when she walks in the door promptly at 9:00 a.m. and out the door promptly at 5:00 p.m. If they ask her to come early or stay late to help open or close the office or complete other tasks, she states, "That's not my job. I was hired to answer phones and make appointments. After all, I don't want to be a workaholic like some of you." She further states that setting these clear boundaries is an important part of her self-care so that others do not take advantage of her. What advice might you offer to Olivia so that she can develop better relationships with her colleagues?

2. Gloria Chatzi is a coworker in the medical office where you work. You like her but are beginning to tire of her many stories about all of her personal problems. Her life always seems to be in turmoil and she wants to fill you in on every detail. You find yourself trying to avoid her, which is difficult because the office is fairly small. You realize that your growing resentment is beginning to impact your attitude toward her and your enjoyment of your job. In addition, you notice that patients sometimes overhear bits of Gloria's stories and worry about the impression they get from this. Finally, you realize that you cannot tolerate the situation any longer and must resolve this problem. Describe what you will do and say to address this issue.

Resources

- AAMA information on continuing education: *www.aama-ntl.org/viewceus.aspx*
- AMT information on continuing education: *www.amt1.com/site/epage/9360_315.htm*
- Information on professionalism in the workplace: *www.sideroad.com/Human_Resources/professionalism.html*

Health Care Yesterday and Today

Learning Objectives

Upon completion of this chapter, the student will be able to:

- define key terms
- describe ancient beliefs about health and illness
- list key people in the history of medicine and describe their contributions to the profession
- discuss at least five significant developments in the medical profession during the past century
- differentiate between acute, long-term, subacute, home, and ambulatory care settings
- compare the sole proprietorship, partnership, and corporation forms of business organization and list the potential benefits and disadvantages of each
- describe the role and education of medical doctors
- list and describe the characteristics of at least 10 different areas in which physicians may specialize
- list and describe four types of nonmedical physician specialties
- describe the role of each member of the health care team.

CAAHEP Competencies

General
Identify community resources

ABHES Competencies

Communication
Serve as liaison between physician and others

Chapter Outline

Brief History of Medicine
Ancient Health Care
Early Development of Medicine
Current Medicine
Future of Medicine
Health Care Settings
Hospitals
Long-Term Care
Subacute Care
Home Care
Ambulatory Care
Types of Medical Practices
Sole Proprietorship
Partnership
Corporation
Health Care Team
Physicians
Other Practitioners
Nurses
Physician Assistants
Medical Technologists

Therapists
Physical therapist
Occupational therapist
Respiratory therapist
Speech therapist
Registered Dietitian
Prehospital Care Specialists
Emergency medical technicians
Paramedics
Technicians
Phlebotomist
Radiologic technicians
Medical laboratory technicians
Administrative Specialists
Medical coding specialist
Medical transcriptionist
Chapter Summary
Team Work Exercises
Case Studies
Resources

Key Terms

acute care
Setting in which short-term health care is delivered to patients who are experiencing sudden illness or injury

ambulatory care
Facility, such as a medical clinic, that provides medical care to nonresidential patients, who arrive and leave on the same day

assisted living
Residential facilities with minimal health care, common dining and social activities, and usually transportation assistance

associate practice
Sole proprietors who share resources, such as office space, equipment, and employees

caduceus
Ancient symbol of the Greek god Hermes that consists of a staff with two serpents entwined around it, surmounted by two wings, and used today by some medical groups to symbolize medical care

cloning
Creation of cells, tissue, or an embryo without the fertilization of an egg

corporation
Body that is granted legal status with rights, privileges, and liabilities separate from those of its members

dissection
Separation and delineation of animal or human tissues for study

ether
Organic compound once used for anesthesia; also called *diethyl ether*

genome
Complete set of chromosomes and, thus, the complete genetic information present in a cell

group practice
Medical group with three or more licensed, full-time physicians

Hippocratic oath
Oath of medical ethics created by Hippocrates

histologist
Specialist in the study of cells and microscopic tissues

home care
Health care assistance for a person living in his or her own home

hospital privileges
Permission granted by a hospital that allows a physician to see patients and practice medicine within that hospital

humor
Term created by Claudius Galen that refers to any fluid or semifluid substance in the body

long-term care
Health care setting that provides care for people who are deemed medically stable, yet unable to provide for their own needs, or people who require end-of-life care

medical asepsis
Practice that frees a specific environment from microorganisms that might cause disease

partnership
Creation of a legal agreement between two or more licensed physicians that specifies the rights, obligations, and responsibilities of each

pasteurization
Process of heating a fluid to a moderate temperature to destroy bacteria without changing the chemical composition of the fluid

resident
Physician who obtains further medical training after internship, usually as a member of the house staff of a hospital

roentgenography
Practice of using radiation technology to examine the bones and other dense structures of a patient's body; also called *radiology* and *x-ray*

sole proprietor
Physician in a solo practice

staff of Asclepius
Ancient symbol of the Greek god Asclepius that consists of a staff with a single serpent entwined around it and used today as a symbol of medical care

subacute care
Health care setting in which temporary care is provided with the goal of helping the patient to regain strength, mobility, and function in order to return home or to an assisted-living setting

teaching hospital
Hospital that is affiliated with a medical school, where residents provide much of the physician-related care under the supervision of licensed physicians

Brief History of Medicine

To better understand the role of medical assistants within the profession of medicine, it is helpful to understand the medical profession itself, its origins, history, and present-day culture.

Ancient Health Care

Earliest records indicate that the first health care professionals were priests and other religious leaders. At that time, human anatomy was poorly understood and microorganisms had yet to be discovered. For these reasons, the prevailing belief of the time was that illness and disease were caused by evil spirits or were punishment from the gods for sinful behavior. Consequently, treatment commonly involved rituals and ceremonies that combined religion, mythology, and nature. For example, early priests in Greek temples believed in the power of nonpoisonous snakes and commonly used them in their healing rituals. Drawings of the **staff of Asclepius** depicting the god of healing, Asclepius, holding a staff with a serpent coiled around the shaft are thought to be the origins of one of the symbols used today in the medical profession. Another symbol, the **cadeceus**, which is a staff with two serpents entwined around it surmounted by two wings, comes from the Greek god Hermes, who was the protector of alchemists (among others). Although the caduceus is sometimes used to symbolize the medical profession (for example, as a symbol of the U.S. Army Medical Corps), the staff of Asclepius is usually considered the more appropriate symbol. (See Figure 4-1.)

Some ancient healing techniques are still practiced today. For example, Greek priests were known to use exercise, massage, and hygiene treatments. In such countries as India and China, extensive use of drugs is recorded as early as 1500 to 3000 B.C. The technique of acupuncture was also introduced by the Chinese during this same time period. These therapies have evolved over the years, but they have withstood the test of time and are still widely used today.

The most notable figure in ancient medical history was Hippocrates (460–377 B.C.). He was born in Greece at a time when medical scholars were beginning to reject many of the teachings of the past. He embraced the newer practice of observing the sick and studying the human body with the goal of identifying the cause of disease and illness. For example, one of his observations included listening to an ill person's chest to help learn about and understand the course of the illness. Perhaps he noticed sounds of lung congestion and correlated it with patients' coughing and difficulty breathing. In any case, his technique was validated and refined over 2000 years later by Rene Laennec (1781–1826), who invented the first stethoscope. Based on his findings, Hippocrates rejected the traditional explanations of priests and philosophers that illness had a spiritual cause and asserted that illness was caused by physical factors. His belief that a healthy diet, hygiene, rest, and fresh air provide healing properties is still relevant today. Hippocrates, who became known as the *Father of Medicine*, traveled throughout Greece teaching others his methods and is best remembered for writing the Oath of Medical Ethics, known today as the **Hippocratic oath**. (See Figure 4-2.)

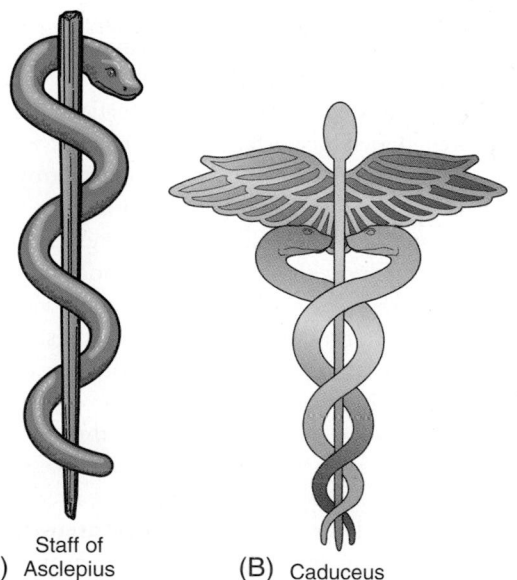

FIG 4-1 Ancient symbols used in medicine today. (A) Staff of Asclepius. (B) Caduceus.

(A) Staff of Asclepius   (B) Caduceus

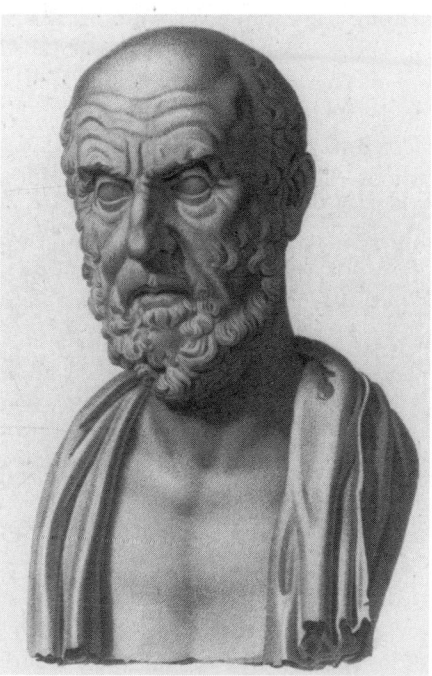

FIG 4-2 Hippocrates, the Father of Medicine. (Used with permission from The Library of Congress.)

Claudius Galen (c. A.D. 129–c. A.D. 216) was a Greek physician who followed the teachings of Hippocrates. Galen furthered his understanding of anatomy and the physiology of traumatic injuries while serving as a surgeon at a school for gladiators, where his study subjects often suffered traumatic injury. However, because Galen lived in a time when human **dissection** (surgical separation and delineation of tissues for study) was not acceptable, much of his research involved the dissection of animals. He subsequently produced numerous writings and illustrations based on his research. Unfortunately, much of his teaching was flawed, because it was based on animal anatomy. Galen became famous for his theory that disease and illness were caused by an imbalance of the four **humors**: black bile, yellow bile, phlegm, and blood. Although Galen used the term *humor* to describe only these four fluids, it came to be used to describe any fluid or semifluid substance in the body. Even now such medical terms as *aqueous humor,* which is a fluid substance found in the eye, carry this meaning. Galen's teachings were generally accepted for the next 1300 years.

Early Development of Medicine

After the Catholic church relaxed its control over scientific and intellectual activities, human dissection became legal and was given a measure of respectability when practiced by classical artists such as Leonardo da Vinci (1452–1519) and Michelangelo (1475–1564), who desired to draw the human body and human anatomy accurately. Human dissection was also practiced extensively by Andreas Vesalius (1514–1564), a Belgian anatomist and physician, who became known as the *Father of Modern Anatomy* after he published a book titled *De Corporis Humani Fabrica* in 1541. This book contained hundreds of anatomical illustrations and corrected many of Galen's erroneous theories.

The advent of the printing press in the 15th century revolutionized medical education by allowing widespread dissemination of information and illustrations. Significant contributions that might otherwise have been ignored were now widely accessible by other like-minded persons. For example, the discoveries of Antoni van Leeuwenhoek were widely distributed by the Royal Society of England (a scientific organization) and subsequent discoveries were made based on such work. Antoni van Leeuwenhoek (1632–1723) was a Dutch linen draper and manufacturer of men's clothing whose hobby was grinding lenses. (See Figure 4-3, A.) He eventually developed magnifying lenses that allowed him to observe microorganisms. (See Figure 4-3, B.) His observations and descriptions led to the development of bacteriology and protozoology. Because of his skill in grinding lenses that were superior to any of his time, he made a significant contribution to the continued evolution of the microscope. Building on van Leeuwenhoek's studies, Marcello Malpighi (1628–1694), an Italian, was the first person to study and identify the link between veins and arteries. As a result of his work, Malpighi became known as the first **histologist** (a specialist in the microscopic study of cells and tissues).

During the 18th century, Edward Jenner (1749–1823) saved the world from the devastating effects of smallpox by developing a smallpox vaccine. He developed the vaccine by observing that a dairymaid seemed to be immune to smallpox because of her previous infection with cowpox. His colleagues initially scoffed at this idea, but he subsequently proved his theory correct when he inoculated a young boy with the cowpox virus and then exposed him to smallpox. When the young boy failed to contract the deadly smallpox disease, Jenner's theory was validated.

Significant contributions to the medical profession during the 19th and 20th centuries were so numerous that they cannot all be described in this text. However, here are a few key events:

- Crawford Williamson Long (1815–1878) was with a group of medical students at a party, known as an "ether frolic," when he observed that people under the influence of **ether** (a gas used as an early inhalation anesthetic) did not seem to feel pain. Subsequently, his successful surgery on a patient anesthetized with ether led to its common use as a general anesthetic.

- Elizabeth Blackwell (1821–1910), who was initially refused admittance to medical school because of her sex, eventually became the first woman in the United States to receive a medical degree. She subsequently established the New York Infirmary for Indigent Women and Children, a hospital staffed entirely by women. She later returned to her native England to become professor of gynecology at the London School of Medicine for Women. (See Fig. 4-4.)

- Louis Pasteur (1822–1895) became known as the *Father of Bacteriology* as a result of his work in recognizing the relationship between bacteria and infectious disease. He discovered that if a substance such as milk was heated during processing, bacteria would be destroyed. This process became known as **pasteurization.**

- Joseph Lister (1827–1912) applied Pasteur's findings to the area of surgery. He developed methods of sterilizing instruments and even washed his own hands with carbolic acid prior to performing surgical procedures. Until that time, other physicians had accepted postsurgical infection as an unfortunate but inevitable part of the healing process. However, Lister's patients exhibited a much lower rate of infection and much greater success in recovery. Therefore, others began following Lister's example, and the practice known today as **medical asepsis**, or trying to eradicate an environment of disease-causing microorganisms, was born. Lister has since been remembered as the *Father of Sterile Surgery.*

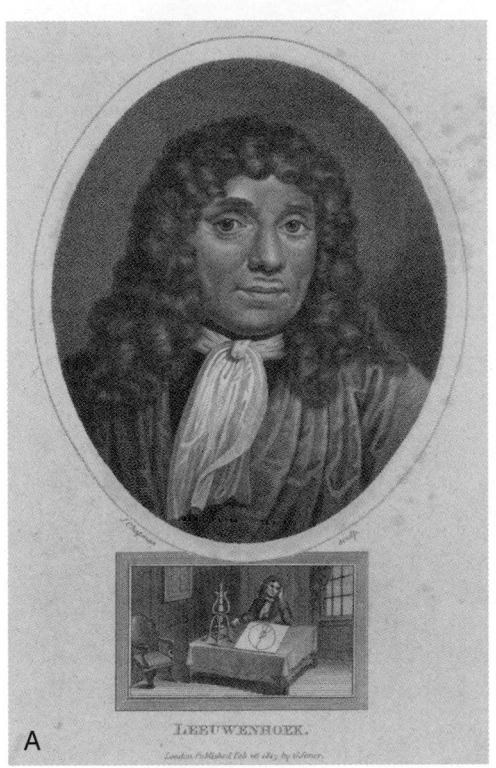

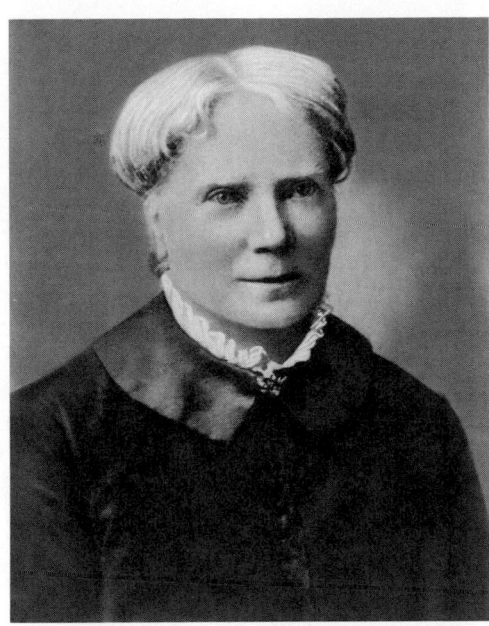

FIG 4-4   Elizabeth Blackwell. (Used with permission from Bettmann/ CORBIS.)

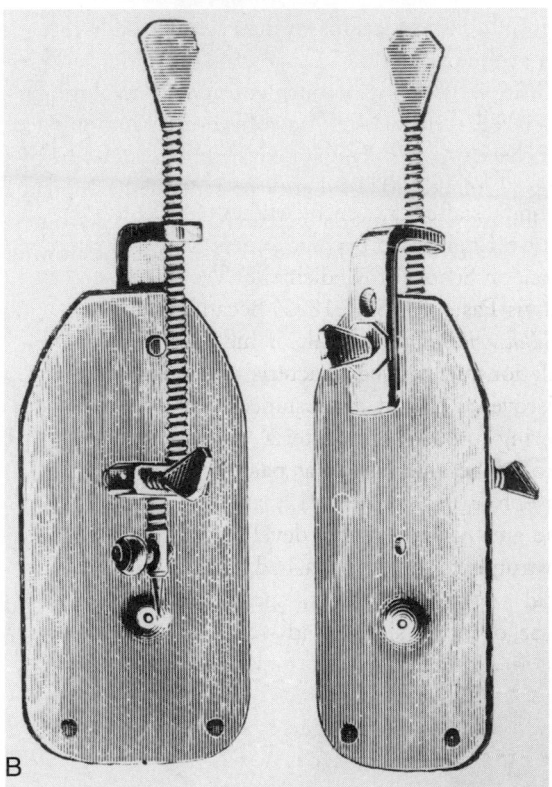

FIG 4-3   (A) Antoni van Leeuwenhoek (Used with permission from The New York Public Library) (B) and his microscope (Used with permission from Bettmann/CORBIS).

- Wilhelm Konrad Roentgen (1845–1922) was a German professor of physics who discovered electromagnetic radiation as a result of his experiments involving electrical currents passed through sealed glass tubes. (See Figure 4-5, A.) This radiation, which he called *x-rays,* eventually became known as **roentgenography** and is most commonly known today as *radiology.* (See Figure 4-5, B.)
- Florence Nightingale (1820–1910) is considered the founder of modern nursing. During the Crimean War, Nightingale was in charge of a core of 38 volunteer nurses who provided care to wounded British troops. Through her determination and keen medical understanding, she greatly improved the deplorable conditions in which she found the soldiers living. She earned the title of The Lady with the Lamp because of her habit of making late-night rounds to check on her patients with a small lamp to light her way. After the war, she continued to advocate for sanitary living conditions for patients and is credited with significantly lowering the death rate of soldiers during war and peacetime. She then turned her attention to the design of hospitals, continuing to stress the importance of sanitation, hygiene, and ventilation. In 1860, she started the Nightingale Training School for nurses, which set the example for nursing schools that followed. (See Figure 4 6.)

✳ *Current Medicine*

Over the past century, the frequency of medical breakthroughs has increased dramatically. Many of these breakthroughs involved the development of new drugs, including

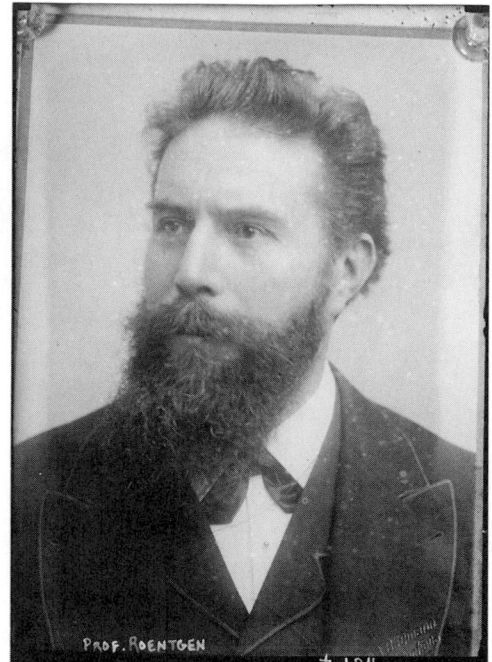

A

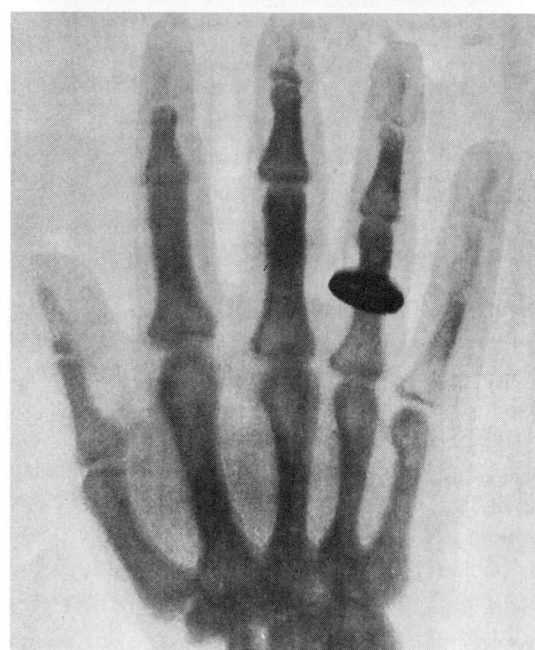

B

FIG 4-5 Wilhelm Konrad Roentgen (A) (Used with permission from The Library of Congress) and one of his first x-rays (B) (From McKinnis: *Fundamentals of Musculoskeletal Imaging*, 2nd ed. FA Davis, Philadelphia, 2005, p. 5, with permission).

vaccines, antibiotics, antivirals, insulin, and thousands of others. Medical advancements have included such diagnostic procedures as magnetic resonance imaging (MRI), computerized axial tomography (CAT), ultrasonography, and countless others. The number of highly technological medical devices, such as pacemakers, implantable defibrillators,

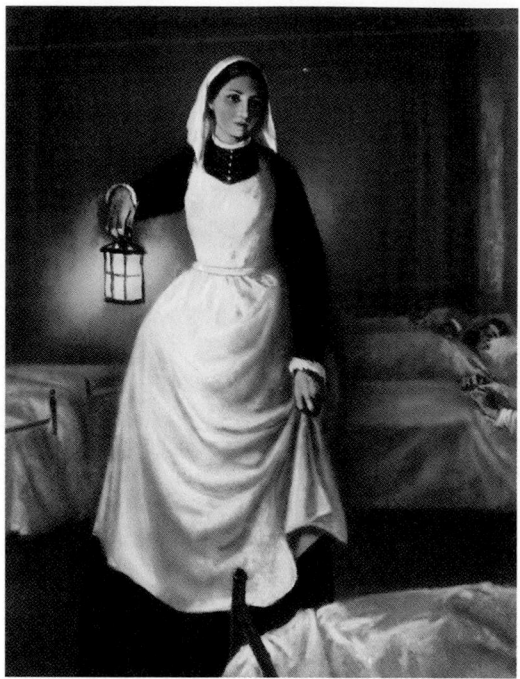

FIG 4-6 Florence Nightingale. (Used with permission from Bettmann/ CORBIS.)

and insulin pumps, seems to increase at a daily rate. Procedures such as organ and tissue transplantation and in vitro fertilization, which were once considered revolutionary, not to mention controversial, have become commonplace. Scientists have successfully mapped the human **genome** by identifying all of the 30,000 genes present in the human body. (See Figure 4-7.) Current research is underway on human stem cells and even in the controversial area of **cloning**.

Future of Medicine

What medicine and science will accomplish in the next 100 years is anyone's guess, given the phenomenal increase in the growth of science, technology, and medicine in the recent past. However, it is safe to say that science, technology, and medicine will continue to develop at a rapid rate. Stem cell research, while currently a subject of some controversy, will likely continue as well. Robotics in medicine has already proven useful and will likely develop further. For all of these reasons, hope for cures or remedies for many diseases and disorders that currently plague the human race is not unfounded.

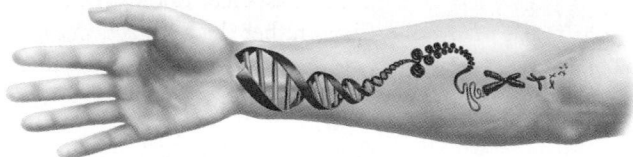

FIG 4-7 The human genome.

Health Care Settings

Physicians and other health care practitioners provide health care to people in a variety of settings depending on their needs. Common health care settings include hospitals and long-term, subacute, home, and ambulatory care facilities.

Hospitals

Hospitals are **acute care** settings, in which health care professionals deliver care to patients who are experiencing sudden illness or injury. Patients may be treated in the emergency department or admitted for medical and nursing care on a 24-hour basis. Depending on the size and type of hospital, it may include a number of specialty units, such as orthopedics, medical, oncology, pediatrics, maternity, surgery, and intensive care. Hospitals may be designated as providing Level I, II, or III trauma care, depending on the types of injuries they are equipped to deal with. Some hospitals, designated as **teaching hospitals**, are affiliated with medical schools. Teaching hospitals employ medical school **residents**, who are physicians in the process of obtaining further clinical training after internship, usually as a member of the hospital staff. These residents provide much of the physician-related care in these hospitals under the supervision of licensed physicians. A growing number of hospitals have day-surgery units where uncomplicated surgeries are performed. Patients generally are admitted and discharged from such units in the same day. Hospitals are further designated as *private* or *nonprofit*. Private hospitals are commonly owned by stockholders and run by companies. Nonprofit hospitals have a community-service focus and are generally run by a board of directors. While these hospitals may make a profit, all such monies must be reinvested in the hospital.

Physicians must possess **hospital privileges** in order to see patients in a hospital. Before a hospital grants such privileges, it will consider such factors as the physician's education, licensure, experience, and prior revocation of privileges or actions against the physician's license.

Long-Term Care

Long-term care (LTC) facilities, also known as *nursing homes,* provide skilled nursing care for people who are deemed medically stable yet unable to attend to activities of daily living (ADLs) without assistance. Such people are generally referred to as *residents* rather than patients because the LTC facility is their home. Sometimes, a person's stay at an LTC facility may be temporary; however, it is more commonly permanent. While nurses and nurses' aides provide care for the residents, the aim of care is to create a homelike atmosphere to the greatest extent possible, where residents have opportunities for social, physical, and creative activities.

Subacute Care

Subacute care facilities provide a level of care somewhere between that of the acute care and long-term care facilities. A patient's stay in such a facility is usually longer than in acute care, but still temporary. The purpose of the patient's stay is commonly rehabilitation activities with the goal of supporting the patient in regaining enough strength, mobility, and function to return home or to a semi-independent assisted-care setting.

Home Care

Home care is a setting in which individuals are able to remain in their own private homes with the help of private nurses, trained aides, chore services, and other types of assistance. Another setting that falls under the umbrella of home care is the increasingly popular adult family homes that are becoming more common in many communities, also known as **assisted living** facilities. The owners of such facilities are generally licensed by the state to provide housing, meals, and limited health care services to a specified number of residents. Most adult family homes accept only private-pay patients and do not provide intensive nursing care. However, they are an attractive option for people who are unable to live independently yet are not in need of LTC placement.

Ambulatory Care

The term *ambulatory* means "to walk or move about freely." An **ambulatory care** facility is one that provides medical care to nonresidential patients who do not stay overnight. Most medical assistants work in ambulatory care settings, such as physicians' offices and medical clinics.

Types of Medical Practices

Physicians have a number of options when choosing the type of medical practice in which they wish to participate. Choices include sole proprietorships, partnerships, and corporations. All types of medical practices are likely to employ medical assistants.

Sole Proprietorship

Historically, physicians worked as **sole proprietors** within their own offices. They were in charge of their practices and could operate them as they wished. Being self-employed, they enjoyed a certain level of independence and flexibility. Patients liked knowing that they could count on seeing their own doctors and appreciated the personal nature of health care. As sole proprietors, physicians were the owners of their practices and could employ whomever they wished, even other physicians.

However, sole proprietorships are becoming less common as physicians these days are more aware of the disadvantages in this type of arrangement. Such disadvantages include potential liability for acts of all employees, long work hours, and being on call virtually 24 hours per day, 7 days per week. Furthermore, physicians must bear all financial responsibility of the practice and, unless they sell them to someone else, their practices end when they retire or die.

In recent years, many physicians began joining together to form **associate practices**. This arrangement allows them to enjoy the benefits of a sole proprietorship while sharing resources, such as office space, equipment, and employees. While associate practices help alleviate the burden of a sole proprietorship somewhat, physicians still must deal with issues of liability, long hours, and continuous on-call time.

Partnership

Because sole proprietorships and associate practices require such a substantial commitment, many physicians are finding **partnerships** to be more attractive. A medical partnership is created when two or more physicians create a legal agreement that specifies the rights, obligations, and responsibilities of each. There are many advantages of a partnership, including an increased potential profit because physicians share expenses and pool such resources as office space, equipment, employees, and insurance. They can also enjoy more freedom because they alternate taking calls for all patients in the practice. (See *On-call system*.) The main disadvantage of a partnership is the potential liability for a partner's debts. A partnership with three or more licensed, full-time physicians is known as a *group practice.*

Patient Education

On-call System
Patients usually hope to talk with their own physicians when they contact the call service on weekends or evenings. Furthermore, they usually expect their own physician to provide care should they be hospitalized. However, physicians in a group practice or corporation usually share on-call duties and, if a physician is out of town, hospital visitation as well. Dealing with a different physician can be disconcerting to patients who have their heart set on seeing or speaking to their own doctor. Therefore, the medical assistant should carefully explain the practice's policy regarding after-hours calls and hospital care to patients at the time that care is established.

Corporation

A **corporation** is an artificially created body with legal and business status that is regulated by the state. The corporation exists independently of shareholders or employees and has a continuous life that does not end or change with a change in the shareholders or employees. Physicians in the corporation are usually shareholders as well as employees of the corporation. This status provides them with significant income and tax advantages, along with attractive benefit packages. Furthermore, as professional employees of the corporation, they are not liable for the acts or debts of other employees of the corporation. Therefore, their personal assets are not in jeopardy if others are involved in litigation. A health maintenance organization (HMO) is one type of a corporation in which physicians commonly practice.

Health Care Team

There are many members of a general health care team. Medical assistants should familiarize themselves with each of these specialties so they can communicate with others in an informed and effective manner. (See *Members of the team.*)

Physicians

Physicians, or medical doctors (MDs), are qualified to diagnose and treat patients for illness and disease, prescribe medication, and perform surgery. Their education usually involves 4 years of "premed" undergraduate coursework, 4 years of medical school, and then 3 to 8 years of an internship or residency, commonly in a specialty area. Many physicians also earn board certification in their chosen specialty by passing a certification examination. Physicians must have a license in the state in which they practice medicine and must participate in continuing education for license renewal.

Patient Education

Members of the Team
Just as with medical specialties, most patients are confused by the many types of therapists, technicians, and other health providers who are members of the health care team within a medical office or clinic. To reduce this confusion and increase patient understanding about who the members of the health care team are and what they do, the medical assistant should consider creating a pamphlet that describes the members of the team as well as their education and role.

Because medical assistants may assist with patient referrals to other physicians, they should become familiar with the many areas in which physicians specialize. (See *Medical specialties.*) Furthermore, such knowledge may be useful to medical assistants as they decide in which areas they are most interested in working. (See *Explaining specialties,* page 37.)

Other Practitioners

There are some health care practitioners whose education and specialty differs from that of medical physicians. These practitioners include chiropractors, dentists, optometrists, and, in some cases, naturopathic physicians. Although these practitioners are specialists in their own right, their practice

Medical specialties

This table lists and describes common medical specialties along with their titles.

Specialty and Title	Description
Allergy and Immunology *Allergist, Immunologist*	Diagnosis and treatment of patients with allergies and immune system disorders
Anesthesiology *Anesthesiologist*	Administration of anesthetics to patients during surgery; pain management intervention for patients with severe, intractable pain
Cardiology *Cardiologist*	Diagnosis and treatment of patients with heart disorders
Dermatology *Dermatologist*	Diagnosis and treatment of patients with skin disorders
Emergency Medicine *Emergency Physician*	Diagnosis, stabilization, and initial treatment of patients with traumatic injury or acute illness in the emergency department or in urgent care centers
Endocrinology *Endocrinologist*	Diagnosis and treatment of patients with endocrine system disorders
Family Practice *Family Practitioner*	Care for members of the whole family, from newborn to elderly, focusing on health maintenance and illness prevention
Gastroenterology *Gastroenterologist*	Diagnosis and treatment of patients with disorders of the stomach and intestines
General Surgery *Surgeon*	Diagnosis and treatment of patients with diseases, disorders, or injuries by using surgical procedures
Geriatrics *Gerontologist*	Diagnosis and treatment of patients with diseases and disorders associated with aging
Gynecology *Gynecologist*	Diagnosis and treatment of patients with diseases and disorders of the female reproductive system
Hematology *Hematologist*	Diagnosis and treatment of patients with diseases and disorders of the blood and blood-forming tissues
Infertility *Infertility Specialist*	Diagnosis and treatment of patients with fertility problems
Internal Medicine *Internist*	Diagnosis and treatment of patients with diseases and disorders of the internal organs
Medical Genetics *Geneticist*	Diagnosis and treatment of patients with genetic diseases and disorders, possibly including genetic screening and genetic counseling

Continued

Medical specialties—cont'd

Specialty and Title	Description
Nephrology *Nephrologist*	Diagnosis and treatment of patients with diseases and disorders of the kidneys
Neurology *Neurologist*	Diagnosis and treatment of patients with diseases and disorders of the nervous system
Nuclear Medicine *Nuclear Medicine Specialist*	Diagnosis and treatment of patients with various disorders by using radiation and imaging technology
Obstetrics *Obstetrician*	Care and treatment of women during pregnancy, childbirth, and the postpartum period
Occupational Medicine *Occupational Medicine Specialist*	Diagnosis and treatment of patients with diseases and disorders related to their occupation
Oncology *Oncologist*	Diagnosis and treatment of patients with cancer
Ophthalmology *Ophthalmologist*	Diagnosis and treatment of patients with diseases and disorders of the eye
Orthopedics *Orthopedist*	Diagnosis and treatment of patients with diseases, disorders, or injuries of the bones, muscles, tendons, and ligaments
Osteopathy *Doctor of Osteopathy*	Treatment of patients using medicine, surgery, and osteopathic manipulative therapy (OMT), with a strong focus on a conservative holistic approach
Otorhinolaryngology *Otolaryngologist*	Diagnosis and treatment of patients with diseases and disorders of the ears, nose, and throat (ENT)
Pathology *Pathologist*	Analysis of tissue samples to confirm diagnosis of various disorders or performance of autopsy to determine cause of death
Pediatrics *Pediatrician*	Diagnosis and treatment of children's disorders with a strong focus on health promotion and illness prevention
Physical Medicine and Rehabilitation *Physiatrist*	Diagnosis and treatment of patients with physical disabilities or musculoskeletal disorders or those who are suffering from chronic pain secondary to injury with the goal of restoring optimal function
Plastic Surgery *Plastic Surgeon*	Performance of surgical procedures for reconstruction in patients who have suffered disfiguring injuries as well as elective enhancement procedures
Podiatry *Podiatrist*	Diagnosis and treatment of patients with diseases and disorders of the feet
Psychiatry *Psychiatrist*	Diagnosis and treatment of patients with mental health disorders
Pulmonology *Pulmonologist*	Diagnosis and treatment of patients with diseases and disorders of the lungs
Radiology *Radiologist*	Diagnosis and treatment of patients with various disorders using radiologic procedures (x-rays)
Sports Medicine *Sports Medicine Specialist*	Diagnosis and treatment of patients with athletic-related injuries
Urology *Urologist*	Diagnosis and treatment of patients with diseases and disorders of the urinary system in females and the genitourinary system in males

Patient Education

Explaining Specialties

Most patients are confused by the many types of physicians and specialty practices. Therefore, a medical assistant who works in an office that provides primary care services should provide pamphlets for patients that list and explain who the specialists are and what type of services they offer.

differs from that of traditional medical doctors and they may have limited authority to prescribe medications and treatments. (See *Nonmedical physician health care providers.*)

Nurses

Nurses are licensed professionals who are closely involved in patient care. Their practice is dictated by the state board of nursing in each state and is legally independent of physicians. However, nurses commonly work closely with physicians in the provision of patient care. Their role and duties include, but are not limited to, patient assessment, nursing care plan design, implementation of physician orders, communication of data about patient status with physicians as well as other members of the health care team, and education of patients and family members. Nursing titles and legal designations vary depending on the nurse's education and legal credential earned. Nurses practice in a wide variety of areas in public, private, acute, long-term, and home care settings. (See *Nursing credentials,* page 38.)

Nonmedical physician health care providers

This table lists some of the most common nonmedical physician health care specialties along with titles, a brief description, and education and licensure requirements.

Specialty and Title	Description of Specialty Area	Education and Licensure
Chiropractic *Chiropractor*	Treatment through manipulation of the spine for patients who suffer disorders related to misalignment of the vertebrae	• Undergraduate degree plus 3 years of chiropractic school • Licensed by state, with a continuing education requirement for renewal
Dentistry *Dentist*	Diagnosis and treatment of patients with diseases and disorders of the teeth and gums	• Undergraduate degree plus 4 years of dental school • Licensed as a doctor of dental medicine (DDM) or Doctor of Dental Surgery (DDS) • Continuing education required to maintain the license, generally 10 to 25 hours per year, depending on the state
Optometry *Optometrist*	Evaluation and measurement of visual acuity and prescription of corrective lenses	• Undergraduate degree plus 4 years at a school of optometry • Licensed by the state (sometimes confused with *ophthalmologists,* who are licensed medical doctors) • Continuing education required to maintain the license, generally 8 to 50 hours per year, depending on the state and the specific type of license
Naturopathy *Naturopathic Physician*	Treatment of patients using natural means, such as nutrition, sunlight, dietary supplements, herbal medicine, homeopathy, acupuncture, and massage	• Licensed in some states

Nursing credentials

This table lists the most common nursing credentials along with a description and the education requirements and degree for each.

Credential	Role Description	Education and Degree
Certified Nursing Assistant (CNA) or *Nursing Assistant, Certified (NAC)*	• Assists nurses with basic patient care activities such as feeding, dressing, toileting, and hygiene	• 120 hours of coursework, including 16 hours of supervised clinical training • Nursing assistant certificate
Licensed Practical Nurse (LPN) or *Licensed Vocational Nurse (LVN)*	• Assists registered nurse with care of noncritical patients • Delegates appropriate tasks to nursing assistants	• Prerequisite coursework (1 to 2 years) • 1 year of nursing education • Certificate in nursing

Registered Nurse (RN)	• Designs plan of nursing care and provides care for all types of patients with a strong focus on leadership, commonly working in management roles
	• Delegates appropriate tasks to LPNs and nursing assistants
		• Associate's Degree in Nursing (ADN)
		  • Prerequisite coursework (1 to 2 years)
		  • 2 years of nursing education
		• Bachelor of Science in Nursing (BSN)
		  • 4 years of liberal arts and sciences coursework, including 2 years of nursing curriculum

Advanced Practice Nurse (Nurse Practitioner [NP], Clinical Nurse Specialist [CNP], Certified Nurse-Midwife [CNM], and Nurse Anesthetist [CRNA], among others)	• Provides advanced care to patients in designated specialty areas, which may include diagnosis, medication prescription, and treatment • In many states, practices legally as an autonomous practitioner (without association of a physician)	• 4-year liberal arts and sciences degree, including 2 years of nursing curriculum • 1 to 3 years of graduate school in nursing area of specialty • Master of Science in Nursing (MSN) (graduate degrees and titles vary with specialty)

Physician Assistants

The role of the physician assistant (PA) was created by physicians to provide them with assistance in the evaluation, diagnosis, and treatment of patients. Historically, the first PAs were selected for their experience as medics in the military, nurses, or some other health care field. Further training was then provided by physicians in certificate programs. Currently, there are more than 130 PA programs in the United States. Some programs provide a 2-year Associate's degree; however, most are now 4-year Bachelor of Science degree programs. In addition, Master's degree programs are now available in some states. After completing their education, PAs must pass a certification examination, which earns them the right to list the PAC (physician assistant, certified) credential after their name. PAs can work in more than 60 specialty areas. Their specific duties are determined by state law and their supervising physician. They have prescriptive authority based on this relationship. Most PAs are directly involved in patient assessment, diagnosis, and treatment in the ambulatory care setting, and some PAs are trained to assist physicians in specialty settings such as surgery.

Medical Technologists

Medical technologists (MTs) earn a Bachelor of Science degree. They are credentialed with a license or certificate to perform diagnostic testing on blood and body fluids to aid in the diagnosis of diseases and disorders. Those who pass the certification examination earn the right to list the ASCP (American Society for Clinical Pathology) credential after their name. Medical technologists work in laboratories of clinics, hospitals, or universities performing a full range of simple and complex laboratory tests. They work with and may supervise medical laboratory technicians. In the course of their work, they operate electronic equipment, computers, and precision instruments in five laboratory areas:

● blood banking
● chemistry

- hematology
- immunology
- microbiology.

Therapists

All therapists work with clients to help them regain or achieve an optimal level of function. However, their education, training, and roles vary greatly. Some of the most common types of therapists found in the health care setting are physical therapist, occupational therapist, speech therapist, and respiratory therapist.

Physical Therapist

A physical therapist (PT) earns a Master of Science degree and may earn a doctorate as well. The PT is a licensed professional and must graduate from an accredited program. Some states require continuing education for license renewal. A PT designs individual therapy programs for clients of all ages in order to restore strength, mobility, and function; decrease pain; and promote overall fitness and health. The overall goal of care is to increase the patient's ability to function at work and at home. Physical therapy treatment methods include exercise, stretching, heat or cold application, ultrasound, electrical stimulation, and massage. PTs teach patients to use such assistive devices as wheelchairs, walkers, crutches, and prosthetics. They may specialize in a variety of areas, including pediatrics, geriatrics, sports medicine, orthopedics, cardiopulmonary rehabilitation, and aquatic therapy. They supervise and delegate tasks to physical therapy assistants (PTAs), who are also valuable members of the therapy team.

Occupational Therapist

An occupational therapist (OT) is a licensed professional who may earn the OTR (registered) credential upon passing a certification examination. A Master's degree is required for entry into practice as an OT. OTs work with patients with a variety of disabilities from physical or natural causes. An OT designs an individual therapy program for each patient that helps him or her achieve an optimal level of function in the performance of his or her ADLs, such as bathing, dressing, and eating. OTs may also assist patients in regaining optimal function in their occupational setting. Such a program may include designing or prescribing special equipment to help a patient function at home or at work or developing computer-aided adaptive equipment and teaching a patient to use it. OTs may specialize in specific patient populations, such as pediatrics, geriatrics, or mentally handicapped patients.

Respiratory Therapist

A respiratory therapist (RT) treats patients with a variety of pulmonary disorders and works with patients of all ages.

RTs also work in a variety of settings, including acute care, ambulatory care, home care, and private businesses. RT duties include helping patients experiencing breathing problems in emergency situations, setting up ventilators, and assisting in the care of patients on life support. RTs may assist physicians with diagnosis by performing pulmonary function tests (PFTs), provide oxygen therapy via various delivery devices, administer such breathing treatments as nebulizers and chest percussion therapy (CPT), teach patients to use respiratory equipment, and deliver and set up oxygen equipment in patients' homes and teach them to use it. Their goal is to help clients achieve and maintain an optimal level of respiratory function. Educational preparation for respiratory therapists is an Associate's degree.

Speech Therapist

A speech therapist (ST) diagnoses and treats patients with speech, voice, or language disorders. STs develop and implement individualized therapy programs based on input from and consultation with other professionals, such as physicians, nurses, and social workers. STs are uniquely qualified to evaluate patients experiencing swallowing difficulties and recommend appropriate dietary and safety modifications accordingly. Requirements to practice speech therapy include a Master's degree in speech pathology plus 375 hours of supervised clinical practice, passing a national examination, and 9 months of postgraduate experience.

Registered Dietitian

A registered dietitian (RD) is an expert in the area of food and nutrition. An RD acts as a consultant in hospitals, long-term care facilities, HMOs, community and public health organizations, and medical centers. RDs also work in sports nutrition, food- and nutrition-related businesses, and research. They may specialize in working with pediatric, renal, and diabetic patients. A Bachelor's degree is required for entry to practice. However, many RDs earn their Master's or Doctorate degrees as well. After graduation, RDs must complete a supervised practice program and pass a national examination. Continuing education is required to maintain registration.

Prehospital Care Specialists

Some health care providers are educated and trained to provide emergency care and transport for those who experience injury or illness. Such individuals generally are employed by fire departments or ambulance companies. Examples of prehospital care specialists are emergency medical technicians and paramedics.

Emergency Medical Technicians

Emergency medical technicians (EMTs) are trained members of the emergency management services (EMS) team and assist paramedics in the stabilization and transportation of patients to the hospital. They are usually dispatched to the scene of an emergency by the 911 operator and may work with police or fire department personnel. They must know how to evaluate the scene to identify potential hazards; provide emergency, lifesaving interventions such as CPR; control bleeding; and possess other first aid skills. There are several levels of certification that may be obtained to increase the EMT's skills and responsibilities. Such skills include obtaining IV access, administering IV fluids, and using defibrillators. EMTs work for ambulance services, fire departments, police departments, and hospitals. Training includes completion of an accredited EMT program, usually 6 months in length. However, training may take longer, depending on the level of certification. EMTs are certified or registered by passing an examination.

Paramedics

Paramedics are trained to provide emergency interventions for ill or injured patients with the goal of stabilizing them enough for transport to the hospital. They are usually dispatched to the scene of an emergency by the 911 operator and work with and supervise EMTs and, possibly, police or fire department personnel. They must know how to evaluate the scene to identify potential hazards; provide emergency, lifesaving interventions such as CPR; control bleeding; and perform other basic and advanced lifesaving skills. Paramedic programs vary in length by state and whether they are full-time or part-time. Training includes advanced cardiac life support (ACLS), pediatric advanced life support (PALS), and other emergency care courses.

Technicians

A variety of technicians work in the hospital and clinic settings to aid in the diagnosis and treatment of illness or injury. Some of these technicians include phlebotomists, radiologic technicians, and medical laboratory technicians.

Phlebotomist

Phlebotomists are trained to draw blood from patients for laboratory testing or from blood donors for blood banks. They spend time working directly with patients, taking blood, and monitoring the patient's response. They also assist the laboratory technologists by helping prepare and process the tests. Other tasks may include updating records, preparing stains and reagents, and cleaning and sterilizing equipment. Phlebotomists work in the laboratories of hospitals, clinics, and blood banks. They may be trained on the job or may complete an accredited 1-semester or 1-year program, earning a diploma or certificate.

Radiologic Technicians

Radiologic technicians help physicians diagnose a patient's disorder by creating images of internal organs, tissues, and bones. Common procedures include x-rays, which show bones, and fluoroscopies and sonograms, which show soft tissues by using sound, magnetic, and radio waves. Radiologic technicians analyze the images and consult with physicians about their significance. They take special precautions to protect themselves and patients from unnecessary radiation exposure. Training usually consists of an Associate's degree in a professional technical program or a Bachelor's degree. People with experience in another health care field may be able to complete a 1-year certification program.

Medical Laboratory Technicians

Medical laboratory technicians (MLTs) assist in the diagnosis and treatment of patients by performing tests on blood, body fluids, or tissue specimens using microscopes, computers, and complex laboratory equipment. They work under the supervision of a medical laboratory technologist (MT), pathologist, or other professional. They may specialize in one of five different areas, including chemistry, blood banking, hematology, immunology, and microbiology. Other MLT duties include equipment and records maintenance and results reporting. Most MLTs work in laboratories of hospitals, public health organizations, universities, pharmaceutical companies, biomedical companies, or the armed forces. MLTs must complete an Associate's degree program and pass a national certification examination.

Administrative Specialists

Administrative specialists help with such administrative duties as coding, transcription, data entry, and medical records. Two types of administrative specialists are medical coding specialist and medical transcriptionist.

Medical Coding Specialist

A medical coding specialist reads and analyzes documentation of physicians and other health care providers to gather data about diseases, injuries, and procedures and translates it into diagnostic and procedural codes. Accuracy in assigning correct codes is critically important for compliance with federal regulations and insurance reimbursement. The medical facility may also use this data for planning and marketing as well as the preparation of management reports. Medical coding specialists work in hospitals, clinics, long-term care facilities, home health agencies, dental offices, insurance companies, and government agencies. Training may be available on-the-job or through continuing education; however, an Associate's degree is recommended. To become a certified medical coder, an individual must pass examinations offered by the American Health

Information Management Association (AHIMA) and the American Academy of Professional Coders (AAPC).

Medical Transcriptionist

Medical transcriptionists work in partnership with health care providers to document patient care. They are health care professionals with expertise in medical language who translate a physician's dictation of a patient's medical history, diagnosis, treatment, and prognosis into written form. Transcriptionists must use common sense and sound judgment, knowing when to seek clarification and verify information in order to ensure the accuracy of the medical record, which is considered a legal document. Certification may be earned by passing an examination and is maintained through continuing education. Medical transcriptionists work in physician's offices, hospitals, clinics, laboratories, insurance companies, government facilities, legal offices, and research centers. Some medical transcriptionists also work out of their homes as independent contractors.

Chapter Summary

- To better understand their role within the profession of medicine, medical assistants should understand the origins, history, and present-day culture of medicine.
- Earliest records indicate that the first health care professionals were priests and other religious leaders. The prevailing belief of the time was that illness and disease were caused by evil spirits or were punishment from the gods for sinful behavior.
- Some ancient healing techniques, such as massage and acupuncture, are still practiced today.
- Hippocrates (460–377 B.C.) is known as the *Father of Medicine* and was the author of the Hippocratic oath. As a result of his studies of the sick and the human body, he rejected historical explanations that illness had a spiritual cause and thought the cause was instead a physical one. His beliefs that a healthy diet, hygiene, rest, and fresh air provide healing properties are still relevant today.
- Claudius Galen (A.D. 129) was a Greek physician who wrote and illustrated numerous studies of animal anatomy. He became famous for his theory that disease and illness were caused by an imbalance of "humors."
- Once human dissection became legal, Andreas Vesalius (1514–1564) was able to create many accurate illustrations of human anatomy based on his studies.
- During the 15th century, the advent of the printing press revolutionized medical education by allowing widespread dissemination of information and illustrations.

- The first microscope was developed through the efforts of Antoni van Leeuwenhoek (1632–1723), a Dutch linen draper.
- Marcello Malpighi (1628–1694), an Italian scientist used van Leeuwenhoek's discoveries to study capillaries and was the first to determine the link between arteries and veins. As a result of his work, Malpighi subsequently became known as the first histologist.
- During the 18th century, Edward Jenner (1749–1823) developed the smallpox vaccine after noting that a dairymaid was immune to smallpox because of her previous infection with cowpox.
- Significant contributions to the medical profession during the 19th and 20th centuries included the development and use of ether as a general anesthetic by Crawford Williamson Long (1815–1878); the first woman physician, Elizabeth Blackwell (1821–1910); development of the process now known as pasteurization by Louis Pasteur (1822–1895), who became known as the *Father of Bacteriology;* methods of sterilizing instruments prior to performing surgery by Joseph Lister (1827–1912); and the discovery of x-rays by Wilhelm Konrad Roentgen (1845–1922).
- Over the past century, the number of medical breakthroughs has increased at a dramatic rate. Just a few examples include the development of many new drugs, diagnostic procedures, and highly technical medical devices. It is safe to say that science, technology, and medicine will continue to develop at a rapid rate in the years ahead.
- Common health care settings include hospitals and long-term, subacute, home, and ambulatory care facilities.
- Physicians have a number of options when choosing the type of medical practice in which they wish to participate. Choices include sole proprietorships, partnerships, and corporations. All types of medical practices are likely to employ medical assistants.
- There are many members of the general health care team. Medical assistants should familiarize themselves with each of these specialties so they can communicate with others in an informed and effective manner. Physicians may specialize in any number of areas. Other health care providers whose education and specialty differ from that of the medical physician include chiropractors, dentists, optometrists, and naturopathic physicians.
- Nurses are licensed professionals who are closely involved in patient care. Their practice is dictated by the state board of nursing in each state and is legally independent of physicians. However, nurses commonly work closely with physicians in the provision of patient care.
- The role of the physician assistant (PA) was created by physicians to provide them with assistance in the evaluation, diagnosis, and treatment of patients.

- Medical technologists (MTs) are credentialed with a license or certificate to perform diagnostic testing on blood and body fluids to aid in the diagnosis of diseases and disorders.
- All therapists work with clients to help them regain or achieve an optimal level of function. Their education, training, and roles vary greatly. Some of the most common types of therapists found in the health care setting are physical therapists, occupational therapists, speech therapists, and respiratory therapists.
- Registered dietitians (RDs) are experts in food and nutrition. They act as consultants in hospitals, long-term care facilities, HMOs, community and public health organizations, and medical centers as well as in other areas.
- Prehospital care specialists include emergency medical technicians (EMTs) and paramedics. They provide emergency care to ill and injured individuals and transport them to the hospital for further care.
- A variety of technicians work in the hospital and clinic settings to aid in the diagnosis and treatment of illness or injury. Some of these technicians include phlebotomists, radiologic technicians, and medical laboratory technicians.
- Administrative specialists help with such administrative duties as coding, transcription, data entry, and medical record keeping. Two types of administrative specialists are the medical coding specialist and medical transcriptionist.

Team Work Exercises

1. Divide into teams of three or four students. Each team will select or be assigned one of the providers listed below and create a brochure or pamphlet that describes that provider's specialty area.
   a. nurse
   b. medical laboratory technician
   c. respiratory therapist
   d. physical therapist
   e. speech therapist
   f. occupational therapist
   g. medical coding specialist
   h. transcriptionist
   i. dietitian
   j. radiologic technician.
   Be sure to include:
   a. typical education
   b. job description

   c. whether they are licensed, certified, or otherwise credentialed
   d. settings in which they typically work
   e. average wages
   f. any other data of interest.
2. Divide into teams of three or four. Each team will select or be assigned one of the physician specialists listed in the *Medical specialties* table on pages 35 and 36 and design a brochure or pamphlet that describes their specialty area. Be sure to include:
   a. typical education
   b. job description
   c. type of patients seen
   d. settings in which they typically work
   e. any specialty credentials required other than a medical license
   f. any other data of interest.

Case Studies

1. Atsuko Katsumi is an elderly woman who fell and broke her hip. Describe the type of health care settings she may experience in the course of her recovery and give a brief description of the type of care she would receive in each.
2. Elsa Yager has been a medical assistant for the past 4 years and is considering going back to school. She would like to become a nurse but isn't sure how long that will take or what type of setting she would prefer to work in. What advice can you give her?

Resources

- American Dietetic Association: *www.eatright.org*
- Association for Healthcare Documentation Integrity (AHDI): *www.aamt.org*
- Information on medical technologist careers: *www.ascp.org/Careerlinks/LabCareers/default.aspx*
- Information on naturopathic medicine and careers: *www.aanmc.org/car_prac/index.php*
- Information on paramedics: *www.uihealthcare.com/depts/emslrc/paramedics.html*
- Information on physician assistant programs: *paprogram.medicine.uiowa.edu/*
- Information on physical therapists: *www.apta.org* and *www.bls.gov/oco/ocos080.htm*
- Information on miscellaneous health care careers: *www.mshealthcareers.com* and *www.allalliedhealthschools.com*

Therapeutic Communication

Learning Objectives

Upon completion of this chapter, the student will be able to:

- define and spell key terms
- list, define, and describe eight parts of the communication cycle
- discuss the impact of nonverbal communication on verbal communication
- describe examples of nonverbal behaviors that may enhance the effectiveness of communication
- demonstrate active listening through role playing
- demonstrate various communication patterns through role playing and include passive, passive-aggressive, assertive, and aggressive communication patterns
- define and give examples of seven defense mechanisms that impede effective communication
- describe six strategies for effectively dealing with difficult people

CAAHEP Competencies

General Competencies
  Professional Communications
    Recognize and respond to verbal communications
    Recognize and respond to nonverbal communications

ABHES Competencies

  Professionalism
    Be courteous and diplomatic
    Be attentive, listen, and learn
  Communication
    Be impartial and show empathy when dealing with patients
    Recognize and respond to verbal and nonverbal communication
    Principles of verbal and nonverbal communication

Chapter Outline

  First Impressions
  Communication Cycle
    Referent
    Message
    Sender and Receiver
    Channels
    Feedback
    Interpersonal Variables
    Environment
  Verbal Communication
  Nonverbal Communications
  Active Listening
  Giving Advice
  Communication Patterns
    Passive
    Passive-Aggressive
    Assertive
    Aggressive
  Communication Challenges
    Defense Mechanisms
      Rationalization

      Compensation
      Regression
      Repression
      Displacement
      Denial
      Projection
    Strategies for Dealing with Difficult People
      Focusing on the patient
      Acknowledging the patient
      Validating the patient's feelings
      Using "I" language
      Moving to a solution
      Setting boundaries
  Cultural Variables
  Chapter Summary
  Team Work Exercises
  Case Studies
  Resources

Key Terms

aggressive
Quality of striving to meet one's own needs while disregarding the rights and needs of others

articulate
To verbally express oneself clearly and easily

assertive
Quality of advocating for one's own rights while respecting the rights of others

boundary
Physical or psychological space that indicates the limit of appropriate versus inappropriate behavior

channel
Mode of conveying a message, including vision, hearing, and touch

communication
Process of sending and receiving information between two or more individuals

compensation
Psychological response in which a person offsets feelings of inadequacy in one aspect of that person's life by achievement in another aspect

congruent
Consistent or matching

decoding
Process by which the receiver of a message extracts its meaning

defense mechanism
Unhealthy coping strategy that a person may employ when feeling emotionally threatened in some way

denial
Psychological response by which a person refuses to acknowledge the validity or reality of something that is obvious to others

displacement
Psychological response by which a person expresses anger or another emotion at a person or object that is not the cause of those feelings

environment
Setting in which a communication experience occurs

feedback
Message returned by a receiver as a response to the sender's message

interpersonal variables
Factors that impact a receiver's interpretation of a message

message
Content of a communication, including verbal, nonverbal, and symbolic language

norms
Unwritten rules of socially acceptable behavior

passive
Quality of submitting or yielding without offering resistance

passive-aggressive
Manipulative behavior that appears initially passive but seeks to control by retaliation in the form of procrastination, stubbornness, and "forgetfulness"

projection
Psychological response in which a person accuses others of that person's own feelings, attitudes, or behaviors

proxemics
Study of how much personal space people prefer and how it relates to culture and environment

rationalization
Psychological response in which a person makes excuses to justify inappropriate behaviors

receiver
Person who receives a message and decodes it

referent
Stimulation or motivation to communicate

regression
Psychological response in which a person reverts to behaviors associated with earlier (younger) developmental stages

repression
Psychological response in which a person eliminates from conscious thought traumatic experiences or certain impulses that the person believes are unacceptable

sender
Person who delivers a message

First Impressions

Because a first impression is so important, a medical assistant must help ensure that each patient's first impression of the medical office is a positive one. Good communication is one of the most essential skills for ensuring a positive first impression. Communication is a complex, continuous, multidimensional process. The **message**, or content, of communication includes not only what a person says but also the nonverbal and symbolic language of facial expressions, body language, and vocal inflections. Thus, a medical assistant must be sure the message she sends with her body language is **congruent**, or consistent, with the message she sends with her words.

Communication Cycle

Communication, or the process of sending and receiving information between two or more individuals, occurs in a cycle. The main features of the communication cycle include the referent, sender, receiver, message, channels, feedback, interpersonal variables, and environment. (See Figure 5-1.)

Referent

The **referent** is what stimulates or motivates the communication. It might be an object, a sight, a sound, an idea, a sensation, or anything that prompts a person to communicate.

Message

The message is the content of the communication. It includes verbal communication through words, nonverbal communication through gestures such as head nodding, and communication through symbolism, as with such commonly understood symbols as ♂ for male and ♀ for female. When a person receives a message, the message also becomes a referent for that person, who in turn may respond with another message.

Sender and Receiver

The person who delivers the message is the **sender**. This person is responsible for the emotional tone and accuracy of the message. The sender can increase the effectiveness of the communication experience by using clear speech, simple language, and adequate volume as well as facial expressions and body language that are congruent with the spoken message. The sender should observe the person to whom he is sending the message for signs of understanding or confusion.

A **receiver** is the person who receives the message and **decodes** it, or extracts the meaning of the message. The accuracy with which the receiver understands the message depends, in part, on how well the receiver pays attention to the sender. Paying close attention involves focusing, listening, and noting verbal and nonverbal cues.

The roles of sender and receiver are fluid, meaning they change back and forth as the communication cycle continues. Compatibility, familiarity, and commonality between sender and receiver enhance their communication and understanding.

Channels

Channels are the means of conveying messages, such as vision, hearing, and touch. Such channels may incorporate facial expressions, voice volume, vocal inflection, touching a person's shoulder, and so on. The more channels a sender uses, the more clearly he conveys the message—as long as all of the channels are consistent with the message he or she is sending.

Feedback

Feedback is the message returned by the receiver, which reflects his or her level of understanding. It also may include the receiver's response to the original message.

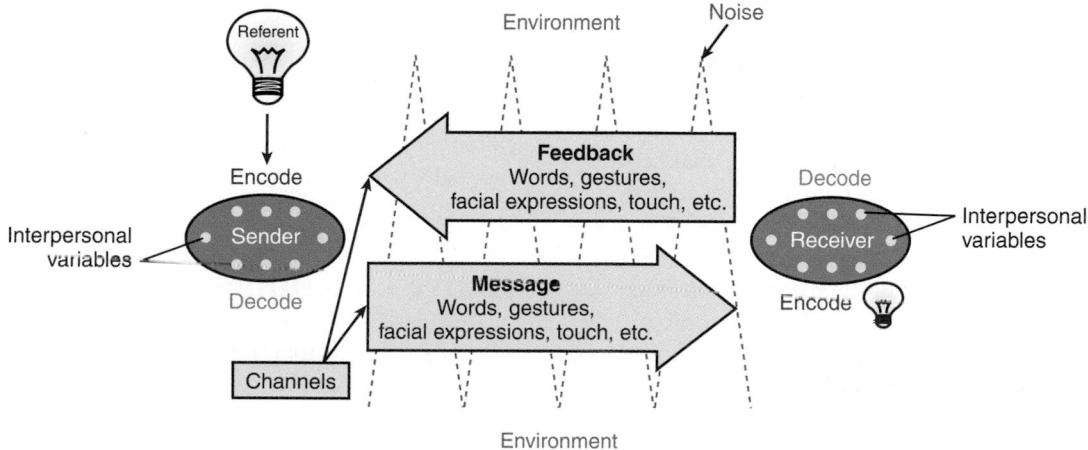

FIG 5-1 Communication cycle.

Interpersonal Variables

Communication is greatly impacted by **interpersonal variables**, or factors that influence the receiver's interpretation. Such factors include personal biases, education, developmental level, sociocultural background, values, beliefs, emotions, gender, health issues, roles, relationships, and prior experiences.

Environment

The communication **environment** is the setting in which the communication experience occurs. A number of environmental factors can interfere with the accuracy of communication, including pain, medication effects, room noise, temperature, humidity, lack of privacy, and inadequate space. In the medical office, a medical assistant is responsible for ensuring accurate communication with patients and coworkers. Therefore, she must address environmental and patient comfort issues in order to minimize distractions and maximize the patient's ability to focus, listen, and understand.

Verbal Communication

Spoken language is a key means of communication. However, the meaning of words can change, depending on vocal pitch and inflection, word emphasis, and pauses. Therefore, the medical assistant must consistently speak clearly, enunciate carefully, use a pleasant tone of voice, and keep her mind on the messages she is conveying. She must also remember that many patients, especially the elderly, may have some degree of hearing loss. When speaking to such individuals, she should face toward them so that they can see her lips and use adequate volume without shouting.

Nonverbal Communications

When a discrepancy exists between verbal and nonverbal messages, a listener will tend to believe the nonverbal message. Therefore, the medical assistant must pay careful attention to her body language. Body language encompasses many components, including hand gestures, mannerisms, facial expressions, posture, touch, and the use of personal space. A medical assistant in a closed stance with her arms crossed, who is looking away from the person and wearing a solemn expression, conveys disinterest or displeasure. To help patients feel welcome and at ease and to project the message of concern, caring, and openness, the medical assistant should use an open body stance, make frequent eye contact, and maintain a pleasant expression, punctuated by an occasional, genuine smile.

An important feature of body language is personal space. The study of how much personal space people prefer and how it relates to cultural and environmental factors is known as **proxemics**. Proxemics of people in the United States reveal a preference for public space up to 25', social space between 4' and 12', personal space from $1^1/_2'$ to 4', and intimate space as 0' (direct touch) to $1^1/_2'$. People are generally reluctant to give up these barriers without a compelling reason. For example, most people are willing to stand closer than usual to a stranger in a crowded elevator or when exiting a crowded concert hall. Even so, there are commonly additional unspoken rules that dictate acceptable behavior in such situations. For example, when riding in crowded elevators, people rarely speak to one another, always face forward, and avoid making eye contact. In waiting rooms, patients rarely choose to sit directly next to a stranger if other options exist. Some may even choose to remain standing in order to maintain control over personal space.

Most people do not invite others into their personal space until a degree of trust and rapport has been established. Yet the health care arena necessitates some exceptions to the rules of personal space. When a patient seeks medical care, he or she generally expects a certain amount of touching to be involved. However, because the touching is extremely personal in some cases, as with a female pelvic examination, the knowledge that such touch is necessary does not automatically make patients feel comfortable with it. Therefore, the medical assistant and other members of the health care team must treat each patient with respect and sensitivity. Most patients feel vulnerable in such situations and want to trust that all touching is appropriate and professional. To earn and maintain such trust, the medical assistant must protect the patient's privacy and dignity.

Touch can be used in an emotionally therapeutic manner to convey interest, sincerity, and empathy. Examples of such touch might include a warm, firm handshake; a pat on the arm; or gently assisting someone as they stand to their feet or get off an examination table. Many patients welcome such forms of appropriate touch and report that it helps them to feel acknowledged and cared for. However, because not all patients welcome such touch, the medical assistant must learn to read the body language of the patient and follow his or her cues. It is always best to err on the side of caution, using less, rather than more, touch when unsure—especially when dealing with the opposite sex.

Active Listening

One of the most important parts of effective communication is active listening. Active listening involves 90% listening and 10% speaking. Most people overestimate their skills as a listener. When a person should be attending to what a speaker is saying, most are thinking about what they want to say next. Additionally, people sometimes become distracted and let their minds wander to other matters. Some, in an effort to be active listeners, jump in and finish the speaker's sentences. Others interrupt the speaker to get in their own thoughts and opinions. In these examples, the listeners are not listening well at all. Rather, they are attending to what they want to say, or even their desire to end the conversation and move on to other things. As a result, a speaker can feel unheard, unacknowledged, and uncared for. True active listening requires more energy than most people realize. It entails attending to the speaker's words and body language, allowing the speaker adequate time to formulate and **articulate** the message, and then reflecting, or paraphrasing, the message that was heard to verify understanding and seek clarification as needed.

Giving Advice

Medical assistants are commonly asked for medical advice by family and friends as well as patients. As much as a medical assistant may feel tempted to respond with advice, she must proceed cautiously. She must diligently avoid the appearance of dispensing medical advice outside of her scope of practice. Such action could put herself and her employers in legal jeopardy. While on the job, the medical assistant must take care to dispense information that is appropriate and consistent with her level of education and role within the medical practice. While away from her job, the wisest policy she can follow is to avoid dispensing any medical advice at all and, instead, suggest that people contact their own health care providers.

Communication Patterns

To become an effective communicator, a medical assistant must understand the different communication styles. These styles include:

- passive
- passive-aggressive
- assertive
- aggressive.

Passive

People who are **passive** come across to others as weak and submissive. They commonly lack self-confidence and usually defer to others, while keeping their own opinions and needs to themselves. Passive patients may be too embarrassed to admit they are confused and too reluctant to ask questions or seek clarification. As a result, they might leave the office feeling frustrated with unmet needs. A passive medical assistant lacks the confidence needed to ask the physician questions and advocate for her patients when the need arises.

The passive communication pattern is sometimes described as a "lose-win" pattern, which means the individual sacrifices her needs in order to defer to the needs of others. However, in reality, neither party wins.

Passive-Aggressive

People who have a **passive-aggressive** communication style usually present themselves in a passive manner. However, this presentation is actually an attempt to manipulate others by deferring initially but then seeking revenge or finding ways to meet their needs by undermining others. They are commonly critical and sarcastic behind the backs of those people to whom they behave passively. They seek control through indirect means, such as sabotage, procrastination, stubbornness, or feigning forgetfulness. Such behaviors may be conscious or unconscious. For example, a passive-aggressive person who is afraid to say "no" when asked to work late and close the office, might later "get revenge" by "forgetting" end-of-shift duties and leaving them for the morning shift. Also, a person who behaves nicely when talking with a supervisor might then be critical of the supervisor to coworkers. A simple way to describe the passive-aggressive communication style is that it is a pseudo (false) lose-win style. Because the person defers her needs to the needs of others in the short-term but then seeks revenge, she ultimately undermines everyone.

Assertive

People who are **assertive** come across as clear, professional, and articulate. They are not afraid to share their opinion or to speak up and ask for help. Even so, they are able to keep their feelings and opinions to themselves when common sense and professionalism dictate. An assertive medical assistant understands that her priority at work is to meet the needs of her patients and her physician employers, which sometimes means that her own needs take a back seat. She is willing to listen to the opinions and ideas of others and is interested in learning and growing on a personal and professional level. A simple way to describe the assertive communication style is that it is win-win. An assertive communicator understands how to attend to the needs of others without completely sacrificing herself in the process. She is able to set appropriate limits with others when necessary and attend to her own self-care needs, while keeping her professional focus where it belongs: on the patient.

Aggressive

People who are **aggressive** come across to others as angry, pushy, bossy, selfish, or insensitive. They rarely hesitate to voice their opinions, regardless of the situation. They disregard the feelings and opinions of others in order to get their own needs met. A medical assistant who is aggressive is not afraid to speak up and advocate on behalf of her patients when she recognizes the need. Unfortunately, because of her insensitivity, she can miss subtle but important cues from her patients (and everyone else) and commonly ends up offending or otherwise alienating others. In defense of aggressive communicators, most of them have no idea how aggressive they are. Rather, they usually view themselves as being assertive and commonly think they are great communicators. Sadly, they are the only ones who think so. A simple way to describe the aggressive communication style is that it is win-lose. These people are so concerned with getting their own needs met that they commonly do it at the expense of others.

Communication Challenges

Most individuals are not nearly as good at communication as they believe. This misperception sets the stage for miscommunication and misunderstanding, even in the best circumstances. In addition, many people unintentionally block effective communication without realizing it. However, the medical assistant who understands these challenges to communication and has strategies for dealing with them will be a successful communicator.

Defense Mechanisms

Defense mechanisms are unhealthy coping strategies that people employ to protect themselves when they feel emotionally threatened. Some of the most common types of defense mechanisms include:

- rationalization
- compensation
- regression
- repression
- displacement
- denial
- projection.

Rationalization

When a person makes excuses to justify inappropriate behavior, that person is making **rationalizations** for her behavior. For example, when an employee steals supplies from the workplace, she might rationalize such actions by stating, "They don't pay me enough anyway."

Compensation

Compensation is a psychological response in which a person attempts to offset feelings of inadequacy in one aspect of life by achieving success in another. This response is not always unhealthy, but certainly may be. For example, a parent who feels guilty for not spending time with his or her child might attempt to compensate by buying the child expensive toys.

Regression

When a person reverts to behavior associated with earlier (younger) developmental stages, he or she is exhibiting signs of **regression**. For example, a 12-year-old child might regress to thumb-sucking behaviors when hospitalized or when dealing with family trauma, such as death or divorce. Self-limiting regressive behaviors provide emotional protection and comfort during a time of emotional trauma. The behavior usually disappears when the emotional turmoil ends. However, prolonged periods of regression may signal serious adjustment difficulties and the need for therapy.

Repression

Repression occurs when a person eliminates from conscious thought traumatic memories or painful or conflictual thoughts or impulses that the person believes are unacceptable. For example, an adult who forgot for many years about experiencing sexual abuse as a child has repressed those memories. Yet the experience has the potential to have a lasting impact on his or her ability to form healthy relationships. A man who finds himself physically attracted to his wife's best friend and recognizes his impulse to act on these feelings as unacceptable may continually forget the woman's name.

Displacement

When a person expresses anger or another emotion at a person or object that is not the cause of those feelings, he or she is employing the defense mechanism of **displacement**. For example, a man who is angry at his boss goes home and vents his anger on his family by picking a fight with his wife and yelling at his children. In the workplace, this behavior sometimes manifests in coworkers mistreating one another, rather than addressing issues they have with the manager.

Denial

When a person refuses to acknowledge the validity or reality of something that is obvious to everyone else, he or she is said to be in **denial**; for example, a person who suffers health problems, relationship problems, and professional problems due to chronic alcoholism but refuses to acknowledge that he or she has an alcohol problem. Friends, family and coworkers are usually well aware of the problem that the individual himself or herself refuses to acknowledge. In some cases, those persons closest to the individual join in the denial. For example, the wife of an abusive alcoholic who makes excuses for her husband's actions is also in denial.

Projection

When a person accuses others of having certain feelings, attitudes, or behaviors that he or she has, he or she is **projecting**. For example, a man who projects feelings of guilt about cheating on his wife might accuse her of being unfaithful to him.

Strategies for Dealing with Difficult People

For most medical assistants, working with and helping people is the most rewarding part of the job. However, working with people can also be the most challenging part of the job. Because of pain or illness, patients do not always behave at their best. They may be upset with their lowered quality of life or feeling frustrated and angry over their lack of improvement. They sometimes seem to have unrealistic expectations of what the physician and medical science are able to offer. They may be feeling frightened, vulnerable, angry, or confused. As a result, patient behavior can sometimes be unpredictable and unpleasant. During such times, a medical assistant can become a convenient target and can find it challenging to maintain her professional demeanor. However, it is especially during such times that her degree of professionalism becomes apparent. To help during such times, a medical assistant can employ several strategies, including:

- focusing on the patient
- acknowledging the patient
- validating the patient's feelings
- using "I" language
- moving to a solution
- setting boundaries.

Focusing on the Patient

It is not easy to avoid taking personal offense at criticism or other negative comments from a patient. However, the medical assistant must remind herself to keep her focus on the patient's needs, rather than on herself. By doing so, she is less likely to feel personally upset or offended by the patient's words or behaviors. In addition, the medical assistant who tries to treat others as she would want to be treated maintains the ability to empathize with her patients. This empathy makes her less likely to react in anger and more likely to respond with compassion.

Acknowledging the Patient

All people like to feel acknowledged, and no one likes to be treated as if they were a number or an object. If patients believe they are being treated as an object rather than a person, they will be offended, angry, and frustrated. A medical assistant may be extremely busy dealing with multiple patients, ringing telephones, physicians, coworkers, and numerous other demands. However, she must never fall into the habit of viewing patients as an inconvenience. Patient care is at the heart of the profession of medical assisting. Regardless of how busy a medical assistant is, it takes no more time to look a patient in the eyes, speak in a kind voice, and smile than it does to deal with that patient in a harried, distracted manner.

Validating the Patient's Feelings

When a patient feels upset, they do not want someone to argue with them or trivialize her feelings. Such treatment will simply further upset the patient. On the other hand, if the medical assistant responds with a calm voice and validates the patient's feelings in a kind, empathetic manner, her response will most likely have a soothing effect that deescalates the situation. However, it can be difficult for a medical assistant to validate a patient's feelings without implying agreement with the patient's statement. For example, a patient complains to the medical assistant, saying, "I can't believe that I wasted $65 on a worthless medication. You people are incompetent!" The medical assistant can simply validate the patient's feelings by saying, "You are feeling concerned that the medication was ineffective." Then, she can offer a temporary solution by saying, "Since you are not feeling better, you should probably speak with the physician." (See *Teaching strategy.*)

Using "I" Language

Communication with others is vital in reaching agreements, resolving conflicts, and creating a positive work environment. However, when people's emotions rise and tempers flare, their efforts at communication may quickly deteriorate into accusations and arguments. In order to avoid such a situation, people should try to plan such conversations for a time when the persons involved are not feeling angry or upset. They should also remind themselves that the goal is to achieve a positive resolution for everyone. When attempting to address a conflict or disagreement, the medical assistant who uses "I" language, rather than "you" language, can help ensure a successful conversation that does not make the other persons involved feel as though they must defend themselves. For example, the medical assistant who is

---

📓 Patient Education

Teaching Strategy

Health care providers sometimes dispense what they believe is good patient education without first taking the time to inquire about the patient's concerns. A patient who is preoccupied with fear and anxiety may hear and remember little of what she "taught." A more effective teaching strategy is to ask the patient to identify his or her greatest concerns. Doing so can help her feel acknowledged and that his or her concerns have been validated. When the patient is able to address these issues, he or she is then better able to hear, understand, and remember other information provided. More importantly, the patient will leave the office feeling cared about and having his or her needs met.

feeling annoyed with her coworker for always returning from lunch late might yell at her as she comes in the door, "You are always late and messing up our schedule, and I've had it!" Doing so will probably put her coworker on the defense and start an argument. A better approach would be to wait until feelings of anger subside and then find an opportunity to have a private conversation where patients cannot overhear. She then might state something like "I've noticed that you've been taking 45 minutes for lunch lately. Because we are each supposed to take 30-minute lunches, this is affecting patient scheduling. I am feeling frustrated but do not want this to hinder our working relationship. I would like to find a solution that meets both of our needs." Of course, there is no guarantee that the coworker will respond as desired, but he or she is much more likely to do so when he or she realizes the impact his or her behavior is having on others and when he or she does not feel that his or her personal character is being attacked.

Moving to a Solution

A medical assistant is most effective when she learns to avoid getting stuck in argumentation with patients, coworkers, or physicians. When she is in a conversation involving conflict, the medical assistant should direct the conversation toward clarifying the problem without pointing blame. Then she can begin discussing possible solutions. If an upset colleague or patient seems intent on laying blame, the medical assistant should tactfully, yet assertively, change the subject by asking a question such as "What solution to this problem do you have in mind?" In addition, the medical assistant should learn to monitor her own behavior. When she notices herself feeling upset or starting to assign blame, she should refocus her attention on finding a positive solution instead.

Setting Boundaries

While a medical assistant should always behave in a tactful, professional manner, she is not obligated to subject herself to verbal or physical abuse. Whether the aggressor is a patient, colleague, or even a physician, the strategies above should be employed. Medical assistants must sometimes set or enforce **boundaries**, or physical or psychological space that indicates the limit of appropriate versus inappropriate behavior. If such interventions fail to work and the behavior escalates, the medical assistant should solicit the intervention of the department or office manager. This person may have the ability to provide a fresh, unbiased perspective and also has a greater level of authority to help identify a solution to the problem. The medical assistant should report any threats of physical violence per office policy. If a patient or another person becomes physically violent, the medical assistant should immediately summon help, such as calling security or even calling the police, per office policy. (See *Resolving conflict in the office.*)

Front office–Back office connection

Resolving Conflict in the Office

In a medical office, conflict can occur even in the best circumstances. In most cases, the underlying cause is miscommunication. To help enhance communication and resolve conflict, office staff, including administrative and clinical workers, should get together on a regular basis for staff meetings. Not only is this a great time to share announcements and discuss changes in policies or procedures but it is also a great time to resolve any identified problems.

Discussions will be most productive if everyone uses the same therapeutic communication skills with one another that they use with their patients. They should also agree to follow common ground rules, such as keeping language and behaviors professional, using "I" language, and moving toward finding solutions rather than staying "stuck" on the problem.

Cultural Variables

Body language and verbal communication takes on different meanings depending upon the cultural **norms** of those involved. Medical assistants should familiarize themselves with cultural norms of the ethnic groups most commonly seen in their facility. (See *Cultural variations in communication.*) Familiarity with this information helps them interact more knowledgeably with others and decreases the likelihood of communication mishaps. (See *Cultural competence in the medical office*, page 51.)

Patient Education

Cultural Variations in Communication

Well-intended efforts to educate patients can sometimes be wasted energy if medical assistants unintentionally offend or confuse patients through cultural insensitivity. For example, use of direct touch, prolonged eye contact, or an overly casual greeting can be so offensive to some individuals that they cannot adequately attend to the message of the speaker. Medical assistants should strive to become culturally competent and, when unsure of how to proceed, should err on the side of addressing their patients in a more conservative, formal manner.

Front office–Back office connection

Cultural Competence in the Medical Office

No one has the time or resources to fully understand the variations in communication styles for every culture. However, the medical office team should meet to brainstorm about ways they could all increase their knowledge and understanding of cultures common to their patient population. For example, each member could take responsibility for choosing a culture of interest, learning about it, and then teaching coworkers about it. That person could serve as the office "expert" and a resource for coworkers.

Before getting started, the team should agree on what information is most valuable to know. Clinical and administrative medical assistants may have different ideas, depending on the needs they have observed in their areas. Therefore, the team should collaborate in creating the "must-have" list of information. Then the office could distribute "cheat sheets" for each cultural group researched, which could be kept on hand as a quick reference for all office staff.

Chapter Summary

- Good communication skills are essential for the medical assistant to ensure that each patient's first impression of the medical office is a positive one.
- Communication includes the sending and receiving of information between two or more individuals. Factors in the communication cycle include the referent, sender, receiver, message, channels, feedback, interpersonal variables, and environment.
- A medical assistant must take care that her verbal and nonverbal communication is congruent with the message she is trying to convey. Otherwise, listeners will believe the nonverbal communication.
- Most people are not comfortable letting others enter their personal space and touch them until a degree of trust has been established. Therefore, the medical assistant must treat patients with respect and sensitivity.
- Touch can be used in a therapeutic manner to convey interest, sincerity, and empathy. Patients commonly welcome appropriate touch and report that it helps them to feel acknowledged and cared for.
- Body language and verbal communication take on different meanings in different cultures. The medical assistant should strive to become familiar with the cultural norms of her patient population.

- One of the most important parts of effective communication is active listening. Most people overestimate their skills as a listener. Active listening involves reflecting or paraphrasing the message that was heard and seeking clarification as needed.
- The medical assistant should resist the temptation to offer medical advice outside her scope of practice. Such action could put her and her employers in legal jeopardy.
- To communicate effectively and develop positive professional relationships, the medical assistant must understand the differences between passive, passive-aggressive, assertive, and aggressive communication styles.
- Common roadblocks to effective communication include the defense mechanisms of rationalization, compensation, regression, repression, displacement, denial, and projection.
- Communicating effectively can be especially challenging in certain situations. Patients may be ill, in pain, upset, angry, or otherwise unhappy. Therefore, the medical assistant must learn specific strategies to help her maintain her professionalism during trying times. Such strategies include focusing on the patient's needs, acknowledging the patient, validating the patient's feelings, using "I" language, directing the conversation toward finding a solution, and setting appropriate boundaries.

Team Work Exercises

1. Divide into groups of five or six students. Create a poster or presentation that identifies common roles within a group, such as the leader, peacemaker, antagonist, clown, and so forth. Assign each team member a role to research. Make sure that the presentation describes how each role can help or hinder effective group processes.
2. Divide into pairs and designate one person as partner A and the other as partner B. Partner A should think of a problem that he or she is comfortable sharing and then begin describing it. Partner B's job is to practice active listening, meaning the focus must remain on partner A and cannot shift to partner B. Incorporate eye contact, body language, paraphrasing, and other active listening strategies. After 10 minutes or so, the partners may trade roles and repeat the exercise. Afterwards, partners should give each other feedback about their listening skills along with suggestions for improvement.

Case Studies

1. A new family has come to the clinic for health care. During the initial interview, the receptionist learns that they are Jewish. What information will the staff need to know to communicate effectively without causing offense?
2. Mrs. Kamell has recently emigrated from the Middle East to live with her son and daughter-in-law. The Kamell family just started coming to the clinic for health care 2 months ago. You have noticed that they have

arrived late again today and seem reluctant to answer many of the questions that are asked. Furthermore, Mrs. Kamell seems content to let her son speak for her. Based on preliminary testing, the physician is concerned that Mrs. Kamell may have cancer, but must do further diagnostic testing to be sure. What information should the medical staff be aware of to help them interact effectively with this family? What guidelines should they follow?

Resources

- Communication Improvement Free Resource Center: *www.work911.com/communication/index.htm*
- Cultural competency articles from the American Medical Student Association: *www.amsa.org/programs/gpit/cultural .cfm* and *www.amsa.org/div/cstudies.cfm*
- Mind Tools: *www.mindtools.com/page8.html*

Legal Considerations

Learning Objectives

Upon completion of this chapter, the student will be able to:

- define and spell key legal terms
- define licensure and certification as well as their purposes
- define the scope of practice and its importance
- discuss the standard of care for health care professionals
- describe negligence and the "4 Ds" of malpractice
- compare and contrast the three main business structure forms for medical offices
- discuss implied consent and informed consent and when they are appropriate
- compare and contrast intentional and unintentional torts
- compare and contrast civil and criminal law as it applies to health care
- explain how the Good Samaritan law protects individuals in cases where consent cannot be obtained
- describe procedures used to release a noncompliant patient and how such a release can help prevent a charge of abandonment
- describe the purpose of a durable power of attorney and a living will
- describe a patient release of information and how it is obtained
- list the circumstances where patient authorization to release information is not necessary
- describe reporting requirements for child and elder abuse.

CAAHEP Competencies

General Competencies

Professional Communications

Respond to and initiate written communications

Legal Concepts

Identify and respond to issues of confidentiality

Perform within legal and ethical boundaries

Establish and maintain the medical record

Document appropriately

Demonstrate knowledge of federal and state health care legislation and regulations

ABHES Competencies

Professionalism

Conduct work within scope of education, training, and ability

Communication

Fundamental writing skills

Legal Concepts

Determine needs for documentation and reporting

Document accurately

Use appropriate guidelines when releasing records or information

Follow established policy in initiating or terminating medical treatment

Maintain licenses and accreditation

Monitor legislation related to current health care issues and practices

Perform risk management procedures

Chapter Outline

Legal Relationship of the Patient and Physician

Medical Practice Act

Licensure

Revoking a License

Scope of Practice

Standard of Care

Consent

Implied consent

Informed consent

Malpractice

The Lawsuit Process

Subpoenas and Depositions

Trial

Malpractice Insurance

Intentional torts

Criminal versus Civil Law

Patient Noncompliance

Statute of Limitations

Risk Management

Documentation

Confidentiality

Exceptions to disclosure rules

Durable Power of Attorney and Living Wills

Reporting Abuse

Child Abuse

Neglect

Emotional abuse

Physical abuse

Sexual abuse

Elder Abuse

Neglect

Physical abuse

Chapter Summary

Team Work Exercises

Case Studies

Resources

Key Terms

abandonment
Failure to make arrangements for a patient's continued medical care

age of majority
Legal status of adulthood, as recognized by the state

against medical advice (AMA)
Designation for a patient who leaves the hospital even though his doctor disagrees with the decision to leave

agent
Representative of a facility, hospital, or doctor's office who represents in word and action the supervising physician

assault
Threat or perceived threat to do bodily harm to another person

battery
Intentional act of touching another person in a socially unacceptable manner without her consent

breach of contract
Failure to comply with an established agreement as specified in a written contract

civil law
Branch of private law that deals with accidental, rather than intentional, injury to a person or personal property

criminal law
Branch of public law that deals with the rights and responsibilities of the government to maintain public order

damages
Monetary award paid by the physician to the patient as directed by the court

defamation
Providing false information (written or spoken) that causes harm to the reputation of another

defendant
Person accused in a court of law

deposition
Formal method of gathering information in which a person testifies to the actions of herself and coworkers

durable power of attorney
Written legal designation of a person to make medical decisions on behalf of another person

emancipated minor
Person under the age of majority who has been declared by a court to be independent and responsible for his own debts

expert witness
Person who is called to testify in court due to her status as an expert on a given subject or in a specialty

felony
Serious crime against the public that is punishable by serving time in prison

fraud
Intentional misrepresentation of a situation for financial gain

gross negligence
Intentional failure to provide care or the commission of an act by an individual with reckless disregard for consequences that endanger a patient

implied consent
Acceptance of treatment expressed through a patient's actions, such as rolling up his sleeve for blood pressure measurement

informed consent
Document that a patient signs, which is a written agreement for treatment

libel
Dishonoring or defaming a person through written documents

licensure
Designation signifying that a person has met the standards and requirements of her profession and is legally able to offer specific services for monetary reimbursement

litigation
In medicine, a legal action that determines the rights and remedies a patient can pursue in the event of suspected medical malpractice

living will
Written directions to a physician that instruct the physician about whether or not to maintain life-support systems in the event of a patient's terminal illness

malfeasance
Unlawful act that causes harm

malpractice
Action by a health care professional that injures a patient and fails to meet reasonable standards of professional care

negligence
Unintentional failure of a health care professional to meet his responsibilities to a patient, resulting in injury to the patient

noncompliance
Failure of a patient to follow his physician's treatment plan

nonfeasance
Failure of a health care professional or organization to perform a task or deliver a service, resulting in harm or injury to a patient

perjury
Act of lying in court, despite taking an oath to tell the truth

plaintiff
Person bringing charges in court

res ipsa loquitur
Latin phrase meaning "the thing speaks for itself" and used in legal situations when negligence is clearly evident

respondeat superior
Latin phrase meaning "let the master answer," a legal doctrine that places responsibility on a physician for the actions of her employee

restitution
Monetary compensation for a loss or injury

risk management
Proactive management that seeks to reduce potential risks of a lawsuit before it occurs

scope of practice
Range of services a professional can offer, based on training, ability, and licensure

slander
Dishonoring or defaming a person through verbal attacks

statute
Law

statute of limitations
Law that sets a time limit within which a person can bring a lawsuit

subpoena
Legal document that notifies a person that he is required to appear in court or be available for deposition

subpoena *duces tecum*
Latin phrase meaning "bring with you under penalty of punishment," a legal document that requires a person to appear in court with specified documents, such as patient records

tort
Wrongful act committed by a person that causes harm to another person or property

vicarious liability
Liability of an employer for the wrongdoing of an employee while on the job

Legal Relationship of the Patient and Physician

A patient's relationship with her physician is complex, not only from the standpoint of her health care but also in the many legal implications that arise from such a relationship. A person who seeks care from a licensed professional is entering a contract with that professional. Once a relationship between the patient and the physician is established, the parties have entered a contract. The contract is the agreement by the physician to provide services and the patient to pay for services, either out of her own pocket or by using a third-party payor (health insurance). Failure of either party to abide by the contract is a **breach of contract**. The patient must pay for services, and the physician must provide services. In addition, if the physician fails to attempt to provide continuous health care to a patient, such as by moving to another city or retiring without forwarding medical records, such an action is considered **abandonment** and is a form of breach of contract. Because medical care of patients must be continuous, it is the responsibility of a physician to provide care or offer an alternative, such as forwarding medical records to another physician. To enter a contract, individuals must be competent adults or **emancipated minors**. Minors can enjoy the same rights and responsibilities as adults, including being responsible for their own debts if declared independent by a court. Teenagers who are married or parents commonly can become emancipated minors and, therefore, enter into contracts. In such situations, responsibility to pay for services is that of the minor, not a parent or guardian.

It is the responsibility of everyone in the physician's office to follow legal and ethical principles that safeguard a patient's privacy and physical safety and keep a patient informed regarding her health care. The medical assistant acts as an **agent** of the physician by representing in actions and words the intention of the physician. Recognition of the physician's responsibility to supervise her medical assistants is called *respondeat superior*. This Latin phrase translates to "let the master answer," which means that if a medical assistant injures a patient, it is the responsibility of the physician to make **restitution**, or monetary compensation for the injury. *Respondeat superior* is a form of **vicarious liability**, in which the employer is responsible for the actions of an employee. For example, if a bus is in an accident, injured passengers seek restitution from the bus company, not the individual driving the bus. Although responsible for her actions as a professional, a medical assistant who accidentally injures a patient is not the liable party—the supervising physician is.

Medical Practice Act

As an agent of the physician, the medical assistant must act within the laws of the state when performing health care procedures, maintaining medical records, and disclosing personal medical information to third parties for treatment, payment, or operations. All 50 states have a Medical Practice Act, which is a **statute**, or law, that regulates the practice of medicine. Failure to follow her state's Medical Practice Act can result in the medical assistant committing a **tort**. A tort is a wrongful act for which a patient can request compensation or other legal remedies (but does not involve a breach of contract). Harm associated with a tort commonly results in a lawsuit. Although harm caused to the patient may be unintentional, penalties can be severe and can range from suspension or revocation of a physician's license, monetary fines, or imprisonment for more serious violations. Following legal and ethical standards of care protects the medical assistant and the physician as well as the patient.

Licensure

Most health professions have some form of regulation to ensure the competence of their members. A license is a legal document that allows an individual to offer a set of services to the public for compensation (payment). **Licensure** is obtained by passing an oral and a written examination. To be eligible to take a medical physician licensing examination, an individual must:

- complete education requirements through an approved medical school.
- complete an approved residency program.
- attain an **age of majority**, which is a legal recognition of adulthood as defined by an individual state so that a person can enter legally binding contracts with others (something a child is not legally allowed to do).

When a person passes the licensure examination in a given state, she can obtain a license to practice medicine in another state by a process of *reciprocity*. Simply stated, reciprocity is one state accepting the current license of a practitioner from another state. When a physician obtains a license to practice medicine, she is able to practice within the scope of her specialty for compensation. Licenses must be renewed every two years and state dues must be paid each year. Proof of continuing education as well as proof of 5 hours of risk management training is required in all states. If the license is not renewed by the deadline, it becomes invalid, medical malpractice insurance becomes inactive, and the individual cannot practice medicine. Practicing medicine without a license by failing to renew a license but continuing to treat patients is a **felony**, a serious crime that usually carries a stiff penalty, such as imprisonment. The law makes no distinction between a physician who lets her license expire and a person who never went to medical school and represents herself as a physician. Each individual is committing a felony and can be punished in a court of law under the guidelines for a felony conviction.

Revoking a License

A state may revoke a physician's license for just cause, including:

- conviction of a crime
  - *felony*—murder, rape, practicing without a license, selling prescription drugs or signed prescription pads
  - *fraud*—billing for treatments never provided, changing dates of service, falsifying medical records.
- unprofessional conduct
  - addiction to drugs or alcohol
  - breach of confidentiality
  - false advertising
  - unethical behaviors toward patients
  - inability to perform duties
  - fee splitting or other inappropriate billing practices.

In addition to maintaining her own licensure and continuing education, a physician is legally responsible for the actions of her employees while on the job. Because a physician is directly responsible for the actions of her medical assistant employee, a physician employer depends on credentialing of medical assistants to ensure proper training. Medical assistants can become certified through the AAMA or the AMT. Certification of a medical assistant can be a deciding factor in a physician's choice of which candidate to hire as an employee and patient care agent.

Scope of Practice

Whether the health care provider is licensed (such as a medical doctor, chiropractor, osteopath, or registered nurse) or certified (such as a medical assistant), that professional must practice within her **scope of practice**, or the range of services a professional can offer, based on training, ability, and licensure. For example, a pediatrician may not fill cavities in a patient's teeth. A dentist is not licensed to give immunizations to a patient. The medical assistant who performs medical procedures that she is untrained or unlicensed to do is putting the practice at risk for a lawsuit, or **litigation**. In such a suit, a patient can seek legal action against the practice or medical assistant. Such action may result in monetary compensation to the patient for harm done by the unlawful actions of the medical assistant or the physician's failure to oversee her actions appropriately. Even if injury to the patient does not occur, the consequences may still be significant, including legal expenses, damage to the reputation of the practice, and even loss of licensure. For example, medical assistants can be trained to assist in minor office surgery but cannot perform the surgery itself. If a physician were to allow an unlicensed employee to perform an office surgery, the physician's license would be revoked or suspended.

Standard of Care

A standard of care, or the minimum safe professional conduct under specific conditions as determined by professional peer organizations, must be maintained at all times. Failure to perform to the standard of care is called **negligence**. If negligence results in harm to a patient, it is considered an *unintentional tort* and the patient can file a lawsuit against the physician or physician's agent, such as the medical assistant. An act of negligence can involve:

- **nonfeasance**, or failure to do what a prudent person would do that results in harm to a patient—for example, failure to monitor a patient's warfarin (Coumadin) levels, which results in the patient being hospitalized for internal bleeding (also called *omission*)
- **malfeasance**, or performance of an improper act that results in harm to a patient—for example, prescribing a medication to a patient with a known allergy, which results in the patient's death (also called *commission*)
- *res ipsa loquitor*, a Latin phrase that means "the thing speaks for itself," indicating an unintentional tort that is an obvious mistake in which negligence is clearly evident—for example, a patient with a tumor on the right leg is brought to the operating room where surgeons amputate the left leg. The negligence "speaks for itself."

Consent

In addition to performing procedures in accordance with the standard of care, the medical assistant or physician must also obtain the patient's consent to perform the procedure. There are the two types of consent that may be obtained when providing care to a patient: *implied* and *informed*.

Implied Consent

Implied consent occurs when a patient consents to treatment through her actions, such as rolling up her sleeve to have her blood pressure checked. A medical assistant must *never* force a patient to have a procedure performed. If a patient declines a procedure, such as drawing blood or a blood pressure check, the medical assistant must note the refusal in the patient's chart. Facility policy may also require her to report the refusal of care to the physician.

Informed Consent

When a patient is scheduled to undergo invasive treatment, such as surgery, the physician must obtain **informed consent**, which involves a written form that is signed by the patient. The physician must ensure that the patient understands:

- the procedure
- why the procedure is being performed
- who will perform the procedure
- expected results of the procedure
- risks of performing the procedure and of doing nothing
- available alternative treatments and how the risks and benefits compare to those of the recommended procedure.

The medical assistant may ask the patient if he has any further questions for the physician. If she suspects that the patient does not understand the procedure, she should inform the physician immediately.

Barriers to Informed Consent

An interpreter may be required to obtain informed consent from a patient who is hearing impaired or speaks a different language than her physician.

Sometimes, the physician may not be able to obtain informed consent. In an emergency situation, a patient may be unconscious or in too much pain to comprehend the physician's explanation of care. In such a situation, where the life, health, and safety of a patient depend on the physician's quick response, the Good Samaritan law protects the physician from litigation. The Good Samaritan law extends to anyone who offers emergency help within the scope of their training and abilities, including anyone who administers CPR or first aid while waiting for emergency services personnel to arrive at the scene of an accident. If a patient regains consciousness during the course of administering first aid, the prudent rescuer should ask, "May I continue?" For example, lifeguards are trained not only to rescue swimmers in trouble but also to administer CPR and first aid. They are, therefore, covered under Good Samaritan laws. (Note that Good Samaritan laws vary by state but always cover aid given in good faith by a person trained to do so.)

Malpractice

Malpractice, the medical form of negligence, is proven by four criteria, commonly known as the "four Ds." If the prosecution can prove that all of these criteria apply in a certain case, the physician will be found guilty of malpractice and a monetary settlement will be awarded:

- *Duty*—The prosecution must prove that a patient-physician relationship existed. A medical chart can be used to show proof of a physician's duty to care for a patient.
- *Dereliction of duty*—The prosecution must prove that the physician failed to meet the standard of care. In court, the prosecution can produce an equally trained physician to testify as an **expert witness**. Commonly, an expert witness in a malpractice case practices the same specialty as the defendant. The expert witness can testify that she would act differently than the accused physician (defendant) and that the result to the patient would be better, resulting in no damage or less damage to the patient.
- *Direct cause*—The prosecution must prove that the damage suffered by the patient is a direct result of the actions of the physician.
- *Damage*—The prosecution must prove that omission or commission by the physician caused the patient injury or harm.

The Lawsuit Process

A patient who brings a lawsuit against the physician is the **plaintiff**, the person who seeks monetary damages for the tort allegedly committed against him. The plaintiff will hire a lawyer to represent him in court. The accused physician is the **defendant**, the person who must defend or explain her actions before the court. She will also hire an attorney to defend her actions and notify the malpractice insurance carrier.

Subpoenas and Depositions

During the collection of information, the medical assistant may be issued a **subpoena**, which is a legal document that requires a person to appear in court or be available for **deposition**. A *deposition* is a formal gathering of information during which the individual who has received the subpoena must answer questions. It is important to remember that, while giving a deposition (also called *being deposed*), the individual is under oath. The medical assistant is bound by law to tell the truth. To lie or omit information in a deposition is a crime, called *perjury*, and is punishable by law. Another method used to gather information is a **subpoena duces tecum**, which requires that the individual appear in court with specific documentation, usually the patient's medical record.

✦ TIP Preparing for a Deposition

Many medical assistants will never be deposed or called as a witness in a medical malpractice lawsuit. If a medical assistant is called, however, she should be prepared by:

- reviewing the medical record, to be sure that her recollection of events is as accurate as possible

- only responding to questions to which she knows the answer, being brief in her answers, and answering only what is asked
- making eye contact with the attorneys, judge, and jury and maintaining a professional demeanor
- dressing appropriately for court (business attire).

Trial

In preparation for a trial, attorneys for the defense and the prosecution will gather necessary information. Patient medical records and depositions from witnesses are collected. Expert witnesses are contacted to give testimony during the trial and a trial date is set by the court. The lawyers from both sides choose a jury, and the trial begins. Each attorney makes opening statements and then calls witnesses. Both attorneys are given the opportunity to question the witnesses through examination and cross-examination. Both attorneys make closing statements explaining to the jury how they proved their argument. The judge will give instructions to the jury and ask them to reach a verdict based on the evidence presented. The jury deliberates or discusses what they saw and heard in the courtroom and reaches a decision. If the jury finds the defendant (physician) not guilty, the case is dismissed. If the jury finds that the physician is guilty of malpractice, a monetary settlement is awarded.

Malpractice Insurance

Most physicians have malpractice insurance out of which the settlement and legal fees are paid in the event of a malpractice lawsuit. Many states have mandatory malpractice laws that require physicians to have a minimum dollar amount of malpractice insurance. If a physician has no malpractice insurance or limited coverage, his personal assets may be seized, depending on how his practice is structured. (See *Medical practice business structures*.)

Intentional Torts

Malpractice insurance does not cover intentional torts. An *intentional tort* is considered **gross negligence**, a form of negligence that involves an intentional act or failure to act that causes harm. Harm done to a patient by a physician or an agent that is determined intentional results in a monetary award, or **damages**, paid to the patient and can also result in criminal charges filed against the physician, agent, or both. Intentional torts include:

- **assault**—An assault is a threat or perceived threat of bodily harm to another person. An assault can involve hitting and punching or just threatening to hurt another person. This situation is easily avoided by maintaining professional decorum.

Medical practice business structures

Incorporating a medical practice as a business offers protection to the individual provider against losing his personal property as a result of a malpractice lawsuit. Each state has its own incorporation procedures and costs. The table below outlines possible business structures for a medical practice, along with a description, legal implications, advantages, and disadvantages.

Business Structure	Description	Legal Malpractice Implications	Advantages	Disadvantages
Sole proprietorship	One owner-operator physician	Person can be sued for personal assets in malpractice.	• Owner-operator makes all the decisions. • Overhead is low. • Owner keeps all the profits.	• Personal financial liability for malpractice claims
Partnership	Two or more partners acting as owner-operators	Individual doctors can be sued for personal assets and may be liable for damage incurred by partners.	• Partners share costs of medical office personnel and overhead. • Partners cover each other for vacation and on-call times.	• Personal financial responsibility for conduct of self and partners • Consultation with partners necessary for business decisions

Medical practice business structures—cont'd

Business Structure	Description	Legal Malpractice Implications	Advantages	Disadvantages
Limited Liability Corporation (LLC) OR Personal corporation (PC)*	Corporation that acts as an independent business entity	Physician cannot be sued for personal assets in malpractice.	• No personal financial liability in case of malpractice • Many people available to cover vacation and on-call hours • Some tax advantages to incorporation	• Costs incurred to form corporation, such as attorney fees • More difficulty dissolving a corporation than a partnership • Corporation taxes due in addition to personal income taxes of physicians • Consultation with large group for business decisions

*Titles of small corporations vary from state to state.

- **battery**—Battery involves touching someone in a socially inappropriate way without her permission. The prudent medical assistant must obtain consent before touching a patient.
- **defamation**—To cause harm to a person's reputation by providing false information in writing (**libel**) or by spoken word (**slander**) is considered a crime. The medical assistant must be careful not to talk about a physician, colleague, or patient in an unprofessional manner. If a physician's practice suffers a loss of patients due to slander, a lawsuit for defamation can be brought against the medical assistant or her employer. Writing derogatory comments in a patient's chart can be considered libel, so care should be used in describing a patient's demeanor. Gossiping about a patient can be considered slander and the patient can bring a lawsuit against the medical office. Disclosing or discussing a patient's sexual history, human immunodeficiency virus status, or drug treatment history could compromise his job, marriage, and mental health. The patient may also feel that the staff is not attentive to his needs and that the gossiping created an atmosphere in which he received substandard care. (See *Libelous charting,* page 60.)
- **false imprisonment**—Holding a patient against her will is considered false imprisonment. Hospital patients are not required to stay for treatment and are always free to leave. Forcing a patient to stay in the hospital is an imprisonment that, without due process of law, is illegal (or *false*). An inpatient should always be able to leave the hospital, even

if it is against the recommendation of her physician. In such a situation, a patient is allowed to sign out of the hospital **against medical advice (AMA)**. The patient indicates that she is aware that she is AMA by signing a document in which she acknowledges that the physician does not recommend that she leave the hospital but that she has decided to disregard the physician's advice.
- **fraud**—Fraud is the intentional misrepresentation of facts for financial gain. For example, charging an insurance company for services not performed or changing dates of service to accommodate eligibility of benefits is fraud.
- **invasion of privacy**—The public release of a patient's information without his consent is considered an invasion of the patient's privacy. If a practice wants to use pictures of a patient for an office brochure or advertisement, the office must obtain the patient's consent to use the photo. Without the patient's consent, a physician's office cannot release medical information. For example, if a physician treats a celebrity, no personal medical information can be released to the media without consent.

Criminal Versus Civil Law

Criminal law is enacted to protect the welfare and safety of the public by determining what is legal and illegal. A person charged with a felony is brought to court and is charged by the state. If a person is accused of murder, the court record will show, for example, *Thomas Jones vs. State of Illinois.* Although the defendant is accused of murdering an individual, the crime is considered to be perpetrated against

Libelous charting

Writing derogatory statements about a patient in her chart can be seen as libel. To avoid the risk of a lawsuit, the medical assistant should always use professional, objective language when documenting care, as in the first charting example below. If the patient were to see charting example #2, she would be offended. She may feel so offended that she would bring charges against the author.

Date	
02/17/08: 10:30 a.m.	Patient describes "deep aching pain in my lower belly." She appears to be in acute distress; she states that she "hasn't slept in a week." ----------------------------------- C. Smith, CMA

Charting example #1

Date	
02/17/08: 10:30 a.m.	Patient describes "deep aching pain in my lower belly." She appears to be faking acute distress (again drug-seeking); she smells of tobacco and has not showered or bathed for what smells like at least 3 days. She claims that she "hasn't slept in a week."------------------------- C. Smith, CMA

Charting example #2

society or the state. Offenses that are criminal are most commonly punishable by imprisonment. Examples of criminal offenses include murder, robbery, larceny, kidnapping, rape, and arson.

Civil law, also called *private law,* is enacted to protect the rights of individuals, as in contract disputes, divorce, family law, inheritance law, contract law, and tort law (which covers malpractice lawsuits). Civil law is the most commonly exercised type of law in ambulatory care. The punishment for civil offenses is usually payment of a monetary award to the individual whose rights were violated. Criminal charges are brought by the state; civil claims are brought by individuals. In civil law, the dispute is considered to be between individuals and the state is not represented as the accuser in the court docket. If a physician is accused of malpractice, the court record will show, for example, *Jayne A. Veins, MD vs. Marjorie Wells.* The accuser is the individual patient. If found guilty, the physician owes monetary compensation to the patient, not to the state where she holds a license to practice medicine. The physician may, however, be investigated by the state if the state suspects that the physician has engaged in criminal behavior.

Patient Noncompliance

Patients who fail to comply with treatment recommendations cannot expect the treating physician to be responsible for the outcome of care. The patient's failure to comply, called **noncompliance,** can compromise his health. Physicians are responsible for treating a patient once a medical chart has been established. A contract is in effect when a patient seeks and receives treatment. The physician, by agreeing to treat the patient, fulfills his portion of the contract by:

- diagnosing and treating the patient to the best of his ability
- being available to the patient for care and return phone calls
- arranging for a different physician to be available in the event of the physician's absence.

The patient is responsible for his portion of the contract in that he agrees to pay copayments, provide insurance information to the office, and comply with treatment recommendations. If a physician suggests treatment and the patient refuses that treatment, the patient's chart should reflect that the patient has been informed of the physician's recommendations but has decided not to comply. Patients have the right to refuse treatment, but the physician is no longer responsible for the outcome. It is reasonable for a physician to expect a patient to:

- truthfully relate his medical history
- follow treatment recommendations, including medication, physical therapy, and lifestyle changes
- keep scheduled appointments
- pay copayments or deductibles as agreed.

Either party may end the patient-physician relationship. If a physician feels that the relationship must end, the medical assistant should send a registered letter to the patient to document the severing of the physician-patient relationship. (See Figure 6-1.)

If a physician were not to write a letter of formal discharge to the patient, but merely refused to see the patient again, the physician can be charged with abandonment and could be held responsible for the poor outcomes of the patient's condition due to a lack of care.

Statute of Limitations

Each state determines the length of time during which an individual can bring a lawsuit, called the **statute of limitations**. Malpractice statutes of limitations vary from state to state and can dictate how long medical records should be kept. If the statute of limitations is 10 years, it would be unwise to destroy medical records prior to that length of time. The information contained in the medical record may exonerate the physician from liability. If a patient was noncompliant in her care and the noncompliance is well documented, that information would help defend the physician from being held responsible for a poor medical outcome.

Risk Management

The best defense against a malpractice lawsuit is to avoid being accused. The medical staff and physician can prevent lawsuits from occurring by following risk management guidelines, which outline appropriate behaviors and procedures that decrease the risk of patient dissatisfaction during an office visit. Proper documentation, presenting reasonable expectations, and being kind and empathetic toward patients all decrease the risk of a malpractice lawsuit being brought against a medical practice. (See *Risk managment do's and don'ts*, page 62, and *Best face forward*, page 62.)

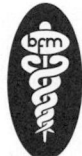

BLUEVILLE FAMILY MEDICINE
15 MAIN STREET
BLUEVILLE, CONNECTICUT 06000
860-555-3212

June 20, 2008

Dear Mr. Nicewicz,

It is unfortunate that I must withdraw my services as your physician. As stated at your office visit on May 16, 2008, you continue to ignore my recommendations regarding your multiple medical problems.

I will be available to you on an emergency basis only until July 15, 2008, which should give you time to find a new physician. In the meantime, you should call your insurance provider to find a cardiologist to care for you. I will forward all of your records upon request, and speak to your new physician regarding your past care.

At this time your physical problems include: hypertension, decreased kidney function, chronic obstructive pulmonary disease, and decreased heart function. These are serious medical conditions that require immediate attention.

Thank you for your anticipated cooperation.

Sincerely,

Robert Greer, MD
Robert Greer, MD

FIG 6-1 Withdrawal of care letter.

Risk management do's and don'ts

A patient who feels judged or disrespected is more likely to file a lawsuit than the patient who enjoys a professional relationship with her physician's office. The "nice factor" is a well-known theory suggesting that patients don't sue physicians who are "nice" to them. The medical assistant, as an agent of the physician, can also influence the patient's experience at the office by being friendly and respectful.

The guidelines below list some of the most common "do's and don'ts" that will help the medical assistant, physician, and other medical staff decrease their risk of a medical malpractice lawsuit.

Do's

• Treat all patients with respect and courtesy.

• Document performed procedures accurately and in a timely manner. Putting off charting procedures increases the risk that you will forget to do so. A court of law considers an undocumented procedure to be one that was never done at all.

• Use the patient's words in the chart, as in example B below.

11/07/08: 3:10 p.m.	The patient complains of dyspnea. ——————————————— ————————————————————————————————Sharon Lind, MA

Charting example A

11/07/08: 3:10 p.m.	The patient states "I can't get my breath, especially on the stairs." ————————————————————Sharon Lind, MA

Charting example B

• Document phone calls and chart missed appointments in the patient's chart. Advice given to a patient on the phone, such as stopping medication and answering questions pertinent to the patient's care, should always be added to the chart. Failed appointments should be charted so that the patient cannot claim that he was not given an appointment and that the physician therefore failed to treat him.

• Follow up with test results and promised phone calls in a timely manner.

• Practice safe work habits. Use gloves and other personal protective equipment (PPE) when appropriate. Keep the environment safe for yourself and your patients.

• Recheck patient release of information before releasing medical information to attorneys or other physicians.

Don'ts

• Never promise a specific outcome to a treatment. For example, never say something like, "You'll be completely cured—no pain, no stiffness. My sister had the procedure last year and she's fine now."

• Never complain about the physician or other members of the medical staff to a patient. For example, do not say, "Dr. Ramirez is so slow, I hope he doesn't make you wait too long."

• Never give medical advice or a diagnosis; do not represent yourself as something you are not, such as a doctor or nurse. Always perform within your scope of training and abilities. For example, do not say, "I wouldn't take that medication, it can damage your liver. I would try this herbal remedy."

• Never use corrective ink to correct errors in a chart. Instead, cross out the error with a line and initial the change.

• Never leave test result information on an answering machine.

• Never gossip about patients or divulge personal or medical information. For example, do not say, "Mrs. Jones is having a gastric bypass; how about just bypassing the spoon and fork!"

• Do not judge the decisions your patient makes regarding his health. For example, do not say, "I can't believe you still smoke. Do you want to die?"

Front office–Back office connection

Best Face Forward

The receptionist is the first person that the patient sees and sets the tone of the visit. An abrupt, rude, or judgmental receptionist makes the work of the clinical medical assistant harder. The patient will expect the same rude behavior from the clinical staff and may not be forthcoming with medical information. By being pleasant to your patients, you make your coworkers' jobs easier.

Documentation

In order to maintain complete, accurate records, each procedure must be recorded in the patient's medical record. Remember, if a lawsuit were to be brought, the patient's medical record could be used against the physician. If a medical assistant took a patient's blood pressure but did not record it in the medical record, there is no legal proof that the blood pressure was ever measured. (For more information on proper procedure documentation, see Chapter 20, "The Patient Interview," page 307.)

Confidentiality

Personal medical information is confidential and should never be released without proper patient consent or establishment of the receiver's "need to know." In general, a patient's medical and personal information can be used for payment, treatment, and administrative operations. A medical assistant can release a patient's name, address, diagnosis, and other necessary information to an insurance company in order to receive payment for services. Medical assistants and physicians can share information in a patient's chart with other health care professionals in order to treat the patient. A medical assistant can refer to a patient's chart and disclose information to a hospital in order to schedule a surgery or computed tomography (CT) scan. For all of these disclosures, the patient must sign authorization to release her personal and medical information. The physician's office will have release of records forms available for patients to sign. Release forms for minor children and incompetent adults, such as mentally retarded patients and Alzheimer's patients, must have the signature of a parent or legal guardian. Disclosures to others, such as an attorney for use in an automobile accident claim or worker's compensation claim, must be requested and documented. See Chapter 7, "HIPAA and a Patient's Rights," for samples of release of information forms used by attorneys. (See *Authorization to release health care information,* page 64.)

Exceptions to Disclosure Rules

There are some circumstances where patient authorization to release medical information is not necessary. It is wise to check each circumstance to ensure that patient privacy is not violated. The following situations permit disclosure without the individual's authorization:

- if the requesting party has a court order, such as in a worker's compensation hearing when a patient's medical file is needed to determine injury and award monetary compensation
- if an impact on public health or safety is possible, for example:
  - reporting communicable diseases and work-related illnesses and accidents
  - identifying missing persons or a suspect, such as disclosing to the police the identity of a gunshot victim in the emergency department (ED)
  - alerting the police to the death of a suspect, such as disclosing the identity of a person who died in a violent manner and whose body is brought to the ED
  - when protected health information (PHI) is evidence of a crime or can be used as such, as in the identity of a severely beaten woman brought to the ED, which can be disclosed to social services against the woman's wishes

  - reporting victims of abuse, neglect, or domestic violence (health care providers are legally responsible for reporting such cases to social services and law enforcement)
  - when there is a perceived serious threat to the patient
- if "organ donor" is indicated on the deceased patient's driver's license, which allows access to medical records without the consent of the next of kin only for the purpose of organ and tissue transplant or donation
- to track vital statistics, such as births and deaths, which are recorded by town and city clerks without consent.

Durable Power of Attorney and Living Wills

Sometimes a patient is unable to speak for himself and make medical decisions. A document such as a **durable power of attorney**, or *designation of health care surrogate*, allows a patient to name another person to make medical decisions on his behalf. These documents may allow another person to manage finances and personal matters or solely to make medical decisions. Each state has standard forms used to designate a medical spokesperson. In addition to these documents, a patient can also outline what type of care he would want in the event of severe injury. Choices for life support, feeding tubes, and ventilators can be outlined in a document called a **living will**. (See *Durable power of attorney for health care,* pages 65 to 67, and *Living will,* page 68.)

Reporting Abuse

Medical assistants are required by law to report all suspected child abuse, spousal abuse, elder abuse, and drug abuse. Procedures and reporting forms will vary from state to state. The medical office will have information regarding the reporting procedure in the office's policies and procedures manual. The medical assistant can give information to adult patients who are suspected of being drug abusers or victims of domestic violence regarding drug treatment programs or battered women's shelters. As adults, they are legally entitled to accept or refuse care. The state's Department of Social Services can take elders and children who are suspected victims of abuse from their abusers. After the medical assistant notifies Social Services, who then notifies the police, custody of the victims is decided by state authorities. There are several signs and symptoms that will help the medical assistant detect suspected abuse of a child or an elder.

Authorization to release health care information

Because information regarding human immunodeficiency virus (HIV) status, mental health, and substance abuse is considered highly sensitive, authorization to release that information must be explicitly outlined. Below is an example of an authorization form that outlines information to be released.

AUTHORIZATION TO RELEASE HEALTH CARE INFORMATION

Patient _Jillian Marecki_   Date _October 09, 2008_

Patient ID# _5150308_

I request and authorize _Blueville Family Medicine_ office to release the health care

information of _Jillian Marecki_ to:

> NAME OF MEDICAL PRACTICE

> PATIENT'S NAME

Carla J. Simmons
Attorney at Law
211 Main Street
Lovely, CT 06111

> THE PERSON OR AGENCY (LAW OFFICES) WHERE THE INFORMATION IS TO BE RELEASED IS SPECIFIED AND THE ADDRESS OF THE AGENCY IS INCLUDED.

Blueville Family Medicine

15 Main Street

Blueville, CT 06000

> NAME AND ADDRESS OF THE DESTINATION OF THE MEDICAL INFORMATION

This request and authorization applies to:
(please sign appropriate lines)

1. All health care information EXCLUDING specific information relating to sexually transmitted diseases, HIV/AIDS diagnosis and treatment, alcohol and/or drug history, and any care related to psychiatric disorders and mental health.

Jillian Marecki

2. All health care information INCLUDING specific information relating to sexually transmitted diseases, HIV/AIDS diagnosis and treatment, alcohol and/or drug history, and any care related to psychiatric disorders and mental health.

_____

I understand that my expressed consent is required for release of information relating to diagnosis and treatment of sexually transmitted diseases, HIV/AIDS, drug and alcohol abuse, and psychiatric disorders and mental health care. If I have been tested, diagnosed, or treated for the aforementioned, permission by my signature at the item authorizes you to release information regarding that testing, diagnosis, and/or treatment.

Jillian Marecki   _Self_
SIGNATURE OF PATIENT OR AUTHORIZED REPRESENTATIVE   RELATIONSHIP TO PATIENT

October 09, 2008
DATE

Child Abuse

Child abuse can occur as neglect, emotional abuse, physical abuse, or sexual abuse. Each form of abuse has many possible signs and symptoms.

Neglect

Suspect that a child is neglected if you see any of these signs or symptoms:

- young child left unattended
- child not fed or bathed
- manner of dress of the child inappropriate for cold weather
- failure to seek medical attention for the child
- failure to child-proof house, such as locking up poisons and cleaners.

Emotional Abuse

Suspect that a child is the victim of emotional abuse if you see any of these signs or symptoms:

- caregiver yells at child, calls child names, or curses the child
- caregiver does not comfort the child by hugging, touching, or showing concern for the child's welfare.

Physical Abuse

Suspect that a child is the victim of physical abuse if you see any of these signs or symptoms:

- bruises on face, buttocks, back, chest, abdomen, or inner thighs
- welts that take the shape of an object, such as a belt, chain, hanger, bat, or rope

- immersion burns (where child is placed into boiling water)
- cigarette burns
- fractures of the nose, skull, legs, or arms
- leg fractures in babies who do not yet walk
- bite marks on any area of the body
- child's fear of the caregiver.

Sexual Abuse

Suspect that a child is the victim of sexual abuse if you see any of these signs or symptoms:

- bruising or bleeding of the genitalia, rectum, or mouth
- stains in underwear
- difficult or painful urination

Durable power of attorney for health care

The following form shows a standard type of durable power of attorney for health care.

DURABLE POWER OF ATTORNEY FOR HEALTH CARE

I, _Walter Mayhew_, am of sound mind, and I voluntarily
(PRINT OR TYPE YOUR FULL NAME)
make this designation.

I designate _Eleanor Mayhew_, my _spouse_,
(INSERT NAME OF PATIENT ADVOCATE) (SPOUSE, CHILD, FRIEND, ETC.)
living at
27 Ridgemont Ave. Blueville, CT 06000
(INSERT ADDRESS OF PATIENT ADVOCATE)
as my patient advocate to make care, custody, and medical treatment decisions for me in the event I become unable to participate in medical treatment decisions. If my first choice cannot serve, I designate

Brenna Kramer, my _Daughter_,
(NAME OF SUCCESSOR)
living at
15 Longfellow Drive Lovely, CT 06111
(ADDRESS OF SUCCESSOR)
to serve as patient advocate.

The determination of when I am unable to participate in medical treatment decisions shall be made by my attending physician and another physician or licensed psychologist.

In making decisions for me, my patient advocate shall follow my wishes of which he or she is aware, whether expressed orally, in a living will, or in this designation.

My patient advocate has authority to consent to or refuse treatment on my behalf, to arrange medical services for me, including admission to a hospital or nursing care facility, and to pay for such services with my funds. My patient advocate shall have access to any of my medical records to which I have a right.

OPTIONAL
I expressly authorize my patient advocate to make decisions to withhold or withdraw treatment that would allow me to die, and I acknowledge such decisions could or would allow my death.

Walter Mayhew
(SIGN YOUR NAME HERE IF YOU WISH TO GIVE YOUR PATIENT ADVOCATE THIS AUTHORITY)

Continued

Durable power of attorney for health care—cont'd

My specific wishes concerning health care are the following: (if none, write "none")

None

I may change my mind at any time by communicating in any manner that this designation does not reflect my wishes.

It is my intent that my family, the medical facility, and any doctors, nurses, and other medical personnel involved in my care shall have no civil or criminal liability for honoring my wishes as expressed in this designation or for implementing the decisions of my patient advocate.

Photostatic copies of this document, after it is signed and witnessed, shall have the same legal force as the original document.

I sign this document after careful consideration. I understand its meaning and I accept its consequences.

Signed _____ *Walter Mayhew* _____ Date: _*October 09, 2008*_

Address:

_____ *27 Ridgemont Ave. Blueville, CT 06000* _____

NOTICE REGARDING WITNESSES

You must have two adult witnesses who will not receive your assets when you die (whether you die with or without a will), and who are not your spouse, child, grandchild, brother or sister, an employee of a company through which you have life or health insurance, or an employee at the health care facility where you are a patient.

STATEMENT OF WITNESSES

We sign below as witnesses. This declaration was signed in our presence. The declarant appears to be of sound mind and to be making this designation voluntarily, without duress, fraud, or undue influence.

Signed by witness: _____ *Eric VanOrden* _____ Date: _*October 09, 2008*_

_____ *Eric VanOrden* _____
(PRINT OR TYPE FULL NAME)

Address:

_____ *10 Apple Hill Drive, Lovely, CT 06111* _____

Signed by witness: _____ *Susan Bancroft* _____ Date: _*October 09, 2008*_

_____ *Susan Bancroft* _____
(PRINT OR TYPE FULL NAME)

Address:

_____ *22 Ridgemont Ave. Blueville, CT 06000* _____

Durable power of attorney for health care—cont'd

ACCEPTANCE BY PATIENT ADVOCATE

(A) This designation shall not become effective unless the patient is unable to participate in treatment decisions.

(B) A patient advocate shall not exercise powers concerning the patient's care, custody, and medical treatment that the patient, if the patient were able to participate in the decision, could not have exercised on his or her own behalf.

(C) This designation cannot be used to make a medical treatment decision to withhold or withdraw treatment from a patient who is pregnant that would result in the pregnant patient's death.

(D) A patient advocate may make a decision to withhold or withdraw treatment which would allow a patient to die only if the patient has expressed in a clear and convincing manner that the patient advocate is authorized to make such a decision and that the patient acknowledges that such a decision could or would allow the patient's death.

(E) A patient advocate shall not receive compensation for the performance of his or her authority, rights, and responsibilities, but a patient advocate may be reimbursed for actual and necessary expenses incurred in the performance of his or her authority, rights, and responsibilities.

(F) A patient advocate shall act in accordance with the standards of care applicable to fiduciaries when acting for the patient and shall act consistent with the patient's best interests. The known desires of the patient expressed or evidenced while the patient is able to participate in medical treatment decisions are presumed to be in the patient's best interests.

(G) A patient may revoke his or her designation at any time or in any manner sufficient to communicate an intent to revoke.

(H) A patient advocate may revoke his or her acceptance to the designation at any time and in any manner sufficient to communicate an intent to revoke.

(I) A patient admitted to a health facility or agency has the rights enumerated in Section 20201 of the Public Health Code, Act No. 368 of the Public Acts of 1978, being section 333.20201 of the Connecticut Compiled Laws.

I understand the above conditions and I accept the designation as patient advocate for

Walter Mayhew
_____

Date: _October 09, 2008_ Signed *Eleanor Mayhew*
_____

- vaginal discharge, odor, or evidence of a sexually transmitted disease
- pregnancy
- unusual sexual knowledge for the child's age.

Elder Abuse

Elder abuse can occur as neglect or physical abuse. Each form of abuse has many possible signs and symptoms.

Neglect

Suspect that an elderly person is neglected if you see any of these signs or symptoms:

- unclean or unsafe living conditions
- preoccupation of patient with money (for example, "My daughter won't want to pay the $5 copayment for the visit.")

- poor personal hygiene
- weight loss from poor food and fluid intake
- medications that are not taken properly and prescriptions that are not filled.

Physical Abuse

Suspect that an elderly person is the victim of physical abuse if you see any of these signs or symptoms:

- frequent injuries or trips to the emergency department
- bruises or broken bones (due to injury, not osteoporosis)
- patient's fear of the caregiver.

Living will

The following form shows a standard type of living will.

LIVING WILL OF

Jennifer L. Chen

I, _____*Jennifer L. Chen*_____ a resident of the City of __*Lovely*__,

__*Barrington*__ County, State of __*Connecticut*__, being of sound and disposing mind, memory, and understanding, do hereby willfully and voluntarily make, publish, and declare this to be my LIVING WILL, making known my desire that my life shall not be artificially prolonged under the circumstances set forth below, and do hereby declare:

1. This instrument is directed to my family, my physician(s), my attorney, my clergyman, any medical facility in whose care I happen to be, and to any individual who may become responsible for my health, welfare, or affairs.

2. Death is as much a reality as birth, growth, maturity, and old age. It is the one certainty of life. Let this statement stand as an expression of my wishes now that I am still of sound mind, for the time when I may no longer take part in decisions for my own future.

3. If at any time I should have a terminal condition and my attending physician has determined that there can be no recovery from such condition and my death is imminent, where the application of life-prolonging procedures and "heroic measures" would serve only to artificially prolong the dying process, I direct that such procedures be withheld or withdrawn, and that I be permitted to die naturally. I do not fear death itself as much as the indignities of deterioration, dependence, and hopeless pain. I therefore ask that medication be mercifully administered to me and that any medical procedures be performed on me which are deemed necessary to provide me with comfort or care or to alleviate pain.

4. In the absence of my ability to give directions regarding the use of such life-prolonging procedures, it is my intention that this declaration shall be honored by my family and physician as the final expression of my legal right to refuse medical treatment and accept the consequences for such refusal.

5. In the event that I am diagnosed as comatose, incompetent, or otherwise mentally or physically incapable of communication, I appoint _____*Benjamin Chen*_____ to make binding decisions concerning my medical treatment.

6. If I have been diagnosed as pregnant and that diagnosis is known to my physician, this declaration shall have no force or effect during the course of my pregnancy.

7. I understand the full import of this declaration and I am emotionally and mentally competent to make this declaration. I hope you, who care for me, will feel morally bound to follow its mandate. I recognize that this appears to place a heavy responsibility upon you, but it is with the intention of relieving you of such responsibility and of placing it upon myself, in accordance with my strong convictions, that this statement is made.

IN WITNESS WHEREOF, I have hereunto subscribed my name and affixed my seal at __*Blueville Savings*__

__*Bank*__, this __*9th*__ day of __*October*__, 20__*08*__, in the presence of the subscribing witnesses whom I have requested to become the attesting witnesses hereto.

Jennifer L. Chen
DECLARANT

Living will—cont'd

The declarant is known to me and I believe him/her to be of sound mind.

Gina DeCarlo
WITNESS SIGNATURE

Gina DeCarlo
PRINT NAME OF WITNESS

24 North Ridge Road, Lovely, CT
WITNESS ADDRESS

October 09, 2008
DATE

Subscribed and acknowledged, before me by *Jennifer L. Chen* and subscribed and sworn before the witnesses, on the _____ *9th* _____ day of _____ *October* _____ ,20 *08* .

MY COMMISSION EXPIRES
NOVEMBER 2010
STATE OF CONNECTICUT
NOTARY PUBLIC

Copies of this instrument have been given to: *Jennifer Chen, Benjamin Chen*

Receipt and acknowledged & date: *October 09, 2008*

Chapter Summary

- Failure to follow the Medical Practice Act can result in suspension or revocation of a physician's license, monetary fines, and imprisonment (for more serious violations).
- Documents such as a durable power of attorney and a living will outline who can make medical decisions or inform the health care staff of the patient's own wishes. These documents should be honored and followed as directed by the physician.
- The medical assistant must:
  - follow legal and ethical principles to safeguard a patient's privacy and physical safety and keep the patient informed of her health care
  - maintain complete patient records, disclose information only when appropriate, and treat patients with respect and kindness
  - help avoid lawsuits by avoiding such hazards as gossiping, promising a cure, and being disrespectful
  - report incidents of suspected child or elder abuse as mandated by the state
  - avoid violating the Medical Practice Act of her state by always practicing within the scope of her training and ability.

Team Work Exercises

1. Role-play physician, patient, and family members in explaining the uses of a durable power of attorney and a living will.
2. Research child abuse reporting laws for your state. Create a guide for a physician's office to use as a reference for

reporting child abuse. Discuss with the class how to handle a suspected abusive caregiver who brings a child in for care. When should the police be contacted? When can you let the child go home with the suspected abuser?

Case Studies

1. Your sister tells you that she has begun dating a great guy. When she introduces you to him, you recognize him as a patient in the medical office where you work. The man has a long history of drug and alcohol abuse and is currently receiving treatment. He has been arrested several times for drunk driving. What information (if any) can you disclose to your sister? Is it appropriate for you to speak to the man directly about his alcoholism and the fact that he is dating your sister? Discuss your thoughts with classmates.

2. Mike Jones calls the office and asks for the results of a pregnancy test on his wife, Ann Jones, who came in earlier today. What circumstances would allow you to release that information? Discuss your thoughts with your classmates.

Resources

- Durable power of attorney form (printable version): *www.med.umich.edu/1libr/aha/umlegal02.htm*
- Good Samaritan law: *pa.essortment.com/goodsamaritanl_redg.htm*
- Living will (printable version): *www.med.umich.edu/1libr/aha/umlegal04.htm*

HIPAA and a Patient's Rights

Learning Objectives

Upon completion of this chapter, the student will be able to:

- define the words presented in the key terms table
- describe the two components of HIPAA Public Law 104-191
- describe the three components of the security standard
- describe who may be listed as a "covered entity" and the responsibilities of the various entities
- describe treatment, payment, and operations (TPO)
- describe how to obtain consent to disclose protected health information (PHI) for TPO
- describe the patient's rights to PHI and how it is obtained
- describe the PHI that a patient does not have the right to access
- discuss the roles and responsibilities of a HIPAA compliance officer
- list at least four safeguards of PHI in each category
- list at least seven components of a medical record
- discuss the importance of a written release of PHI
- list the required privacy policy documents and their purposes
- describe the PHI that may be verbally disclosed
- discuss the penalties of failing to comply with HIPAA guidelines.

CAAHEP Competencies

Administrative Competencies
 Perform Clerical Functions
  Organize a patient's medical record
 Process Insurance Claims
  Apply managed care policies and procedures
  Apply third-party guidelines
General Competencies
 Legal Concepts
  Identify and respond to issues of confidentiality
  Perform within legal and ethical boundaries
  Establish and maintain the medical record
  Document appropriately
  Demonstrate knowledge of federal and state health care legislation and regulations
ABHES Competencies
 Professionalism
  Maintain confidentiality at all times
  Be cognizant of ethical boundaries
  Conduct work within scope of education, training, and ability
 Communication
  Be impartial and show empathy when dealing with patients
  Adapt what is said to the recipient's level of comprehension
 Administrative Duties
  Locate resources and information for patients and employers
 Legal Concepts
  Determine needs for documentation and reporting
  Document accurately

Procedures

 Release of PHI for non-TPO purposes
 Providing and explaining the NPP

Chapter Outline

 HIPAA
  Title I: Insurance Reform
  Title II: Administrative Simplification
   Reduced cost
   Privacy protection
   Patient's right to access
 HIPAA Compliance
  HIPAA Compliance Officer
  Safeguards for PHI
   Administrative
   Technical
   Physical
 HIPAA Documents
 HIPAA Noncompliance
 Chapter Summary
 Team Work Exercises
 Case Studies
 Resources

HIPAA

The Health Information Portability and Accountability Act of 1996 (HIPAA) mandates privacy for health information, standards for electronic transactions of health information and claims, security of electronic health information, and national identifiers for the parties in health care transactions. HIPAA privacy principles pertain to what is called **protected health information (PHI)**, which is information from a patient's medical record that contains details that could be used to identify the patient to whom it relates. Per HIPAA, it is the responsibility of the physician and other parties handling this information to protect it from misuse, regardless of the form of media it is in (such as electronic or print copy) and whether it is at rest (such as in a file that is accessed, stored, processed, or maintained) or in transit (such as sent through the U.S. mail or via fax or e-mail). Information included on the new patient registration, or intake, form is considered PHI, along with many other components of a person's medical record. (See Figure 7-1.) Thus, a practice must monitor its **disclosure**—its process of releasing, transferring, providing access to, or divulging information in any manner to a second party—of PHI for health care practices (business activities of the practice, including employee training, marketing, fund-raising, licensing, and quality assessments) to ensure compliance with HIPAA. (See *PHI in the medical record.*)

PHI in the medical record

In addition to the patient registration form, protected health information (PHI) in the medical record includes:

- insurance information
- consent forms
- HIPAA forms
- health history form
- physical examination notes
- progress notes
- laboratory reports
- diagnostic reports (such as x-rays, scans, and electro-cardiograms)
- medication record
- physical and occupational therapy reports
- home care reports
- hospital documents (operating room report, discharge notes, pathology reports)
- correspondence (medical and financial)
- consultation reports.

CONFIDENTIAL PATIENT INFORMATION

BLUEVILLE FAMILY MEDICINE
15 MAIN STREET
BLUEVILLE, CT
860-555-3212

Name_____ Date of birth_____ Full-time student ☐ Yes ☐ No
Address_____ City_____
Home phone_____ Cell phone_____
Insured name_____ Insured date of birth_____ Relationship to patient_____
Insured employer_____ Employer address_____
Insurance carrier_____ ID#_____ Group #_____

HEALTH HISTORY

Have you ever suffered from:

☐ Asthma	☐ Fainting	☐ Muscle weakness	☐ Lower back pain
☐ Diabetes	☐ Anxiety	☐ Difficulty sleeping	☐ Difficulty swallowing
☐ High blood pressure	☐ Bleeding disorder	☐ Allergies	☐ Neck pain or stiffness
☐ Migraine headaches	☐ Constipation	☐ Stomach upset	☐ Diarrhea
☐ Fatigue	☐ Stress	☐ Mental disorder	☐ Infection

☐ Cancer (If so, what kind?)_____ ☐ Chronic pain (If so, where?)_____

FAMILY HISTORY

☐ Cancer (Who?)_____ What type?_____
☐ High blood pressure (Who?)_____
☐ Diabetes (Who?)_____

MEDICATIONS AND SUPPLEMENTS

Do you take any medications? Do you take any nutritional supplements?
If so, please list (include dosages): If so, please list:

_____ _____
_____ _____
_____ _____
_____ _____
_____ _____

REASON FOR TODAY'S VISIT

☐ Check up
☐ Physical for school, sports, or employment
☐ Other (please explain)_____

Women only

Date of last menstrual period_____
Number of pregnancies_____ Miscarriages?_____
Number of children_____ Difficult or painful menstruation?_____

Men only

Have you ever had erectile difficulty?_____ Prostate problems?_____
Do you get up at night frequently to urinate?_____

I understand that Blueville Family Medicine will file my insurance for payment of services rendered. I also understand
that I am responsible for any amount due Blueville Family Medicine if my Insurance is denied.

Signature of patient or guardian_____ Date_____

Relationship to patient_____

Robert Greer, MD • Sharon Piecek, APRN • Hector Rodriguez, MD • Henry Lee, MD • Anne Wilson, MD

FIG 7-1 New patient registration form.

HIPAA, Public Law 104-191, contains two main parts:

- Title I—Insurance Reform
- Title II—Administrative Simplification.

Title I: Insurance Reform

The primary purpose of the insurance reform portion of HIPAA is to provide continuous insurance coverage for workers and their insured dependents when they change or lose a job. Prior to the reform act, if an employee left or lost a job and changed insurance coverage, a "preexisting condition" clause could be added to their new medical insurance. This clause would allow the new insurer to deny coverage for a chronic condition, such as diabetes or heart disease, leaving the patient without any medical insurance for these costly conditions. HIPAA now limits the use of preexisting condition exclusions and prohibits discrimination for past or present poor health. In addition, HIPAA ensures that, upon renewal of an existing health insurance policy, the insurer cannot reduce coverage to exclude previously covered services. In other words, patients never become too sick to receive health insurance.

Title II: Administrative Simplification

The goals of the administrative simplification portion of HIPAA are to reduce administrative costs, ensure privacy, and ensure a patient's right to his own health information.

Reduced Cost

To reduce administrative costs, Title II mandates the implementation of standards for electronic and print **transactions** involving PHI. The word *transaction* is used to describe any exchange of information between parties that contains PHI. Thus, any communication between the medical office and, say, a billing office or insurer that contains PHI would be considered a transaction. The standards for these transactions as outlined in HIPAA fall into four categories:

1. *Standard codes* are codes that identify diagnoses, procedures, services, drugs, and supplies. For example, ICD-9 and CPT-4 codes are standard code sets used to describe diseases and procedures, respectively. These code sets are used throughout the United States to communicate details of the medical record. Because these code sets are universally used, they help avoid misinterpretation by persons who use this information for financial and administrative duties.

2. *Unique identifiers* are numeric and alphanumeric strings attached to a transaction that identify a specific provider, employer, health plan, patient, facility, and so forth. That patient's name is not used, which further ensures privacy protection.

3. *Transaction code sets* are standardized codes used to represent health care concepts and procedures for healthcare-related financial and administrative purposes. These sets identify the type of information contained in the transaction. There are 10 transaction sets in HIPAA. Each is identified by a three-figure code:

- 270—eligibility, coverage, or benefit inquiry (in which the medical office inquires about a patient's eligibility on a certain date, coverage for a certain service, or how much the insurance company will pay for that service)
- 271—eligibility, coverage, or benefit information (in which the insurance company responds to the medical office's inquiry about a patient's eligibility on a certain date, coverage for a certain service, or how much they will pay the medical office for that service)
- 276—health care claim status request (in which a medical office or affiliated billing agency inquires about the status of a claim previously sent to the insurance company for payment)
- 277—health care claim status notification (in which the insurance company responds to the medical office or billing agency regarding acceptance or rejection of the claim, whether the claim is pending receipt of more information, or if incorrect information was supplied for the claim)
- 278—request for a health care services review (in which the medical office asks the insurance company to authorize payment for a service before that service is delivered, such as hospital admission, nursing home placement, and referrals for specialized care)
- 278—response to a request for a health care services review (in which the insurance company will respond to a medical office's request for preauthorization for services)
- 820—payment order or remittance advice (in which a sponsor, who is usually an employer, would provide payment to or request payment advice from the insurance company for an employee who is or will be enrolled in the health plan)
- 834—benefit enrollment and payment (in which a sponsor, who is usually an employer, enrolls, updates, or cancels enrollment of employees and dependents in a health care plan)
- 835—health care claim payment or advice (in which the insurer provides payment or an explanation of benefits [EOB] to a medical office)
- 837—health care claim, professional, institutional, dental, and retail pharmacy (in which a medical office, hospital or other institution, dentist's office, or retail pharmacy sends a claim for payment to an insurance company).

4. *Electronic data interchange (EDI)* standards are the standards for encrypting the data in a transaction when sent electronically. For example, the medical assistant might use a computer program (or e-mail) to send details of an office visit to an insurer for payment for services. In order to send the information in such a manner, the medical office must comply with EDI standards for such electronic transactions, including using a software program that adequately encrypts, or scrambles, the information so that it is unreadable if intercepted by a third party before arriving at its destination. Several encryption software programs are available. Manufacturers of medical software comply with the HIPAA EDI standards, as enforced by the American National Standards Institute (ANSI).

By standardizing the exchange of health care data and increasing the efficiency of computer-to-computer transactions of medical data, analysis costs and data use decrease. In addition, standardized formats for diagnosis and procedure codes and identifiers for providers and health plans reduce the time otherwise needed by the administrative medical assistant to determine what is written in a document. Standardization of information also improves the accuracy of data and decreases revenue cycle time. Claims for payment can be analyzed and paid more quickly.

Privacy Protection

HIPAA allows disclosure of PHI for the purposes of treatment, payment, and operations of the medical practice and mandates that all other disclosures must be specifically authorized by the patient. Patients can share PHI with other parties, such as an attorney, by requesting the disclosure and signing an **authorization**, which is written permission to disclose PHI when a consent form does not apply or another exception is evident.

Privacy and security procedures, mandated in the HIPAA act under Title II, ensure confidentiality and prevent the unauthorized disclosure of PHI. However, this component of HIPAA is commonly misunderstood. Unfortunately, these misconceptions have led many health care workers to think, "I can't tell anyone anything about a patient." (See *Disclosure: What can I say?*) While the act's language may be confusing, the intent of the legislation is to keep patient information confidential and secure without limiting access in a way that prevents medical staff from treating patients or receiving payment for care. The **security standard** in HIPAA, Title II, protects three important elements of PHI:

- *confidentiality*—prevention of unauthorized disclosure of data
- *integrity*—prevention of unauthorized modification to data
- *availability*—prevention of loss of access to resources and data. (See Procedure 7-1: *Release of PHI for non-TPO purposes*, page 76.)

An exception to privacy protection is the release of **de-identified information**, which is PHI with all personal identifiers removed from the data set, making it impossible to connect the information to an individual. A medical assistant will rarely be involved in transmitting de-identified information. (Such instances may include newborn screening for human immunodeficiency virus.) Typically, information that relates to communicable diseases becomes de-identified when a state reports the incidence of disease in that state to the Centers for Disease Control and Prevention.

Disclosure: What can I say?

The processes for written disclosure of PHI are exact and the medical office's policies and procedures manual can be used as a guide for following the rules of disclosure. However, disclosure is commonly given verbally and less formally, so the medical assistant must know what type of information she is allowed to disclose. The table below identifies situations in which disclosure of protected health information (PHI) is acceptable and unacceptable and examples of what the medical assistant should say in those situations.

Situation	Disclose	Example	Don't disclose	Example
If a friend or family member asks for information regarding a specific patient *by name,**	Patient's location and general condition	• "She is in room 1133, in stable condition." • "He is in ICU, in critical condition."	Specific conditions	• "Her fractured leg has been casted and she has been sedated." • "Inoperable tumors were found during his surgery."

Continued

Disclosure: What can I say?—cont'd

Situation	Disclose	Example	Don't disclose	Example
Medical assistant from another office calls seeking information on a patient's treatment	PHI for the purpose of treatment at another office	• "We removed the cast on the leg yesterday; the physical therapist can proceed with re-habilitation per the physician's order."	Treatment given for an unrelated condition	• "The patient has a sub-stance abuse history."
Billing company asks for information to receive payment from insurance	Dates of service and codes for payment inquiry	• "I can resend the dates of service, diag-noses, and CPT codes."	Payments made by the patient when she had no coverage	• "Her coverage began on July 1, 2007, prior to that she was self-pay."
Local newspaper calls asking if the mayor of the city has been admitted to the hospital	No information	• "I am not permitted to disclose any infor-mation to the press. I can refer you to our community relations department."	Any information that would lead the caller to assume that the person was admitted	• "The mayor was admitted this morning. You can speak to his wife for details."
State Department of Health reports cases of tuberculosis to the Centers for Disease Control and Prevention	Only de-identified infor-mation (name of infec-tion and number of cases)	• "We received reports of 27 cases of tuber-culosis in the state of Connecticut in 2007."	Any information that would lead to the iden-tity of the individual patients	• "Most of the reported cases are employees of the Department of Transporta-tion's Tolland County Office."

* Confirm the identity of the friend or family member.

PROCEDURE 7-1

Release of PHI for non-TPO purposes

Task
Ensure that protected health information (PHI) released for purposes other than treatment, payment, or operations (TPO) is performed with proper patient authorization.

Conditions
• Authorization to Release PHI form
• Patient's medical record
• Pen

Standards
In the time specified and within the scoring parameters determined by the instructor, the student will successfully perform a release of PHI for non-TPO purposes.

Performance Standards
1. Check the Authorization to Release form's informa-tion for completeness, including:

a. patient's name, date of birth, and Social Security number to ensure that the authorization is for the correct patient and is not mistakenly used for another patient

b. patient's initials next to the notice of the right to revoke permission to disclose to ensure that the patient understands his rights

c. patient's or legal guardian's signature (original, not a photocopied or faxed signature) to prevent the possibility of forgery

d. date signed to ensure that the request is recent and pertains to current information

e. information requested for reasonable length of time (for example, not entire record spanning 54 years)

PROCEDURE 7-1—cont'd

f. HIV, mental health, and substance abuse information specifically requested by the patient (separately indicated with initials or signature) to ensure confidentiality and protection of personal health information

g. indication of recipient of information, including name, address, and other contact information to ensure that the information is released to an individual who has the authority to view the information.

2. Retrieve the patient's medical record.

3. Photocopy the documentation requested.

4. Recheck the authorization and photocopied documentation to ensure that *only* the information requested and authorized is released because a release of

unauthorized information can result in fines to the medical office.

5. If a courier is picking up the information, check the identification of the courier to prevent the release of information to the wrong courier. If you are mailing the information, recheck the name and address of the recipient before sending it to ensure the identity and location of the recipient is correct.

6. Document the release of information in the patient's medical record to maintain a complete medical record.

7. File the Authorization to Release form in the patient's medical record or designated file to ensure that proper documentation is available if a question about the release arises at a later time.

PHI Outside the Office

Some medical practices hire a billing company to file health care claims electronically. HIPAA mandates that the practice must treat that billing company as a **business associate**, a person or organization who, on behalf of the medical practice, performs or assists in the performance of a function or activity involving the use of **individually identifiable health information (IIHI)**, or medical information contained in a patient's record that could be used to identify the patient. The physician's office and the billing company must have a written **business associate contract**, which is a legal document that specifies that the physician's office is releasing PHI for the purposes of reimbursement and that the billing company may not use the information for any other purpose. The billing company may be required to sign a **data use agreement** that limits its use of PHI. The names and addresses of the patients, for example, cannot be sold to a marketing company. If the billing company, acting in an effort to collect payment, transmits PHI electronically, the billing company and the physician's office are covered entities and must comply with HIPAA. A transfer of information between the physician's office and the billing company related to health care may include:

- health care claim forms
- health care payment and explanation of reimbursement
- coordination of benefits (secondary insurance)
- health care claim status (denials and requests for further information)
- enrollment and disenrollment in health care plans
- eligibility for enrollment in a health care plan
- health care plan premium payments
- referrals and preauthorizations for treatment
- first report of injury
- narrative notes.

✦ **TIP** HIPAA in the Mail

If an office files billing via U.S. mail, does it have to comply with HIPAA? YES! Although the target of HIPPA is electronic information, all forms of PHI—whether written by hand, stored in a computer and transmitted to another agency, or photocopied and put into an envelope for a courier to pick up—are personal and confidential and should only be disclosed with proper authorization. Note: Providers with 10 or more employees were required to convert to electronic transactions to Medicare by October 16, 2003. Therefore, HIPAA compliance is now mandatory.

Patient's Right to Access

In addition to preventing unauthorized use of PHI, the administrative simplification provisions also specify a patient's right to his own PHI. Prior to HIPAA, health care providers could deny access to medical records and refuse to share a patient's health information with him. A patient now has the right to request:

- access to his health information
- amendment of PHI
- additional restriction of information
- alternative means of communicating health information
- accounting of disclosures of his PHI.

Access to Information

A patient has the right to access, inspect, and obtain a copy of their medical records. The provider may require the request in writing and must fulfill it within 30 days. Reasonable fees may be charged for copies and should be cost-based. In general, copy costs and postage are reasonable. If the patient agrees to a summary in lieu of the complete chart, the cost of preparing the summary may be included but should be disclosed to the patient prior to preparation.

An office can deny a patient access for certain reasons without giving the patient the right to review the denial. Under the HIPAA privacy regulations, a patient does not have the right to access:

- psychotherapy notes
- information compiled in reasonable anticipation of, or for use in, legal proceedings
- information exempted from disclosure under the Clinical Laboratory Improvements Amendment (CLIA)
- information that would reveal the identity of and therefore endanger a person other than the health care provider who is a source of information.

HIPAA specifically excludes psychotherapy notes from disclosure. Although such notes as medication records, start and stop dates of sessions, diagnoses, test results, and frequency and types of treatment are considered PHI, psychotherapy notes are not stored in the general medical record, nor are personal notes. A psychologist or psychiatrist has the right to deny patient access if she feels that release of the information would be detrimental to the patient's health. Denial of release of records by a psychologist or psychiatrist is not subject to any review process.

Access to PHI obtained from an individual source other than the health care provider under a promise of confidentiality can also be denied if that information would compromise the identity of the source of the information or could be used for legal proceedings. For example, if the medical chart of Mr. Jones refers to his wife's disclosure of domestic violence or evidence of wounds incurred during an attack on his wife, releasing the chart to Mr. Jones could endanger Mrs. Jones.

Amendment of PHI

Patients have the right to request an amendment of their PHI if they feel that information contained in the medical record is inaccurate. The provider can require that the request for amendment be in writing and can deny the amendment for these reasons:

- The provider who is requested to amend the PHI is not the originator of the information. If medical records were transferred from one medical office to a second medical office, the receiving medical office is not responsible for the accuracy of the documents. The patient could then request that the originator amend the document.
- The provider believes that the PHI is accurate and complete without amendment.
- HIPAA does not require that the provider make the information accessible to the patient. The information must be one of the four types outlined above in the denial of access to records, including psychotherapy notes, information compiled for a legal proceedings, information exempted by CLIA, and information that could compromise the identity of a source other than the health care provider.

A medical office must respond to a patient's request for amendment within 60 days. Denial of amendments must be accompanied by reasons for the denial. The office must also give the patient an opportunity to file a statement of disagreement.

Additional Restriction of Information

A patient has the right to ask for restrictions on how the medical office will use and disclose PHI for TPO. A patient may have a previous medical history that is not applicable to current treatment and can request that this information not be shared. Such information as abortions, successful treatment of sexually transmitted diseases (STDs), and cosmetic surgery may be embarrassing to a patient and its disclosure would not effect treatment outcomes. The medical office is not required to agree to the requests, but must have a process to review the request in the case of a denial. In some situations, PHI is disclosed for reasons other than TPO. (See *PHI and public health and safety*.)

Alternative Communications

Patients have the right to request confidential communications by alternative means. A patient may request that the medical office call her only at work, not at home. A request that an answering machine not be used for sensitive information is also appropriate. The alternative communications request must be reasonable; the patient cannot request that she receive phone calls only between 2 a.m. and 5 a.m. The patient does not need to explain her reasons for the alternative communication request; however, if domestic violence is suspected, the medical assistant should follow reporting laws as indicated by her state.

PHI and public health and safety

Occasionally, a patient's protected health information (PHI) may be disclosed if such a disclosure could positively impact public health or safety. Such situations include:

- disclosure of psychiatric notes or drug use history of an individual seeking a day care license, teaching certification, or gun permit (requires a court order)
- sharing information on communicable diseases and work-related illnesses and accidents
- reporting victims of abuse, neglect, or domestic violence
- law enforcement purposes, such as allowing investigators to view photographs of wounds taken in the course of treating a person who may have incurred those wounds while committing a violent crime
- births and deaths.

Accounting of Disclosures

Patients have a right to request an accounting of any disclosures of PHI for purposes other than TPO. Patients are entitled to one accounting of disclosures per calendar year, free of charge. Additional requests for disclosures can be granted at a reasonable cost. A log of disclosures, computerized or written, should be maintained in anticipation of a patient's request for an accounting. The disclosure log should include:

- date of disclosure
- name of the agency or individual who received the PHI, including the agency's address (for example, *Child Protective Services, Elaine Mendenhall, MSW*)
- brief description of the PHI disclosed (for example, *office treatment notes 1/15/06 through 4/15/06; x-ray left humerus 2/11/06*)
- brief statement of the purpose of the disclosure (for example, *child abuse investigation*).

HIPAA Compliance

Because HIPAA requires physician's offices to change the way that information is stored, transferred, and utilized, a time frame for compliance with HIPAA was specified. All time frames for compliance are past, with the latest deadline falling on April 21, 2005. Therefore, compliance with HIPAA in transaction and code set standards (October 2003), Medicare electronic claims (October 2003), privacy rules (April 2003), unique identifiers for employers (July 2004), and security standards (April 2005) is mandatory. By these dates, physician offices were required to comply with each of the portions of HIPAA.

HIPAA Compliance Officer

The medical office must have a person who assumes the responsibilities of ensuring compliance with HIPAA regulations regarding security, disclosure, and use of PHI. The compliance officer, or *privacy officer*, is typically the office manager and is responsible for:

- providing training for all personnel regarding the release and use of PHI
- ensuring that privacy and security rules are outlined in a policy and procedures manual and that this manual is available to personnel for reference
- providing patients and personnel with a process to register a complaint regarding the misuse of PHI
- providing disciplinary guidelines for failure to comply with **privacy standards** (policies and procedures in a facility that determine who has access to PHI), such as verbal and written warnings, employee termination, and a referral to federal agencies for criminal prosecution (if applicable)

- providing information to patients regarding the proper procedures for requesting amendments, appeals, and rebuttals (See *Seven components of a compliance plan.*)
- instituting administrative, technical, and physical measures that ensure reasonable safeguards to PHI from unauthorized use or disclosure. (See *HIPAA compliance: Everyone's job,* page 80.)

Safeguards for PHI

There are three types of safeguards that a medical practice should institute to avoid the misuse of PHI:

- administrative
- technical
- physical

Administrative

Administrative safeguards for PHI include:

- verifying the identity of an individual picking up health records
- verifying a patient's identity on the telephone after putting the caller on hold and returning to the call
- immediately reporting a suspected breach of confidentiality to the HIPAA compliance officer
- making sure that each patient signs a **Notice of Privacy Practices (NPP)**, a document that explains how the patient's medical information will be used to perform duties related to treatment, payment, or operations (TPO), before releasing information for TPO
- checking a patient's medical record for special instructions regarding contacting the patient before making the call

---

Seven components of a compliance plan

The Office of the Inspector General recommends the following steps for individual and small-group practices to follow to ensure compliance with HIPAA guidelines:

1. Conduct periodic internal monitoring and audits.
2. Implement compliance and practice standards.
3. Designate a HIPAA compliance officer.
4. Conduct training and education.
5. Respond appropriately to detected offenses and develop a corrective action plan.
6. Develop open lines of communication for staff to ask questions and refer to the policies and procedures manual.
7. Enforce disciplinary standards through well-publicized guidelines. (Disciplinary rules should be included in the policies and procedures manual.)

Front office–Back office connection

HIPAA Compliance: Everyone's Job

The HIPAA compliance officer is responsible for training front and back office staff. The staff is responsible for understanding the policies and procedures that protect a patient's protected health information (PHI) in both areas. The front desk staff must have an understanding of how test results are kept private and how to release them to a patient. The clinical staff must also have an understanding of how to release PHI and the required paperwork that must accompany the release.

When considering patient privacy and patient's rights, clinical and administrative staff must be well versed in the laws and adhere to them. They should work together to educate patients, while making PHI available to the patient in a manner that does not violate HIPAA privacy standards. For example, a patient may tell the front desk medical assistant that she cannot accept phone calls at work and ask why the clinical staff cannot call her husband at work with her test results. The front desk medical assistant must be able to explain to the patient that doing so would violate HIPAA privacy standards. The medical assistant should suggest other methods of relaying the information, such as leaving a message (with the patient's permission) on her home phone or cell phone.

- placing fax machines in private areas, away from patients; making sure personnel never leave information at the fax machine
- designating a private area for physicians to dictate notes and return phone calls; patients should not be able to hear dictations or phone calls.

Technical

Technical safeguards for PHI include:

- requiring a unique username and password for each staff member to use to access patient computer records and setting passwords to expire periodically so that staff members must choose a new password to gain access
- instituting firewall protection to prevent a compromise in security from an outside source (such as a computer "hacker")
- deleting usernames and passwords when staff members discontinue employment with the practice
- utilizing practice management software that tracks users and their activities
- ensuring that staff members always log off when leaving a computer station

- periodically running virus protection software
- not allowing personnel to use computers to check e-mail or send personal e-mails to prevent potential corruption of data from viruses acquired through home e-mail addresses.

Physical

Physical safeguards for PHI include:

- storing patient files away from patient-accessible areas
- locking patient files when the office is closed
- ensuring that staff members never leave a patient file open at the reception desk
- filing medical records before the cleaning staff comes in at night and placing items to be filed in a folder
- making staff aware that conversations at the front desk could be overheard; instructing all staff to close the privacy window and be careful of their voice volume when talking on the telephone.
- not posting providers' schedules with names of patients in an area that can be seen by other patients
- although patient sign-in sheets are acceptable, making sure to require a patient to sign their name only, without listing a reason for the visit.

HIPAA Documents

HIPAA compliance can be obtained through proper training and adherence to mandated rules. All personnel who have a need to use PHI should undergo training and have access to documents that outline disclosure regulations and patients' rights. The documents should be kept in a policies and procedures manual and available for personnel to review. The policies and procedures manual should contain these HIPAA documents:

- *Notice of privacy practices* describes the use of PHI for carrying out treatment, payment, or **health care operations** (TPO). (See Procedure 7-2: *Providing, explaining, and obtaining acknowledgment of the NPP.*) A written acknowledgement is recommended, rather than a verbal one. (See *Acknowledgment of NPP.*)
- *Consent for use or disclosure for TPO* is a patient's consent to the use of and disclosure of health information for TPO (optional).
- *Authorization to use or disclose PHI* must be obtained when a consent form does not apply or another exception otherwise permitting use or disclosure of PHI does not apply. (See *Outside release form*, page 82.)
- *Business associate contract*, or *data use agreement*, describes privacy protection for a patient's PHI when using outside entities that provide services for your organization whose access to PHI is necessary.

PROCEDURE 7-2

Providing, explaining, and obtaining acknowledgment of the NPP

Task

Use the Notice of Privacy Practices (NPP) to ensure that a patient understands the right to protected health information (PHI) and how the office will use the information for treatment, payment, and operations (TPO) and obtain the patient's signature on the acknowledgment form.

Conditions

- Notice of Privacy Practices
- New Patient Registration form
- Acknowledgment of Receipt of NPP form
- Patient's medical record
- Pen

Standards

In the time specified and within the scoring parameters determined by the instructor, the student will successfully provide and explain the NPP and obtain the patient's signature on the acknowledgment form.

Performance Standards

1. Give the patient the Notice of Privacy Practices (NPP) along with the New Patient Registration form so that the patient can read the NPP along with the registration form.
2. Ask the patient to read the NPP and answer any questions that he may have.
3. Ask the patient to sign the acknowledgment of receipt and understanding of NPP.
4. File the acknowledgment in the patient's medical record to maintain a complete medical record and ensure proper documentation if questions about privacy arise at a later time.

Patient Education

Acknowledgment of NPP

When a new patient comes to the office, he should be given a copy of the Notice of Privacy Practices (NPP) from HIPAA. This document will tell the patient how his protected health information (PHI) will be used for treatment, payment, and operations (TPO). The NPP is usually given to the patient the first time he receives instructions from the office. The first experience with patient education at the office can set the tone for subsequent patient teaching. The medical assistant should create a rapport with the patient, encourage the patient to ask questions, and answer questions as they arise. If this first experience is positive, the patient may feel more comfortable about asking other staff members medical, financial, or administrative questions in the future.

Because the NPP is about seven pages long, many medical practices laminate a few copies to use for new patient registration. Regardless of how the office distributes the NPP, it must include:

- who within the practice will comply with privacy practices
- who outside of the practice will comply with privacy practices
- outline of the practice's responsibilities for protecting health information

- ways in which the practice may use or disclose PHI
- patient's rights regarding PHI, along with the procedure for exercising those rights
- procedure for changing policies outlined in the notice (or the notice itself)
- contact information for questions or complaints a patient might have regarding the practice's disclosure of PHI (including information for contacting the practice and the appropriate government agencies)
- question-and-answer section outlining the most common questions regarding the NPP.

Acknowledgment form

The patient must sign an acknowledgement form (as shown below) to indicate that he has read the notice and understands the implications such privacy restrictions will have on the handling of his medical record. This signed document will allow the office to use PHI for TPO. The medical assistant may have to explain components of the document to the patient. A written, rather than verbal, acknowledgment of this notice is recommended.

Continued

Patient Education—cont'd

ACKNOWLEDGMENT FORM

I _____Beryl Travalian_____ have read and understand the Notice of Privacy Practices Policy.

_____Beryl C. Travalian_____   _____08/27/07_____
Signature of patient or guardian   Date

- *HIPAA compliance officer job description* is a written description of the officer's roles and responsibilities.
- **Termination policy** is a written statement that mandates termination of an employee who fails to comply with internal privacy policies and procedures.

HIPAA Noncompliance

Failure to comply with HIPAA regulations can result in serious civil and criminal penalties. The HIPAA legislation required the U.S. Department of Health and Human Services (HHS) to establish and implement national standards and identifiers for electronic transactions and handle ongoing issues involving transaction code sets and security. The HHS developed sample documents for physicians' offices to download and use. The authority to enforce the transaction code set requirements was given to the Centers for Medicare and Medicaid (CMS), formerly the Health Care Financing Administration (HCFA). The Office of Civil Rights (OCR) was given the responsibility for ongoing enforcement of the privacy standards and the handling of complaints. The

Patient Education

Outside Release Form

Attorneys will commonly have their clients sign a release of medical information form. The medical assistant should insist that the patient provide an original signature on the form. She should never accept a duplicated or faxed copy of a form requesting the release of protected health information (PHI). Most attorneys' offices will send a letter to the physician requesting release of PHI, along with a release request form signed by the patient. The medical assistant should never release information to an attorney if the request is made without the required release form. When accepting a release of records form that is not generated by the medical office, the medical assistant should be sure to inspect the request for completeness, including the elements noted below.

The medical office can generate the request for release of information and can specify the agency to receive the PHI. By generating the request "in house," the medical assistant knows that the documentation is complete and that the patient understands the purpose of the release of information. When asking a patient to sign a release of information document, the medical assistant should explain to the patient where the information will go and for what purposes.

Patient Education—cont'd

AUTHORIZATION FOR RELEASE OF PROTECTED HEALTH INFORMATION

Josefina Marie Simms   _8/16/54_   _876-32-1234_
Patient name   Date of birth   Social security #

> PATIENT'S NAME, DATE OF BIRTH, AND SOCIAL SECURITY NUMBER ARE INCLUDED.

I, _Josefina Marie Simms_ , authorize the use or disclosure of my protected health information by
     PATIENT NAME

Dr. Robert Greer as specified below. I understand that signing this authorization is voluntary and that Dr. Greer may not require me to sign this authorization before Dr. Greer provides me with treatment. I understand that I have the right to revoke this authorization at any time by providing a signed, written notice of such revocation to Dr. Greer. I understand that a description of my rights to revoke my authorization is set forth by Dr. Greer.

> RIGHT TO REVOKE THE PERMISSION TO DISCLOSE IS INCLUDED.

Notice of Privacy Practices: I understand that information is being released pursuant to this authorization at my request and that the information may no longer be protected by law or regulation and may be redisclosed by the recipient.

Please use or disclose the following information:
☒ The entire medical record
☐ The following limited health information

_____

_____

> INFORMATION TO BE DISCLOSED IS SPECIFIED AND THE REQUEST IS REASONABLE. (FOR EXAMPLE, A REQUEST FOR 45 YEARS OF A MEDICAL RECORD IS AN UNREASONABLE REQUEST.)

The following information cannot be disclosed without specific authorization. Please initial next to each item below that you specifically authorize the release of health information relating to the testing, diagnosis, or treatment for:

JMS HIV or AIDS

JMS Drug and alcohol abuse

JMS Mental health or psychiatric disorders

> BECAUSE INFORMATION REGARDING HUMAN IMMUNODEFICIENCY VIRUS (HIV) STATUS, MENTAL HEALTH HISTORY, AND SUBSTANCE ABUSE HISTORY ARE CONSIDERED HIGHLY SENSITIVE, AUTHORIZATION TO RELEASE THAT INFORMATION MUST BE EXPLICITLY OUTLINED.

Please specify the time period for the information you described to be disclosed:
☐ All information maintained at this time by Dr. Greer
☒ Information maintained by Dr. Greer from _10/8/2004_ to _2/28/2005_

Please specify who may receive the information requested by this authorization:

Carla J. Simmons
Attorney at Law
211 Main Street
Lovely, CT 06111

> THE PERSON OR AGENCY (LAW OFFICES) WHERE THE INFORMATION IS TO BE RELEASED IS SPECIFIED AND THE ADDRESS OF THE AGENCY IS INCLUDED.

By signing below, I understand and acknowledge the following:
• I have read and understand this authorization
• I am authorizing Dr. Greer to use or disclose the health information to the person(s) identified in this authorization.
If I have any questions about disclosure of my protected health information pursuant to this authorization, I may contact Anthony Campbell, Paralegal, law offices of:

Carla J. Simmons
Attorney at Law
211 Main Street
Lovely, CT 06111

> THE DOCUMENT IS SIGNED AND DATED.

Josefina Marie Simms   _Josefina Marie Simms_   _5/24/2008_
Printed name of patient   Signature of patient   Date

OCR refers more serious issues to the Office of the Inspector General (OIG). The OIG refers criminal cases to the FBI and other agencies.

Penalties for noncompliance include:

- *privacy, security, and transaction violation*—$100 to $25,000 fine per person for identical violations in a calendar year
- *knowingly obtaining and disclosing IIHI*—$50,000 fine
- *obtaining IIHI under false pretenses*—$100,000 fine
- *obtaining IIHI under false pretenses with the intent to sell, transfer, or use for commercial advantage, personal gain, or malicious harm*—$250,000 fine and up to 10 years in prison.

In addition to safeguarding PHI, the OIG is also responsible for prosecuting fraud, abuse, and waste in claims submission. Health care providers and staff must be aware of the potential liability of submitting fraudulent claims. Patterns of claims submission that result in excessive reimbursement can result in prosecution under HIPAA guidelines. Deliberate unethical behavior can result in prosecution under the Criminal False Claims Act (18 US Code). Such behavior includes:

- charging insurance companies for procedures not performed
- submitting claims for equipment, medical supplies, and services that are not reasonable or necessary
- willfully omitting or providing misleading information to promote reimbursement of a claim
- billing for each component of a service, called *unbundling*, when all-inclusive codes are available and would result in lower reimbursement
- knowingly using the wrong provider identification numbers so that a nonparticipating physician is paid at the participating physician rate
- changing dates of service to fit patient eligibility.

Chapter Summary

- The Health Information Portability and Accountability Act of 1996 (HIPAA) was enacted to safeguard patients' privacy and the security of protected health information (PHI).
- Following HIPAA mandates ensures the confidentiality, integrity, and availability of PHI.
- Patients have the rights to access their PHI, request an amendment of their PHI, impose additional restrictions on disclosure of their PHI, request alternative communication regarding their PHI, and obtain an accounting of all disclosures of their PHI.

- The medical assistant may be required to act as a HIPAA compliance officer, providing training to personnel and creating and maintaining administrative, technical, and physical safeguards for PHI.
- Failure to comply with HIPAA mandates can result in serious civil and criminal penalties.

Team Work Exercises

1. In groups of three to eight students, create a HIPAA training session to present to classmates or another class on campus. Include such items as release of PHI, amendments to PHI, and role of the HIPAA compliance officer. Include a brief quiz at the end of your presentation.
2. In groups of two students, role-play a medical assistant explaining the purpose of the Notice of Privacy Practices form to a patient.

Case Studies

1. Mrs. Li Chuan Chu is a new patient. She speaks limited English and was unable to have her daughter come with her to the physician's office to interpret. Can Mrs. Chu be treated? Can she sign the Notice of Privacy Practices if she doesn't understand the document? Can her PHI be released for TPO? Discuss solutions to the dilemma with your classmates.
2. You receive a faxed authorization for release of PHI to a patient's attorney for use in a worker's compensation claim case. Can you accept the document? If not, how can you comply with the patient's request for release of information?

Resources

- American Medical Association: *www.ama-assn.org/ama/pub/category/424.html*
  Health Insurance Portability and Accountability Act (HIPAA) of 1996: Title 1 Statutory Text: *www.cms.hhs.gov/hipaa1/content/HIPAASTA.pdf*
- HIPAA Academy: *www.HIPAAacademy.net*
- HIPAA Administrative Simplification, Dept. of HHS: *www.aspe.os.dhhs.gov/adminsimp*
- HIPAA EDI implementation guide: *www.wpc-edi.com/hipaa_40.asp*
- Samples of downloadable release forms: *www.cms.hhs.gov*

Bioethics

Learning Objectives

Upon completion of this chapter, the student will be able to:

- define and spell key terms in the glossary
- compare morals and ethics
- differentiate between law and ethics
- define bioethics
- discuss the seven ethical principles described in this chapter
- differentiate between utilitarianism and deontology
- describe the features of an ethical dilemma
- explain the purpose of an ethics committee
- discuss the purpose of a code of ethics
- identify two codes of ethics relevant to the profession of medical assisting.

CAAHEP Competencies

General Competencies

Legal Concepts
  Identify and respond to issues of
    confidentiality
  Perform within legal and ethical
    boundaries

ABHES Competencies

Professionalism
  Maintain confidentiality at all times
  Be cognizant of ethical boundaries
  Evidence a responsible attitude
  Be courteous and diplomatic

Chapter Outline

Ethics and Morals
Law and Ethics
Bioethics
Ethical Principles
  Nonmaleficence
  Beneficence
  Autonomy
  Distributive Justice
  Paternalism
  Veracity
  Fidelity
Ethical Philosophies
  Deontological Philosophies
  Teleological Philosophies
  Philosophical Divide
Anatomy of an Ethical Dilemma
  Ethical Decision Making
  Ethics Committee
**Ethics and the Medical
  Professional**
  Code of Ethics
  Ethical Behavior in the Medical Office
    Trust and loyalty
    Confidentiality

Respect and dignity
*Commitment to professional
  development*
Chapter Summary
Team Work Exercises
Case Studies
Resources

Key Terms

ambiguity
State of uncertainty or vagueness

autonomy
Right to self-determination

beneficence
Duty to provide a good or benefit

bias
Unfair or incorrect belief that stems from prejudice and inhibits impartial judgment or action

bioethics
Study of the ethical implications of discoveries and advances in modern medicine and health care

consent
To agree or give permission

deontology
Ethical philosophy concerned with duties and rights

distributive justice
Principle regarding the fair distribution of scarce resources

ethics
Study of human behavior and moral choices based on a set of principles; rules or standards governing professional conduct

fidelity
Concept of loyalty or faithfulness

justice
Concept of fairness or equity

morals
Judgment regarding the value of certain behaviors based on personal belief

nonmaleficence
Duty to do no harm

norm
Unwritten rules of socially acceptable behavior

paternalism
Practice of providing for people without giving them rights or responsibilities

teleological philosophies
Philosophies that focus on consequences or the ends, more than on actions or the means, in determining value

utilitarianism
Ethical philosophy concerned with achieving the greatest good for the greatest number of people

veracity
Quality of truthfulness

Ethics and Morals

Morals and *ethics* are terms that are sometimes used interchangeably because they are based on values regarding human conduct. However, there are some subtle differences. **Morals** are deeply held personal beliefs about what constitutes right or wrong behavior. Such beliefs stem from a variety of sources, including religion, family customs, culture, and past experiences.

Ethics goes further than a simple pronouncement of moral judgment and involves thoughtful analysis, commonly at a philosophical level. Ethics evaluates human behavior in light of specific ethical principles and looks at the impact of such behavior on individuals and society as a whole. Stated more simply, when one is behaving ethically, one is concerned with the big picture as well as the immediate situation.

Law and Ethics

Although a behavior may be deemed unethical by some individuals, it is not necessarily illegal. Conversely, a behavior that has been designated as illegal is not necessarily considered unethical by all. All cultures have beliefs about what is considered right and wrong behavior. Actions that are considered most harmful or offensive by the majority may be designated as illegal. Individuals who commit such acts, if caught, will be subject to some form of fine or punishment. For example, in the United States, killing another person for personal gain or other selfish reasons is considered by most people to be morally and ethically wrong. Therefore, the act of murder has been legally designated a crime. Penalties for those convicted of murder are quite severe. Yet killing another individual in self-defense or as part of a government-sanctioned military action is deemed acceptable, in some cases perhaps even honorable.

However, people do not always agree about what constitutes right or wrong behavior. In such cases, there is usually not enough agreement to support legislation making such behavior illegal. For example, consensual sex between unmarried adults is legal in the United States. Some people believe this is wrong, yet others do not. When there is lack of agreement, formation of laws to prohibit such behaviors is unlikely. In some cases, rules may be enacted to regulate, rather than prohibit, specific acts. Such regulation generally specifies where, when, and by whom such acts may be performed. For example, therapeutic abortion has been legal since the 1973 *Roe v. Wade* Supreme Court ruling. However, there are specific rules that regulate where such procedures may be performed and by whom. Although abortion is deemed immoral or unethical by some, such beliefs are not sufficient to make the act illegal. An act only becomes illegal when specific action, such as the passage of a law by a governing body, makes it so.

On the other hand, some people might argue that some acts, though illegal, are not morally or ethically wrong. For example, the legal age to buy and consume alcohol varies between states and countries. An 18-year-old who buys or drinks alcohol in one place might be breaking the law, while the same person could travel a few miles over the border to a different state or country and legally commit the same act. Even so, some might argue that even though the issue of legality changed from one place to the other, the issue of morality did not. Some individuals believe that drinking alcohol is wrong regardless of the individual's physical location or age. Others would disagree.

Bioethics

Biomedical ethics, or *bioethics,* is a specialized branch of ethics that concerns itself with human behavior within the context of modern medicine. In recent years, modern science has provided humankind with an amazing number of new treatment options. Human cloning, in vitro fertilization, stem cell research, and some forms of organ transplantation once made good topics for science fiction novels but were not considered realistic. Today, however, organ transplantation and in vitro fertilization are commonplace. Stem cell research, though still controversial, is currently underway. Animal cloning is currently being done in a limited way. Human cloning, though not common practice, is the subject of much debate. It seems only a matter of time before some form of human cloning takes place, authorized or otherwise. The topics of abortion and euthanasia are not new. Yet our struggle to understand and agree upon standards for human conduct are exemplified by continuous debate on both issues.

In addition to these controversial topics are the more common, yet equally difficult, situations that patients and families face on a daily basis. The explosion of medical research has necessarily compounded the complexity of decision making required of patients and family members. In many situations, the "right" choice is not readily apparent, leaving everyone to agonize and, perhaps, disagree about what ought to be done in any given situation.

The number and variety of situations that confront health care providers are infinite. Therefore, it is not possible to predict them or to explain what ought to be done in each and every case. So what are health care workers to do? At worst, they can keep their heads in the sand, refusing to discuss and deal with these difficult and painful topics. Doing so tends to result in responses dictated by fear and prejudice when touchy topics arise and difficult decisions must be made, which is not helpful to anyone. A far better plan is for health care workers to become educated and prepared with information and tools that can help them navigate these difficult waters and provide better guidance to their patients. These tools include an understanding of key ethical principles, ethical philosophies, and a thoughtful plan for responding to ethical dilemmas when they arise.

Ethical Principles

Ethical principles are rules about how people ought to behave. An understanding of these principles is necessary to understand the ethical reasoning process. Upon initial examination, ethical principles may seem simple and straightforward. However, they commonly come into conflict with one another, sometimes creating complicated situations. Some of the most common ethical principles applied to health care include:

- nonmaleficence
- beneficence
- autonomy
- distributive justice
- paternalism
- veracity
- fidelity.

Nonmaleficence
Nonmaleficence refers to the duty of health care providers to "do no harm." This principle was first mentioned in the Hippocratic oath and has since been repeated in one form or another in various professional ethical codes. Few would argue the merit of such a principle. However, the reality of most forms of medical treatment is that there is always the potential for harm. Even something as simple as prescribing an antibiotic to a patient with an infection has some potential to cause harm. Although potential adverse effects of most antibiotics are minor, some could be life-threatening.

Beneficence
The principle of **beneficence** goes a step beyond nonmaleficence. It states that health care providers must aim to *provide benefit* for their clients in addition to avoiding doing harm. This principle has served to guide some of the changes that have occurred over the past century regarding the regulation of medications. Years ago, virtually anyone could sell their own version of a remedy, sometimes called "snake oil," wherever and to whomever they wished. They could make unsubstantiated claims about its curative powers. In most cases, these "remedies" provided no benefit and, worse yet, were sometimes harmful. Since that time, laws have been enacted

in the United States that require medications to be proven safe as well as beneficial before they are approved for sale. Such regulation is an example of the principle of beneficence at work.

With beneficence in mind, physicians are obligated to provide medications and treatments that have a reasonable likelihood of helping patients. As a patient faces a decision regarding possible surgery, a diagnostic procedure, or a new medication, the physician must provide information regarding potential risks and benefits. In every case, there is some element of risk, because no procedures or medications are totally risk free. In this decision-making process, the health care provider and patient strive to make a choice that minimizes potential harm (nonmaleficence) while maximizing potential benefit (beneficence).

Autonomy

The principle of **autonomy** refers to the right of individuals to self-determination. This principle includes the notion of freedom of choice that is so highly valued by all Americans. The right to autonomy allows people to make choices about lifestyle, work, education, and many other issues, such as religion, political affiliation, marriage, and more. Autonomy also includes the right to choose or reject forms of health care treatment. Respecting a patient's right to autonomy means that the physician and other health care workers must enable the patient to make informed choices. For invasive and otherwise risky treatments, health care providers must, therefore, obtain **consent** (agreement or permission) from patients.

Distributive Justice

The principle of **distributive justice** comes from the broader principle of **justice,** which most Americans hold so dear. The principle of justice is founded on the concept of *fairness*. The principle of distributive justice then concerns itself with the fair allocation, or distribution, of scarce resources. This principle is especially relevant in the realm of health care, where resources are always scarce. For example, there is a chronic need for transplantable organs, which raises the difficult question of how fair decisions might be made about who receives a transplant and who does not. Furthermore, such difficult decisions must be made to maximize good (beneficence) for the greatest number of people, while minimizing harm (nonmaleficence) to all.

Paternalism

Paternalism may arise in situations where the ethical principles of autonomy and beneficence are in conflict with one another. In this setting, a dominant "paternal" role is taken by a health care provider, judge, or other person or entity who makes a decision for the good of another person, possibly against that person's wishes. In doing so, the person's right to autonomy is denied. For example, a parent is allowed to give consent for the medical treatment of her child who is a minor, or an adult is the surrogate decision maker for an elderly parent who has been deemed incapable of making her own decisions because of dementia.

Veracity

The principle of **veracity** refers to the quality of truthfulness. This simple principle is generally understood and valued by most individuals, although it is not always an easy one to follow. For example, a physician may need to find a kind but honest way to tell a patient that she has cancer, or the office manager must find a tactful way to talk with an employee about her unacceptable behavior. On the other hand, there may be times when complete honesty is not needed or even appropriate to the situation. Consider the following questions: What should a medical assistant say if a patient asks her for the results of a tissue biopsy? Knowing that such information should only be relayed by the physician, how should the medical assistant respond? What should the medical assistant say when a parent asks about the purpose of her 15-year-old daughter's appointment with a gynecologist? Should the medical assistant's response be any different if the parent happens to be a very good personal friend?

Fidelity

The principle of **fidelity** refers to faithfulness, the duty to keep reasonable promises and meet obligations. An example of reasonable expectations includes the patient's right to expect health care providers to respect privacy and maintain confidentiality. A patient also has the right to expect that health care providers will do what they say they will do (keep promises). For example, if a medical assistant states that a phone call will be made or a message conveyed, then the patient is reasonable in expecting that the medical assistant will carry out these tasks. However, at times patients may have unreasonable expectations. For example, a patient who expects a 100% cure rate with every treatment or medication and becomes angry when results do not meet expectations is not reasonable.

Ethical Philosophies

All people operate from the foundation of one or a combination of ethical philosophies, whether or not they are aware of it. Understanding ethical philosophies and identifying which one feels most "true" helps individuals understand why they view issues as they do and why they may seem unable to understand others who have opposing viewpoints. Understanding ethical philosophies also helps a person understand why she analyzes ethical dilemmas as she does. Two of the most common types of ethical philosophies are deontological and teleological.

Deontological Philosophies

Deontological philosophies operate from the belief that all human beings are of equal worth. This type of philosophy focuses on individual behaviors, rights, and duties. According to deontological philosophies, ethical principles are absolute and exceptions are rarely, if ever, justified. Thus, some actions are considered intrinsically immoral or wrong, regardless of any good or useful consequences that might result from them. For example, a person who believes it is wrong to kill and views that doctrine in a deontological way will not tolerate exceptions to that rule. So, for example, if a person adheres to this doctrine, he may be opposed to capital punishment, military action, and abortion because each of these can be considered a mode of killing. A person with such a deontological view believes that violating the doctrine in any way will cause greater harm to humanity than any immediate harm that may be caused by adhering to it.

On the other hand, some persons may use their deontological perspective to override their usual beliefs about appropriate behavior. For example, they may feel a great obligation to serve their country by joining the military, regardless of their feelings about killing others, or may feel compelled to commit a crime, such as bombing an abortion clinic.

Teleological Philosophies

Teleological philosophies focus more on the consequences of actions, rather than actions themselves. **Utilitarianism** is one of the most common teleological philosophies. The name of this philosophy is taken from the idea of *utility* or *usefulness*. Developed by two English philosophers, Jeremy Bentham and John Stuart Mill, this philosophy interprets the rightness or wrongness of actions according to their consequences. Similar to deontology, utilitarianism also values duty and obligation and regards all human beings of equal value. However, utilitarianism rarely views particular issues or behaviors as strictly right or wrong; rather, it allows for **ambiguity,** or a state of uncertainty or vagueness. This emphasis on the "shades of gray" in a particular issue steers a person to consider the consequences or end result of an action as an integral component in determining its ethical rightness. Examining the end result, then, demands that the needs of many people supersede the needs of a few, and values highly the greater good for humankind as a whole. For example, a person who adheres to utilitarianism may believe that a pregnant woman's right to *autonomy* supersedes whatever rights her unborn fetus may have. For

the legal system to rob the woman of her autonomy, even temporarily, may be viewed by some as a greater harm to her and to society as well, for in this country the right to self-determination (autonomy) is prized above nearly everything else.

Philosophical Divide

No one ethical philosophy is right or wrong. Each person operates from a philosophical foundation consistent with her own religious beliefs, personal values, and life experiences. Individual actions may be supported or rejected by others based on their different philosophical foundation. If two persons are operating from different ethical philosophies, they may never agree on issues as controversial as abortion or capital punishment and will probably never understand one another's viewpoints. Sadly, without such understanding social debate commonly deteriorates into name-calling and other unproductive argumentation.

Learning about ethical philosophies such as utilitarianism and deontology promotes understanding of why people tend to disagree so heatedly about some issues and may further explain why some social debates never see resolution. Regardless of the ethical philosophy used and the specific decisions made, some situations have the potential for profound, long-term consequences.

Anatomy of an Ethical Dilemma

In many cases, what first seems to be an ethical dilemma is really just a situation in which miscommunication has occurred or inadequate information is available. Therefore, the first steps in addressing a potential ethical dilemma are to gather data and seek clarification of all relevant issues. Interested parties must put emotion aside long enough to really communicate and gather the data. When they do so, they are generally able to agree about a course of action. However, if parties are in perpetual disagreement, a true ethical dilemma may exist. How can anyone know for sure? The defining criteria of an ethical dilemma include:

1. A decision must be made.
2. The outcome will have profound consequences.
3. There is disagreement among involved parties about the right course of action.

Ethical Decision Making

In the case of a true ethical dilemma, decision making may be extremely difficult. So how is a reasonable decision finally achieved? Unfortunately, in most cases, a person responds based on emotion and personal beliefs, rather than careful reflection. Sometimes a person's response is based on a previous experience that has little bearing on the current situation. Making such judgments is known as **bias.** Sadly, this type of response commonly leads to conflict.

On the other hand, thoughtful decision making based on a solid understanding of ethical principles and careful reasoning, called the *ethical reasoning process,* will generally lead to consensus among key parties and result in sound decisions. A person must learn this type of decision making; it does not come naturally to most people. When people follow this process, they are able to think their way through a situation systematically, considering all relevant issues and arriving at a thoughtful conclusion. Use of the ethical reasoning process does not guarantee an easy resolution to any problem. However, careful, thoughtful reasoning supports decision makers in making the best decision possible under difficult circumstances. (See *Ethical reasoning process.*)

Ethics Committee

An ethics committee serves several functions within a health care organization and the larger community. Such a committee usually helps formulate institutional policies and provides education for health care staff and, possibly,

---

Ethical reasoning process

There are many systems that employ an ethical reasoning process to analyze ethical dilemmas. Here are the most common features included in most of them:

- *Identify and clarify the problem(s).* Putting the problem(s) in writing is commonly helpful.

- *Gather all relevant data.* Avoiding tunnel vision in gathering data will enable the inclusion of data that may initially seem unimportant but may actually be relevant.

- *Identify issues in conflict.* Beginning with the examination of differing opinions and views may help as well as identifying relevant ethical principles and personal bias.

- *Brainstorm.* Allow a free flow of ideas without making judgments about whether ideas are valuable.

- *Identify the most promising choices.* Narrow down the options from brainstorming to the most reasonable courses of action and examine the potential consequences of each.

- *Negotiate or recommend a final course of action.* Determine a course that maximizes benefit and minimizes harm.

- *Evaluate.* Consider the value of the final outcome as well as the effectiveness of the overall problem-solving process.

---

community members. Such education can aid staff members in putting aside personal bias in order to support clients and families most effectively as they navigate difficult situations. An ethics committee serves a consultative role as well. For example, disagreement between family members and health care providers on decisions regarding patient care is common. A member of an ethics committee may act as a guide for interested parties and help them through the decision-making process. Alternatively, the entire committee may meet to conduct a more formal analysis of a case. Recommendations from the committee are not legally binding but can be helpful to staff who are in conflict and to family members who are paralyzed by confusion, grief, or guilt.

Ethics and the Medical Professional

A solid understanding of health care ethics can help a medical assistant in several ways. It can help her identify and clarify her own personal values, behave in a manner consistent with the values of her profession, and respond to situations in the medical office in a thoughtful, consistent manner.

Code of Ethics

All health care providers, including medical assistants, must demonstrate behavior that is legal and ethical. The medical assistant should have an understanding of ethical principles and be familiar with codes of ethics that pertain to her profession. The AAMA has adopted a code of ethics that embodies the core values agreed upon by the members of the profession and sets the standards for personal and professional conduct. Not surprisingly, the AAMA Code of Ethics and the related Medical Assistant's Creed share themes that are consistent with the American Medical Association code of ethics. (See *AAMA Code of Ethics and Medical Assistant's Creed.*)

Ethical Behavior in the Medical Office

Medical assistants are obligated to behave professionally and ethically in the medical office. They must act and respond to all situations in a manner consistent with their own professional code of ethics and with the expectations of their employer. A medical assistant will fulfill this obligation easily if she takes the time to clarify her own values and seeks understanding regarding health care ethics. (See *Ethical conflicts.*) Issues of importance in the clinical setting are the same as those touched on in the AAMA Code of Ethics, including trust and loyalty, confidentiality, respect and dignity, and commitment to professional development.

AAMA Code of Ethics and Medical Assistant's Creed

The American Association of Medical Assistants (AAMA) Code of Ethics and Medical Assistant's Creed* touch on themes of service, trust, loyalty, confidentiality, respect for others, desire to benefit others, and commitment to professional development.

AAMA Code of Ethics

The Code of Ethics of AAMA shall set forth principles of ethical and moral conduct as they relate to the medical profession and the particular practice of medical assisting.

Members of AAMA dedicated to the conscientious pursuit of their profession, and thus desiring to merit the high regard of the entire medical profession and the respect of the general public which they do serve, do pledge themselves to strive always to:

A. Render service with full respect for the dignity of humanity.

B. Respect confidential information obtained through employment unless legally authorized or required by responsible performance of duty to divulge such information.

C. Uphold the honor and high principles of the profession and accept its disciplines.

D. Seek to continually improve the knowledge and skills of medical assistants for the benefit of patients and professional colleagues; participate in service activities aimed toward improving the health and well-being of the community.

Medical Assistant's Creed

The AAMA Medical Assistant's Creed reads:

- I believe in the principles and purposes of the profession of medical assisting.
- I endeavor to be more effective.
- I aspire to render greater service.
- I protect the confidence entrusted to me.
- I am dedicated to the care and well-being of all people.
- I am loyal to my employer.
- I am true to the ethics of my profession.
- I am strengthened by compassion, courage, and faith.

*Copyright by the American Association of Medical Assistants, Inc. Used with permission.

Ethical conflicts

Clinical or administrative medical assistants are obligated to provide education and information to patients as directed by their employer on a wide range of subjects. If a medical assistant has religious, moral, or ethical beliefs that prohibit her from providing information about contraception, pregnancy termination, blood transfusion, or other subjects, she should inform her potential employer during the job interview process. Failing to do so is a form of dishonesty and may eventually prove a hardship to the medical assistant's coworkers, who may need to cover for her.

Trust and Loyalty

A person rarely grants another trust automatically. Usually, a person earns the trust of another through behaving in a trustworthy manner, such as by demonstrating loyalty and commitment to high-quality work. A medical assistant should seek to earn the trust of her employer and the physicians and others with whom she works as well as her patients. A medical assistant who is dependable in attendance, punctuality, and work effort as well as respectful in her behavior toward others will quickly earn the trust of most people. Further trust is developed as a medical assistant demonstrates that she can be trusted with sensitive information and increasing responsibility.

Confidentiality

The importance of confidentiality in health care is a common theme, because a medical assistant has no more important duty than to protect her patient's privacy, keeping all information confidential. When tempted to share personal health care information about a patient with another party, a medical assistant must always ask herself these questions first:

- Is this party a health care professional directly involved in this patient's care?
- Has legal documentation been provided that grants this party legal access to this information?
- How would the patient feel about me sharing this information with this party?
- Will my sharing of this information benefit or harm this patient?
- If I were in this patient's shoes, how would I feel about my personal health information being shared in this way and with this party?

Respect and Dignity

Few persons would argue against being treated with respect and dignity, and most would agree that treating others with respect and dignity is desirable. Why, then, does disrespectful behavior seem to be so prevalent? Because humans are emotional beings, they commonly act and react based on how they are feeling at the moment without carefully considering the potential ramifications of their actions. As a result, their words may be poorly chosen, their behaviors may be interpreted by others as offensive, and the emotions they are feeling may cause them to communicate in an overly aggressive manner.

A medical assistant may feel that her patients, coworkers, or even the physicians and supervisors, on occasion, treat her disrespectfully. She may even be tempted to respond in kind. However, the truly professional medical assistant does not let such events influence her behavior. A medical assistant is never justified in treating a patient or member of the health care team in a disrespectful manner, regardless of how that person behaves. Even so, if the medical assistant really believes her coworker's behavior was out of line, she should find an appropriate time and place to discuss the issue privately with her coworker. She can let her coworker know that she found that person's words or behavior to be unprofessional and unacceptable. She should then suggest an alternative way in which the person might convey the message in the future. The medical assistant must behave tactfully and professionally throughout the conversation to set an example of professionalism and decrease the risk of causing the person to react defensively.

Commitment to Professional Development

A hallmark of a true professional is the commitment to lifelong learning. Nowhere is this commitment more important than in the health care field, where the knowledge base changes rapidly, seemingly on a daily basis. A medical assistant must make a commitment to continue her education in some fashion for the duration of her career. Opportunities for continued education are numerous. For example, a medical assistant committed to professional development can attend in-house educational offerings at work; take formal college classes; attend regional, state, or national medical assistant conferences; read medical assistant and other health care journals; and study topics of interest on her own.

Chapter Summary

- Morals and ethics are based on values regarding human conduct. Morals are deeply held personal beliefs about what constitutes right or wrong behavior. Ethics involve thoughtful analysis and evaluate human behavior in light of specific ethical principles and look at the impact of such behavior on individuals and society as a whole.

- Although a behavior may be deemed unethical by some individuals, it is not necessarily illegal. Conversely, a behavior that has been designated as illegal is not necessarily considered unethical by all.

- Bioethics is a specialized branch of ethics that concerns itself with human behavior within the context of modern medicine. The number and variety of situations that confront health care providers are limitless. Therefore, health care providers should become educated and be prepared with information and tools that can help them navigate these difficult waters and provide better guidance to their patients.

- Ethical principles are rules about how people ought to behave. Common ethical principles include nonmaleficence, beneficence, autonomy, distributive justice, paternalism, veracity, and fidelity.

- Understanding ethical philosophies and identifying which one feels most "true" to them helps individuals understand why they view issues as they do and why they may seem unable to understand others who have opposing viewpoints. The two key ethical philosophies include deontology and utilitarianism. Knowledge of these philosophies helps promote understanding about why people tend to disagree so heatedly about some issues and may further explain why some social debates seem never to be resolved.

- The defining criteria of an ethical dilemma include the need for a decision, an outcome with profound consequence, and disagreement among interested parties.

- In the case of a true ethical dilemma, decision making may be extremely difficult. However, thoughtful decision making based on a solid understanding of ethical principles and careful reasoning will generally lead to consensus among key parties and result in sound decisions.

- The ethical reasoning process includes problem clarification, data gathering, identification of relevant ethical principles, brainstorming, identification of options, negotiation of a course of action, and evaluation.

- An ethics committee serves as a resource within the health care organization and the larger community. It helps formulate institutional policies, provides education, and may serve as a consultant when a difficult decision must be made.

- A solid understanding of health care ethics can help a medical assistant identify and clarify her own personal values, behave in a manner consistent with the values of her profession, and respond to situations in the medical office in a thoughtful, consistent manner.

- All health care providers, including medical assistants, must demonstrate behavior that is legal and ethical. The medical assistant should have an understanding of ethical principles and be familiar with codes of ethics that pertain to her profession.

- The AAMA Code of Ethics and Medical Assistant's Creed include themes of service, trust, loyalty, confidentiality, respect for others, desire to benefit others, and commitment to professional development.
- Medical assistants must demonstrate the qualities of trust, loyalty, confidentiality, respect and dignity, and commitment to professional development.

Team Work Exercises

1. Divide into teams of three to five students. Read the following scenario with the members of your team. Then discuss the ethical issues involved, according to the guidelines that follow the scenario.

   Madge is an 82-year-old African American female who lies in a coma on life support. She was admitted to the hospital two weeks ago after falling, hitting her head, and suffering a severe intracranial bleed. Initially, her family urged health care providers to do everything possible to keep Madge alive. They stressed that she had recently been living independently in her own home and was an avid gardener. They were hopeful that she could return to a similar quality of life. After many tests and procedures and minimal improvement in Madge's' condition, the family now faces a heart-wrenching decision. Should they continue to push for aggressive care, knowing that the prognosis is poor yet hoping for the chance of a miracle? Or should they make the difficult decision to withdraw all aggressive forms of care, provide comfort measures only, and "allow nature to take its course"?
   a. Discuss this scenario and reach a consensus among team members about what recommendation you think should be made in this case.
   b. Now picture in place of Madge your own mother or child. Does the choice still seem as simple? Discuss your thoughts and feelings with your teammates.
   c. Now consider the same scenario with the following changes:
      - Madge is now a 4-year-old, blond-haired, blue-eyed little girl.
      - Madge is now a 32-year-old Asian American widowed nurse with four young children at home.
      - Madge is now a 57-year-old Native American woman who is an alcoholic, has no family, and is on public assistance.
      - Madge is now Miguel, a 33-year-old, unmarried Mexican American man who does seasonal work.
      - Madge is now Michael, a 45-year-old white male who is a stockbroker with good insurance and a wife and two teenagers at home.
      - Madge is now Marvin, a 33-year-old artist who has been diagnosed with HIV and is openly gay.
   d. The purpose of changing the patients in this scenario is to help you notice any potential biases you may have. While it may be easy to agree in theory that all humans are of equal worth and deserve equal treatment, we may, in fact, react differently based on personal values, beliefs, and biases when faced with each situation. We commonly don't even realize our biases until confronted with such a scenario. Does your opinion about the "right" decision change in any of these scenarios? Discuss your thoughts with your teammates.

2. Divide into teams of three to five students. Over the course of the next week, watch a medical movie or television show, making note of any ethical dilemmas that are presented. Then get together with your team to describe your findings. Describe the situation presented in the movie or show and identify the ethical principles you believe were upheld or violated and why.

Case Studies

1. A coworker has come to you for advice. She feels that some of the comments that one of the physicians has made to her are demeaning and rude. She didn't say anything at the time because there were other people around, including a patient. However, this has been bothering her and she cannot seem to let it go. What advice do you have to offer her?

2. A coworker comments one day that she just noticed in her patient's chart a comment about a history of four pregnancy terminations. She is angry that this patient "obviously has such low respect for human life." She is further frustrated that "hardworking people like us have to pay for these welfare patients to clean up their mistakes." You are concerned that you coworker is making such comments about a patient and wonder if she is jumping to some possibly inaccurate conclusions. What is most concerning about this person's comments? What assumptions does she seem to be making? How will you respond to her?

Resources

- *The American Journal of Bioethics: www.bioethics.net*
- Bioethics news and issues: *www.bioethics.com*
- Ethical guidelines for conducting research on human subjects at the National Institutes of Health, Office of Human Subjects Research: *www.nihtraining.com/ohsrsite/index.html*

Patient Education

Learning Objectives

Upon completion of this chapter, the student will be able to:

- define key terms
- describe the medical assistant's role in patient education
- compare and contrast the three domains of learning
- list teaching methods that appeal to each of the learning domains
- describe a plan for assessing the learning needs of a patient
- differentiate between short- and long-term learning objectives
- describe the role of self-efficacy in motivating behavior changes
- create a plan to increase a patient's feelings of self-efficacy
- describe the stages of grief and loss according to theorist Elizabeth Kubler-Ross
- list at least ten potential barriers to effective patient education and a possible solution to each
- discuss age-related teaching considerations and list appropriate teaching methods for patients of various ages
- describe three different teaching strategies that might be used for patient education
- list at least five different teaching tools along with considerations for each
- describe a plan for evaluating medical literature to determine its appropriateness for patient education
- discuss two methods of evaluating patient learning
- create a tool to document patient education
- discuss the patient medical record as a legal document.

CAAHEP Competencies

General Competencies

Professional Communications

Recognize and respond to verbal communications

Recognize and respond to nonverbal communications

Patient Instruction

Instruct individuals according to their needs

Provide instruction for health maintenance and disease prevention

ABHES Competencies

Communication

Adaptation for individualized needs

Legal Concepts

Use appropriate guidelines when releasing records or information

Follow established policy in initiating or terminating medical treatment

Instruction

Instruct patients with special needs

Teach patients methods of health promotion and disease prevention

Chapter Outline

Medical Assistant's Role in Patient Education

Learning Styles

Learning Domains
  Cognitive Domain
  Affective Domain
  Psychomotor Domain

Assessing Learning Needs

Identifying Learning Objectives

Organizing the Teaching Session

Motivation to Learn
  Locus of Control
  Self-Efficacy

Barriers to Effective Patient Education
  Emotional Response to Illness and Disability
  Physical and Personal Barriers to Learning

Age-Related Teaching Considerations

Teaching Strategies
  Verbal Lecture
  Conversational
  Group

Patient Education Literature

Evaluation of Learning

Legal Implications of Patient Education

Chapter Summary

Team Work Exercises

Case Studies

Resources

Key Terms

acceptance
Stage of grief and loss when a person acknowledges the reality and permanence of life changes

affective domain
Thought processes involving emotions, values, and attitudes

anger
Stage of grief and loss when a person experiences feelings of rage

bargaining
Stage of grief and loss when a person makes irrational attempts to negotiate for unlikely or impossible changes

cognitive domain
Thought processes that involve the intellect and include thinking on several levels

compliance
Patient's adherence to the plan of care as instructed by the health care provider

denial
Stage of grief and loss when a person refuses to accept the reality of a situation

empathy
Understanding of the emotions and thoughts of another

jargon
Technical, specialized language used by professionals that is generally confusing to other people

learning domains
Modes of learning conducted by different parts of the brain

learning objectives
Goals or outcomes to be achieved in the learning process

locus of control
Person's belief about the degree of control that he has over events in his life

psychomotor domain
Processes that involve physical activity and the senses (sight, sound, touch, smell, and taste)

resolution
Stage of grief and loss when a person expresses emotions more freely and begins to identify changes in life caused by the loss

self-efficacy
Person's perception of how capable and confident he feels about being able to make a specified change or accomplish a goal

Medical Assistant's Role in Patient Education

As important players on the health care team, medical assistants should collaborate with physicians, nurses, and others in the provision of patient education. Because time and resources are usually limited, the medical assistant may find it a challenge to provide good quality teaching. To make the most of the time available, the medical assistant should view every patient contact as an opportunity for some type of teaching. Receptionists might provide literature on appropriate topics for patients to read while they are waiting. Nurses and medical assistants can provide teaching and encouragement that reinforce the physician's instructions. Other members of the health care team, such as therapists and dietitians, can provide focused teaching in their areas of expertise that is consistent with identified goals. If everyone makes the most of every available teaching moment, patients will receive comprehensive education in a manner that also conveys the message that the health care team is cohesive and unified in their approach. (See *Handy literature*.)

Learning Styles

Patient education is most effective when teaching methods are adapted to a patient's individual learning style. (See Chapter 1, "Succeeding as a Student," on page 3 for more information on learning styles.) When possible, a medical assistant should ask the patient how he prefers to learn. Some patients will not know and children will probably not even know what the term *learning style* means. An adult may or may not know his learning style, but the medical assistant can ask about prior experiences with learning and the patient's preferred studying

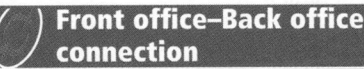

Front office–Back office connection

Handy Literature

Administrative and clinical medical assistants should make sure that an assortment of patient teaching literature is available in any areas where patients will be waiting. The administrative medical assistant can make sure that literature racks in the reception area remain fully stocked with appropriate literature. The clinical medical assistant should make sure that appropriate educational literature is available in examination and treatment rooms. Doing so provides patients with multiple opportunities to access this information and read through it while they are waiting to be seen.

method to determine his style. When the medical assistant is unsure of a patient's learning style, she should use methods that address multiple styles. She should also ask the patient about learning or sensory disabilities so she can modify teaching tools and methods appropriately.

Learning Domains

A medical assistant will be most effective in helping patients learn if she has a general understanding of the learning process. An important first step is to learn about the **learning domains**. Learning domains are the different parts of the brain that are involved in the learning process. Understanding them can help the medical assistant modify her instruction to appeal to these domains. There are three learning domains:

- cognitive
- affective
- psychomotor. (See Figure 9-1.)

Cognitive Domain

The **cognitive domain** involves the intellect and includes thinking on several levels. The lowest level involves simple memorization and data recall. Other levels involve understanding, meaningful application to new situations, sorting trivial details from significant ones, and determining the overall value of an idea or concept. Teaching strategies that utilize the cognitive domain include lecture, active discussion,

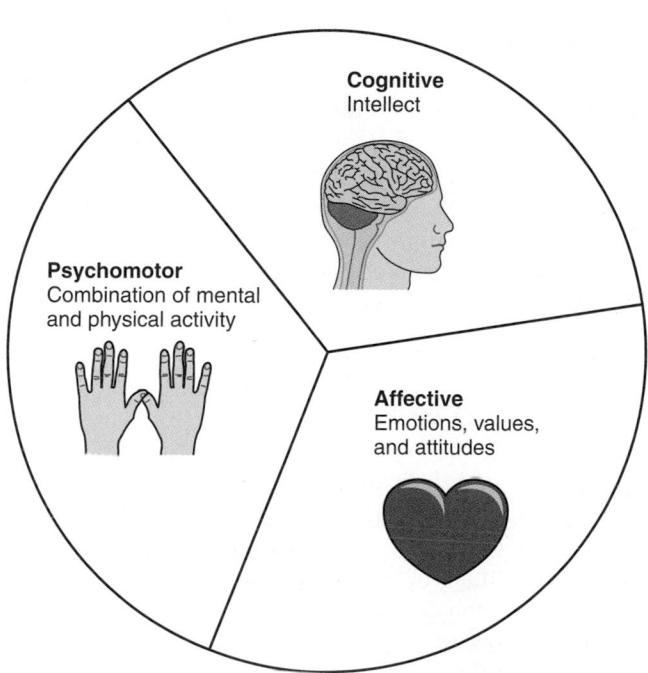

FIG 9-1 Three learning domains.

role playing, and independent projects. These activities utilize all levels of cognitive function in a way that permits a patient to raise and address her own concerns, learn from others, and participate in active problem solving.

Affective Domain

The **affective domain** involves emotions, values, and attitudes. This domain enables a person to listen and pay attention to what others have to say and to become actively engaged in conversation by responding verbally and behaviorally. The affective domain enables a person to choose behaviors based on her value system. Teaching methods that utilize the affective domain include discussion and role playing with a focus on feelings, beliefs, and values. Private one-on-one discussion is appropriate for personal issues. Group discussion allows group members to exchange ideas, learn from the experiences of others, and feel supported by them.

Psychomotor Domain

The **psychomotor domain** enables a person to learn skills that require a combination of mental and physical activity. A person uses the sense of sight, sound, touch, smell, and even taste as she learns by manipulating physical objects. Performance of new skills under the guidance of instructors increases the person's confidence in her abilities. Further practice allows the beginner to move from minimal competence to a higher degree of proficiency. As the person becomes more skilled and confident, she is able to adapt when unexpected problems occur. The most effective teaching strategies for the psychomotor domain include demonstration, practice, and return demonstration. Most people learn best by first watching the teacher demonstrate the behavior or skill. Doing so allows them to see the steps from start to finish. They can then perform skills with instructor guidance to obtain coaching and feedback in a safe, structured setting. After sufficient practice, a person can then perform a demonstration of the skills she has mastered. Demonstration is the most accurate and effective means of evaluating that learning has occurred. (See *Skill demonstration tips*, page 98.)

Assessing Learning Needs

One of the most common mistakes that health care providers make when delivering patient education is failing to assess the patient's learning needs. In an effort to quickly check patient education off the "to-do" list, many health care providers quickly recite a brief set of verbal instructions and believe that they have done a good job of teaching. In fact, this type of teaching commonly leaves patients thinking "What did she just say?" or "I already knew all of that." In

Patient Education

Skill Demonstration Tips

When the medical assistant is demonstrating a new skill to a patient, she should follow these steps:

- Assemble the supplies and equipment.
- Ensure adequate lighting and privacy.
- Review the purpose and rationale with the patient.
- Perform the steps of the skill in the same sequence that the patient must perform them.
- Explain the key rationale for each step without overanalyzing.
- Adapt the speed, timing, and techniques to the patient's abilities.
- Allow time for questions.
- Guide the patient as she performs and practices the skill.

either case, the teaching session was probably much less effective than the teacher thought.

To be an effective teacher, a health care provider should first take time to talk with the patient, ask questions, and *listen* to determine the patient's current level of knowledge and understanding about the issue at hand. Doing so provides opportunities to correct misinformation or misunderstandings and lets the provider know where to begin in the process of providing new information. It also allows the provider to begin identifying the patient's concerns and potential barriers to learning or **compliance**. Compliance is the patient's adherence to the plan of care as instructed by the health care provider and is a key goal in good patient education. Other goals throughout the assessment and teaching process include identifying the patient's resources. Examples of resources include finances, insurance, living situation, and help from family or friends. Appropriate referrals may be necessary if significant lack of resources is identified.

Identifying Learning Objectives

Learning objectives identify goals or outcomes to be achieved and help guide the teaching session. The medical assistant should invite the patient to participate in and contribute to goal setting. Doing so will help the medical assistant understand the issues of greatest concern to the patient and help the patient feel included. Short-term learning objectives address immediate survival needs—for example, ensuring that a newly diagnosed diabetic patient knows how to use a glucometer to check his blood glucose levels. Long-term learning objectives focus on knowledge and skills that a patient may need to adapt to permanent health changes and achieve optimal health and well-being over the long term. An example of long-term learning objectives would be teaching the diabetic patient how to perform daily examination of his feet and how to care for his skin in order to prevent complications of wound infection that could lead to amputation. Learning objectives should be clear and measurable so that the medical assistant and the patient can identify when they have been accomplished. Furthermore, learning objectives must be realistic so that the medical assistant and patient can feel confident about the chances of success. Finally, learning objectives should be stated in terms of what the patient will accomplish, not what the medical assistant will do.

Organizing the Teaching Session

Experienced teachers know that effective learning rarely happens by accident. Careful thought and preparation are necessary. The medical assistant must be clear about the purpose and goal of the teaching session. The session is where the time invested in assessing learning needs and determining learning objectives pays off. When the medical assistant determines the content of the session, she should create an outline to organize the session into a logical sequence, progressing from simple to complex subjects. She can reinforce learning by repeating key points throughout the teaching session and then summarizing all key points again at the end.

To hold the patient's attention, the medical assistant should infuse energy into the session by varying vocal tone and using culturally appropriate eye contact and gestures. She should engage the patient in the conversation as fully as possible. She might accomplish this task by inviting the patient to ask questions, having him repeat key steps or key points, and having him employ as many senses as possible. She should address all learning domains.

Motivation to Learn

While knowledge is helpful in motivating people to make health changes, knowledge alone is not typically enough. If it were, then nearly everyone would achieve and maintain an optimal weight, participate in regular exercise, eat a healthy diet, never use tobacco or drink to excess, and manage stress effectively. However, many people simply are not motivated enough to make lifestyle changes based on information alone, and no amount of lecturing will change the situation.

Such people are commonly labeled *noncompliant.* However, health care providers who find themselves feeling frustrated or angry with such patients should remember that they themselves are rarely 100% compliant in their own recommended health care activities.

In reality, virtually everyone could be labeled as non-compliant at one time or another. Therefore, health care providers should remember that such labeling may be unfair to a patient who desires to make changes but who may feel powerless to do so. The health care provider's job is to help the patient identify barriers that hinder success and support him in getting the results that he, the patient, wants. In general, a patient can identify barriers, because most people have tried and failed to make health changes in the past. Instead of arguing with the patient, the provider might create a list of obstacles as a starting point. When the patient identifies obstacles, the discussion can center around identifying potential solutions. Some obstacles, such as lack of money or inability to drive, may be very real. However, they can also usually be resolved through identification of community resources or encouraging the patient to utilize his own personal support system. The most effective approach involves gentle prompting by the provider to enable the patient to identify solutions. In many cases, the true obstacles to patient success in making lasting lifestyle changes is the locus of control and a struggle with feelings of low self-efficacy.

Locus of Control

Locus of control describes a person's beliefs about the degree of control (or lack of control) that he has over events in his life. A person who believes that everything that happens to him is up to fate, chance, luck, God, or another external source is said to have an *external* locus of control. On the other hand, a person who believes that he is in control of the events in his life and that his destiny is largely up to him is said to have an internal locus of control. Of course, many people believe in a mix of the two. Even so, studies have shown that, in general, people whose locus of control is more internal than external are more goal-oriented and get higher-paying jobs. They are more likely to devote the study and work necessary to get ahead and earn promotions because they believe their efforts will pay off. People who believe their success is up to fate or some other external power are less likely to see the value of such efforts.

Understanding the concept of locus of control helps health care providers better understand patients. Patients with an internal locus of control are more likely to "take charge" of their health and demonstrate willingness to invest time and effort into self-care activities because they believe they can alter their own destiny. On the other hand, those with an external locus tend to be more fatalistic and are less

likely to adopt lifestyle changes or alter their self-care practices. Those with an external locus also tend to feel more helpless and victimized by God, fate, luck, or even their medication or their health care provider.

Health care providers who attempt to influence these life-long beliefs and patterns will find themselves up against a challenge. The development of locus of control happens over a lifetime but is most influenced during the early formative years. Such influences include family, culture, religion, and life experiences. Efforts to influence patients are best aimed at education combined with activities that help foster the patient's feelings of self efficacy.

Self-Efficacy

An important factor that determines how likely patients are to successfully institute behavior changes is their feeling of **self-efficacy**. Self-efficacy is a patient's perception of his capability to make changes and his confidence in his ability to do so. A number of factors impact a patient's feelings of self-efficacy, such as self-esteem and past experiences with success and failure. Helping increase patient's self-efficacy is the key to helping them make changes. A medical assistant can do a number of things to help boost a patient's feelings of self-efficacy:

- Identify and address the patient's beliefs and concerns regarding health issues and needed changes.
- Determine the patient's definitions of health, exercise, healthy eating, or whatever the key issues are.
- Prompt the patient to identify small steps that he feels sure he can successfully make now. Success with small steps leads to increased feelings of confidence and increased self-efficacy. Future steps will feel easier.
- Encourage realistic short-term and long-term goals. Losing 50 pounds in 1 month is not realistic or healthy. On the other hand, a short-term goal of losing 5 pounds each month for a total of 50 pounds over the next 10 to 12 months is realistic and healthy.
- Focus on permanent changes toward a healthier life, rather than quick fixes that have little chance of lasting.
- Help the patient understand the *whys.* Most people become more enthusiastic about making changes once they truly understand how and why they are beneficial.
- Ask the patient to identify his own reasons for making changes. For example, the medical assistant might ask a patient, "What do *you* think the value is in taking your blood pressure medicine every day?" Notice that this question is not a closed question that permits a "yes" or "no" response. The patient will feel obligated to think of a response. If he happens to say, "I don't know," then a good follow-up questions is, "If you *did* know an

answer, what would it be?" This sounds like a silly question but it is amazingly effective. When a patient identifies the value himself, he is more likely to "buy in" to the plan.

- Design a plan that is flexible yet specific. For example, the patient with a hectic schedule may need to vary the days and times that she exercises. A specific goal may be to exercise a minimum of three times each week by briskly walking for 20 minutes.
- Put the plan into writing and make sure that the patient and health care provider keep a copy. Be sure the patient has made a verbal commitment to the plan.
- Suggest adding new healthy behaviors to the patient's life before eliminating unhealthy ones. For example, many people fail at weight loss because they eliminate food, thus feeling deprived, without bothering to increase physical activity. Success is more likely if exercise is added first with a gradual change in eating patterns to follow. As people begin to experience positive results from exercise, many find they feel more motivated to eat a healthy diet.
- Work new behaviors into the existing routine. Most people do not want to make drastic lifestyle changes. Review the patient's normal daily routine and help her identify where the new behavior will fit. Perhaps she watches a favorite television show each evening and could watch it while walking on a treadmill rather than sitting in her recliner.
- Express concern and caring. A persuasive statement from a professional medical assistant can be influential. For example, the medical assistant might say, "I am concerned about you. Your blood pressure and cholesterol levels have been pretty high. I would very much like to see you bring them both down so that you can be healthier, feel better, and live to see your grandchildren grow up."
- Employ the shotgun approach to teaching by using a variety of strategies and tools to teach and encourage.
- Consult with physicians about appropriate referrals for professional consultation. Examples include registered dietitians, diabetic educators, physical therapists, and psychologists. (See *Total team approach*.)
- Refer the patient to support groups when appropriate where he can meet other people who are dealing with similar issues.
- Monitor the patient's progress through future office visits or even by calling him at home. A patient is much more likely to stick with behavior changes when he knows that the health care provider is interested in him enough to follow up. (See *Key interventions for self-efficacy*.) Small successes build self-efficacy, which leads to permanent changes. (See Figure 9-2.)

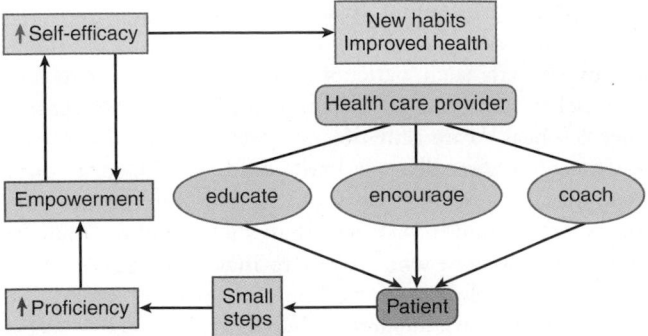

FIG 9-2 Path to self-efficacy.

Front office–Back office connection

Total Team Approach

For the most effective patient education, all members of the office staff should get involved using the total team approach. Although everyone in the office is busy and no one has a lot of time, everyone can do something to create a positive impact on patient education. The staff should consider creating a committee with representatives from all areas of expertise (physicians, nurses, administrative and clinical medical assistants, and so on) to brainstorm about what each member of the team can do to contribute to effective patient education. They can then create a plan agreeable to all so that everyone knows his or her role.

Patient Education

Key Interventions for Self-Efficacy

Here are the most essential, or key, interventions for increasing a patient's feelings of self-efficacy:

- Invite her to identify her own learning goals.
- Start with small realistic steps that she believes are achievable.
- Link new behaviors to old.
- Ask her for a commitment.
- Connect her to a support person or support group.
- Identify a plan for follow-up and let her know that the provider will be monitoring her progress.
- Express confidence in her ability to succeed.

Barriers to Effective Patient Education

Most patients want to make positive changes in their lives, including changes in their health practices. However, they commonly encounter barriers that impede their ability to do so. To help patients make needed changes, medical assistants must do more than simply dispense information. They must help patients identify barriers and move beyond them. Examples of common barriers include emotions, such as denial and anger; sensory deficits, such as hearing loss; or physical issues, such as pain or decreased mobility.

Emotional Response to Illness and Disability

Many people respond to permanent health loss in a manner similar to the way they respond to other significant losses in their lives. Typical stages of grief and loss as identified by researcher Elizabeth Kubler-Ross include denial, anger, bargaining, resolution, and acceptance. Such a grief reaction is normal and, to a certain extent, even healthy. However, effective patient education may be hindered while patients are in the early stages of grief and may not be possible for patients who get permanently stuck in the grief process.

The medical assistant should evaluate the patient for signs of grieving and note which stage the patient is in. The medical assistant must understand that the stages of grief are fluid, meaning that a patient may fluctuate between stages and even exhibit signs of multiple stages at once. However, over time, the patient should progress to the point of acceptance. The medical assistant can help the patient by noting where the patient is in this process and modifying educational methods accordingly.

A patient who is experiencing the initial stage of **denial** refuses to accept the reality of the changes in his life, health, or situation. He may appear withdrawn and refuse to discuss the health issue. He tends to misunderstand and distort information or ignore it completely. The medical assistant should respond with **empathy**, which means that she is able to understand and identify with the patient's feelings. She should also be available to answer questions. Her attempts to teach the patient should include simple, careful explanations that focus on the present. The medical assistant's explanations to family or friends should be aimed at helping them understand the impact of the grieving process on their loved one.

As a patient begins to progress though the stages of grief, he may feel and express **anger**, which is rage that masks the pain and grief hiding behind it. Initially, it manifests in the form of emotional outbursts and statements of blame directed at others. The medical assistant must not take such expressions personally or argue with the patient. Rather, she should respond with empathetic listening. She should also offer reassurance to family members and significant others with an explanation that such a response is normal.

Bargaining is an irrational attempt to negotiate for unlikely or impossible changes. As the patient displays signs of the bargaining stage, he may offer to make behavior changes in exchange for a promise of better health. The medical assistant must take care not to offer false reassurance in these situations. She should emphasize the reality of the present situation and encourage setting realistic short-term goals. For example, a patient with metastatic lung cancer most likely has a poor long-term prognosis. Therefore, the medical assistant should not promise a remission of the cancer or make guesses at life expectancy. However, after consulting with the physician and nursing staff, it may be realistic for the medical assistant to encourage the patient to plan to attend an upcoming family reunion or grandchild's birthday party.

Many patients will enter a period of depression as they face the inevitability of their health loss. During this time, the patient may exhibit typical depressive symptoms, such as fatigue, apathy, loss of interest in usual activities, and insomnia. He may not feel the interest or energy required to learn or make behavior changes. The medical assistant should provide empathetic support and acknowledge the patient's feelings as normal, while gently reminding him that he may not feel this way indefinitely. In cases of severe depression, the physician may wish to prescribe antidepressant medications or refer the patient for psychological counseling.

As the patient enters the **resolution** phase of the grieving process, he expresses emotions more freely and begins to identify the changes caused by the health loss. As this happens, the medical assistant may acknowledge and validate the patient's feelings and begin to share information needed for the near future. **Acceptance** is the stage in which the patient acknowledges the reality and permanence of the changes and begins to actively move forward. More formal teaching sessions may be scheduled as the patient expresses acceptance of the health change and displays more interest in learning. Patients are commonly motivated by a desire for an optimal degree of independence and normalcy in their daily lives. At that point, the medical assistant may focus on information and skills the patient will need in the short- and long-term future. (See Figure 9-3.)

Physical and Personal Barriers to Learning

A number of physical and personal barriers may hinder effective patient education. Some issues of physical discomfort, such as heat, cold, or pain may be modifiable. The medical assistant should address those issues before attempting

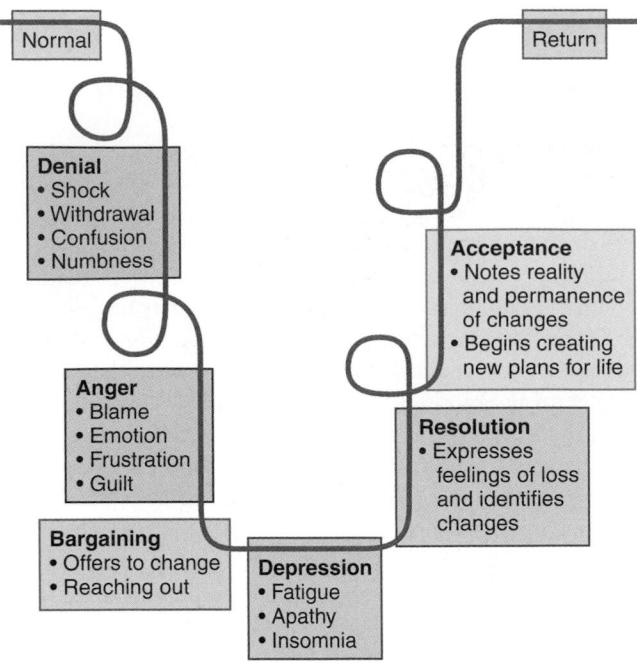

FIG 9-3 Stages of grief and loss.

Age-Related Teaching Considerations

Teaching methods and tools should be appropriate for the age of the patient. A child's ability to learn depends on his developmental maturity. A young child needs information presented in a more concrete manner. Therefore, the use of tangible objects that appeal to the senses will be the most effective. As a child gets older, the medical assistant can present information in a more abstract, less tangible manner, based on concepts that involve thoughts, feelings, and creative components, rather than concrete narration or pictures.

Most teenagers have an aversion to being "lectured to" but enjoy working on computers. Therefore, they are the ideal candidates for programmed computer instruction. This form of instruction involves sequential presentation, interaction, feedback, and correction and allows learners to work at their own pace. In addition, teenagers and adults usually enjoy teaching that includes the use of audiovisual technology, such as CDs, television, or videos. These tools are also useful for patients with reading comprehension or illiteracy problems or those with sensory deficits.

The medical assistant should ask an adult patient to identify his own learning needs based on the issues he wishes to address. The medical assistant should respond to such issues first. This approach not only helps to resolve concerns that will distract the patient from other learning but also lets the patient know that the medical assistant genuinely cares about his needs and concerns. Depending on a patient's learning style, he may find visual data in the form of diagrams, graphs, pictures, or illustrations to be helpful. The

patient education. Other issues may be less readily solved; however, the medical assistant can add modifications in the teaching plan to address those issues. For example, a patient has limited energy and tires easily. The administrative medical assistant might schedule the patient's appointment for early in the day, when the patient's energy level is at its highest, to avoid impacting the patient's ability to learn. (See *Common barriers to learning*.)

Common barriers to learning

This table lists common barriers to learning along with potential solutions the medical assistant and other office staff may employ to address them.

Barriers	Solutions
Physical or environmental • Room is too hot, cold, or drafty • Environmental noise • Poor lighting • Uncomfortable seating • Poorly arranged furnishings	• Ask the patient about comfort issues and adjust the thermostat if necessary. Open or close windows. • Adjust lighting. • Take measures to minimize background noise.
Patient limitations • Pain • Low energy, fatigue • Decreased strength	• Medicate for pain or anxiety per the physician's order or encourage the patient to take her own medications as appropriate.* • Adjust seating for the patient's comfort. • Limit the length of teaching sessions according to the patient's tolerance.

Common barriers to learning—cont'd

Barriers	Solutions
• Impaired mobility • Impaired coordination or agility • Impaired memory • Dementia • Anxiety	• End the teaching session or allow a rest period when the patient displays signs of fatigue or loss of concentration (poor eye contact or slumped posture). • Schedule teaching for a time when the patient's energy is greatest (such as early in the day). • Schedule several short sessions, rather than one long one. • Help the patient problem-solve physical barrier issues (such as stairs). • Use an unhurried approach. • Provide frequent encouragement and reassurance. • Include family or significant others in the teaching session (if appropriate and the patient agrees). • Write lists or instructions for the patient to take with her. • Use multiple strategies that appeal to as many senses as possible. • Refer the patient, as appropriate, for specialized information or counseling.
Illiteracy (functional illiteracy is defined as reading comprehension below fifth-grade level)	• Avoid slang or medical language. • Use simple language. • Provide material written at fourth-grade level or below. • Read instructions to the patient.
Sensory deficit: Diminished hearing or deafness	• Face the patient so he can see lips and facial expressions. • Speak at an adequate volume for the patient to hear but do not shout. • Speak in a clear, unhurried manner using a low tone of voice. (Elderly patients commonly have difficulty hearing high-pitched vocal tones.) • Use visual aids, including illustrations and pictures. • Employ a sign language interpreter if appropriate.
Sensory deficit: Poor vision or blindness	• Speak clearly but do not shout. (Poor vision does not equal deafness.) • Use large-print materials for the patient with poor vision. • Announce your presence when entering the room and introduce yourself. • Evaluate the color use on visual teaching aids if the patient is color-blind.
Language and cultural barriers	• Avoid stereotyping. • Collaborate with health care providers of other cultures and languages to learn from them. • Consider communications patterns, time perception, and gender roles. • Adapt the teaching approach to the patient's religious or cultural beliefs, as appropriate. • Employ an interpreter, if appropriate. • Use a courteous, formal approach, addressing the patient by his last name. • Use culturally appropriate eye contact, touch, and gestures. • Use visual aids, including illustrations and pictures. • Monitor the patient's facial expression and body language for signs of confusion. • Use simple language and wording. • Demonstrate procedures and have the patient do a return demonstration to ensure learning. • Provide written instructions in the patient's primary language.
Lack of privacy	• Close doors or install insulated screens to minimize noise and ensure privacy. • Avoid discussing confidential information within the hearing of others.
Lack of time	• Focus on the immediate "survival" needs first. • Use the team approach, including all members of health care team as appropriate. • Provide prehospital education prior to hospital admission (for elective procedures). • Integrate teaching with medical care.

* Note that some medications may cause sedation or otherwise impair the patient's ability to learn and remember new information.

medical assistant can use such visual aids to help show relationships between numbers and concepts, summarize and clarify key concepts, and help learners grasp information quickly. Throughout the teaching process, the medical assistant should invite the adult patient to collaborate in identifying goals, topics, and strategies. (See *Age-appropriate teaching strategies.*)

Teaching Strategies

There are three main teaching strategies, or formats, that a medical assistant can employ when providing patient education:

- verbal lecture
- conversational
- group.

Verbal Lecture

The verbal lecture format is efficient for giving instructions. The medical assistant may use this format when time is limited and the subject matter is simple. For example, a medical assistant tells a patient to take her antibiotic capsules three times each day with a full glass of water until all the capsules are gone. This format does not encourage discussion but does allow patients to ask questions and seek clarification if needed. This format is more effective if the medical assistant also gives the patient

Age-appropriate teaching strategies

This table lists age appropriate teaching strategies and the tools needed to employ them.

Patient Age	Strategies	Tools
Infant	• Consistency • Secure handling • Soft, soothing voice • Smile • Make eye contact	N/A
Toddler and preschooler	• Play allowing the patient to touch equipment, such as a stethoscope, before using it on him • Provide a toy stethoscope and let the patient listen to a doll's heart or even yours • Role playing	• Pictures • Books • Blocks • Dolls • Toys
School-age child	• Simple explanations • Question and answer • Demonstration	• Age-appropriate books • Pamphlets • Videos • Toys
Teen to middle-age adult	• Allowing choice • Inviting collaboration and expression of feelings • Providing information	• Age appropriate books • Pamphlets • Videos • Computer-aided instruction
Older adult	• Allowing choice • Inviting collaboration • Teaching when the patient is rested and mentally alert • Limiting the length of teaching sessions • Focusing on realistic goals of optimal strength and independence • Adapting strategies to sensory deficits	• Books (considering use of large-print materials for those with poor vision) • Pamphlets • Videos

instructions or important information in writing. Simple instructions for taking her pill three times a day could be quickly put into writing. In addition, most medical offices keep a variety of pamphlets, brochures, and booklets on hand that cover various topics of concern for their patient population. Giving these to the patient affords her the opportunity to review the information as many times as necessary after she leaves the office.

Conversational

A conversational approach encourages the patient to participate and collaborate. It also fosters an environment in which the patient feels comfortable asking questions and giving feedback. Such an approach is useful for helping the patient understand a new diagnosis and take ownership of a treatment plan that he has helped design.

As the patient becomes more knowledgeable about his health care issue, the medical assistant should encourage him to take more responsibility for managing his own self-care. The medical assistant helps the nurses and physicians in monitoring the patient's progress and should be available for consultation. Her role is to clarify information for the patient and reinforce positive behaviors.

Group

The group format can be effective for some teaching situations. It allows discussion and brain storming and encourages general interaction. Patients often find emotional support in such groups when they realize that they are not alone in dealing with their health issue. Effective group process requires a trained leader who is able to facilitate group discussion and guide the group in a positive and productive direction. (See *Analogy and role play*.)

Patient Education Literature

The medical assistant should evaluate the patient education literature used in the medical office for currency, accuracy, clarity, and appropriate reading level. Research indicates that most literature currently used in health care is above the reading level of most patients. It is recommended that all literature be written below the sixth-grade level. Some sources recommend that it be at fourth-grade level or lower. Medical assistants should avoid using medical terms and **jargon**, or the technical specialized language of medicine, or translate it into common language to avoid confusing patients.

 Patient Education

Analogy and Role Play
When providing patient education, the medical assistant will find the use of analogy and role play valuable.

Analogy
An analogy is a comparison between two partially similar things. It can be used to translate a complex idea into a simpler, more easily understood concept that the patient can understand. However, the medical assistant should be familiar with the patient's background, experience, and culture to select an appropriate analogy. Examples of analogies that may be useful include the following:

- The heart is like a pump.
- An aneurysm is like an inner tube with a weak, bulging spot.
- Blood flowing through veins and arteries is like water flowing through pipes.
- Skin is like a rubber band, it loses elasticity with age and exposure to sunlight.
- Having an asthma attack feels like trying to breathe through a straw.

- Insulin is like a tiny key that must unlock tissue cells before glucose can enter.

Role play
Role play allows the patient to try out actions, words, and responses to see what works best for him. It gives the patient a chance to consider and practice the most effective means of coping with difficult situations and allows the patient and medical assistant to evaluate the session and try out other variations. Examples of role play that might benefit the patient are:

- The medical assistant pretends to be one of a diabetic teenager's friends and teases him about his dietary practices and insulin use. This scenario gives the teen the chance to think about and practice different responses.

- The medical assistant pretends to be a pushy friend or relative who keeps trying to get the patient to overeat or to drink too much alcohol. The patient tries out different responses.

Literature should also be available in other languages and have reputable Internet sites listed for patients who wish to do further research on their own.

Evaluation of Learning

Health care providers commonly make assumptions about patient learning without taking the time to determine if patients really understand specific information or if they are capable of performing certain skills. The medical assistant should always conduct some type of evaluation to determine whether the patient has really achieved the desired learning goals. Evaluation also provides useful feedback about the effectiveness of teaching methods. Furthermore, it provides opportunities to reinforce key points and clarify areas of confusion. Including a tool, such as a checklist, in the patient's chart allows various members of the health care team to keep track of what subjects have been covered and what they still must address. It also provides a simple way to track evaluation of learning or skills.

Return demonstration performed by the patient is the best method of verifying whether the patient is truly able to perform skills, such as administering their own insulin or using a metered dose inhaler, accurately and safely. (See Figure 9-4.)

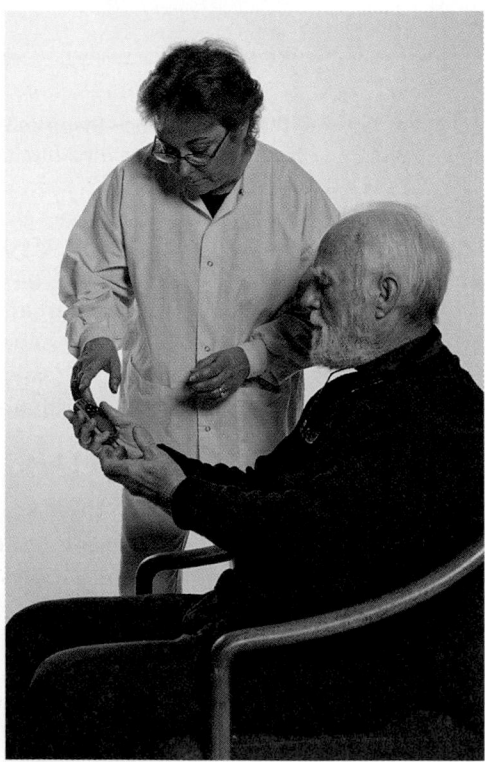

FIG 9-4 Return demonstration.

To evaluate other forms of learning, the medical assistant may ask the patient to describe or summarize key concepts. The medical assistant may also administer more formal tools, such as simple posttests or questionnaires. She can send such tools home with the patient to help him remember how to perform the skill. She can also file such aids in the patient's chart to document learning. In addition, she may ask the patient to provide a self-report in the form of a simple journal.

Legal Implications of Patient Education

Patient education is important for a number of reasons. First and foremost, patients are entitled to information about their health and to understand any issues related to their condition. In addition, the medical record also serves as a legal record. Therefore, documentation about patient education must be thorough, accurate, and timely.

The old saying "not charted, not done" applies to patient education as well. Because medical records are legal documents, from a legal perspective, any care or education that goes undocumented never occurred. Attorneys or insurance personnel may review medical records years after care was provided. After that length of time, it is unlikely that anyone involved in a patient's care would remember any of the details. Therefore, the medical record must speak for itself. It is not unusual for litigation to hinge on whether a patient was adequately informed about his diagnosis, prognosis, treatment, medications, or other aspects of care. Therefore, the medical assistant must carefully document all patient education.

Chapter Summary
- As important members of the health care team, medical assistants should collaborate with physicians, nurses, and others in the provision of patient education.
- Patient education is most effective when the medical assistant adapts her teaching methods to the patient's individual learning style. When the medical assistant is unsure of a patient's learning style, she should address multiple styles.
- The medical assistant should ask the patient about learning or sensory disabilities so that she can modify teaching tools and methods appropriately.
- Medical assistants will be most effective in helping patients learn if they have a general understanding of the learning domains, including cognitive (intellect), affective

(emotions, values, and attitudes), and psychomotor (senses of sight, sound, touch, smell, and taste).

- The medical assistant should assess the patient to determine what his learning needs are before beginning teaching.
- Learning objectives identify goals or outcomes to be achieved and help guide the teaching session. The medical assistant should invite the patient to participate and contribute to goal setting. Learning objectives should involve short-term and long-term goals.
- The medical assistant must be clear about the purpose and goal of the teaching session. The medical assistant should create an outline to organize the session into a logical sequence that progresses from simple to complex subjects.
- The medical assistant should infuse energy into the session by varying vocal tone and using culturally appropriate eye contact and gestures.
- While knowledge is helpful in motivating people to make health changes, knowledge alone is commonly not enough. The medical assistant should help the patient identify barriers that hinder his success and support him in getting results.
- Self-efficacy is an important factor in determining patient success in instituting changes.
- Many people respond to permanent health loss in a manner similar to how they respond to other significant losses in their lives. Typical stages of grief and loss include denial, anger, bargaining, resolution, and acceptance.
- The medical assistant should evaluate the patient for signs of grieving and note which stage he is in. It is important to understand that the stages of grief are fluid, meaning that patients may fluctuate between stages and even exhibit signs of multiple stages all at once.
- A number of physical and personal obstacles may hinder effective patient education. Some issues of physical discomfort may be heat, cold, or pain. The medical assistant should address those issues before attempting patient education. Other issues may be less readily solved; however, the medical assistant can add modifications in the teaching plan to address those issues.
- A child's ability to learn depends on his developmental maturity. A young child needs information presented in a more concrete manner. As a child gets older, the medical assistant can present information in a more abstract manner.
- Teaching strategies for conveying information include the verbal lecture format, conversational approach, and group format.
- As a patient becomes more knowledgeable about his health care issue, the medical assistant should encourage him to take more responsibility for managing his own self-care. The medical assistant helps the nurses and physicians in monitoring the patient's progress and should

be available for consultation. Her role is to clarify information for the patient and reinforce positive behaviors.

- The medical assistant should evaluate patient education literature used in the medical office for currency, accuracy, clarity, and appropriate reading level. It is recommended that all literature be written below the sixth-grade level. Some sources recommend that it be at fourth-grade level or lower. Medical assistants should avoid using medical terms and jargon or translate it into common language to avoid confusing patients.
- The medical assistant should always conduct some type of evaluation to determine whether the patient has met established outcomes. Evaluation also provides useful feedback about the effectiveness of teaching methods. Furthermore, it provides opportunities to reinforce key points and clarify areas of confusion.
- Return demonstration performed by the patient is the best method of verifying whether patients are truly able to perform skills, such as administering their own insulin or using a metered dose inhaler, accurately and safely.
- Patient education is important because patients are entitled to information about their health and to understand any issues related to their condition. In addition, the medical record also serves as a legal record. Therefore, documentation about patient education must be thorough, accurate, and timely.

Team Work Exercises

1. Divide into teams of three to five students. Visit one or more medical offices in your area. Identify all of the places where patient education literature is kept, and collect at least five samples of patient education literature. Evaluate this literature for target audience, attractiveness and creativity, and reading level. Report your findings to the class.
2. Divide into teams of three to five students. Select one of the following patients and role-play a teaching session where you utilize age-appropriate teaching strategies that appeal to all three learning domains. Incorporate at least one age-appropriate analogy into your teaching session.
   a. 5-year-old child; teach him about why hand washing will help him keep from getting sick.
   b. 11-year-old; teach her about why it is important to wear a seatbelt in the car and a helmet when riding her bicycle.
   c. 16-year-old; teach her about safe, effective use of oral contraceptives.
   d. 45-year-old; teach him about lifestyle modifications to reduce his risk of cardiovascular disease.
   e. 65-year-old; teach her about smoking cessation.
   f. 75-year-old; teach him about how to care for the surgical incision on his arm and how to prevent infection.

Case Studies

1. Anthelia is a clinical medical assistant who works in an allergy clinic. The physician has asked her to teach a 17-year-old boy how to administer his own injection of epinephrine, which comes in his emergency "bee sting kit." Describe the approach that Anthelia should take. Include:
   a. learning domains
   b. assessment of learning needs
   c. identification of learning objectives
   d. how to organize the teaching session
   e. motivation to learn
   f. identification of potential barriers
   g. specific age-appropriate teaching strategies
   h. evaluation of learning.
2. Kaelee is a medical assistant who works in an internal medicine clinic. She has been asked to teach a 61-year-old man who has recently had his left foot amputated due to complications of a diabetic foot ulcer about lifestyle modifications to reduce his blood pressure. He seems fatigued and apathetic. Describe how Kaelee might design one or more teaching sessions with this patient. Discuss the following:
   a. potential barriers to learning and how they can be overcome
   b. self-efficacy issues
   c. age-appropriate teaching strategies
   d. how teaching sessions will be organized
   e. evaluation of learning.

Resources

- Extensive list of medical analogies: *www.altoonafp.org/analogies.htm*
- Five stages of grief and loss: *www.davidkessler.org/items-of-interest/5-stages-of-grief*
- Patient education information: *www.medicalcenter.osu.edu/patientcare/patient_education*
- Printable patient education information: *www.familydoctor.org*

UNIT II

Administrative

The Office Environment

Learning Objectives

Upon completion of this chapter, the student will be able to:

- define the key terms presented in the glossary
- describe an inviting and comfortable reception area
- discuss how the facility environment can help ensure patient privacy
- discuss office compliance with the Americans with Disabilities Act
- list at least five items to include in an office to make patients feel comfortable and at ease
- describe the personality characteristics of an effective receptionist
- discuss strategies for managing unexpected delays that cause patients to wait for long periods of time in the reception area

CAAHEP Competencies

General Competencies
Professional Communications
  Recognize and respond to nonverbal communications
Legal Concepts
  Identify and respond to issues of confidentiality
Patient Instruction
  Explain general office policies

Instruct individuals according to their needs
Provide instruction for health maintenance and disease prevention
Identify community resources

ABHES Competencies

Professionalism
  Project a positive attitude
  Maintain confidentiality at all times
  Be cognizant of ethical boundaries
  Project a responsible attitude
  Be courteous and diplomatic
Communication
  Be attentive, listen, and learn
  Be impartial and show empathy when dealing with patients
  Adapt what is said to the recipient's level of comprehension
  Use appropriate medical terminology
  Recognize and respond to verbal and nonverbal communication
  Use correct grammar, spelling, and formatting techniques in written works
  Observe principles of verbal and nonverbal communication

Chapter Outline

Welcoming New Patients
  Americans with Disabilities Act
Office Design
  Privacy
  Workflow
  Ergonomics

Reception Area
  Managing Office Space
  Lighting
  Colors
  Reading Materials
  Music
  Cleanliness
Educational Resources
  Marketing Materials
Office Safety
  Other Precautions
Chapter Summary
Team Work Exercises
Case Studies
Resources

Key Terms

accessibility
Degree of a person's ability to gain entrance to a facility when using a wheelchair or other assistive device

asepsis
State of cleanliness that is free from disease-causing microorganisms

disability
Deficiency, especially physical, that prevents or restricts normal performance

ergonomics
Science of equipment or workplace design that aims to minimize operator fatigue

marketing
Process of letting customers or potential customers know of a product or service

productivity
Extent of a person's ability to perform a job function

repetitive motion injury
Physical injury caused by a specific repeated motion

workflow
Physical space that facilitates accomplishment of work-related duties

Welcoming New Patients

When a patient enters the physician's office for the first time, the impression of the office surroundings and staff can welcome or alienate the new patient. A warm, professional, pleasant reception staff and environment will welcome a patient and inspire confidence in patients about the care they will receive. An office staff's **productivity**, or their ability to perform their job duties efficiently and effectively, will continue that first impression of capability and patients will feel encouraged to stay with the practice.

Americans with Disabilities Act
The design of a clinic, physician's office, or hospital must be functional and easy to maintain. In addition, it must be in compliance with the Americans with Disabilities Act (ADA). A **disability**, which is a physical or mental impairment that may limit an individual's access to or use of facilities, must be considered. The ADA is legislation passed in 1990 to ensure the rights of persons with disabilities in many areas. It provides enforceable standards to ensure **accessibility** and prohibit discrimination in employment, public services, transportation, public accommodation, communications, and other areas. ADA regulations insist that all persons be able to enter and use the facility, regardless of their physical limitations. Doorways must be wide enough to accommodate wheelchairs, ramps must be available, and bathrooms must be designed so that sinks and toilets are accessible to all. Ensuring easy access to the office and examination rooms for such patients will promote ease of use and establish a workflow that increases overall productivity.

Office Design

The layout or design of the office can promote comfort and ease of use for staff, physicians, and patients. A new building or one that was originally designed as a physician's office lends itself better to easy delineation of work areas, reception areas, and treatment rooms than a building that was once a bank or retail store. However, with proper planning, a design team or even medical office personnel can create an appropriate environment for a medical practice from any space.

Privacy
Clinical and office staff need areas in which to convey private, personal information to patients. An office design that includes adequate space between the reception window and seating area ensures that conversations are not overheard by other patients. The medical assistant at the reception window should be able to receive insurance cards and co-payments,

answer billing questions, and make follow-up appointments without disturbing patients or other office staff. Computer screens should face only the office staff and not be visible to patients at the reception window. When speaking on the phone, the reception staff should shut the privacy window so that patients in the waiting room do not hear the exchange. Conversation in the reception area should be limited. The medical assistant should call the patient into the examination room by name and wait to ask medical questions until the patient is in the treatment room.

When a patient reaches the examination or treatment room, privacy is vital. A patient is commonly naked under a paper gown and feels vulnerable. Closing doors for privacy and knocking before entering show the patient that he is respected and his dignity is important to the staff. Having a mirror and a hook or hanger in the examination room for patients to hang clothing are thoughtful touches.

A physician will commonly speak to a patient in an office after the examination. Doing so allows the patient to be fully clothed and discuss treatment options with the physician across a desk, rather than in a paper gown on an examination table.

Workflow

The office environment that is designed to allow easy access to work materials and enough space for all workers to perform their tasks greatly increases work productivity. Adequate **workflow** is achieved by providing enough physical space for employees to perform job duties. Office and clinical staff must have access to telephones and areas to unpack newly ordered items and place patient charts for later filing. Workflow is disrupted when there is inadequate space for one or more staff members or if staff fail to return materials to their proper location due to insufficient space. If a staff member cannot answer the phone because too many patient files are on the desk, that staff member cannot do her job. The office staff should always keep the work area neat and

orderly with a place for all items when not in use. In addition, equipment and supplies that are not properly stored present a danger if fire exits are blocked or staff members need to step over items in a hallway. Also, the unorganized office appears unprofessional and does not inspire patients' confidence.

The office with a successful workflow will ensure that each work station is located in an area from which the person working there can easily access the items needed to perform that job. For example, reception staff should be able to answer telephones, retrieve patient charts, create new patient charts, and use the computer and copier without having to run around the office. Clinical staff should be able to retrieve examination and treatment items in close, secure storage areas, rather than in a hallway outside of the office where clinical staff would have to walk through the reception area to retrieve items. (See Figure 10-1.)

The expansion of a practice, hiring more medical assistants or physicians, may disrupt workflow. The office manager will need to reevaluate storage options and work stations. Staff members feeling cramped and disrupted workflow decrease overall productivity. Anything that decreases productivity can lead to frustration.

Ergonomics

Ergonomically designed equipment and work spaces prevent injury, reduce fatigue, and promote productivity. **Ergonomics** ensure that equipment and work spaces fit the needs of individuals. For example, chairs should fit the height of the user, and desks, computers, and files should be accessible with comfort. To reduce eyestrain, staff should position the computer screen in an area where glare is minimal. The height of desks and computer tables should allow workers to sit straight with elbows bent on the desk or table. Poorly designed work spaces cause employees to move into awkward positions. If the employee must constantly move into uncomfortable positions, a repetitive motion injury can

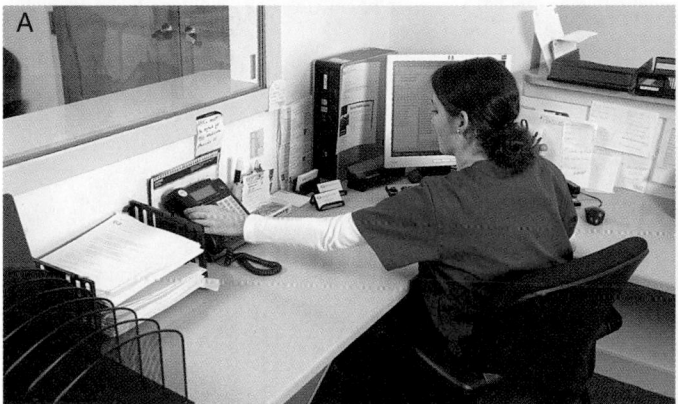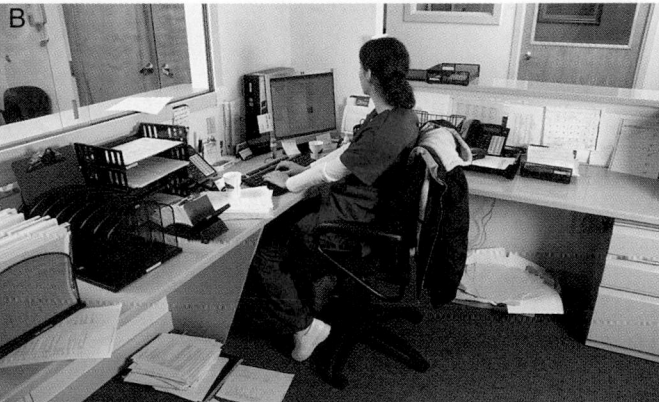

FIG 10-1 Successful workflow practices. (A) Successful workflow. (B) Insufficient work space.

occur. **Repetitive motion injuries** are injuries sustained from constant repeated strain on muscles. For example, a table that is too high will cause wrist strain, such as carpal tunnel syndrome; a table that is too low will cause the worker to look down and can cause neck strain. (See Figure 10-2.)

Because staff members in physicians' offices and hospitals commonly retrieve and file many medical reports and other records, step stools for upper shelves should be available. For safety, step stools should have rubber tips. If step stools have rollers, they should have locks for added safety. Employees should never improvise using a chair, bucket, or other object to reach high shelves.

Equipment used frequently for clinical purposes should be stored in accessible areas; physicians and medical assistants should be able to comfortably and privately interview patients in examination rooms.

Reception Area

A patient enters a medical office through the reception area. While it is commonly referred to as a *waiting room,* waiting should be minimized as much as possible. Proper scheduling can prevent lengthy waiting. (See Chapter 12, "Appointment Scheduling," on page 133.) Because the reception area is the first room that a new patient will see, it should be inviting and comfortable. Seating should be

comfortable and adequate for the size of the practice. There should be enough seats for all people and enough space between the seats that patients feel comfortable and have their own space. (See Figure 10-3.) Chairs can also be arranged into groups so that people entering with family members or friends can sit together. Chairs should be supportive and easy to get in and out of. Chairs that are too low may be difficult for elderly patients or patients with lower back problems. Dividing the reception room into two separate areas for healthy people and those who may be sick with a communicable illness is also a way to show consideration to patients. (See *Sick child area.*)

Managing Office Space

Having enough chairs in the reception area and enough examination rooms to accommodate the physician's schedule is only beneficial if employees can manage the flow of patients, physicians, and employees within the space. Medical assistants must be able to keep the flow of patients steady and avoid crowding in high-use areas. For example, having patients check in and then enter a hallway to treatment rooms where a scale is located in the hallway can help medical assistants take height and weight measurements prior to showing the patient into the examination room. To avoid crowding in high-traffic areas, the office design can include a separate exit in a hallway opposite the entrance for patients coming out of

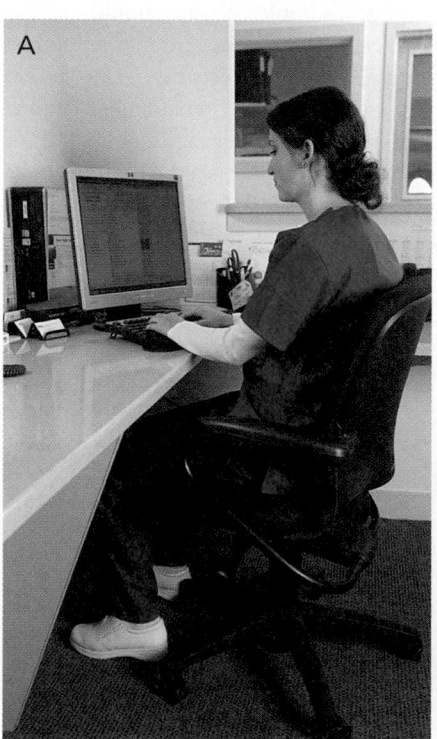
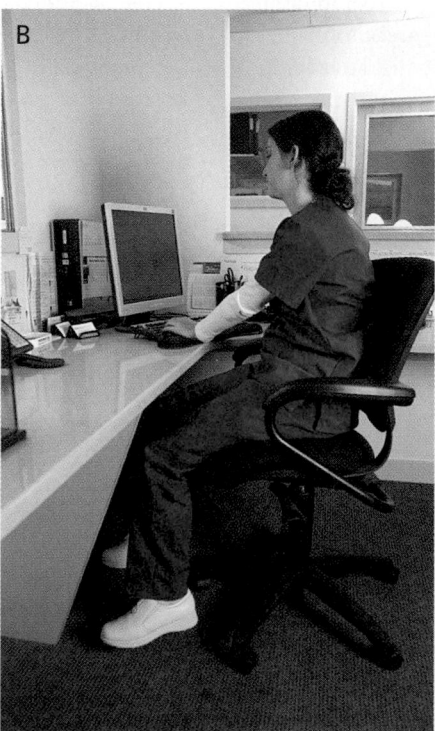
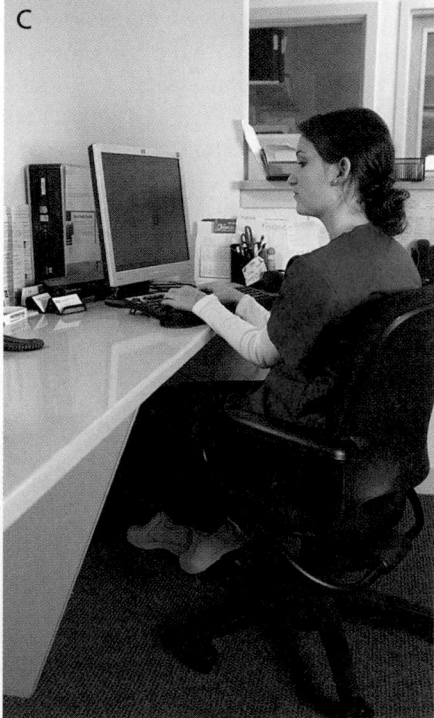

FIG 10-2 Proper and improper ergonomics. (A) Desk at proper height. (B) Desk set too high. (C) Desk set too low.

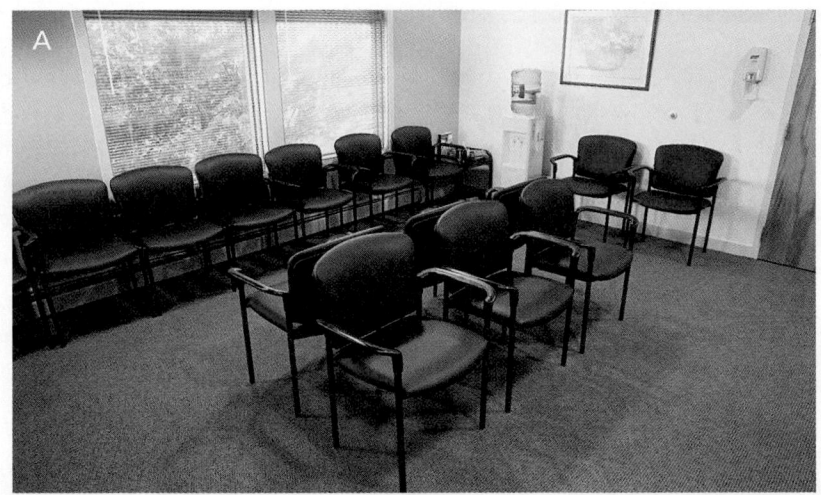

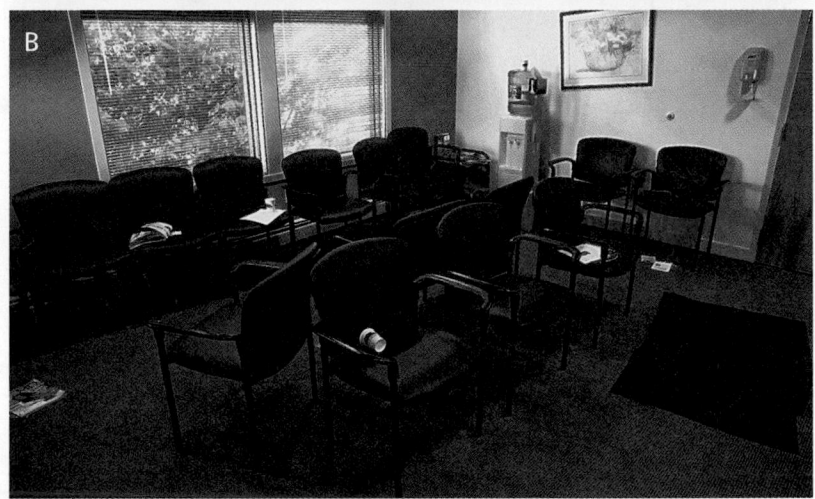

FIG 10-3 Acceptable and unacceptable reception areas. (A) Acceptable area that is spacious and clean with comfortable furniture and good lighting. (B) Unacceptable area that is poorly lit, crowded, and dirty.

Front office–Back office connection

Sick Child Area

Pediatric offices commonly have a separate waiting area for sick children. These children may be contagious and are usually uninterested in playing with toys. A comfortable couch where a caregiver can hold a sick child away from healthy, noisy children is appreciated. Be sure to keep tissues and a wastebasket in the area in case a child becomes ill in the waiting area.

The administrative medical assistant should advise the clinical medical assistant that sick children are in the sick child waiting area. The two medical assistants should work together to get such children into treatment rooms quickly to prevent further exposure of healthy children to pathogens in the waiting area.

the examination rooms. This hallway can also include a station for scheduling future appointments. Because checking in and out are on opposite sides of the front desk, patients aren't backing up in the hallway creating a bottleneck. (See Figure 10-4.) In addition to providing a flow of patients entering and exiting the treatment areas, medical assistants must be able to act quickly if a patient in the reception area needs immediate attention. If all examination rooms are filled, an emergency patient can be seated in an office or the laboratory if the medical assistant determines that the patient should not be left alone. A patient who arrives at the office in acute distress must be attended to immediately. (See Chapter 47, "Office Emergencies," page 967.)

Lighting

Since patients may read in the reception area, lighting should be bright but not glaring. High illumination in the

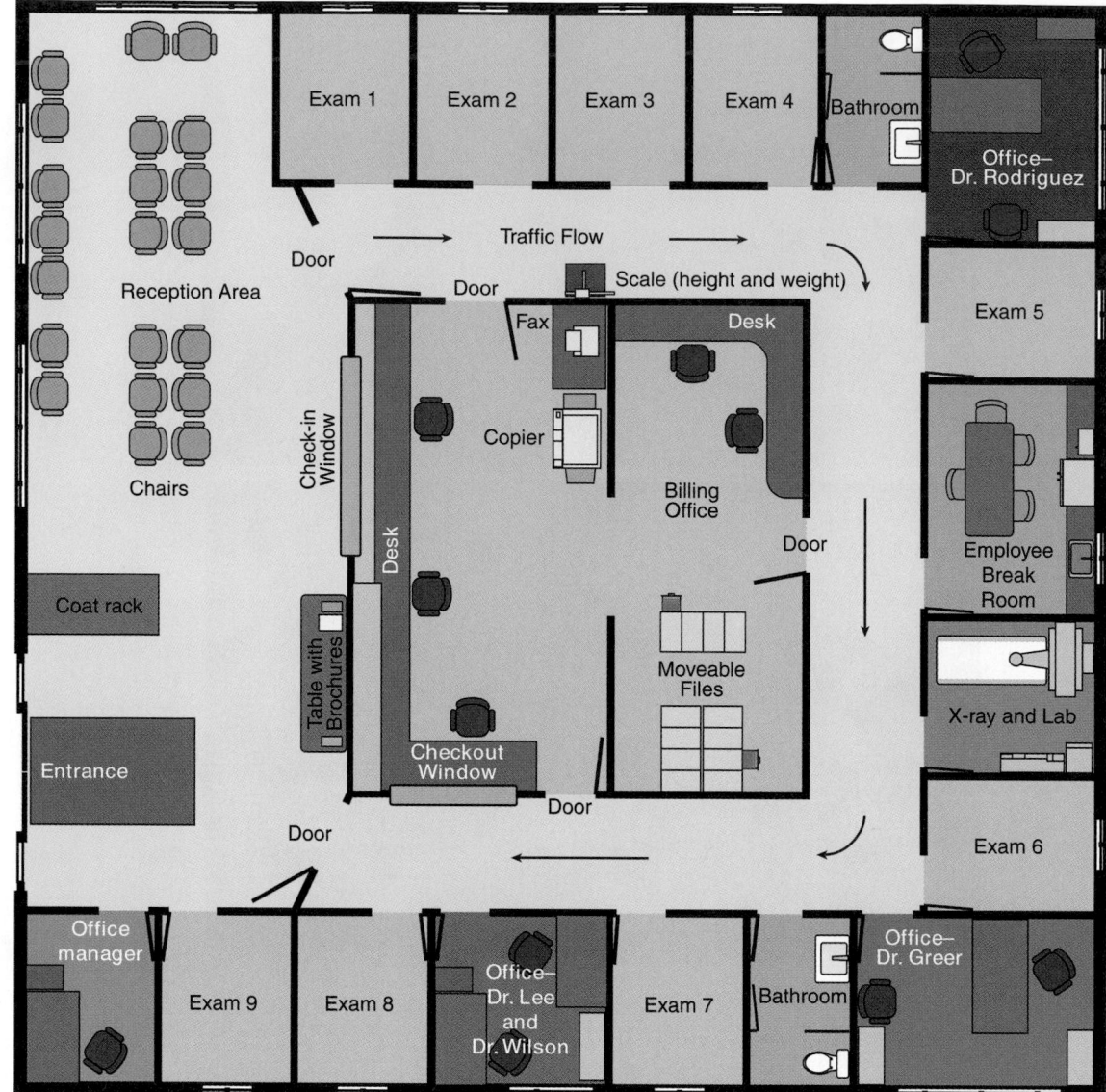

FIG 10-4 Diagram of a medical office designed for efficiency and optimal flow.

form of ceiling lights makes the room appear larger and inviting. Low lighting from table lamps can be added for extra light near chairs but should be used in conjunction with ceiling lights. (See Figure 10-5.)

Colors

Neutral tones are a better choice than bright colors in a reception area or examination room. Colors that are too bold or bright might seem aggressive and make patients feel ill at ease. Off-white or cream is a better choice than bright white, and paint should be a flat finish rather than a glossy finish to avoid glare. Colors can match or coordinate with chairs, paint, and carpet. Framed artwork, such as paintings and posters, can complement the furniture and overall look of the room. When updating the paint, carpeting, or furniture of a reception room, the office manager or designer should ask, "Would I feel comfortable sitting or reading in this room?" Although flowers and plants are generally an attractive addition to a room, the office manager or designer should be careful to choose plants that are nontoxic and not common allergens. Silk flowers and plants are a safer choice; however, even these need dusting and regular maintenance.

Reading Materials

The office manager or other staff member should make a variety of reading materials available for patients and remove

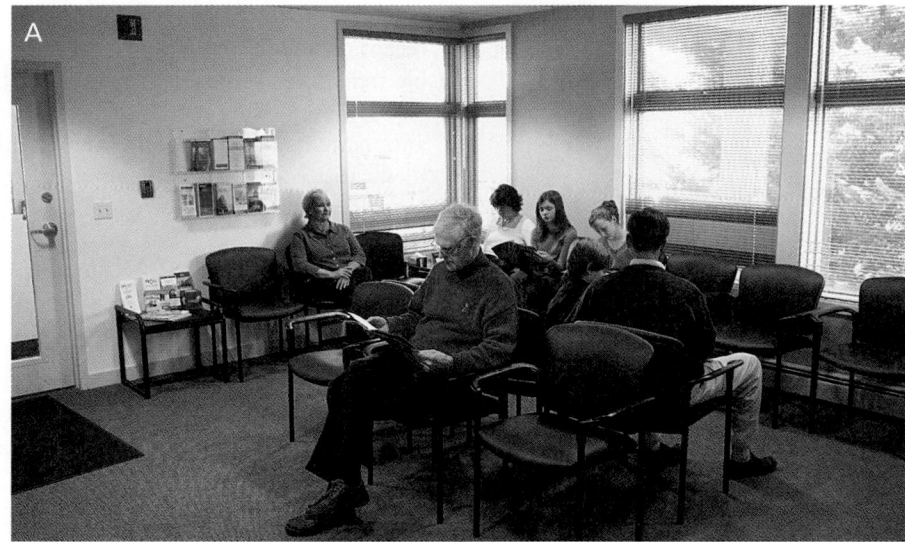

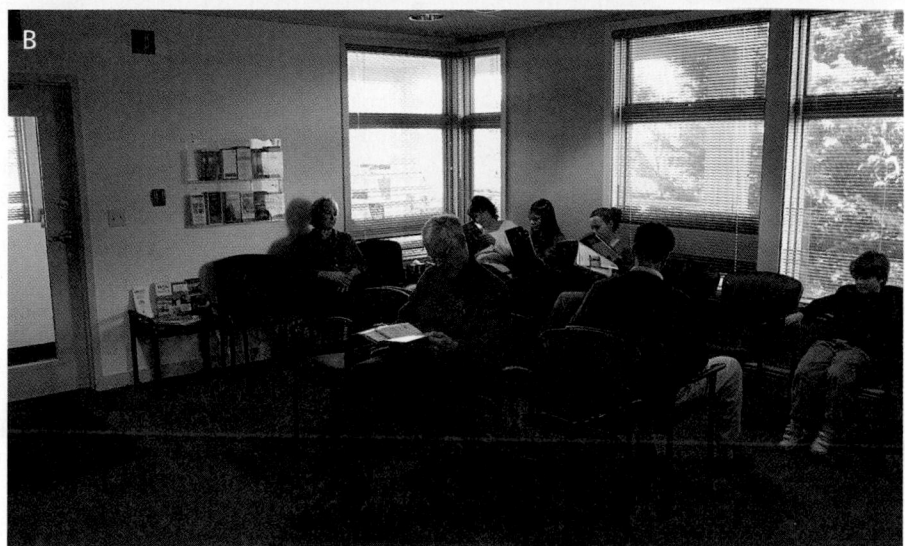

FIG 10-5 Effects of correct lighting. (A) Successful lighting plan. (B) Inadequate lighting.

outdated magazines from the reception area. Although it remains unproven, patients commonly associate outdated magazines in the reception area with longer waiting periods. Pediatric offices should have children's books and magazines as well as reading material for adults. An orthodontic practice, which will see many teenagers, should offer reading materials for that age group. Reading materials should never include items that could be offensive to patients; sexually explicit or politically charged materials should be avoided.

Music

Music can be incorporated into the reception area but should never be intrusive. A radio can be used, but speakers that spread the music throughout the room are preferred. It should never be so loud that it is intrusive to people who may want to read or simply relax. If a television is on in the waiting room for entertainment or information, the radio should be turned off to avoid competing with the sound from the television.

Cleanliness

Cleanliness in the clinical areas is vital to maintaining medical **asepsis**, or a state of cleanliness that is free from disease-causing microorganisms. It is also vital to maintain cleanliness in the reception area. If the reception area has cobwebs, dust, or dirty carpeting or bathrooms, patients may infer that the clinical areas are also dirty. Most offices have a cleaning service to clean these areas; however, it is the responsibility of all employees to maintain a clean environment at all times. Although eating and drinking is usually prohibited in reception areas, the medical assistant may have to pick up garbage or clean a spill if it occurs.

Educational Resources

Patient education is always important in the clinical setting. The reception area can offer pamphlets that identify specific diseases and disorders and possible treatments offered at the office. A rack of educational pamphlets should be kept filled with a variety of offerings. Patients can choose the materials, or staff members can give patients specific pamphlets to read.

These educational pamphlets can aid physicians in educating patients about their medical condition. If patients have read about a condition in the reception area, they may already be familiar with its physiology and treatment options. These educational pamphlets may also be available in examination rooms for physicians and patients to review.

The office can also use a television in the reception area as an educational resource. A television and DVD player can provide patients with information specific to the practice's area of specialty. Because a DVD is viewed by all people in the reception area, it should not contain graphic material (such as surgery or infected wounds). Educational companies that create these DVDs provide a variety of topics depicted in a manner that is appropriate for a reception area. While most of these materials include sound, some are pictures only (or the sound can be turned off).

Marketing Materials

The receptionist can offer office brochures or make them available in the reception area. Because patients may be unaware of all the services offered by the practice, brochures can encourage them to seek additional services or to recommend the practice to others. Patients and staff members can also give office brochures to friends or family members. Insurance and billing practices, HMO participation, hours of practice, and scope of services are types of information to include in a brochure.

In addition to a brochure for the practice, the office might offer **marketing** materials for other local physicians that accept referrals from the office. Services that are not offered in the office can be referred and endorsed by the office. Marketing materials for services that contribute to improved patient health, such as local health clubs, diet centers, smoking cessation clinics, and health food and vitamin stores, can be presented in the office.

In addition, pharmaceutical representatives will commonly leave brochures outlining the benefits of specific medications for specific diseases. At the discretion of the physician, these brochures can be placed in the reception area for patients to read and consider as a possible treatment option. It is important that patients understand that medication decisions are made by physicians and patients, not merely by marketing materials. If a medication is taken off the market for safety concerns, the marketing materials for that drug should be removed immediately.

Office Safety

Safety in the office should be maintained by attending to possible hazards and avoiding risky behaviors. Some hazards to avoid include:

- exposed electrical cords
- hallways blocked with boxes or equipment
- defects in carpeting that may cause trips and falls
- fire hazards such as long, flammable curtains
- broken equipment that may electrocute or cause fires
- spilled liquids that could cause falls
- broken furniture or sharp edges on tables.

Behaviors to avoid include:

- standing on tables or chairs to reach high objects
- items that are stacked in cabinets or closets and may fall when cabinet doors are opened
- leaving coffee makers or other appliances on when not in use
- smoking anywhere inside the building.

Other Precautions

In addition to avoiding hazards and risky behaviors, there are many precautions that will ensure a safe office environment, including:

- using surge protectors to protect computers and other electrical equipment from power surges that may accompany thunderstorms
- unplugging televisions and microwaves in the event of a thunderstorm
- installing smoke detectors and sprinkler systems or asking the landlord to do so (the landlord and tenant benefit from the added safety; owners and renters can receive a discount on property insurance for having and maintaining smoke detectors and sprinklers)
- disposing of broken jars or plastic bottles that may leak
- clearly marking steps in areas that people may not see with such words as "step down" or "watch your step"
- inspecting the office periodically for safety hazards, because the best way to ensure safety is to prevent hazards before they occur.

Chapter Summary

- The appearance of the physician's office, clinic, or hospital environment can influence a patient's opinion before treatment begins.
- A professional, pleasant, clean environment inspires patient confidence and allows staff to work efficiently.
- Properly chosen colors and lighting, attention to privacy needs, comfortable chairs, and appropriate reading materials show patients that the physicians and staff are interested in patient comfort and delivering quality health care.
- Attention to workflow and ergonomics increases productivity, reduces employee frustration, and prevents repetitive motion injuries, such as carpal tunnel syndrome and neck strain.
- Office staff should immediately address such safety concerns as blocked exits, faulty wiring, or other hazards such as spills to avoid injury to staff, physicians, or patients.
- Patient education through the use of practice brochures, disease and disorder pamphlets, and DVDs helps patients understand their specific conditions as well as the overall offerings of the practice.

Team Work Exercises

1. With a group of classmates, choose five appropriate topics for educational materials in each of the following settings:
   a. obstetrics and gynecology
   b. pediatrics
   c. dermatology

   Research the conditions and select educational materials—pamphlets and DVDs. Discuss with the remainder of the class why you chose the materials that you did. Who is your audience for each of the topics? How readable is the material that you chose?

2. With a group of classmates, design an office. Be sure to include a reception area, a front desk, examination rooms, a bathroom, and offices. You may include a break room for employees as well. Think about the flow of patients and staff. Decide on a budget, using local vendors, and choose furniture. Discuss comfort, durability, and maintenance of the furniture. What materials will you use for flooring, walls, countertops, and file storage? Why?

Case Studies

1. The physician's office you have been working in for the past 5 years has grown tremendously. Two new medical assistants and a physician's assistant were hired recently to meet the increasing needs of the practice. What was once your desk is now quickly becoming a dumping site for charts in need of filing, x-rays, HMO treatment request forms, and faxes. While you appreciate the new employees, you are beginning to resent the changes in the practice. You ask the physician-owner for a staff meeting to address your concerns. Make a list of items to discuss at the staff meeting and determine possible solutions to the problem. For example, has the practice grown to the point where more space is needed? Are there too many inactive patient medical records in the files that could be moved to a storage area? Can an area be designated for items that need to be filed? Should employee hours be expanded to keep up with filing and organizing medical records? Discuss these issues with classmates. Have you experienced changes in your work environment that are similar to the scenario? If so, discuss.

2. Mrs. Chen comes to the office for an examination with Dr. Rodriguez. She approaches your desk in the reception area and explains in a loud voice that she experienced chest pain the night before and is quite upset. She does not appear to be in an immediate physical crisis but is emotionally needy. You don't want to have the conversation with her in the reception area, but the examination rooms are all full. How can you help Mrs. Chen? Discuss options with classmates.

Resources

- Ergonomics: *www.usernomics.com/ergonomics.html*
- The benefits of working in a healthy environment: *www.ghchealth.com/healthy-office-environment.html*
- Office environment concerns for obese patients: *www.ama-assn.org/ama1/pub/upload/mm/433/officeenvironment.pdf*

Telephone Techniques

Learning Objectives

Upon completion of this chapter, the student will be able to:

- define the key terms presented in the glossary
- discuss why etiquette, tone, speed, and volume are important components in the use of the phone
- describe the proper procedure for taking incoming calls
- describe the acceptable way to place someone on hold
- describe the proper procedure for making outgoing calls
- describe the types of phone calls that should be taken by the medical assistant, the registered nurse, and the physician
- list four questions to ask when triaging a phone call and the appropriate action based on the response
- describe how to contact emergency services by phone and direct them to the caller's location
- describe useful techniques in managing a problem call.

CAAHEP Competencies

Administrative
Perform Clerical Functions
Schedule and manage appointments

General
Professional Communications
Recognize and respond to verbal communications

Recognize and respond to nonverbal communications
Demonstrate telephone techniques

Legal Concepts
Identify and respond to issues of confidentiality
Perform within legal and ethical boundaries
Document appropriately

Patient Instruction
Explain general office policies
Instruct individuals according to their needs

ABHES Competencies

Communication
Be attentive, listen, and learn
Adapt what is said to the recipient's level of comprehension
Serve as a liaison between physician and others
Use proper telephone techniques
Receive, organize, prioritize, and transmit information expediently

Administrative Duties
Schedule and monitor appointments
Perform telephone and in-person screening

Procedures

Demonstrating telephone techniques

Chapter Outline

Essential Tool
Telephone Etiquette
Answering Incoming Calls
Hold
Volume and tone

Clarity and speed
Multilingual callers
Making Outgoing Calls
Ending Calls
Time Zones
Call Handling
Taking Messages
Triaging Calls
Difficult Callers
Automated Routing Units
Documentation
Answering Service or Machine
Chapter Summary
Team Work Exercises
Case Studies
Resources

Key Terms

bilingual
Capable of conversing in two languages

call forwarding
Technology that enables a telephone call to reach a specific person, department, or desk

confidentiality
Principle of keeping personal medical and financial information private and avoiding divulgence of such information to any unapproved party

empathy
Understanding the emotions and thoughts of another

enunciation
Act of pronouncing words distinctly

etiquette
Rules for socially acceptable behavior

fluent
Able to speak and write well

jargon
Abbreviated versions or slang for terms used in a specialized profession or trade

multilingual
Proficient in several languages

pronunciation
Generally accepted sound of a spoken word

slang
Unconventional word or phrase used in place of a conventional word that is commonly clinical or complex in some way

triage
Process of screening patients to determine which need immediate medical treatment and in what order each patient must be seen

voice mail
System that enables a caller to leave a recorded message for the recipient

Essential Tool

The telephone is the communication tool most used in the clinical setting. New patients who call for information and to make an initial appointment will form an impression of the office based on that first phone call. The medical assistant must be professional, helpful, and clear in communicating over the telephone. Medical assistants also use the telephone to follow up on insurance claims, confirm patient appointments, and order supplies. The medical assistant ensures **confidentiality**—or the principle of keeping medical, financial, and personal information private and avoiding disclosure to unauthorized persons—by following the guidelines set by the Health Information Portability and Accountability Act (HIPAA). Regardless of how often the medical assistant uses the telephone, she must always adhere to confidentiality rules when conducting telephone communications to ensure that medical, financial, and personal information remains private. (For more information on HIPAA, see Chapter 7, "HIPAA and a Patient's Rights," page 71.) Physicians, nurses, and clinical medical assistants use the telephone to give instructions to patients, explain test results, and answer questions. Without the use of the telephone, no physician's office could remain open for long.

Telephone Etiquette

A telephone call should be handled in a professional and courteous manner. Adhering to telephone **etiquette,** or socially accepted rules for using the telephone, includes saying "please" and "thank you" and allowing your caller to speak. The caller may perceive interruptions, abruptness, or discourteous behavior as not only rude but also unprofessional. **Enunciation,** which is the practice of pronouncing words clearly and at a speed that affords the listener the opportunity to hear and understand the message, is essential for clear communication. Using proper **pronunciation,** the generally accepted sound of words, also helps the recipient understand the message. Pronouncing words in a way that is appropriate to the region helps the listener understand the message. A medical assistant who moves from Boston to Houston will need to change how she pronounces words to accommodate the difference in regional accents. In addition, the medical assistant should avoid using **jargon,** which is the use of abbreviations or medical terms that the patient might not be familiar with, so that the patient will understand the message. A medical assistant who uses medical jargon on the telephone may intimidate recipients and cause them to avoid asking questions that might aid in comprehension. As with jargon, the medical assistant should avoid using **slang,** or unconventional words or phrases to describe clinical conditions, because the patient may not understand the true meaning. When answering the phone, the medical assistant should speak clearly, in a pleasant tone, and at a comfortable volume. The patient calling the office should never feel that he is interrupting work and that the medical assistant is too busy to answer his questions and concerns. The caller must feel that the medical assistant answering the phone has **empathy,** which is an understanding of the caller's emotions and needs. Telephone communication is an integral part of the job; full attention must be given to the caller.

Answering Incoming Calls

The medical assistant must identify the practice and herself. Examples of telephone greetings include:

- "Doctor Warner's office, Louise speaking. How may I help you?"
- "Middletown Orthopedics, this is Sharon. Can you hold please?"

Stating the practice name helps callers know that they dialed the correct number. Stating the receiving person's name lets them know the name of the person with whom they are speaking and that the medical assistant is listening and ready to help. Using this type of greeting puts the caller at ease and helps ensure a successful call.

Hold

If the medical assistant wants to put a caller on hold to answer another line or to speak to a patient at the reception desk, she should ask the caller *if* she may put the patient on hold, such as "Can you hold, please?" Although most people will agree to be put on hold, the medical assistant must wait for the caller's response before putting him on hold. A caller may say, "No you can't put me on hold, this is an emergency!" The medical assistant must then triage the call to assess emergency status. She should never put a caller on hold who tells her there is an emergency.

Volume and Tone

When speaking on the telephone, the medical assistant should use a level of volume appropriate to the caller. An elderly patient may have trouble hearing, so speaking more loudly may be helpful. However, speaking too loudly and overemphasizing words can be irritating and perceived as condescending or patronizing. The medical assistant's tone, or sound of her voice, should be pleasant and convey a helpful attitude. A monotone voice tells the caller "I am bored and don't care about your call." A varied pitch with inflection raised at the end of sentences engages the caller.

Clarity and Speed

The medical assistant should speak clearly and distinctly. A medical assistant with a heavy accent should speak slowly and work toward using commonly accepted word pronunciations. Medical assistants for whom English is a second language should list and practice speaking the commonly used terms that are difficult to pronounce. Clear communication also includes using terms that the receiver is familiar with and avoiding terms that are too technical. The medical assistant should be sure to know the caller; if she is speaking to a patient who is a physician, nurse, medical assistant, or other health care provider, the use of technical medical terms or medical jargon is appropriate. If the caller is an attorney, a college president, or an accountant, despite being highly educated, they will most likely be less familiar with medical terminology.

The speed of speech should be appropriate to the caller's needs. When given directions to the office, the caller may be taking notes, so the medical assistant should allow the caller time to catch up. Speaking too slowly, however, will frustrate the caller and he will disengage from the dialogue. Speaking too rapidly causes confusion; the caller may have to ask the medical assistant to repeat her statements. Speaking too fast also conveys the message "I am too busy to give my time to you."

✦ **TIP** Language Choice

Take cues from the caller's use of terms. A caller who says, "My last UA showed gram-negative rods" has more medical knowledge than the caller who says, "Last time the MA tested my pee and I had a bladder infection." Speak to the caller in terms that she will understand.

Multilingual Callers

Because English may not be the caller's first language, many physician's offices practice in a multilingual environment. Medical assistants who are **bilingual,** speaking two languages, or even **multilingual,** speaking three or more languages, should offer to speak to the caller in the language most comfortable for the caller. However, the medical assistant offering to speak in another language must be fluent in that language, that is, able to speak and write in that language so that the communication is complete. A medical assistant offering to speak in a language that she has limited knowledge of can cause confusion and misinterpretation. If a caller is most comfortable speaking Spanish and the medical assistant is fluent in Spanish, the phone call can be conducted in Spanish. If a Spanish-speaking physician is part of the practice, offering to make an appointment with that physician will be helpful. If no Spanish-speaking physician is available, the medical assistant should tell the caller that she recommends bringing a family member to interpret if the office does not have an interpreter available.

✦ **TIP** Avoid Slang

The use of slang terms may confuse people. "Are you feeling sick?" is a clear statement, understood by the recipient. "Are you under the weather?" is not only unprofessional but can be taken literally by people for whom English is a second language. The receiver may wonder what the weather has to do with her health concern.

Making Outgoing Calls

When making outgoing calls, the medical assistant should identify herself and the practice name, just as she would when receiving a call. She should then ask to speak to the patient. For example:

- "This is Louise from Doctor Warner's office. May I speak to Greg Ramirez, please?"
- "Hello, Mr. Lynch? This is Sharon from Middletown Orthopedics."
- "Hi, Bill? This is Doug from Associated Internists."

The medical assistant may recognize the patient when he answers the phone; however, confirming his identity is vital. Speaking to a person without confirming his identity could result in a breach of confidentiality. Discussions of and references to personal or medical information on the telephone are protected under HIPAA mandates. The medical assistant can continue the call only when she is sure of the recipient's identity.

The recipient of the call will also need the identity of the caller (the medical assistant) and the office that she represents. When the recipient acknowledges the medical assistant and identifies himself, the medical assistant can give the reason for the call—for example, "I am calling to confirm your 10 a.m. appointment with Dr. Wilson for tomorrow, April 7th, at 3:30." (See *Example of an outgoing call.*) By clearly identifying herself, confirming the identity of the recipient, and identifying the office and the reason for the call, the medical assistant sets the tone for a successful call.

Ending Calls

At the conclusion of a phone call, the medical assistant should repeat important information from the phone call, such as confirmation of appointment date and time or patient instructions. For example, the medical assistant could say, "Mrs. Martin, so you understand that if Cindy's fever or rash returns, you need to call the office and bring her in for Dr. Wilson to examine her again." If the patient is unsure of instructions, the medical assistant must try to explain further. Patient understanding of the results of the phone call will ensure proper follow-up care. (See *Procedure 11-1: Demonstrating telephone techniques.*)

Example of an outgoing call

Here is an example of an appropriate outgoing telephone call by a medical assistant. The medical assistant uses all of the rules of telephone etiquette when calling the home phone number for Mr. James O'Reilly.

Recipient: "Hello"

Medical assistant (caller): "Hello, Mr. O'Reilly?"

Recipient: "Yes, this is he."

Medical assistant: "Hello, Mr. O'Reilly, this is Janice from Rockridge Endocrinology."

Recipient: "Oh, hello, I meant to call to make another appointment when I left last Wednesday, but I was running late and had to pick up my son at soccer practice."

Medical assistant: "That's fine, Mr. O'Reilly, I can help you schedule the follow-up right now."

When the recipient says, "Oh, hello," his response tells the medical assistant that she is speaking to Mr. O'Reilly and that she can discuss medical or personal information if necessary.

Time Zones

Patients will live in the same time zone as the office, but vendors of office and clinical supplies, insurance companies, or HMO accrediting agencies may be located several states away, so the medical assistant should be aware of different time zones and take into account office hours in those areas. For example, a New York office should not expect to reach a California office until noon Eastern Standard Time (9 a.m. Pacific time). (See *North American time zones,* page 126.)

Call Handling

Appointment scheduling, driving directions, and insurance and billing questions can be answered by the medical assistant. Medical questions regarding diagnosis and treatment should be handled by a physician or registered nurse. Because the medical assistant is usually the person who answers the phone, deciding who needs to speak with the patient will be her responsibility. (See *Incoming calls and actions,* page 127.)

✦ **TIP** ID the Caller

To confirm the identity of a caller and therefore establish "need to know," caller ID technology can be helpful. If the

PROCEDURE 11-1

Demonstrating telephone techniques

Task

Demonstrate proper telephone answering, screening, and message-taking techniques.

Conditions

- Telephone
- Message pad
- Appointment schedule
- Appropriate patient chart
- Pen or pencil

Standards

In the time specified and within the scoring parameters determined by the instructor, the student will successfully demonstrate proper telephone techniques by answering incoming calls, performing patient screening, and taking messages in an efficient, professional manner.

Performance Standards

1. Gather all necessary supplies and have them handy near the telephone area. Being organized before answering the telephone allows you to take a message accurately and efficiently.

2. Promptly answer the telephone on the third ring or sooner to avoid causing anxiety or annoyance to the caller waiting on the line.

3. Greet the caller by identifying your office and yourself to assure the caller that he has dialed the correct number.

4. Listen to the caller and obtain the caller's name and reason for the call to assist the caller appropriately and efficiently.

5. If necessary, place the caller on hold and obtain the medical record to access necessary patient information in the medical record or to pass along to the appropriate staff member who can assist the caller.

6. If you need to transfer the caller to another staff member, let the caller know the name and occupation of the person to whom you will be transferring him so the caller can get connected to the person quickly in the event that there is an error in transferring the call.

7. If the caller wishes to speak with a person who is unavailable, take a message, being sure to include:
   a. person or patient's name and contact phone numbers
   b. date and time of the call
   c. detailed message
   d. your name or initials as the person taking the call.

Phone Message

For: *Dr. Greer*   Date: *12-4-09*   Time: *11:13 am*

Name: *Tammy Connery*
Contact information
Phone: *564-860-4321*   ☐ home ☐ work ☒ cell
Fax:
Email:

Message:
Tammy missed two doses of her birth control pills
and wants to know what she should do?

Call taken by: *Ann Chapin, CMA*
Date: *12/04/09*   Time : *11:15 am*

---

8. Tell the caller that you will be giving the message to the appropriate person and explain the office's policy for return calls, if appropriate. Some offices have special times of the day in which return calls are made to patients.

9. If the call is appropriate for a medical assistant to take, perform a screening, asking appropriate questions to determine if the call is an emergency situation.

10. If you must put the caller on hold to get an answer to his question, ask the caller if he can hold. Be sure to wait for the caller's answer to avoid offending the caller who does not wish to wait on hold.

11. When you take the caller off hold, be sure to confirm the identity of the caller to avoid a breach of confidentiality and identify yourself again to avoid causing confusion and then provide the caller with the requested information.

12. Be sure to identify and respond professionally to issues of confidentiality during the conversation because some callers may be providing sensitive information or results.

13. Perform within all legal and ethical boundaries during the conversation. Medical assistants and all health care providers must avoid taking phone calls that are not within their scope of practice.

14. If the call is related to a patient, document the phone call in the patient's chart as necessary to maintain an accurate medical record.

North American time zones

When calling a different time zone, the medical assistant must determine if it is too early or late to make the call by adding one hour for each zone change to the east (right) and subtracting one hour for each time zone to the west (left). The map below shows the time zones for the United States and Canada.

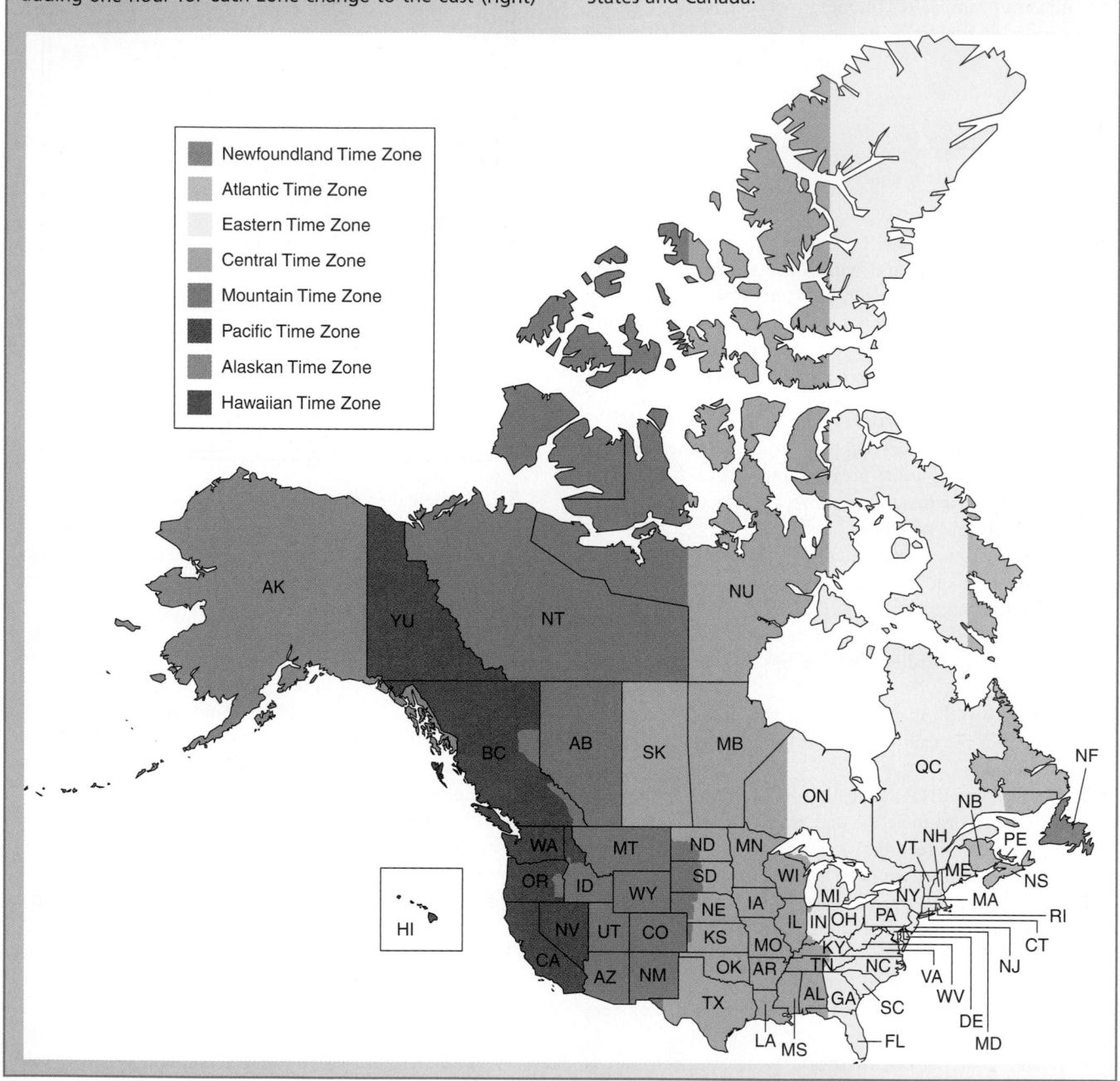

Newfoundland Time Zone
Atlantic Time Zone
Eastern Time Zone
Central Time Zone
Mountain Time Zone
Pacific Time Zone
Alaskan Time Zone
Hawaiian Time Zone

Incoming calls and actions

The medical assistant can help many patients who call the office. However, she must ask the physician or registered nurse (RN) to handle some situations. The table below outlines possible phone requests from patients and who should handle the call.

Type of call	Action taken by MA	Who handles the call?
Patient calls to make or change an appointment	Schedule a nonemergency appointment or reschedule appointments as needed.	• Medical assistant
Patient calls to confirm an appointment	Confirm the time and date of the appointment.	• Medical assistant
Patient calls for a prescription refill	Take a message for the physician, including the patient's name, pharmacy name, and prescription number. Put the patient's chart and message on the physician's desk.	• Physician calls the pharmacy to order the refill. • Medical assistant calls the patient to indicate that the refill has been ordered. • If no refill is granted, the medical assistant or physician calls the patient to explain.
Patient calls seeking medical advice	Take a message and put it and the patient's chart on the physician's or RN's desk.	• Physician or RN
Patient calls with a question about billing or insurance	Identify the caller as a patient or guardian and then answer billing or insurance questions.	• Medical assistant
Patient calls with a complaint	Ask "Is there anything I can help with?" If the complaint is medical, take a message for the physician or RN. If the problem is related to scheduling, attempt to reschedule and better accommodate the patient's schedule. If it is a billing problem, record the information, call the insurance company, and get information to the patient as soon as possible.	• Physician or RN for medical complaints • Medical assistant for administrative (scheduling or billing) complaints
Patient asks to speak to the physician	Ask the patient "Is there something I can help with?" If the patient says no, the medical assistant should ask if the nurse or physician can help and give the message to the RN or physician as appropriate.	• Medical assistant, RN, or physician, based on information needed
Patient calls with a question about medication, illness, or injury	Take information from the patient, including the patient's name, the nature of the injury or illness, and the patient's question and put the message and the patient's chart on the RN's or physician's desk.	• RN or physician
Patient calls for test results	Identify the caller as the patient or guardian of the patient and then take a message and put it and the patient's chart on the physician's or RN's desk.	• RN or physician
Outside laboratory calls with patient test results	Write down the laboratory test results as dictated over the phone or give the phone to a clinical medical assistant or another designated person and confirm the laboratory fax number if results must be faxed.	• Medical assistant or RN

Continued

Incoming calls and actions—cont'd

Type of call	Action taken by MA	Who handles the call?
Insurance company calls for information to process a claim on a patient	Identify the caller and give the required information about the patient (only the information needed to process the claim).	• Medical assistant
Attorney's office calls for information regarding a patient's claim, such as worker's compensation or an auto accident	Identify the caller and check to see that the patient has signed an authorization to release the information to the attorney's office (releasing only the information related to the claim).	• Medical assistant
Another physician calls to speak to the physician	Ask if the call is regarding a specific patient, retrieve the patient's chart, and transfer the call to the physician.	• Physician
Pharmaceutical sales representative calls to talk to the physician or RN about new medications or how existing medications are working for patients	Make appointment for the sales representative to see the physician or RN (scheduled as office policy dictates).	• Medical assistant
Office or clinical supply sales representative calls to ask if the office needs products or to notify the office about sales and special products	Take message for appropriate staff member.	• Medical assistant or office manager
Person calls to speak with a staff member about a personal matter	Direct the call to the appropriate staff member, following office guidelines regarding personal calls during office hours.	• Staff member

phone shows the telephone number of the caller, check that number, for example, against the letterhead of the attorney's office or a list of insurance company numbers kept at the desk for quick reference. If you cannot confirm the identity of the caller, offer to call the caller back at her office. Other methods that are considered a legitimate confirmation of a caller are having spoken with the individual in past conversations and recognizing her voice or the caller referring to a previous conversation.

Taking Messages

When taking messages for physicians, nurses, or fellow medical assistants, the medical assistant should try to include as much information as possible, including:

- name of the caller
- date and time of the call
- return phone number and when the person can be reached

- action requested (such as if the caller wants a call back or if the caller will call again later)
- message, including the patient's question with reference to specifics, such as medication and dosage
- initial or signature of the medical assistant taking the message.

Triaging Calls

Triaging a call is deciding if *immediate* medical attention is required and assisting the caller in getting the appropriate attention. Many patients who call the office feel that their situation demands immediate attention through speaking to a physician or getting an immediate appointment. The medical assistant must accurately assess the priority of the situation. Having a list of questions by the telephone will guide the medical assistant in assessing the urgency of the call. (See *Emergency dialogue*.)

If a phone call is an immediate emergency, the medical assistant can assist the caller by taking the following actions:

Emergency dialogue

While all calls are not emergencies, the medical assistant's job is made easier when she has these questions and associated actions at hand by the phone when calls arrive.

(Keep in mind, not all questions will be appropriate in a given situation.)

Question	Reason	Follow-up Questions
What happened?	It is most important to find out the nature of the injury first.	When did the injury take place?
What is the patient's name? How old is the patient?	If the patient is a child, it is necessary to determine if the caller is a parent or guardian who has the legal right to make medical decisions for the child.	If the caller is a parent, the call can continue with specific questions as outlined below. If the caller is not a parent or guardian, the parent should get on the phone. If the parent is not available, the medical assistant is able to provide only emergency care without the consent of a parent or guardian.
Is the patient breathing?	Difficulty breathing is a life-threatening emergency. Direct the caller to use an inhaler (if available) and to call 911.	If caller answers "Yes" to the question, "Do you want me to call 911?" then the medical assistant should use another telephone line to call 911, give the location of the caller, and stay on the line until emergency medical services arrive.
Is there bleeding? From where? How much?	Arterial bleeding requires immediate medical attention, but venous or capillary bleeding does not.	If the caller answers "Yes," to the question, "Can you stop the bleeding?" then the medical assistant should instruct the caller to put pressure on the wound to control bleeding. If the caller cannot stop the bleeding, the medical assistant should instruct the caller to continue applying pressure and call 911.
What is the patient's temperature?	Fevers of 100°F or higher in adults and 101°F in children should be seen in the office immediately.	How long has the patient had the fever? If the patient has had a high fever for more than 12 hours, the medical assistant should ask the caller to bring the patient to the office immediately.
Did the patient take a medication? What is the name and how much?	Overdoses of some medications are life-threatening and require a 911 call.	Are there instructions on the bottle for overdose? If there are not instructions on the bottle, the medical assistant should instruct the caller to call the Poison Control Center at 1-800-222-1222.

1. Establish the nature of the emergency, such as breathing difficulty, injury, heart attack, seizure, or diabetic coma.
2. Stay on the line with the caller and get the exact location of the caller.
3. From another telephone line, call emergency medical services (EMS) or have another medical assistant or employee make the call.
4. Give EMS the location of the caller and the nature of the injury or illness.
5. Stay on the line with the caller until EMS arrives.
6. Document the phone call and actions taken.

In nonemergency situations, asking questions on the phone is used to determine the action to be taken. Patients calling for an appointment should be asked some questions to determine when they should be seen. These questions include:

- How long have you had the pain or symptoms?
- Are you taking any medications? Are you in need of refills?
- Do you need a blood sugar (glucose), thyroid, or lipid (cholesterol) panel? (Patients who are taking maintenance medications will be familiar with the blood tests that are monitored for their condition.)

If the medical assistant determines that no immediate emergency exists, an appointment can be made at the patient's earliest convenience.

Difficult Callers

Not all callers to the physician's office will be pleasant and cooperative. Patients with complaints regarding billing and insurance or the progress of their medical condition may be angry or even abusive. The medical assistant must always remain calm and professional and never argue with a patient or return abusive comments. She should be careful never to yell at the patient, even if the patient is yelling at her. Asking questions of the caller for clarification of the complaint can help to calm the patient and show that the medical assistant is attentive to his needs. If the physician, nurse, or office manager must handle the call, the medical assistant should take a complete message from the caller. When giving the message to the recipient, she should be sure to include that the caller was upset, abusive, or angry. The medical assistant should give the message and the patient's chart to the physician, nurse, or office manager *in person,* rather than leaving it on the desk.

If a caller is so abusive that no constructive outcome of the phone call is possible, the medical assistant should tell the patient that she will hang up if the abuse (such as swearing, screaming, or threatening) continues. She should hang up on the caller only after she has made it clear that she will do so if they do not calm down. She should then immediately report any abusive behavior to the physician or office manager and document abusive language in the patient's chart.

Automated Routing Units

Large practices, clinics, and hospitals commonly use automated systems for directing calls. When a caller is connected, a recorded voice gives a greeting and options for connecting to specific departments or staff members. With the use of a touch-tone phone, the caller is directed to the appropriate recipient.

When calls are directed to individual phones, the receiver should answer and identify the department and give her name. For example, "Scheduling, this is Shannon. How may I help?"

If the phone rings and goes unanswered, the calls go back to an operator. The operator can give the caller the option of using **voice mail** to leave a recorded message for the department or individual. For example, "Hello this is Joanne, the operator. No one is available in the billing department. Would you like to leave a message for them?" The operator can then connect the caller to a voice mail box that can hold messages to be returned later.

Documentation

Proper documentation of phone calls in a patient's chart can clarify questions that may occur later. (See *Examples of phone call documentation.*)

Documenting phone calls can help physicians when speaking with patients in the office. If a patient calls with questions regarding medication, the medical assistant or nurse can document the call and any instructions given, such as blood glucose testing and insulin levels. At the patient examination, the physician can refer to the chart and say, "So, you had some questions on the use of the blood glucose meter? Are you comfortable with the machine and managing your blood sugar?" The physician can confirm that patient education is established or that the patient needs more help using the machine.

Abusive phone calls made by angry patients should be documented in the patient's chart as well. Physicians and staff need to know if a patient might be unruly in the office during the visit or abusive on the phone in the future. Documenting angry and abusive phone calls can also prompt a physician to refuse to continue to see a patient, severing the doctor-patient relationship.

Answering Service or Machine

Many practices use an answering service to answer incoming calls when the office is closed. The practice should give the answering service instructions on directing calls to on-call physicians in the case of emergency, taking messages for the office, and telling the caller the office hours. Answering services do not answer questions or make patient appointments.

If the physician practice does not want to hire an answering service, **call forwarding** is an option. With this technology, when a patient calls the office phone, the call is forwarded to the on-call physician's cellular phone. The medical assistant may be required to change the on-call number as the physicians rotate their on-call duty. The practice may also elect to designate one cellular phone for the on-call service and the physicians will take turns keeping the phone. In either scenario, the medical assistant can assist the physicians by charging the cellular phone and reminding the physicians of the on-call schedule.

Examples of phone call documentation

Occasionally, notations made in a patient's chart regarding a phone call can be useful at a later date when questions arise. For example, why did Mrs. Wilson wait two years for

her checkup? Looking in the chart might show that the patient had an appointment last year but called to cancel it. The administrative medical assistant would have written:

Date	
12/10/05; 9:45 a.m.	*Patient called. Canceled appt. of 12/19. Will call to reschedule.* ———————————————— *A. Chapin, CMA*

This piece of information can be useful if Mrs. Wilson were to claim that she was not told to make an appointment or that lack of attention to her needs caused her harm (such as a late diagnosis of cancer). Documentation of the cancelled appointment can show that the physician

was not negligent in offering care, but that the patient refused care.

In addition, the physician will document phone calls in the patient's chart if medication dosages are changed or if he instructs the patient to discontinue a medication.

Date	
12/19/05; 2:45 a.m.	*Spoke to patient. She says she no longer feels nauseated. medication makes her constipated. I told to discontinue use of compazine.* ———————————————— *A. Wilson, MD*

When opening the office in the morning, the medical assistant should call the answering service to get messages and tell the service that the office is open and will be answering the phone. When closing the office, the medical assistant will call the answering service and alert them to answer incoming calls and the physician who will be receiving any emergency calls that arise.

Offices that might not offer 24-hour phone coverage, such as optometrists, chiropractors, physical and occupational therapists, and radiology groups, may use an answering machine when the office is closed. The answering machine message should include the name of the office and when the office will reopen. The message may also include instructions for emergency care. Emergencies may be referred to 911 or the nearest emergency room—for example, "You have reached Middlefield Chiropractic Associates. The office is now closed. Our office hours are Monday through Thursday 8:30 a.m. to 7:00 p.m. and Friday and Saturdays from 8:30 a.m. to 2:00 p.m. If this is a medical emergency, please call 911 or go to the nearest emergency room. To leave a message for the office, please wait for the tone. Thank you for calling Middlefield Chiropractic Associates." Alternatively, the message may provide a physician's cell phone number—for example, "You have reached Middlefield Chiropractic Associates. The office is now closed. Our office hours are Monday through Thursday 8:30 a.m. to 7:00 p.m. and Friday and Saturdays from 8:30 a.m. to 2:00 p.m. If this is an emergency, please call 911. To speak to the on-call physician, please dial 123-555-9708. To leave

a nonemergency message for the office, please wait for the tone. Thank you for calling Middlefield Chiropractic Associates."

Chapter Summary

- Using courteous, clear communication on the telephone helps promote understanding and good relationships with patients, insurance companies, and vendors.
- Accurate appointment scheduling, driving directions, and billing questions are the responsibility of the medical assistant; medical questions should be directed to the physician or registered nurse.
- The medical assistant must assess emergency versus routine patient needs on the phone in a methodical, calm manner and take appropriate actions.
- Taking accurate and complete messages for physicians and coworkers allows patient questions and concerns to be addressed properly and shows patients that their needs are important to staff and physicians.
- Proper documentation of phone calls ensures complete, accurate records of telephone exchanges.
- The use of answering services or machines allows access to the office when it is closed. Understanding the telephone system and protocols will help the medical assistant perform her job duties.

Team Work Exercises

1. Assume that your class is in charge of answering the phones at a busy pediatric office. Create roles for class members, including:
   a. administrative medical assistants
   b. clinical medical assistants
   c. registered nurses
   d. physicians
   e. billing staff
   f. office manager
   g. parent or guardian
   Take turns playing the part of the parent or guardian who calls with a request, including:
   a. scheduling an appointment
   b. asking about an emergency medical situation
   c. changing the time of an existing appointment
   d. parent new to the area scheduling an appointment for a child (new patient) and needing directions to the office
   Discuss as a group what the appropriate responses are to the various calls.

2. In groups of three to five, create lists of medical jargon and slang that could be confusing to patients when spoken over the phone. Create a dialogue using these terms and try to confuse the other groups with your use of jargon and slang.

Case Studies

1. Mr. Kraft calls the office and is very angry. His insurance denied a claim for an office visit saying that the visit was not medically necessary. The physician's office has not yet billed Mr. Kraft, but he tells you, "You had better not bill me for that visit, or I'll sue you." Mr. Kraft does not want to hear that you can appeal the denial if he is willing to fill out the form that was sent to him. He tells you, "Paperwork is your *&¢$*& job, not mine!" What should you do? Should you alert the physician or the office manager? Discuss the scenario with your classmates.

2. Sadie Collins calls to cancel her follow-up appointment for her clavicle fracture of 10 weeks ago. She states that she feels fine and does not need to come in. What documentation should you write in Sadie's chart? Why?

Resources

- Revamping your telephone technique: *www.nfib.com/object/IO_27174.html*
- Telephone technique self-test: *www.ompersonal.com.ar/selftests/telephonetechnique.htm*
- Belding, S.: *Winning with the Caller from Hell: A Survival Guide for Doing Business on the Telephone.* Toronto: ECW Press, 2006.
- Evenson, R.: *Customer Service Training 101: Quick and Easy Techniques That Get Great Results.* Albany, N.Y.: AMACOM Publishing, 2005.

Appointment Scheduling

Learning Objectives

Upon completion of this chapter, the student will be able to:

- define and spell key terms related to appointment scheduling
- compare and contrast the various types of scheduling
- create an appointment matrix for a practice
- prepare a daily appointment sheet
- describe six considerations in scheduling appointments
- discuss the importance of triage in scheduling patient appointments
- create proper cancellation documentation and describe its importance
- create a reminder system and discuss the three types of reminder systems
- discuss how practice policies regarding appointments can be applied
- schedule and monitor appointments
- schedule inpatient and outpatient hospital procedures
- triage phone calls, giving priority to patients who need immediate care
- maintain confidentiality in appointments on a computerized or manual system
- communicate effectively with patients, giving directions and instructions when needed.

CAAHEP Competencies

Administrative
  Perform Clerical Functions
    Schedule and manage appointments

Schedule inpatient and outpatient admissions and procedures
Clinical
  Patient Care
    Perform telephone and in-person screening
General
  Professional Communications
    Recognize and respond to verbal communications
    Demonstrate telephone techniques
  Operational Functions
    Utilize computer software to maintain office systems

ABHES Competencies

Communication
  Use proper telephone techniques
  Interview effectively
  Use appropriate medical terminology
  Recognize and respond to verbal and nonverbal communication
Administrative Duties
  Apply computer concepts for office procedures
  Schedule and maintain medical records
  Schedule inpatient and outpatient admissions

Procedures

  Creating appointment cards
  Creating an appointment matrix and scheduling appointments using the rules of triage
  Documenting appointment cancellations and no-shows and rescheduling appointments
  Scheduling inpatient and outpatient procedures

Chapter Outline

Key Terms

appointment matrix
Grid or schedule (computerized or manual) that shows the times available for scheduling patients and the days and hours the practice is open (excluding lunches and breaks)

catch-up time
Time in the schedule that is not booked with appointments to let doctors and staff catch up on paperwork, return phone calls, or catch up with appointments if patient visits take longer than anticipated

cluster booking
Scheduling technique that involves consecutive booking of patients who have similar problems or are undergoing similar procedures

double booking
Scheduling technique in which several patients are scheduled for the same appointment time and are attended to at the same time in different rooms

established patient
Patient who has previously received care at the office

modified wave
Scheduling technique in which two or three patients are scheduled at the beginning of each hour and then one patient is scheduled every 10 to 20 minutes into the hour

new patient
Patient who has not previously received care at the office

no-show
Patient who has a scheduled appointment but fails to appear

open hours
Block of time in which patients are seen by the physician on a first-come, first-served basis

practice-based
Scheduling technique that designates special days for common treatments based on time limits and staff and equipment availability

stream
Most common scheduling technique in which patients are seen in a steady stream at set appointment times of 15-, 30-, 45-, or 60-minute intervals

triage
Process of determining if a patient has an emergency and needs to go to the emergency room or if he can be worked into the physician's schedule for the day

wave
Scheduling technique in which patients are scheduled in the first half-hour of each hour

Challenges in Appointment Scheduling

The success of an office and quality of care depend on consistent scheduling to create a workflow. If scheduling is done haphazardly, patients will be required to wait for long periods of time or be rushed through an appointment, which may compromise the quality of care. To allow profitable use of the physician's and staff's time, matching the scheduling system to the type of practice and ability of the staff is vital. Imagine a psychologist having five patients arrive at the same time! However, a general practitioner with several clinical medical assistants may consider five patients at once an easily workable schedule. Proper planning ensures that equipment in specific rooms is not needed for more than one patient at the same time. If the practice has one x-ray machine, five patients cannot be scheduled for an x-ray at the same time.

The most common complaint among patients is the amount of time spent in the waiting room. Patients appreciate when the staff recognizes that their time is valuable and works to reduce waiting time. Overall patient satisfaction is increased when attention to scheduling prevents long waiting.

Types of Scheduling Systems

The type of patient scheduling used in the ambulatory care office depends on many factors. How many doctors, nurses and clinical medical assistants are available to care for patients? How many treatment rooms are available? What type of equipment is used and what procedures are performed in the treatment rooms? Because all of these issues must be considered, there are several scheduling systems an office can choose as the best for that practice.

Practice–Based Scheduling

Most specialty groups develop their own method for scheduling patients based on time limits and staff and equipment availability. Such a system is called *practice-based* *scheduling*. For example, an orthopedist might schedule a recheck in the morning on a patient who needs physical therapy (PT) so that the patient can go to PT immediately after the appointment. An obstetrician's office may schedule all ultrasounds on Thursdays, when the technician is scheduled to work; an orthodontist may restrict scheduling fittings for new braces to Monday and Wednesday mornings to cluster the times that she will be unavailable to see other patients.

Stream Scheduling

If equipment is portable or available in all treatment rooms, a simpler system to utilize would be the **stream** system.

Offices using this system see patients in a steady stream at set appointment times of 15-, 30-, 45-, or 60-minute intervals. The type of appointment dictates how much time is reserved for each patient—for example, 60 minutes for a **new patient** (someone who has never been seen at the office before), 45 minutes for a stress test, and 15 minutes for a checkup.

Cluster Booking

When patients with similar problems or procedures are booked consecutively, it is called *cluster booking*. Examples of cluster booking include pediatric vaccines and routine gynecologic appointments, which might be booked on a specific day or only in the afternoon to allow equipment and supplies to be prepared ahead in anticipation of these patients.

Double Booking

Sometimes, several patients are scheduled for the same appointment time and are attended to at the same time in different rooms. This technique is called *double booking*. Large and small practices can double book; however, in a small office, "juggling" patients can get hectic. Double booking works best for short visits. For example, a chiropractic office may schedule several patients for the same time who need a maintenance adjustment and no therapy at the time of the visit.

Wave Scheduling

In the **wave** scheduling system, patients are scheduled in the first half-hour of each hour. Because there will be some early, some late, and some **no-show** patients (patients who do not cancel but simply fail to appear for their appointments), the hour will fill. This system works best in a larger practice; a small office runs the risk of doctors waiting with no patients to be seen. A variation of this system is called the *modified wave* system. In this system, two or three patients are scheduled at the beginning of each hour and then one patient is scheduled every 10 to 20 minutes into the hour. This modification to the wave system may ensure a more consistent patient flow.

Open Hours

Emergency rooms and clinics commonly use the **open hours** scheduling method. Patients are seen by the physician on a first-come, first-served basis. This system may cause patients to wait several hours to be seen, but no appointment is necessary. Of course, any life-threatening or urgent condition is treated immediately.

Catch-up Time

No matter the scheduling system, **catch-up time,** when no patients are scheduled, should be incorporated to let doctors get current with paperwork or return phone calls. After an office surgery, the room must be thoroughly cleaned, taking up the clinical medical assistants' time and attention. This time also allows the schedule to run on-time if patient visits take longer than anticipated. Short breaks in the schedule can also allow doctors and staff to take a break, make a personal phone call, or use the restroom.

Patient Scheduling

Scheduling appointments with patients can happen over the telephone or when the patient checks out of the office after an appointment. When scheduling a patient over the phone or in person, the medical assistant should be sure to include all necessary information to avoid confusion on the part of the patient or the office staff.

Scheduling Patients by Phone

When scheduling a patient for an appointment over the telephone, the medical assistant must first determine if the patient is a new patient or an **established patient** (someone who has been seen in the office previously and whose medical record is kept at the office).

New Patient

When scheduling a new patient, the medical assistant will need to gather information from the patient prior to the visit. This information will include the patient's:

- name
- address and phone number
- insurance carrier and policy number
- reason for the appointment.

The medical assistant may also ask the patient to bring copies of previous medical records, recent x-rays, or laboratory results. The medical assistant should always remind a new patient to bring her insurance card to the visit so that a copy can be made. A new patient may need information from the medical assistant regarding insurance coverage, office hours, and copayment fee policies as well as directions to the office. It may be the policy of an office to mail an informational brochure to a new patient prior to her appointment. (See *Informational office brochure*, page 136.)

✦ TIP New Patient, More Time

A new patient must complete Confidential Patient Information and HIPAA forms. Thus, the administrative medical assistant should be sure to schedule extra time for the patient to fill out paperwork before the examination.

◢ Patient Education

Informational Office Brochure

The informational office brochure is an opportunity for the medical office staff to assist a new patient in achieving a smooth transition to a new health care provider and ensuring continuity of care for that patient. Brochures can be given to patients in the office or mailed to them upon making their first appointment. Such a brochure could include:

- hours of practice

- scheduling and cancellation procedures

- insurance participation

- services offered.

Brochure as referral

The office brochure can also act as a patient referral tool. Specialty practices can send copies of the brochure to primary care providers to indicate what services the office can provide to their patients.

Blueville Family Medicine
15 Main Street
Blueville, CT
860-555-3212

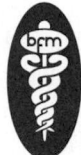

Robert Greer, MD
Family Medicine

Hector Rodriguez, MD
Family Medicine

Anne Wilson, MD
School and Sports Physicals

Sharon Piecek, APRN
Nutritional Counseling and Weight
Loss, Diabetes Management

Henry Lee, MD
Acupuncture

Services Include:

- Routine physicals, including well-child, well-adult, and sports physicals

- All childhood immunizations, including HPV

- In-office x-ray and physical therapy departments

- Acupuncture

- Nutritional counseling, including weight loss and diabetes management

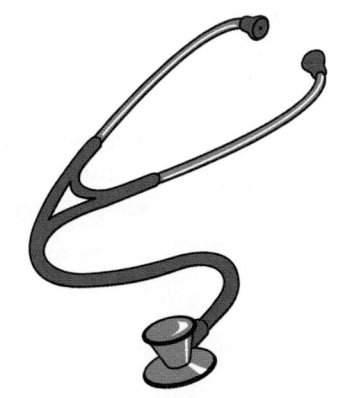

- Emergency, 24-hour on-call service

- Affiliated with Hartell Memorial Hospital

- Most insurance accepted

Conveniently located next to
Johnson Auto Body

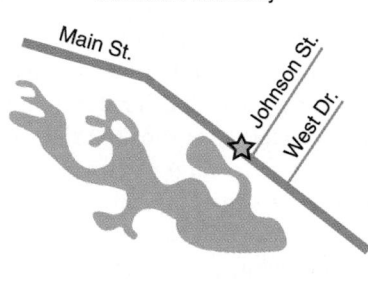

Ample parking at side of
building

Established Patient

Scheduling an appointment for an established patient by phone will be shorter because less information is needed. However, the medical assistant should ask a patient who has not been seen for a while if any personal information, such as address, phone number, and insurance carrier, has changed. If the patient has changed insurance, the medical assistant should explain differences in coverage or copayment and ask that the patient bring the insurance card at the time of the visit.

✦ TIP Confirm, Confirm, Confirm

The medical assistant should conclude all appointment phone calls by confirming the information. For example, she should say, "Okay, Mrs. Jones, we will see you on Wednesday, February 4th, at 3:30 p.m."

Scheduling Patients During In-Office Checkout

After patients see the physician, they must check out and schedule a follow-up appointment, if necessary. Scheduling a follow-up appointment should include offering an appointment card. An appointment card is a courtesy to the patient, and many offices create them on the computer. (See *Procedure 12-1: Creating appointment cards*, page 138.) It helps them remember the date and time of the appointment and provides the office telephone number if the patient needs to reschedule. (See Figure 12-1.) The copayment may be taken before or after the patient visit, based on office policy. Also, remember to offer a receipt based on office policy.

✦ TIP Offer All Options

When offering an appointment to patients on the phone or in person in the office, ask them if they would like a morning or afternoon appointment and then offer specific times. For example:

Medical Assistant: "Is the morning of the 17th better or the afternoon?"
Patient: "Afternoon, please."
Medical Assistant: "I have a 3 p.m. or a 4:30 p.m. on the 17th."
Rather than asking, "What time is good on the 17th?" prompting the patient with specific times will expedite the scheduling process by offering only available appointments.

Appointment Matrix

An **appointment matrix** is a grid or schedule of appointments that shows time slots for scheduling patients and the practice's days and hours of operation. The matrix is organized to show rooms, doctors and other personnel, and hours of use. The matrix can be created in advance and show blocked time for holidays, vacation time, lunches, and breaks. Scheduled machine maintenance can be included to reflect rooms that may be unavailable at a given time. (See *Procedure 12-2: Creating an appointment matrix and scheduling appointments using the rules of triage*, page 138.) The appointment matrix may be computerized or in a book form.

Computerized Appointment Systems

Most offices are fully computerized and patient appointments are made using a computer. The system will allow the user to jump from various days and times while viewing the other appointments that have already been scheduled. (See Figure 12-2.)

If the system is not working, the medical assistant can make tentative appointments for patients and then call them back with changes (if necessary) when the system is working again. The new administrative medical assistant may be familiar with the software from school or will need to be trained on the specific software program. The differences among the various programs are minor and the student who is proficient in one software program should easily adapt to the office software.

✦ TIP Appointment Analysis

An office may generate appointment reports by day, week, month, or specific doctor to track trends and identify busy times. Analysis of the appointment trends can be used to adjust staff scheduling to meet the needs of the practice. For example, if Wednesdays after school are particularly popular

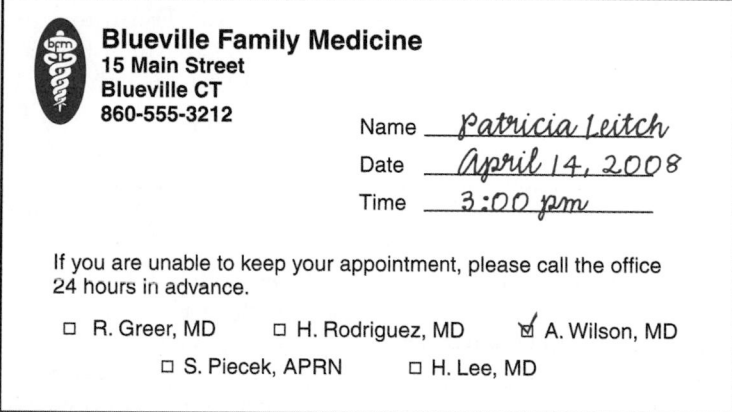

FIG 12-1 Appointment card given to patients making follow-up appointments in the office.

PROCEDURE 12-1

Creating appointment cards

Task
Create appointment cards and give to five patients at the front desk after scheduling.

Conditions
- Computer
- Card stock
- Scissors or paper cutter
- Pen

Standards
In the time specified and within the scoring parameters determined by the instructor, the student will successfully create appointment cards to give to patients during appointment scheduling.

Performance Standards
1. Using your computer, card stock, and scissors, create appointment cards that are the size of a business card so that it can fit into the patient's wallet.

2. Be sure to include the following information when creating cards:
   a. name and telephone number of the practice so patients can easily call the office if they need to reschedule the appointment.
   b. line for the patient's name so that the family member with the appointment is identified for the patient.
   c. line to write in the date and time of the appointment for patient reference.
3. Print appointment cards.
4. During the front-desk appointment role-play procedure, write out an appointment card and give it to the patient.

PROCEDURE 12-2

Creating an appointment matrix and scheduling appointments using the rules of triage

Task
Create an appointment matrix and manage appointments.

Conditions
- Computer and printer
- Pen

Standards
In the time specified and within the scoring parameters determined by the instructor, the student will successfully create an appointment matrix and perform scheduling procedures as instructed.

Performance Standards

1. Using your computer, create an appointment matrix for Drs. Greer, Rodriguez, Wilson, Lee, and Sharon Piecek, APRN, for the week of September 15, 2008 through September 19, 2008. Use the following information when creating the matrix:
   a. The office is open from 8:30 a.m. to 7 p.m. on Monday, Tuesday, and Thursday.
   b. The office is open from 8:30 a.m. to 4:30 p.m. on Wednesday and Friday.
   c. Create the matrix in 15-minute intervals. Appointments are based on 15-, 30-, 45-, and 60-minute intervals.

   d. The providers' hours are: Dr. Greer—Monday from 8:30 a.m. to 3 p.m., Tuesday none, Wednesday from 8:30 a.m. to 4:30 p.m., Thursday from 1 p.m. to 7 p.m., Friday from 8:30 a.m. to 1 p.m.; Dr. Rodriguez—Monday from 12:30 p.m. to 7 p.m., Tuesday from 8:30 a.m. to 4 p.m., Wednesday none, Thursday from 8:30 a.m. to 4 p.m., Friday from 8:30 a.m. to 1 p.m.; Dr. Wilson—Monday none, Tuesday from 11 a.m. to 7 p.m., Wednesday from 8:30 a.m. to 3 p.m., Thursday from 8:30 a.m. to 4 p.m., Friday from 10 a.m. to 4:30 p.m.; Dr. Lee—Monday from 8:30 a.m. to 4 p.m., Tuesday from 12:30 p.m. to 7 p.m., Wednesday from 8:30 a.m. to 4:30 p.m., Thursday from 1 p.m. to 7 p.m., Friday from 8:30 a.m. to 4:30 p.m.; Ms. Piecek—Monday from 8:30 a.m. to 4:30 p.m., Tuesday from 8:30 a.m. to 1 p.m., Wednesday from 8:30 a.m. to 4:30 p.m., Thursday none, Friday from 8:30 a.m. to 4:30 p.m.
2. Block time for lunches for each provider. Providers working a late shift should be given a break later in the day. Blocking provider times for lunch and breaks allows them to respond to phone messages, eat, and catch up if they get behind schedule.
3. Print the appointment matrix to use at the front desk.

PROCEDURE 12-2—cont'd

4. Practice telephone procedures by taking five appointments on the phone (role-play with other students).
5. Two of the patients are new patients (NPs). To ensure complete records, obtain the appropriate information from these patients on the telephone:
   a. full name
   b. date of birth to check insurance coverage
   c. daytime phone number to contact them in case you need to change appointment or they are a no-show
   d. complete address to send practice information to the patient
   e. source of referral for marketing purposes
   f. insurance coverage to check insurance eligibility prior to patient visit
   g. reason for appointment to schedule the appropriate amount of time for the visit.

6. Role-play the remaining five appointments with students at the front desk to practice face-to-face appointment scheduling.
7. Schedule the following appointments:
   a. Candace Burns—flu
   b. John Howard—NP
   c. Lynn Littel—sore throat
   d. Gary O'Neil—NP smoking cessation
   e. Jeff Ramirez—suture removal
   f. Cindy Pantarella—adult PE
   g. Hannah Collins—BP check
   h. Sadie Hernandez—cast removal
   i. Christopher Evans—sports PE
   j. Jill Evans—sports PE.

Appointment Sheet

Friday, January 22nd

Time	Name	Room	Duration	Reason
9:00	Maria Ortiz	Room 1	30 minutes	Sports physical
9:15	Joe Kramer	Room 2	45 minutes	New patient
11:15	Susan Howard	Room 1	30 minutes	URI
11:30	Tara Olsen	Room 2	45 minutes	New patient
11:45	Walter Sims	Room 1	30 minutes	BP & heart check
12:00		**LUNCH**		
1:30	Hannah Collins	Room 2	45 minutes	PE/Laboratory work
1:45	Les Collins	Room 1	15 minutes	BP check
2:15	Sarah Goren	Room 1	45 minutes	New patient
2:30	Jessica Vente	Room 2	30 minutes	Sports physical
3:00	Nora Williams	Room 1	30 minutes	Sports physical
3:15	Mike Williams	Room 2	30 minutes	Sports physical
3:30	Chris O'Connell	Room 1	15 minutes	BP check
4:00	Joe Hart	Room 2	45 minutes	New patient

FIG 12-2 Computerized appointment system day sheet.

with patients, an extra assistant can be added to accommodate school physicals or vaccinations.

Manual Appointment Book System

A manual appointment book serves as a written record of patient appointments for each day. Books are organized by time, room, or physician as in a computerized system. Although most offices are computerized, the manual appointment book system is always available and can be the primary schedule or used as a backup to a computerized system. As in a computerized system, the manual daily appointment sheet, which is generally a photocopy of that day's page of the appointment book, shows the names of patients scheduled for the day, the treatment room for each, and the length and purpose of the appointment. Each day, the medical assistant should make copies of the sheet and post them in the administrative and clinical areas so that staff can anticipate the schedule. In addition, an appointment sheet can be used as a legal record of patient appointments. (See Figure 12-3.)

Daily Worksheet

In a manual or computerized system, the medical assistant may use a daily worksheet to show patient appointments as well as meetings with pharmaceutical representatives, physician or assistant time out of the office, staff meetings, and equipment maintenance. Although computerized appointment systems allow the medical assistant to input patient appointments and block time for other purposes, they will rarely allow her to add other notes without specific modifications to the software package. In any case, the medical assistant should print a hard copy of the computerized worksheet or photocopy the appointment book and add notes for the staff. Such a worksheet provides a complete picture of staff activities for the day. (See Figure 12-4.)

Appointment Changes and Cancellations

Patients are commonly busy people who may need to cancel or reschedule appointments to fit their work schedule and various commitments. When a patient cancels an appointment, it must be noted in the patient's chart. In the event that the patient does not come in for follow-up care and her health suffers, the cancelled appointment can show that the physician's office was not negligent in scheduling follow-up visits. If applicable, it is also wise to indicate that the office offered the patient a new appointment, but that she failed to reschedule. (See *Procedure 12-3: Documenting appointment cancellations and no-shows and rescheduling appointments,* page 144.)

Computerized Changes and Cancellations

Rescheduling or cancelling appointments in the computerized system commonly does not leave a record of the appointment change. The appointment is removed from the system to accommodate a new appointment in that time slot. The recording of the appointment change in the patient's chart is, therefore, the only record of the cancelled appointment. No-show appointments, also called *failed appointments,* may be noted in the computerized system because that time slot cannot be used for another patient.

Charging for Cancelled Visits or Denying Future Visits

Because revenue is lost when a patient's time slot is not filled, some offices have charge policies for no-show or cancelled appointments. If a patient is a no-show or cancels within 24 hours of the appointment time, the office may choose to charge the patient for the copayment amount. The charge policy of the office must be in accordance with state and insurance guidelines. The office may also deny future appointments to a patient who chronically cancels or fails to appear for appointments. When dealing with this type of patient, it is imperative that the medical assistant be clear about the policy of the office regarding charges or denials of visits. (See *Why do some patients cancel?*)

Triage for Setting Appointments

When a patient calls the office for an appointment, the medical assistant must conduct **triage**, or an evaluation of the urgency of the patient's condition. A patient calling for a routine checkup or physical is not an emergency and the medical assistant can schedule this patient at any time that

---

Why do some patients cancel?

Some patients may have "chronic cancelitis"; that is, they repeatedly cancel their appointments. A patient may repeatedly cancel appointments because of:

- fear of a diagnosis or bad news
- financial constraints
- fear of needles or pain
- shame about mental illness or sexually transmitted disease
- fear that the office staff will mock or judge him.

Treating chronic "cancelitis"

Patients who chronically cancel may benefit from a conversation with a staff member about payment plans or sliding-scale fees as well as the physician's obligation to keep information confidential and educate patients as needed. The medical assistant plays an important role in ensuring that patients understand the professional obligations of the medical staff.

Appointment Sheet

Friday, January 22nd

9:00	Maria Ortiz	Room 1	30 minutes	Sports physical
9:15	Joe Kramer	Room 2	45 minutes	New patient
9:30				
9:45				
10:00				
10:15				
10:30				
10:45				
11:00				
11:15	Susan Howard	Room 1	30 minutes	URI
11:30	Tara Olsen	Room 2	45 minutes	New patient
11:45	Walter Sims	Room 1	30 minutes	BP & heart check
12:00	LUNCH			
12:15	LUNCH			
12:30	LUNCH			
12:45	LUNCH			
1:00	LUNCH			
1:15	LUNCH			
1:30	Hannah Collins	Room 2	45 minutes	PE/Laboratory work
1:45	Les Collins	Room 1	15 minutes	BP check
2:00				
2:15	Sarah Goren	Room 1	45 minutes	New patient
2:30	Jessica Vente	Room 2	30 minutes	Sports physical
2:45				
3:00	Nora Williams	Room 1	30 minutes	Sports physical
3:15	Mike Williams	Room 2	30 minutes	Sports physical
3:30	Chris O'Connell	Room 1	15 minutes	BP check
3:45				
4:00	Joe Hart	Room 2	45 minutes	New patient

FIG 12-3 Manual appointment sheet.

is convenient for the office and the patient. If, however, the medical assistant determines that the patient needs immediate attention, she can direct the patient to come in immediately or go to the emergency room. When questioning patients on the phone, the medical assistant must be careful to get the needed information without panicking the patient or trivializing the situation. Asking clear, concise, open-ended questions will elicit the information needed. Examples of items to ask include:

- How long have you had the symptoms?
- Where is the pain? How intense is the pain? Does it radiate?
- Where is the origin of the bleeding or discharge? How profuse?
- If fever, how high? (See *Phone triage notes,* page 145.)

This type of appointment triage is for phone appointment requests only. If a patient appears in the office without an appointment but is a possible emergency situation, it is considered an office emergency. (See Chapter 47, "Office Emergencies," page 967, for more information.)

✦ **TIP** Tele-Triage

Each medical office should have a triage "what-to-do" sheet near every phone. The list should contain questions to ask if the call is a medical emergency; for example:

- "Who is the patient?"
- "Is the patient conscious?"
- "Is the patient breathing?"
- "Where are you calling from?"

Daily Worksheet

Friday, January 22nd

Time	Name	Room	Duration	Reason
9:00	Maria Ortiz	Room 1	30 minutes	Sports physical
9:15	Joe Kramer	Room 2	45 minutes	New patient
10:00	Dr. Greer out of office – dentist appointment			
11:15	Susan Howard	Room 1	30 minutes	URI
11:30	Tara Olsen	Room 2	45 minutes	New patient
11:45	Walter Sims	Room 1	30 minutes	BP & heart check
12:00	Meet with pharmaceutical rep regarding new lipid-lowering drug			
1:30	Hannah Collins	Room 2	45 minutes	PE/Laboratory work
1:45	Les Collins	Room 1	15 minutes	BP check
2:00	Centrifuge calibration – call ABC Electronics to confirm			
2:15	Sarah Goren	Room 1	45 minutes	New patient
2:30	Jessica Vente	Room 2	30 minutes	Sports physical
2:45	UPS pickup for broken hemocytometer			
3:00	Nora Williams	Room 1	30 minutes	Sports physical
3:15	Mike Williams	Room 2	30 minutes	Sports physical
3:30	Chris O'Connell	Room 1	15 minutes	BP check
3:45	Sarah's husband is coming in to change light fixture in room 1			
4:00	Joe Hart	Room 2	45 minutes	New patient

FIG 12-4 Daily worksheet. (A) Computerized daily worksheet.

Daily Worksheet

Friday, January 22nd

9:00 _Maria Ortiz   Room 1   30 minutes   Sports physical_

9:15 _Joe Kramer   Room 2   45 minutes   New patient_

9:30 _____

9:45 _____

10:00 _Dr. Greer out of office – dentist appointment_

10:15 _____

10:30 _____

10:45 _____

11:00 _____

11:15 _Susan Howard   Room 1   30 minutes   URI_

11:30 _Tara Olsen   Room 2   45 minutes   New patient_

11:45 _Walter Sims   Room 1   30 minutes   BP & heart check_

12:00 _Meet with pharmaceutical rep regarding new lipid-lowering drug_

12:15 _LUNCH_

12:30 _LUNCH_

12:45 _LUNCH_

1:00 _LUNCH_

1:15 _LUNCH_

1:30 _Hannah Collins   Room 2   45 minutes   PE/Laboratory work_

1:45 _Les Collins   Room 1   15 minutes   BP check_

2:00 _Centrifuge calibration – call ABC Electronics to confirm_

2:15 _Sarah Goren   Room 1   45 minutes   New patient_

2:30 _Jessica Vente   Room 2   30 minutes   Sports physical_

2:45 _UPS pickup for broken hemocytometer_

3:00 _Nora Williams   Room 1   30 minutes   Sports physical_

3:15 _Mike Williams   Room 2   30 minutes   Sports physical_

3:30 _Chris O'Connell Room 1   15 minutes   BP check_

3:45 _Sarah's husband is coming In to change light fixture in room 1_

4:00 _Joe Hart   Room 2   45 minutes   New patient_

(B) Manual daily worksheet.

PROCEDURE 12-3

Documenting appointmet cancellations and no-shows and rescheduling appointments

Task
Document cancellations and no-shows and reschedule appointments.

Conditions
- Appointment matrix created in Procedure 12-1 on page 138
- Pen

Standards
In the time specified and within the scoring parameters determined by the instructor, the student will successfully document three cancelled appointments and reschedule these appointments and document a no-show appointment in the appointment matrix and call the no-show patient to reschedule.

Performance Standards
Telephone role-play several scenarios with a classmate.

Scenario 1
1. Lynn Littel has a sore throat and needs to reschedule her appointment for Wednesday after 3:30 p.m.
2. Mark Ms. Littel's appointment as cancelled in the appointment matrix to allow that time slot to be used by another patient and reschedule her appointment.
3. Repeat the new date and time of the appointment to Ms. Littel to ensure that the patient has the correct date and time.

Scenario 2
1. Mrs. Evans calls regarding Christopher and Jill's appointments. She needs to bring Jill on Tuesday (any time) and Christopher on Thursday or Friday when he is home from soccer camp.
2. Mark Christopher and Jill's appointments as cancelled and reschedule their appointments. Repeat the new dates and times to Mrs. Evans to ensure communication.

Scenario 3
1. John Howard did not show up for his appointment with the nurse practitioner (NP). Call Mr. Howard and identify yourself and the practice to ensure that the patient knows who is calling.
2. Tell him that he had an appointment on the date and at the time specified in your appointment matrix to inform him of the purpose of your call.
3. Ask him to reschedule. If he chooses to do so, reschedule the appointment.
4. Inform him of the no-show policy of the office (if a charge applies to no-show appointments) so that he will be less inclined to fail to appear for another appointment.
5. If he chooses not to reschedule, tell him to call in the future if he needs care from the office. Remaining pleasant and professional may result in a future appointment.
6. Mark the no-show appointment in the matrix to ensure a complete record.
7. Mark the new appointment for Mr. Howard (if necessary) and add the new patient information for the new appointment to ensure a complete record.

Referral Procedures

A specialty office may require a referral from the patient's primary care provider for insurance reimbursement. When the medical assistant is scheduling an appointment over the phone, she must tell patients if they are required to bring a referral form at the time of the visit or if their primary care practitioner will be faxing a referral form. When working for a primary care practitioner, faxing referral forms or handing the referral form to the patient for specialty care happens during the office checkout procedure. The medical assistant may need to schedule appointments for hospital services for patients and should remember to include referral information to ensure eligibility for medical insurance payment. (See *Procedure 12-4: Scheduling inpatient and outpatient procedures.*)

✦ TIP HIPAA TIP
Because faxing a referral form is considered a transmission of patient identifiable information, the record of each transmission must include a confirmation that the fax was received by the correct fax machine. The medical assistant should print the receipt and keep it in a designated fax transmission file for future reference.

Phone triage notes

Each office will have specific phone triage guidelines; the table below shows what scenarios need immediate attention and if the patient should go to the emergency room or call 911.

Scenario	Action
Difficulty breathing	Patient calls 911* or goes immediately to the emergency room.**
Chest pain	Patient calls 911* or goes immediately to the emergency room.**
Bleeding	Depending on the extent of bleeding: • patient comes to the office immediately. • for arterial bleeding, patient calls 911* or goes to the emergency room.**
Rash or fever	Patient comes in to the office ("work-in" patient appointment).
Possible allergic reaction	Medical assistant evaluates the reaction's severity on the phone: • patient with breathing difficulty goes to the emergency room.** • patient with minor allergic reaction (such as swelling or rash) comes to office immediately.
Wounds or possible fractures	Patient comes to the office if the medical assistant determines that the wound or fracture is minor. (An orthopedic office may see a possible fracture in the office or direct the patient to the emergency room** and send the on-call physician to meet them.)

* When directing a patient to call 911, the office policy may be to stay on the line with the patient while another employee calls 911 and reports the emergency and the address. A child or hysterical adult would never be directed to place the 911 call without help. Discussing these potential situations with all staff members ensures that policies for emergency phone calls will be consistent.

** Only direct people to drive to the emergency room if there is a driver *other than the patient* available.

PROCEDURE 12-4

Scheduling inpatient and outpatient procedures

Task

Schedule a patient for one inpatient and two outpatient procedures using the physician's orders and obtain proper precertification and referrals.

Conditions

- Physician's orders
- Two copies of a blank referral form
- Hospital precertification form
- Patient's medical record (office notes)
- Reminder card
- Pen

Standards

In the time specified and within the scoring parameters determined by the instructor, the student will successfully complete a referral form for hospital admission precertification and outpatient specialty referrals and schedule related procedures.

Performance Standards

1. Make an extra copy of the blank referral form provided on page 148.

2. Refer to the physician's order for MRI, arthroscopic surgery, and physical therapy for Lynn Olsen. Carefully read the physician's orders to avoid errors or confusion. Role-play the following steps with another student.

MRI referral

3. Call the patient's insurance carrier for referral approval and a referral number to ensure that the insurance carrier will pay for the procedure.

4. Using the information gathered from the order, the photocopy of the insurance card, Ms. Olsen's office notes, and the insurance phone call, complete the referral form for an MRI scan, according to managed care policies and procedures to ensure third-party guidelines are followed and reimbursement is not compromised.

5. Check the referral for spelling and completeness to ensure accuracy.

6. Call the MRI scheduler with Ms. Olsen at the desk and coordinate between the hospital's schedule and the patient to avoid scheduling conflicts.

Continued

PROCEDURE 12-4—cont'd

7. Give Ms. Olsen a reminder card with the scheduled appointment to remind the patient of the date and time of the scan.

8. Ask Ms. Olsen if she needs directions to the MRI facility and provide them as needed.

Arthroscopic surgery precertification

9. Refer to treatment notes from 10/03/08.

10. Call the patient's insurance carrier for precertification to ensure payment for the procedure.

11. Using the necessary documentation, complete the hospital precertification for surgery according to third-party guidelines, being sure to include a precertification number to ensure payment.

12. Check the precertification for completeness and accuracy to ensure proper documentation and payment.

13. Schedule the surgery with the patient and the hospital scheduler to avoid scheduling conflicts for the patient.

Physical therapy referral

14. Refer to the patient's office notes from 10/14/08, post-surgical checkup.

15. Refer to the second outpatient services referral form for Lynn Olsen's postsurgical care.

16. Using the physician's orders, operative notes, and treatment notes, complete the referral form for physical therapy (according to the managed care policy), being sure to check for completeness and accuracy.

17. Call the PT office to schedule the first PT visit while the patient is present to avoid scheduling conflicts.

18. Submit all forms to your instructor for approval.

Physician's Orders

Blueville Family Medicine
15 Main Street
Blueville CT
860-555-3212

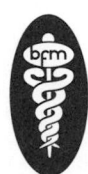

Robert Greer, MD
Hector Rodriguez, MD
Anne Wilson, MD
Sharon Piecek, APRN
Henry Lee, MD

Patient: *Lynn Olsen*

Date of Birth: 05/01/88

Arthroscopic repair of meniscal tear right knee. Patient to be seen in office 3 days postop. Arrange physical therapy to begin after postop check.

Preop Labs: *CBC*

Diagnosis: *Torn right medial meniscus; suspected lateral meniscal tear*

Hector Rodriguez, MD

PROCEDURE 12-4—cont'd

Patient treatment notes (from patient file)

09/28/08 – Patient presents with knee pain, limping favoring right leg. She states she was playing soccer yesterday and felt "something move inside my knee." Patient complains that after soccer game, the knee "locked." Pain is intermittent, sharp, and sometimes debilitating. Positive orthopedic findings: palpable click upon extension, + McMurray's test, pain upon compression and rotation, negative anterior draw test. Order MRI to confirm tear. H. Rodriguez, MD

10/03/08 – MRI of right knee 10/01/08 confirms medical meniscal tear; suspected lateral tear, cannot be confirmed. Order arthroscopic repair. H. Rodriguez, MD

10/14/08 – Postop check – arthroscopic procedure to right knee of 10/09/08. Repair of medial meniscal tear; no lateral tear was noted. Healing well, no postop swelling, no fever, no infection at scope sites. Schedule PT - 3X per week for 2 weeks, active ROM and strengthening. Return in 2 weeks for check. H. Rodriguez, MD

Photocopy of patient's insurance ID card:

ANTHEM BLUE CROSS AND BLUE SHIELD

Lynn Olsen
IDENTIFICATION NO: XJF0099888888
State Blue Care POE, $10.00

PCP: *Hector Rodriguez, MD*

Group Number: *8089933X*

Continued

Termination of Services

In addition to a verbal denial of appointments to a patient who chronically fails to appear for or cancels appointments, written communication is also necessary. Such a letter should indicate that the physician will no longer care for the patient. (For more information on such a letter, see Chapter 6, "Legal Considerations," page 53.)

Chapter Summary

- Appointment scheduling can impact quality of care and should follow a consistent system that creates an efficient workflow.
- Scheduling patients to fit the type of practice, space constraints, and availability of staff and equipment enables the best use of resources and profitable use of physician and staff time.
- Patients appreciate when scheduling decreases waiting time but does not require patients to be rushed through appointments.
- The medical assistant must obtain such standard information as the patient's name, telephone number, insurance carrier, and insurance ID number (as determined by the practice) to prepare adequately for patient visits.
- Patients should be scheduled by phone in a clear, concise, courteous manner. Phone calls should end with the medical assistant repeating the appointment time and date for extra clarification.
- Appointments scheduled in the office should include issuing a reminder card, collecting a copayment, and answering administrative questions as needed.

Team Work Exercises

1. Discuss which form of scheduling will be most efficient for the following types of practices:
   a. pediatrician (two physicians, two medical assistants, and one RN)

PROCEDURE 12-4—cont'd

Outpatient Services Referral

Blueville Family Medicine
15 Main Street
Blueville CT
860-555-3212

Robert Greer, MD
Hector Rodriguez, MD
Anne Wilson, MD
Sharon Piecek, APRN
Henry Lee, MD

Patient: _____

Date of Birth: _____   Gender: _____

Insurance Carrier: _____   Group #: _____

ID #: _____   Referral #: _____

Referred to _____

Facility address _____

Facility phone _____

First appointment date _____

Reason for referral _____

Physician orders _____

_____

_____

_____

---

b. ophthalmologist (one physician and two medical assistants)

c. psychologist (one therapist and one medical assistant)

d. chiropractor (one physician and one medical assistant).

2. You work at a busy multiphysician office that is fully computerized. The schedule for the day has been printed and posted at the front desk and in the clinical area. At 3:00 p.m., the computer system stops working. Technical support has been called but the problem will not be resolved until at least 5:00 p.m. Discuss as a group solutions to your scheduling dilemma.

Case Studies

1. Kevin Donohue is scheduled for a stress test and heart checkup with Dr. Greer. He calls to cancel the appointment and says that he doesn't want to reschedule since he is "feeling great," and doesn't "want to waste the 10-dollar copayment." What should the medical assistant say to Kevin? What documentation should she send as a follow-up to the phone call? Should she speak to Dr. Greer?

2. Wendy O'Leary has just failed to appear for the fourth appointment in a row. The medical assistant calls her

PROCEDURE 12-4—cont'd

Hospital Precertification – Verification for Admission

Blueville Family Medicine
15 Main Street
Blueville CT
860-555-3212

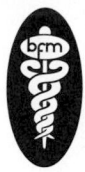

Robert Greer, MD
Hector Rodriguez, MD
Anne Wilson, MD
Sharon Piecek, APRN
Henry Lee, MD

Patient: _____

Date of Birth: _____ Gender: _____

Insurance Carrier: _____ Group #: _____

ID #: _____ Referral #: _____

Referred to _____

Facility address _____

Facility phone _____

Date of admission _____

Diagnosis _____

Approved length of stay _____

Surgical procedure(s) _____

Other procedure(s) _____

Copayment _____

---

house but only the answering machine answers. What type of message (if any) should the medical assistant leave? What should she say to Wendy if she calls for another appointment? Discuss with classmates and the instructor the various reasons patients fail to appear for or cancel multiple appointments.

Resources

These web sites are vendors for medical office scheduling software and include demonstration software:

- Appointment Quest: *www.appointmentquest.com/scheduling/healthcare*
- Leonardo MD Online Medicine: *www.LeonardoMD.com*
- Schedule View: *www.scheduleview.com/medicalscheduling-software.htm*

Written Office Communications and Mail

Learning Objectives

Upon completion of this chapter, the student will be able to:

- define the key terms as presented in the glossary
- describe the functions of written communications in the ambulatory care setting
- identify the various types of letters, notes, faxes, and e-mails that may be written by the medical assistant
- identify the parts of a letter in the four major letter styles
- compose business letters to patients, attorneys, and insurance companies
- identify the various types of incoming mail to the office
- proofread documents for grammar, spelling, and content
- address envelopes consistent with postal regulations
- transcribe medical documents from audiotapes and written notes.

CAAHEP Competencies

General Competencies
Professional Communications
  Respond to and initiate written communications
Legal Concepts
  Identify and respond to issues of confidentiality

Perform within legal and ethical boundaries
Establish and maintain the medical record

ABHES Competencies

Communication
  Receive, organize, prioritize, and transmit information expediently
  Use correct grammar, spelling, and formatting techniques in written works
  Apply electronic technology
  Master fundamental writing skills
Administrative Duties
  Perform basic secretarial skills
  Locate resources and information for patients and employers
Legal Concepts
  Follow established policy in initiating or terminating medical treatment

Procedures
  Responding to written communications
  Initiating written communications

Chapter Outline
  Communications and the Medical Office
  Business Letters
    Four Styles for Letters
    Letters to Patients
    Letters to Physicians
    Letters to Attorneys

Faxed Documents
Preparing an Envelope
Internal Marketing
  Reminder Notes
  Birthdays and Holidays
  Generating Referrals
E-mail Guidelines
Incoming Mail
Transcription of Medical Documents
Chapter Summary
Teamwork Exercises
Case Studies
Resources

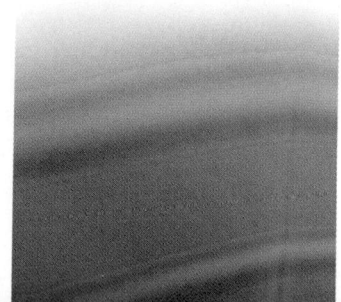

Key Terms

business letter
Formal document sent by mail that contains information related to business, rather than personal, affairs

dictation
Creation of a tape or computer voice file to be transcribed

internal marketing
Method used to stimulate business with existing patients through mailings and other means

proofread
Check of a written document for accuracy in spelling, punctuation, grammar, word choice, and sentence structure

summary of care
Written description of assessment, services (procedures), and outcomes of care provided to a patient

transcription
Creation of a written document from dictated tapes or computer voice files

Communications and the Medical Office

Written communication in the medical office is an important responsibility of the administrative medical assistant. Clear, concise, professional communications reflect the professionalism of the medical assistant and the medical office. Correspondence to patients, referring physicians, attorneys, and insurance carriers should be thoughtfully composed and mailed in a timely and cost-effective manner. To ensure professionalism, the medical assistant should **proofread** these communications, which involves checking for accuracy in spelling, punctuation, grammar, word choice, and sentence structure. Health Information Portability and Acountability Act (HIPAA) guidelines must be considered when choosing letters, faxes, and e-mail as the appropriate form of written communication. Confidentiality of written communications is important to safeguard a patient's medical and financial information.

Business Letters

The **business letter** is used when a formal document is needed. Copies of letters to patients, referring physicians, or attorneys should be placed in the patient file. Electronic backup on USB drives or CD-ROM ensures that the correspondence is recorded.

Business letters include:

- *date*—date on which the letter is written (Position the date according to the style of letter used.)
- *inside address*—name, address, and zip code of the letter's recipient
- *attention line*—specific person to whom the letter should be delivered (If the recipient's name is not known, a title or specific department can be used.)

    Example: MEDICAL DIRECTOR
    BILLING DEPARTMENT

- *salutation*—greeting that begins the letter by addressing the recipient (Capitalize the first letter of each word. Use *Miss* or *Ms.*, as preferred by recipient, if known; use *To Whom it May Concern* if name is not known.)

    Example: Dear Mrs. Smith

- *subject or regarding line*—brief explanation of the purpose of the letter

    Examples: ACCOUNT OVERDUE
    PHYSICAL THERAPY SERVICES

- *body*—message of the letter
- *closing*—ending of the letter

- *signature line*—name and title of the person who signs the letter
- *reference notation*—abbreviation at the bottom of the last page of the letter that is used to identify the person who typed the letter
- *enclosure notation*—indication for the reader of any materials enclosed with the letter
- *copy notation*—list of the people that received the letter in addition to the addressee. (See *Elements of a business letter.*)

Elements of a business letter

The following letter includes the different elements that can be included in a business letter.

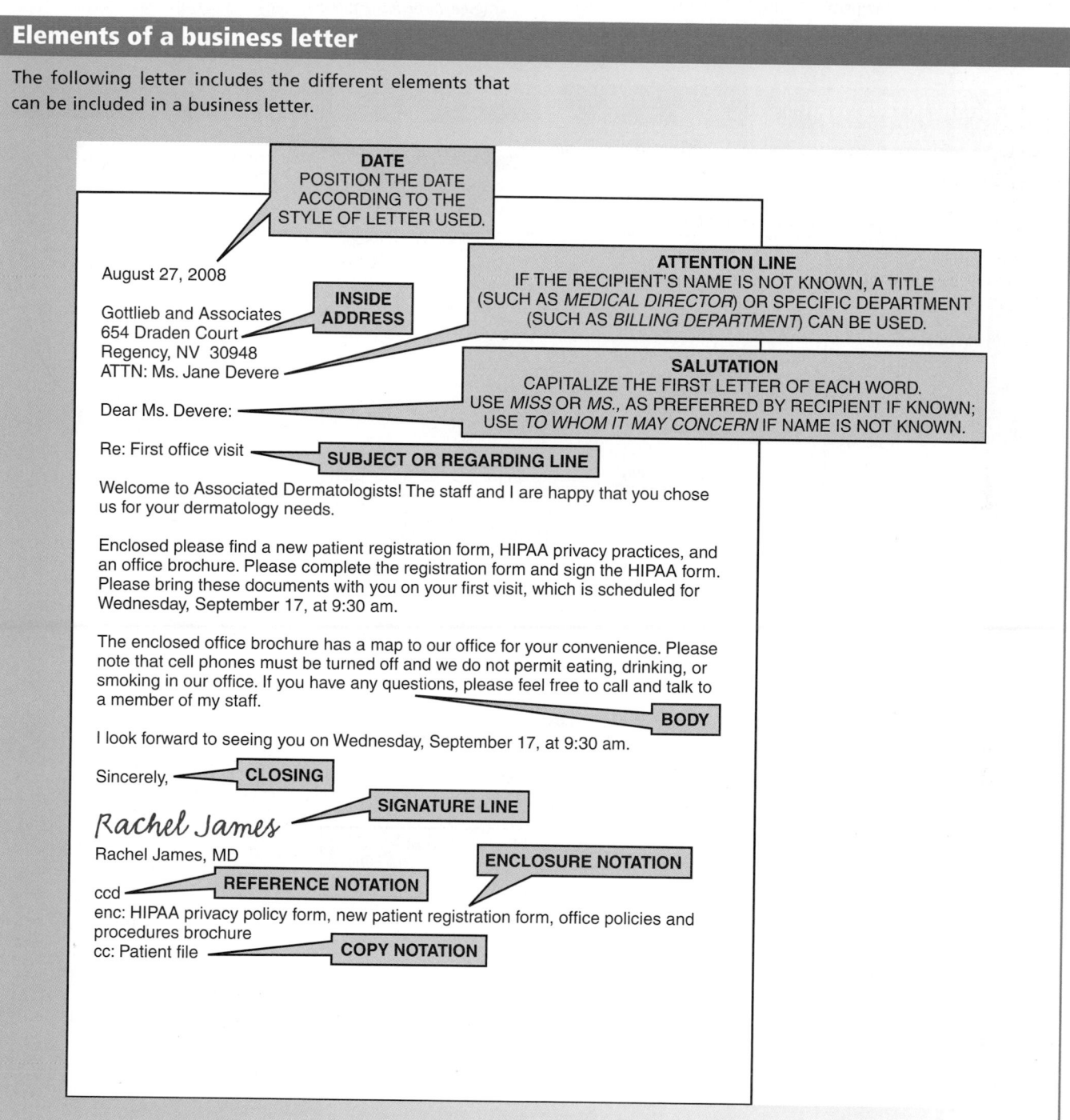

Four Styles for Letters

Letters can be written in four basic styles:

- *full-block*—most common format for business letters, with all lines in standard letter format, flush left
- *modified-block*—typed with all lines beginning at the left margin, with the exception of the date line, complimentary closing, and the keyed signature, all of which are aligned with each other, flush left with the left margin set in the center of the document
- *indented*—typed with the first line of each paragraph indented 5 spaces
- *simplified*—typed with all lines flush with the left margin but omitting the salutation and complimentary closing. (See *Four basic letter styles*.)

Four basic letter styles

Following are examples, using the same letter, of the four basic letter styles.

FULL-BLOCK LETTER

April 28, 2008

John Taylor
123 Main Street
Abraham, ME 54321

Dear Mr. Taylor,

Re: Lions Club Meeting — ALL LINES FLUSH LEFT

Thank you for inviting me to speak at the Willington Lions Club Meeting on July 14 at 7 pm as requested. My topic will be the use of statin drugs versus alternative methods of lowering cholesterol. I will discuss with the group what cholesterol is (both "good" and "bad"), how it affects the body, and how it is assessed. I will explain to the group the role of the liver in cholesterol production and alternatives to statins and other medications.

Since the Lions were very active in the town basketball tournament to raise money for the school, I will include some statistics on exercise and cholesterol that I hope the group finds interesting.

I will need a projector and a screen. I can bring my laptop, as my PowerPoint presentation is on a USB drive. I will provide handouts.

I look forward to seeing you on July 14th.

Sincerely,

FOUR LINE SPACES TO LEAVE ROOM FOR SIGNATURE

Wendy Janick, ND

Four basic letter styles—cont'd

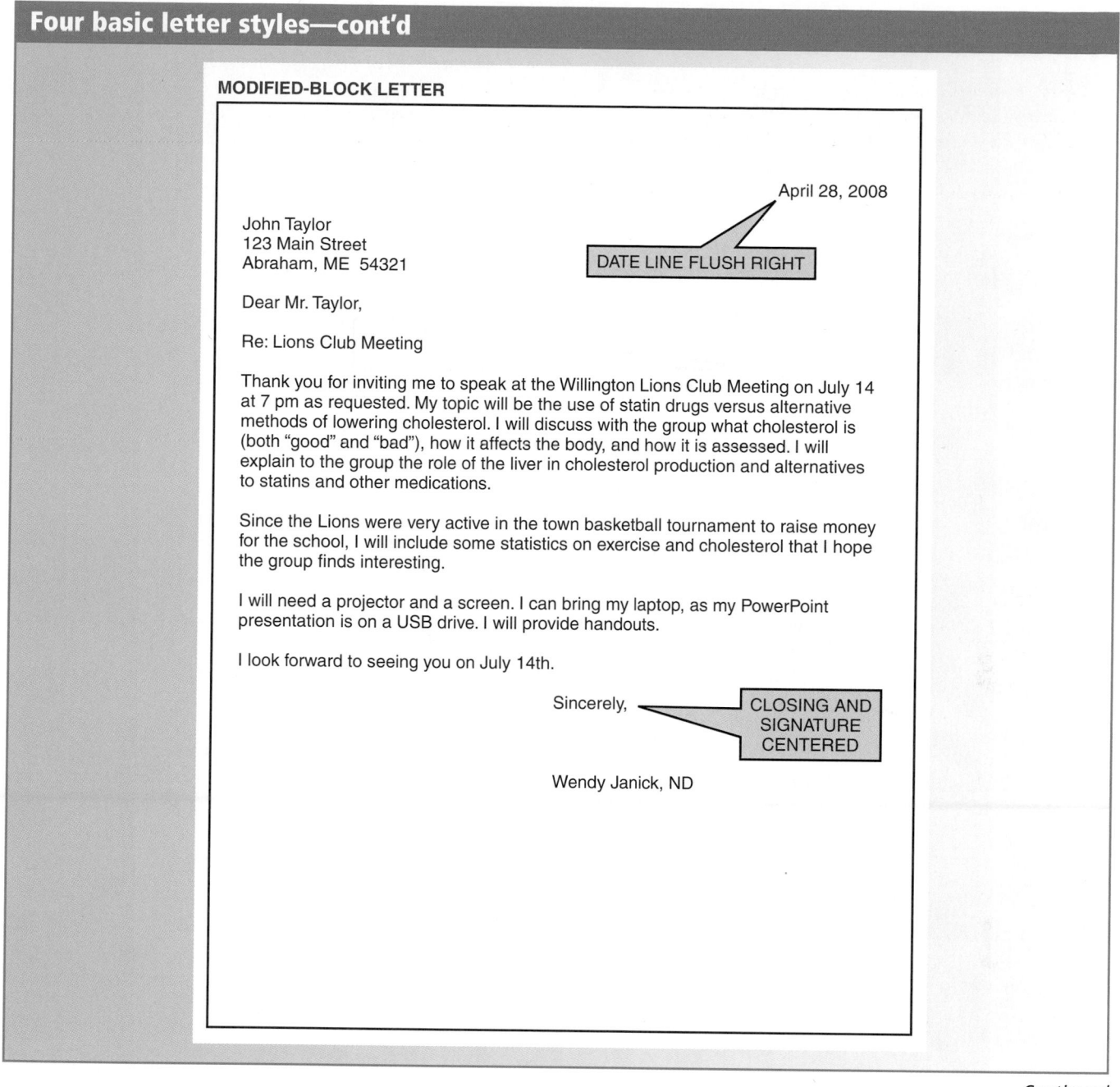

MODIFIED-BLOCK LETTER

April 28, 2008

DATE LINE FLUSH RIGHT

John Taylor
123 Main Street
Abraham, ME 54321

Dear Mr. Taylor,

Re: Lions Club Meeting

Thank you for inviting me to speak at the Willington Lions Club Meeting on July 14 at 7 pm as requested. My topic will be the use of statin drugs versus alternative methods of lowering cholesterol. I will discuss with the group what cholesterol is (both "good" and "bad"), how it affects the body, and how it is assessed. I will explain to the group the role of the liver in cholesterol production and alternatives to statins and other medications.

Since the Lions were very active in the town basketball tournament to raise money for the school, I will include some statistics on exercise and cholesterol that I hope the group finds interesting.

I will need a projector and a screen. I can bring my laptop, as my PowerPoint presentation is on a USB drive. I will provide handouts.

I look forward to seeing you on July 14th.

Sincerely,

CLOSING AND SIGNATURE CENTERED

Wendy Janick, ND

Continued

Letters to Patients

Written correspondence to patients is common and can serve many functions. The administrative medical assistant can send bills, medical information, or discontinuance of care notification. Here are the different types of letters sent to patients:

- *Financial*—The medical assistant may bill a patient monthly for outstanding copayments or unpaid portions of insurance billings. (See Chapter 17 for a full discussion of this form of written communication to patients.)

- *Medical information*—The medical assistant may send written documentation of a patient's condition to him in a letter—but only after the physician has spoken to the patient and explained his condition. The letter serves as confirmation of the conversation with the patient and is never used alone to convey medical information. (See *Procedure 13-1: Responding to written communications*, pages 157 and 158.)

Four basic letter styles—cont'd

INDENTED LETTER

April 28, 2008

John Taylor
123 Main Street
Abraham, ME 54321

Dear Mr. Taylor,

Re: Lions Club Meeting

PARAGRAPHS INDENTED 5 SPACES

Thank you for inviting me to speak at the Willington Lions Club Meeting on July 14 at 7 pm as requested. My topic will be the use of statin drugs versus alternative methods of lowering cholesterol. I will discuss with the group what cholesterol is (both "good" and "bad"), how it affects the body, and how it is assessed. I will explain to the group the role of the liver in cholesterol production and alternatives to statins and other medications.

Since the Lions were very active in the town basketball tournament to raise money for the school, I will include some statistics on exercise and cholesterol that I hope the group finds interesting.

I will need a projector and a screen. I can bring my laptop, as my PowerPoint presentation is on a USB drive. I will provide handouts.

I look forward to seeing you on July 14th.

Sincerely,

Wendy Janick, ND

- *Discontinuance of care*—Patients who don't comply with treatment recommendations can be released from care if notice is given in writing. A certified letter ensures that the patient has received notification and that the doctor is no longer responsible for caring for the patient. (See *Letter to discontinue care,* page 159.) Be sure to place a copy of the release of care letter in the patient's file for permanent record keeping. (See Chapter 6 for a full discussion of the physician's legal obligations of care to the patient and how to suspend such obligation if necessary.)

Letters to Physicians

A physician may write to another physician to thank her for referrals, convey patient information, or inform her of new procedures offered at his office in order to solicit referrals. (See *Procedure 13-2: Initiating written communications,* page 160.)

Letters to Attorneys

Attorneys will correspond with a physician's office if the patient's injuries were the result of an accident or a

Four basic letter styles—cont'd

SIMPLIFIED

April 28, 2008

John Taylor
123 Main Street
Abraham, ME 54321   → OMIT SALUTATION

Re: Lions Club Meeting

Thank you for inviting me to speak at the Willington Lions Club Meeting on July 14 at 7 pm as requested. My topic will be the use of statin drugs versus alternative methods of lowering cholesterol. I will discuss with the group what cholesterol is (both "good" and "bad"), how it affects the body, and how it is assessed. I will explain to the group the role of the liver in cholesterol production and alternatives to statins and other medications.

Since the Lions were very active in the town basketball tournament to raise money for the school, I will include some statistics on exercise and cholesterol that I hope the group finds interesting.

I will need a projector and a screen. I can bring my laptop, as my PowerPoint presentation is on a USB drive. I will provide handouts.

I look forward to seeing you on July 14th.

Wendy Janick, ND   → OMIT CLOSING
                     → SIGNATURE (TYPED OR HANDWRITTEN)

PROCEDURE 13-1

Responding to written communications

Task

Respond to a written communication.

Conditions

- Correspondence from an outside party
- Patient chart
- Paper
- Computer

Standards

In the time specified and within scoring parameters determined by the instructor, the student will successfully respond to written correspondence by creating a response letter.

Performance Standards

1. Read the correspondence received by the office from an outside party to determine what kind of response is required.

Continued

> **Law Offices of Mark Gesmond, JD**
> **27 Crandon Way**
> **Blueville CT 06000**
>
> May 19, 2008
>
> Dr. Hector Rodriguez
> Blueville Family Medicine
> 15 Main Street
> Blueville, CT 06000
>
> RE: David Swartz
> DOI: January 13, 2008
>
> Dear Dr. Rodriguez,
>
> Please be advised that this office represents Mr. David Swartz for injuries sustained in an automobile accident on 01/13/08. Please send reports and notes related to Mr. Swartz's treatment at your office. If you have any questions, please call my office at 555-0989.
>
> Thank you,
>
> *Tina Sawyer*
>
> Paralegal

2. Choose the appropriate letter style for the required response.

3. Construct a response letter. Use information from the patient's chart to ensure accuracy as well as appropriate language, grammar, and spelling to convey professionalism in the letter.

Date	
01/17/08; 9:40 a.m.	Patient entered with sharp, stabbing pain in the neck and left shoulder. He states that he was in an auto accident on 01/13/08 where he was hit from the right front and collided with a guard rail on the opposite side. He states that the pain has gotten progressively worse over the past few days. He has been unable to sleep; Tylenol and hot packs give minimal relief. X-rays at ED are negative for fracture or pathology. Rx - Motrin 800 mg PRN for pain. ——————————————————— C. Smith, CMA

Date	
01/22/08; 10:05 a.m.	Patient states that the pain is less, continuing Motrin allows him to sleep. He will return if necessary. ——— Released from care. ———————————— C. Smith, CMA

4. Proofread the letter so you can catch errors before sending it.

5. Place the letter on the physician's (instructor's) desk for her review and signature.

6. Photocopy the signed letter and put a copy in the patient's chart.

7. Using the computer and printer, address the envelope and indicate on the envelope the amount of postage that you would affix in the correct area for postage.

Letter to discontinue care

The following is an example of a letter written to a patient to discontinue providing medical care for that patient. The medical assistant should be sure to place a copy of the letter in the patient's file.

May 5, 2008

Mr. Hank Thomas
10 Elm Street
Hartford, CT 06100

Dear Mr. Thomas,

Due to your continued lack of concern for your high blood pressure, diabetes, and obesity, I am withdrawing my services as your physician. You have consistently cancelled appointments, failed to take prescribed medications, and refused to follow the weight-loss diet that was outlined for you in the office on January 14, 2008.

I will forward your medical records to another physician upon your request.

Sincerely,

Michael Jones, MD

Michael Jones, MD
MJ: cb

PROCEDURE 13-2

Initiating written communications

Task
Initiate a written letter thanking a physician for a patient referral.

Conditions
- Patient chart
- Paper
- Computer

Standards
In the time specified and within the scoring parameters determined by the instructor, the student will successfully initiate written correspondence relating to patient care.

Performance Standards
1. Refer to the patient's chart, as needed, to obtain accurate information about the referral.
2. Choose the appropriate letter style for the required correspondence.
3. Construct a letter thanking a physician for a patient referral using appropriate language, grammar, and spelling to convey professionalism in the letter.
4. Proofread the letter so you can catch errors before sending it.
5. Place the letter on the physician's (instructor's) desk for her review and signature.

Dr. Daniel Greenberg
198 Ferguson Drive
Blueville, CT 06000

Name _Amanda Combs_

Date _10/14/08_

Acupuncture for chronic neck pain
× 5 weeks

---

worker's compensation injury. The physician's office is required to release information to attorneys only with the written authorization of the patient. Attorneys may request a physician to write a **summary of care** and perform a disability examination. (See *Summary of care letter.*)

✦ TIP Misspelling = Unprofessional
Misspelled words in written correspondence appear unprofessional and sloppy. The medical assistant should use the spellcheck function on the computer or a dictionary when unsure of a word's correct spelling. The medical assistant may also want to ask a coworker to **proofread** the letter before sending it to prevent embarrassment. (See *Commonly misspelled words*, page 162.)

Faxed Documents

Faxing documents that contain protected health information poses a risk of inappropriate disclosure. While it is permissible to transfer data via fax, the medical assistant should:

1. recheck the fax number before hitting send
2. recheck for authorization to release the information (See the Authorization to Release Protected Health

Summary of care letter

The following is an example of a summary of care letter written by a physician for use by the patient's attorney.

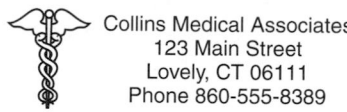

Collins Medical Associates
123 Main Street
Lovely, CT 06111
Phone 860-555-8389

August 19, 2008

Walter Simmons
Attorney at Law
14 Main Street
Lovely, CT 06111

RE: My Patient, Your Client, David Kowalski
Date of Injury: 08/15/08

History:

The patient entered this office on 08/18/08 stating that he had been in an auto accident on 08/15/08 where he struck another vehicle in the front right side. He relates the following complaints: neck pain and stiffness, headaches, dizziness, and intermittent numbness about the head. He reports that the symptoms have progressively worsened since the accident on 08/15/08.

After reviewing x-rays taken at the emergency room on 08/15/08, I note the following radiographic findings: No fracture or dislocation of the cervical and upper thoracic spine. Loss of cervical lordosis; no osseous pathology is noted.

Examination:

The patient's movements about the neck and upper body appear to be slow, stiff, and guarded. There is loss of cervical lordosis, with a slight head tilt to the right and the right shoulder is held higher than the left. Spasm and active tender trigger points are noted in the trapezius, levator, rhomboids, and posterior cervical musculature, most noted on the patient's right side. The patient's upper extremity deep tendon reflexes and dermatomes appear to be symmetrical and intact. Range of motion about the cervical spine is as follows: flexion, 25 degrees with pain and dizziness; extension, 10 degrees with pain at end range; right rotation, 50 degrees with pain and dizziness; left rotation, 60 degrees with mild discomfort; right lateral flexion, 15 degrees with pain; and left lateral flexion, 20 degrees with pain on the right side. Foraminal compression, Jackson's cervical compression to the right, and Soto Hall's test all exacerbate the patient's complaints.

Clinical Impression:

The patient is suffering from acute whiplash syndrome, myofascitis, radiculitis, and cephalgia as a result of the motor vehicle accident of 08/15/08.

Treatment Plan:

The patient will be treated with acupuncture, myofascial release, and range of motion exercises. He will be treated in this office 3 times per week for 3 weeks and then reevaluated. Updates to follow.

Sincerely,

Carol Jennings, D.O.
CJ:sg

Commonly misspelled words

The following list includes some of the most commonly mis-spelled words in medical correspondence. Knowing the correct spelling of these words will help ensure that correspondence from your office is clear and professional.

abscess	asthma	defibrillator	fissure	humerus	parenteral	specimen
aerobic	benign	desiccation	glaucoma	ischium	parietal	surgeon
aneurysm	capillary	dissect	hemorrhoid	occlusion	perineum	vaccine
asepsis	chancre	epididymis	homeostasis	osseus	peritoneum	

Information in Chapter 7, "HIPAA and a Patient's Rights," page 71.)

3. always use a cover sheet with an attention line. (See *Fax cover sheet*.)

Incoming faxes that contain protected health information should be taken from the fax machine and filed or covered as soon as possible. Leaving protected health information in a fax machine violates HIPAA regulations and increases the chance that the documents will be lost.

Preparing an Envelope

Envelopes should be printed on the computer. The printer paper tray can be adjusted to accommodate envelopes. (See the printer instructions for specific information.) The envelope should include a return address as well as a send-to address. Addresses should be keyed in all uppercase letters. (See *Addressing an envelope* and *Abbreviations for mailing addresses*.)

Fax cover sheet

Following is an example of a typical fax cover sheet used when sending health information via fax.

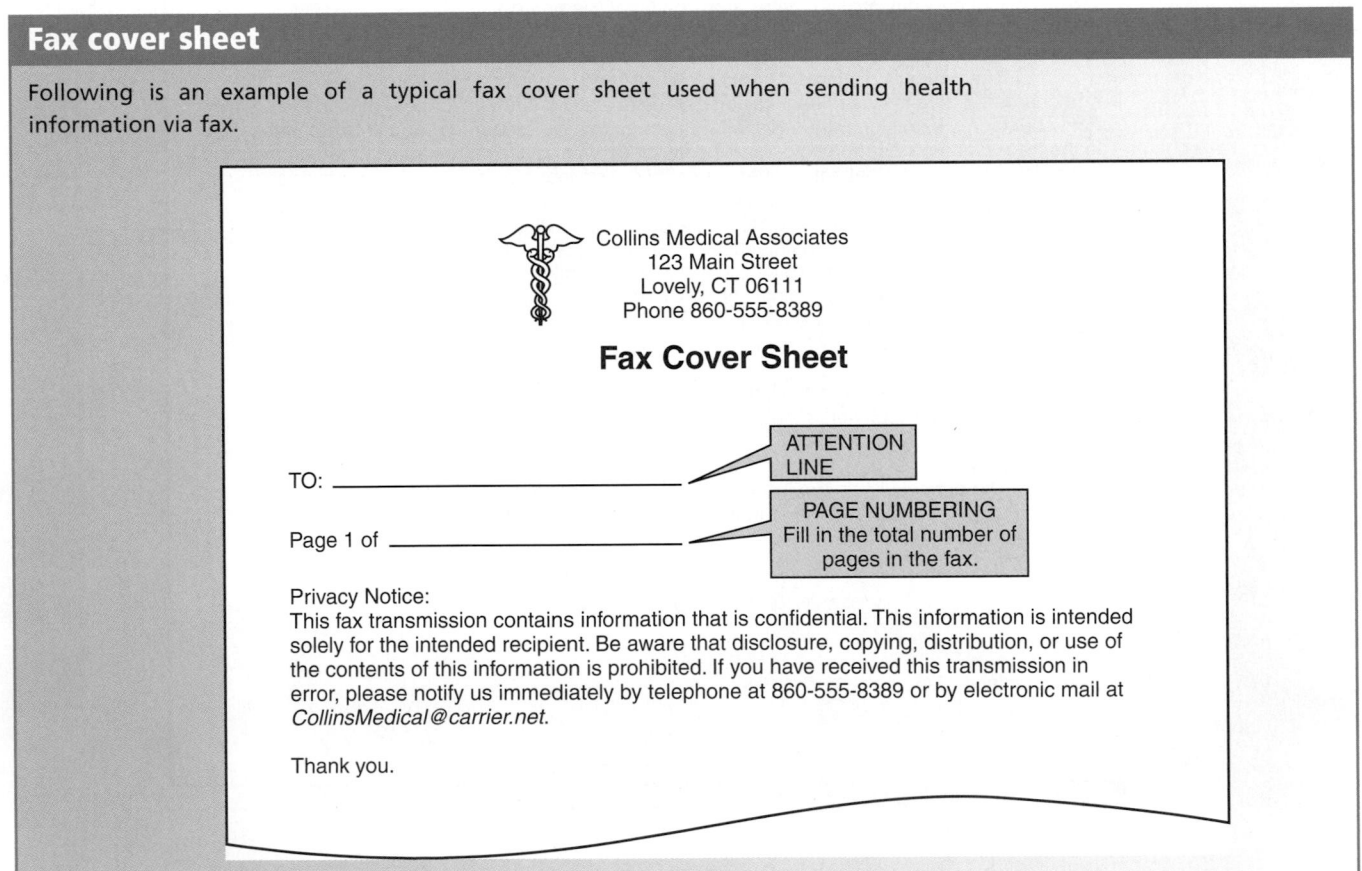

Collins Medical Associates
123 Main Street
Lovely, CT 06111
Phone 860-555-8389

Fax Cover Sheet

TO: _____   ATTENTION LINE

Page 1 of _____   PAGE NUMBERING
Fill in the total number of pages in the fax.

Privacy Notice:
This fax transmission contains information that is confidential. This information is intended solely for the intended recipient. Be aware that disclosure, copying, distribution, or use of the contents of this information is prohibited. If you have received this transmission in error, please notify us immediately by telephone at 860-555-8389 or by electronic mail at *CollinsMedical@carrier.net*.

Thank you.

Addressing an envelope

The following illustration shows how to address an envelope according to United States Postal Service regulations.

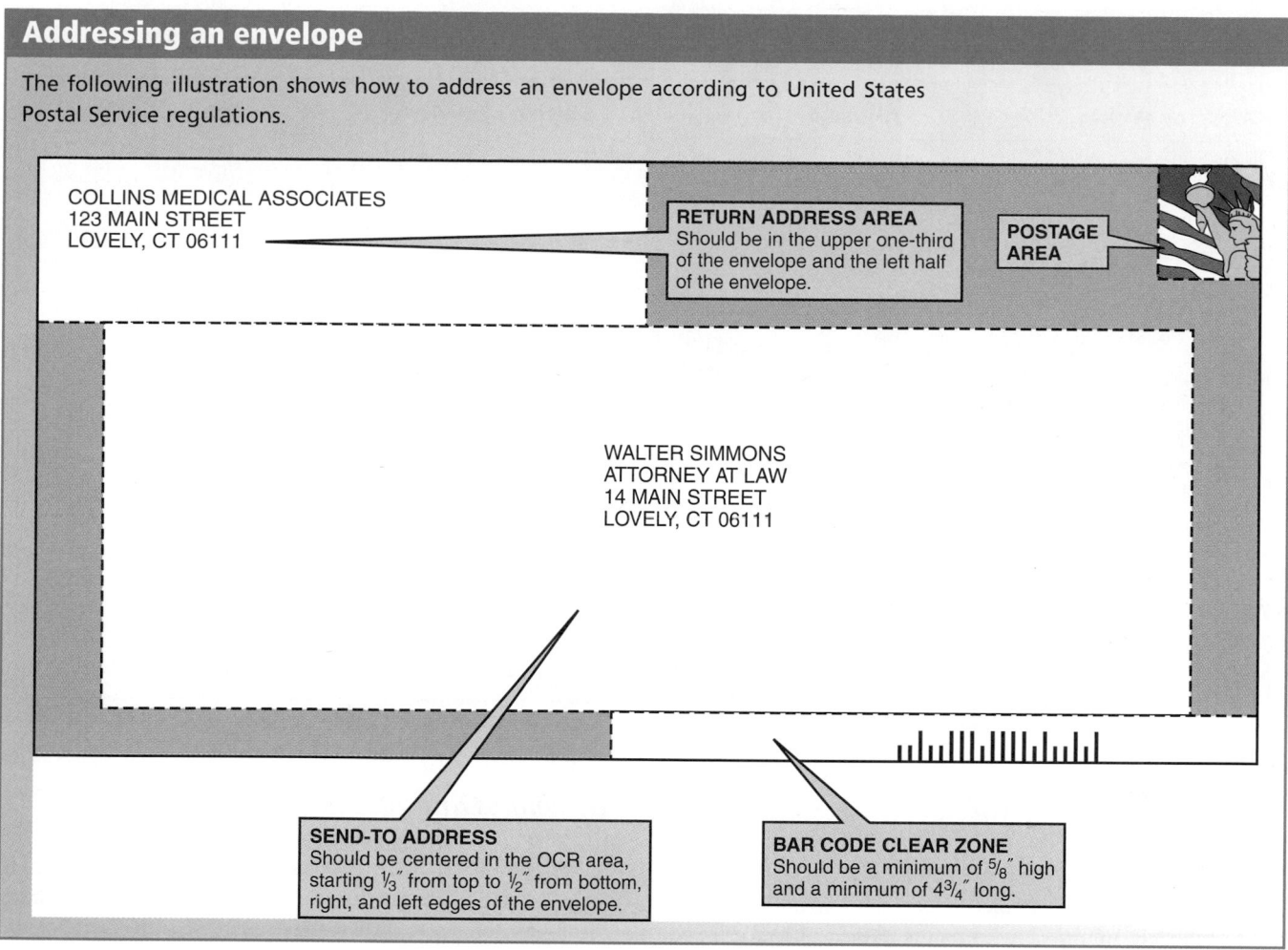

Abbreviations for mailing addresses

The table lists the states and provinces in the United States along with their postal abbreviations.

State or Province	Abbreviation	State or Province	Abbreviation
Alabama	AL	Montana	MT
Alaska	AK	Nebraska	NE
Arizona	AZ	Nevada	NV
Arkansas	AR	New Hampshire	NH
California	CA	New Jersey	NJ
Colorado	CO	New Mexico	NM
Connecticut	CT	New York	NY
Delaware	DE	North Carolina	NC
District of Columbia	DC	North Dakota	ND

Continued

Abbreviations for mailing addresses—cont'd

State or Province	Abbreviation	State or Province	Abbreviation
Florida	FL	Ohio	OH
Georgia	GA	Oklahoma	OK
Guam	GU	Oregon	OR
Hawaii	HI	Pennsylvania	PA
Idaho	ID	Puerto Rico	PR
Illinois	IL	Rhode Island	RI
Indiana	IN	South Carolina	SC
Iowa	IA	South Dakota	SD
Kansas	KS	Tennessee	TN
Kentucky	KY	Texas	TX
Louisiana	LA	Utah	UT
Maine	ME	Vermont	VT
Maryland	MD	Virgin Islands	VI
Massachusetts	MA	Virginia	VA
Michigan	MI	Washington	WA
Minnesota	MN	West Virginia	WV
Mississippi	MS	Wisconsin	WI
Missouri	MO	Wyoming	WY

Internal Marketing

Internal marketing is a way to remind patients to come into the office for care. For example, patients who are busy may forget to schedule routine appointments. Also, patients may be unaware of a new doctor in the practice, and internal marketing is a way to tell them about the services she will offer as well as other new services that the practice is offering. If the physicians purchase a new piece of equipment, such as an x-ray machine, patients can have their x-rays taken at the office, rather than having to go to a separate imaging facility. New HMO affiliations may enable patients to come back to the practice if they had previously left due to noncoverage of services. Specific medical updates, new medications, or procedures offered at the office can encourage patients to make an appointment. Having the patient receive information from the practice puts the practice name and phone number in the patient's hands, which can increase appointments. A gentle, friendly reminder helps patients make time for health care.

Reminder Notes

Written reminders tell busy patients that it is time to call the office to schedule their teeth cleaning, yearly physical, Pap smear, or other routine care appointments. These reminders are usually postcards. The postcards can reflect the upbeat atmosphere of the office by using cartoons and pictures. (See Figure 13-1.)

Birthdays and Holidays

Birthday and holiday greetings will also remind patients of their relationship to the office and may prompt them to make an appointment. Receiving birthday cards or holiday cards promotes a friendly relationship with the patient and the gesture is generally appreciated. Patients may refer friends and family to the "nice doctor who always remembers my birthday." (see Figure 13-2.)

✦ TIP Holiday Marketing

If the office decides to send holiday cards, be sure to send the appropriate religious card (such as for Christmas, Hanukkah, or Ramadan). Some offices opt to send Thanksgiving cards because most Americans celebrate Thanksgiving and fewer cards are received at that time. Thus, the card "stands out" in the patient's mail. (See Figure 13-3.)

Generating Referrals

In addition to internal marketing to the office's existing patients, the office may receive referrals from other health care professionals. When new services, new equipment, or new providers are added to the practice, letters to fellow professionals can stimulate referrals from those offices. (See *Letter to solicit referrals*, page 167.) After receiving a referral, a letter of thanks to the referring physician shows appreciation and good will.

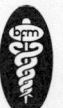 Blueville Family Medicine
15 Main Street
Blueville, CT 06000
860–555–3212

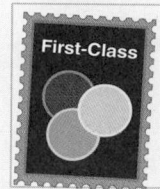 First-Class

Dear Lamar,

This is to remind you of your physical exam.
If you are unable to keep this appointment, please
give the office at least 24 hours notice.

Lamar - 09-22-08 at 3:30 pm

Lamar Shatner
15 Spellings Lane
Blueville, CT 06000

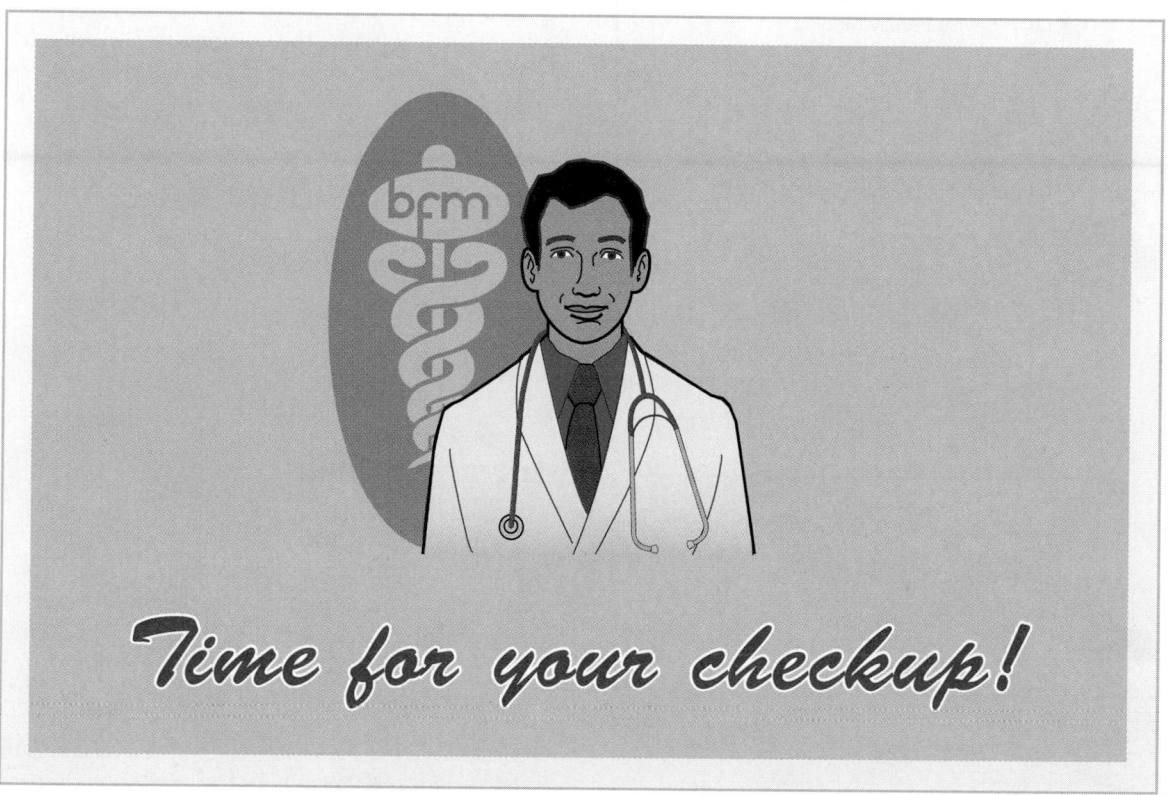

Time for your checkup!

FIG 13-1 Reminder postcard.

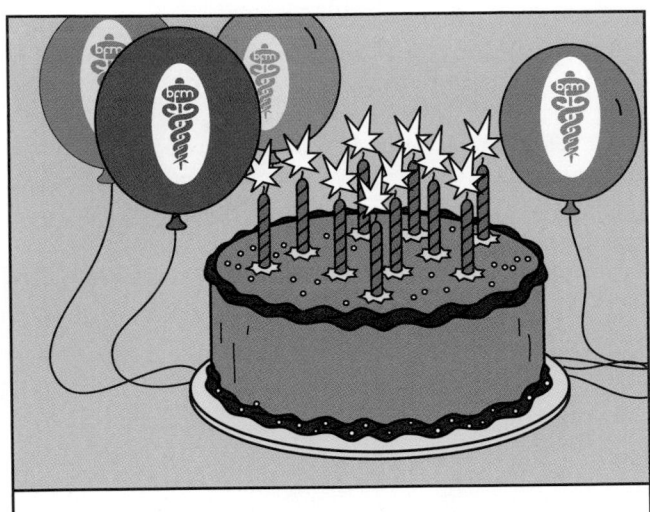

Dear Jacob,

Wishing you health and happiness on your birthday.

 Sincerely,
The Doctors and Staff
at Blueville Family Medicine

FIG 13-2 Birthday card from office to patient.

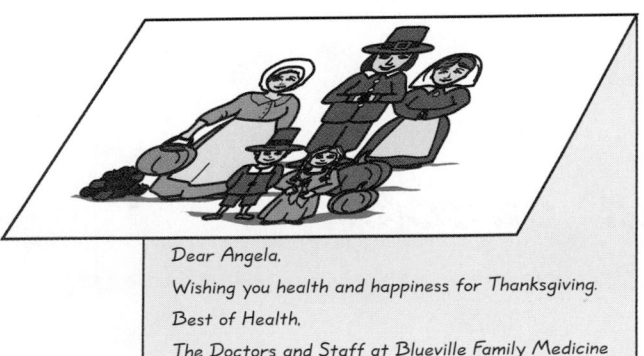

Dear Angela,
Wishing you health and happiness for Thanksgiving.
Best of Health,
The Doctors and Staff at Blueville Family Medicine

FIG 13-3 Thanksgiving card from office to patient.

E-mail Guidelines

Electronic mail (e-mail) is an informal type of correspondence. E-mail outside of an intranet system in an office cannot be considered private. No protected patient information should be disclosed in an e-mail message outside of the hospital or physician's office because the identity of the recipient cannot be confirmed. E-mail within a hospital or physician's office from one department to another can be considered private. Here are some other guidelines for using e-mail:

- *Language*—E-mail messages that are written by a medical assistant are a reflection of the medical office. The language should be friendly yet professional.
- *Formality*—When sending e-mail messages to coworkers or familiar personnel at other offices, you can use the recipient's first name. When sending messages to unfamiliar recipients, always use a more formal address (such as *Ms., Mr.,* or *Dr.*).
- *Punctuation*—Professional e-mail messages should read professionally. E-mail slang (such as "LOL" for "laugh out loud") doesn't belong in a professional e-mail message. Other e-mail conventions, such as omitting punctuation or writing in all capital letters, may be perceived as sloppy or rude. If the medical assistant has a friendly relationship with the recipient, she should use her personal e-mail account for nonbusiness correspondence. Professional e-mail accounts should be used for professional correspondence only.

✦ TIP Professional E-Mail Address

Some people pick a goofy, funny, or suggestive e-mail address. If you send a resume to an office for a job opening, don't send it from an e-mail account with such an address. How can an office take you seriously if you call yourself "GiveMeChocolate" or "SexyGuy"?

Incoming Mail

The medical office will receive mail from patients, vendors, attorneys, and various businesses. (See *Types of mail,* page 169.) The administrative medical assistant may be responsible for opening the mail each day and directing it to the appropriate person or department within the office. This list explains the various types of mail the office may receive:

- *Insurance reimbursements*—Checks to physicians from insurance companies for medical services should be recorded on the patient's financial records in a computerized system or on a manual ledger card system. Explanation of benefits documentation that accompanies a payment explains which services provided by the physician are included in the reimbursement. The administrative medical assistant should post the checks or forward them to the billing department for posting.

- *Patient correspondence*—Patients may write to the physician to thank her for care or communicate other information of a personal nature. Mail that looks like personal correspondence, such as a greeting card or personal letter, should not be opened by the medical assistant but given unopened to the physician.

- *Payments*—Patients may not make a copayment at the time of their visit and instead mail the copayment to the office. Also, patients may send checks to pay for charges for services that were not paid in full. As in the case of insurance checks, the administrative medical assistant should post the checks or forward them to the billing department for posting.

- *Medical records*—Other medical providers, such as doctors' offices, hospitals, and rehabilitation centers, may forward patient medical records to the office at the request of

Letter to solicit referrals

The first example is a letter written to a physician to introduce a new colleague in the practice in order to solicit referrals for new services offered.

The second example is a letter thanking a physician for referring a patient to the practice.

LETTER TO SOLICIT REFERRALS

October 1, 2008

Dr. Susan Spencer
Main Street Rheumatology
1212 Main Street
Townington, UT 98098

Dear Susan,

PHYSICAL THERAPY SERVICES → INTRODUCTION OF NEW SERVICES IN SUBJECT OR REGARDING LINE

I am pleased to announce the addition of Michelle Garner, RPT, to our staff. Michelle is a graduate of UCONN school of physical therapy and has years of experience in the care of patients with chronic joint pain from her tenure at the Madison Pain Clinic.

Michelle is available to come meet with you and discuss treatment options and modalities that will benefit your patients. She has had great success with reflex sympathetic dystrophy and chronic neuralgia. Enclosed is a brochure from the Pain Clinic highlighting Michelle's success with chronic neuralgia as well as her resumé.

If you need therapy for your RA patients, please consider referring them to Michelle for physical therapy. Our office participates with BC/BS, Healthnet, and Mediplan, so services for physical therapy are covered under these plans.

I hope to hear from you soon.

Sincerely,

Michael Jones

Michael Jones, MD

MJ:cb → MICHAEL JONES IS THE AUTHOR OF THE LETTER; CINDY BROWN, CMA, TYPED THE LETTER.
Enc:2 → REFERS TO THE NUMBER OF ENCLOSURES IN THE LETTER

Continued

Letter to solicit referrals *(Cont.)*

LETTER OF THANKS FOR REFERRALS

November 11, 2008

Dr. Susan Spencer
Main Street Rheumatology
1212 Main Street
Townington, UT 98098

Dear Susan,

Thank you for your referral of RA patients this past month. Michelle, our PT, has had some good progress with several of the patients; they are delighted with their care. I am sure they will convey to you their happiness with their therapy programs.

Sincerely,

Michael Jones

Michael Jones, MD

---

the patient or physician. These materials should be filed in the patient's chart and given to the physician. Because medical records are protected information, you must follow HIPAA privacy procedures when opening this type of mail. Patient medical records should be placed out of view of other patients entering the office and should be viewed only by personnel who need to access the information for treatment, payment, or operations (TPO).

- *Continuing education*—Advertisements for seminars and classes for continuing education for physicians, nurses, medical assistants, therapists, and office personnel should be forwarded to the appropriate personnel.
- *Financial*—Bills for equipment leases, office or medical supplies, rent of office space, and state and federal tax information should be forwarded to the personnel who handle the office finances. Bank statements should be forwarded unopened to the financial department or the physician.
- *Advertising*—Medical offices receive mail from vendors of office supplies, medical supplies, x-ray supplies, and even magazines. This mail should be forwarded to the person responsible for ordering such supplies.
- *Personal and Confidential*—Any mail marked "personal and confidential" should be given unopened to the addressee.

Transcription of Medical Documents

Medical reports can be **transcribed** from **dictation** tapes or computer voice files. The administrative medical assistant working in the hospital setting may be required to transcribe various medical documents, including history and physical examinations, consults, operative reports, pathology reports, radiology reports, and discharge summaries. The medical assistant in the ambulatory care center may be asked to transcribe letters, memos, history and physical reports, or disability ratings. Transcribing equipment consists of a tape player or voice recognition computer software. When using a tape player, the transcriptionist operates a pedal to hear the dictation at a speed that is comfortable. The machine allows the transcriptionist to rewind the tape, increase or decrease the volume, and adjust the tone, or pitch, higher or lower to ensure that all words are heard and transcribed accurately. In the case of voice recognition software, a transcriptionist or proofreader must review the document for errors. Because transcribed documents contain patient identifiable information, HIPAA privacy guidelines must be maintained. The contents

Types of mail

The table defines various types of mail and some examples of situations where these types of mail would be used. Where applicable, examples of correspondence both sent and received are included.

Type	Definition	Example
Certified mail	Proof of receipt of mail through a return receipt signed by the recipient to verify delivery	• Send: Letter of discontinuation of care sent to patient • Receive: Letters from attorneys requesting patient records
Collect on delivery (COD)	Collection of payment for merchandise or postage from the recipient upon delivery of mail	• Send: Medical equipment, vitamins/herbal supplements, or other items not covered by insurance can be sent COD to patients from the office • Receive: Merchandise ordered by office
Express mail	Guaranteed overnight delivery within the U.S.	• Send: Summary of care or other documentation to the patient's attorney for court proceedings • Receive: Documentation from another physician regarding a patient
First class mail	Sealed and unsealed letters (up to and including 11 oz), statements, bills, and business letters	• Send: Statements to patients, letters to patients, attorneys, insurance carriers, other physicians • Receive: Correspondence from attorneys and other physicians, checks from insurance companies and patients
Second class mail	Newspapers, journals, magazines	• Receive: Newspapers and magazines for the waiting room, journals for the medical staff or coding department
Third class mail	Circulars and advertising materials that weigh less than 16 oz	• Receive: Advertising for medical and office supplies
Fourth class mail	Packages weighing 1 to 70 lb with a combined girth of 108″	• Receive: Medical and office supplies ordered online or by phone
Priority mail	First class mail weighing more than 11 oz and up to 70 lb; fastest method of delivering heavier mail within 2 to 3 days	• Receive: Patient medical records sent by referring physician • Send: Patient medical records to physician upon request of patient, documents sent to attorneys
Registered mail	Method for shipping items with a declared monetary value that are sent first class; can be insured for a maximum amount of $25,000	• Send: Equipment to manufacturer for repair or maintenance • Receive: Equipment from vendor such as small laboratory machines—glucometers, hemocytometers, or medical equipment such as stethoscopes, reflex hammers, otoscopes ordered online or by phone
Restricted delivery	Mail delivered to a specific addressee or someone authorized in writing to receive the mail for the addressee	• Send: Protected health information sent to physician, patient, or attorney • Receive: Protected health information from any source may be sent to the office to the specific care of a staff member

of transcribed documents are not to be shared with anyone who does not demonstrate the "need to know." (see Figure 13-4.)

✦ TIP Professionalism and Privacy Protection

The medical assistant can emphasize to patients that she will always protect their confidential medical and personal information by presenting professional documentation and adhering to HIPAA guidelines that protect information. The medical assistant can demonstrate the professional tone and attitude of the office via these written communications. Patients will understand that the office personnel take the responsibility of guardianship of medical records, legal correspondence, and personal information seriously not only by the restrictions of disclosure but by the voice and professional tone of written office correspondence.

✦ TIP What She Said: Transcribing Accuracy

Use the physician's words when transcribing documents. While it is acceptable to correct minor grammatical errors, never change the MEANING of the document. If a document seems incomplete or does not seem clear, ask the dictating physician for clarification.

Elm Street Orthopedics
134 Main Street
Anytown, USA

July 14, 2008

Patient Name: Patricia Wilson
Date of Birth: 06/16/1964
Date of Evaluation: 07/11/2008

SUBJECTIVE: Mrs. Wilson is a 44-year-old white female who slipped and fell at home on 05/12/2008, landing on her right wrist. She was seen at Thomaston Walk-in Clinic on 05/12/2008 where x-rays of the right wrist, forearm, and elbow were negative for fracture or pathology. The patient was placed in a volar splint in the position of function and sent to this office for followup. Today she presents with minimal pain. Pain and range of motion is much improved in the right wrist.

Review of x-rays from 05/12/2008 confirms no fracture, pathology or structural abnormality.

OBJECTIVE: The splint was removed and the wrist examined. No swelling or discoloration is noted. No tenderness to palpation in the anatomical snuffbox was noted. There was no pain with axial pressure on the thumb. No tenderness over the scaphoid tubercle was noted. There was slight tenderness of the radial styloid. No ulnar styloid tenderness was noted, and there was full ROM of the elbow. The wrist had a decreased ROM of flexion and extension secondary to slight pain.

ASSESSMENT: Contusion of the right wrist.

PLAN: The plan is to discontinue the splint and range of motion with resumption of normal activities. The patient may resume lifting and/or working on a prn basis. She is instructed to return if symptoms return.

Michael Jones, MD

MJ: cb
D: 07/12/2008
T: 07/14/2008

FIG 13-4 Transcribed document.

Chapter Summary

- The medical assistant must recognize the importance of professionalism and confidentiality when communicating with patients, insurance carriers, attorneys, and other physicians' offices.
- Letters, e-mails, and faxes must always be written in a professional and accurate manner that represents the office.
- All written communications must be clear and concise and use language that is appropriate to the recipient.
- Spelling, grammar, and punctuation should be checked before sending written documentation or correspondence.
- Adherence to HIPAA confidentiality laws and confirmation of authorization to release protected information is vital.

Team Work Exercises

1. Role-play faxing protected health information with a classmate. Create a fax cover sheet and fill it out appropriately. Confirm the identity of the recipient before you fax the information.
2. Create a business letter and envelope. Exchange business letters with classmates. Read each other's letters for clarity and proofread them for errors. Check each other's business envelopes for completeness and accuracy.

Case Studies

1. Brenda Nunez is a patient who has been with the practice for many years. She has filled in as a receptionist on several occasions when one of the office staff is ill or on vacation. Brenda has always been a professional worker and has made the transition from patient to staff and back to patient with ease. She has asked you for a letter of recommendation for a permanent job with another physician. While you are disappointed that Brenda will no longer be available to fill in, you understand her need for a full-time position. Draft a letter to a prospective employer on Brenda's behalf. What items would you consider important to include in the letter?
2. Attorney Michael Liebowitz has handled many worker's compensation cases involving the office. Mr. Liebowitz is a professional who always adheres to the rules of confidentiality. However, his new assistant, Jayne, does not seem to understand the importance of confidentiality. She yelled at you on the phone for not forwarding a medical record even after you explained that you cannot disclose such records without permission. When you ask to speak to Mr. Liebowitz, Jayne gets defensive and hangs up on you. Write a letter to Mr. Liebowitz outlining the problem. Remember that you are friendly with Mr. Liebowitz, but be firm in your objections to his new assistant.

Resources

- How to write a business letter: *owl.english.purdue.edu/handouts/pw/p_basicbusletter.html* and *www.wisc.edu/writing/Handbook/BusinessLetter.html*
- Examples of reminder cards (dental): *www.bracesinfo.com/cards/*
- Examples of holiday cards and internal marketing: *www.medicalartspress.com.*

unit3

Medical Records Management

Learning Objectives

Upon completion of this chapter, the student will be able to:

- define the key terms presented in the glossary
- list and discuss the equipment and supplies necessary for a filing system
- discuss and have an understanding of the four basic filing systems
- create a paper medical record using appropriate supplies and systems
- use indexing rules to arrange a list of patient names alphabetically
- arrange a group of patient numbers in filing sequence for consecutive-, middle-, and terminal-digit filing systems
- assign correct color tabs to a list of patient names
- discuss the pros and cons of color, alphabetical, numeric, and accession log filing in a physician's office and a hospital
- discuss the advantages of electronic health records
- discuss the process of converting from paper-based records to electronic health records
- discuss the appropriate procedure and documentation for release of a medical record or information contained in the medical record.

CAAHEP Competencies

Administrative
  Perform Clerical Functions
    Organize a patient's medical record
    File medical records

ABHES Competencies

Administrative Duties
  File medical records
Legal Concepts
  Use appropriate guidelines when releasing records or information

Procedures

Creating a medical record
Filing a medical record using the alphabetical system

Chapter Outline

Importance of Medical Records Management
File Storage
  Vertical Files
  Open-Shelf Lateral Files
  Moveable Files
File Folders
  Fasteners
  Tabs
  Units
Filing Systems
  Alphabetical System
    Simple alphabetical filing
    Color-coded alphabetical filing
  Numeric Filing

    Consecutive filing
    Nonconsecutive filing
    Accession log filing
Other Information on the File Folder
Locating and Tracking Medical Records
  Tracking Medical Records
  Cross-Referencing Medical Records
Electronic Health Record
  Increased Access
  Cost Reduction
  Reduced Medical Errors
  Barriers to EHR Conversion
Medical Record Maintenance
  Medical Records Archives
  Medical Records Purging
  Release of Medical Records
Chapter Summary
Team Work Exercises
Case Studies
Resources

Key Terms

accession log
Record of numbers assigned to each new patient record

active files
Medical files of patients who are currently seen in the office

alphabetical filing
Organizing system based on the alphabet, usually using the patient's last name

archives
Storage place for records that are no longer in use but are kept for legal purposes

closed records
Medical records of patients who no longer seek treatment in the office

color coding
Alphabetical filing system that adds colored stickers to the open end of a file to facilitate a visual maintenance of files.

consecutive filing
Filing system that uses sequential numbers to order medical records

cross-reference
Guide placed where a medical record could be misfiled to indicate the correct location of the file

inactive records
Records of patients who have not been seen for an extended period of time (usually 1 to 6 years) but who may return for care

middle-digit filing
Numeric system that uses the middle digits of an identification number as the primary indexing unit

nonconsecutive filing
Numeric system that does not use consecutive ordering for medical records

numeric filing
System that assigns an identification number to each patient file

out guide
Marker used to indicate that a medical record has been taken from the filing system

purge
Permanent removal of medical records that are no longer in use

terminal-digit filing
System that uses the last digits of an identification number as the primary indexing unit

unit
Each part of a patient's name or identification number used in a filing system

Importance of Medical Records Management

Medical records must be organized in a way that makes them retrievable and accessible to health care workers who need them. A well organized, easy-to-use records management system includes rules for:

- creation of the medical record or patient record
- where it is stored, or *filed*
- how it is maintained
- how medical information within the medical record is released.

Maintaining the integrity of the filing system is necessary to ensure privacy and accessibility to patient information. All health care workers who access files must understand and utilize the system correctly. When a filing system is misused, valuable time is wasted searching for important information and the information could be permanently lost. Because a physician's medical decisions can be based on data in the patient's file, the well-being of a patient depends on appropriate access to his file.

File Storage

There are three primary types of filing cabinets that can be used in medical offices. Depending on availability of storage space, the size of the practice, and the need for access, an office may choose to use vertical files, open-shelf lateral files, or moveable files, or a combination of those types.

Vertical Files

File cabinets that have pull-out drawers and stand vertically can be used to store restricted access files. Restricted access files may include psychiatric notes or information on treatment of substance abuse and human immunodeficiency virus (HIV). Cabinets can be locked for extra security. Some offices may store financial documents, such as bank statements, and legal documents, such as rental agreements and malpractice insurance policies, in the locked files to ensure that they will not be lost.

Open-Shelf Lateral Files

Open-shelf lateral files are most commonly used for color-coded files because they enable easy viewing of the right side of each file (with color-coded labels). Because the side of the folder is visible, these shelves should not be in an area where patients can see them. Although no medically sensitive information is written on the outside of the file, the patient's name could be read by unauthorized individuals.

The open-shelf file system would, therefore, be inappropriate for clinics that treat patients with acquired immune deficiency syndrome (AIDS), sexually transmitted diseases (STDs), or substance abuse.

Moveable Files

Moveable shelving allows access to a large number of medical records without taking up a lot of space. Moveable shelving can be rolled on rollers, moved with a crank handle, or operated electronically. (See Figure 14-1.) Hospitals commonly use moveable file storage because of the large number of patient records and the infrequent access to individual records.

File Folders

File folders are designed for different types of labels and organizational systems. (See Chapter 20, "The Patient Interview," on page 307, for information on organizing items within the medical record.) The makeup of a file folder varies slightly from practice to practice. However, most folders contain several elements, including:

- fasteners
- tabs
- units.

Fasteners

Fasteners allow the medical assistant to secure papers (such as charting notes and laboratory results) to the file folder. Fasteners are usually long strips of metal that are bent around the back of the file folder and through holes punched near the edge of the file. Corresponding holes punched in the pages to be inserted in the medical record enable the medical assistant to thread the pages through the long metal prongs of the fastener. After threading the pages on, the medical assistant must bend the prongs so that they lie flush with the pages in the record, thus keeping them fastened in place in the file. (See Figure 14-2.) A file folder may contain fasteners on one or both sides of the folder.

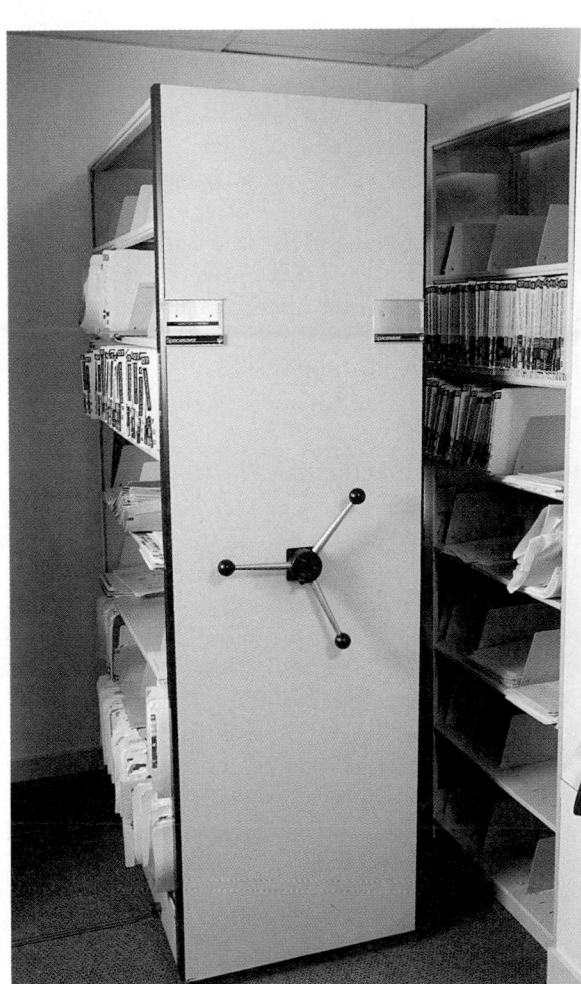

FIG 14-1 Movable shelving with crank handles.

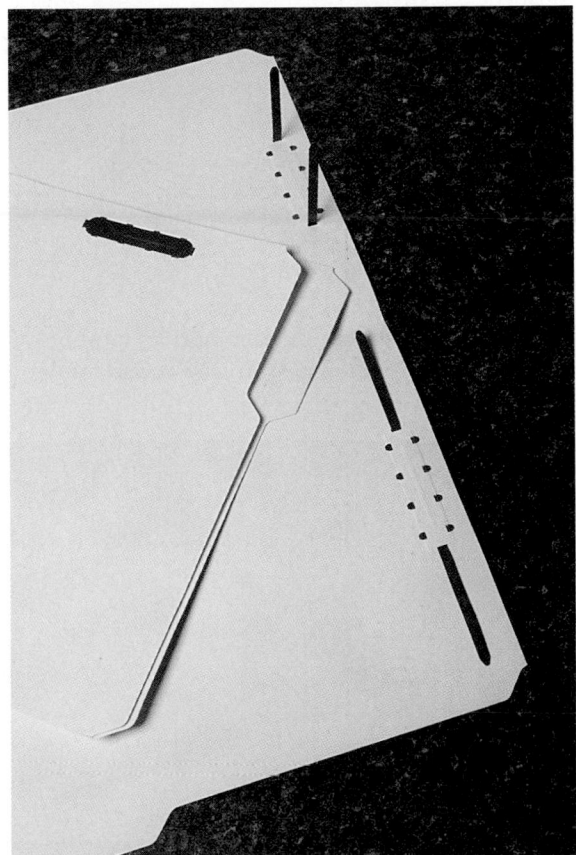

FIG 14-2 File folder with fasteners and a tab.

Tabs

Tabs are a small section of the folder that projects beyond the other side of the folder. On the tab, the medical assistant can place color-coded or printed letter labels. A tab commonly extends along the top edge of the file folder. Such tabs vary in position and size to facilitate easy viewing of files in a pull-out drawer. Tabs that extend along the entire right edge of folders accommodate color-coded stickers for use in open-shelf systems. (See Figure 14-3.)

Units

Rules for filing medical records follow the unit system. **Units** are any portion of a patient's name, accession number, or other numerical filing designation that is used to order and identify the medical record. The medical assistant who creates a new medical record file must attach labels to the file tab to identify the patient using the units designated by that filing system.

Filing Systems

There are two main types of filing systems:

- alphabetical systems
  - by patient's last name
  - color coded by patient's last name
- numerical systems
  - consecutive
  - middle digit
  - terminal digit
  - accession log.

Regardless of the system used, filing rules must be easy to follow. In addition, personnel who have access to files must be sure to use the system consistently to ensure that files can be found easily. Disregarding filing rules will lead to inefficiency and may compromise the quality of patient care.

Alphabetical System

Files in an alphabetical system are organized using the patient's name. One alphabetical system simply files folders in alphabetical order by the patient's last name. Another system uses color-coded labels with letters of the patient's name.

Simple Alphabetical Filing

Although the simple **alphabetical filing** system is easy to use, it does not afford patients anonymity because their names must be prominently displayed on the file folder. This system depends on some simple rules:

- Use the units in order:
  - last name (For hyphenated last names, omit the hyphen and file as if one name.)
  - first name
  - middle name or initial
  - title (if applicable).
- Follow the basic alphabetical ordering rule of "nothing before something." (For example, R. Dailey is filed before Robert Dailey and Smith is filed before Smith-Diaz.)
- Prefixes are treated as part of the name. Omit the punctuation and file accordingly. (For example St. Michel is filed as Saintmichel and McDonald is filed as Mcdonald.)
- Titles without a surname are considered the first indexing unit. (For example, Sister Angela is filed alphabetically by "Sister.")
- Seniority units are filed alphabetically. (For example, Gary Henderson, Jr., is filed before Gary Henderson, Sr.)

Color-coded Alphabetical Filing

Color-coded alphabetical systems can be designed for open lateral files or vertical file drawers. In this system, each letter of the alphabet is assigned a colored label that is placed on the side or top of the file folder for ease of use. (See *Alpha-Z color-coding system*.) The labels are placed down the right side of the file in a lateral system and on the top of the file for a vertical drawer system. (See Figure 14-4.)

Adding colors to the side or top of the file does not affect the alphabetical filing rules. The color coding helps keep files in alphabetical order and prevents misfiled records by creating a visual block of color when files are correctly placed. If a file is misplaced, the colors will not match, easily identifying the misfiled record. (See Figure 14-5.)

A commonly used system includes three stickers, one for each of the first two letters of the patient's last name and one for the first letter of their first name. Other systems use the first three letters of the last name. (See Figure 14-6.) The three labels should be placed along the top or side of the

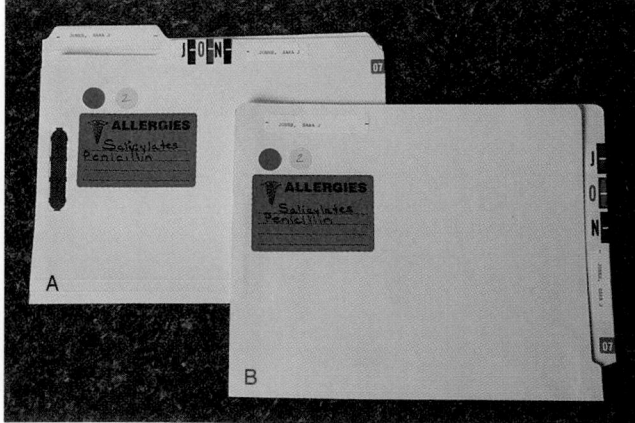

FIG 14-3 File folders with tabs. (A) Top tabs for drawer filing. (B) Side tabs for open-shelf filing.

FIG 14-4 Color-coded alphabetical filing. (A) Labels on right side for lateral system. (B) Labels across top for vertical drawer system.

Alpha-Z color-coding system

The Alpha-Z system is one system for color-coded alphabetical filing. This system uses a combination of 13 colors with white letters for the first half of the alphabet and the same colors with white stripes and white letters for the remaining 13 letters of the alphabet. Because letters next to each other in the alphabet are assigned very different colors, filing errors are easily identified. The accompanying photograph shows the labels used in the Alpha-Z color-coding system.

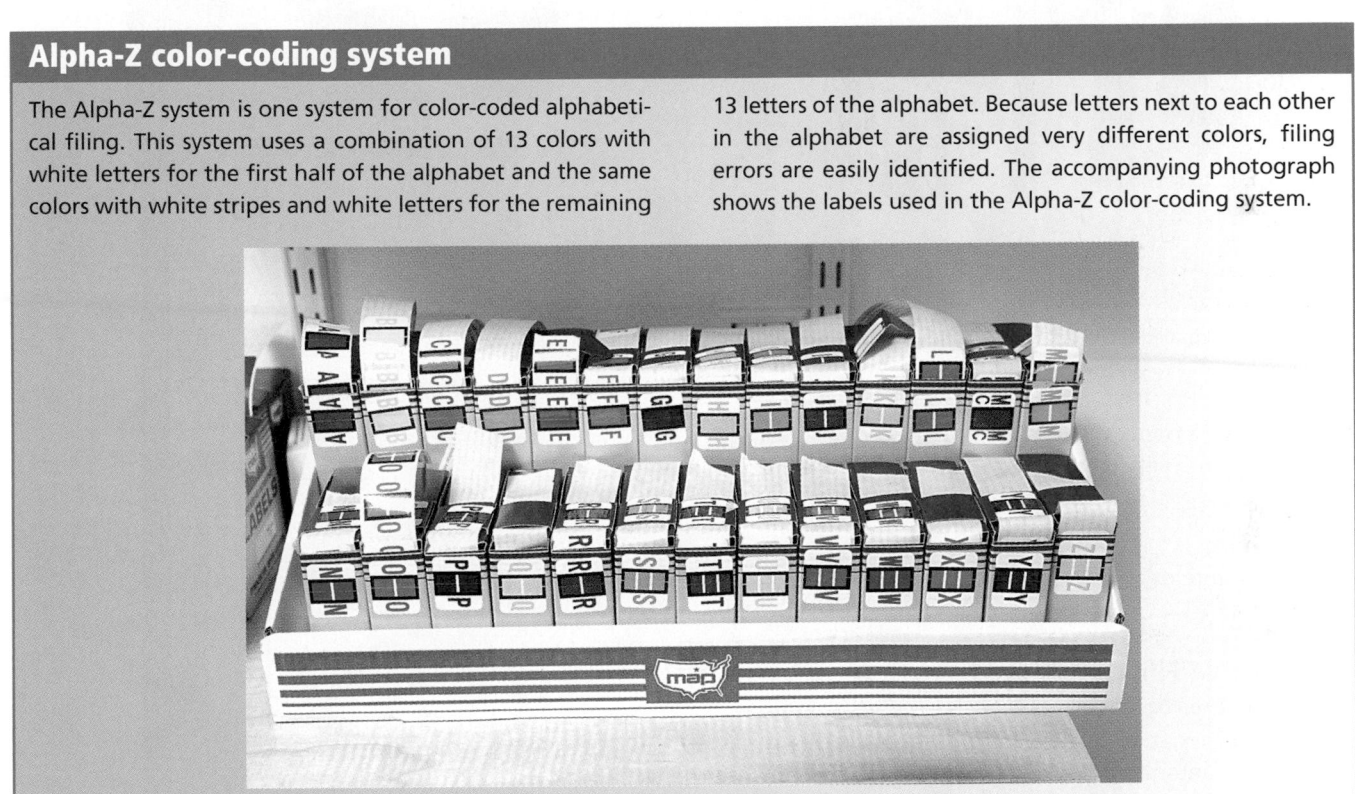

folder in a uniform fashion. (See *Procedure 14-1: Creating a medical record,* page 179.)

Numeric Filing

Numeric filing is a system of organizing medical records by number. While the numeric filing system affords greater confidentiality, a record of the chart number for each patient must be maintained. The increased privacy afforded by using a numeric system makes it a good choice for psychiatric offices, drug rehabilitation clinics, and social services agencies. However, when a computer system is not functioning, medical record retrieval is difficult. If an office uses a

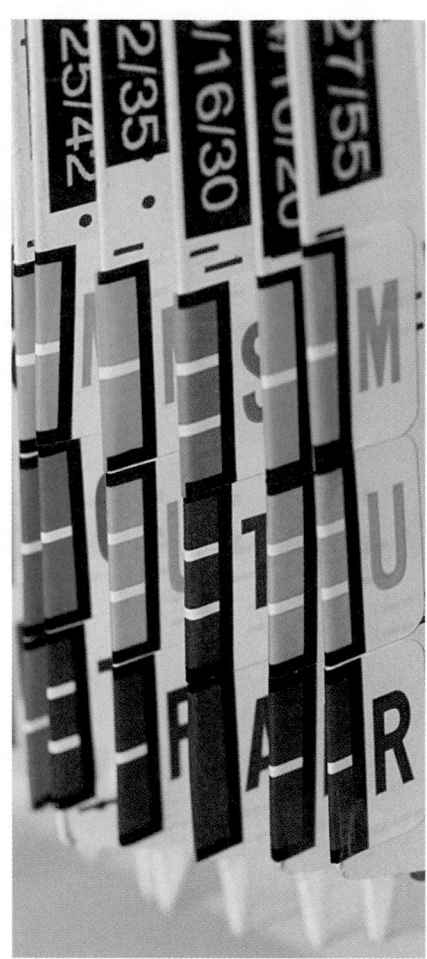

FIG 14-5 Misfiled medical record with colored labels for easy identification.

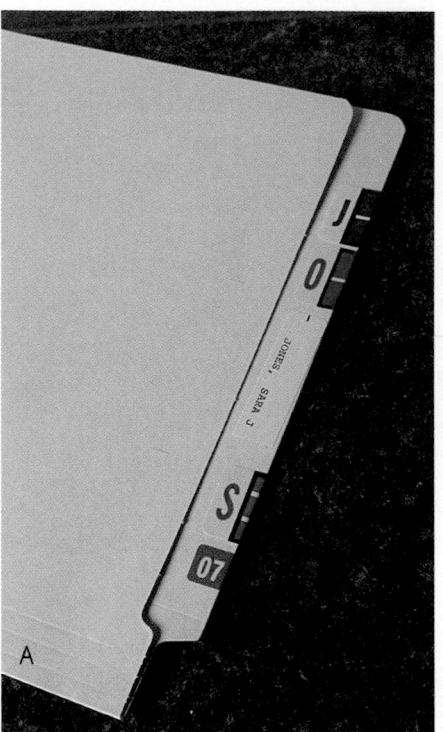

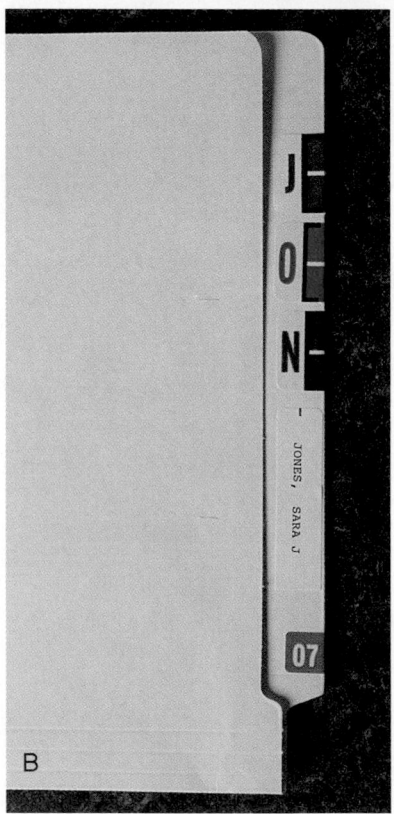

FIG 14-6 Three-sticker systems. (A) File using first two letters of last name and first letter of first name. (B) File using first three letters of last name.

numeric filing system, the office staff must establish backup systems to find patient records. There are three types of numeric filing systems:

- consecutive
- nonconsecutive
- accession log.

Consecutive Filing

Also called *straight numerical filing* or *serial filing,* **consecutive filing** is a system of filing records that uses six digits, broken down into three two-digit segments. The records are filed in ascending order from smaller to larger numbers—for example, record number 849932 is filed before record number 849942. (See Figure 14-7.)

Nonconsecutive Filing

A **nonconsecutive filing** system is another numerical filing system that uses six digits, broken down into three two-digit segments. Offices will commonly use numbers for these

Creating a medical record

Task
Create a medical record.

Conditions
- File folder
- Colored letter labels
- Patient intake form
- Signed HIPAA statement
- Pen
- Other stickers (provided by the instructor, such as allergy indicators)

Standard
In the time specified and within scoring parameters determined by the instructor, the student will successfully create a medical record.

Performance Standards
1. Fill out the patient intake form. (You can use your name or make up a patient as directed by your instructor.)
2. Explain the HIPAA information to a patient (by role playing with a classmate) and have the patient sign the HIPAA form to indicate that the patient has received, read, and understood the document.
3. Insert the patient intake form into the medical record by using the fastener to attach it to the right inside of the medical record. (Note: Each medical office has its own guidelines for how to file a signed HIPAA statement in the medical record.)
4. Place the correct colored letter labels on the outside right edge of the folder, folding the label over the edge so that the letter is visible from both sides.
5. Place the allergy alert, insurance, or physician labels on the outside of the folder (as indicated by your instructor).

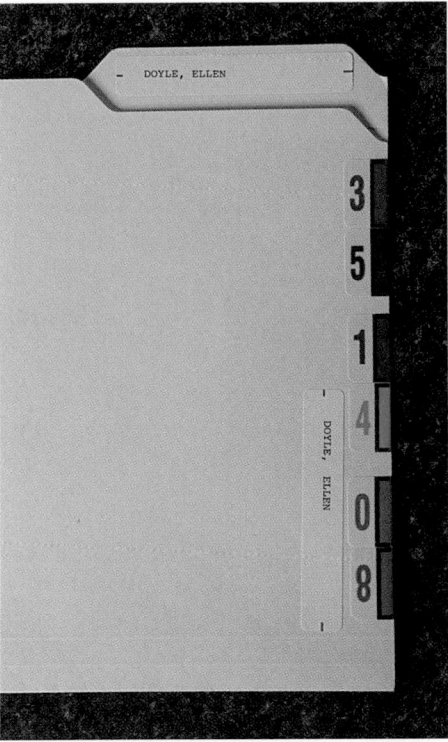

FIG 14-7 Medical record filed using consecutive filing system.

units from patient information, such as telephone numbers, dates of birth, or the treating physician. However, use of Social Security numbers as file numbers is not recommended for privacy reasons and the risk of identity theft.

The two basic forms of nonconsecutive filing are **middle-digit** and **terminal-digit filing**. In a middle-digit nonconsecutive filing system, the medical assistant must use the numbers designated as the middle unit as the primary unit used to file the medical record. In terminal-digit filing, she must use the unit designated as the terminal unit. Middle- and terminal-digit filing may be used to group files by common characteristics. For example, terminal-digit

filing may be used for files where the last two digits indicate the patient's year of birth. In a pediatric office, these files could then be easily accessed to send reminders for vaccinations or school physicals (See *Consecutive and non-consecutive filing systems,* page 180.)

Accession Log Filing
Accession log filing assigns the next number in a sequence to each medical record created. The records are filed consecutively by accession number and the office staff keeps a log of all patient names and number assignments in a book or computer database. However the log is maintained, it is confidential information, so the office staff must ensure that only those persons who need to use the log for treatment, payment, or operations (as dictated by HIPAA guidelines) have access to it. Although the system ensures confidentiality, it can create problems when searching for a file because the medical assistant must look up the patient's accession number in the log every time the patient visits the office. In addition, because the accession number is the only number used in this filing system, the only information that the accession log provides is how old the medical record is in relationship to other medical records. Thus, the number is not helpful for sending reminders or organizing other patient demographic information. A computerized database that searches for the file number by the patient's name will allow

Consecutive and nonconsecutive filing systems

The table shows the order of medical records filed using the consecutive filing system, the middle-digit nonconsecutive filing system, and the terminal-digit nonconsecutive filing system.

In consecutive filing, the first digit is the primary unit used for filing, then the middle digit, then the terminal digit. In middle-digit filing, the middle digit is the primary filing unit, then the first digit, then the terminal digit. In terminal-digit filing, the terminal digit is the primary filing unit, then the middle digit, and then the first digit.

Consecutive (1, 2, 3)	Middle digit (2, 1, 3)	Terminal digit (3, 2, 1)
01 07 09	02 01 11	03 04 01
02 01 11	03 01 08	03 01 08
02 04 10	04 02 10	01 07 09
02 06 10	02 04 10	04 02 10
03 01 08	03 04 01	02 04 10
03 04 01	04 05 12	03 04 10
04 02 10	04 05 13	02 01 11
04 02 12	01 07 09	04 05 12

KEY:
- = primary filing unit
- = secondary filing unit
- = tertiary filing unit

location of the medical record. The accession log gives the patient's name and the date of the first visit along with the accession number needed to find the medical record. If a manual log book is used, an alphabetical log by patient's name may also be maintained for cross-reference. It is imperative to keep such a log locked securely in a drawer or filing cabinet and a computerized database must have password protection. (See Figure 14-8.)

The accession log number can also be used as the patient's financial account record. Because the accession number gives an idea of how old the file is, outstanding balances of financial records with lower accession numbers can be identified to pursue payment.

Other Information on the File Folder

In addition to labeling a folder according to a specific filing system, the outside of the medical record can also be used to display other important information. For example, the file may have a colored label that indicates the primary care practitioner for each patient or a numbered label that indicates medical insurance coverage. Drug and

Accession #	Patient Name	Date of First Visit
503	Cheryl White	8/5/04
504	Julia Wells	8/5/04
505	Hector Ramirez	8/5/04
506	Alison Andrews	8/6/04
507	John Phelps	8/6/04

FIG 14-8 Accession log book.

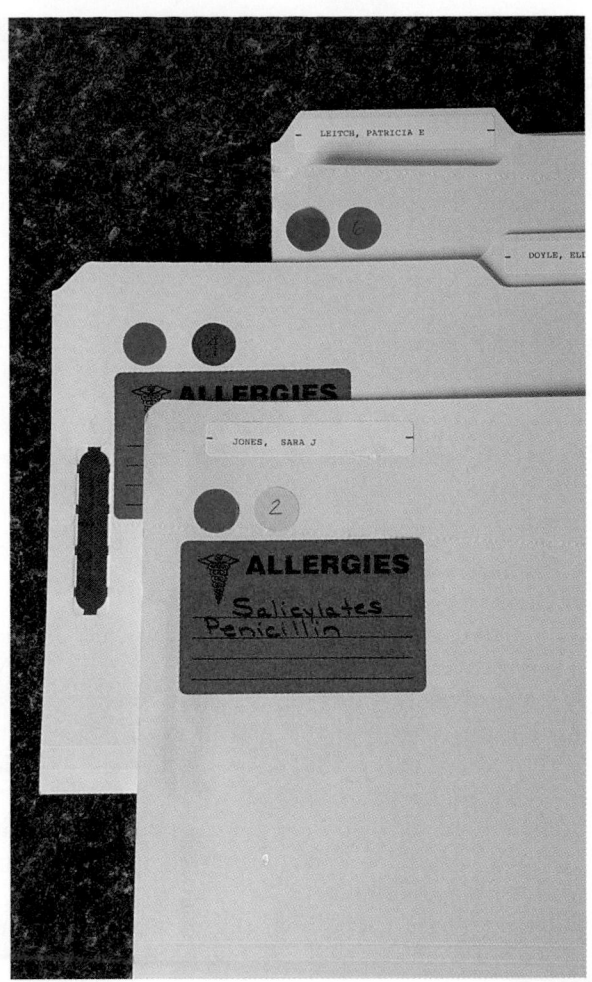

FIG 14-9 Important information indicated on the exterior of the medical record.

significant food allergies are commonly indicated by a red sticker on the outside of a patient's file. (See Figure 14-9.) If a patient changes insurance carriers or primary care practitioners, the medical assistant can easily replace the labels.

No medically sensitive information such as disease status or treatments received can be written on the outside of a medical record. This information is confidential and protected and must be retained within the interior of the medical record.

Locating and Tracking Medical Records

In addition to following the filing system in place in a medical office, the medical assistant must be familiar with the ways in which the office keeps track of medical records that are in use. In addition, the medical assistant must be familiar with methods used to avoid common misfiling errors.

Tracking Medical Records

Regardless of the filing method used, a system must indicate that a medical record has been taken from the filing system. When taking a medical record from a filing system, the medical assistant must put an **out guide** in its place, which indicates that the medical record has been removed as well as the present location of that record. When the record is replaced, the out guide is removed. The medical assistant can cross out the previous entry and reuse the out guide. Out guides are usually made of lightweight cardboard or stiff paper. (See Figure 14-10.)

Cross-Referencing Medical Records

Locating medical records can become a bit confusing when patients change names. When a patient changes her name, the medical assistant must make a new folder and file the medical record according to the new name. Marriage, divorce, adoption, or taking religious vows are some reasons a patient may change names. In addition, differentiating the last name from the first may also be difficult—for example, John James, Jim Paul, or Mei Le Huan. As a result, a staff person may search for or file the record in the wrong place. A **cross-reference** guide is a good way to remedy such a situation. A cross-reference guide is similar to an out guide,

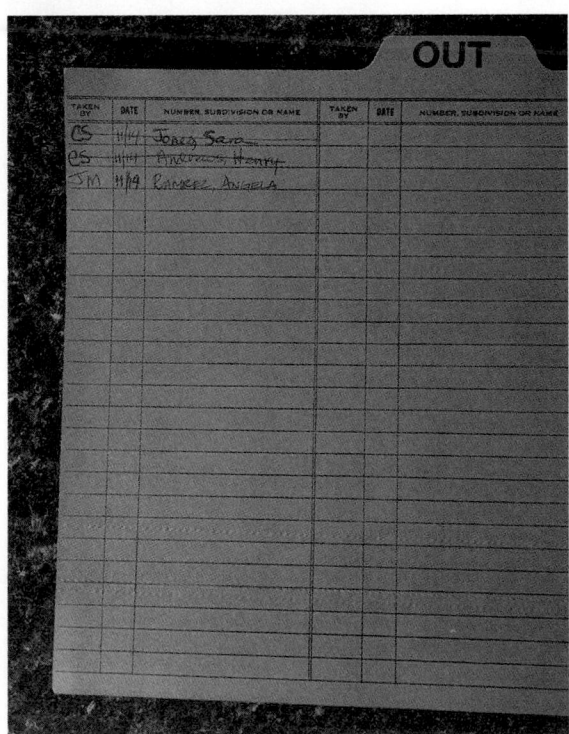

FIG 14-10 Out guide.

but is placed where a medical record may be misfiled. When a staff member attempts to file the record in the incorrect spot, the cross-reference guide will point out the error immediately and will also indicate the correct location for the record. (See Figure 14-11.)

One of the most common reasons for name changes is marriage. When a patient changes her name, the medical assistant should ask her what legal name she will use. For example, if Ann Jones married Hector Ramirez, the medical assistant should ask Ms. Jones if she plans to take her husband's name. If Ms. Jones does take her husband's name, the medical assistant should make necessary changes to her medical record, file the record according to the name *Ramirez,* and create a cross-reference guide to insert where the record would have been filed under *Jones.* It is common practice to ask patients at each visit if there are any changes in their address, insurance coverage, or name. (See *Procedure 14-2: Filing a medical record using the alphabetical system.*)

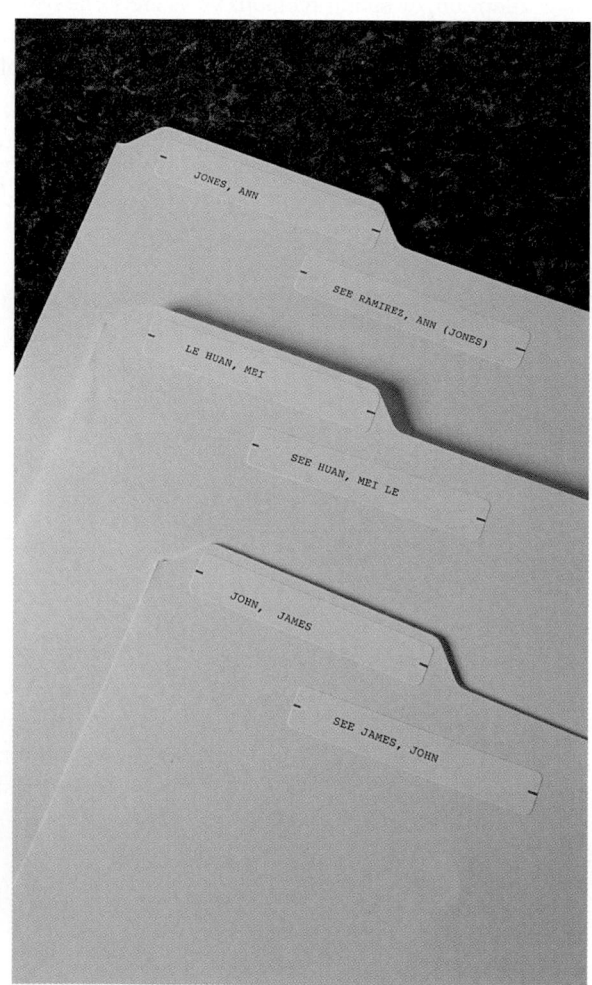

FIG 14-11 Cross-reference guide.

▮ PROCEDURE 14-2

Filing a medical record using the alphabetical system

Task
File a medical record using the alphabetical filing system.

Conditions
- Set of mock patient charts
- File storage unit
- Out guide, if needed

Standard
In the time specified and within scoring parameters determined by the instructor, the student will successfully file a medical record using the alphabetical filing system.

Performance Standards
1. Gather charts to be filed.
2. File each chart by placing it between files in the correct alphabetical order.
3. Cross-reference names if necessary to ensure accuracy.
4. Place the charts in the proper storage unit with color-coded tabs facing forward so that the letter is visible from both sides.
5. Review charts and observe for color-coded tabs that may be out of order and, if detected, refile the chart in the correct order.
6. If removing a patient's chart, put an out guide in place of the file to help staff find missing charts.

Electronic Health Record

An electronic health record (EHR) is a comprehensive computerized health record for a patient that includes data from multiple providers who have diagnosed and treated the patient. The data can be stored and updated throughout the patient's life. The advantages of an EHR rather than a traditional paper medical or health record include:

- increased access to medical data
- cost reductions
- reduction in medical errors.

Increased Access
Most patients receive health care services from multiple providers. During a patient's lifetime, he may see many providers. For example, a patient may see the following providers for the conditions listed:

- cardiologist—for high blood pressure and arrhythmia
- endocrinologist—for diabetes or a thyroid dysfunction

- chiropractor—for lower back or neck pain
- orthopedic surgeon—for carpal tunnel syndrome and athletic injuries
- physical therapist—for rehabilitation of athletic injuries
- primary care provider—for routine physicals.

In this scenario, the patient may be taking multiple medications and having multiple therapy sessions with a chiropractor and a physical therapist and progress toward the resolution of each problem may vary. When using EHR, each of the patient's providers can access medication records, examination notes, and treatment records from all the providers. The cardiologist, who recommends to the patient that he exercise to lose weight, can see that the orthopedic surgeon has requested that the patient not stress a hip or knee joint. The chiropractor can see that the orthopedic surgeon has prescribed a narcotic pain killer for the knee pain and that explains the patient's decreased neck or back pain. The providers can also access imaging studies, x-rays, and blood test results in the EHR and discuss these results with the patient during an office visit. In addition, the information stored within the EHR can be accessed by multiple people simultaneously. For example, the billing department can access treatment notes for insurance carrier requests while the physician is simultaneously accessing the EHR during a patient visit. The billing department does not have to wait to access a paper file after the physician has seen the patient.

Cost Reduction

Patients in the United States spend 2 trillion dollars per year on health care; approximately 30% of that money is spent on administrative costs. In a paper-based system, referrals to specialists, requests for further information, copies of medical records, and copies of x-rays and other imaging studies incur the costs of copying and mailing. Storage space for paper medical records, climate control for file rooms, security measures, and personnel costs for file management add to the overall cost of doing business.

Treatment and diagnostic testing costs are also increased in a paper-based system because lack of access to data leads to repeated procedures. The endocrinologist does not have the blood chemistry panel that the cardiologist ordered 2 weeks ago. The patient's blood must be retested and additional costs to the insurer and the patient are incurred. The orthopedic surgeon must x-ray the patient's hip because the low back and hip x-rays taken by the chiropractor last week are not accessible. The patient is exposed to unnecessary radiation as well as unnecessary costs.

Reduced Medical Errors

Medical errors, the eighth leading cause of death in the United States, are defined as adverse events that could have been prevented based on current medical knowledge.

Prescribing a medication that the patient is allergic to or that is contraindicated based on the patient's concurrent medications can cause injury or even death. Surgical errors are caused when the wrong procedure is performed or the wrong surgical site is chosen, such as amputating the wrong leg. Most medical errors are caused by a failure of communication among the many providers caring for the patient. Communication failures can include:

- *Misfiled or lost paper medical records.* Medical assistants, nurses, and physicians cannot provide adequate care without a complete history of the patient's allergies, previous surgeries, or past diagnoses. Trying to provide care without this information can impact medical decision making.
- *Unreadable information.* Poorly written charts or prescriptions may lead to medical errors, such as the wrong medication or dosage.
- *Mishandled or mislabeled laboratory specimens.* If the testing order is illegible, the laboratory cannot conduct the test. Because the EHR system submits electronic testing orders, the information is typed into the patient's record, thus ensuring readability.

Barriers to EHR Conversion

Although the reasons to convert paper-based medical records to EHR are compelling, there are many barriers to the conversion process. Many offices use paper-based medical records because the conversion process is expensive and time-consuming. (See *EHR conversion methods,* page 184.)

In addition to the expense of converting old files, it is expensive to purchase an EHR system and train personnel to use it. At the American Health Information Management Association conference in October 2006, panelists estimated that purchasing and installing EHR would cost over $32,000 per physician, with ongoing monthly maintenance costs of around $1,200. These costs make EHR systems unattainable for some practices. Thus, the medical assistant must be prepared to work in a paper-based or electronic environment.

✦ TIP Terminology Tip

Electronic records are new and the terms to describe them are commonly confused. EHR and EMR (electronic medical record) are used interchangeably to describe the patient care records or files. EHR, however, is typically used to describe the concept and EMR is generally used to describe a specific record. In addition, a reference to an EHR system is also commonly abbreviated as *EHR* or *EMR*.

Medical Record Maintenance

When an office develops a filing system, it must be sure to safeguard the medical records in that system. Files should

EHR conversion methods

In converting paper medical records to electronic health records (EHRs), an office must choose one of several conversion methods, each having problems and considerations.

Method	Advantages	Potential Problems
Key all data into EHR	No handwritten material is used, reducing errors	• Errors introduced while inputting information into EHR • Increased cost of inputting all information from lengthy medical records
Use optical character reader (OCR) to convert files	Possibly cheaper than hand keying documents	• Generally only 90% to 95% accurate
Scan paper medical record	Cheaper and faster than other methods	• Continued illegibility of poorly written charts • Compared to new EHR, inconsistency in appearance and organization, which can cause confusion, frustration, and inefficiency

never be stored in areas that provide public access. Paper medical records must be stored behind a reception area or in separate file rooms. EHR must be stored in a password-protected environment that includes logs to record the individuals who are accessing the record and which portions in order to ensure that medical personnel access records only for necessary functions of treatment, payment, and operations (TPO). In addition, staff using computers should make sure that the computer screens are not in view of patients in front office areas and computer screens in treatment rooms show the EHR of the patient being seen, not the previous patient that was treated in that room. The office staff should also ensure that the office is locked whenever it is empty, including during lunch and coffee breaks. Locking files, if feasible, is an excellent added security measure.

Medical Records Archives

Medical files of patients who are currently being seen in the office are called *active files*. These files should be accessible for use and cover patients who have been seen within the past 1 to 6 years, depending on office policy and availability of storage space. EHRs of patients who have not been seen in the office within 6 years may be removed from the active system and transferred to electronic storage and kept in a secure, locked area.

Records of patients who have not been seen for over 6 years may be designated as **closed** or **inactive**. A *closed* medical record indicates a patient who no longer seeks treatment in the office, including a patient who has moved from the area, changed doctors (commonly for insurance coverage), or died. An *inactive* record indicates a patient who has not been seen for a given period of time but may return for future care.

Closed and inactive paper medical records should be **archived** in a safe location that is not accessed frequently, such as a locked back storage room, basement, or off-site storage facility, to protect the confidentiality of the records. Closed and inactive EHR can be saved on compact discs (CDs) and locked in a secure area of the office.

Medical Records Purging

The Medical Practice Act of each individual state determines record-keeping requirements in that state. Most states require medical offices to **purge** their paper records, which is the permanent removal of medical records that are no longer in use. When purging paper medical records, an office must destroy them by shredding or burning them in order to ensure that they cannot be accessed by unauthorized personnel. Some offices will opt to maintain large numbers of inactive files in order to reduce the risk of inappropriately destroying medical records. However, some offices may opt to transfer paper-based medical records to CDs to reduce storage space needs. Because EHRs do not require much storage space, office staff can maintain such records on CDs and store them in a secure location, rather than dealing with the expense and security risks of destroying medical records. As more providers convert to EHR and become accustomed to its use, archiving EHR will become more common than purging.

Release of Medical Records

A medical record or a portion of it can be released to persons who demonstrate a "need to know." Examples of a legitimate "need to know" include consultation by another physician, legal action, or insurance processing. (See Chapter 7, "HIPAA and a Patient's Rights," on page 71, for a release of records procedure.) Physicians, attorneys, insurance companies, government agencies, and the patient may request copies of medical records. In general, the medical assistant will release copies of a medical record. However, she can release original x-rays and magnetic resonance imaging (MRI) scans with the stipulation that they be returned to the original medical record. As the guardians of sensitive personal health information, medical assistants and other health care providers are responsible for maintaining patient confidentiality. Remember the rule, "when in doubt, do not give it out." (See *Special circumstances for records release.*)

Chapter Summary

- The medical assistant is responsible for the creation, filing, storage, and appropriate release of medical records.
- Depending on the needs of the office or hospital, an alphabetical or numeric filing system will dictate how medical records are kept.

- EHR systems are being introduced into many offices and can reduce errors and costs due to increased accessibility and readability.
- Color coding of records may also be used to provide added protection against misfiling records.
- Consistently applying the rules for creation, storage, and release of medical records will ensure that records are accessible when needed and released only when appropriate.

Team Work Exercises

1. Discuss with your instructor and classmates converting from paper-based medical records to EMR. Research some software that can be used to create medical records. Should your "practice" scan the old records? Key the old records? Create a timeline for training the office personnel and converting records. How should you design a system that will allow the conversion to take place without interrupting the physician's and billing staff's access to the medical records?
2. Using the paper medical records created by the class in Procedure 14-1, discuss the filing system and storage requirements for your medical records. Create a storage area in the classroom or clinical laboratory. Create out guides and cross-reference guides for medical records (if necessary).

Special circumstances for records release

In general, a patient has a right to privacy for his health records. The medical assistant will be required to obtain the patient's consent to release information in the record before doing so. However, there are some special circumstances in which consent requirements vary from the normal requirements.

Court cases

When a medical record is subpoenaed by a court of law, the medical assistant may release those medical records without the patient's consent. The medical assistant must release original documents (photocopied documents are not acceptable in court) unless the judge specifies that copies are acceptable. The medical assistant should release the original documents with the stipulation that the court return all the documents after use. She should also note the absence of the documents in the patient file, including the date they were taken and the date the court returned the records.

Specific consent

Because release of some medical information could impact a patient's ability to lead his life, the medical assistant must obtain specific permission from the patient to release these types of information:

- references to diagnosis and treatment of HIV or AIDS
- sexually transmitted diseases
- psychiatric disorders and mental health records
- drug and alcohol abuse history.

Guardianship

Custodial and noncustodial parents, foster care providers, and guardians must sign a release form authorizing transfer of medical records for children under age 18.

Emancipated minors

Children who are under the age of 18 and living on their own, married, a parent, or in the armed services can become emancipated by a judge. These persons have exclusive access to their medical records, and a parent cannot request the record without the patient's consent.

Case Studies

1. Which of the following filing systems would be appropriate for a pediatric office? A mental health clinic? A substance abuse center? Support your answer.
   a. Alphabetical
   b. Alphabetical with color coding
   c. Numeric
   d. Accession log
2. You are working in an office that uses an alphabetical color-coded system. Sally Jenkins has recently married Henry O'Leary. Sally has decided to hyphenate her name. Where should you file Sally's medical record? Will you need to make a new file folder for her? Where should a cross-reference guide be placed? How would you change the record if Sally were to take her new husband's name? Where would you file her medical record? Do you need to file a cross-reference guide? If so, where?

Resources

- Health and Human Services discussion of EHR adoption: *www.hhs.gov/healthit/ahic/healthrecords*
- Electronic medical records software: *www.actimedical.com, http://www.edgemed.com/, www.purkinje.com/ehr/home.cfm,* and *www.lighthousemd.com*
- Medical filing supply vendors: *megastarsystems.com/docs/officeprod/,www.ancom-filing.com/medical_page.html?source= overture,* and *oifilingsystems.reachlocal.com*
- Adam, A.: *Implementing Electronic Document and Record Management Systems.* Philadelphia: CRC Press, 2007.
- Hamilton, B., and Hamilton, L.: *Electronic Health Records.* New York: McGraw-Hill, 2008.
- Lehmann, H. P., et al.: *Aspects of Electronic Health Record Systems,* 2nd ed. New York: Springer-Verlag, 2006.

Office Management

Learning Objectives

Upon completion of this chapter, the student will be able to:

- define the key terms as presented in the glossary
- discuss the roles and responsibilities of an office manager and a human resources director
- describe at least three key qualities of an effective office manager or human resources director
- list at least three benefits of teamwork
- describe the purpose of staff meetings, brainstorming, and employee participation in decision making
- discuss the uses of a policies and procedures manual
- describe the purpose of marketing and tracking
- describe the various forms of internal and external marketing and their uses.

CAAHEP Competencies

General Competencies

Professional Communications
  Recognize and respond to verbal communications

Legal Concepts
  Identify and respond to issues of confidentiality
  Perform within legal and ethical boundaries

Operational Functions
  Perform an inventory of supplies and equipment

Perform routine maintenance of administrative and clinical equipment
Utilize computer software to maintain office systems

ABHES Competencies

Professionalism
  Project a positive attitude
  Be a "team player"
  Exhibit initiative
  Evidence a responsible attitude

Communication
  Be attentive, listen, and learn
  Interview effectively

Administrative Duties
  Manage physician's professional schedule and travel

Office Management
  Maintain physical plant
  Operate and maintain facilities and equipment safely
  Inventory equipment and supplies
  Evaluate and recommend equipment and supplies for the practice
  Maintain liability coverage
  Exercise efficient time management

Instruction
  Orient and train personnel

Procedures

Training new personnel using the policies and procedures manual
Taking and reordering inventory, performing maintenance, and checking safety
Preparing physician travel

Chapter Outline

Qualities of Leadership
  Praising While Problem Solving

Office Management Roles and Responsibilities
Dealing with Employees
  Conducting an Interview
  New Employee Orientation
    Policies and procedures manual
  Conducting a Staff Meeting
  Conducting an Employee Evaluation
    Disciplinary actions and terminations
Taking an Inventory and Ordering Supplies
    Maintaining laboratory equipment and supplies inventory
  Selecting Computer Hardware and Software
    Using computers in the medical office
Assisting with Physician Travel Arrangements
Marketing in the Medical Office
  Internal Marketing
  External Marketing
  Tracking Marketing
Chapter Summary
Team Work Exercises
Case Studies
Resources

Key Terms

agenda
Items of business to be addressed at a staff meeting

brainstorming
Process in which individuals in a group offer ideas to solve a specified problem

constructive criticism
Method of instruction that focuses on actions that can improve an employee's job performance rather than focusing on the negative aspects of the person's performance

external marketing
Methods of informing people who have not been patients of the practice about the practice and its services

internal marketing
Method used to stimulate business with existing patients through mailings and other means

job description
Written description of the qualifications and duties of a position

policies and procedures manual
Handbook that provides detailed information about regulations regarding tasks and how to perform the tasks

Qualities of Leadership

An effective manager possesses qualities of leadership that help her lead her team effectively and efficiently. Such leadership qualities include the ability to empower others, gain experience in a multitude of tasks, have enthusiasm for her job, and work hard. The office manager of a medical practice can empower her employees by respecting their skills and abilities and trusting their judgment in their areas of expertise. She can also use her varied experience to support the office staff with whatever help is necessary. A willingness to do so not only creates an efficient workplace but also fosters a spirit of teamwork.

The group that feels appreciated and connected as a team will work together toward common goals. Such strategies as **brainstorming,** in which a group of people think of possible solutions to problems and discuss them, promote an open dialogue between the office manager and office staff and show employees that the manager values their opinions. When supervising medical assistants, the office manager must remember that medical assistants are educated professionals who take their jobs seriously.

In general, an employee appreciates a manager who understands the employee's job responsibilities and role in the organization. A manager who "worked her way up" is commonly in touch with the employee because she once performed the tasks of that employee. An enthusiastic, hardworking manager will help out when a department is busy and does not consider any job "beneath" her. If the manager has not done the work of the employee, she should ask the employee to teach her how to perform each of her job functions in order to gain an understanding of the responsibilities of all of the personnel that she supervises.

✦ TIP Know What They Do
A medical assistant who would like to become a supervisor should learn the responsibilities of a clinical and administrative medical assistant. Although she may never want to work at the front desk or work as a clinical medical assistant, she may supervise both positions. Having an understanding of all of the jobs in the office will make her more effective as a supervisor.

Praising While Problem Solving
An effective manager is also able to express appreciation for her employees' successes and does not merely focus on solving problems. For example, if the front desk runs smoothly except for copayment collections, the effective supervisor will discuss the good points as well as the problem. The manager can express her appreciation for the jobs that are well done, such as smooth appointment scheduling, accurate record

keeping and filing, and professional telephone techniques. The employees feel appreciated, not threatened, when the manager then asks for input on the copayment problem. When the manager voices appreciation and praise for the employees' good work, they are more willing to accept some **constructive criticism** on problem issues. (See *Attributes of a quality manager*.)

Office Management Roles and Responsibilities

Physicians spend most of their time and energy caring for their patients. They will, in turn, rely on the expertise of an office manager (OM) to ensure that the office operations run smoothly and effectively. The OM will commonly serve as the HIPAA compliance officer as well as function as the supervisor of personnel. In general, the role of the OM includes:

- creating and updating the office's policies and procedures manual
- supervising office personnel
- supervising externship students
- conducting regular staff meetings
- supervising the purchase of equipment and supplies
- arranging for maintenance and calibration of equipment
- supervising the purchase and locked storage of controlled substances
- ensuring that Material Safety Data Sheets are kept on all necessary chemicals, cleaning solutions, and supplies
- approving financial transactions, including payroll and accounts payable and receivable, and creating financial reports as needed
- maintaining malpractice insurance and developing risk management strategies
- reattesting and maintaining physician participation in managed care.

Some larger medical practices and all hospitals employ a human resources director and HIPAA compliance officer in

Attributes of a quality manager

The table below lists common attributes of a quality manager along with questions that the medical assistant can ask herself to determine if she already possesses these attributes or should seek to obtain them.

Attribute	Question
Appreciative	• Do I thank and respect others for their hard work?
Approachable	• Am I easy to talk to?
	• Am I willing to listen to others?
	• Can I set a friendly and professional tone in the office?
Detail-oriented	• Do I recheck my work for errors?
	• Do I pay attention to small details?
Effective communicator	• Can I communicate effectively in oral and written form?
Flexibile	• Am I willing to try new ideas and seek solutions to problems?
Honest and truthful	• Do I admit my errors?
	• Will I give honest feedback to employees?
Objective	• Will I treat all employees equally and fairly?
	• Will I try to find solutions to problems that benefit everyone?
Organized	• Can I lead by example by being organized in my work?
	• Do I prioritize tasks?
Skilled in dealing with people	• Do I enjoy working with people?
	• Can I build the confidence and self-esteem in others to bring out the best in them?
Optimistic	• Am I generally an optimistic person?
	• Do I assume things will go right or wrong?
Perceptive	• Can I understand nonverbal cues that give me insight into a person?
	• Do I know when someone needs my help?
Realistic	• Will I demand too much or too little from employees?
Knowledgeable in the field	• Do I have an understanding of the job descriptions for the people I will supervise?

addition to the OM. At a large facility, such as a hospital, an OM could not perform all of the duties required of all three positions. In general, the role of the HR director includes:

- creating and updating the office policies and procedures manual
- recruiting and hiring office personnel
- orienting and training new personnel and externship students
- providing continuing education for employees as needed
- performing evaluations and salary reviews
- dismissing employees and conducting exit interviews
- maintaining confidential personnel records
- complying with state and federal regulations regarding employees.

Because the job duties of the OM and the HR director overlap, an individual office will delineate the roles of the personnel. As with any position in the physician's office or hospital, a **job description** is necessary so that employees know what their responsibilities are and no functions of the office are unattended to.

Dealing with Employees

As a supervisor, you will have to interact with different people with varying personalities. It will be your job to get everyone working toward common goals. Employees must communicate with each other and cooperate in getting tasks accomplished. An effective leader leads by example. Communicate and work with each employee to delineate roles in the tasks of the office. Through training, make sure that employees have an understanding of the roles of other members of the team and their jobs. When employees know who performs tasks in the office, they can troubleshoot and ask for help if necessary.

✦ TIP Getting Rid of Gossip

Gossip can be a destructive force in an office. If people are developing personal animosity towards one another, take steps to end the negative comments. Never take sides or participate in the gossiping. Treat all employees with respect and they will in turn treat each other with respect. If you feel that you cannot get people to work together in a positive fashion, you may need to fire an employee or ask the advice of the physician owner.

Conducting an Interview

When looking to hire a new employee, the office manager will conduct an interview of the applicant. The office manager should conduct the interview in a private office and ask not to be disturbed during the interview. The OM should ask the applicant about:

- ability to perform the job functions
- transportation to work
- availability of hours
- last job
- duties of the previous job
- clinical and administrative skills
- strengths and weaknesses.

In addition, the OM should take note of the applicant's appearance, eye contact, vocabulary, and general nature. The OM should let the applicant do most of the talking and should wait until the end of the interview to discuss salary questions.

An interview worksheet helps ensure that the OM asks all applicants the same questions. She can then add the worksheet to the applicant's folder along with the application and resume. The interview worksheet includes information that will help the interviewer decide which candidate is best suited to the job. Items will include the candidate's skills, hours of availability, and expected salary range. (See Figure 15-1.)

When conducting an interview, the OM is not legally allowed to ask about the applicant's home life, such as if she is married or single, cares for an elderly relative, has children and good day care arrangements. If the OM were to ask these questions and the applicant was not offered the position, she could assume that she was a victim of discrimination and could file a lawsuit against the medical practice. Although the OM cannot ask these questions, an applicant will commonly offer information in an effort to show that she is a good candidate for the position. An applicant may inform the OM that, while she does have two children, the day care is only a 5-minute drive from the home of her mother, who frequently helps out with childcare. Although the OM cannot ask the questions, she can base hiring on information offered by the applicant during the interview. The OM is allowed to ask the applicant to disclose any felony convictions, and the applicant is required, by law, to answer truthfully. If the applicant discloses a felony conviction, the OM can ask for details about the crime committed. The decision to hire an individual with a felony conviction should be thought out carefully and should never compromise patient safety.

The Americans with Disabilities Act of 1990 ensures the rights of persons with disabilities. Persons with disabilities can be asked if they need accommodation to perform job duties, such as a big-screen computer for a visually impaired applicant, a telephone amplifier for a hearing-impaired applicant, or wheelchair access to a work area for an applicant in a wheelchair.

Name ___Jean Martinez___   Interview date and time ___10/16/08, 4:30 p.m.___

Position ___front desk/reception_____ (front office, clinical, float, etc.)

Ask the applicant if he/she can perform:

Vital signs _____✓_____   Hgb, glucose _____

Height & weight _____✓_____   Assisting with surgery _____

Injections _____   Patient education _____

Scheduling _____✓_____   Billing & coding _____✓_____

Preauthorization _____✓_____   Specialty referrals ✓ _at previous job in ortho office_

Hospital scheduling _____   Financial reports ✓ _familiar with Medisoft_

Appearance ___Professional, well dressed_____   Eye contact ___good___

Work experience ___3 years front desk/billing dept. at Williamsville Orthopedics;___

___needs work closer to home; she moved to Blueville___

Availability – MTWTFS ___Days and evenings except Wed after 5 pm___

Overall impression ___Professional, confident, experienced___

Salary discussion ___states she was making $14.50 at previous position___

NEVER ASK
"Do you have children?"
"Are you planning to get pregnant?"
Any personal questions about age, national origin, religion, sexual orientation, marital status.

FIG 15-1 Interview worksheet.

The OM should keep the application and resume of applicants private and avoid sharing the information with other personnel. Only the individuals who are responsible for making the hiring decision, such as the OM and physician-owner, should have access to these materials. Upon hiring, the OM should file the applicant's application and resume in the employee's personnel file. Personnel files are private; only the employee and supervisors should be viewing the personnel file.

After the interview, the OM should check professional and, if applicable, personal references. The OM should call the reference and ask about the employee's work ethic, ability to perform the job, and interactions with employees. The OM should ask if the employee:

- was on time every day for work
- had a pleasant attitude
- was empathetic towards patients
- was flexible in job duties.

Some companies allow only the HR manager to take reference calls. This person may not have worked directly with the applicant and may only offer the dates of employment as a matter of policy. The OM should not consider such a policy as a mark against an applicant. Instead, the OM should try to contact another reference who can speak more freely about the applicant.

The physician-owner may interview applicants or review the OM's interview notes to make a decision. The OM should meet with the physician-owner to suggest that the most impressive applicant be hired, considering the personalities of the people the new employee will work with. Once an applicant is chosen, the OM should call the applicant to offer the position and agree on a starting date.

✦ TIP Giving a Reference
If an employee is seeking a new job and asks the OM for a reference, the OM should find out what she can and cannot

say. Some employers will only allow an OM to give the dates of employment, while others will allow a more detailed reference. The OM may need to keep the identity of the employee confidential from the supervisor or physician-owner. Maintaining confidentiality extends beyond patient files. An OM who can be trusted by her employees maintains this confidentiality and, in turn, gains her employees' respect.

New Employee Orientation

The first day of a new job is full of excitement as well as uncertainty. The OM should introduce the new staff member to her coworkers and welcome her to the team. Many offices have a new employee follow another employee through the workday. The new person will watch the work being performed and have the opportunity to ask questions. Once the new employee is comfortable with the job duties, she is allowed to perform tasks.

Policies and Procedures Manual

In addition to the new employee orientation, a **policies and procedures manual** is a powerful tool for learning a new job. Employees can refer to the manual as new tasks or situations arise. The policy portion of the manual refers to the "rules" of the office.

For example, the office charges 5 cents per page for photocopying records for patients. That is the *policy*. The *procedure* outlines how to carry out the photocopying of the medical records and collecting payment:

1. Verify the patient's identity with a photo driver's license.
2. Have the patient sign and date a release form.
3. Photocopy pages from the patient's medical record.
4. Document the copying of pages in the notes and attach the signed release form.
5. Put the records into a large, sealed envelope.
6. Collect the 5 cents per page fee and give the records to the patient.

A policies and procedures manual should be available for all employees to refer to. The OM should update the manual as needed. When in doubt about a policy or procedure, the manual should instruct employees to check with the OM or physician.

An OM commonly gives a copy of the manual to a new employee to take home and review. The OM can direct the new employee to areas of the manual that specifically relate to her job. For example, the newly hired billing and coding specialist will need to review the procedures for electronic transmission of billing and the policies for resubmitting rejected claims. The OM should not assume that reading the manual will give adequate information to the new employee; conducting a discussion with the new employee allows her to ask questions and ensures understanding of the policies and procedures. (See *Procedure 15-1: Training new personnel using the policies and procedures manual*.)

Conducting a Staff Meeting

Staff meetings are a great way for the team to discuss the effectiveness of work procedures, communicate concerns or changes to policies, and appreciate jobs well done. The staff meeting should begin with an agenda. The **agenda** is an outline of topics to be discussed and the order in which they will be presented. All employees appreciate organized meetings that are held in a reasonable amount of time. Staff meetings that run too long are counterproductive, and staff will begin to resent the meetings. (See Figure 15-2.)

The OM should take steps to make the meeting successful, including:

- e-mailing the agenda to staff members prior to the meeting and providing copies at the beginning of the meeting
- holding the meeting in the office when no patients are scheduled
- turning on the answering machine or answering service so that no one has to leave to answer phones
- offering beverages and snacks (optional).

The staff meeting helps make the staff aware of each individual's job and what gets accomplished on a daily basis. Hearing about coworkers' responsibilities and accomplishments helps an employee understand that every person in the office is an important member of the team. If the administrative staff does not schedule appointments, the clinical staff will have no patients to see. If the clinical staff does not complete charting, the billing department cannot obtain payment for services. When employees realize that their jobs impact the ability of others to complete tasks, they will feel an obligation to others in the organization to do a good job. At the end of a busy day, the front office staff, clinical personnel, physicians, and office managers can feel a sense of pride in their accomplishments. For example, during the day, Amy, the front desk medical assistant, may help an elderly patient into a treatment room. Steve, who is a clinical assistant, calls an insurance company on behalf of a patient who has a billing question. Wendy, who works in the billing department, helps Steve find a lost patient chart. Amy, Wendy, and Steve can appreciate the help that coworkers offer.

Conducting an Employee Evaluation

As a supervisor, it is the OM's job to give employees feedback on their work. The OM should praise their good

Training new personnel using the policies and procedures manual

Task

Orient new personnel to the information contained in the policies and procedures manual.

Conditions

- Policies and procedures manual
- New employee personnel file

Standards

In the time specified and within the scoring parameters determined by the instructor, the student will successfully train new personnel using the policies and procedures manual.

Performance Standards

1. Role-play the supervisor and then the new employee with a classmate. The new employee will read a section of the policies and procedures manual. The supervisor then answers questions posed by the new employee. The supervisor ensures that the new employee understands the policies and procedures by asking questions.

2. Ask the new employee to read a section of the policies and procedures manual (as directed by the instructor) to promote understanding.

3. Ask the new employee to relate the policy and procedure outlined and give a rationale for the item to ensure that the employee not only knows how to do the procedure but has an understanding of why the procedure is conducted in this manner, which helps promote compliance with the procedure.

4. Give the new employee an opportunity to ask questions to demonstrate the importance of understanding the policies and procedures.

5. Answer the employee's questions and be sure to ask if the explanation is clear to ensure proper understanding.

6. Ask the new employee to sign a statement in her personnel file to indicate that she has read and understands the policies and procedures manual (or designated section) to promote adherence to policies and procedures.

POLICIES AND PROCEDURES MANUAL REVIEW STATEMENT

I _____ have read and understood the P&P manual, section(s) _____ and will adhere to these policies and procedures. I understand that if I have questions regarding specific procedures, I can refer to the P&P manual or ask supervising personnel.

_____   _____
Signature of employee   Date

_____   _____
Signature of manager   Date

---

work and show appreciation for their efforts. Periodic raises and promotions for exceptional work encourage good employees to stay with the office. Adding additional responsibilities or supervisory functions to an employee's job description shows the employee that competence and attention to detail is appreciated. Suggesting cross-training to the employee and steps to expand her knowledge base can further the employee's career. (See *Cross-train for success,* page 194.)

If necessary, constructive criticism is always preferred to merely criticizing an employee's efforts. Suggesting how the employee could do the work better, more efficiently, or in a more timely manner allows the employee to strive toward an attainable goal. If necessary, the OM should give the employee a corrective action plan. For example, if the employee is chronically late for work, the OM should explain that the employee must be on time 15 consecutive workdays or face dismissal. If misfiling is a

```
                          AGENDA
              Staff meeting-November 12, 2008
                     3:00 to 5:00 p.m.

    1. Introduce new clinical medical assistant - Wendy Jones

    2. Front desk - collection of copayments

    3. Scheduling MRIs at hospital - changes to procedure

    4. New hemocytometer - training schedule

    5. Carpet cleaning next Friday - reminder to move furniture
       into storage closet

    6. Schedule changes for Dr. Greer

    7. Employee of the month award

    8. Items from you

    9. Next month's meeting date and time
```

FIG 15-2 Sample agenda for staff meeting.

problem, the OM should give the employee some resources on how to file, such as a medical assisting textbook with exercises for the employee to do. The OM should offer to help the employee as needed in the corrective action plan.

✦ TIP The Sandwich Approach

An OM conducting an evaluation should consider the "sandwich" approach. Begin the evaluation with praise, then discuss areas that need improvement, and end the evaluation with more praise. The OM will be able to address the need

---

Front office–Back office connection

Cross-train for success

The office manager should encourage employees to cross-train in order to be available to help departments that are busy. A multiskilled medical assistant is valued by the office. The clinical medical assistant who learns how to submit electronic insurance claims and answer patient billing questions can cover the billing department if someone is ill or on vacation. The administrative medical assistant who keeps up with clinical skills such as taking vital signs can assist busy clinical staff at a moment's notice.

---

for improvement, and the employee will feel encouraged by the praise.

Disciplinary Actions and Terminations

A negative employee can make the whole office feel bad and produce a counterproductive environment. If corrective action is possible, the OM should meet with the employee and devise a plan for improvement that includes a timeline. The OM should document the employee's efforts towards corrective action.

In the event that such corrective action does not succeed, the OM may need to fire an employee. To protect the office legally, the OM should keep a written file on an employee who is a problem. In the file, the OM should:

- document the employee's unacceptable behavior, such as tardiness, rudeness to patients or coworkers, and an inability or unwillingness to perform job duties
- date the incidents and include the names of other personnel who may be involved
- directly quote any inappropriate statements made by the employee to patients or other staff members.

When the physician-owner and the OM decide that the employee will be terminated, they should be prepared for the employee to react angrily. They should keep the dialogue as short as possible and tell the employee that they have chosen to terminate her employment and that she should leave the office. To avoid a scene, the OM may want to fire the employee when patients are not in the office.

Taking an Inventory and Ordering Supplies

The OM may take an inventory of supplies and order the clinical and administrative supplies needed to run the office. Alternatively, the clinical staff may order clinical supplies and the administrative staff, the front desk supplies. In such a case, the OM should supervise staff members who are responsible for taking inventory and placing orders. Written or computerized inventory sheets can help determine the need for supplies. (See *Clinical cabinet inventory*.)

Maintaining Laboratory Equipment and Supplies Inventory

The OM commonly has the task of inventorying and ordering supplies and maintaining equipment or directing a staff member to do so. These tasks must be performed on a weekly, monthly, or quarterly basis as needed. An inventory of frequently used supplies, such as bandages, syringes, and thermometer covers, is commonly necessary each week, because the office cannot run without these needed items. The OM or staff can take an inventory on a monthly basis for items that are used less frequently or kept in large supply, such as tongue depressors and examination table paper. The equipment manufacturers recommend maintenance schedules for equipment. They may base these recommendations on the number of times the machine is used or the time period between maintenance inspections. The policies and procedures manual should contain instructions for maintaining laboratory and office safety. The OM should organize and maintain the laboratory and office contents to promote optimal function and ensure safety. (See *Procedure 15-2: Taking and reordering inventory, performing maintenance, and checking safety*, pages 196 and 197.)

Selecting Computer Hardware and Software

The OM may be required to update computer hardware and software or computerize an office that has previously recorded all information on paper. Because protected health information (PHI) is available on office computers, the OM must ensure that logins and passwords are used to protect patient privacy and that virus and spyware protection are installed and periodically updated. Failure to safeguard PHI could result in fines.

Many software programs offer physician office management tools, including programs for:

- creating a patient database
- appointment scheduling
- insurance billing (electronic submission or U.S. mail claims)
- patient billing (with dunning notices for overdue bills)
- financial reports (daily, weekly, or monthly revenues)
- sorting revenue by doctor or department
- online banking
- taking inventory.

Vendors who sell software packages to physician offices may customize programs to fit specific needs. Because

---

Clinical cabinet inventory

A clinical cabinet inventory sheet can be taped to the inside of the cabinet. When items are used, the medical assistant should change the quantity listed to reflect usage. This type of inventory can also be tracked using a computer spreadsheet. The medical assistant must remember to update the item's quantity in the inventory spreadsheet. The figure below shows an example of a printed clinical cabinet inventory sheet. As disposable items are used, the amount of remaining items is updated.

ITEM	AMOUNT	ORDER DATE
MMR vaccines	35 units 29	9/15/07 (exp 6 months)
DPT vaccines	25 units	9/15/07 (exp 6 months)
Band-aids	6 boxes	5/12/07
Alcohol pads	8 boxes (500 units/box)	5/12/07
Gauze pads	10 boxes (1000 units/box)	7/11/07
Exam table paper rolls	2 boxes (6 rolls per box)	8/12/07
HGB slides	1 box (100 units/box)	8/12/07
Lancets	2 boxes (100 units/box)	8/12/07

PROCEDURE 15-2

Taking and reordering inventory, performing maintenance, and checking safety

Task

Take an inventory of equipment and supplies and reorder supplies, perform routine equipment maintenance, and check laboratory safety.

Conditions

- Various equipment and supplies in the classroom and laboratory
- Inventory log
- Reorder form
- Equipment safety and maintenance instructions (provided by the manufacturer)
- Equipment quality control log
- Pen

Standards

In the time specified and within the scoring parameters determined by the instructor, the student will successfully perform an inventory of equipment and supplies in the classroom and laboratory, fill out the reorder form, perform routine maintenance on equipment as directed by the instructor, check the condition of the laboratory and classroom for safety violations, and correct any violations.

Performance Standards

1. Your instructor will assign a section of the laboratory or classroom for you to take an inventory. Using the inventory log and reorder form, count supplies and equipment and note items that need to be reordered. Be sure to check the contents of open packages to get an accurate count of items and ensure proper reorder.

2. Inspect the equipment for missing or broken parts, frayed electrical cords, or other safety hazards to ensure laboratory safety.

3. Report the condition of the equipment, noting the serial number on each item so that you can get the equipment repaired at no cost if a service contract is in place and to clearly identify each machine if the laboratory contains more than one of the same machine. Equipment to examine includes:
   a. autoclave
   b. ECG machine
   c. computers
   d. height and weight scale
   e. wall-mounted sphygmomanometer (blood pressure cuff)
   f. wall-mounted ophthalmoscope-otoscope unit
   g. glucometer
   h. cholesterol meter.

4. Run a quality control check on a machine (as directed by your instructor). Fill out the results in the quality control log. Date and initial your work to show when the machine was last tested and ensure timely testing.

5. Clean the autoclave as directed by the manufacturer's instruction manual to promote proper sterilization of instruments.

6. Check the entire laboratory for safety hazards and mark the laboratory safety inspection sheet to

REORDER FORM		
Supply Item	Quantity	Reorder Date
Band-aids	6 boxes	5/12/08

PROCEDURE 15-2—cont'd

QUALITY CONTROL LOG

Name of Equipment

Date	Time	Strip #	QC Reading	Initials
7/14/08	8:51 a.m.	2	104	KM

prevent injury to staff and patients. Be sure to inspect:

a. electrical cords for fraying or malfunctioning
b. electrical outlets for loose covers or damage
c. computer keyboards, monitors, towers, other components, and wiring
d. light sources and rechargeable batteries
e. ECG leads and wires
f. other equipment (as directed by the instructor).
7. Initiate repairs to the equipment (as directed by the instructor).

LABORATORY SAFETY INSPECTION SHEET

Equipment	Status	Repair needed	Initials
Electrical cords: computers	One loose connection – to the monitor	Tightened connection	LZ
Electrical cords: lights	OK		LZ

customized software can be expensive, the OM should compare prices and options that best fit the needs of the office. The OM should consult the office staff who will be using the software. If vendors come to the office to demonstrate software packages, the OM should include the staff in the presentation. In addition, the OM should provide training to all staff—clinical and administrative, if possible. (Many software companies will include staff training as a service for purchasing their software package.)

Computer hardware—the computer monitor, tower, printer, and keyboard—must be replaced and updated periodically. Service contracts are available on most computer equipment as well as trade-in allowances. If the OM is responsible for choosing computer hardware, she must do some research. Comparing prices, warranties, and service contracts could save the office money and save the staff from the aggravation of computer malfunction.

Using Computers in the Medical Office

Because computers in a medical office contain PHI and other sensitive information, the OM should train employees to:

- turn off a computer screen when moving away from the computer
- place monitors so that patients cannot see the screen, to ensure privacy
- be sure that the patient at the front desk cannot see the computer screen (if necessary, by shielding the screen or positioning her body to prevent the patient from viewing the screen) (See Figure 15-3.)
- take printouts from the printer right away and not leave sensitive information in the printer or in a visible spot at the front desk

- log off the computer when away from it. (In addition, the OM should be sure to deactivate the login and password of an employee who leaves the practice.)

Assisting with Physician Travel Arrangements

The OM will be charged with arranging the travel of physicians or staff members who attend seminars, continuing education courses, and lectures. The physician and staff members rely on the OM to arrange transportation, hotel accommodations, and registration for these events. The OM may need to call the provider of the seminar to determine the registration procedures at arrival time. The OM can help the physician or staff member by creating an itinerary that includes such items as flight information (including check-in time and flight time), registration time and location of seminar events, and hotel reservations (including a confirmation number). By reviewing the itinerary with the physician or staff member prior to departure, the OM can help the attendees have a positive experience. (See *Procedure 15-3: Preparing physician travel*.)

Marketing in the Medical Office

A successful medical office uses marketing to inform its patients of the services it offers. As the office expands, it should inform patients of new services, expanded office

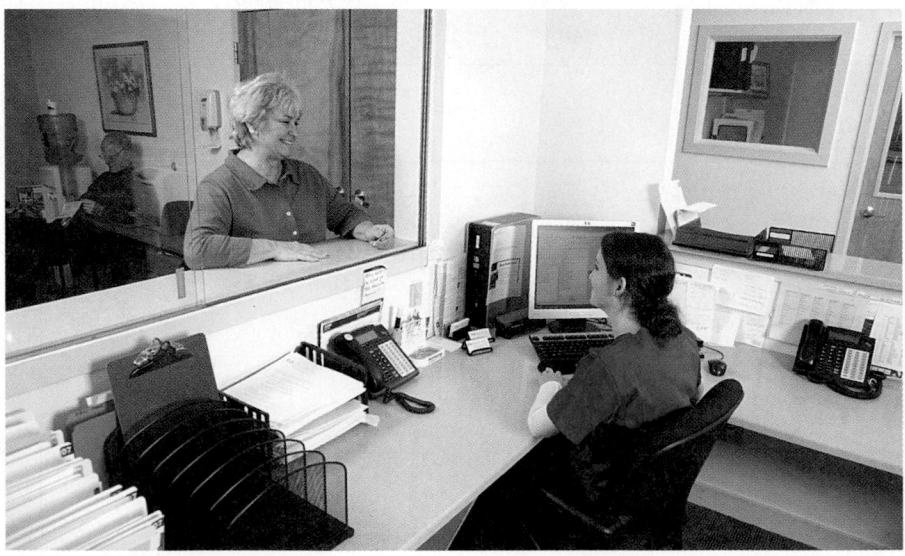

FIG 15-3 Shield the computer monitor from the view of patients.

Preparing physician travel

Task

Prepare the physician's itinerary for travel arrangements, hotel and rental car reservations, and seminar registration.

Conditions

- Computer with access to the Internet
- Physician or company credit card

Standard

In the time specified and within the scoring parameters determined by the instructor, the student will successfully arrange travel plans for the physician, including travel arrangements, hotel and rental car reservations, and seminar registration.

Performance Standards

1. Discuss with the physician (role-played by the instructor) what city she needs to fly to, the dates of the flight, and her preference for rental car, plane seating, and hotel accommodations to save time in deciding on options when making arrangements.

2. Research flights from your local airport to the destination.

3. Research hotels that are near the seminar and that meet the physician's criteria.

4. Find a rental car at the destination airport that meets the physician's criteria.

5. Print the travel information and confirm it with the physician to ensure that the physician is comfortable with the arrangements before purchase.

6. Create a confirmation notification for the physician that confirms travel reservations.

```
Dr. Wilson,

Here is your information for travel:

Air: Southwest Airlines
leaves Bradley airport 8:48 a.m. on flight 708
connect in Chicago to flight 412 to San Diego
arriving at 11:22 a.m.

Shuttle to hotel - call on Radisson courtesy phone

Hotel: Radisson Harbor San Diego
Dates: April 17th thru April 22nd
confirmation # ACF6790045

Conference - "Pain management in reflex sympathetic dystrophy"
Conference registration confirmation #29888RSD

Air: Southwest Airlines
leaves San Diego airport 7:05 a.m. on flight 307
connect in Chicago to flight 1198 to Bradley
arriving at 4:12 p.m.
```

hours, or changes to insurance policies. There are two types of marketing: internal and external.

Internal Marketing

Informing existing patients of changes in the practice is called *internal marketing.* If a patient regularly sees one of the doctors in the practice, she may not be aware of the services of the physical therapist or the acupuncturist. Mailing announcements to the existing patients can create business for a new service being offered. In addition, they may tell friends and family about the expanded services. (See Figure 15-4.)

Reminder cards and newsletters are other tools for internal marketing. Patients may not remember to call to schedule their yearly physical; sending reminder cards generates office visits. Sending periodic newsletters can keep the office name in a patient's mind. Marketing companies create newsletters that the office can send to existing patients. The topics of the newsletters can vary from vaccine schedule

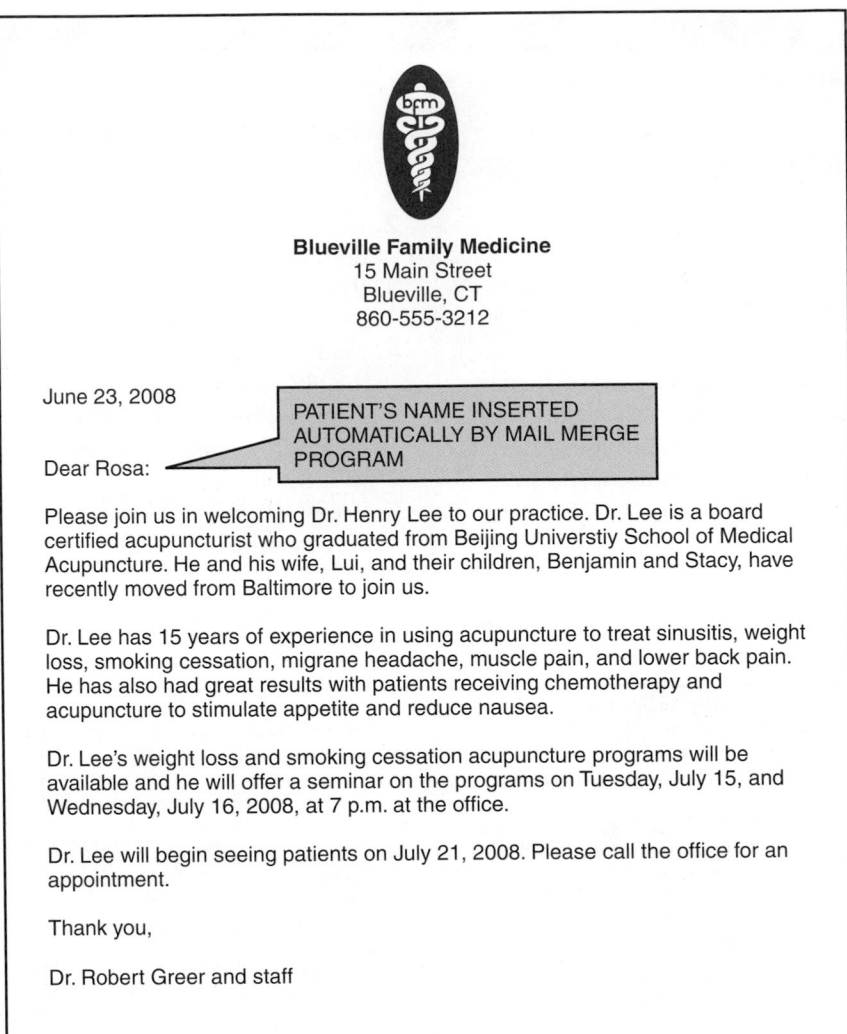

Blueville Family Medicine
15 Main Street
Blueville, CT
860-555-3212

June 23, 2008

Dear Rosa:

> PATIENT'S NAME INSERTED AUTOMATICALLY BY MAIL MERGE PROGRAM

Please join us in welcoming Dr. Henry Lee to our practice. Dr. Lee is a board certified acupuncturist who graduated from Beijing Universtiy School of Medical Acupuncture. He and his wife, Lui, and their children, Benjamin and Stacy, have recently moved from Baltimore to join us.

Dr. Lee has 15 years of experience in using acupuncture to treat sinusitis, weight loss, smoking cessation, migrane headache, muscle pain, and lower back pain. He has also had great results with patients receiving chemotherapy and acupuncture to stimulate appetite and reduce nausea.

Dr. Lee's weight loss and smoking cessation acupuncture programs will be available and he will offer a seminar on the programs on Tuesday, July 15, and Wednesday, July 16, 2008, at 7 p.m. at the office.

Dr. Lee will begin seeing patients on July 21, 2008. Please call the office for an appointment.

Thank you,

Dr. Robert Greer and staff

FIG 15-4 Internal marketing letter to an existing patient.

reminders to handwashing for infection prevention. (See Figure 15-5.)

✦ TIP Referral Requests

A great marketing tool is to ask people to refer their friends and family to the office. When patients express gratitude for quality care, the medical assistant should tell them that the best compliment is a referral. The office manager should make sure that the medical assistant is trained in how to appropriately ask for referrals.

External Marketing

External marketing refers to marketing that targets people who have not been patients of the practice. Yellow page, newspaper, radio, and television advertising can be used to let the public know the services the office provides, where it is located, and how to contact the office. (See Figure 15-6.)

Tracking Marketing

Because the office will use many forms of marketing, the OM should keep a record of which forms of advertising and marketing yield patients and which do not. A list of promotional codes can be created to track effective marketing practices. The OM can create a simple database that tells her the source of each referral—for example, A for yellow pages, B for patient referral, C for physician referral, D for newsletter, E for HMO listing, and F for other. The OM can review the database periodically to determine which forms of marketing are most effective. In addition, the new patient intake form should include the question, "How did you hear about us?" The medical assistant can add the source of the referral to a marketing tracking file. Marketing sources that can be included in the marketing tracking file might include a yellow pages advertisement, a patient referral, an HMO listing, or a newspaper advertisement. If

Blueville Family Medical News
July 2008
Keeping in touch with all your health needs

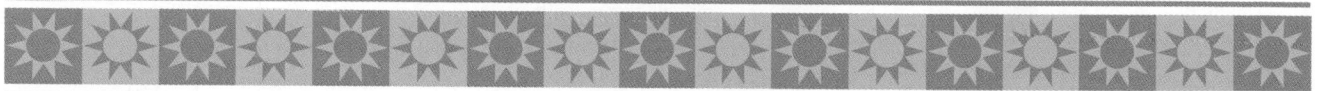

Blueville Family Medicine
15 Main Street
Blueville, CT
860-555-3212

Robert Greer, MD
Hector Rodriguez, MD
Anne Wilson, MD
Sharon Piecek, APRN
Henry Lee, MD, L.A.C.

New Happenings in our office

Expanded Office Hours

In an effort to make our office hours convenient to our busy patients, we have expanded our hours to include Monday and Thursday evenings until 7:30 p.m. and Saturdays from 8:30 to 1 p.m. Call the office for an appointment.

Welcome Dr. Henry Lee

Please join us in welcoming Dr. Henry Lee to our practice. Dr. Lee is a board certified acupuncturist who graduated from Beijing University School of Medical Acupuncture. He and his wife, Lui, and their children, Benjamin and Stacy, have recently moved from Baltimore to join us.

Dr. Lee has 15 years of experience in using acupuncture to treat sinusitis, weight loss, smoking cessation, migraine headache, muscle pain, and lower back pain. He has also had great results with patients receiving chemotherapy and acupuncture to stimulate appetite and reduce nausea.

Dr. Lee's weight loss and smoking cessation acupuncture programs will be available and he will offer seminars on the programs on Tuesday, July 15, 2008, at 7 p.m. and Wednesday, July 16, at 6 p.m. Call the office to reserve a seat at one of the seminars.

Dr. Lee will begin seeing patients on July 21, 2008. Please call the office to schedule an appointment.

Welcome, New Baby!

Please join us in congratulating Kelly Manera, our billing coordinator, and her husband Ken on the birth of their daughter, Kathryn Elizabeth, on June 11, 2008. Mom and baby are doing fine and Kelly will return to work in September. Welcome Kathryn Elizabeth!

Nutrition Notes from Sharon Piecek, APRN, RD

Preventing Cataracts with Good Nutrition

A cataract is an age-related thickening of the lens of the eye that impairs vision. Surgical removal of the cataract will prevent blindness, but good nutrition can reduce your chances of developing cataracts. Oxidative stress plays a big role in the development of cataracts. A diet rich in antioxidant foods can reduce your risk of cataracts. Specifically, foods high in vitamin A, vitamin C, and vitamin E have been known to decrease cataract development.

To reduce your risk of cataracts, include the following foods in your diet:

Sweet potatoes	950 mcg of vitamin A per ½ cup cooked serving
Carrots	320 mcg of vitamin A per ½ cup raw serving
Broccoli	60 mg of vitamin C per ½ cup serving
Fresh strawberries	70 mg of vitamin C per ½ cup serving
Almonds	36 mg of vitamin E per 1 cup serving
Sunflower seeds	13 mg of vitamin E per ¼ cup serving

In addition to reducing your risk for cataracts, vitamins A, C, and E are antioxidants that protect the body against all forms of oxidative stress and, therefore, help you fight infection. Remember A, C, and E are your ACE against infection!

For more nutritional counseling, call the office and make an appointment to see me. I am happy to assist you in making healthy food and lifestyle choices.

Best of Health,
Sharon

Human Papilloma Virus Vaccines Are Available

HPV vaccines are available for female patients who are age 12 and older. Although the vaccine is not mandated by the state for public school attendance, the vaccine has been shown to reduce susceptibility to HPV infection. Ask Dr. Rodriguez or Dr. Wilson for more information.

Don't Miss out on Fall Sports!

High school and junior high school sports physicals are available with Dr. Rodriguez, Dr. Wilson, or Sharon Piecek, APRN. Without a signed physical form, athletes cannot participate in school sports teams and clubs. Physicals take approximately 45 minutes; call the office for an appointment.

FIG 15-5 Sample newsletter.

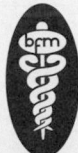

Blueville Family Medicine
15 Main Street
Blueville, CT
860-555-3212

Robert Greer, MD.....Family medicine
Hector Rodriguez, MD.....Family medicine
Anne Wilson, MD.....School and sports physicals
Sharon Piecek, APRN.....Nutritional counseling,
weight loss, and diabetes management
Henry Lee, MD, L.A.C......Acupuncture

FIG 15-6 Sample Yellow Pages advertisement.

the source of the referral is another patient, sending a note thanking the patient for the referral is a friendly gesture and might engender more referrals.

Chapter Summary

- The role of the office manager is to create a constructive working environment for all employees.
- Creating a positive environment that promotes teamwork and mutual respect is essential.
- Conducting staff meetings enables the office manager to update procedures, address staff concerns, and recognize employees for exceptional performance.
- Periodic performance reviews give employees feedback so that they can continuously improve their work.
- When the office manager leads by example with hard work and dedication, she shows that she cares about patients, coworkers, and physicians.

Team Work Exercises

1. Discuss with classmates your favorite supervisor or teacher. How did this person use the strategies of good leadership to create a team environment?
2. Discuss with your classmates a situation where leadership was lacking. How did that lack affect the outcomes of the group or work team?
3. Divide into groups of four to seven persons. Each group should discuss five tasks that can be included in a policies and procedures manual. For each item, create a policy regarding conditions for the task and a procedure that outlines how the task should be performed. When all five tasks have been addressed, the groups should exchange their policies and procedures and critiques those of the other

group. Are the policies stated in understandable terms? Are the policies reasonable and enforceable? Are the procedures outlined in a step-by-step manner? Are the steps easy to follow? Each group should provide constructive comments.

Case Studies

Role-play the following scenarios with classmates.

1. Barbara is chronically late for work. Although she is expected to be in the office by 8:30 a.m. to call the answering service and get messages from the previous day, she has not arrived at the office before 8:45 a.m. on any day for the past 2 weeks. Two other staff members have complained to the office manager that the telephone and scheduling have been compromised due to Barbara's tardiness. How should the office manager approach the problem with Barbara? One student should role-play as the office manager and another role-play as Barbara and then switch roles and repeat the exercise.
2. Jayne and Kelly do a great job running the front desk and processing insurance claims. They usually collect between $6000 and $7000 per week. In the past week, however, the billing department collected a record $9737.12. Sarah, the office supervisor, plans to mention the week's record collections at the staff meeting on Friday. Brainstorm with classmates what types of incentives and recognition Jayne and Kelly deserve. Then role-play the staff meeting.
3. A student extern will be starting to work in the office next week. The student medical assistant will need to spend time in each department learning the roles and responsibilities of many of the employees. The office manager, receptionists, billing coordinator, and clinical medical assistants must meet to discuss how teaching a student will impact their busy work schedule and why teaching externs is important to the practice. Role-play the meeting.
4. In pairs, classmates should play the roles of interviewer and interviewee. Create interview worksheets to guide questions during the interview. After conducting the interviews, discuss the strengths and weaknesses of the interviewer and interviewee. Then switch roles and repeat the exercise.

Resources

- Medical practice manager's network: *www.mpmnetwork.com/*
- Professional Association of Health Care Office Management: *www.pahcom.com/*
- Newsletter for Physician Office Administrators: *www .ardmorepublishing.com/mompage1.html*
- Moghadas, K.I.: *Medical Practice Policies and Procedures.* Chicago: American Medical Association, 2005.
- Rainer, C.: *Practice Management: A Practical Guide to Starting and Running a Medical Office.* Lima, OH: Wyndham Hall Press, 2004.

Coding and Insurance

Learning Objectives

Upon completion of this chapter, the student will be able to:

- define the key terms in the glossary
- describe how a claim travels through the medical office
- describe the different types of insurance products
- explain how a resource-based relative value system impacts claims coding
- explain how an effective superbill can help achieve a quick, clean claim processing
- apply skills to locate CPT codes
- apply skills to locate an ICD-9-CM code
- discuss how effective communication among the front desk, medical assistant, and physician is vital to the accurate processing of an insurance claim
- explain how to process a referral to a specialist or from a primary care physician
- accurately complete a CMS-1500 form
- describe the registration process for a new patient
- explain fraud and abuse and their consequences.

CAAHEP Competencies

Administrative Competencies

Process Insurance Claims

Apply managed care policies and procedures

Apply third-party guidelines

Perform procedural coding

Perform diagnostic coding

Complete insurance claim forms

Operational Functions

Utilize computer software to maintain office systems

ABHES Competencies

Administrative Duties

Apply managed care policies and procedures

Obtain managed care referrals and precertification

Perform diagnostic coding

Complete insurance claim forms

Use physician fee schedule

Financial Management

Implement current procedural terminology and ICD-9-CM coding

Analyze and use current third-party guidelines for reimbursement

Procedures

Coding procedures and diagnoses

Submitting a CMS-1500 form to a third-party payor

Communicating with a third-party payor

Chapter Outline

Health Insurance and Payment Coding

Procedural Coding

  CPT-4 coding

  HCPCS

Diagnostic Coding

  ICD-9-CM coding

  Multiple diagnosis codes

  Conventions

Superbill

Insurance in the Physician's Office

Employer Insurance Programs

Managed Care

  Health maintenance organization

  Independent practice association

  Preferred provider organization

Traditional Insurance

Consumer-Driven Health Plans

  Health savings account

  Health reimbursement account

  Flexible spending account

Government Programs

  Medicare

  Medicaid

  CHAMPUS

  CHAMPVA

Worker's Compensation

Multiple Insurance Policies

COBRA

Self-Pay Patients

Insurance Claims

  HIPAA

  Submitting a claim Life cycle of an insurance claim

  Obtaining referrals

Payment Systems

  Usual, customary, and reasonable

  Fee-for-service

  Resource-based relative value scale

  Capitation

Payment Processing

Payment Denials and Appeals Process

Fraud and Abuse

Chapter Summary

Team Work Exercises

Case Studies

Resources

Health Insurance and Payment

Health insurance is a contract between an insurance provider and the **policyholder**, the person who buys the insurance. A policyholder can also include dependent children, a spouse, and, in some states, a domestic partner as **beneficiaries**, or additional persons insured on the plan. The policyholder pays a **premium**, which is a monthly payment to the insurance company that guarantees the policyholder and his beneficiaries will receive the benefit of insurance coverage according to the coverage plan. A plan commonly includes coverage by the insurance company for some portion of medical expenses, including diagnostic and therapeutic procedures, for the policyholder and his beneficiaries. The list of covered services varies with the insurance carrier and the specific plan that the policyholder selects.

Health insurance benefits are paid by the insurance company after submission of a medical insurance claim, which is a request from the health care provider for payment. The administrative medical assistant submits this claim to the insurance company by coding the claim, which involves assigning alphanumeric codes to the diagnostic procedures used to identify the patient's condition and the procedures performed to treat it. All claims must be submitted on a CMS-1500 form, the claim form created by the U.S. Department of Health and Human Services. The coding system and the CMS-1500 form are recognized internationally and are written in the language used for reimbursement of medical claims.

In addition, the patient may be responsible for a portion of the payment, known as coinsurance. The patient's responsibility may be a percentage of the total fee charged or a **copayment**, which is a set amount paid at each office visit.

Coding

The medical assistant must include on an insurance claim a procedural code and a diagnostic code for each service provided to the patient in order to receive reimbursement from an insurance company or other third-party payor. The process of coding claims is complex and commonly requires a person who is professionally trained as a coder. This text introduces the medical assistant to basic coding. Medical assistants interested in developing more advanced coding skills should pursue certification through the American Academy of Professional Coders.

Procedural Coding

In order to obtain payment for a physician from an insurer, the medical assistant must tell the insurer what services the physician provided to the patient. These services, or procedures, are not described using words, but by assigning specific codes. In the physician's office, the medical assistant will use codes from *Current Procedural Terminology*, 4th edition, and health care procedural coding systems.

CPT-4 Coding

Current Procedural Terminology, **4th edition, (CPT-4)**, is a coding system that converts descriptions of medical, surgical, and diagnostic services delivered by providers into five-digit numeric codes. The first edition of CPT was published by the American Medical Association in 1966 and was revised three times during the late 1960s and early 1970s. Because procedures and technologies in medicine are always changing, updates to the CPT manual are published annually. The medical assistant must use the most current manual. (See *CPT-5*.) There are several types of CPT-4 codes:

- category I codes
- category II codes
- category III codes
- modifiers.

Category I

Category I codes are the primary codes used to describe procedures. They are divided into six sections in the CPT manual:

1. Evaluation and Management—codes 99201 through 99499
2. Anesthesia—codes 00100 through 01999 and codes 99100 through 99140
3. Surgery—codes 10021 through 69990
4. Radiology—codes 70010 through 79999

CPT-5

Insurers and practitioners anticipate a new edition of the *Current Procedural Terminology* (CPT) manual, CPT-5, to be published by 2011. The major changes to the CPT manual will be the use of terminology that more clearly describes procedures and services. The descriptions in the CPT-4 edition commonly include such phrases as "with or without," "and/or," or "by any method." The fifth edition will contain more precise definitions for procedures. Such phrases as "with or without" will no longer accompany one code; rather, two separate codes will be used to describe each procedure. The fifth edition of CPT, with its more precise language, will also conform more to HIPAA standards that require common, concise coding language.

5. Pathology and Laboratory—codes 80048 through 89356
6. Medicine—codes 90281 to 99199 and codes 99500 through 99602.

Within the six sections, procedures and services are described by subsections, subheadings, categories, and subcategories. Reading the full description of the procedure code enables the medical assistant to choose the appropriate code. (See *Coding options for leg casts*.) An insurance company can charge a medical office for **upcoding**, or using a code that yields a higher reimbursement than the actual service performed. If a pattern of upcoding is established, the insurer may accuse an office of intentional fraud.

Coding options for leg casts

Because CPT-4 coding is very specific, the medical assistant must ensure that she uses the correct code for the service provided. For example, the following list demonstrates the many different options for coding a leg cast application.

Code	Description
29345	Application of a long leg cast (thigh to toes)
29355	walker or ambulatory type
29358	Application of long leg cast brace
29365	Application of cylinder cast (thigh to ankle)
29405	Application of short leg cast (below knee to toes)
29425	walker or ambulatory type

INDENTED CODE MUST INCLUDE STATEMENT DIRECTLY ABOVE IT.

The medical assistant must code for the specific type of cast applied to the patient to ensure correct payment. Coding a cast incorrectly could delay payment or lead to fines for inappropriate coding. In the example above, a medical practice would be in error if it coded for a long leg cast when a short leg cast was actually applied. The medical office may be reimbursed at a higher rate for the application of a long leg cast and would therefore receive reimbursement for services that they did not actually provide.

Evaluation and Management Codes

Evaluation and management (E/M) codes (99201 through 99499) are used to describe physician services based on three main factors:

- place of service, such as a hospital (inpatient) or office visit (outpatient)
- type of service, such as a consultation, admission to a hospital, newborn care, or office visit for primary management of the patient's health care status
- patient status, including:
  - new patient (patient who has not previously received professional face-to-face services from the physician or other provider of the same group within the past 3 years)
  - established patient (patient who has received professional face-to-face services from the physician or other provider of the same group within the past 3 years)
  - outpatient (patient who is not formally admitted to a health care facility)
  - inpatient (patient who has been formally admitted to a health care facility).

In addition to the three categories, the E/M codes are further divided by such factors as patient history, physical examination, and the complexity of the decision-making process. To choose the appropriate E/M code, the medical assistant should read the description in the CPT manual to ensure that she chooses the correct code. (See *Common E/M code criteria*.)

Common E/M code criteria

The following chart shows the criteria for some common evaluation and management (E/M) codes for new and established patients.

Code	History	Examination	Medical Decision Making
New patients			
99201	**Problem-focused**	**Problem-focused**	**Straightforward**
	• Chief complaint • Brief history of present illness or problem	• Limited examination of the affected body area or organ system	• Minimal number of diagnoses or management options • Minimal amount or complexity of data to be reviewed • Minimal risk of complications, morbidity, or mortality
99202	**Expanded problem-focused**	**Expanded problem-focused**	**Straightforward**
	• Chief complaint • Brief history of present illness • Problem-pertinent system review	• Limited examination of the affected body area or organ system and other symptomatic or related organ system(s)	
99203	**Detailed**	**Detailed**	**Low complexity**
	• Chief complaint • Extended history of present illness • Problem-pertinent system review extended to include a review of limited number of additional systems • Pertinent past, family, and social history directly related to the patient's problems	• Extended examination of the affected body area(s) and other symptomatic or related organ system(s)	• Limited number of diagnoses or management options • Limited amount or complexity of data to be reviewed • Low risk of complications, morbidity, or mortality

Common E/M code criteria—cont'd

Code	History	Examination	Medical Decision Making
New patients			
99204	**Comprehensive**	**Comprehensive**	**Moderate complexity**
	• Chief complaint • Extended history of present illness • Review of systems that are directly related to the problem(s) identified in the history of present illness plus a review of all additional body systems • Complete past, family, and social history	• General multisystem examination or a complete examination of a single organ system	• Multiple number of diagnoses or management options • Moderate amount or complexity of data to be reviewed • Moderate risk of complications, morbidity, or mortality
99205	**Comprehensive**	**Comprehensive**	**High complexity**
			• Extensive number of diagnoses or management options • Extensive amount or complexity of data to be reviewed • High risk of complications, morbidity, or mortality
Established patients			
99212	**Problem-focused**	**Problem-focused**	**Straightforward**
99213	**Expanded problem-focused**	**Expanded problem-focused**	**Low complexity**
99214	**Detailed**	**Detailed**	**Moderate complexity**
99215	**Comprehensive**	**Comprehensive**	**High complexity**

Category II

Category II codes are a set of supplemental tracking codes used for performance measurement. Category II codes are optional, but their use will decrease the likelihood that the insurance company will want to examine all of the claims for the patient, called *record abstraction*. The additional information offered by the category II codes includes results from laboratory testing or clinical findings from evaluation and management. These codes support the need for further services. When these codes are included on a claim, the insurer does not need to ask the physician for more documentation to support the claim. Category II codes are not reimbursable and should never be used without a category I code. (See *Added information from category II*, page 208.)

Category III

In 2002, category III was added to the manual. Category III is a listing of temporary codes used to identify new technologies. Because emerging technologies in medicine are common, the category III codes allow physicians to be reimbursed for new procedures. Category III codes are located after the medicine section of the coding manual. Codes can remain in the category III section for a maximum of 5 years. At that point, the AMA must decide to move them up to category I or delete them from the list.

CPT Modifiers

CPT **modifiers** are two-digit numeric codes that are added to a CPT-4 code. The addition of the modifier indicates that the service or procedure has changed. The modifier is indicated on the CMS-1500 form on line 24, box D, to the right of the CPT code. (See Figure 16-1.) While many CPT-4 codes do not require a modifier, they are necessary to describe special circumstances during procedures. (See *Examples of CPT modifiers*, page 209.)

Added information from category II

Category II codes are CPT code descriptors. They are not stand-alone procedure codes, but rather additional codes that give information to support the need for a procedure. To choose the appropriate category II codes, the medical assistant should carefully review the medical record.

For example, the physician sees a patient with COPD for a physical examination. During the examination, the physician discusses the patient's smoking habit with her and, based on the patient's response, prescribes acupuncture as a smoking cessation treatment. He documents these details in the patient's medical record.

The medical assistant can use this additional information to support services aimed at smoking cessation, such as a prescription for acupuncture or nicotine replacement therapy. Use of category II codes can save time because it gives additional information without narrative documentation.

Thus, the medical assistant can add category II codes 1000F (the patient was asked about her tobacco use) and 1034F (the patient reports she is a current tobacco user) to support the prescription of acupuncture treatment.

Date	
10/15/08: 7:09 a.m	PE - BP - 140/88, T-98.4, R-22, HEENT-WNL. Resp-wheezing, cough. The patient reports smoking 1½ to 2 packs of cigarettes per day. The patient states that "I want to quit, I just don't have the willpower." Acupuncture for smoking cessation prescribed with Dr. Lee. ——— ——————————————————————————— R. Green, MD

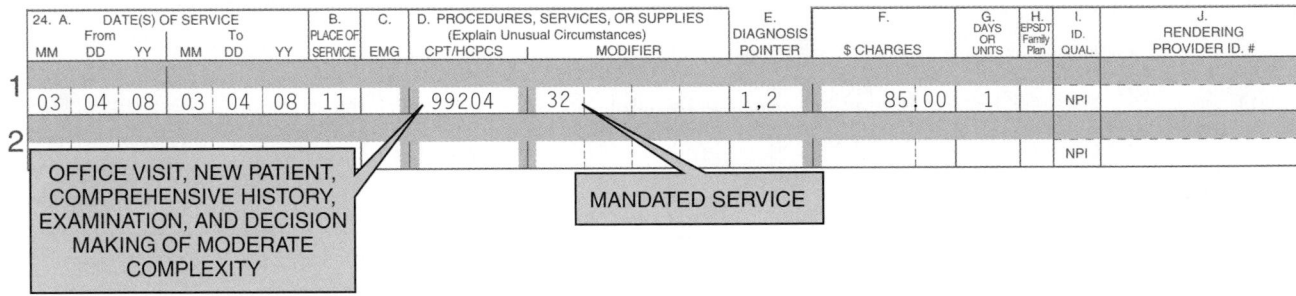

FIG 16-1 CMS-1500 form with CPT code and modifier.

HCPCS

In addition to CPT codes that identify examinations and procedures, medical assistants must translate medical equipment and transport services provided to patients into codes for reimbursement. Health care procedural coding system (HCPCS) is a standardized coding system used for this purpose. These codes primarily identify products, supplies, and services not included in CPT coding, such as ambulance services, durable medical equipment, prosthetics, orthotics, and supplies when used outside a physician's office. HCPCS codes are found in the CPT or ICD-9-CM manual and can be used with CPT codes for examinations and procedures. HCPCS codes are comprised of a single alpha character and then 4 numerical digits, for example:

- A0021—ambulance service, outside state per mile, transport

- A4211—supplies for self-administered injections
- E0130—walker, rigid (pickup), adjustable or fixed height.

Diagnostic Coding

In order to receive payment for procedures and services, the medical office must prove that the patient needed those procedures or services. The medical office establishes the necessity for procedures by determining a diagnosis. Diagnoses, just like procedures, are communicated to the insurer using a code. These diagnostic codes are numeric or alphanumeric codes called *ICD-9-CM codes.*

ICD-9-CM Coding

The *International Classification of Diseases,* 9th edition–Clinical Modifications, is the coding manual used to report the patient's diagnosis. The medical office must assign an

(Text continues on page 212.)

Examples of CPT modifiers

The following table lists CPT modifier codes along with a description and example.

Code	Description	Example	
		Scenario	Code and meaning
21	**Prolonged evaluation and management (E/M) services** Assigned when E/M services provided are greater than the highest reportable level of service. (Providing documentation of the service with the claim is recommended.)	A patient being evaluated for anxiety is upset. The provider spends an hour counseling the patient.	**99215-21** Comprehensive E/M
22	**Unusual procedural service** Assigned when a procedure requires greater than usual services. (Documentation is required for reimbursement.)	A patient needs a revision of an external fixation device under anesthesia. During the procedure, the provider determines that the fracture is not healing and requires more pins, wires, and rings than expected.	**20693-22** Adjustment of external fixation device requiring anesthesia
23	**Unusual anesthesia** Assigned for anesthesia administered for services that usually require local or no anesthetic	A patient who has a history of anxiety needs a suspicious dermal lesion removed. Although this procedure is usually done with a local anesthetic, the provider determines a need for a general anesthetic.	**11302-23** Shaving of epidermal lesion diameter 1.2 to 2.0 cm
24	**Unrelated E/M service by same physician during postoperative period** Assigned when an E/M service is performed in the standard postoperative period for a condition unrelated to a surgical diagnosis	Two weeks after knee surgery, a patient falls and breaks his radial shaft. Provider performs a reduction of a wrist fracture.	**25500-24** Closed treatment of radial shaft fracture
25	**Significant, separate, identifiable E/M service by the same physician on the same day of the procedure or other service** Assigned when E/M service was performed on the same day as another procedure. (Requires additional documentation.)	During a well-child visit, a physician notes bruising on the child that suggests abuse. The physician decides to examine and interview the patient more thoroughly.	**99215-25** Comprehensive E/M
26	**Professional component** Assigned when an interpretation of an x-ray, magnetic resonance imaging (MRI) scan, or other diagnostic test is performed by another physician	A chiropractor interprets x-rays of a patient's lower back taken at the hospital.	**72100-26** Radiologic examination; spine, lumbosacral; 2 or 3 views
32	**Mandated services** Assigned when services were mandated by a third party (such as a payor, attorney, or court order)	A patient wants to have a gastric banding procedure for weight loss. The insurer requires two physicians to recommend the procedure.	**99203-32** New patient E/M detailed history; detailed examination

Continued

Examples of CPT modifiers—cont'd

Code	Description	Example	
		Scenario	Code and meaning
47	**Anesthesia by surgeon** Assigned when a surgeon administers anesthesia while performing surgery	A patient has an abscess on the wall of his scrotum. The surgeon administers anesthesia and drains the abscess.	**55100-47** Drainage of scrotal wall abscess
50	**Bilateral procedure** Assigned when a procedure is performed bilaterally during the same session	A patient has an arthroscopic surgical repair of the anterior cruciate ligament (ACL) in both knees.	**29888-50** Arthroscopically aided anterior cruciate ligament repair/ augmentation or reconstruction
51	**Multiple procedures** Assigned when multiple procedures are performed during the same session	A patient has an arthroscopic repair to her left ACL and a meniscectomy of her right knee.	**29888** Arthroscopy with meniscus repair (medial or lateral) **AND** **29880-50** Arthroscopically aided anterior cruciate ligament repair/ augmentation or reconstruction
52	**Reduced services** Assigned when service is reduced and does not match the CPT code	During an upper GI series with a barium swallow, a patient vomits and can no longer continue the examination.	**74246-52** Radiologic examination, GI tract, upper air contrast, with specific high-density barium
53	**Discontinued procedure** Assigned when a physician terminates the procedure for the well-being of the patient	A patient is anesthetized and prepared for a heart transplant, but the heart arrives in damaged condition.	**33945-53** Heart transplant, with or without recipient cardiectomy
54	**Surgical care only** Assigned when a surgeon performed only the surgical portion of a surgical package	A patient has a car accident while on vacation 300 miles from home, requiring a repair of a fractured femoral shaft. Emergency surgery will be followed by care from a specialist near the patient's home.	**27506-54** Open treatment of femoral shaft fracture, with or without external fixation
55	**Postoperative management only** Assigned when a physician cares for a patient after surgery performed by another physician	A patient has a car accident while on vacation. A specialist near the patient's home monitors his postoperative progress.	**99024-55** Postoperative follow-up visit normally included in the surgical package
56	**Preoperative management only** Assigned when a physician clears a patient for surgery (nonemergency)	A physician examines a patient with severe heart disease and determines that the patient is healthy enough to undergo a heart transplant by a cardiac surgeon.	**99214-56** Detailed E/M
57	**Decision for surgery** Assigned when a physician examines a patient and recommends surgery that will be performed by another physician	A patient arrives in the emergency department (ED) after a car accident with a ruptured spleen. The ED physician diagnoses the rupture and sends the patient to surgery.	**99283-57** Emergency department visit, expanded problem-focused history

Examples of CPT modifiers—cont'd

Code	Description	Example	
		Scenario	*Code and meaning*
58	**Related procedure or service by the same physician during the postoperative period** Assigned for services that a physician provides during the postoperative period that are related to the surgery that physician performed earlier	A patient has an infection at a previous surgical site. The patient must undergo debridement of the surgical wound and removal of the mesh inserted on his abdominal wall.	**11008-58** Removal of prosthetic material or mesh, abdominal wall for necrotizing soft tissue infection
62	**Two surgeons** Assigned when two primary surgeons are required for a surgical procedure	A patient falls, breaking his left hip and damaging his right hip, which had previously been replaced. Both hips require surgical repair.	**27130-62 (left, initial)** **27134-62 (right, revision)** Initial hip replacement, left, and revision of hip replacement on the right; done by two surgeons at the same time to reduce anesthesia time
63	**Procedure performed on infant less than 4 kg** Assigned when a procedure is performed on a premature baby	An infant weighing less than 4 kg has an abnormal passageway between his stomach and intestines, requiring repair.	**43880-63** Closure of gastrocolic fistula
66	**Surgical team** Assigned when a highly complex surgery is performed that requires more than two surgeons. (Each surgeon reports the same procedure using the 66 modifier.)	A patient with severe chronic obstructive pulmonary disease (COPD) requires a double lung transplant. During the procedure, another surgeon will bypass the heart.	**32854-66** Lung transplant, double, with cardiopulmonary bypass
76	**Repeat procedure by same physician** Assigned when a physician repeats a surgical procedure originally performed by that same physician	A patient has a vasectomy, but follow-up sperm count indicates that the vas deferens has reattached. The surgeon who initially performed the surgery repeats the procedure.	**55250-76** Vasectomy, unilateral or bilateral, including postoperative semen examinations
77	**Repeat procedure by another physician** Assigned when a physician repeats a surgical procedure originally performed by a different physician	A patient who has a vasectomy but experiences reattachment of the vas deferens schedules a repeat of the procedure with a different surgeon.	**55250-77** Vasectomy, unilateral or bilateral, including postoperative semen examinations
78	**Return to operating room for related procedure during postoperative period** Assigned when a physician must perform a procedure during the postoperative period that is related to the original surgical procedure that the physician performed	A patient has a repair to the meniscus of his left knee. Four days after the surgery, he falls off of his crutches and ruptures his patellar tendon.	**27380-78** Suture of infrapatellar tendon

Continued

Examples of CPT modifiers—cont'd

Code	Description	Example	
		Scenario	*Code and meaning*
79	**Unrelated procedure or service by the same physician during the post-operative period** Assigned when the same physician performs two surgical procedures on a patient but the second procedure is unrelated to the first	A patient has a repair to the meniscus of his left knee. Four days after the surgery, he falls off of his crutches and fractures his right femur.	**27500-79** Closed treatment of femoral shaft fracture, without manipulation
80	**Assistant surgeon** Assigned when surgery requires an assistant surgeon due to the complexity of the procedure or its duration	A patient has a growing heart tumor. The surgery will take several hours and requires an assistant to perform cardiopulmonary bypass.	**33120-80** Excision of intracardiac tumor, resection with cardiopulmonary bypass, assistant surgeon performs closure
81	**Minimum assistant surgeon** Assigned when surgery is started with one surgeon and a second surgeon is called in for a short time to assist	While a patient is undergoing repair of perforated ulcers of the small intestine, the surgeon becomes ill, requiring a second surgeon to finish the procedure.	**44603-81** Suture of small intestine for perforated ulcers (multiple); assistant surgeon required since more ulcers are found than expected
90	**Reference (outside) laboratory testing** Assigned when a physician requests laboratory test results from an outside laboratory	A physician orders a complete blood count (CBC) for a patient. The medical assistant performs the venipuncture but does not test the blood. She sends the blood to an outside laboratory to perform the CBC.	**85025-90** **and 36415 (venipuncture)** Physician reports CBC
91	**Repeat clinical diagnostic laboratory test** Assigned when a clinical diagnostic test is repeated on the same day for multiple test results	A patient undergoes a glucose tolerance test. During the test, three samples are taken at 1-hour intervals.	**82951-91** Glucose tolerance testing
99	**Multiple modifiers** Assigned to report use of more than one modifier. (Must list modifier 99 first and then other related modifier codes in numerical order.)	Premature infant (weight 3.8 kg) undergoes surgical repair of a fistula joining the trachea and esophagus. Because of the complexity of the surgical case, it requires two primary surgeons.	**43305-99** **43305-62** **43305-63** Two primary surgeons needed for repair of tracheoesophageal fistula in infant weighing less than 4 kg

ICD-9-CM code to every claim that is processed by an insurance carrier. The coding system provides a numeric or alphanumeric code for every illness, injury, and condition. ICD-9-CM codes are updated yearly, so the medical assistant must be sure to use the current codes when filing claims. If the medical office does not provide an accurate diagnostic code with each procedural code, the insurance company will deny the claim and withhold payment for those services.

✦ TIP The Importance of Accurate Diagnostic Coding

Because the diagnostic code (ICD-9-CM) must support the medical necessity of a procedure to garner reimbursement, it is essential for the medical assistant to check and recheck claims coding. A common error in coding claims is transposing two or more digits in a code. Thus, checking the codes for errors in transposition is a good way to ensure accurate coding and swift reimbursement.

For example, in order to receive reimbursement for a throat culture done in the medical office, the diagnostic code on the claim must support the procedure code. If the claim lists the diagnostic code 463 (for acute tonsillitis) to support the procedure code 87650 (for a throat culture), the medical office is sure to receive speedy payment. However, if the medical assistant transposes digits in, say, the diagnostic code and codes acute tonsillitis as 436 (which is actually the code for ill-defined cerebrovascular disease), she will fail to support the procedure code 87650 for throat culture, because the diagnosis of cerebrovascular disease does not support the medical necessity of a throat culture.

ICD-9-CM Coding Manual

The ICD-9-CM coding manual provides a listing of all diagnostic codes as well as instructions on how to code diagnoses. The medical assistant should be sure to read the instructions at the beginning of the book to understand the correct procedure for choosing an accurate code. She must understand that the ICD-9-CM manual should be used as a resource book. All of the information needed to accurately code diagnoses is contained in the book itself. While diagnostic coding is complex, with practice, the medical assistant can become a confident, efficient diagnostic coder.

The ICD-9-CM coding manual is divided into two sections:

1. The introduction offers instructions to the reader on how to code diseases and disorders. Because the introduction includes the latest updates to the coding guidelines, it is imperative that the medical assistant use the most current manual.
2. The second section is divided into three volumes:
   - Volume 1 is a tabbed list of codes, arranged in numerical order and divided into chapters by diseases or disorder. (See *ICD-9-CM, Volume I chapters,* page 214.)
   - Volume 2 begins with an alphabetical listing of diseases and disorders with their corresponding numeric codes. It also contains a Table of Drugs and Chemicals and an Index to External Causes of Injuries and Poisonings.
   - Volume 3 is a tabbed alphabetical listing of hospital procedures. The medical assistant should not use these codes for physician's office procedures. (Coding procedures in the physician's office requires the use of CPT-4 codes.)

The medical assistant should use Volumes 1 and 2 of the ICD-9-CM coding manual to code diagnoses in the physician's office. The only exception to this rule is coding for psychiatric disorders. Psychiatric disorders are listed in the *Diagnostic and Statistical Manual of Mental Disorders,* 4th edition (DSM-IV), which is not discussed in this text.

V Codes

V codes are used to describe a patient's health status and identify the reason for the medical care other than for a disease process or an injury. V codes fall into three categories:

- *Problem-oriented V codes* identify risk factors that may affect the patient but are not an injury or illness—for example, V02, which indicates a carrier or suspected carrier of an infectious disease, and V69.0, which indicates lack of physical exercise.
- *Service-oriented V codes* identify services for patients who are not currently sick but are seeking medical services for other reasons, such as injury aftercare and routine examinations—for example, V67.4, which indicates a follow-up examination of a healed fracture after treatment, and V20.2, which indicates a routine infant or child health check.
- *Fact-oriented V codes* simply identify the patient's condition—for example, V27.0, which indicates the outcome of delivery of a single newborn, and V09.0, which indicates infection with a microorganism that is resistant to penicillins.

E Codes

E codes are used to establish medical necessity, identify causes of injury and poisoning, and identify medications. Certain rules apply when using E codes:

- E codes can never be a primary code; they will not support medical necessity for a procedure.
- E codes will not affect the *amount* of reimbursement
- E codes can speed up the process of reimbursement by providing additional information to the insurance company, such as liability.
- If multiple E codes are used, the following priority is given:
   - child abuse (E967.0 to E967.9)
   - cataclysmic events (E908.0 to E909.9)
   - transportation accident (E800 to E848).

✦ TIP Where Do I Start?

Although the tabbed numeric list of codes is called *Volume 1* and the alphabetical list is *Volume 2,* Volume 2 appears in most manuals before Volume 1. When searching for a code, the medical assistant will usually need to search Volume 2 (alphabetical) first, then Volume 1. The alphabetical listing of codes in Volume 2 enables the medical assistant to look up a diagnosis by several listings. For example, *osteogenesis imperfecta* is also called *Adair-Dighton syndrome* with an

ICD-9-CM, Volume 1 chapters

The following table lists the chapters and appendices included in Volume I of the *International Classification of Diseases,* 9th edition–Clinical Modifications (ICD-9-CM) manual.

Chapters and Appendices	Diagnostic Code Range
1. Infectious and Parasitic Diseases	001 through 139
2. Neoplasms	140 through 239
3. Endocrine, Nutritional, and Metabolic Diseases and Immunity Disorders	240 through 279
4. Diseases for the Blood and Blood-Forming Organs	280 through 289
5. Mental Disorders	290 through 319
6. Diseases of the Nervous System and Sense Organs	320 through 389
7. Diseases of the Circulatory System	390 through 459
8. Diseases of the Respiratory System	460 through 519
9. Diseases of the Digestive System	520 through 579
10. Diseases of the Genitourinary System	580 through 629
11. Complications of Pregnancy, Childbirth, and the Puerperium	630 through 677
12. Diseases of the Skin and Subcutaneous Tissue	680 through 709
13. Diseases of the Musculoskeletal System and Connective Tissue	710 through 739
14. Congenital Anomalies	740 through 759
15. Certain Conditions Originating in the Perinatal Period	760 through 779
16. Symptoms, Signs, and Ill-Defined Conditions	780 through 799
17. Injury and Poisoning	800 through 999
V codes—Supplemental Classification of Factors Influencing Health Status and Contact with Health Services	V01 through V83
E codes—Supplemental Classification of External Causes of Injury and Poisoning	E800 through E999
Appendix A—Morphology of Neoplasms	M codes (M8000 through M9970)
Appendix B—Glossary of Mental Disorders (glossary)	No codes provided
Appendix C—Classification of Drugs by the American Hospital Formulary Service List Number and their ICD-9-CM Equivalents	4:00 through 92:00
Appendix D—Classification of Industrial Accidents According to Agency (used for statistical purposes only)	111 through 690
Appendix E—Three-Digit Categories (all three-digit ICD-9-CM codes, V codes, and E codes)	001 through 999; V01 through V82; E800 through E999

ICD-9-CM code of 756.51. The code is listed in Volume 2 under both names for the disorder. In Volume 1, the code is only listed once, with the disorder name *osteogenesis imperfecta.* (See *Basics of diagnostic coding.*)

Multiple Diagnosis Codes

If more than one diagnosis code is used, the codes must be prioritized and entered on the CMS-1500 form in order of significance. The codes must also be linked to the appropriate procedures on the CMS-1500 form. For example, a patient is seen for a sore throat and a well-child visit. The procedures are an office visit (CPT-4 code 99213) and a throat culture (CPT-4 code 87650). Because the main purpose of the visit was the well-child visit, the medical assistant should code that procedure first on the CMS-1500 form and code the sore throat second. When relating the procedures to the diagnoses, the medical assistant should match the office visit with the diagnosis of well child and the throat culture with the sore throat. A maximum of four diagnostic codes are allowed per CMS-1500 form. (See Figure 16-2.)

Conventions

The ICD-9-CM manual contains symbols, abbreviations, punctuation, and notations that are collectively called *conventions.* Conventions and their corresponding definitions are listed in the front of the ICD-9-CM manual. Many of

Basics of diagnostic coding

For a medical assistant to determine the correct diagnostic code for a condition (diagnosis), she must refer to the *International Classification of Diseases*, 9th edition–Clinical Modifications (ICD-9-CM) manual and follow these steps:

• Find the patient's condition in Volume 2, the alphabetical index of the manual, which is arranged by condition. Some conditions have multiple entries.

• Find the numeric code listed with the condition in the alphabetical index.

• Go to the tabbed code list, which is arranged numerically, and find the code.

• Read the additional information in the tabbed listing for the code to choose the most appropriate code for the condition.

• If a fifth digit is required (indicated by a range or series of numbers set in brackets under the numeric code), refer to the listing of symptoms with assigned digits at the beginning of the group of codes describing the condition.

For example, to find the ICD-9-CM code for *spastic hemiplegia, dominant side,* the medical assistant should first look in the alphabetical index under *hemiplegia* and take the three-digit base code from that listing.

Hemiparesthesia (*see also* Disturbance, sensation)   782.0

Hemiplegia   342.9

   acute (*see also* Disease, cerebrovascular, acute)   436

   alternans facialis   344.89

   apoplectic (*see also* Disease, cerebrovascular, acute)   436

Next, the medical assistant should look up the code *342* in the tabbed numeric listing. There, she will find the coding list for *Hemiplegia and hemiparesis*, which includes the four-digit code for *spastic hemiplegia: 342.1*. To find the fifth-digit code, the medical assistant must look at the symptoms listing at the beginning of the group of codes. There, she will find that *affecting dominant side* is indicated with a *1*. So, the complete code she must use is *342.11*.

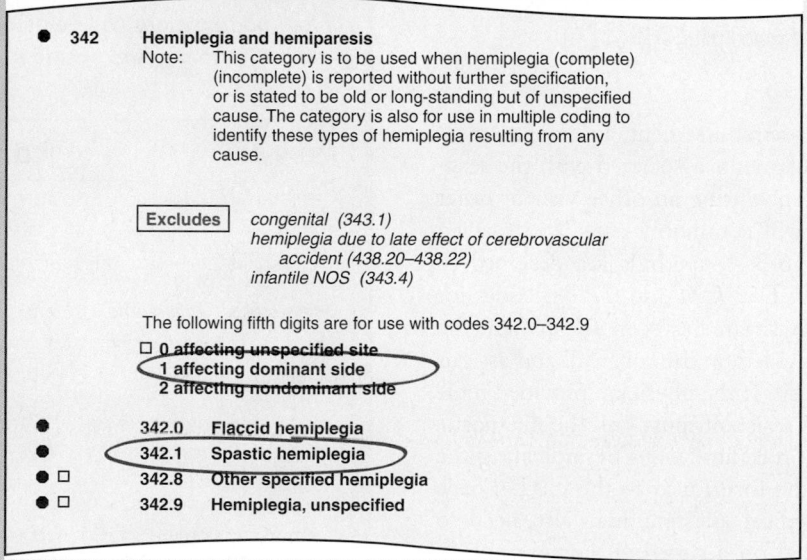

●   **342**   **Hemiplegia and hemiparesis**
    Note: This category is to be used when hemiplegia (complete) (incomplete) is reported without further specification, or is stated to be old or long-standing but of unspecified cause. The category is also for use in multiple coding to identify these types of hemiplegia resulting from any cause.

    | Excludes | congenital (343.1)
                  hemiplegia due to late effect of cerebrovascular accident (438.20–438.22)
                  infantile NOS (343.4)

    The following fifth digits are for use with codes 342.0–342.9
       □ 0 affecting unspecified site
         1 affecting dominant side
         2 affecting nondominant side

●   342.0   **Flaccid hemiplegia**
●   342.1   **Spastic hemiplegia**
● □   342.8   **Other specified hemiplegia**
● □   342.9   **Hemiplegia, unspecified**

Continued

Basics of diagnostic coding—cont'd

Coding guidelines for the CMS-1500

In addition to determining the coding, the medical assistant must understand the best way to record that information on the CMS-1500 form. Here are some guidelines on the best way to list the coding on the form:

- When the medical assistant determines the primary reason (diagnosis, condition, problem) for the visit, procedure, service, or supply provided as documented in the patient's medical record, she should list the corresponding ICD-9-CM code for this reason first on the CMS-1500 form. She should then list additional ICD-9-CM codes that describe current, coexisting conditions. She should *not* code conditions that were previously treated and no longer exist.

- The medical assistant should be sure to list all ICD-9-CM codes at their most specific level. The insurance carrier may choose to return claims submitted with three- or four-digit codes if four and five digits are available.

- The medical assistant should be sure to avoid coding diagnoses documented as *probable, suspected, questionable,* or *rule out* as if the diagnosis is confirmed. She should code the condition to the physician's highest degree of certainty at the encounter described, such as

describing symptoms, signs, abnormal test results, or other reasons for the encounter.

- The medical assistant should code and report a chronic disease treated on an ongoing basis as many times as the patient receives treatment for the condition.

- When a patient receives only ancillary diagnostic or therapeutic services during an encounter, the medical assistant should first list the code for the diagnosis or problem associated with the procedures and then list the appropriate V code for the service second.

- For surgical service, the medical assistant should use the ICD-9-CM code that corresponds to the diagnosis for which the surgery was performed. If the postoperative diagnosis is different from the preoperative diagnosis at the time the claim is filed, the medical assistant should use the ICD-9-CM code for the postoperative diagnosis.

- The medical assistant should be sure to list codes for all documented conditions that exist at the time of the visit and require or affect patient care, treatment, or management.

- Conversely, the medical assistant should *not* list codes for conditions that were previously treated and no longer exist.

---

these conventions will be used in the ICD-10 manual, which will replace ICD-9-CM in 2010 or 2011. (See *A look to the future.*) The conventions give information that is used to help the medical office find the diagnostic code that relates most closely to the written description of the diagnosis. (See *Conventions in ICD-9-CM codes,* page 218.)

Superbill

In order to file a claim for reimbursement, a physician must indicate diagnoses and treatments associated with the services he provides to a patient during an office visit or other encounter. To do so, he will commonly use a form called a *superbill.* (See Figure 16-3.) Superbills are designed to include commonly used ICD-9-CM and CPT-4 codes for that office. When the physician has seen the patient, he checks off the services provided on the superbill and assigns a diagnostic code to the visit. If the physician provided multiple services, the medical assistant must link the diagnostic codes to their respective procedure codes by indicating the ICD-9-CM code (from the form) next to the CPT-4 code where appropriate. A medical assistant may also need to check off services provided on a superbill. For example, a clinical medical assistant provides gait training for a patient who has crutches for a sprained ankle. She must then check

A look to the future

The *International Classification of Diseases,* 9th edition–Clinical Modifications (ICD-9-CM) will be replaced with a newer classification system, ICD-10, by 2011 and the term *clinical modifications* will be deleted. The following table outlines the changes expected in the ICD-10 manual.

ICD-9-CM	ICD-10
International Classification of Diseases, 9th edition–Clinical Modifications	*International Statistical Classification of Diseases and Related Health Problems*
Diseases of the Nervous System and Sense Organs (one chapter)	• Diseases of the Nervous System • Diseases of the Eye and Adnexa • Diseases of the Ear and Mastoid Process (three chapters)
Mental Disorders (appendix)	Mental and Behavioral Disorders (appendix)
Fourth- and fifth-digit requirements	Fourth-, fifth-, and sixth-digit requirements

(Text continues on page 219.)

1500

HEALTH INSURANCE CLAIM FORM

APPROVED BY NATIONAL UNIFORM CLAIM COMMITTEE 08/05

☐☐ PICA   PICA ☐☐

| 1. MEDICARE ☐ (Medicare #)   MEDICAID ☐ (Medicaid #)   TRICARE CHAMPUS ☐ (Sponsor's SSN)   CHAMPVA ☐ (Member ID#)   GROUP HEALTH PLAN ☒ (SSN or ID)   FECA BLK LUNG ☐ (SSN)   OTHER ☐ (ID) | 1a. INSURED'S I.D. NUMBER   (For Program in Item 1) XXHL129973534 |

2. PATIENT'S NAME (Last Name, First Name, Middle Initial)
OLESNEVICH   JUSTIN

3. PATIENT'S BIRTH DATE   MM 03 DD 08 YY 1998   SEX M ☒ F ☐

4. INSURED'S NAME (Last Name, First Name, Middle Initial)
OLESNEVICH   MARY

5. PATIENT'S ADDRESS (No., Street)
277 WESTON ROAD

6. PATIENT RELATIONSHIP TO INSURED
Self ☐ Spouse ☐ Child ☒ Other ☐

7. INSURED'S ADDRESS (No., Street)
277 WESTON ROAD

CITY BLUEVILLE   STATE CT

8. PATIENT STATUS
Single ☒ Married ☐ Other ☐

CITY BLUEVILLE   STATE CT

ZIP CODE 06100   TELEPHONE (Include Area Code) (860) 111 7736

Employed ☐ Full-Time Student ☒ Part-Time Student ☐

ZIP CODE 06100   TELEPHONE (Include Area Code) (860) 111 7736

9. OTHER INSURED'S NAME (Last Name, First Name, Middle Initial)

10. IS PATIENT'S CONDITION RELATED TO:

11. INSURED'S POLICY GROUP OR FECA NUMBER
678844

a. OTHER INSURED'S POLICY OR GROUP NUMBER

a. EMPLOYMENT? (Current or Previous) YES ☐ NO ☒

a. INSURED'S DATE OF BIRTH MM 07 DD 17 YY 1974   SEX M ☐ F ☒

b. OTHER INSURED'S DATE OF BIRTH MM DD YY   SEX M ☐ F ☐

b. AUTO ACCIDENT? YES ☐ NO ☒   PLACE (State)

b. EMPLOYER'S NAME OR SCHOOL NAME
BLUEVILLE FAMILY SERVICES

c. EMPLOYER'S NAME OR SCHOOL NAME

c. OTHER ACCIDENT? YES ☐ NO ☒

c. INSURANCE PLAN NAME OR PROGRAM NAME
UNITED HEALTH SYSTEMS

d. INSURANCE PLAN NAME OR PROGRAM NAME

10d. RESERVED FOR LOCAL USE

d. IS THERE ANOTHER HEALTH BENEFIT PLAN? YES ☐ NO ☒   *If yes*, return to and complete item 9 a-d.

READ BACK OF FORM BEFORE COMPLETING & SIGNING THIS FORM.

12. PATIENT'S OR AUTHORIZED PERSON'S SIGNATURE I authorize the release of any medical or other information necessary to process this claim. I also request payment of government benefits either to myself or to the party who accepts assignment below.

SIGNED _____   DATE _____

13. INSURED'S OR AUTHORIZED PERSON'S SIGNATURE I authorize payment of medical benefits to the undersigned physician or supplier for services described below.

SIGNED SIGNATURE ON FILE

14. DATE OF CURRENT: MM 06 DD 07 YY 09   ILLNESS (First symptom) OR INJURY (Accident) OR PREGNANCY(LMP)

15. IF PATIENT HAS HAD SAME OR SIMILAR ILLNESS. GIVE FIRST DATE MM DD YY

16. DATES PATIENT UNABLE TO WORK IN CURRENT OCCUPATION FROM MM DD YY   TO MM DD YY

17. NAME OF REFERRING PROVIDER OR OTHER

WELL-CHILD VISIT; USE 99212 (E/M)

18. HOSPITALIZATION DATES RELATED TO CURRENT SERVICES FROM MM DD YY   TO MM DD YY

19. RESERVED FOR LOCAL USE

20. OUTSIDE LAB? YES ☐ NO ☒ $ CHARGES

21. DIAGNOSIS OR NATURE OF ILLNESS OR INJURY (Relate Items 1, 2, 3 or 4 to Item 24E by Line)
1. V20.2 _____   3. _____
2. 693.9 _____   4. _____

22. MEDICAID RESUBMISSION CODE   ORIGINAL REF. NO.

23. PRIOR AUTHORIZATION NUMBER

24. A. DATE(S) OF SERVICE From MM DD YY / To MM DD YY	B. PLACE OF SERVICE	C. EMG	D. PROCEDURES, SERVICES, OR SUPPLIES (Explain Unusual Circumstances) CPT/HCPCS / MODIFIER	E. DIAGNOSIS POINTER	F. $ CHARGES	G. DAYS OR UNITS	H. EPSDT Family Plan	I. ID. QUAL.	J. RENDERING PROVIDER ID. #
1	07 17 09 / 07 17 09	11		99212	1	85 00	1		NPI	
2	07 17 09 / 07 17 09	11		95004	2	104 00	1		NPI	
3									NPI	
4									NPI	
5									NPI	
6									NPI	

DERMATITIS (RASH) DUE TO UNSPECIFIED SUBSTANCE; USE 95004 (PERCUTANEOUS ALLERGY TESTING)

25. FEDERAL TAX I.D. NUMBER 865623498

26. PATIENT'S ACCOUNT NO.

27. ACCEPT ASSIGNMENT? (For govt. claims, see back) YES ☒ NO ☐

28. TOTAL CHARGE $ 189 00

29. AMOUNT PAID $

30. BALANCE DUE $ 189 00

31. SIGNATURE OF PHYSICIAN OR SUPPLIER INCLUDING DEGREES OR CREDENTIALS (I certify that the statements on the reverse apply to this bill and are made a part thereof.)
HECTOR RODRIGUEZ, MD

SIGNED _____ DATE _____

32. SERVICE FACILITY LOCATION INFORMATION
a. NPI   b.

33. BILLING PROVIDER INFO & PH # (860) 555 3212
HECTOR RODRIGUEZ, MD
15 MAIN STREET
BLUEVILLE CT 06100
a. 1077358914   b.

NUCC Instruction Manual available at: www.nucc.org   **PLEASE PRINT OR TYPE**   APPROVED OMB-0938-0999 FORM CMS-1500 (08-05)

FIG 16-2 CMS-1500 form with linked procedure and diagnosis codes.

Conventions in ICD-9-CM codes

The following table lists the symbols, abbreviations, punctuation marks, and notations known as *conventions* in the *International Classification of Diseases,* 9th edition–Clinical Modifications (ICD-9-CM) manual along with the meaning and examples of each.*

Convention	Meaning	Example
● (octagon)	Must use additional digits (fourth and sometimes fifth digits for ICD-9-CM; ICD-10 will have some codes with a sixth digit)	The full code **642.52 Severe pre-eclampsia; delivered, with mention of postpartum complication** is broken down as: ● **642 Hypertension complicating pregnancy, childbirth, and the puerperium** ● **642.5** Severe pre-eclampsia **642.52** delivered, with mention of pospartum complication
◀ (triangle pointing left)	New code; changed from previous edition of ICD-9-CM manual	● **783.2** Abnormal loss of weight and underweight • **783.21** Loss of weight ◀
• (solid circle) with italic text	Not a principal diagnosis; must be used with other primary code	• *774.0 Perinatal jaundice from hereditary hemolytic anemias* *Code first underlying disease (282.0-282.9)*
☐ (empty box)	Unspecified code used only if additional information is not yet available (for example, in the emergency department); changed to more specific code when further information becomes available	● **802 Fracture of face bones** ● **802.2** Mandible, closed ☐ **802.20** Unspecified site
: (colon)	Used after an incomplete term that needs one or more of the descriptions listed to make it assignable to a code	● **686.0** Pyoderma Dermatitis: purulent septic suppurative
} (brace)	Used to enclose a series of terms, each modified by a statement to the right of the brace	☐ **537.3** Other obstruction of duodenum cicatrix stenosis } of duodenum stricture volvulus
[ ] (brackets)	Used to enclose synonyms or to indicate range or series of possible diagnoses for fifth digit	**443.1** Thromboangiitis obliterans [Buerger's disease]
( ) (parentheses)	Used to enclose supplementary words or nonessential modifiers that can be used but are not required in the code and do not affect the code	**Jaksch (-Luzet) disease or syndrome** ☐ (pseudoleukemia infantum) 285.8
Excludes	Cannot be used if associated condition is present	● **690 Erythematosquamous dermatosis** Excludes *eczematous dermatitis of eyelid (373.1)*

Conventions in ICD-9-CM codes—cont'd

Convention	Meaning	Example
Includes:	Used to further define or give an example	● **280 Iron deficiency anemia** **Includes:** anemia asiderotic hypochromic-microtic sideropenic
With	Two conditions included; both must be present	● **487 Influenza** **487.0** With pneumonia
And	One of two descriptors must be present	**Adair-Dighton syndrome** (brittle bones and blue sclera, deafness) 756.51
NOS	Not otherwise specified; used if no further information is given	☐ **378.9** Unspecified disorder of eye movementsOphthalmoplegia NOS Strabismus NOS
NEC	Not elsewhere classified; used if information at hand indicates a specific condition that has no separate code	☐ **459.0** Hemorrhage, unspecified Rupture of blood vessel NOS Spontaneous hemorrhage NEC
See	Cross reference to look elsewhere; code not listed	**Actinomyces** israelii (infection)—*see* Actinomycosis
See also	Cross reference to look under another main term; code is listed	**Adaptation reaction** (*see also* Reaction, adjustment) 309.9

* The conventions and symbols listed are common. However, some manuals vary in the use of one or more symbols. The medical assistant should be sure to check the symbol key in whatever manual she uses to ensure correct coding.

off the box for gait training and the amount of time spent with the patient on the superbill.

The medical assistant then sends the superbill to the coding department. The coder will review the superbill to make sure all of the essential information has been included and that modifiers are applied appropriately in order to submit an accurate claim. If the physician has written in a diagnosis or a procedure instead of checking off a box, the coder must determine the appropriate code for the diagnosis or procedure.

At one time, superbills, also called *encounter forms,* could be sent directly to insurance companies with a request for payment. However, now superbills are used only as a communication tool within the office. (See *Procedure 16-1: Coding procedures and diagnoses,* page 221.)

Insurance in the Physician's Office

In the physician's office, the medical assistant will work with various forms of insurance to obtain payment for services rendered to the patient. The most common form of health insurance is a policy obtained through an employer. However, people who are self-employed or work for a small company that does not offer health insurance can buy individual policies. In addition, government programs provide health insurance to people ages 65 and older, people with disabilities, people of low income, active duty military and their families, and veterans. Accidental injuries, depending on their cause, may be paid through worker's compensation insurance or through a homeowner's, commercial, or automobile liability policy.

The various forms of insurance all have specific rules for obtaining payment for services but share some common rules. Insurance claims processing is a complex task, but the medical assistant will become proficient as she processes the various forms of insurance. When filing any form of insurance claim, accuracy and completeness of the claim is vital.

Employer Insurance Programs

Employers will negotiate with health insurance carriers to obtain health insurance for their employees. It is extremely expensive for an individual to buy health insurance; the

Blueville Family Medicine
15 Main Street
Blueville CT
860-555-3212

Patient Name: _____

Date: _____

Provider: ☐ Robert Greer, MD
☐ Hector Rodriguez, MD
☐ Anne Wilson, MD
☐ Sharon Piecek, APRN
☐ Henry Lee, MD

CPT-4 Codes

Examinations		Laboratory	
Exam brief (New Pt)	99201	Urinalysis	81000
Exam intermediate (New Pt)	99202	Pregnancy test	81025
Exam detailed (New Pt)	99203	UA volume	81050
Exam comprehensive (New Pt)	99204	Allergy test - skin extracts	95004
Exam comp, high complex (New Pt)	99205	Allergy - biologicals	95010
Exam brief (Est Pt)	99211	Allergy - patch test	95044
Exam intermediate (Est Pt)	99212	PTT	85002
Exam detailed (Est Pt)	99213	Hematocrit	85014
Exam comprehensive (Est Pt)	99214	Hemoglobin	85018
Exam comp, high complex (Est Pt)	99215	Diff WBC	85004
		Occult blood	82270
X-rays		Throat culture	87650
Chest - one view	71010		
Chest - 4 views	71030		
Spine - single view (specify level)	72020	ECG	93270
X-ray - shoulder 1 view	73020	ECG - 24-hour monitor	93224
X-ray elbow	73085		
X-ray wrist (2 views)	73100		
X-ray hip (1 view)	73500	**Physical Medicine**	
X-ray knee	73560	Acupuncture	97780
X-ray ankle (3 views)	73610	Acupuncture with ES	97813
X-ray foot (2 views)	73620	Gait Training	97116
		Nutritional counseling (subsequent)	97803

ICD-9-CM Codes

Well-child visit	V20.2	Myofascitis	729.1
Prenatal visit	V22	Sinusitis	473.9
Prenatal visit - high risk	V23	Tonsillitis	474.0
Allergy exam	V72.7	Otitis media	382.9
Anemia	285.9	Otitis externa	380.10
Lower back pain	724.2	Otitis interna	386.30
Neck pain	723.1	Urinary tract infection	599.0
Hypertension	642.2	Conjunctivitis	077.99
Fatigue	789.79	Angina	413.9
HF	428.0	COPD	496

FIG 16-3 Superbill.

risk to the insurer that one person will become very ill and require expensive services is high. The insurer must charge a high monthly premium for an individual or individual family policy. For this reason, many employers offer health insurance to their employees at a group rate. A large employer can negotiate a lower cost with a health insurer because the more people who enroll in the insurance program, the lower the risks and, therefore, the costs to the insurer. The risk of high-cost care to the insurer decreases if a large number of people enroll because, although a few people within the group may become ill and require expensive care, others in the group will remain healthy and cost

PROCEDURE 16-1

Coding procedures and diagnoses

Task
Using a superbill and CPT-4 and ICD-9-CM coding manuals, choose the correct procedural and diagnostic codes for a patient visit and correctly fill out the appropriate fields on the CMS-1500 form.

Conditions
- Pen
- Superbill
- CMS-1500 form (obtained from instructor)
- CPT-4 and ICD-9-CM coding manuals

Standards
In the time specified and within the scoring parameters determined by the instructor, the student will accurately choose codes for a patient visit and correctly fill out the appropriate fields on the CMS-1500 form.

Performance Standards
1. Refer to the patient superbill (below) and note the procedures and diagnosis written by the physician.

Blueville Family Medicine
15 Main Street
Blueville CT
860-555-3212

Patient Name: _Christine Vanover_

Date: _07/17/09_

Provider: ☐ Robert Greer, MD
☐ Hector Rodriguez, MD
☒ Anne Wilson, MD
☐ Sharon Piecek, APRN
☐ Henry Lee, MD

CPT-4 Codes

Examinations		Laboratory	
Exam brief (New Pt)	99201	Urinalysis	81000
Exam intermediate (New Pt)	99202	Pregnancy test	81025
Exam detailed (New Pt)	99203	UA volume	81050
Exam comprehensive (New Pt)	99204	Allergy test - skin extracts	95004
Exam comp. high complex (New Pt)	99205	Allergy - biologicals	95010
Exam brief (Est Pt)	99211	Allergy - patch test	95044
Exam intermediate (Est Pt)	99212	PTT	85002
Exam detailed (Est Pt)	99213	Hematocrit	85014
Exam comprehensive (Est Pt)	99214	Hemoglobin	85018
Exam comp. high complex (Est Pt)	99215	Diff WBC	85004
Bartholin's gland I & D		Occult blood	82270
X-rays		Throat culture	87650
Chest - one view	71010		
Chest - 4 views	71030		
Spine - single view (specify level)	72020	ECG	93270
X-ray - shoulder 1 view	73020	ECG - 24-hour monitor	93224
X-ray elbow	73085		
X-ray wrist (2 views)	73100		
X-ray hip (1 view)	73500	**Physical Medicine**	
X-ray knee	73560	Acupuncture	97780
X-ray ankle (3 views)	73610	Acupuncture with ES	97813
X-ray foot (2 views)	73620	Gait Training	97116
		Nutritional counseling (subsequent)	97803

ICD-9-CM Codes

Well-child visit	V20.2	Myofascitis	729.1
Prenatal visit	V22	Sinusitis	473.9
Prenatal visit - high risk	V23	Tonsillitis	474.0
Allergy exam	V72.7	Otitis media	382.9
Anemia	285.9	Otitis externa	380.10
Lower back pain	724.2	Otitis interna	386.30
Neck pain	723.1	Urinary tract infection	599.0
Hypertension	642.2	Conjunctivitis	077.99
Fatigue	789.79	Angina	413.9
HF	428.0	COPD	496
Bartholin's gland cyst			
Interstitial cystitis			

Continued

PROCEDURE 16-1—cont'd

2. Using the CPT-4 coding manual, assign the appropriate office visit code, laboratory code, and office surgical procedure code.

3. Using the ICD-9-CM coding manual, assign the appropriate diagnosis codes for the patient. Write the procedure and diagnostic codes on the superbill to ensure that the superbill reflects all of the diagnoses and procedures related to the visit.

4. Fill out the appropriate fields on the CMS-1500 form, being sure to link the diagnosis and procedure codes.

5. Recheck the CPT-4 and ICD-9-CM codes against each coding manual to prevent transposition of digits and other errors.

the insurer little while still paying their premiums. Thus, the risk to the insurer is spread across a larger group. Low-cost health insurance is a benefit that will attract employees to a company. Employers offer health insurance as a benefit to help employees stay healthy and productive.

Large employers will commonly offer their employees several different insurance plans, covering varying services at varying premium costs. Employees who have children may choose a policy that covers more pediatric services than do employees whose children are grown. Employees who take expensive medications may choose a policy that offers the most medication benefit. The medical assistant must be aware that people working for the same employer may have different policies and, therefore, different benefits. Dental insurance is commonly offered by the employer as a separate policy that employees can choose to buy. Dental services are generally not covered by health insurance, with the exception of procedures requiring general anesthesia, which may be covered as a medical service. Employer insurance plans can include managed care, indemnity plans, health savings accounts, and health reimbursement accounts.

Managed Care

Managed care is a way of providing health insurance while controlling costs and involves a contract between an insurer and a physician to provide services to insurance members at predetermined rates. Managed care encompasses a variety of methods of integrating the financing and delivery of health care, including:

- hiring providers as employees
- offering a flat-rate payment per patient
- offering a **fee-for-service** arrangement, in which payment for each service is provided using a discounted scale.

Commonly, the managed care system includes a **primary care provider** (PCP), a physician who is responsible for referring the patient to a specialist when appropriate. A

referral is essentially the PCP's request to the specialist to examine the patient. The insurance company requires a referral to be in written form; if not, the insurer will not pay for the specialist's services. The insurance company encourages the PCP to refer patients to specialists within the managed care system who have agreed to the predetermined rates.

While PCPs strive to maintain clinical objectivity in diagnosing and treating patients, managed care administrators will commonly attempt to steer the clinical decision-making process in order to control costs. One way the insurers have of controlling costs involves subjecting the services a physician offers to a **utilization review**, which is an evaluation of the necessity, quality, and effectiveness of a medical service. The PCP requesting services for her patient must prove the necessity of those services to the utilization review staff of the managed care organization to obtain payment. Insurers may also give PCPs financial incentives, such as a bonus, to reduce costs.

Insurers with managed care plans offer provider relations representatives to answer questions that staff members filing insurance claims may have or to update the office on changes to policies and procedures for reimbursement or referral. Managed care websites, seminars, and newsletters also offer providers and staff information on covered services, fee schedules, and reimbursement procedures. The medical assistant filing claims to managed care plans must keep up with changes to the plans and inform patients of their changes to insurance coverage as needed. Several forms of managed care include health maintenance organizations (HMOs), independent practice associations (IPAs), and preferred provider organizations (PPOs).

Health Maintenance Organization

A health maintenance organization (HMO) is a form of managed care offered by many insurers. Because varying strategies to control the cost of health care are employed, out-of-pocket expenses to the patient can vary. Patients can select the plan that offers the most services that their family will use at the lowest cost. Small copayments are common in HMOs. Several forms of HMOs are available, including:

- staff model
- group model
- open-ended
- point-of-service.

Staff Model HMO

A staff model HMO employs salaried providers who provide services only to plan members; they do not see patients outside of the HMO plan. A wide variety of services that include radiology, pediatrics, internal medicine, obstetrics, gynecology, endocrinology, physical therapy, and oncology are offered by HMO employees at a clinic or hospital. A medical doctor is designated as the patient's PCP, who is responsible for preventive and routine care. If the patient needs the services of a specialist, the patient must obtain a referral from the PCP and see one of the specialists within the staff model HMO. Life-threatening emergencies do not require a referral. If a patient is traveling outside of the HMO service area, he must obtain preauthorization for nonemergency care. Other than emergency and out-of-area preauthorized care, no coverage is offered if the patient sees a provider outside of the HMO network of providers.

Group Model HMO

Physicians working in a group model HMO are paid a set fee each month per patient. The physician's fee does not change with the number of office visits or services provided to the patient. This form of payment is called *capitation*. The physician is not an employee of the group model HMO and can see patients outside of the HMO. Physicians are commonly members of several group model HMOs while also seeing patients with other forms of health insurance. A group model HMO requires a referral from the PCP for specialty care. No benefits are paid to nonparticipating providers with the exception of life-threatening emergencies.

Open-ended HMO

Physicians working in an open-ended HMO are not employees of the HMO. They are paid on a fee-for-service basis. Patients do not select a PCP and do not need a referral to see a specialist. Patients must choose providers from a list of providers on the HMO panel, the physicians that agree to the HMO reimbursement contract. Patients may also choose a nonparticipating provider but will need to pay a larger deductible before the insurer will pay benefits. Benefit payments to nonproviders are generally paid at 80% of HMO rates after the patient has paid the deductible.

Point-of-service HMO

Physicians working in a point-of-service HMO are not employees of the HMO but are contracted to provide services to HMO members at discounted rates. Payments are made on a fee-for-service system. Patients must choose a PCP from a list of providers and obtain referrals for specialty care. Pediatric well-child visits and annual gynecological examinations do not require referrals. Because insurance companies are paying discounted rates, they can offer attractive rates to employers, which makes point-of-service HMOs extremely popular. The insurance company, the employer, and the employee all pay a lower cost for care. The point-of-service plan is also attractive to physicians because large companies have many employees, which means many patients for the physician. In this type of HMO, the insurer pays no benefits to nonparticipating providers.

Independent Practice Association

An independent practice association (IPA) is a group of individual health care providers who join in an agreement with an insurer to provide health care to patients enrolled in the IPA plan. The physicians and providers are not financially connected to each other but do agree to refer to one another within the group. IPA physicians hire their own staff and maintain their own offices. IPA physicians can also see patients who are not enrolled in the IPA plan. Insurers pay a primary care physician on a capitated fee system and specialists on a fee-for-service basis. They require referrals and utilization reviews for specialty services and pay benefits only to providers in the IPA program. Thus, patients enrolled in this type of program must see physicians within the group.

Preferred Provider Organization

A **preferred provider organization** (PPO) is a managed care plan that contracts with local physicians. Physicians agree to accept a set fee for each service provided, instead of the fee that the physician usually bills. Patients will pay a copayment upon arrival at the physician's office. Some plans will require that the patient also have a referral to see a specialist. PPO plans can be purchased at group rates through employers or purchased by an individual. Benefits to nonparticipating providers are subject to deductibles and are generally paid at 80% of the accepted fee contract.

Traditional Insurance

In addition to managed care, patients can choose a traditional insurance policy, called an indemnity plan. An indemnity plan is more expensive than managed care products but offers the most flexibility to patients. Providers are paid a percentage of the charges, and the patient pays the remainder. This form of payment is also called *fee-for-service* and covers many procedures. The most common plans pay 80% and the patient then pays 20%. The insurance company does not set the fees, as in an HMO or PPO. Instead, the physician determines the fee using the standard of *usual, customary, and reasonable* (UCR) rates. UCR payments are determined by examining the physician's usual fee, the fee customarily charged by physicians in the same locality, and what is considered to be a reasonable fee for the service. In order to reduce the premium costs of the indemnity plan, the patient commonly assumes responsibility for a deductible, which is a set amount of money that must be paid by the patient for services before the insurance company will begin paying the 80% reimbursement. Indemnity plans can be purchased at group rates through employers or purchased by an individual. (See *What type of insurance should I choose?*.)

Consumer-Driven Health Plans

Consumer-driven health plans (CDHPs) offer options for health care insurance in addition to managed and traditional care plans. People may elect to save for their own health expenses or pay more out-of-pocket for services rather than pay higher premiums for more comprehensive insurance coverage.

All of the plans are used in conjunction with high-deductible health policies (HDHPs). The HDHPs are designed to provide coverage for routine care after a high deductible is paid. After a maximum out-of-pocket expense paid by the patient, the HDHP covers most health costs, including prolonged hospitalization, surgery, and long-term care. The focus of the HDHP is to insure the patient for high-cost care while he pays out-of-pocket for lower-cost care. The HDHP can be an HMO, a PPO, or an indemnity plan as long as it meets the requirements. A plan is defined by the federal government as an HDHP if:

- The minimum deductible is $1,100 per individual or $2,200 per family (or higher).
- The annual out-of-pocket expense is $5,500 per individual and $11,000 per family (or higher).
- Only first-dollar coverage (no deductible) is provided for qualified preventive care, such as well-child visits, usually with a copayment.

▱ Patient Education

What Type of Insurance Should I Choose?

Because of the range of insurance options available, a patient may ask the medical assistant for advice about what type of policy would be best for him and his family.

The following table compares managed care and traditional coverage options.

Policy Type	Provider Payment Method	Referral Required from PCP	Patient's Choice of Provider
Staff model HMO	Primary care providers (PCPs) as salaried employees of the HMO	Yes	No, all covered providers are HMO employees.
Group model HMO	Capitation	Yes	No, only in-network providers are covered.
Open-ended HMO	Fee-for-service at HMO rates	No	Nonparticipating providers are paid at 80% of HMO rates.
Point-of-service HMO	Fee-for-service at HMO rates	Yes	No, only in-network providers are covered.
Independent provider association (IPA)	Capitation (for PCPs) or fee-for-service at HMO rates (for specialists)	Yes	No, only in-network providers are covered
Preferred provider organization (PPO)	Fee-for-service at HMO rates	Some	Nonparticipating providers are paid at 80% of usual, customary, and reasonable (UCR) rates.
Indemnity policy	80% of UCR fee-for-service basis	No	All providers are eligible for payment at 80% of UCR rates.

The three forms of CDHPs are the health savings account, health reimbursement account, and flexible spending account.

Health Savings Account

A health savings account (HSA) is a tax-sheltered savings account that can be used to pay for medical expenses not covered by many insurance plans. Qualified expenses covered by an HSA include remodeling done to a home to accommodate patients with disabilities, ambulance services, orthopedic appliances, and telephone and TV modifications to assist patients with vision and hearing impairments. High deductibles apply to HSA plans and must be paired with a qualified health plan to cover the costs of routine care. Money in the account that is not used for medical care earns interest and remains in the account, similar to an independent retirement account (IRA). Contributions to the account are made by the employee, employer, or both. Contributions made by the employee are taken from the employee's paycheck before federal and state taxes are calculated. Maximum contributions allowed by law are set yearly. Beginning in 2007, individuals can make a one-time transfer from their IRA to their HSA, subject to the maximum allowed contribution of $2,850 for an individual and $5,650 for a family. Every year, the U.S. Treasury Department determines the maximum allowable contributions to a health care plan for that year. If the employee changes jobs, the HSA account can be moved to a new employer.

Health Reimbursement Account

A health reimbursement account (HRA) is designed to reimburse an employee for medical expenses incurred by high deductibles and copayments associated with HDHPs. HRAs are funded exclusively by the employer; employees do not make any salary contribution to pay for the HRA. Expenses covered by the HRA are any medical care expenses covered by the primary medical insurance but not paid by the insurance company because of a deductible or copayment. The HRA operates on a calendar-year basis. The employer establishes the annual maximum reimbursement to employees on January 1 of each year. An employee may qualify for reimbursement from the HRA only while employed by the employer. The employer may cancel or amend the HRA program at any time. (See *HSA and HRA differences.*)

Flexible Spending Account

A **flexible spending account (FSA)** is funded by the employee and is not subject to federal, Social Security, or state taxes on the contributions. Employers may contribute a small amount to the plan. The spending account accumulates interest for one calendar or benefit year, but unused money is returned to the employer at the end of that period. The

HSA and HRA differences

The following table outlines the different characteristics of a health spending account (HSA) and a health reimbursement account (HRA).

HSA	HRA
• Payments to the account may be made by the employee, employer, or both.	• Payments to the account are made only by the employer.
• The employee can take the account from job to job.	• The employee forfeits all benefits when he leaves the employer.
• The account may operate on a benefit-year or calendar-year basis.	• The account operates on a calendar-year basis only.
• The account may reimburse for home remodeling and accommodations related to health needs.	• The account reimburses only for qualified medical expenses.

employee must consider how much money he wants to contribute since the money will not accumulate from year to year. The amount of contribution can be adjusted each year in anticipation of expenses. Funds can be used to pay for qualified medical expenses and dependent-care expenses, such as day care. Many people with children elect to contribute to an FSA to pay for day-care expenses with pretax dollars.

Government Programs

While many people buy health insurance for themselves and their dependents through their employer or through an individual policy, many others are covered by government plans designed to offer health insurance to people who are retired, have a low income, or are active or retired military personnel and their dependents. Government plans that cover these people are Medicare, Medicaid, CHAMPUS, and CHAMPVA.

Medicare

Medicare is a government health insurance program for:

- people age 65 or older
- people under age 65 with certain disabilities
- people of all ages with end-stage renal disease (permanent kidney failure requiring dialysis or a kidney transplant)
- people of all ages with amyotrophic lateral sclerosis (Lou Gehrig's disease).

Medicare offers four parts:

- part A—hospital insurance
- part B—physician services

- part C—"Medicare Advantage," in which patients can elect to have part A and B services provided through an HMO provider with reduced copayments and out-of-pocket expenses
- part D—prescription drug services.

Medicare is financed by a portion of the payroll taxes paid by workers and their employers. It is also financed in part by monthly premiums deducted from Social Security checks. The program helps with the cost of health care, but it does not cover all medical expenses or the cost of most long-term care. Patients can elect to buy long-term care insurance, which will cover expenses of nursing facilities and home care. The Centers for Medicare and Medicaid Services is in charge of the Medicare program. Patients apply for Medicare at their Social Security office.

The physician must decide if she is going to participate in the Medicare program. If the physician chooses to participate, Medicare will send payments directly to the physician's office, rather than to the patient. Medicare distributes a copy of its fee contract to every medical office each November in paper or electronic format. Medicare also posts this fee system, or *schedule,* online at its website, listed by region. Medicare will pay 80% of the posted fee, and the patient or her supplemental insurance pays the remaining 20% of the allowed amount. Also, if the physician participates in Medicare and the patient has a Medigap plan, a supplemental plan that picks up what Medicare does not pay, Medicare will automatically forward the claim on to the Medigap payor for payment. Although a nonparticipating physician must still file Medicare claims, Medicare will send the payment directly to the patient, who is then responsible for paying the physician. If a patient also has Medigap insurance, the nonparticipating physician's office must file the Medigap insurance claim for supplemental payment. In addition, the Medicare payment is 5% less for a nonparticipating physician than a participating physician. Pharmacies and laboratories are required to accept Medicare assignment and cannot elect to be a nonparticipating provider. (See *Services not covered by Medicare.*)

Medicaid

Title XIX of the Social Security Act is a federal and state entitlement program that pays for medical assistance to certain individuals and families with a low income and limited resources. This program, known as *Medicaid,* became law in 1965 as a cooperative venture jointly funded by federal and state governments to assist states in furnishing medical assistance to eligible people. Medicaid is the largest source of funding for medical and health-related services for America's poorest people. Every state has different criteria for billing Medicaid, but the federal government institutes standards for states to obtain matching funds for the program. To obtain federal funding, a state's Medicaid program must include medical coverage for the following:

- inpatient hospital services
- outpatient hospital services
- prenatal care
- vaccines for children
- physician services
- nursing facility services for persons age 21 or older
- family planning services and supplies
- rural health clinic services
- home health care for persons eligible for skilled-nursing services
- laboratory and x-ray services
- pediatric and family nurse practitioner services
- nurse-midwife services
- federally qualified health-center (FQHC) services, and ambulatory services of an FQHC that would be available in other settings
- early and periodic screening, diagnostic, and treatment (EPSDT) services for children under age 21.

States may also receive federal matching funds to provide certain optional services. The most common of the currently approved optional Medicaid services are:

- diagnostic services
- clinic services
- intermediate-care facilities for the mentally retarded
- prescribed drugs and prosthetic devices
- optometrist services and eyeglasses
- nursing facility services for children under age 21
- transportation services
- rehabilitation and physical therapy services
- home and community-based care to certain persons with chronic impairments.

Although individual states vary, people are generally eligible for Medicaid if they are members of the following groups:

- children under age 6 whose family income is at or below 133% of the federal poverty level (FPL)
- pregnant women whose family income is below 133% of the FPL (services to these women are limited to those related to pregnancy, complications of pregnancy, delivery, and postpartum care)
- recipients of Supplemental Security Income (SSI), which is a federal program that supplements the income of persons who have disabilities, providing money for basic needs (Some states use more restrictive Medicaid eligibility requirements that predate SSI.)
- recipients of adoption or foster care assistance under Title IV of the Social Security Act
- special protected groups (typically, individuals who lose their cash assistance due to earnings from work or from increased Social Security benefits, but who may keep Medicaid for a period of time)

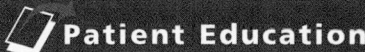

Patient Education

Services not Covered by Medicare

Sometimes Medicare patients will request services that may not be covered by Medicare. For example, if a patient wants to have his cholesterol checked every week, Medicare will say such measures are "not medically necessary." If the patient still wants to have the test run, the medical assistant must require the patient to sign a notice called the *advanced beneficiary notice (ABN)*. This notice explains to the patient that, according to Medicare, the test is not needed; Medicare will not reimburse for it, and the patient agrees to pay for the test in full.

Patient's Name: __Walter Simmons__   Medicare # (HICN): __987-65-4321A__

ADVANCE BENEFICIARY NOTICE (ABN)

NOTE: You need to make a choice about receiving these health care items or services.

We expect that Medicare will not pay for the item(s) or service(s) that are described below. Medicare does not pay for all of your health care costs. Medicare only pays for covered items and services when Medicare rules are met. The fact that Medicare may not pay for a particular item or service does not mean that you should not receive it. There may be a good reason your doctor recommended it. Right now, in your case, **Medicare probably will not pay for –**

Items or services:

   Acupuncture

Because:

   Maximum number of visits allowed per calendar year has been met.

The purpose of this form is to help you make an informed choice about whether or not you want to receive these items or services, knowing that you might have to pay for them yourself. Before you make a decision about your options, you should read this entire notice carefully.
- Ask us to explain if you don't understand why Medicare probably won't pay.
- Ask us how much these items or services will cost you (Estmated cost: $ __65.00__).

PLEASE CHOOSE **ONE** OPTION. CHECK **ONE** BOX. **SIGN & DATE** YOUR CHOICE.

☒ **Option 1. YES. I want to receive these items or services.**

I understand that Medicare will not decide whether to pay unless I receive these items or services. Please submit my claim to Medicare. I understand that you may bill me for items or services and that I may have to pay the bill while Medicare is making its decision. If Medicare does pay, you will refund to me any payments I made to you that are due to me. If Medicare denies payment, I agree to be personally and fully responsible for payment. That is, I will pay personally, either out of pocket or through any other insurance that I have. I understand I can appeal Medicare's decision.

☐ **Option 2. NO. I have decided not to receive these items or services.**

I will not receive these items or services. I understand that you will not be able to submit a claim to Medicare and that I will not be able to appeal your opinion that Medicare won't pay.

__07/30/08__   __Walter Simmons__
Date   Signature of patient or person acting on patient's behalf

---

NOTE: Your health information will be kept confidential. Any information that we collect about you on this form will be kept confidential in our offices. If a claim is submitted to Medicare, your health information on this form may be shared with Medicare. Your health information which Medicare sees will be kept confidential by Medicare.

OMB Approval No. 0938-0566   Form No. CMS-R-131-G   (June 2002)

- all children born after September 30, 1983, who are under age 19 and come from families with incomes at or below the FPL.

Providers agreeing to participate in Medicaid must accept Medicaid payment rates as payment in full but may charge a copayment to some patients. The provider is not allowed to charge a copayment to Medicaid beneficiaries who are pregnant women, children under age 18, and hospital or nursing home patients who are expected to contribute most of their income to institutional care. In addition, all Medicaid beneficiaries are exempt from copayments for emergency services and family planning services.

States may pay health care providers directly on a fee-for-service basis or through various prepayment arrangements, such as health maintenance organizations (HMOs). Each state, for the most part, has broad discretion in determining the payment methodology and payment rate for services within federally imposed upper limits and specific restrictions. Generally, payment rates must be sufficient to enlist enough providers to care for the needs of the patients in the geographic region. States must make additional payments to qualified hospitals that provide inpatient services to a disproportionate number of Medicaid beneficiaries or other low-income or uninsured persons under what is known as the *disproportionate share hospital (DSH) adjustment.*

CHAMPUS

The Civilian Health and Medical Program of the Uniformed Services (CHAMPUS) was enacted by Congress in 1956. The purpose of CHAMPUS was to provide civilian health care to dependents of military service members. The plan covered care supplemental to that available in military facilities. It provided authorized inpatient and outpatient care from civilian physicians and hospitals when deemed medically necessary. All CHAMPUS beneficiaries who have retired from the military are moved to the Medicare program at age 65. In keeping with the cost savings associated with HMO plans, CHAMPUS was revised in 1993 to offer lower-cost options to patients in the form of Tricare. Tricare offers three programs to eligible participants:

- Tricare Standard, which most resembles an indemnity plan, allows beneficiaries to use any civilian health care provider who is eligible under Tricare regulations. The beneficiary is responsible for payment of an annual deductible and coinsurance. There is no fee for enrollment in Tricare Standard.
- Tricare Extra, which is a PPO-style plan, allows a beneficiary to elect to use civilian providers within a regional contractor's provider network. Fees are paid to providers on a fee-for-service basis at HMO (discounted) rates. The coinsurance for the patient is at least 5% less than

with Tricare Standard. There is no fee charged to the individual to use Tricare Extra benefits.
- Tricare Prime, which is an HMO-style plan, requires the beneficiary to choose a PCP and obtain referrals for specialty care. However, it charges lower copayments to the patient. The patient is charged an annual enrollment fee for Tricare Prime.

CHAMPVA

The Civilian Health and Medical Program of the Department of Veterans Affairs (CHAMPVA) is a health benefits program in which the Department of Veterans Affairs (VA) shares the cost of certain health care services and supplies with eligible beneficiaries. CHAMPVA operates like an indemnity plan; patients choose their own physicians and deductibles and copayments may apply. CHAMPVA pays providers on a fee-for-service basis in which fees are determined by a formula using UCR and federal guidelines. In general, the CHAMPVA program covers most health care services and supplies that are medically necessary. To be eligible for CHAMPVA, patients cannot be eligible for Tricare (CHAMPUS) and must be in one of these categories:

- spouse or child of a veteran who has a disability rating determined by a Veterans Administration (VA) regional office of permanently and totally disabled for a service-connected disability
- surviving spouse or child of a veteran who died from a VA-rated service-connected disability
- surviving spouse or child of a veteran who was, at the time of death, rated permanently and totally disabled
- surviving spouse or child of a military member who died in the line of duty, not due to misconduct. (In most of these cases, these family members are eligible for Tricare [CHAMPUS], not CHAMPVA).

Worker's Compensation

Every state mandates that employers carry worker's compensation insurance. This insurance covers medical costs related to injuries or illnesses sustained by employees as a result of their job. Employers pay premiums to an insurer based on the risk of injury or illness to employees. A construction company whose workers use power tools and must climb onto roofs will pay higher premiums than a company whose workers sit at a desk all day. Physicians who treat patients under worker's compensation must register annually with their state Worker's Compensation Board. Services are reimbursed to physicians on a fee-for-service basis and no copayment or deductible is charged to the patient.

A worker's compensation claim must include a first report of injury notice, which describes the accident or injury and its date, time, and location. (See Figure 16-4.) This notice is initiated by the employer and sent to the physician. The

Form 122

For your protection Connecticut Law requires notice that worker's compensation fraud is a crime. Please see next page for the full fraud statement

WORKER'S COMPENSATION EMPLOYER'S FIRST REPORT OF INJURY OR ILLNESS
STATE OF CONNECTICUT - THE LABOR COMMISSION - DIVISION OF INDUSTRIAL ACCIDENTS
HARTFORD, CT 06555

GENERAL

EMPLOYER (Name & Address Incl. Zip)	CARRIER/ADMINISTRATOR CLAIM NUMBER	OSHA CASE/FILE #	REPORT PURPOSE CODE

Barry Manufacturing
2589 Industrial Drive
Presley, CT 06001

JURISDICTION — JURISDICTION CLAIM NUMBER

INSURED REPORT NUMBER
87TYM5673472

EMPLOYERS LOCATION ADDRESS (IF DIFFERENT)	LOCATION #
Same	Same

SIC CODE	EMPLOYER FEIN	PHONE # 860-123-3876

CARRIER / CLAIMS ADMIN

CARRIER (NAME, ADDRESS & PHONE #)	POLICY PERIOD	CLAIMS ADMINISTRATOR (NAME, ADDRESS & PHONE #)

Worker Compensation Fund
P.O. Box 1195
Presley, CT 06001
Telephone: 1-800-123-4786

POLICY PERIOD: TO 12/31/10

CHECK IF APPROPRIATE
☐ SELF INSURANCE

CARRIER FEIN	POLICY/SELF-INSURED NUMBER	ADMINISTRATOR FEIN

AGENT NAME & CODE NUMBER
Baldwin Insurance Agency, Code #96360

EMPLOYEE

NAME (LAST, FIRST, MIDDLE) Hansen, Craig, William	DATE OF BIRTH 12/30/71	SOCIAL SECURITY NUMBER 000-00-0000	DATE HIRED 01/14/98	STATE OF HIRE active

ADDRESS (INCL ZIP)	SEX	MARITAL STATUS	OCCUPATION/JOB TITLE

42 Wilshire Ave.
Blueville, CT 06100

SEX: ☒ MALE ☐ FEMALE ☐ UNKNOWN

MARITAL STATUS: ☐ UNMARRIED SINGLE/DIVORCED ☒ MARRIED ☐ SEPARATED ☐ UNKNOWN

OCCUPATION/JOB TITLE: machinist

EMPLOYMENT STATUS: active

PHONE 860-543-2100	# OF DEPENDENTS 3	NCCI CLASS CODE

WAGE

RATE $680.00 PER: ☒ WEEK ☐ DAY ☐ MONTH ☐ OTHER:	# OF DAYS WORKED/WEEK 5	FULL PAY FOR DAY OF INJURY? ☒ YES ☐ NO DID SALARY CONTINUE? ☐ YES ☒ NO

OCCURRENCE

TIME EMPLOYEE BEGAN WORK ☒ AM ☐ PM 8:00	DATE OF INJURY/ILLNESS 09/15/08	TIME OF OCCURRENCE 4:22 ☐ AM ☒ PM	LAST WORK DATE 09/15/08	DATE EMPLOYER NOTIFIED 09/15/08	DATE DISABILITY BEGAN 09/15/08

CONTACT NAME/PHONE NUMBER Henry Watanabee 860-555-7400 ext 43	TYPE OF INJURY/ILLNESS lower back sprained	PART OF BODY AFFECTED Lower back

DID INJURY/ILLNESS EXPOSURE OCCUR ON EMPLOYER'S PREMISES? ☒ YES ☐ NO	TYPE OF INJURY/ILLNESS CODE	PART OF BODY AFFECTED CODE

DEPARTMENT OR LOCATION WHERE ACCIDENT OR ILLNESS EXPOSURE OCCURRED Loading dock	ALL EQUIPMENT, MATERIALS, OR CHEMICALS EMPLOYEE WAS USING WHEN ACCIDENT OR ILLNESS EXPOSURE OCCURRED dolly

SPECIFIC ACTIVITY THE EMPLOYEE WAS ENGAGED IN WHEN THE ACCIDENT OR ILLNESS EXPOSURE OCCURRED unloading boxes from truck	WORK PROCESS THE EMPLOYEE WAS ENGAGED IN WHEN ACCIDENT OR ILLNESS EXPOSURE OCCURRED shipping

HOW INJURY OR ILLNESS/ABNORMAL HEALTH CONDITION OCCURRED, DESCRIBE THE SEQUENCE OF EVENTS AND INCLUDE ANY OBJECTS OR SUBSTANCES THAT DIRECTLY INJURED THE EMPLOYEE OR MADE THE EMPLOYEE ILL

CAUSE OF INJURY CODE

slipped on water on loading dock while carrying heavy box

DATE RETURN(ED) TO WORK 10/22/08	IF FATAL, GIVE DATE OF DEATH	WERE SAFEGUARDS OR SAFETY EQUIPMENT PROVIDED? ☒ YES ☐ NO WERE THEY USED? ☒ YES ☐ NO

TREATMENT

PHYSICIAN/HEALTH CARE PROVIDER (NAME & ADDRESS)	HOSPITAL (NAME & ADDRESS)	INITIAL TREATMENT

Robert Greer, MD
15 Main Street
Blueville, CT 06100

860-555-3212

Hartell Memorial
773 Carson Street
Blueville, CT 06100

INITIAL TREATMENT:
☐ NO MEDICAL TREATMENT
☐ MINOR: BY EMPLOYER
☐ MINOR CLINIC/HOSP
☒ EMERGENCY CARE
☐ HOSPITALIZED >24 HRS
☐ FUTURE MAJOR MEDICAL/LOST TIME ANTICIPATED

OTHER

WITNESS (NAME & PHONE #) Sarah Kramer   860-555-7868

DATE ADMINISTRATOR NOTIFIED 09/16/08	DATE PREPARED 09/16/08	PREPARER'S NAME & TITLE Rebecca Stavola, Legal Counsel	PHONE NUMBER 860-555-7400 ext 62

SEE NEXT PAGE FOR IMPORTANT INFORMATION

White: Labor Commission   Yellow: W.C. Insurance Carrier   Pink: Employee   Goldenrod: Employer's File

FIG 16-4 First report of an injury.

physician's office must include a copy of this report with all claims sent to the insurance carrier for payment.

In addition to covering the cost of medical care, worker's compensation insurance must cover the cost of lost wages while the patient is unable to work. If an employee dies as a result of a work-related accident or illness, the employee's dependents become eligible for payment of benefits.

Some limitations apply to worker's compensation coverage. Thus, submission of a claim for worker's compensation must be agreed to by the employer and employee. (See *Worker's compensation claims* below.) Employees are not covered if they are reckless in their job performance, arrive at work drunk, use illicit drugs, injure themselves purposely, or fight at work. Employees who fail to use safety equipment, such as steel-tipped boots or protective eyewear, may also forfeit their benefits.

Multiple Insurance Policies

Patients may have more than one health insurance policy and payment can be obtained from a primary (billed first) and a secondary policy. When gathering insurance information, the medical assistant should ask the patient which insurance is primary and which is secondary. Minor children covered by two policies of their parents are covered using the **birthday rule**. The birthday rule states that the primary coverage for children is the policy of the parent with the birthday that is first in the calendar year. For example, if Mary is born on January 12 and John is born on March 8,

the mother's policy (Mary's) is primary for all of the children. The parents can elect, however, to have primary coverage with either policy. So, in the example, if John's coverage had better obstetric services than Mary's, she could elect to use John's policy as her primary policy. However, she would have to use that policy as primary for all medical coverage, not just obstetrics. John would have to pay for the primary coverage for his wife, Mary, through his employer.

Multiple insurance policies require that the medical assistant have an understanding of coordination of benefits. **Coordination of benefits** means that the medical office bills the primary insurance company and then the medical assistant notes the amount paid on the bill sent to the secondary insurance company. The secondary insurance company then pays all or a portion of the remaining bill. Medicare will forward claims to a secondary insurance company for claims from participating providers. All other secondary claims must be filed by the physician's office. The patient pays a copayment at the time of the office visit (if applicable) and is responsible for the unpaid portion after all insurance companies have paid their portions.

COBRA

In 1986, Congress passed the Consolidated Omnibus Budget Reconciliation Act (COBRA). This act provides continuation of group health insurance coverage for subscribers and their dependents when they leave employment. Prior to the act, an individual and his family would be without health insurance coverage upon termination of employment by the employer or the employee. COBRA coverage allows a subscriber and his dependents to stay on the group health insurance of the employer for a maximum of 18 months after termination of employment. Many people use COBRA coverage to ensure that they and their dependents are not without medical insurance for any period of time between jobs. The COBRA coverage is subject to the following restrictions:

- The originating health insurance plan must provide coverage for 20 or more employees.
- Private-sector and state government employers must provide coverage, but federal government and some church-related organizations are exempt.
- The employer must allow the former employee and his dependents to remain on the group plan at the group rates. However, the employer is no longer obligated to pay any portion of the premium.

Under COBRA, a group health insurance plan is defined as a plan providing medical benefits to employees through insurance, such as an HMO (any form) or an indemnity policy. Medical benefits under the plan may include:

- physician care
- inpatient and outpatient hospital care

📖 Patient Education

Worker's Compensation Claims

If the employer and employee cannot agree on the nature of an injury, the physician's office cannot file the claim as worker's compensation. The medical assistant should explain to the patient that he must discuss the status of the injury with his employer and come to an agreement so that the medical office can file his claim appropriately.

When a claim has been established as a work-related injury, the medical assistant should make sure that the patient keeps a copy of the first report of injury for his records. If the employee is unable to work, the physician will provide him with a notice of limitation to show his employer. When the physician determines that the patient is able to return to work, he will issue a return-to-work order. The medical assistant must make copies of the physician's order, placing one copy in the medical record and giving two copies to the patient (one for the patient to give to his employer and another for the patient to keep for his records). Without the return-to-work order, the employer will not allow the patient to return to his job.

- surgery
- prescription drug benefits
- dental and vision care.

Self-Pay Patients

Although most people have some form of insurance that covers a portion of their health care costs, some patients do not have any insurance coverage. A patient who does not have health insurance through their employer may not be eligible for a government health insurance plan. In 2007, the reported number of uninsured Americans varied from 8.2 million, according to the Kaiser Family Foundation, to 47 million, as reported by the National Coalition on Healthcare. Some patients may be temporarily without health insurance during job changes or divorce. Uninsured patients can be seen by the physician and a payment plan can be arranged to spread the cost of care over several months. Many physicians will offer services at a reduced rate to help their uninsured patients. Each physician practice will have policies regarding payment arrangements for self-pay patients.

Insurance Claims

Processing an insurance claim is a central operation in a medical office. Many guidelines, restrictions, and requirements are involved in such a procedure.

HIPAA

One of the most important requirements in filing an insurance claim involves the Health Insurance Portability and Accountability Act (HIPAA), a law passed in 1996 that protects the privacy and security of a patient's protected health information (PHI). HIPAA allows disclosure of PHI only for the purposes of treatment, payment, and operations (TPO) of the medical practice and mandates that all other disclosures be specifically authorized by the patient. Under these rules, insurance claims can be filed for payment without additional authorization from the patient. (For more information on HIPAA, see Chapter 7, "HIPAA and a Patient's Rights," page 71.)

Life Cycle of an Insurance Claim

The medical assistant must gather information from the patient and the physician to process insurance claims for payment. From the point that a patient enters the physician's office until the bill is finally paid, the medical assistant must take steps to gather the necessary information and submit the claim accurately to ensure fast payment. The cycle of processing an insurance claim follows these steps:

1. A new patient enters the office for treatment and begins the **registration** process, which involves filling out a new patient registration form with his personal and insurance information. The registration form aids in the collection of **demographics**, which is information that the medical assistant needs to complete the claim. Demographic information includes the patient's address, telephone number, employer, and insurance coverage information. For children, information also includes the names and addresses of both parents. (See Figure 16-5.) The patient's or guardian's signature on the registration form authorizes the release of the patient's demographic information for the purposes of TPO. After the patient is registered, the medical assistant should collect the insurance copayment from the patient, because a patient might not stop back to see the front desk after completing the visit. When the payment is collected, the medical assistant should give the patient a receipt.

2. The medical assistant creates a medical record for the patient and inserts the new patient intake form.

3. The medical assistant makes a photocopy of the medical insurance card provided by the patient and keeps the copy in the patient's medical record. The insurance card contains the details about the patient's insurance policy, including the insurance identification number, the group number (if there is one), and the amount of the copayment. The back of the card contains the claim address, phone numbers to verify coverage and benefits and, possibly, a website address for the insurance company. At this point, it is extremely important for the medical assistant to collect all the information relating to the patient's insurance. One of the major reasons for nonpayment of insurance claims is incorrect information, such as transposed numbers or misspelled names. Copying the insurance card helps eliminate some of these problems and ensures that the patient's name, identification number, and group number are accurate. (See Figure 16-6.)

4. The medical assistant verifies the patient's benefits. **Verification** is confirming with the insurance company that the patient is covered by the policy and determining the extent of the patient's benefits under that policy. Verifying benefits prior to providing services to the patient can avoid nonpayment of a claim by the patient. Because of long hold times on the phone, many front desk personnel will use the insurance company's website to verify benefits. A password and identification number are required to access the data.

5. The physician examines the patient.

6. The physician provides the diagnosis and treatment for the service, commonly on the superbill.

7. The medical assistant uses the information on the superbill to complete the CMS-1500 form for reimbursement.

8. The medical assistant fills out the CMS-1500 form by using a billing software program and submits the claim

---

CONFIDENTIAL PATIENT INFORMATION

BLUEVILLE FAMILY MEDICINE
15 MAIN STREET
BLUEVILLE, CT
860-555-3212

Name _Michelle Calabrese_ Date of birth _6/21/1984_ Full time student ☐ Yes ☒ No
Address _88 West Road_ City _Presley, CT_
Home phone _123-9674_ Cell phone _203-998-5633_
Insured name _self_ Insured date of birth _01/11/1984_ Relationship to patient _self_
Insured employer _Aloisio Advertising Associates_ Employer address _33 Park Ave, Presley, CT_
Insurance carrier _United Health Systems_ ID# _XGA00443_ Group # _4488_

HEALTH HISTORY

Have you ever suffered from:

☐ Asthma	☐ Fainting	☐ Muscle weakness	☐ Lower back pain
☐ Diabetes	☐ Anxiety	☒ Difficulty sleeping	☐ Difficulty swallowing
☐ High blood pressure	☐ Bleeding disorder	☐ Allergies	☐ Neck pain or stiffness
☒ Migraine headaches	☐ Constipation	☒ Stomach upset	☐ Diarrhea
☐ Fatigue	☒ Stress	☐ Mental disorder	☐ Infection

☐ Cancer (If so, what kind?) _none_ ☒ Chronic pain (If so, where?) _neck and right shoulder_

FAMILY HISTORY

☒ Cancer (Who?) _mother_ What type? _breast cancer (died last year)_
☒ High blood pressure (Who?) _father, mother_
☒ Diabetes (Who?) _father, grandmother_

MEDICATIONS AND SUPPLEMENTS

Do you take any medications? Do you take any nutritional supplements?
If so, please list (include dosages): If so, please list:
Tylenol for headaches _none_
Synthroid - 5 mg a day

REASON FOR TODAY'S VISIT

☒ Check up
☐ Physical for school, sports, or employment
☒ Other (please explain) _painful urination_

Women only

Date of last menstrual period _4/2/09_
Number of pregnancies _0_ Miscarriages? _0_
Number of children _0_ Difficult or painful menstruation? _sometimes_

Men only

Have you ever had erectile difficulty? ___ Prostate problems? ___
Do you get up at night frequently to urinate? ___

I understand that Blueville Family Medicine will file my insurance for payment of services rendered. I also understand that I am responsible for any amount due Blueville Family Medicine if my insurance is denied.

Signature of patient or guardian _Michelle Calabrese_ Date _04/15/09_

Relationship to patient ___

Robert Greer, MD • Sharon Piecek, APRN • Hector Rodriguez, MD • Henry Lee, MD • Anne Wilson, MD

FIG 16-5 New patient registration form.

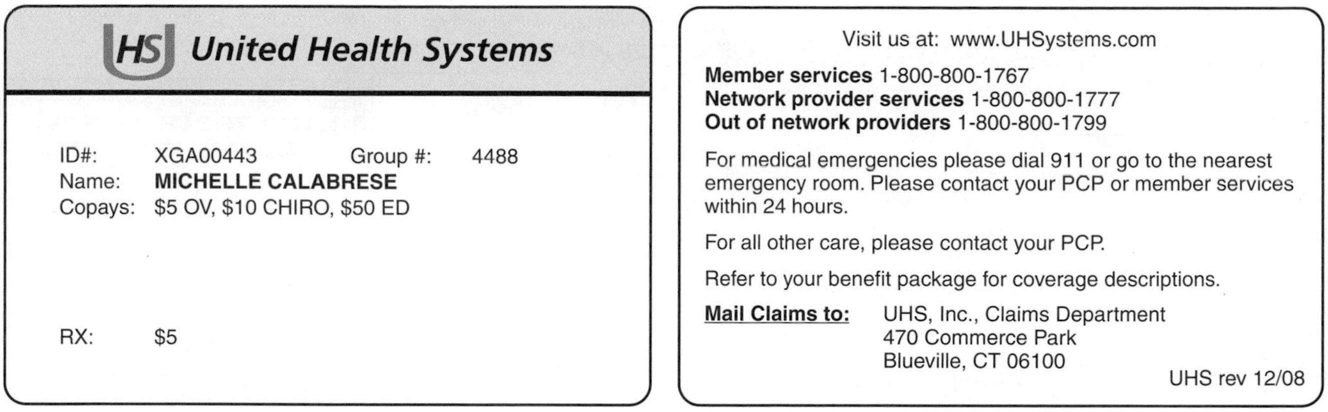

HS United Health Systems

ID#:   XGA00443   Group #:   4488
Name: **MICHELLE CALABRESE**
Copays: $5 OV, $10 CHIRO, $50 ED

RX: $5

Visit us at: www.UHSystems.com

Member services 1-800-800-1767
Network provider services 1-800-800-1777
Out of network providers 1-800-800-1799

For medical emergencies please dial 911 or go to the nearest emergency room. Please contact your PCP or member services within 24 hours.

For all other care, please contact your PCP.

Refer to your benefit package for coverage descriptions.

Mail Claims to: UHS, Inc., Claims Department
                       470 Commerce Park
                       Blueville, CT 06100
                                           UHS rev 12/08

FIG 16-6 Front and back of insurance card.

electronically or via U.S. mail. (See Figure 16-7.) This process is also referred to as *posting the claim.*

9. The insurance company processes the claim and sends payment for services to the provider.

Submitting a Claim

When a claim is ready, the medical assistant will submit, or *post,* the claim. This process is made simple by computer billing software. In the billing software, dictionaries are set up to hold all the data that is referenced over and over again. There are dictionaries to hold physician billing information as well as a listing of all the physicians who might refer patients to the practice. There are dictionaries that hold all of the CPT codes, another one for modifiers, and another for ICD-9-CM codes. Insurance companies are in another dictionary. An office will also usually create a master patient index and add to it every new patient when the patient registers. The report function of the billing software includes the CMS-1500 form. It also includes management reports that the office manager and billing supervisor can use to track payments, denials, and outstanding bills.

The medical assistant will usually submit the day's claims in batches. When a batch is completed, or *closed,* the claims are ready to submit. Some software will allow you to submit the claims through an edit check. The edit check looks for incorrect data and will print out a report that lists incorrect claims that the medical assistant must fix before submitting them. Once the claims pass the edit check, they are ready to be submitted to the insurance company.

The medical assistant may have to submit some claims by paper, most commonly third-party liability claims, such as worker's compensation and motor vehicle accidents. Billing software typically allows the user to print these claims by flagging them in the program. Once printed, the medical assistant can mail the claims to the insurance company. Insurance companies generally require the medical office to submit copies of office visit notes along with these claims.

In addition to the electronically submitted claim, Medicare may ask that the medical office mail a copy of the CMS-1500 form if it contains any surgical claims for unusual services (identified by the modifier 22).

Electronic Claim Submission

The majority of medical practices file claims electronically. After keying claims, the medical assistant sends the claims via an encrypted claims submission program. Some practices send claims directly to the insurance company; other practices use a clearinghouse. The clearinghouse is a company that processes the claims through additional edits, or *scrubs,* to make sure the claims contain no errors, designated as *clean.* Once the claims are determined to be error-free, the clearinghouse submits them to the various insurance carriers for processing and payment. (See *Procedure 16-2: Submitting a CMS-1500 form to a third-party payor,* page 235.)

✦ TIP Effective Communication

Effective communication with insurance companies and patients helps obtain quick, accurate payment. Establishing direct and reliable contacts with insurance provider representatives may help the medical assistant get answers to complex questions. A medical assistant who chooses to be friendly and helpful when assisting patients through difficult claims can also help obtain payment as well as satisfy patients.

Obtaining Referrals

A referral is a request by a PCP for the patient to be seen by a specialist. Most HMOs, PPOs, worker's compensation plans, and Tricare (Extra and Prime) plans require a referral for specialty care to be considered for payment. The medical assistant working in the primary care physician's office will commonly be asked to forward a referral to a specialist. The medical assistant working in a specialty office must typically ask the patient for a referral prior to the patient's visit. The referral can

(Text continues on page 237.)

THE PATIENT'S DATE OF BIRTH IS WRITTEN IN MM/DD/YYYY FORMAT.

THE INSURANCE ID # IDENTIFIES THE EMPLOYEE OR BENEFICIARY.

THE PATIENT'S NAME MUST MATCH THE ID CARD EXACTLY.

INFORMATION ON THE PATIENT'S CONDITION IN BOX #10 IS NEEDED TO DETERMINE IF THE CLAIM IS TO BE FILED AS A WORKER'S COMPENSATION OR OTHER LIABILITY POLICY.

THE INSURED'S NAME IS THE EMPLOYEE WHO HOLDS THE CONTRACT.

THE DIAGNOSIS POINTER LINKS THE DIAGNOSIS CODE IN BOX 21 TO THE PROCEDURE CODE IN BOX 24D. LINKING THESE CODES IS REQUIRED TO RECIEVE PAYMENT.

INCLUSION OF THE MEDICAL PRACTICE'S FEDERAL TAX ID NUMBER IS MANDATED BY THE IRS FOR THE INSURANCE COMPANY TO PROCESS CHECKS TO PHYSICIANS.

CHECKING YES TO ACCEPT ASSIGNMENT INDICATES TO THE INSURANCE COMPANY THAT THE CHECK SHOULD BE SENT DIRECTLY TO THE PHYSICIAN.

INCLUSION OF THE PHYSICIAN'S NATIONAL PROVIDER ID NUMBER WAS REQUIRED BY APRIL 2007.

1500

HEALTH INSURANCE CLAIM FORM

APPROVED BY NATIONAL UNIFORM CLAIM COMMITTEE 08/05

MEDICARE (Medicare #) ☐ MEDICAID (Medicaid #) ☐ TRICARE CHAMPUS (Sponsor's SSN) ☐ CHAMPVA (Member ID#) ☐ GROUP HEALTH PLAN (SSN or ID) ☒ FECA BLK LUNG (SSN) ☐ OTHER (ID) ☐	1a. INSURED'S I.D. NUMBER (For Program in Item 1) XGA00443

2. PATIENT'S NAME (Last Name, First Name, Middle Initial)
CALABRESE MICHELLE

3. PATIENT'S BIRTH DATE 01 11 1984 SEX M ☐ F ☒

4. INSURED'S NAME (Last Name, First Name, Middle Initial)
CALABRESE MICHELLE

5. PATIENT'S ADDRESS (No., Street)
88 WEST ROAD   STATE CT

6. PATIENT RELATIONSHIP TO INSURED
Self ☒ Spouse ☐ Child ☐ Other ☐

7. INSURED'S ADDRESS (No., Street)
88 WEST ROAD

CITY PRESLEY   STATE CT

8. PATIENT STATUS
Single ☒ Married ☐ Other ☐
Employed ☒ Full-Time Student ☐ Part-Time Student ☐

TELEPHONE (Include Area Code)
(860) 123 9674

ZIP CODE 06100

10. IS PATIENT'S CONDITION RELATED TO:

a. EMPLOYMENT? (Current or Previous) ☐ YES ☒ NO
b. AUTO ACCIDENT? ☐ YES ☒ NO   PLACE (State) ____
c. OTHER ACCIDENT? ☐ YES ☒ NO

9. OTHER INSURED'S POLICY OR GROUP NUMBER

11. INSURED'S POLICY 4488

a. INSURED'S DATE OF BIRTH 01 11 1984 SEX M ☐ F ☒

b. EMPLOYER'S NAME OR SCHOOL NAME
ALOISIO ADVERTISING ASSOCIATES

c. INSURANCE PLAN NAME OR PROGRAM NAME
UNITED HEALTH SYSTEMS

d. INSURANCE PLAN NAME OR PROGRAM NAME

10d. RESERVED FOR LOCAL USE

d. IS THERE ANOTHER HEALTH BENEFIT PLAN?
☐ YES ☒ NO   If yes, return to and complete item 9 a-d.

READ BACK OF FORM BEFORE COMPLETING & SIGNING THIS FORM.

12. PATIENT'S OR AUTHORIZED PERSON'S SIGNATURE I authorize the release of any medical or other information necessary to process this claim. I also request payment of government benefits either to myself or to the party who accepts assignment below.

SIGNED SIGNATURE ON FILE   DATE

13. INSURED'S OR AUTHORIZED payment of medical services described

SIGNED SIG

14. DATE OF CURRENT: 10 19 08 ILLNESS (First symptom) OR INJURY (Accident) OR PREGNANCY(LMP)

15. IF PATIENT HAS HAD SAME OR SIMILAR ILLNESS. GIVE FIRST DATE MM DD YY

16. DATES PATIENT FROM

17. NAME OF REFERRING PROVIDER OR OTHER SOURCE
17a.
17b. NPI

18. HOSPITALIZATION FROM

19. RESERVED FOR LOCAL USE

20. OUTSIDE ☐ YES ☒ NO $ CHARGES

21. DIAGNOSIS OR NATURE OF ILLNESS OR INJURY (Relate Items 1, 2, 3 or 4 to Item 24E by Line)
1. 722.52
2. 729.1
3. ____
4. ____

22. MEDICAID RESUBMISSION CODE   ORIGINAL REF. NO.

23. PRIOR AUTHORIZATION NUMBER

24. A. DATE(S) OF SERVICE					B. PLACE OF SERVICE	C. EMG	D. PROCEDURES, SERVICES, OR SUPPLIES (Explain Unusual Circumstances) CPT/HCPCS	MODIFIER	E. DIAGNOSIS POINTER	F. $ CHARGES	G. DAYS OR UNITS	H. EPSDT Family Plan	I. ID. QUAL.	J. RENDERING PROVIDER ID. #
From MM	DD	YY	To MM	DD	YY									
2 08	10	22	08		11		99204		1,2	85 00	1		NPI	
													NPI	
													NPI	
													NPI	
5													NPI	
6													NPI	

25. FEDERAL TAX I.D. NUMBER 865623498 SSN ☐ EIN ☒

26. PATIENT'S ACCOUNT NO. 703

27. ACCEPT ASSIGNMENT? (For govt. claims, see back) ☒ YES ☐ NO

28. TOTAL CHARGE $ 85 00

29. AMOUNT PAID $

30. BALANCE DUE $ 85 00

31. SIGNATURE OF PHYSICIAN OR SUPPLIER INCLUDING DEGREES OR CREDENTIALS (I certify that the statements on the reverse apply to this bill and are made a part thereof.)
HECTOR RODRIGUEZ, MD
SIGNED   DATE

32. SERVICE FACILITY LOCATION INFORMATION

33. BILLING PROVIDER INFO & PH # (860) 555 3212
HECTOR RODRIGUEZ, MD
15 MAIN STREET
BLUEVILLE CT 06100
a. 1077358914   b.

NUCC Instruction Manual available at: TYPE   APPROVED OMB-0938-0999 FORM CMS-1500 (08-05)

FIG 16-7 CMS-1500 claim form.

PROCEDURE 16-2

Submitting a CMS-1500 form to a third-party payor

Task
Complete and submit a CMS-1500 form to a third-party payor in electronic or hard copy format.

Conditions
- Patient medical record
- Superbill
- CMS-1500 forms in printer (for mailed claims)
- Computer with CMS-1500 software

Standards
In the time specified and within the scoring parameters determined by the instructor, the student will accurately complete and submit a claim for payment using CMS-1500–compatible software or by referring to the patient's medical record.

Performance Standards
1. Refer to the patient's medical record (containing the patient registration form and photocopy of the patient's insurance card) or the patient database to insert the name, address, telephone number, and insurance information into the CMS form (lines 1 through 13).
2. Recheck all information for accuracy to prevent a denial of the claim due to inaccurate data.
3. Refer to the superbill to fill out the following lines of the CMS form:
   a. #14—illness (first symptom) OR injury (accident)
   b. #15—date patient has had same or similar illness (if applicable)
   c. #16—dates unable to work (if applicable)
   d. #17—referring provider and that provider's national provider identification number (NPI) (if applicable)
   e. #18—dates of hospitalization (if applicable)
   f. #21—diagnosis code(s), using the ICD-9-CM codes from the superbill. (Enter the codes in spaces 1, 2, 3, and 4.)
   g. #24 A—date of service
   h. #24 B—place of service code. (The physician's office code is 11.)
   i. #24 D—CPT codes from the superbill with modifiers (if applicable)
   j. #24 F—charge for the procedure listed
   k. #24G—"1" in the days/units column to indicate that the procedure was performed once.
   l. #25—federal tax identification number or physician Social Security number (as determined by office policy) to provide the insurance company with a record for federal and state income tax purposes
   m. #26—patient's account number (as designated by the practice)
   n. #27—check in box to accept (yes) or reject (no) assignment, as designated by office policy (Checking yes sends payment directly to the physician's office.)
   o. #28—total charges for the procedures entered
   p. #29—amount paid by the patient (if any)
   q. #30—balance due
   r. #31—indication of physician's signature on file. (The medical assistant must include a signature or designation of "signature on file" on each claim she submits for it to be eligible for payment.)
   s. #33—billing provider name, address, and phone number to ensure that payment is submitted to the correct office
   t. #33 a—physician's NPI to ensure that the claim is eligible for payment
4. Save and print the claim form.
5. Make a copy of the completed form for the patient's medical record so that, if the claim is lost, the office can resend it in a timely manner.
6. If filing the claim electronically, save the claim and send it via electronic claims submission protocols. (The password-protected software encrypts the data for secure transmission.) If filing by mail, address the envelope to the claims department, enclose the CMS-1500 form, and seal the envelope to ensure privacy.
7. Document the date of submission of the claim to maintain a record in case of a delay in payment.
8. Back up the data onto a separate data storage device, such as a USB drive, to ensure that data is not lost in case of damage to the computer's memory.

HS **United Health Systems**

ID#: XXHL129973534   Group #: 678844
Name: **MARY OLESNEVICH**
Copays: $5 OV, $10 CHIRO, $50 ED

RX: $5

Visit us at: www.UHSystems.com

Member services 1-800-800-1767
Network provider services 1-800-800-1777
Out of network providers 1-800-800-1799

For medical emergencies please dial 911 or go to the nearest emergency room. Please contact your PCP or member services within 24 hours.

For all other care, please contact your PCP.

Refer to your benefit package for coverage descriptions.

Mail Claims to: **UHS, Inc., Claims Department**
                      283 Commerce Park Drive
                      Blueville, CT 06100
                                        UHS rev 12/08

Continued

PROCEDURE 16-2—cont'd

CONFIDENTIAL PATIENT INFORMATION

BLUEVILLE FAMILY MEDICINE
15 MAIN STREET
BLUEVILLE, CT
860-555-3212

Name _Mary Olesnevich_ Date of birth _07/17/1974_ Full time student ☐ Yes ☒ No
Address _277 Weston Road_ City _Blueville, CT_
Home phone _555-7736_ Cell phone _203-977-8033_
Insured name _self_ Insured date of birth _07/17/1974_ Relationship to patient _self_
Insured employer _Blueville Family Services_ Employer address _115 Washington Street, Blueville, CT_
Insurance carrier _United Health Systems_ ID# _XXHL129973534_ Group # _678844_

HEALTH HISTORY

Have you ever suffered from:

☐ Asthma	☐ Fainting	☐ Muscle weakness	☒ Lower back pain
☐ Diabetes	☒ Anxiety	☒ Difficulty sleeping	☐ Difficulty swallowing
☐ High blood pressure	☐ Bleeding disorder	☒ Allergies	☒ Neck pain or stiffness
☒ Migraine headaches	☒ Constipation	☒ Stomach upset	☐ Diarrhea
☐ Fatigue	☒ Stress	☐ Mental disorder	☐ Infection

☐ Cancer (If so, what kind?) _none_   ☒ Chronic pain (If so, where?) _neck, lower back_

FAMILY HISTORY

☒ Cancer (Who?) _father_   What type? _lung (died in 2005)_
☒ High blood pressure (Who?) _father_
☒ Diabetes (Who?) _grandmother, uncle_

MEDICATIONS AND SUPPLEMENTS

Do you take any medications?   Do you take any nutritional supplements?
If so, please list (include dosages):   If so, please list:
Lipitor 5 mg/day   _Centrum multi_
Zoloft 2 mg/day
Allegra 10 mg/day (not every day)
Prilosec 5 mg/day

REASON FOR TODAY'S VISIT

☐ Check up
☐ Physical for school, sports, or employment
☒ Other (please explain) _extremely tired, my neck and back hurt_

Women only

Date of last menstrual period _2/15/09_
Number of pregnancies _3_   Miscarriages? _1_
Number of children _2_   Difficult or painful menstruation? _sometimes_

Men only

Have you ever had erectile difficulty? _____ Prostate problems? _____
Do you get up at night frequently to urinate? _____

I understand that Blueville Family Medicine will file my insurance for payment of services rendered. I also understand
that I am responsible for any amount due Blueville Family Medicine if my insurance is denied.

Signature of patient or guardian _Mary Olesnevich_   Date _03/12/09_

Relationship to patient _self_

Robert Greer, MD • Sharon Piecek, APRN • Hector Rodriguez, MD • Henry Lee, MD • Anne Wilson, MD

PROCEDURE 16-2—cont'd

Blueville Family Medicine
15 Main Street
Blueville CT
860-555-3212

Patient Name: _Mary Olesnevich_

Date: _March 8, 2009_

Provider: ☐ Robert Greer, MD
☐ Hector Rodriguez, MD
☐ Anne Wilson, MD
☒ Sharon Piecek, APRN
☐ Henry Lee, MD

CPT-4 Codes

Examinations			Laboratory		
Exam brief (New Pt)		99201	Urinalysis		81000
Exam intermediate (New Pt)		99202	Pregnancy test		81025
Exam detailed (New Pt)		99203	UA volume		81050
Exam comprehensive (New Pt)		99204	Allergy test - skin extracts		95004
Exam comp, high complex (New Pt)		99205	Allergy - biologicals		95010
Exam brief (Est Pt)		99211	Allergy - patch test		95044
Exam intermediate (Est Pt)	X	99212	PTT		85002
Exam detailed (Est Pt)		99213	Hematocrit	X	85014
Exam comprehensive (Est Pt)		99214	Hemoglobin	X	85018
Exam comp, high complex (Est Pt)		99215	Diff WBC		85004
			Occult blood		82270
X-rays			Throat culture		87650
Chest - one view		71010			
Chest - 4 views		71030			
Spine - single view (specify level)		72020	ECG		93270
X-ray - shoulder 1 view		73020	ECG - 24-hour monitor		93224
X-ray elbow		73085			
X-ray wrist (2 views)		73100			
X-ray hip (1 view)		73500	**Physical Medicine**		
X-ray knee		73560	Acupuncture		97780
X-ray ankle (3 views)		73610	Acupuncture with ES		97813
X-ray foot (2 views)		73620	Nutritional counseling (initial exam)	X	97802
			Nutritional counseling (subsequent)		97803

ICD-9-CM Codes

Well-child visit		V20.2	Myofascitis		729.1
Prenatal visit		V22	Sinusitis		473.9
Prenatal visit - high risk		V23	Tonsillitis		474.0
Allergy exam		V72.7	Otitis media		382.9
Anemia	X	285.9	Otitis externa		380.10
Lower back pain		724.2	Otitis interna		386.30
Neck pain		723.1	Urinary tract infection		599.0
Hypertension		642.2	Conjunctivitis		077.99
Fatigue	X	789.79	Angina		413.9
HF		428.0	COPD		496

be faxed to the specialist's office or given to the patient to present at the time of the office visit. The referral must include:

- name and NPI of the referring PCP
- type of service(s) requested by the PCP (for example, evaluation by an endocrinologist, psychologist, or nephrologist)

- date of the referral, because referrals expire (although expiration times vary among insurance carriers). (See Figure 16-8.)

When the specialist sees a patient for a referred service, the medical assistant filing the CMS-1500 form must

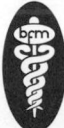

Blueville Family Medicine
15 Main Street
Blueville CT
860-555-3212

Outpatient Services Referral

Blueville Family Medicine
15 Main Street
Blueville CT
860-555-3212

Robert Greer, MD
Hector Rodriguez, MD
Anne Wilson, MD
Sharon Piecek, APRN
Henry Lee, MD

Patient: *Kaitlin Hartley*

Date of Birth: *11/02/1958*   Gender *female*

Insurance Carrier: *Universal HMO*   Group #: *3448*

ID#: *XRV86712984400*   Referral #: *87995443*

Referred to: *Rebecca Roberts, MD Endocrinology Associates*

Facility address: *17 Main Street, Blueville CT*

Facility phone: *860-555-9087*

First appointment date
10/16/09

Reason for referral *increased thirst, excessive urination, enlarging mass in neck*

Physician orders *examination for diabetes and thyroid function testing*

FIG 16-8 Specialty referral.

include the referring PCP's name and NPI number on lines 17 and 17b. (See Figure 16-9.)

Payment Systems

Insurance carriers use several methods to determine payment rates. Because HMOs require providers to enroll as participating physicians in order to provide care to their beneficiaries, rates of payment must be attractive for physicians to apply. Government plans cannot mandate that physicians participate in programs such as Medicare, Medicaid, Tricare, or CHAMPVA; but they also must attract physicians to participate in their programs. While all of the insurers need to attract physicians, they also need to control costs, offering the lowest possible premiums and deductibles to stay competitive. All of these factors add to the complexity of payment calculations. Methods for determining payments include:

- usual, customary, and reasonable (UCR)
- fee-for-service (FFS)
- resource-based relative value scale (RBRVS)
- capitation.

14. DATE OF CURRENT: MM	DD	YY	◄ ILLNESS (First symptom) OR INJURY (Accident) OR PREGNANCY(LMP)	15. IF PATIENT HAS HAD SAME OR SIMILAR ILLNESS. GIVE FIRST DATE MM	DD	YY
03	20	09		
17. NAME OF REFERRING PROVIDER OR OTHER SOURCE			17a.	
LOUISE RENSHAW MD			17b. NPI	7690859444

FIG 16-9   Lines 17 and 17b from CMS-1500 form.

Usual, Customary, and Reasonable

The usual, customary, and reasonable (UCR) payment method is employed in some of the more expensive indemnity plans. It is based on prevailing rates determined by the insurance company. To determine these rates, the insurance company examines typical fees charged by physicians and other medical specialists in the same region or orders a study of a specific region to show the prevailing rates in that area.

Fee-for-Service

In the fee-for-service payment method, the insurance company looks at each line item submitted on the CMS-1500 claim form. It determines eligibility and makes payments for each line item based on an agreed-upon fee schedule (HMO rates) or on the UCR data that are available.

Resource-Based Relative Value Scale

Medicare uses the resource-based relative value scale (RBRVS) to determine payment to providers. An RBRVS system is made up of a set of formulas that take into account the resources needed to provide services. There are three factors considered in determining this need:

- work necessary to provide the service
- expense incurred by the practice in relation to the service
- malpractice insurance expenses.

In addition, a geographical adjustment factor is included for each region. Medicare will supply the fee schedule for each procedure code, but that is only part of the system. The payment rules associated with RBRVS also include:

- Medicare will allow a physician to bill for an evaluation on the same day as a major surgical procedure, but only if the claim includes the modifier 57 with the evaluation procedure code.
- Medicare won't pay for supplies separately, because the value of most of these supplies has already been included in the RBRVS under the practice expense portion of the formula.
- The codes listed in the surgery section include references to the number of follow-up days included in the surgical procedure itself. The days listed will be 0, 10, or 90 days.

Many of the commercial (nongovernment) carriers have also used the RBRVS and adapted it by adding their own reimbursement rules. Rules for those insurance companies are outlined in the provider's billing handbook, usually available on the company's website. Some of these sites require a password, based on participation as a provider with the company.

Capitation

HMOs that offer capitation systems base payment to physicians on the number of patients who are signed up with the physician, called a *panel*. The insurance company pays the physician a set fee each month for each patient in the panel. This fee is referred to as the *per member per month (PMPM) rate*. For example, if a physician is the primary care physician for 2,500 patients enrolled with an insurance company, the insurance company will calculate a rate that fits the age and nature of the panel (depending on the history of usage, or claims, submitted by that group of patients and severity of illness in the patient base). So, if the insurance company agrees to pay the physician $12.85 per member each month, the physician will receive a flat rate of $32,125 per month to provide care for all 2,500 patients. Thus, this system encourages physicians to be judicious when ordering diagnostic tests and treatments for patients. Although $32,125 per month may seem like a substantial sum of money, a physician who is not judicious will quickly lose money.

An insurance company may pay for some services in addition to the PMPM rate. These services may include an annual physical and additional procedures that the physician has contracted to exclude from the PMPM rate, such as a primary care physician who also provides gynecological services.

Payment Processing

Although some medical offices may receive payments automatically (from the insurance company directly into the practice's bank account), most offices still process payments in the form of checks. Larger practices may use lock boxes that are arranged with a bank. The practice indicates payments should be sent to the lock box, and bank personnel deposit the checks and then send the explanation of benefits (EOB) directly to the physician's office. (See *Anatomy of an EOB*, page 240.) Billing personnel in the medical office then post the payments to the patients' accounts, following the itemized information on the EOB, called *remittance advice*. In addition to recording in the patient's account any payments received, the medical assistant must apply any adjustments. Such an adjustment includes a contractual **write-off**, which is the difference between the amount billed by the physician and the amount allowed by the insurance

Anatomy of an EOB

Every health insurer is required to provide the subscriber with an explanation of benefits (EOB), which outlines the response to medical claims filed for reimbursement. The only exception to this rule is that health maintenance organizations (HMOs) are not required to provide an EOB to the patient for services provided by a participating provider who receives full reimbursement directly from the insurer. Even so, the HMO is required to provide an EOB for any payment if the patient requests it. The EOB must include:

• name of the service provider

• dates of service

• identification of the service by CPT-4 code

• provider's charge

• amount or percentage payable after deductibles, copayment, and any other reduction of the amount claimed

• explanation of any reduction in or denial of reimbursement for the amount claimed

• telephone number or address where the insured person may obtain clarification

• information on how to file an appeal of a claim denial and a deadline for submission.

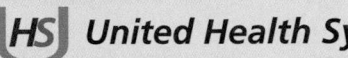 **United Health Systems**

United Health Systems
283 Commerce Park Drive
PO Box 6978
Blueville, CT 06100

Claims 1-800-555-1212

EXPLANATION OF BENEFITS – THIS IS NOT A BILL

Patient name: Steven E. Muzinski
United Health Systems ID# XGA00658   Group # 4388
Provider: Hector Rodriguez, MD   NPI # 12244559988

Patient name	DOS	CPT	Charge	Paid	Allowed	Code	Pt res
Muzinski, Steven E.	04/23/09	99215	95.00	80.00	90.00		10.00

Reason code

To file an appeal of a denial of a claim, send explanation to:

UHS, Inc., Claims Department
283 Commerce Park Drive
PO Box 6978
Blueville, CT 06100

company according to the contract. (See *Why charge more?*.) The billing staff must also apply copayments as well as any insurance deductibles. When the billing staff member finishes posting the payment and determines that all insurance companies have paid, she must bill the patient for any remaining balance.

Payment Denials and Appeals Process

Payment of a claim submitted by a medical office may be denied by an insurance carrier for many reasons. If the insurer denies a claim, that insurer must provide an appeals process. An appeals process involves an opportunity for the medical office to provide additional information regarding the claim to further support the medical necessity for the procedure. Commonly, the narrative notes of patient care will support the treatment and must be submitted to the insurance carrier. The medical assistant must read and refer to the EOB for the denial rationale in order to initiate the appeal process. (See *Procedure 16-3: Communicating with a third-party payor,* page 242.)

Fraud and Abuse

There are two forms of improper claims submission: fraud and abuse. Because the ultimate goal of billing and coding claims is to generate revenue, the medical assistant must be aware of the rules of compliance associated with claim submission. Every claim that leaves the physician's office should be a true, accurate reflection of the services provided to the patient. Claims that are coded improperly so that payment is too high can result in increased scrutiny by insurance companies, possibly inhibiting timely payment on all claims. Alternatively, such improper coding could be identified as fraud or abuse and the medical office may be forced to pay penalties to the insurance company.

The U.S. Department of Justice defines health care fraud as the purposeful misrepresentation or misstatement regarding a medical service's type, scope, or nature that could lead to incorrect payments made to the provider. Victims of health care fraud include private insurance companies as well as Medicare, Medicaid, worker's compensation, and others. Examples of health care fraud include:

- using another person's insurance card to obtain services
- changing dates of service to coincide with dates of insurance coverage
- soliciting or offering a kickback, such as payment for a referral of patients in exchange for ordering diagnostic tests or covered medical equipment
- coding more expensive procedures than those actually performed
- billing for services or equipment never provided
- separate bills for services that should be combined in one fee.

Medicare defines abuse as reimbursement for services where medical necessity is not established. It is not necessarily an intentional act. Examples of insurance abuse include:

- upcoding, in which the severity of the diagnosis is exaggerated in order to support the CPT-4 code. (The physician or coder may not realize that a lesser diagnostic code would be more appropriate.)
- services provided in excess of medical need, such as repeated reevaluations or excessive physical or occupational therapy treatments. (The provider or coder does not necessarily know that the charges are excessive.)

Penalties for fraud and abuse can be imposed on the medical practice by the insurance carrier that made excessive

Why charge more?

Physicians' offices can choose to charge whatever they want for a service, but insurance companies decide what amount they will pay. For example, if a physician charges $100 for a vitamin B_{12} injection, but Medicare allows only $60 for the injection, Medicare will pay 80% of $60 (or $48). The patient or the patient's secondary insurance will pay $12 (the remaining 20% of the $60 approved by Medicare). A Medicare-participating physician is not allowed to bill the patient the remaining $40, and must "write off" the balance.

So why do physicians' offices bill at the higher price? Physicians are obligated to bill a service at the same price to all patients. Another insurance company may pay $75 for the same B_{12} injection, while yet another may allow $80. If the physician charged only the $60 price approved by Medicare, he would lose money by discounting the service to companies that allow a higher reimbursement for that service.

In addition, if a physician's office were to charge varying prices based on the insurance company billed, billing could become very complicated. The medical assistant creating the claims would have to keep up with any changes in allowed charges for all insurance companies. So, to simplify the process, most offices charge a little more than the highest allowed reimbursement for that service across all insurance companies with which they have contracts.

PROCEDURE 16-3

Communicating with a third-party payor

Task
Write a letter to a third-party payor requesting an appeal for a denied claim.

Conditions
- Patient medical record
- CMS-1500 claim form sent to third-party payor for payment
- Denial notification from third-party payor
- Office letterhead
- Computer

Standards
In the time specified and within the scoring parameters determined by the instructor, the student will successfully write a letter of appeal for payment of a denied claim.

Performance Standards
1. Read information from the patient's medical record (below) so that you can understand the claim completely.

2. Reread the CMS-1500 form originally submitted (below) to check for errors.
3. Read the denial notification on the explanation of benefits (below).
4. Compose a letter requesting payment of the claim based on medical necessity as proven by the patient's medical record. Be sure to refute the reasons given for denial of the claim.
5. Reprint the CMS-1500 form because the insurance company will only accept an original form when receiving a resubmitted claim.
6. Sign the letter and submit it to the insurance company (your instructor).

Date	
03/24/09; 11:15 a.m.	Pt complains of neck pain, stiffness, sensitivity to light, and severe right-sided temporal pain. She has been unable to sleep due to pain, did not go to work yesterday or today. Ibuprofen, Tylenol offer limited relief. Points stimulated w/ES- GB 20, GB 21, B11, Si 13, Liv3, Li4, H9, Gv20, Li 18 — for 20 minutes. Pt states pain and sensitivity to light decreased immediately. Tx plan 2x per week for 4 weeks, then re-eval. ------- Henry Lee, MD
03/26/09; 11:30 a.m.	Pt states that she was able to sleep for the past 2 nights, head pain reduced from 10 to 6 on 10 scale. Went to work today, by the end of the day experienced light sensitivity Tx as 3/24 ------------------- Henry Lee, MD
03/30/09; 9:15 a.m.	Pt states pain at 6 on 10 scale, she drank wine last night and headache increased. Suggested no alcohol until pain subsides. Tx as above, increased sensitivity at Liv3 ----- ------------------------- Henry Lee, MD
04/02/09; 4:00 p.m.	Pt states no change in symptoms. Tx as above ----------- ------------------------- Henry Lee, MD
04/06/09; 4:30 pm	Pt states pain 4 on 10 scale, sleeping better, went to gym today, feeling well. Tx as above --------- Henry Lee, MD

HS *United Health Systems*

ID#: XGA00778   Group #: 4488
Name: **CARA COHELO**
Copays: $5 OV $10 CHIRO $50 ED

RX: $5

Visit us at: **www.UHSystems.com**

Member services 1-800-800-1767
Network provider services 1-800-800-1777
Out of network providers 1-800-800-1799

For medical emergencies, please dial 911 or go to the nearest emergency room. Please contact your PCP or member services within 24 hours.

For all other care, please contact your PCP.

Refer to your benefit package for coverage descriptions.

Mail Claims to: UHS, Inc., Claims Department
283 Commerce Park Drive
Blueville, CT 06100

UHS rev 12/08

PROCEDURE 16-3—cont'd

CONFIDENTIAL PATIENT INFORMATION

BLUEVILLE FAMILY MEDICINE
15 MAIN STREET
BLUEVILLE, CT
860-555-3212

Name _Cara Cohelo_   Date of birth _6/21/1984_   Full time student   ☐ Yes   ☒ No
Address _127 West Road_   City _Presley, CT_
Home phone _123-8888_   Cell phone _203-111-2223_
Insured name _self_   Insured date of birth _6/21/1984_   Relationship to patient _self_
Insured employer _Aloisio Advertising Associates_ Employer address _33 Park Ave, Presley, CT_
Insurance carrier _United Health Systems_   ID# _XGA00778_   Group # _4488_

HEALTH HISTORY
Have you ever suffered from:

☐ Asthma	☐ Fainting	☐ Muscle weakness	☐ Lower back pain
☐ Diabetes	☐ Anxiety	☐ Difficulty sleeping	☐ Difficulty swallowing
☐ High blood pressure	☐ Bleeding disorder	☐ Allergies	☒ Neck pain or stiffness
☒ Migraine headaches	☐ Constipation	☒ Stomach upset	☐ Diarrhea
☐ Fatigue	☒ Stress	☐ Mental disorder	☐ Infection

☐ Cancer (If so, what kind?) _none_   ☒ Chronic pain (If so, where?) _neck and right shoulder_

FAMILY HISTORY
☐ Cancer (Who?) _____   What type?_____
☒ High blood pressure (Who?) _grandmother_
☐ Diabetes (Who?) _grandfather_

MEDICATIONS AND SUPPLEMENTS
Do you take any medications?   Do you take any nutritional supplements?
If so, please list (include dosages):   If so, please list:
Clarinex, not every day   _Fem essentials (multi)_
Ibuprofen occasionally for headaches

REASON FOR TODAY'S VISIT
☐ Check up
☐ Physical for school, sports, or employment
☒ Other (please explain) _severe headaches_

Women only
Date of last menstrual period _03/14/09_
Number of pregnancies _0_   Miscarriages? _0_
Number of children _0_   Difficult or painful menstruation? _sometimes_

Men only
Have you ever had erectile difficulty?_____   Prostate problems?_____
Do you get up at night frequently to urinate?_____

I understand that Blueville Family Medicine will file my insurance for payment of services rendered. I also understand that I am responsible for any amount due Blueville Family Medicine if my insurance is denied.

Signature of patient or guardian _Cara Cohelo_   Date _03/27/09_

Relationship to patient _____

Robert Greer, MD   •   Sharon Piecek, APRN   •   Hector Rodriguez, MD   •   Henry Lee, MD   •   Anne Wilson, MD

Continued

PROCEDURE 16-3—cont'd

1500

HEALTH INSURANCE CLAIM FORM

APPROVED BY NATIONAL UNIFORM CLAIM COMMITTEE 08/05

☐☐☐ PICA   PICA ☐☐

1. MEDICARE ☐ (Medicare #)	MEDICAID ☐ (Medicaid #)	TRICARE CHAMPUS ☐ (Sponsor's SSN)	CHAMPVA ☐ (Member ID#)	GROUP HEALTH PLAN ☒ (SSN or ID)	FECA BLK LUNG ☐ (SSN)	OTHER ☐ (ID)	1a. INSURED'S I.D. NUMBER (For Program in Item 1) XGA00778

2. PATIENT'S NAME (Last Name, First Name, Middle Initial) COHELO CARA M	3. PATIENT'S BIRTH DATE MM 06 DD 21 YY 1984 SEX M ☐ F ☒	4. INSURED'S NAME (Last Name, First Name, Middle Initial) COHELO CARA M

5. PATIENT'S ADDRESS (No., Street) 127 WEST ROAD	6. PATIENT RELATIONSHIP TO INSURED Self ☒ Spouse ☐ Child ☐ Other ☐	7. INSURED'S ADDRESS (No., Street) 127 WEST ROAD
CITY PRESLEY	STATE CT	8. PATIENT STATUS Single ☒ Married ☐ Other ☐	CITY PRESLEY	STATE CT
ZIP CODE 06100	TELEPHONE (Include Area Code) (860) 123 8888	Employed ☒ Full-Time Student ☐ Part-Time Student ☐	ZIP CODE 06100	TELEPHONE (Include Area Code) (860) 123 8888

9. OTHER INSURED'S NAME (Last Name, First Name, Middle Initial)	10. IS PATIENT'S CONDITION RELATED TO:	11. INSURED'S POLICY GROUP OR FECA NUMBER 4488
a. OTHER INSURED'S POLICY OR GROUP NUMBER	a. EMPLOYMENT? (Current or Previous) ☐ YES ☒ NO	a. INSURED'S DATE OF BIRTH MM 06 DD 21 YY 1984 SEX M ☐ F ☒
b. OTHER INSURED'S DATE OF BIRTH MM DD YY SEX M ☐ F ☐	b. AUTO ACCIDENT? PLACE (State) ☐ YES ☒ NO	b. EMPLOYER'S NAME OR SCHOOL NAME ALOISIO ADVERTISING ASSOCIATES
c. EMPLOYER'S NAME OR SCHOOL NAME	c. OTHER ACCIDENT? ☐ YES ☒ NO	c. INSURANCE PLAN NAME OR PROGRAM NAME UNITED HEALTH SYSTEMS
d. INSURANCE PLAN NAME OR PROGRAM NAME	10d. RESERVED FOR LOCAL USE	d. IS THERE ANOTHER HEALTH BENEFIT PLAN? ☐ YES ☒ NO If yes, return to and complete item 9 a-d.

READ BACK OF FORM BEFORE COMPLETING & SIGNING THIS FORM.

12. PATIENT'S OR AUTHORIZED PERSON'S SIGNATURE I authorize the release of any medical or other information necessary to process this claim. I also request payment of government benefits either to myself or to the party who accepts assignment below.

SIGNED SIGNATURE ON FILE   DATE _____

13. INSURED'S OR AUTHORIZED PERSON'S SIGNATURE I authorize payment of medical benefits to the undersigned physician or supplier for services described below.

SIGNED SIGNATURE ON FILE

14. DATE OF CURRENT: MM 03 DD 20 YY 09 ◄ ILLNESS (First symptom) OR INJURY (Accident) OR PREGNANCY(LMP)	15. IF PATIENT HAS HAD SAME OR SIMILAR ILLNESS. GIVE FIRST DATE MM DD YY	16. DATES PATIENT UNABLE TO WORK IN CURRENT OCCUPATION FROM MM DD YY TO MM DD YY
17. NAME OF REFERRING PROVIDER OR OTHER SOURCE LOUISE RENSHAW MD	17a. 17b. NPI 7690859444	18. HOSPITALIZATION DATES RELATED TO CURRENT SERVICES FROM MM DD YY TO MM DD YY
19. RESERVED FOR LOCAL USE		20. OUTSIDE LAB? ☐ YES ☒ NO $ CHARGES

21. DIAGNOSIS OR NATURE OF ILLNESS OR INJURY (Relate Items 1, 2, 3 or 4 to Item 24E by Line)	22. MEDICAID RESUBMISSION CODE ORIGINAL REF. NO.
1. 346.01 3.	23. PRIOR AUTHORIZATION NUMBER
2. 4.	

24. A. DATE(S) OF SERVICE From MM DD YY / To MM DD YY	B. PLACE OF SERVICE	C. EMG	D. PROCEDURES, SERVICES, OR SUPPLIES (Explain Unusual Circumstances) CPT/HCPCS / MODIFIER	E. DIAGNOSIS POINTER	F. $ CHARGES	G. DAYS OR UNITS	H. EPSDT Family Plan	I. ID. QUAL.	J. RENDERING PROVIDER ID. #
1	03 27 09 03 27 09	11		97813	1	65 00	1		NPI	
2	03 29 09 03 29 09	11		97813	1	65 00	1		NPI	
3	04 01 09 04 01 09	11		97813	1	65 00	1		NPI	
4	04 04 09 04 04 09	11		97813	1	65 00	1		NPI	
5	04 06 09 04 06 09	11		97813	1	65 00	1		NPI	
6									NPI	

25. FEDERAL TAX I.D. NUMBER 865623498 SSN ☐ EIN ☒	26. PATIENT'S ACCOUNT NO. 1296	27. ACCEPT ASSIGNMENT? (For govt. claims, see back) ☒ YES ☐ NO	28. TOTAL CHARGE $ 325 00	29. AMOUNT PAID $	30. BALANCE DUE $ 325 00

31. SIGNATURE OF PHYSICIAN OR SUPPLIER INCLUDING DEGREES OR CREDENTIALS (I certify that the statements on the reverse apply to this bill and are made a part thereof.) SIGNATURE ON FILE SIGNED DATE	32. SERVICE FACILITY LOCATION INFORMATION a. NPI b.	33. BILLING PROVIDER INFO & PH # (860) 555 3212 HENRY LEE MD 15 MAIN STREET BLUEVILLE CT 06100 a. 8700334239 b.

NUCC Instruction Manual available at: www.nucc.org   **PLEASE PRINT OR TYPE**   APPROVED OMB-0938-0999 FORM CMS-1500 (08-05)

Side labels: CARRIER — PATIENT AND INSURED INFORMATION — PHYSICIAN OR SUPPLIER INFORMATION

PROCEDURE 16-3—cont'd

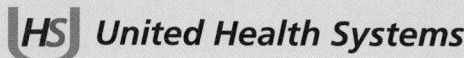

HS **United Health Systems**

United Health Systems
283 Commerce Park Drive
PO Box 6978
Blueville, CT 06100

Claims 1-800-555-1212

EXPLANATION OF BENEFITS – THIS IS NOT A BILL

Patient name: Cara Cohelo
United Health Systems ID# XGA00778   Group # 4488
Provider: Henry Lee, MD   NPI # 8700334239

Patient name	DOS	CPT	Charge	Paid	Allowed	Code	Pt res
Cohelo, Cara	03/27/09	97813	65.00	0.00	0.00	A12	65.00
Cohelo, Cara	03/29/09	97813	65.00	0.00	0.00	A12	65.00
Cohelo, Cara	04/01/09	97813	65.00	0.00	0.00	A12	65.00
Cohelo, Cara	04/04/09	97813	65.00	0.00	0.00	A12	65.00
Cohelo, Cara	04/06/09	97813	65.00	0.00	0.00	A12	65.00

Reason code

A12 – further documentation needed to process claim

To file an appeal of a denial of a claim, send explanation to:

UHS, Inc., Claims Department
283 Commerce Park Drive
PO Box 6978
Blueville, CT 06100

payments. Penalties can include revocation of participating provider status (HMO) or participating physician status (Medicare, Medicaid, Tricare). Other penalties include recovery of overpayments and withholding of pending payments. In cases of fraud, where intentional misrepresentation is evident, criminal prosecution and jail sentences are possible.

Chapter Summary
- Because health insurance products vary, the medical assistant must be aware of the various products and be aware of changes to policies.

- There are various forms of payment to physicians for services, including fee-for-service, UCR, RBVS, and capitation.
- Gathering demographic information from a patient at the first visit is necessary for complete claims submission.
- A patient can elect to self-pay upon arrangement with the physician. Medicare patients electing to self-pay for an uncovered procedure must sign an advance beneficiary notice (ABN) before receiving care.
- Copayments, where applicable, should be collected prior to patient examinations.
- Coding procedures and diagnoses are learned skills that require the medical assistant to understand coding procedures and be aware of coding changes.

- The medical assistant must be able to include referral information on CMS-1500 forms for specialist payment when specialty care requires a referral.
- If claims for payment are denied, the medical assistant can appeal the decision by providing further documentation to support the need for services.
- Fraud and abuse are the intentional or unintentional coding of claims for excessive payment. The medical assistant must have a working understanding of current codes to avoid coding in error.
- Fraud can be prosecuted with civil and criminal penalties; abuse can be prosecuted with civil penalties.

Team Work Exercises

1. Divide into groups of four to six students each. Each group must choose one type of medical office:
   a. pediatrics
   b. obstetrics and gynecology
   c. family practice
   d. orthopedics
   e. dermatology
   f. cardiology.

   Each group must create a superbill for their practice, including the procedures and diagnoses that the group thinks are most commonly used. Using the CPT-4 and ICD-9-CM coding texts, find the codes to include on your superbill. Ask the other groups to comment on your choices.
2. Divide into teams of six to nine students. Each team must create a computer or poster presentation on one of the following topics and present it to the class:
   a. life cycle of an insurance claim
   b. steps for coding a procedure
   c. steps for coding a diagnosis
   d. response to denied claims.

Case Studies

1. Leona Jensen has been a patient for many years. She has just turned 65 years old and has retired from her job as a police dispatcher. She comes in for a visit to see Dr. Rodriguez. What information should you obtain from Mrs. Jensen?
2. Ralph Sawyer, a 38-year-old construction worker who was injured at work, calls the office. He tells you that he must return to work because his compensation benefits are not enough for his family to live on and his wife recently lost her job. He has been out of work for the past 2 weeks, and his salary benefits from worker's compensation have yet to arrive. He is agitated and tells you that he is behind in paying his mortgage. He is scheduled to see Dr. Greer tomorrow. What should you tell Ralph?

Resources

- American Academy of Professional Coders: *www.aapc.com*
- American Health Information Management Association: *www.ahima.org*
- CMS programs and information: *www.cms.gov*
- Complete U.S. Government rules for HSAs: *www.treas.gov/offices/public-affairs/hsa/pdf/all-about-HSAs_051807.pdf*
- Healthcare Billing and Management Association: *www.hbma.com*
- Medicaid eligibility: *www.cms.hhs.gov/MedicaidGenInfo*
- Professional Association of Health Care Office Management: *www.pahcom.com*
- Types of managed care: *www.sbhcs.com/hospitals/monmouth_medical/managed/types.html*

Billing and Collections

Learning Objectives
After reading this chapter the student will be able to:

- define the key terms presented in the glossary
- explain the importance of timely billing and collections in the physician's office
- list the key components of a patient statement
- describe monthly and cycle billing
- describe the various options for collecting overdue accounts
- apply HIPAA principles to billing and collections.

CAAHEP Competencies

Administrative Competencies
Perform Bookkeeping Procedures
Perform accounts receivable procedures
Perform billing and collection procedures

General Competencies
Patient Instruction
Explain general office policies

ABHES Competencies
Administrative Duties
Perform billing and collection procedures
Instruction
Orient patients to office policies and procedures

Procedures
Explaining office financial policies to a patient
Creating a collection letter

Chapter Outline
Patient Billing
Determination of Fees
Explaining Fees to the Patient

Billing Procedures
Aging of Accounts
Computerized Billing and Account Transactions
Monthly and Cycle Billing
Monthly billing
Cycle billing
Credit and Collections
Policies and Procedures
Extending Credit
Collections
Collection strategies
Telephone collections
Collection agency
Chapter Summary
Team Work Exercises
Case Studies
Resources

Patient Billing

Billing patients in an ambulatory setting is a necessary task of the administrative medical assistant. Effective billing practices promote a healthy **cash flow**, the amount of money a business must maintain to ensure that patients can be cared for and overhead expenses and salaries can be paid. While most offices are now computerized, some may still use a manual, or pegboard, system. Regardless of the billing system, accurate, timely billing promotes trust and understanding among staff, patients, and physicians.

Determination of Fees

Providers of health care have many different arrangements with insurance carriers regarding the determination of fees. Providers within an HMO network agree to a fee schedule of services and how much (if any) money can be collected directly from the patient in the form of a copayment, or *copay*. Providers outside of an HMO network may receive a reduced portion of the total fee or no fee at all from the insurance carrier. However, they may bill the patient for the remaining balance.

Explaining Fees to the Patient
Comprehensive communication and understanding of fees between staff and patients will encourage timely payments. It is the responsibility of the administrative medical assistant to explain to the patient:

- which portion of the total bill the patient is responsible for and when this money is due
- when office charges are owed and how much is owed
- fees charged for missed appointments, telephone consultations, copying of reports, and other charges that the patient may be unaware of.

The medical assistant can use various tools to help explain these fees and policies. She can refer to a brochure that outlines the financial policies of the office. (See Figure 17-1.) To explain insurance charges, many offices have a chart at the front desk that shows the names of various insurance plans with their respective copayment amounts, covered services, and exclusions. (See Figure 17-2.) From this chart, the medical assistant can compile and provide a brief outline of the covered services to a patient for clarification. (See Figure 17-3.) The medical assistant can refer to the chart when speaking to a patient on the phone or in person. (See *Procedure 17-1: Explaining office financial policies to a patient,* page 251.)

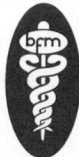

BLUEVILLE FAMILY MEDICINE
15 MAIN STREET
BLUEVILLE, CONNECTICUT 06000
860-555-3212

Robert Greer, MD
Family Medicine

Hector Rodriguez, MD
Family Medicine

Anne Wilson, MD
School and Sports Physicals

Sharon Piecek, APRN
Nutritional Counseling and Weight Loss, Diabetes Management

Henry Lee, MD
Acupuncture

Blueville Family Medicine Financial Policies

Copayments
Copayments are due at time of visit. Please come to your appointment with your copayment in cash, a personal check, or credit card.

Returned check policy
A charge of $20 will be incurred for any check returned for insufficient funds in addition to any charges from the bank. The office reserves the right to deny checks from patients who have had returned checks previously.

Lack of health insurance
If you have little or no health insurance, you can speak with Dr. Rodriguez or Kelly Manera in the billing department about an affordable monthly payment schedule.

Past-due bills
Bills are considered past-due after 30 days of nonpayment. The office bills patient balances each month. Bills that are 90 days late are sent to a collection agency.

FIG 17-1 Office financial policies brochure.

Billing Procedures

Adequate cash flow in the physician's office depends on accurate, timely billing practices. If the total amount of unpaid patient balances increases over time, the practice may not be able to meet the costs of running the office. Physicians' offices usually bill a patient's insurance company first, while the patient pays only a copayment at the time of the visit. After the office receives reimbursement from the insurance company, it *balance bills* the patient, that is, bills for the outstanding balance of unpaid charges.

Aging of Accounts
Aging of accounts begins when the patient receives the first bill. The first bill the medical office sends to a patient is considered *new*. It does not age until it remains unpaid

Insurance plan	Copay	Covered services	Exclusions/limitations
Blue Cross & Blue Shield POE	$5	OV, X-rays, Mamm, PAP, Well Child, UA, Hct, Immunizations, TC	1 checkup per year
Blue Cross & Blue Shield POS	$10	OV, X-rays, Mamm, PAP, Well Child, UA, Hct, Immunizations, TC	2 checkups per year
HealthNet	$10	OV, X-rays, Mamm, PAP, Well Child, UA, Hct, Immunizations, TC	Need referral for x-ray; 1 checkup per year
Physician's Health Network	$15	OV, X-rays, Mamm, PAP, Well Child, UA, Hct, Immunizations, TC	1 checkup per year
Carpenter's Health Fund	$10	OV, X-rays, Mamm, PAP, Well Child, UA, Hct, Immunizations, TC	Will pay for ultrasound breast examination in lieu of mammography with Rx from physician

FIG 17-2 Insurance plans and patient fees chart.

Blueville Family Medicine	15 Main Street Blueville CT	860-555-3212 ask for Kelly Manera for billing inquiries
Your plan is: Blue Cross & Blue Shield POE (Point of Enrollment)	Your copayment for office visits is $5	Your plan covers office visits (2 checkups per year), mammography, pap smears, urinalysis, routine immunizations, and throat cultures. X-rays and most blood tests that we run in the office are covered. If you need to see a specialist, we will write the appropriate referral form but it is your responsibility to confirm coverage of services with the specialist.

FIG 17-3 Outline of covered services.

for 1 month. If the patient does not pay the bill within the first month, it is considered 30 days old. If the office bills each month, bills can age from 30 days to 60 days and even 90 days and beyond. In general, the longer a patient does not pay a bill, the greater the likelihood that he will never pay it.

Computerized Billing and Account Transactions

A vast array of computer software is available to help run a medical office. Most of these software packages can generate patient bills. As with a manual billing system, a computerized patient bill should include:

- patient's name and address
- insurance plan name, identification number, and plan code
- dates of service
- description of services (in words as well as codes)
- payment made by the insurance company (received or pending)
- amount due from the patient
- instructions on how to submit payment, including the address of the practice.

PROCEDURE 17-1

Explaining office financial policies to a patient

Task
Explain the office financial policies to a new patient

Conditions
- Office brochure
- Financial policies document
- Patient's medical record

Standards
In the time specified and within the scoring parameters determined by the instructor, the student will successfully explain the financial policies of the office to the patient as outlined in the financial policies document.

Performance Standards
1. Introduce yourself to the patient and ask her to read the office financial policies brochure.
2. Ask the patient if she has any questions regarding the office policies listed in the brochure to ensure understanding.
3. Ask the patient to sign the financial policies document (below) to document patient's understanding of financial policies.
4. Place the signed financial policies document in the patient's medical record to provide a record of the patient's understanding of financial policies.

Financial Policies Statement

I, _____ , have read and understand Blueville Family Medicine's financial policies as outlined in the office brochure.

The office can generate bills according to the patient's last name, physician, account number, or other identifying information. The method used is significant because it could dictate when the office can send patient bills.

The medical assistant can record payments in the computerized system by inputting the patient's name and the amount of the payment. If a patient makes a partial payment, recording the payment will ensure that the next month's bill reflects the new balance. Recording these account transactions provides a complete record of payments received.

Monthly and Cycle Billing

A medical office commonly determines when to generate and send bills to patients based on the size of the practice and the schedule of the billing staff. The two most common billing systems are monthly billing and cycle billing.

Monthly Billing

Monthly billing is a system of generating bills for all patients at the same time each month. Such a system is convenient for a small practice. In a monthly billing system, billing and mailing statements are generally accomplished in an afternoon or a day. The schedule of the billing staff must accommodate the task of sending out all of the bills. A medical assistant who normally works on insurance claims or telephoning insurance companies for payment may suspend these activities to devote time to billing patients. Monthly billing is sometimes generated and mailed on the 26th or 27th of each month so that patients receive billing statements on the 1st or 2nd of the next month.

Cycle Billing

A larger practice may use a **cycle billing** system, which divides patient bills throughout the month. Because the practice needs a printer to generate the bills, dividing monthly billing into smaller, more frequent batches can free printers for other tasks throughout the day. Systems for cycle billing can vary and include:

- dividing patient accounts by an alphabet system:
  - bill patients with last names beginning with A to F in week 1

- bill patients with last names beginning with G to L in week 2
- bill patients with last names beginning with M to R in week 3
- bill patients with last names beginning with S to Z in week 4
- dividing patients by physician:
  - bill for physician 1 in week 1
  - bill for physician 2 in week 2
  - bill for physician 3 in week 3
  - bill for physician 4 in week 4
- dividing by account numbers:
  - bill even account numbers in week 1
  - bill odd account numbers in week 2
- dividing by office location (for large practices with multiple locations).

Whatever cycle billing system is used, the billing staff must know when patients have received bills in order to accomplish accurate account aging. If the patient fails to pay the balance of the bill within 30 days, it may be considered late. Office policies regarding overdue accounts vary.

Credit and Collections

Unfortunately, sometimes a patient's clear understanding of a balance due does not prompt payment. If a patient ignores a bill, the practice may use a **collection agency**, which is a business hired by the practice to recover bad debts, that is, to collect on overdue accounts. Other times, a patient is temporarily unable to pay the bill because of his own cash flow issues. In such a case, the practice may choose to extend credit to the patient.

Policies and Procedures

Policies and procedures for extending credit and collecting debts should be established by the physician employers or office manager. The role of the administrative medical assistant is to enforce the policies as directed by the physicians or management. Even so, all members of the health care team should be able to assist patients with basic billing questions. (See *Answering billing questions.*) The medical assistant may be required to write a letter asking for payment to avoid collection proceedings. Established guidelines for credit and collections enables the medical assistant to deal confidently with a patient regarding past-due balances.

Front office–Back office connection

Answering Billing Questions

Most commonly, the administrative medical assistant answers a patient's billing questions. However, a patient may ask a clinical medical assistant about a bill while in the examination room. Thus, the clinical medical assistant should have an understanding of the payment policies of the office. Clinical medical assistants should ask the billing personnel how to read the various documents, such as explanations of benefits (EOBs) from insurance companies and statements generated from the office. The clinical medical assistant should be able to answer patient billing questions as they arise.

A good credit and collection policy will address:

- **How is credit extended to a patient?** The office manager or physician may arrange a credit extension to patients or develop a minimum monthly payment system for a patient with high balances.
- **When are payments due from the patient?** Copayments may be due at each visit. For frequent visits, the office and patient may agree upon a maximum outstanding copayment balance.
- **What types of payments are accepted?** Cash and personal checks are the most common forms of payment from patients. Some offices accept credit cards. If a patient pays with cash, the medical assistant should give the patient a receipt for his records. (See Figure 17-4.)
- **When is a patient balance considered overdue?** An office can conduct account aging in 30-, 60-, and 90-day increments, with a bill generated each month to the patient. The office can print past-due messages on bills to prompt patient payment. (See Figure 17-5.)
- **How will patients be reminded of overdue accounts?** In addition to the past-due message on printed patient bills, the office may contact the patient by letter or phone. In a collection letter, the medical assistant should use language that is firm, yet polite. If the account is only 30 days overdue, the medical assistant should refrain from mentioning a collection agency, because it is possible that the patient will make some sort of payment arrangement. If a patient has ignored a bill for 90 days, however, the medical assistant should consider his account as more likely to be sent to the collection agency. (See Figure 17-6.) Depending on the office policy, accounts that are 90 or 120 days past due are usually considered for collection proceedings. (See *Procedure 17-2: Creating a collection letter*, page 256.)

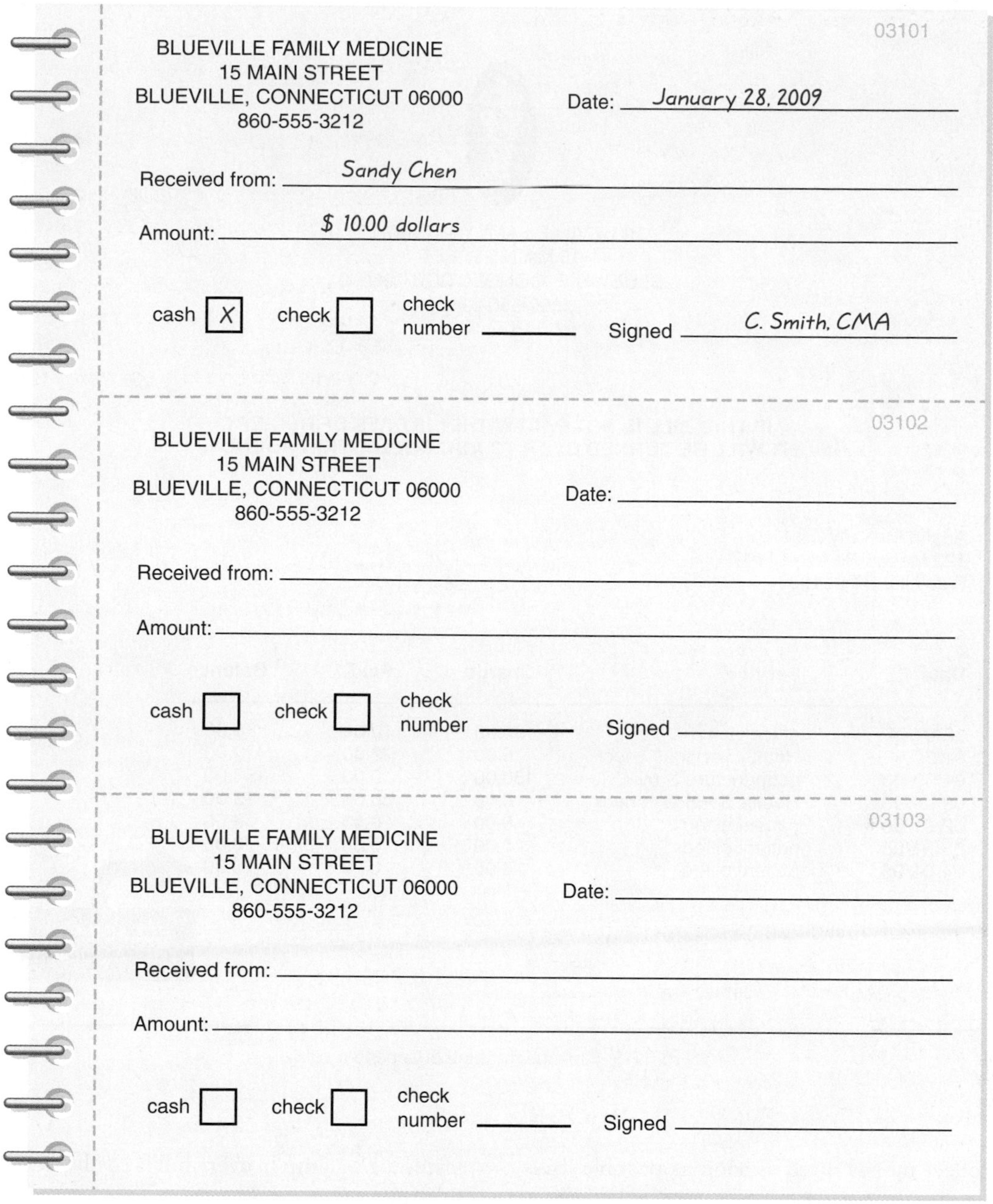

BLUEVILLE FAMILY MEDICINE
15 MAIN STREET
BLUEVILLE, CONNECTICUT 06000
860-555-3212

03101

Date: *January 28, 2009*

Received from: *Sandy Chen*

Amount: *$ 10.00 dollars*

cash [X]   check [ ]   check number _____   Signed *C. Smith, CMA*

BLUEVILLE FAMILY MEDICINE
15 MAIN STREET
BLUEVILLE, CONNECTICUT 06000
860-555-3212

03102

Date: _____

Received from: _____

Amount: _____

cash [ ]   check [ ]   check number _____   Signed _____

BLUEVILLE FAMILY MEDICINE
15 MAIN STREET
BLUEVILLE, CONNECTICUT 06000
860-555-3212

03103

Date: _____

Received from: _____

Amount: _____

cash [ ]   check [ ]   check number _____   Signed _____

FIG 17-4 Cash receipt.

Extending Credit

Physicians may provide special arrangements for patients with financial difficulties or give professional courtesy discounts to colleagues. Patients who cannot pay copayments or pay for uncovered services may reach an agreement with the physician to pay a reduced rate or use a prolonged schedule of payments. Although rare, a physician may agree to a barter system with a housecleaner or lawn care provider or for other services the physician can use to offset the unpaid charges.

Collections

There are numerous ways to collect payment for services provided. Many involve making the payment process as immediate or easy for the patient as possible. Sometimes, however, notifying the patient of a past-due balance is best done over the phone.

Collection Strategies

The best way for a medical office to avoid the stress of collecting on overdue accounts and having to confront angry

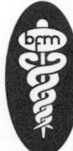

BLUEVILLE FAMILY MEDICINE
15 MAIN STREET
BLUEVILLE, CONNECTICUT 06000
860-555-3212

**IF THIS BILL IS NOT PAID WITHIN 15 DAYS OF RECEIPT,
IT WILL BE TURNED OVER TO ABC COLLECTION AGENCY.**

Austin McNally
122 Mason Road, Apt #17
Blueville, CT 06100

Date	Service	Charge	Paid	Balance
12/07/07	office visit	85.00	0.00	85.00
01/22/08	Health Services check	0.00	72.00	13.00
01/30/08	acupuncture & ov	150.00	10.00	153.00
02/24/08	Health Services check	0.00	80.00	73.00
02/01/08	patient billed	0.00	0.00	73.00
03/01/08	patient billed	0.00	0.00	73.00
04/01/08	patient billed	0.00	0.00	73.00

**PLEASE PAY
THIS AMOUNT.**

FIG 17-5 Past-due message on a patient bill.

patients is to collect money owed as soon as possible. Bills that are not overdue do not cause stress for the patient or the staff.

One way the medical assistant can obtain prompt payment is to ask the patient *how* she will be paying, not *if* she will be paying. For example, at the front desk, the medical assistant says, "Ms. Clifford, your copayment today is $15; will you be paying with cash or check?" In this statement, the medical assistant does not offer the patient the option of *not* paying. Another strategy is to include a return envelope with every bill when mailing bills to patients. If the office includes an addressed envelope with the bill, it is easier for the patient to write the check and simply place it in the envelope. Some offices will actually stamp the return envelope in an effort to increase collections. However, including a stamp in every bill is costly, so offices should use this strategy sparingly.

Telephone Collections

Calling patients with past-due accounts can be stressful but is commonly effective. A patient who is experiencing financial problems may be embarrassed about the status of her account. Another patient may have simply forgotten to pay or thought he mailed a check. These patients are commonly eager to explain their circumstances and come to an amiable resolution.

If a patient is unwilling or unable to pay, however, he may become rude or even verbally abusive. Regardless of the patient's demeanor, the administrative medical assistant must remain respectful and courteous. She should never

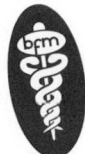

BLUEVILLE FAMILY MEDICINE
15 MAIN STREET
BLUEVILLE, CONNECTICUT 06000
860-555-3212

February 5, 2006

Ms. Lynn Jones
123 Main Street
Blueville, CT

Dear Ms. Jones,

Your account of $203.45 is now 30 days overdue. If you are unable to pay in full, please contact me so that we can arrange a schedule of payments. I can be reached at 555-1444. I look forward to your call.

Sincerely,

Kelly Manera

Kelly Manera
Billing Manager

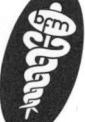

BLUEVILLE FAMILY MEDICINE
15 MAIN STREET
BLUEVILLE, CONNECTICUT 06000
860-555-3212

April 3, 2006

Ms. Lynn Jones
123 Main Street
Blueville, CT

Dear Ms. Jones,

Your account with our office is 90 days past due. Previous requests for payment have been ignored. I have been unable to reach you by telephone to discuss this matter. Please pay your balance of $203.45 by April 20th to avoid collection proceedings. If you have any questions, please contact me at 555-1444.

Sincerely,

Kelly Manera

Kelly Manera
Billing Manager

FIG 17-6 Examples of collection letters.

PROCEDURE 17-2

Creating a collection letter

Task
Create a collection letter for a past-due account.

Conditions
- Record of patient's account
- Computer
- Office letterhead

Standards
In the time specified and within the scoring parameters determined by the instructor, the student will successfully create a letter to a patient regarding his past-due account.

Performance Standards
1. Refer to the patient's financial account (below) to see how old the account is and how much the patient owes.

2. Determine the appropriate collection agency to use (as provided by your instructor or using your local telephone book).
3. Compose a letter to the patient, explaining that his account will be sent to the collection agency (use name in letter) if it remains unpaid.
4. Make a copy of the letter and place it in the patient's medical record to provide a record that the notice of collection was sent to the patient.

Henry Paulson
22 Pinecrest Lane
Blueville, CT

Date	Description	Charge	Note	Balance
April 12, 2007	OV, stress test	140.00		140.00
April 19, 2007	payment – personal ck	10.00		130.00
May 11, 2007	Ins payment	110.00		20.00
May 22, 2007	OV, med ck	85.00		105.00
June 8, 2007	Ins payment	60.00		45.00
July 1, 2007	Patient billed			
August 1, 2007	payment – personal check	20.00		25.00
August 20, 2007	OV, x-ray, meds	330.00		365.00
September 1, 2007	Patient billed			365.00
September 18, 2007	Insurance – no pay, patient called			365.00
October 1, 2007	Patient billed		called pt he will send payment this month	365.00
November 1, 2007	Patient billed		called pt he will send payment this month	365.00
December 1, 2007	Patient billed		called pt he will send payment this month	
January 2, 2008	Patient billed		payment 20.00	345.00
February 1, 2008	Patient billed		called pt – no answer	345.00
March 3, 2008	Patient billed		called pt – no answer	345.00
April 1, 2008	Patient billed		called pt – no answer	345.00

threaten a patient with collection proceedings over the phone; this information must always be conveyed in writing. If the patient is abusive or threatening, the medical assistant must notify the physician or office manager of the patient's behavior. She should also document the phone call and the patient's comments in the patient's medical record.

Financial matters require the same privacy protection as any medical information. The medical assistant should place collection calls in a private area of the office to ensure the confidentiality of the call. She should also refrain from discussing specific patient financial situations with anyone who does not need to know. Finally, she must always document collection calls in the patient's file.

Collection Agency

A medical office can hire a private collection agency to recover past-due payments for a flat fee or a percentage of the recovered amount. Therefore, the office should consider referring only large accounts when hiring a collection agency because the agency charges a minimum fee for its services. In addition, sending a patient's account to collections inhibits a full and open physician–patient relationship that is essential for proper patient care. Thus, the medical assistant should always consult with the physician or office manager before initiating collection proceedings.

When an office is considering collections for a patient account, the medical assistant should mail a final warning to the patient stating that the delinquent account will be sent to collections if no payment is received within a given time period. Because collection proceedings impact credit ratings, this notice will usually prompt the patient to pay the past-due amount before her credit is affected.

Chapter Summary

- Effective billing practices in an ambulatory setting promote healthy relationships between patients and the office staff.
- Consistent, effective billing ensures proper patient care and prompt payment of office expenses, such as employee salaries.
- Billing systems require accuracy and consistency, yet leave room for special arrangements as needed.
- The medical assistant may contact a patient with a delinquent account by letter or telephone. She must always document such contact with the patient.

Team Work Exercises

1. Divide into teams of four to six students. Research local insurance carriers and their copayment and payment policies. Create an informational brochure for an office that outlines the patient responsibility for office visits, routine physicals, mammograms, ECGs, well-child visits, and global surgical packages. Post the brochures in the classroom and discuss your findings with the class.

2. Divide into groups of three to five students. Discuss ways that you might increase patient payments in the medical office. What strategies have you seen employed by your own physician's office? Which ones do you think work, and which ones do not? Create some guidelines for an office based on your discussion. A representative from each group must present the top four strategies for collections that the group feels are most effective.

Case Studies

1. Lynn Jones has a 90-day past-due account with the office. On the phone, she states that she is unable to pay because she is going through a divorce and has yet to collect any child support from her ex-husband. Later the same week, you see Lynn at your hairdresser's getting an expensive manicure and acrylic nail set. What should you do? What are the appropriate places to discuss Lynn's overdue account?

2. Mr. Wallace is a retired brick mason who comes into the office for his physical. He is a great guy and the office staff and physicians all enjoy seeing him. He tells you that he forgot his $10 copayment but he brought in a bag of tomatoes from his garden. He asks that you forgive the copayment. What should you do?

Resources

- Information for patients on understanding medical bills: *www.aafp.org/fpm/20040300/monitor_boxc.html*
- Collection agencies: *www.bad-debts.net,* *www .collectionscheap.com,* and *www.abccompanies.com*
- Caplan, S.: *Streetwise Credit and Collections: Maximize Your Collections Process to Improve Your Profitability.* Avon, MA: Adams Media Corporation, 2007.
- Stanley, K. (ed.): *Maximizing Billing and Collections in the Medical Practice.* Chicago: AMA Press, 2007.
- HCPro (Firm) Staff: *Improve Billing and Collections: Get the Money You Deserve Now.* Marblehead, MA: HCPro, 2006.

Accounting and Banking

Learning Objectives

Upon completion of this chapter, the student will be able to:

- define key terms presented in the glossary
- describe the importance of accurate, complete accounting records in the ambulatory care setting
- describe how cost analysis and cost ratios can be used to make financial decisions
- describe the importance of complete, accurate bookkeeping practices
- describe how payroll is calculated, including deductions
- be able to balance a business checking account against a bank statement.

CAAHEP Competencies

Administrative Competencies

Perform Bookkeeping Procedures
  Prepare a bank deposit
  Post entries on a day sheet
  Perform accounts receivable procedures
  Perform billing and collection procedures
  Post adjustments
  Process a credit balance
  Process refunds
  Post nonsufficient fund (NSF) checks
  Post collection agency payments
General Competencies
Operational Functions
  Utilize computer software to maintain office systems

ABHES Competencies

Administrative Duties
  Apply computer concepts for office procedures
  Prepare a bank statement and deposit record
  Reconcile a bank statement
  Post entries on a day sheet
  Perform billing and collection procedures
  Prepare a check
  Establish and maintain petty cash fund
  Post adjustments
  Process credit balance
  Process refunds
  Post NSF funds
  Post collection agency payments
Financial Management
  Use manual and computerized bookkeeping systems
  Manage accounts payable and receivable
  Maintain records for accounting and banking purposes
  Process employee payroll

Procedures

Preparing a bank deposit slip
Reconciling a bank statement
Posting entries, adjustments, and collection agency payments on day sheet
Processing credit balances
Processing a refund
Posting an NSF check

Chapter Outline

Financial Management
Accounting Practices
  Fixed and Variable Costs
  Cost Ratio
  Income Statement
  Balance Sheet
  Bookkeeping
    Ledger cards
    Adjustments
    NSF checks
  Accounts Receivable Ratio
  Collection Ratio
  Accounts Payable
    Deliveries and supplies
    Writing checks
  Payroll
    Preparing payroll checks
Banking Practices
  Reconciling Bank Statements
  Making Bank Deposits
  Petty Cash
Chapter Summary
Team Work Exercises
Case Studies
Resources

Financial Management

Comprehensive financial management of the physician's office is an important function of the administrative medical assistant or office manager. Having complete and accurate records of what money is coming in and what money is going out allows managers and physician-owners to understand the overall financial health of the practice. Such an analysis gives physician-owners the information needed to make financial decisions, such as expansion of the practice, new equipment purchases, and new employee hiring.

Accounting Practices

Accounting practices can be divided into two main categories: financial and managerial. **Financial accounting** provides data for outside entities such as the federal government. Analysis of net profit provides information needed to pay federal and state taxes. The practice's accounting firm will provide forms for administrative staff to fill out, including total money collected and business expenses, such as salaries, office and medical supplies, license fees, and continuing education expenses. The accounting firm will then use this information to determine what the practice owes for federal and state taxes. The administrative staff should keep copies of receipts in case of an audit.

Managerial accounting provides information for the managers or physician-owners. Where is money being spent? What are the best returns on investment procedures? What does it cost to perform particular services? The practice can determine whether to continue providing certain services or drop them, depending on how costly they are to perform and how much income they generate. Services that generate a larger income and cost less generate a "good return on investment" and should be offered by the practice.

Fixed and Variable Costs

For the office manager to analyze where the practice is spending money and how it is generating income, she must conduct a cost analysis of fixed and variable costs. A **fixed cost** does not vary by the number of patients being seen in the practice. Such expenses as rent or mortgage, equipment leases, or payments are examples of fixed costs. **Variable costs** depend on the number of patients seen in a practice and can include clinical supplies and staff salaries. As patient volume increases, the average cost of treating a patient declines because fixed costs *per patient* decline. (See *Fixed costs and profits*.)

Cost Ratio

By conducting a **cost ratio** analysis, which compares the practice's total expenses to the number of procedures and services provided, an office manager can predict how many

Fixed costs and profits

The following table shows how an increasing volume of patients decreases the fixed cost per patient and, therefore, increases the profit per patient.

It is important to note that in the example above, the additional staff needed to see 100 more patients, from 1,300 to 1,400 patients, actually reduces the profit per patient. The office manager should consider how busy the office should be to be profitable and when the busy office actually decreases profit per patient.

FIXED COSTS	Rent or mortgage on building	6,400	6,400	6,400	6,400	6,400	6,400	6,400
	Equipment leases	1,100	1,100	1,100	1,100	1,100	1,100	1,100
VARIABLE COST BECAUSE IT INCREASES WITH AN INCREASE IN PATIENT VISITS	Staff salaries	49,000	49,500	51,000	55,000	59,000	67,000	69,000
	Clinical and office supplies	1,350	1,400	1,450	1,500	1,550	1,600	1,700
	Total expenses	57,850	58,400	59,950	64,000	68,050	76,100	78,200
	Patient visits per month	900	1,000	1,100	1,200	1,300	1,400	1,500
	Monthly income ($75 average charge/patient)	67,500	75,000	82,500	90,000	97,500	105,000	112,500
TOTAL EXPENSES + TOTAL NUMBER OF PATIENTS	Cost per patient	64.28	58.40	54.50	53.33	52.35	54.36	52.13
$75.00 AVERAGE CHARGE – COST PER PATIENT	Profit per patient	10.72	16.60	20.50	21.67	22.65	20.64	22.87
PROFIT PER PATIENT × NUMBER OF PATIENTS	Monthly net profit	$9,648	$16,600	$22,550	$26,004	$29,445	$28,896	$34,305

patients the office *must* see to generate adequate income (net monthly income) to cover expenses. If the practice must expand by hiring new staff, buying more equipment, or buying or renting a larger office suite, such a cost ratio analysis can show the manager how many more patients must be seen to cover the increase in expenses. In addition, such an analysis reveals the cost-effectiveness of certain procedures and services. (See *Cost ratio analysis: X-ray department*, page 262.)

Income Statement

If an office manager wishes to assess the total profit and expenses for a month of services, she can use an **income statement.** (See Figure 18-1.) This statement is an overall picture of monthly financial obligations and revenue that can be used to predict future earnings and monitor increases or decreases in profits.

Balance Sheet

A **balance sheet** shows the value of the office at a given date. It lists the assets, liabilities, and owner's equity of the office. **Assets** are the values of all of the property owned by the practice. Items considered assets include furniture, equipment, and computers as well as the building if owned by the practice. **Liabilities** are the total money owed to creditors. For example, if the practice owes $8000 in payments for the x-ray machine, that $8000 is a liability.

Owner's equity is the total assets minus the liabilities. For example, if the x-ray machine is worth $20,000 and the practice owes $8,000, the owner's equity for the x-ray machine is $12,000. The balance sheet is updated by adding credit and debit entries. Increases in assets are recorded as debits; increases in liabilities and owner's equity are recorded as credits. (See Figure 18-2.)

Bookkeeping

More than one person in the medical office can do bookkeeping, the day-to-day financial record-keeping. The front desk staff normally records patient procedure charges and payments, in addition to scheduling appointments. Computerized medical office management systems include insurance billing, patient billing, and appointment scheduling functions as well as functions for payroll, accounts payable, and productivity reporting. Most medical offices use a computerized management system for financial records; however, staff can perform all functions manually if necessary.

Each day, the medical assistant must record patient visits, charges, and payments. The medical assistant bills the insurance company by sending a completed CMS-1500 form electronically or via the mail. The insurer sends the medical office reimbursement (payment), usually in the form of a check. The insurance company check commonly

Cost ratio analysis: X-ray department

A medical office has its own x-ray machine and technician. The office manager wants to conduct a cost ratio analysis to determine the cost-effectiveness of the x-ray department. To do so, the office manager must compare the total expenses of the x-ray department to the total number of x-rays (or x-ray services) performed each month.

The cost ratio analysis above indicates that the x-ray department's cost per procedure is low. Thus, the x-ray department has the ability to generate significant income for the practice. If, however, insurance reimbursement for x-rays in the office were reduced and, therefore, the number of x-rays taken each month were to drop to 60, the ratio becomes $43.33 per procedure ($2600 ÷ 60). This increased cost ratio may cause the physician-owners and managers to decide to stop offering x-rays in the office and, instead, refer patients to another facility for x-ray services.

```
X-Ray Department Expenses

        X-ray technician salary              $1500
        Lease/loan on machine                $ 800
        Supplies (film, developer, fixative) $ 300

                         Total Expenses:     $2600

Total number of x-ray procedures per month = 250

Cost Ratio: $10.40/procedure
```

```
Date         Profit description                               Amount
10/01/08     Carpenters Local 896 check                     2,477.08
10/03/08     Allied Health Services check                  17,344.99
10/03/08     Medicare check                                 7,990.44
10/03/08     Aetna Life check                               4,337.01
10/03/08     Guardian Life check                            8,907.45
10/15/08     Carpenters Local 896 check                     3,551.98
10/16/08     Allied Health Services check                  11,445.07
10/16/08     Medicare ceck                                  3,221.08
10/16/08     Aetna Life check                               6,997.07
10/16/08     Guardian Life check                            2,407.09
10/16/08     Mutual of Omaha check                          1,104.56
10/17/08     Casino Workers Local 445 check                   874.22
10/21/08     ABC Collection Corporation                     1,456.02
10/01-10/31  Front desk cash/check copayments               8,800.00
10/01-10/31  Patient balances paid by personal checks       1,759.30
                                                           82,673.36


Date         Expense description                              Amount
10/01/08     Henderson Realty office rent                   6,400.00
10/01/08     Office supplies                                   435.00
10/01/08     Clinical supplies                              1,550.00
10/21/08     Telephone bill and advertising in Yellow Pages   683.44
10/21/08     Payroll taxes                                 16,433.07
10/21/08     Total payroll for October                     45,488.58
                                                           70,989.58



Total income for October 2008       $82,673.36
Total expenses for October 2008     $70,989.58
Net profit for October 2008         $11,683.78
```

FIG 18-1 Income statement.

ASSETS		LIABILITIES	
Current Assets		**Current Liabilities**	
Cash	82,000	Accounts payable	700
Accounts receivable	27,000	Short-term notes	0
(less doubtful accounts)	< 3,000>	Current portion of long-term notes	0
Inventory	11,000	Interest payable	0
Temporary investment	0	Taxes payable	14,000
Prepaid expenses	0	Accrued payroll	12,000
Total Current Assets	117,000	Total Current Liabilities	26,700
Fixed Assets		**Long-term Liabilities**	
Long-term investments	5,000	Mortgage	0
Land	0	Other long-term liabilites	0
Buildings	0	Total Net Fixed Assets	0
(less accumulated depreciation)	0		
Plant and equipment	14,000		
(less accumulated depreciation)	< 3,000>		
Furniture and fixtures	11,000		
(less accumulated depreciation)	< 1,000>		
Total Net Fixed Assets	26,000		
TOTAL ASSETS	143,000	TOTAL LIABILITIES	26,700

FIG 18-2 Balance sheet.

represents payment for services provided to many patients. The medical assistant must use the explanation of benefits (EOB) that the insurance company sends with the payment to apply the payments to the appropriate patient accounts. The medical assistant will also collect copayments from patients at the time of their visits. She must record all payments in the computerized accounting program or on a day sheet. (See *Entering charges and payments on a day sheet,* page 264.)The medical assistant can then generate reports of daily, weekly, monthly, and quarterly charges and payments.

✦ TIP Check the Numbers

Computerized systems calculate accounts receivable balances based on what is keyed into the system. The medical assistant should always review her records for accuracy. In addition, if the medical assistant cannot balance the day sheet, she should check for transposed digits (such as 59 written as 95). If she still cannot get it to balance, she should ask a coworker to check her work. It is possible for anyone to repeatedly overlook a mistake, but a "fresh eye" can usually catch it.

Ledger Cards

A medical practice may use ledger cards, which are used to record each patient's charges and payments. The medical assistant records on the patient's ledger card any charges and copayments she received at the time of service and the date of service. When the practice receives insurance or patient payments in the mail, the medical assistant must also record these payments on the ledger card. If a practice uses a

manual ledger card system, the medical assistant must also record the transactions on the day sheet. If a practice uses a computerized accounting system, individual account statements can be printed that show the same charges and payments as a ledger card.

Adjustments

Adjustments to account balances are "write-offs" of money that the medical practice does not expect to collect, even though it charged the fee. Because a medical practice contracts with many insurance companies and Medicare that have various fee schedules, physicians expect the insurance company to adjust the payment for the service so that it is in line with their contracted fee. Thus, although the practice charges the full fee, it will not collect the full amount. The practice must then make adjustments on the patient's ledger card to discount the fee by the specified amount. (See *Procedure 18-1: Posting charges, adjustments, and payments,* page 264.)

NSF Checks

When a patient pays with a check, the practice may receive that check back from the bank marked *NSF* for "not sufficient funds." This designation means that there is not enough money in the checking account to pay the amount of the check. Usually, such a situation arises unintentionally and the patient will pay the money owed. Office policy may dictate that the patient pay a fine for a returned check. The medical assistant should check her state law regarding returned check fines before imposing a fine. A bank will generally charge a
(Text continues on page 267)

Entering charges and payments on a day sheet

Entering charges and payments into a computerized or manual day sheet helps the medical assistant keep track of the payments received and services provided at the medical office each day. The following example of a computerized day sheet shows how a day sheet tracks patient visits and services provided, charges for those services, and payments received from patients and insurance companies.

Patient name	Description	Charges	Payments	New Balance	Old Balance
Joe Smith	OV, X-ray	150.00	15.00	155.00	20.00
Mike Connors	OV, UA, X-ray	180.00	10.00	340.00	170.00
Maria Sanchez	New Pt OV	210.00	15.00	195.00	0.00
Insurance payment Tina Sawyer	---------	.00	415.00	0.00	415.00
TOTALS		540.00	455.00	690.00	605.00

THE AMOUNTS RECEIVABLE, OR AMOUNT OF MONEY OWED TO THE PRACTICE, WENT FROM $605.00 TO $690.00

A computerized day sheet will include built-in formulas that compute the totals automatically. However, if the medical assistant uses a manual day sheet, she can check the accuracy of the totals by using this formula:

Old balances	605.00
+ charges	+ 540.00
= (subtotal)	1145.00
− payments	− 455.00
= New balance	690.00

PROCEDURE 18-1

Posting charges, adjustments, and payments and balancing a day sheet

Task
Post charges, adjustments, and payments from an insurance company, patients, and a collection agency to a day sheet and balance the day sheet.

Conditions
- Computer and printer or manual day sheet
- Checks (from insurance companies and patients)
- Collection agency payment
- Pen

Standards
In the time specified and within the scoring parameters determined by the instructor, the student will successfully post charges, adjustments, and payments and balance a day sheet.

Performance Standards
1. Post charges and payments to the ledger cards (below) for these patients, who visited the office on April 22, 2008:
   a. Andrew Stevenson came in for an office visit ($40 charge) and paid a $10 copayment in cash.
   b. Jenna Collins came in for an office visit and urinalysis (combined charge of $75) and paid a $15 copayment by check (#534).
   c. Barry Chen came in for an x-ray ($75 charge) and paid a $25 copayment in cash.
   d. John Rivera came in for an office visit and urinalysis and paid a $10 copayment by check (#1766).
   e. Hannah Martin came in for an ECG (charge $105).
2. Create a computerized day sheet according to the format of the daysheet or use a manual day sheet (provided by your instructor).
3. Post entries on the day sheet according to the activities listed above.
4. Post the insurance payment (check below) from United Health Systems to the day sheet and apply payments to the patient accounts on the ledger cards.
5. Apply the amount allowed from the insurance company's explanation of benefits, adjusting the patient balances to reflect only the amount allowed.

PROCEDURE 18-1—cont'd

6. Post the collection agency payment (check below) from ACME Collections, Inc., on the patient ledger card and day sheet.

7. Include the following adjustments to the day sheet and the appropriate patient's ledger card:

a. Hannah Martin—Medicare adjustment $15.00
b. John Rivera—HMO adjustment $15.00
c. Barry Chen—HMO adjustment $47.00

8. Balance the day sheet.

Andrew Stevenson
167 Main Street, Colbrush, CT
860-123-0932

Date	Procedure	Charge	Payment	Balance
	Balance brought forward			170.00
03/06/2008	office surgery	650.00	25.00	795.00

Hannah Martin
36 Gratuity Way, Blueville, CT
860-555-9778

Date	Procedure	Charge	Payment	Balance
	Balance brought forward			0.00
03/08/2008	ECG	105.00	0.00	105.00

Jenna Collins
14 Wayside Drive, Blueville, CT
860-555-9778

Date	Procedure	Charge	Payment	Balance
	Balance brought forward			150.00
03/08/2008	OV-exp. xray. LBP. PT. Acu	404.00	15.00	539.00

John Rivera
83 Pinecrest Road, Blueville, CT
860 555-7695

Date	Procedure	Charge	Payment	Balance
	Balance brought forward			50.00
03/08/2008	PE. stress test	153.00	15.00	188.00

Barry Chen
762 Elm Street, Blueville, CT
860-555-6823

Date	Procedure	Charge	Payment	Balance
	Balance brought forward			100.00
03/07/2008	office surgery	410.00	25.00	485.00

Gary Travini
11 Appleton Drive, Blueville, CT
860-555-7833

Date	Procedure	Charge	Payment	Balance
	Balance brought forward			0.00
10/20/2007	office surgery	404.00	20.00	384.00
11/22/2007	OV. UA. stress test	185.20	20.00	549.00
12/01/2007	check returned NSF	20.00		569.00
12/13/2007	patient check		69.00	500.00
01/05/2008	patient billed			
02/05/2008	patient billed			
03/05/2008	patient billed final notice to collect			
04/01/2008	account sent to ACME collections			500.00

Continued

PROCEDURE 18-1—cont'd

United Health Systems
283 Commerce Park Drive
P.O. Box 6978
Blueville, CT 06100

2349786799943

April 16, 2008   DATE

PAY
TO THE
ORDER OF   Blueville Family Medicine $ 1,453.00

One thousand four hundred fifty–three and ---no/00   DOLLARS

FOR _____

⑈2349786799943⑈ ⑆000000188⑆ 111111883301⑈

Patient	ID#	Date of service	Amount charged	Copay	Amount allowed	Amount paid
Jenna Collins	X1J100990077	03/08/2008	$404.00	15.00	390.00	375.00
Andrew Stevenson	XDD269873888	03/06/2008	$650.00	25.00	610.00	585.00
John Rivera	XLK798639922	03/08/2008	$153.00	15.00	148.00	133.00
Barry Chen	XRS689812544	03/07/2008	$410.00	25.00	385.00	360.00
					Total	1,453.00

ACME Collections, Inc.
456 Underhill Road
Granville, CT 23456
860-234-3456

45978

April 18, 2008   DATE

PAY
TO THE
ORDER OF   Blueville Family Medicine $ 107.55

One hundred seven and -- 55/00   DOLLARS

FOR _____

⑈045978⑈ ⑆000000106⑆ 111111338801⑈

Patient	Account balance	Payment
Gary Travini	500.00	118.30
Collection fee @ 10%		10.75 –
Check amount		$107.55

$15 or $20 processing fee to the practice for every NSF check that it processes. Many offices charge the same fee to the patient to recover that cost. To record an NSF check returned by the bank, the medical assistant should add the check amount (plus any penalty per office policy) to the account as a charge, returning the patient's balance to the amount owed before the payment.

Accounts Receivable Ratio

The **accounts receivable ratio** is a formula the medical office can use to measure the time it takes for bills to be paid. The formula compares the total charges to the monthly collections. (See *Accounts receivable ratio formula*.)

Collection Ratio

A medical assistant can also evaluate **accounts receivable** by determining the **collection ratio,** which is a comparison of an outstanding debt amount to the amount collected. Simply stated, how much of the money billed is actually paid. The goal of the collection ratio for a medical office should be 0.85 to 0.90. (See *Collection ratio evaluation*.)

✦ TIP Rewarding High Collections

Collection ratios that are 90% or higher are a reflection of the hard work of the billing staff. The physician or office manager may offer bonuses, a day off, or a gift certificate to motivate continued success.

Accounts Payable

Accounts payable are financial obligations of the practice to outside vendors or patients and include fixed and variable

---

Accounts receivable ratio formula

The medical practice tracks the total amount charged for services in a given month as well as the total amount collected in payments from patients and insurers. These totals are used to determine the accounts receivable ratio using this formula:

$$\frac{\text{Total accounts receivable (how much money was charged?)}}{\text{Monthly receipts (how much money was collected?)}}$$

$$\frac{\$210,397 \text{ (charges)}}{\$103,455 \text{ (collected)}} = 2.03$$

The accounts receivable ratio is 2.03. Thus, payment turnaround time is approximately 2 months for account payments. An accounts receivable ratio that is 2 or less indicates that the practice collects on outstanding charges in 2 months or less. Such a ratio shows that the office is keeping up with billing and collections.

Collection ratio evaluation

An office manager may want to determine a collection ratio for several reasons. One possibility is when a new physician is hired and, thus, more services are provided to more patients. With the increase in services billed, the billing department is challenged to keep up with collections.

To determine the collection ratio, the medical assistant must determine the total monthly charges and the total amount collected after adjustments (and unpaid patient portions) using this formula:

Total montly charges:	$210,397
Managed care adjustments:	– $10,945
Medicare adjustments:	– $7,833
Total monthly collections:	$191,619

Of the $210,397 in charges, $191,619 is collectable in "real dollars," which provides a collection ratio of 0.91 (191,619 ÷ 210,397).

The formula above assumes that all patients will pay copayments and balances on outstanding bills. If the office determines that there will be an additional $3,000 that will remain uncollected from patients, the ratio drops to 0.896, or (191,619 − 3,000 = 188,619 ÷ 210,397). This ratio is still within the acceptable range for a collection ratio.

---

costs. Accounts payable procedures include receiving and tracking deliveries and other supply purchases for payment, writing checks, and managing payroll.

Deliveries and Supplies

To ensure a good relationship with suppliers, the medical office should pay bills upon receipt. Clinical and office suppliers may deliver supplies to the office, or office staff may pick them up at local suppliers. Items shipped to the office should include a packing slip. The packing slip will identify items (and quantities) sent. Upon receipt of the packages, the medical assistant should check items received against the packing slip to ensure that the delivered items match the items charged to the office. (See Figure 18-3.)

When the medical assistant verifies that all items on the packing slip are included in the package, she can send the packing slip to the accounts payable department. In addition, some bills, such as utilities, office rental or mortgage, and some supply bills, will arrive at the office in the mail. The medical assistant can forward these items to the accounts payable department as well.

Writing Checks

The medical assistant must record all checks written, whether to vendors or employees, in the check register.

PACKING SLIP

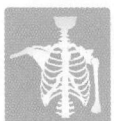

TriCounty X-ray

1867 Commerce Parkway
Presley, CT 06001

Ship to   Attn: Cindy Smith, CMA
                 Blueville Family Medicine
                 15 Main Street
                 Blueville, CT 06000
                 869-555-3212

Bill to   Blueville Family Medicine
            15 Main Street
            Blueville, CT
            860-555-3212

Order Date	Order Number	Shipped Via	Tracking Number
10/02/08	78963	UPS	89BXZ767687134

Quantity	Description	Unit Price
2	Box 100 12 x 14 plain film x-ray	$42.95
3	Box 50 10 x 10 plain film x-ray	$31.95
	Subtotal	$181.75
	Tax	$12.75
	Shipping	$11.45
	TOTAL	**$205.95**

FIG 18-3 Typical packing slip.

The check register is a log of expenses that the medical office can later use for cost analysis, comparing vendor prices, proof of payment, and balancing the checkbook. The check register can be computerized, manual, or both. (See Figure 18-4.) Items to record in the register include:

- name of vendor or patient
- amount of check
- date of check
- items received or packing slip number (if vendor). (See Figure 18-5.)

Occasionally, a patient may pay the practice for services and then the patient's insurance company reimburses the practice for the same service. The patient may do so because he assumes that the service is not covered or that he has not yet met a deductible. In such a case, the medical assistant must refund the money to the patient. A refund to a patient should be processed as soon as the insurance check arrives at the office. The medical assistant should record the payment from the insurance company, noting the credit balance. She must then refund the patient any excess money previously paid to the account,

returning the account balance to zero. (See *Procedure 18-2: Processing a credit balance and refund and posting an NSF check*, page 272.)

Payroll

Paying employees on a weekly or biweekly basis is usually the job of an office manager. The office manager should give all employees a Withholding Exemption (W-4) form at the onset of employment. (See Figure 18-6.) The W-4 shows the total amount of deductions the employee claims and affects the federal taxes withheld from each paycheck.

Preparing Payroll Checks

The office may pay employees at an hourly rate or a salary rate. Salaried employees earn the same amount of money each week and may be paid for overtime, depending on their agreement with the physician-owners. Hourly employees must keep track of hours worked by using a time sheet, time card, or computer log-in system. Regardless of how the hourly information is gathered, the office manager calculates the amount of the paycheck by multiplying the number of

Number	Date	Description of Transaction	C	Debit (-)	Credit (+)	Balance
	12/20/08	Previous balance				$78,590.34
11032	12/21/08	Payroll taxes		$1588.55		$77,001.79
11033	12/22/08	Payroll- Robert Greer		$3014.39		$73,987.40
11034	12/22/08	Payroll- Hector Rodriguez		$2043.22		$71,944.18
11035	12/22/08	Payroll- Ann Wilson		$1325.33		$70,618.85
11036	12/22/08	Payroll- Henry Lee		$1246.67		$69,372.18
11037	12/22/08	Payroll- Sharon Piecek		$734.52		$68,637.66
11038	12/22/08	Payroll- Kelly Manera		$324.11		$68,313.55
11039	12/22/08	Payroll- Cindy Smith		$611.43		$67,702.12
11040	12/22/08	Payroll- Shelly Gonzalez		$476.28		$67,225.84
	12/22/08	Deposit- insurance & personal checks			$22,763.21	$89,989.05
11041	12/22/08	Patterson Office Supply		$136.12		$89,852.93
11042	12/22/08	Henderson Realty- office rent Jan 09		$6400.00		$83,452.93
11043	12/22/08	Yellow Page.com- advertising		$1250.00		$82,202.93

FIG 18-4 Check register.

hours worked by the hourly rate. Commonly, the office manager will use a payroll worksheet to make these calculations. (See Figure 18-7.)

When she has calculated the paycheck amount, she can write the paychecks by hand or in a computer software system. Payroll checks should show the employee all deductions and hours worked. In addition, they should include:

- name of the employee
- number of hours worked (regular, if hourly, and overtime)
- dates of pay period (beginning date and ending date)
- date of check
- gross salary
- itemized tax deductions, including federal income tax, Social Security tax (FICA), and state taxes (if applicable)
- other itemized deductions, such as health insurance and retirement savings
- net salary (gross earnings minus taxes and deductions). (See Figure 18-8.)

✦ TIP On Time or Early

Always pay employees on the same day of the week or every 2-week period. If a payday is changed due to a holiday, pay employees a day early. The employees will appreciate it!

BLUEVILLE FAMILY MEDICINE
15 MAIN STREET
BLUEVILLE, CT 06000
860-555-3212

11041

November 1, 2008 DATE

PAY TO THE ORDER OF Patterson Office Supplies $ 136.12

One hundred thirty six and 12/100 DOLLARS

BLUEVILLE SAVINGS BANK

FOR patient files, alpha stickers Hector Rodriguez, MD

⑆011041⑈ ⑆000000105⑆ 111111333301⑈

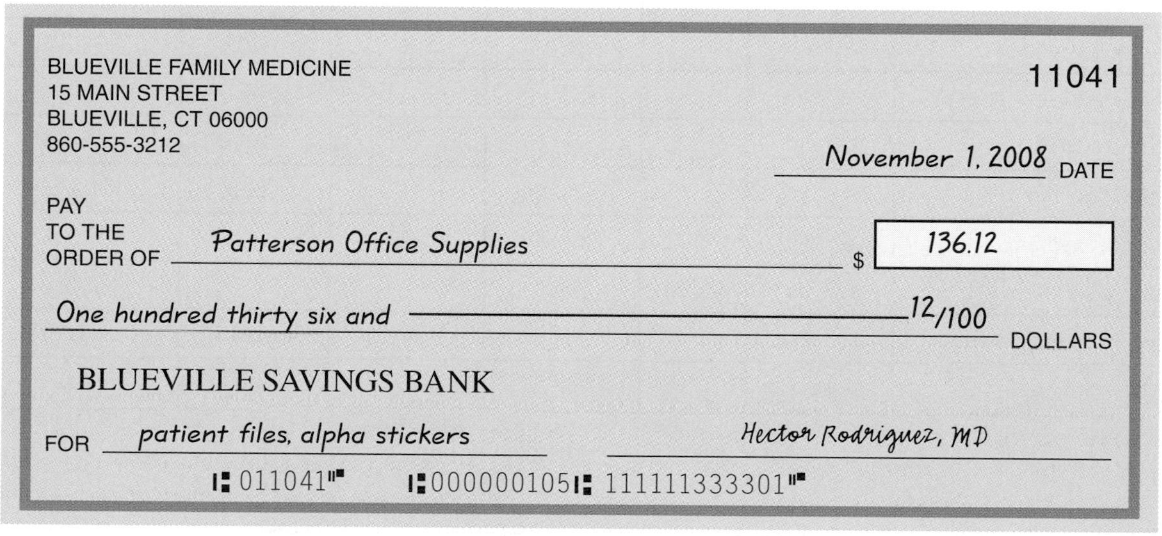

FIG 18-5 Business check.

Form **W-4**	**Employee's Withholding Allowance Certificate**	OMB No. 1545-0074
Department of the Treasury Internal Revenue Service	▶ Whether you are entitled to claim a certain number of allowances or exemption from withholding is subject to review by the IRS. Your employer may be required to send a copy of this form to the IRS.	**20 08**

Cut here and give Form W-4 to your employer. Keep the top part for your records.

1 Type or print your first name and middle initial.	Last name	2 Your social security number

Home address (number and street or rural route)	3 ☐ Single ☐ Married ☐ Married, but withhold at higher Single rate. **Note.** If married, but legally separated, or spouse is a nonresident alien, check the "Single" box.
City or town, state, and ZIP code	4 **If your last name differs from that shown on your social security card, check here. You must call 1-800-772-1213 for a replacement card.** ▶ ☐

5 Total number of allowances you are claiming (from line **H** above **or** from the applicable worksheet on page 2) ... **5** ☐

6 Additional amount, if any, you want withheld from each paycheck . . . . **6** $ ☐

7 I claim exemption from withholding for 2008, and I certify that I meet **both** of the following conditions for exemption.
● Last year I had a right to a refund of **all** federal income tax withheld because I had **no** tax liability **and**
● This year I expect a refund of **all** federal income tax withheld because I expect to have **no** tax liability.
If you meet both conditions, write "Exempt" here . . . . ▶ **7** ☐

Under penalties of perjury, I declare that I have examined this certificate and to the best of my knowledge and belief, it is true, correct, and complete.

Employee's signature
(Form is not valid
unless you sign it.) ▶   Date ▶

8 Employer's name and address (Employer: Complete lines 8 and 10 only if sending to the IRS.)	9 Office code (optional)	10 Employer identification number (EIN)

FIG 18-6 W-4 form.

Employee	Hourly rate	Hours worked	Gross salary	Withholding	Health insurance	Retirement
Robert Greer, MD	salary	-----	$3300.00	4	49.33	$165.00
Hector Rodriguez, MD	salary	-----	$2400.00	5	81.63	$120.00
Anne Wilson, MD	salary	-----	$1500.00	3	40.18	$77.50
Henry Lee, MD	salary	-----	$1400.00	4	49.33	$70.00
Sharon Piecek, APRN	salary	-----	$950.00	4	49.33	$50.00
Kelly Manera	$14.00	32	$448.00	2	24.07	$22.40
Jennifer Morgan	$14.00	38	$532.00	1	24.07	$26.60
Carol Chapin	$15.50	25	$387.00	2	0	$19.38
Wendy Jones	$13.00	20	$260.00	0	0	$13.00
Shelly Gonzalez	$15.50	42	$666.50	2	24.07	$33.32
Cindy Smith	salary	-----	$750.00	3	40.18	$37.50

40 HOURS @ REGULAR TIME ($15.50/HR) + 2 HOURS @ 1½ TIME ($23.25/HR)

FIG 18-7 Payroll worksheet.

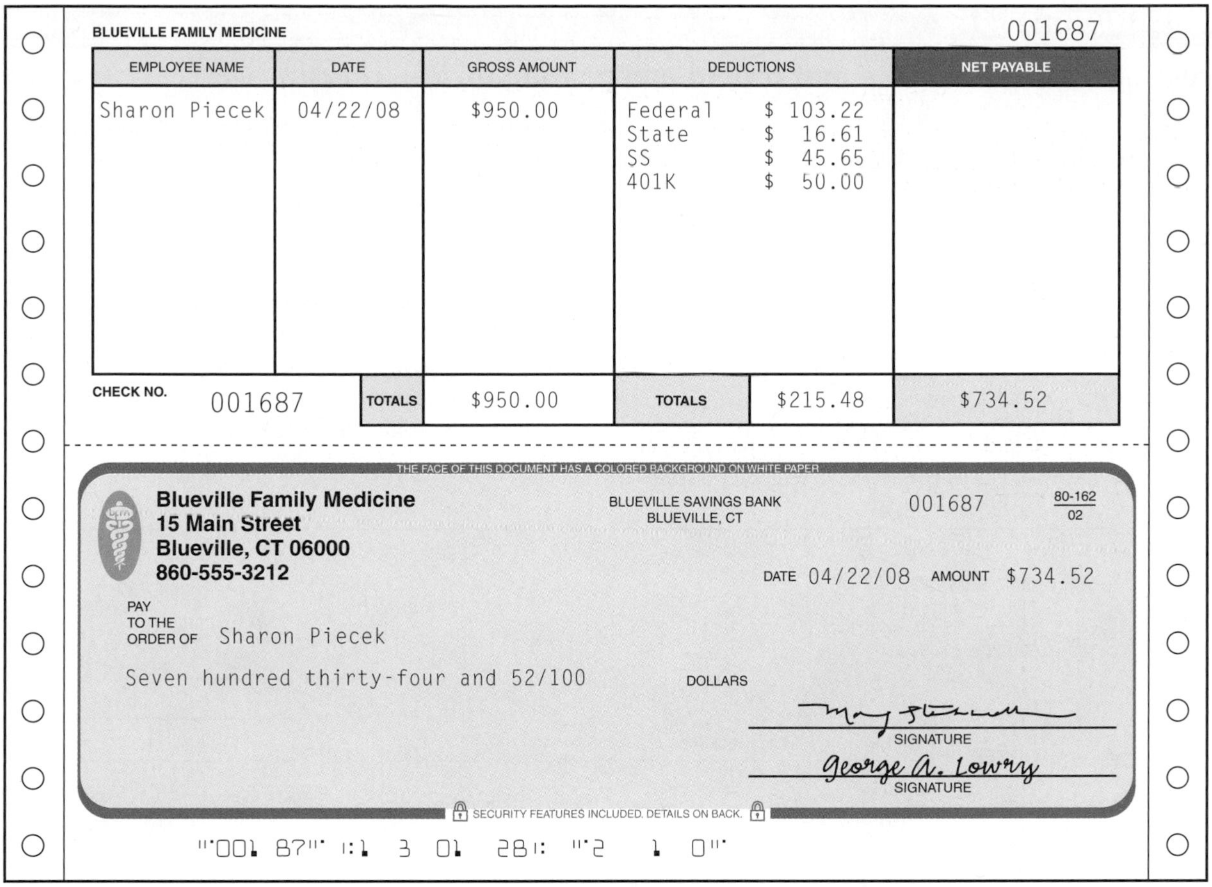
BLUEVILLE FAMILY MEDICINE 001687

EMPLOYEE NAME	DATE	GROSS AMOUNT	DEDUCTIONS		NET PAYABLE
Sharon Piecek	04/22/08	$950.00	Federal	$ 103.22	
			State	$ 16.61	
			SS	$ 45.65	
			401K	$ 50.00	
CHECK NO. 001687	TOTALS	$950.00	TOTALS	$215.48	$734.52

THE FACE OF THIS DOCUMENT HAS A COLORED BACKGROUND ON WHITE PAPER

Blueville Family Medicine
15 Main Street
Blueville, CT 06000
860-555-3212

BLUEVILLE SAVINGS BANK
BLUEVILLE, CT

001687 80-162/02

DATE 04/22/08 AMOUNT $734.52

PAY TO THE ORDER OF Sharon Piecek

Seven hundred thirty-four and 52/100 DOLLARS

SIGNATURE

George A. Lowry
SIGNATURE

SECURITY FEATURES INCLUDED. DETAILS ON BACK.

FIG 18-8 Paycheck.

The medical office must have a federal tax reporting number in order to process payroll checks. On a quarterly basis, the office must pay all federal and state taxes withheld using the appropriate reporting forms. The office manager can use a computer software program to calculate federal and state payroll taxes and determine the amount to deposit in the bank tax account as mandated by federal law. Although this account is just a place to hold tax funds until the practice makes its required quarterly tax payments, the bank does not allow access to this account for any other reason than to pay taxes at the specified payment periods.

At the end of each calendar year, the medical office must generate Wage and Tax Statement (W-2) forms for each employee. (See Figure 18-9.) This form shows total wages, federal income tax withheld throughout the year, Social Security wages and taxes withheld, and Medicare wages and taxes withheld. An employee needs this form to file her personal tax returns. The office manager should give the W-2 form to employees no later than January 31st so that each employee has ample time to meet the April 15th deadline for income tax filing.

Banking Practices

In addition to the many accounting practices performed by the medical assistant or office manager, running a medical office requires an extensive understanding of proper banking practices. Some of the most common and most essential banking practices are:

- reconciling bank statements
- making bank deposits
- managing petty cash.

Reconciling Bank Statements

The bank in which a medical practice keeps its accounts will send a monthly statement to the practice. Many banks also offer online bank statements as an alternative. The office manager can use the account number and password to log in and view the statement. She can also print statements to check against the office's records. On the statement, the bank records all deposits and withdrawals and includes the balance at the end of the statement period. In addition, most offices

PROCEDURE 18-2

Processing a credit balance and refund and posting an NSF check

Task
Process a credit balance, process a refund, and post a *not sufficient funds* (NSF) check.

Conditions
- Day sheet
- Checks (insurance and patient checks)
- Collection agency payment
- Pen

Standards
In the time specified and within the scoring parameters determined by the instructor, the student will successfully process a credit balance and a refund and post an NSF check.

Performance Standards
1. Post the insurance check for Irina Sharapova to her ledger card.
2. Write a refund check to Mrs. Sharapova and record her balance as zero.
3. Post the returned check (below) from Ariana Klieger on the day sheet (from previous procedure) and on the patient's ledger card (below).

Universal HMO
1 Vista Boulevard
Regionville, NY 04321
800-888-8765

0088678721

April 20, 2008 _____ DATE

PAY
TO THE
ORDER OF ___ Blueville Family Medicine _____ $ | 30.00 |

Thirty and -- 00/100 DOLLARS

FOR _____

"∎ 0088678721 "∎   ∎: 000000886 ∎: 7711117354301 "∎

Name	Procedure	Amount charged	Allowed	Copay	Paid
Irina Sharapova	99204	85.00	70.00	40.00	30.00

Irina Sharapova
211 Elm Street, Blueville, CT
860-555-1129

Date	Procedure	Charge	Payment	Balance
	Balance brought forward ——————			0.00
03/07/2008	*OV exp*	85.00	15.00 (writeoff)	70.00
03/07/2008	*Payment, personal check #859*		50.00	20.00

PROCEDURE 18-2—cont'd

BLUEVILLE FAMILY MEDICINE
15 MAIN STREET
BLUEVILLE, CT 06000
860-555-3212

11432

_____ DATE

PAY
TO THE
ORDER OF _____ $ [   ]

_____ DOLLARS

BLUEVILLE SAVINGS BANK

FOR _____   _____

⑈011432⑈   ⑆000000105⑆ 111111333301⑈

Arianna Klieger
769 Elm Street
Blueville, CT 06000

772

April 7, 2008 DATE

PAY
TO THE
ORDER OF _____ *Blueville Family Medicine* _____ $ [45.00]

Forty-five and _____ *no/100*
DOLLARS

PRESLEY SAVINGS AND LOAN

Arianna Klieger

MEMO _____

⑆044008804⑆ 960130629721⑈ 1000

Arianna Klieger
769 Elm Street, Blueville, CT
860-555-9733

Date	Procedure	Charge	Payment	Balance
	Balance brought forward ———	———	———	0.00
04/07/2008	office surgery	410.00	45.00	365.00

a Control number 00000000		OMB No. 1545-0008		
b Employer identification number (EIN) 99-9999999		1 Wages, tips, other conpensation 49400.00	2 Federal income tax withheld 7728.36	
c Employer's name, address, and ZIP code Blueville Family Medicine 15 Main Street Blueville, CT 06000		3 Social security wages 49400.00	4 Social security tax withheld 3380.37	
		5 Medicare wages and tips 49400.00	6 Medicare tax withheld 790.57	
		7 Social security tips	8 Allocated tips	
d Employee's social security number 123-45-6789		9 Advance EIC payment	10 Dependent care benefits	
e Employee's first name and initial Last name Suff. Sharon L. Piecek		11 Nonqualified plans	12a See instructions for box 12	
		13 Statutory employee ☐ Retirement plan ☒ Third-party sick pay ☐	12b	
		14 Other	12c	
			12d	
f Employee's address and ZIP code 1406 Long Pond Road Blueville, CT 06000				

15 State	Employer's state ID number	16 State wages, tips, etc.	17 State income tax	18 Local wages, tips, etc.	19 Local income tax	20 Locality name
CT	5555-5555	49400.00	1275.04	49400.00		Blueville

Form **W-2** Wage and Tax Statement

Department of Treasury–Internal Revenue Service

FIG 18-9 W-2 form.

have a computerized financial management system that can report all deposits and withdrawals as well as the account balance for the statement period. (See *Reconciling office and bank records*.) Whether the office has computerized or manual records, the office manager should compare the bank records to the office records to reconcile them, or ensure that the check and deposit amounts on both statements match and that the account balances match. (See *Procedure 18-3: Reconciling a bank statement*, page 277 to 278.)

✦ TIP Online Banking

Banks send statements at the end of each month. Most banks, however, also offer online banking information that an office manager can access at any time. If questions arise, the online banking information can be useful in answering questions in a timely manner. Usually, the information is accessible using the checking account number and is secured by a pass word.

Making Bank Deposits

The office manager or medical assistant must record and deposit into the practice's checking account checks from insurance companies and personal checks and cash from patients. Depending on the size of the practice, staff may make bank deposits daily, a few times per week, or once per week. The office manager is usually in charge of bank deposits; however, she may ask a medical assistant to prepare the deposit or take it to the bank.

Many offices require the medical assistant to make photocopies of checks for deposit to be kept in a file in case of a discrepancy between the amount of the check and the deposit amount recorded by the bank. Because the medical assistant must write the check number on the deposit slip along with its amount, she can easily identify the check if a discrepancy with the bank occurs. Cash is listed separately on the deposit slip. (See Figure 18-10.) The medical assistant should count cash twice to ensure accuracy. The medical assistant should be sure to get a slip from the bank, confirming the deposit, and file it with the photocopies of checks for complete records. (See *Procedure 18-4: Preparing a bank deposit*, page 279.)

✦ TIP Adding Machines

Some adding machines can produce a printable paper receipt. The office manager can use this capability to print out the computations she has entered to review them for accuracy.

(Text continues on page 282)

Reconciling office and bank records

The office manager should reconcile each monthly bank statement with the office records for that month. To do so, she must print out the office accounting record for that month (commonly called a *deposit and withdrawal report*) and compare it with the bank statement.

The office manager should check off the withdrawals and deposits that appear on the deposit and withdrawal report and the bank statement, and then look for items that do not appear on the bank statement to account for any difference in the final balance. Checks written at the end of the month may be missing from the bank statement if they have not been processed, or *cleared,* by the bank by the statement closing date.

When comparing the two statements, the office manager would find in this case that the final balances do not match. Checks numbered 11041 and 11044 were not yet cashed by the recipients. In addition, check number 11046 does not appear on the statement. To reconcile the statements, then, the office manager must subtract the outstanding withdrawals (in this case, checks 11041, 11044, and 11046) from the bank statement balance.

Using an adding machine with printable tape, the office manager can add the total amount of money from the checks not yet cashed and subtract it from the ending bank balance. That amount should be equal to the office accounting.

Deposit and Withdrawal Report – December 2008

Number	Date	Description of Transaction	C	Debit (-)	Credit (+)	Balance
		Previous balance				$56,315.12
11029	12/05/08	New England Telephone		$670.33		$55,644.79
	12/10/08	Deposit insurance & personal cks			$11,231.44	$66,876.23
11030	12/10/08	CT Light & Power		$311.90		$66,564.33
11031	12/15/08	AMA- conference fee		$750.00		$65,814.33
	12/18/08	Deposit insurance & personal cks			$12,776.01	$78,590.34
	12/19/08	Withdrawal cash- office party supplies		$200.00		$78.390.34
11032	12/19/08	Payroll taxes		$1588.55		$76,801.79
11033	12/19/08	Payroll- Robert Greer		$3014.39		$73,787.40
11034	12/19/08	Payroll- Hector Rodriguez		$2043.22		$71,744.18
11035	12/19/08	Payroll- Ann Wilson		$1325.33		$70,418.85
11036	12/19/08	Payroll- Henry Lee		$1246.67		$69,172.18
11037	12/19/08	Payroll- Sharon Piecek		$734.52		$68,437.66
11038	12/19/08	Payroll- Kelly Manera		$584.11		$67,853.55
11039	12/19/08	Payroll- Cindy Smith		$611.43		$67,242.12
11040	12/19/08	Payroll- Shelly Gonzalez		$476.28		$66,765.84
11041	12/19/08	Payroll- Jennifer Morgan		$492.56		$66,273.28
11042	12/19/08	Payroll- Wendy Jones		$475.87		$65,797.41
11043	12/19/08	Payroll- Carol Chapin		$294.13		$65,503.28
	12/19/08	Deposit insurance & personal cks			$22,763.21	$88,266.49
11044	12/22/08	Patterson Office Supply		$136.12		88,130.37
11045	12/22/08	Henderson Realty- office rent Jan 09		$6400.00		$81,730.37
11046	12/22/08	Yellow Pages.com - advertising		$1250.00		$80,480.37

Continued

Reconciling office and bank records—cont'd

Blueville Savings Bank
122 Main Street
Blueville, CT 06000

860-555-1298
www.bluevillesavings.com

Statement Account# 6869750033
Blueville Family Medicine
15 Main Street
Blueville, CT
860-555-3212

Bank Statement January 1, 2009
Beginning balance $56,315.12   Average balance $72,625.42
Ending balance $82,359.05

Check #	Date of Transaction	Withdrawal	Deposit Date	Deposit Amount
11029	12/15/08	$670.33	12/10/08	$11,231.44
11030	12/19/08	$311.90		
11031	12/19/08	$750.00	12/18/08	$12,776.01
	12/19/08	$200.00		
11032	12/22/08	$1588.55		
11033	12/22/08	$3014.39		
11034	12/22/08	$2043.22		
11035	12/22/08	$1325.33		
11036	12/22/08	$1246.67		
11037	12/22/08	$734.52	12/19/08	$22,763.21
11038	12/22/08	$584.11		
11039	12/22/08	$611.43		
11040	12/22/08	$476.28		
11041	missing in sequence			
11042	12/22/08	$475.87		
11043	12/22/08	$294.13		
11044	missing in sequence			
11045	12/24/08	$6400.00		
Totals	checks and withdrawals	$20,726.73	deposits and interest	$46,770.66

Reconciling office and bank records—cont'd

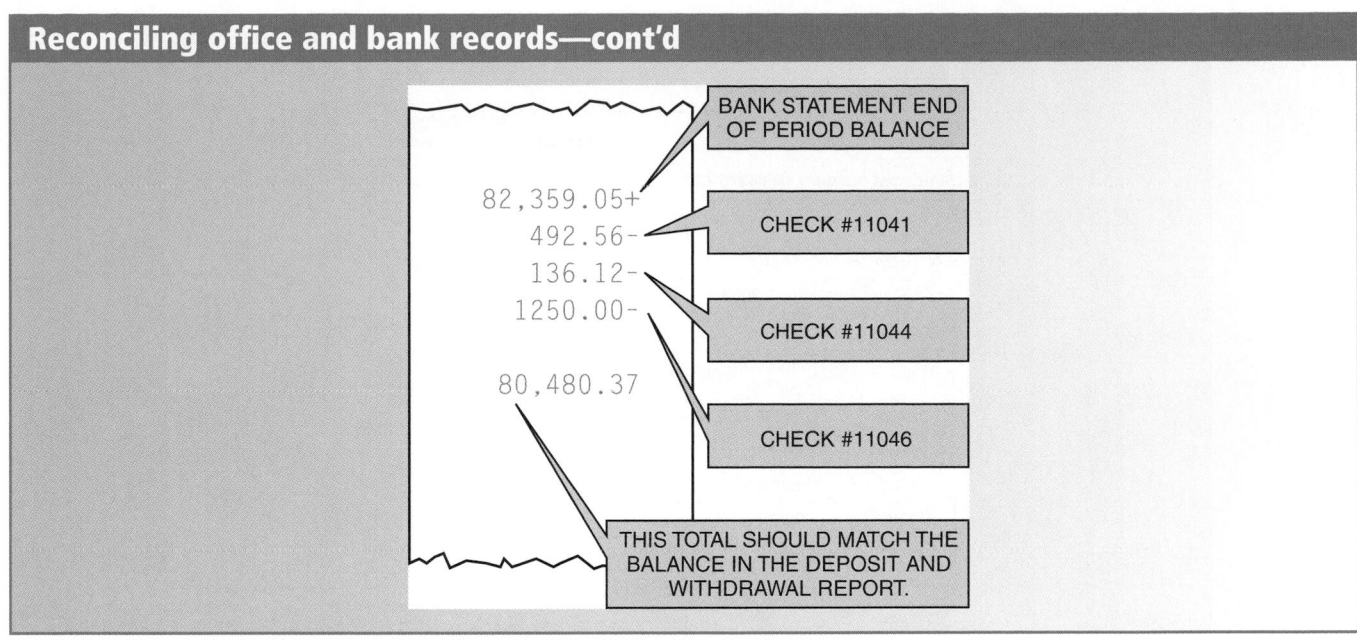

Reconciling a bank statement

Task
Reconcile the monthly deposit and withdrawal report with a bank statement.

Conditions
- Computerized monthly deposit and withdrawal report
- Bank statement
- Adding machine
- Pen

Standards
In the time specified and within the scoring parameters determined by the instructor, the student will successfully reconcile the deposit and withdrawal report with a bank statement.

Performance Standards
1. Using the bank statement dated April 1, 2008, and the deposit and withdrawal report for that same period (below), compare the totals and note the difference in the amounts, if any.
2. Compare each withdrawal and deposit on the bank statement to the report.
3. In comparing each item, be sure to determine if the amounts on the statement and the report match to prevent discrepancies in totals.
4. For each matching item, make a check mark next to the item on the report and the corresponding item on the bank statement to track your progress and ensure no items are missed.
5. Draw a circle around any item on the report that is not also included on the bank statement as well as any item on the statement that is not on the report to determine outstanding checks, uncredited deposits, or errors.
6. Using the adding machine, add all circled withdrawals. Then add all circled deposits on the report.
7. Subtract the total outstanding withdrawals from the bank statement ending balance.
8. Add the total outstanding deposits to the bank statement ending balance.
9. Confirm that the resulting amount matches the balance of the deposit and withdrawal report.

Continued

PROCEDURE 18-3—cont'd

Blueville Savings Bank
122 Main Street
Blueville, CT 06000

860-555-1298
www.bluevillesavings.com

Statement Account s#6869750033
Blueville Family Medicine
15 Main Street
Blueville, CT
860-555-3212

Bank Statement April 1, 2008
Beginning balance $59,008.31
Ending balance $57,778.19

Average balance $55,715.89

Check #	Date of Transaction	Withdrawal	Deposit Date	Deposit Amount
11733	03/08/08	$458.25	03/14/08	$8,231.44
11734	03/09/08	$611.90		
11735	03/09/08	$734.47	03/21/08	$11,772.11
11736	03/09/08	$1248.22		
11737	03/09/08	$3019.39		
11738	03/09/08	$2033.22		
11739	03/09/08	$1338.33		
11740		missing in sequence		
11741	03/09/08	$324.11		
	03/09/08	$250.00		
11742	03/09/08	$475.88		
11743	03/09/08	$294.11		
11744	03/09/08	$1585.55		
11745		missing in sequence		
11746	03/21/08	$6400.00		
Totals	**checks and withdrawals**	**$18,773.43**	**deposits and interest**	**$20,003.55**

Deposit and Withdrawal Report – March 2008

Number	Date	Description of Transaction	C	Debit (-)	Credit (+)	Balance
		Previous balance				$59,008.31
11733	03/07/08	Payroll- Kelly Manera, CMA		$458.25		$58,550.06
11734	03/07/08	Payroll- Cindy Smith, CMA		$611.90		$57,938.16
11735	03/07/08	Payroll- Sharon Piecek, APRN		$734.47		$57,203.69
11736	03/07/08	Payroll- Henry Lee, MD		$1248.22		$55,955.47
11737	03/07/08	Payroll- Robert Greer, MD		$3019.39		$52,936.08
11738	03/07/08	Payroll- Hector Rodriguez, MD		$2033.22		$50,902.86
11739	03/07/08	Payroll- Ann Wilson, MD		$1338.33		$49,564.53
11740	03/07/08	Payroll- Shelly Gonzalez, CMA		$356.08		$49,208.45
11741	03/07/08	Payroll- Jennifer Morgan, CMA		$324.11		$48,884.34
11742	03/07/08	Payroll- Wendy Jones		$475.88		$48,408.46
11743	03/07/08	Payroll- Carol Chapin		$294.11		$48,114.35
11744	03/07/08	Payroll taxes		$1585.55		$46,528.80
	03/09/08	Cash withdrawal for office		$250.00		$46,278.80
	03/11/08	party supplies				
11745		Patterson Office Supply		$136.12		$46,142.68
	03/14/08	Deposit insurance & personal cks			$8,231.44	$54,374.12
11746	03/16/08	Henderson Realty- Office rent for April 2008		$6400.00		$47,974.12
	03/21/08	Deposit insurance & personal cks			$11,772.11	$59,746.23
	03/31/08	Deposit insurance & personal cks			$9,763.07	$69,509.30

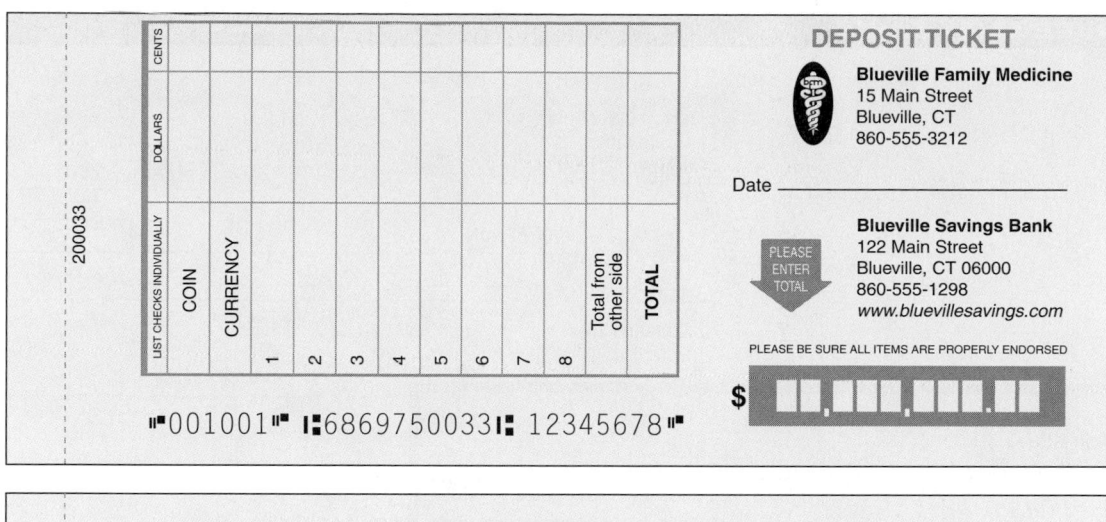

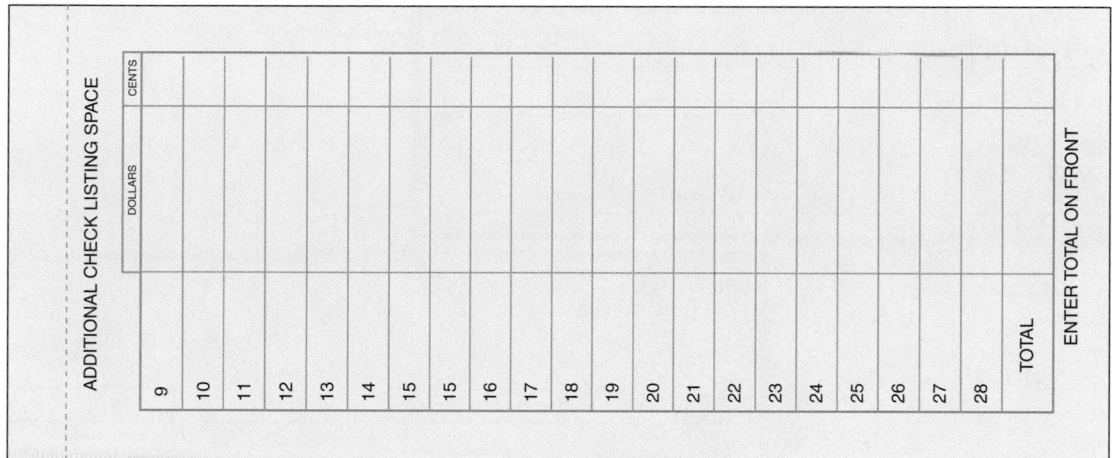

FIG 18-10 Deposit slip.

PROCEDURE 18-4

Preparing a bank deposit

Task

Prepare a bank deposit.

Conditions

- Bank deposit form
- Checks (insurance and patient checks)
- Cash received
- Office checkbook register
- Pen

Standards

In the time specified and within the scoring parameters determined by the instructor, the student will successfully prepare a bank deposit and record the deposit in the office checkbook register.

Performance Standards

1. Using the personal checks from patients (below), the United Health Systems check from Procedure 18-1 on page 264, and the bank deposit form in Figure 18-10 enter the check numbers and amounts of all checks on the deposit slip.

2. Total the cash received from the day sheet on page 264 and enter the amount on the deposit slip in the appropriate section.

3. Total the amount of the checks and cash using an adding machine. Recheck your total to avoid errors.

4. Write the total amount of the deposit in the total column.

5. Write the amount of the deposit in the office checkbook register (below) and add it to the previous balance.

6. Recheck your math before writing the new balance in the register to ensure accuracy.

Continued

PROCEDURE 18-4—cont'd

Brenda Capshaw
1 Circle Drive
Redtown, CT 06111

457

April 19, 2008 DATE

PAY
TO THE
ORDER OF *Blueville Family Medicine* $ 15.00

Fifteen and ———————————————— *no*/100 DOLLARS

Blueville Trust
Blueville, CT

Brenda Capshaw

Michael McGuinniss
7125 Main Street
Blueville, CT 06101

3239

April 19, 2008 DATE

PAY
TO THE
ORDER OF *Blueville Family Medicine* $ 20.00

Twenty and ———————————————— *no*/100 DOLLARS

**Blueville First Bank
Blueville, CT**

FOR ⑆123456780⑆ 0301 123 456⑈ 7⑈

Michael McGuinniss

Charles Ayers
1719 Lake Avenue
Green Lake, CT 06088

466

April 19, 2008 DATE

PAY
TO THE
ORDER OF *Blueville Family Medicine* $ 15.00

Fifteen and ———————————————— *no*/100 DOLLARS

1st Green Lake Bank
Green Lake, CT

Charles Ayers

Alicia Carter
43 East End Avenue
Redtown, CT 06111

337

April 19, 2008 DATE

PAY
TO THE
ORDER OF *Blueville Family Medicine* $ 20.00

Twenty and ———————————————— *no*/100 DOLLARS

1st Green Lake Bank
Green Lake, CT

FOR ⑆123456780⑆ 0301 123 456⑈ 7⑈

Alicia Carter

Kirsten Tremblay
231 Purple Place
Blueville, CT 06000

199

April 19, 2008 DATE

PAY
TO THE
ORDER OF *Blueville Family Medicine* $ 15.00

Fifteen and ———————————————— *no*/100 DOLLARS

Blueville National Bank
Blueville, CT

FOR ⑆123456780⑆ 0301 123 456⑈ 7⑈

Kirsten Tremblay

PROCEDURE 18-4—cont'd

10549

Date __4/16/08__

To _____

_____

Amount _____

Deposit _____ $66,387.45

10550

Date __4/16/08__

To __Clinic One Supply__

Amount __$136.12__ $66,251.33

Deposit __$22,766.21__ $89,017.54

10551

Date __4/22/08__

To __Henderson Realty__

__Office rent May 2008__

Amount __$6,400.00__

Deposit _____ $82,617.54

10552

Date __4/22/08__

To __Yellow Page.com -__

__advertising__

Amount __$1,250.00__

Deposit _____ $81,367.54

10553

Date _____

To _____

_____

Amount _____

Deposit _____

BLUEVILLE FAMILY MEDICINE   10553
15 MAIN STREET
BLUEVILLE, CT 06100
860-555-3212   _____ DATE

PAY
TO THE
ORDER OF _____ $ [   ]

_____ DOLLARS

BLUEVILLE SAVINGS BANK

FOR _____   _____

⑆010553⑆ ⑆ 000000105⑈111111333301⑆

Petty Cash

Patients who pay a copayment at each visit may require change for large bills. Having a petty cash drawer will allow front desk staff to take a $20 bill and give $10 change. The medical assistant can also use petty cash to pay for postage-due items received or supplies that are needed immediately. The medical assistant should reconcile the petty cash drawer each day by using a computerized or manual log. (See Figure 18-11.) When the office manager or medical assistant makes the bank deposit, she can exchange large bills from petty cash for smaller bills (1-dollar bills and 5-dollar bills) so that the petty cash drawer will always have change when needed.

Date	Description	Transaction amount	Total	Initials
04/10/08	Cash drawer– beginning of day	$410.00	$410.00	C.S, CMA
04/10/08	COD delivery Dawson Medical Supply	$230.00	$190.00	C.S, CMA
04/10/08	Total cash copays	$300.00	$490.00	C.S, CMA
04/10/08	Office staff meeting lunches – Deli delivery	$73.00	$417.00	JM, CMA
04/10/08	Take copay cash from drawer to deposit	$300.00	$117.00	C.S, CMA

FIG 18-11 Petty cash log.

Chapter Summary

- Accounting is an important component of any business, including the physician's office.
- Having an understanding of the financial status of the practice, including how money is earned and how it is spent, enables long-term planning.
- Financial success of the business depends on using accounting information to make decisions regarding expenses and services offered.
- Complete, understandable bookkeeping practices ensure that money collected and spent is documented and appropriate.
- Federal and state taxes can be accurately assessed and paid only when complete documentation is available.

Team Work Exercises

1. Divide into teams of four to seven students and create a time sheet for each employee (student). Each employee should fill in the time sheet with hours worked, ranging from 18 to 45 hours, and choose a filing status (married or single and number of dependents). Some employees should receive a salary and some should be paid an hourly rate (plus overtime, possibly). After you have completed your time sheet, swap time sheets with others on the team and calculate the gross pay for the employee whose time sheet you have. Add a section for deducting 5% for retirement and a flat rate (dollar amount indicated by your instructor) for health insurance coverage. Finally, calculate the gross pay amount to which you would apply federal taxes.

2. Divide into groups of three to five students. Each group researches a different procedure for the physician's office to offer to patients. Research the cost of the equipment or supplies and the average charges for the procedure in your area. Create a cost ratio analysis of the procedure. Present your procedure to the class along with its cost ratio analysis.

Case Studies

1. Accounts receivable for your practice has increased over the past 6 months. Why might you see this type of trend? What corrective actions can be taken to increase revenues and therefore decrease accounts receivable?

2. X-ray film costs have risen from $1.10 per 14 × 11 sheet to $2.00 per sheet. Assume a charge of $125.00 per x-ray

and salary and other supply costs per month of $2200. What is the cost ratio if the practice performs 150 x-rays per month? What is the cost ratio at the old film cost? How many additional x-rays are needed to achieve the same cost ratio?

Resources

- American Medical Association: *Maximizing Billing and Collections in the Medical Practice.* Chicago: American Medical Association Press, 2007.
- Brewer, P.C., et al.: *Introduction to Managerial Accounting,* 4th ed. New York: McGraw Hill, 2007.
- Payroll software: *www.paycycle.com, www.adp.com,* and *www.surepayroll.com*
- Up-to-date tax compliance rules: *www.IRS.gov*

UNIT III

Clinical

Infection Control and Medical Asepsis

Learning Objectives

Upon completion of this chapter, the student will be able to:

- define and spell the key terms presented in the glossary
- identify the role of the medical assistant in infection control
- identify disease-producing microorganisms
- list common infectious diseases
- identify the links in the chain of infection
- differentiate between the stages of disease
- describe the body's defense mechanisms
- demonstrate the performance of hand washing with soap and water
- demonstrate the performance of hand sanitization with an alcohol-based hand rub
- explain standard precautions
- list common types of personal protective equipment
- describe strategies to increase health and safety in the workplace
- differentiate medical asepsis and surgical asepsis
- differentiate sanitization, disinfection, and sterilization
- demonstrate equipment and instrument sanitization
- demonstrate equipment and instrument disinfection
- demonstrate wrapping a pack for sterilization
- demonstrate the performance of sterilization using an autoclave
- educate patients regarding methods to reduce disease transmission.

CAAHEP Competencies

Clinical Competencies

  Fundamental Principles

    Perform hand washing

    Wrap items for autoclaving

    Perform sterilization techniques

    Dispose of biohazardous materials

    Practice standard precautions

General Competencies

  Patient Instruction

    Provide instruction for health maintenance and disease prevention

ABHES Competencies

Clinical Duties

  Apply principles of aseptic technique and infection control

  Wrap items for autoclaving

Procedures

Washing hands with soap and water

Sanitizing hands with an alcohol-based hand sanitizer

Sanitizing equipment

Disinfecting equipment

Wrapping a pack for autoclaving

Using an autoclave for sterilization

Chapter Outline

Infectious Disease

Microorganisms and Pathogens

  Bacteria

  Rickettsia

  Virus

  Fungus

  Protozoa

Chain of Infection

  Pathogen

  Reservoir Host

  Means of Exit

  Mode of Transmission

  Means of Entry

  Susceptible Host

Types of Infection

Stages of Disease

  Incubation Stage

  Prodromal Stage

  Acute Stage

  Declining Stage

  Convalescent Stage

The Body's Defense Mechanisms

  Mechanical Defenses

  Chemical Defenses

  Cellular Defenses

    Inflammatory response

  Immunity

    Active natural immunity

    Active artificial immunity

    Passive natural immunity

    Passive artificial immunity

Standard Precautions

  Personal Protective Equipment

  Disposal of Biohazardous Waste

  Vaccinations

  Exposure Control

    Bloodborne pathogen exposure

    Biohazard spill

Asepsis

  Sanitization

    Hand sanitization

    Sanitization of equipment and the environment

  Disinfection

  Sterilization

    Autoclave

    Chemical sterilization

  Types of Asepsis

    Medical asepsis

    Surgical asepsis

Chapter Summary

Team Work Exercises

Cases Studies

Resources

Key Terms

antibody
Immunoglobulin produced by white blood cells in response to a specific antigen

antigen
Marker that identifies a cell as being part of the body (self) or not part of the body (nonself)

asepsis
Practice of maintaining an environment free from pathogens

bacteria
One-celled organism, some of which are capable of producing disease

disease
Any condition characterized by subjective complaints, a specific history, clinical signs or symptoms, and laboratory or radiographic findings

disinfection
Application of a substance to materials and surfaces to destroy pathogens

fomite
Any object that adheres to and transmits infectious material (such as a comb, countertop, or drinking glass)

fungi
Kingdom of organisms that includes yeasts, molds, and mushrooms and is usually not pathogenic to humans

incubation
Interval between exposure to infection and the appearance of the first symptoms

infectious disease
Any disease caused by a microorganism that may be directly or indirectly transmitted between individuals, causing infection

microorganism
Living organism too small to be seen with the naked eye

normal flora
Organisms found on and in a person's body that do not cause disease

parasite
Pathogen requiring another living organism in order to survive

pathogen
Disease-producing microorganism

phagocytosis
Process in which specialized white blood cells (phagocytes) engulf and destroy microorganisms, foreign antigens, and cellular debris

prodromal
Interval between earliest symptoms and appearance of a rash or fever

protozoa
Organism mainly found in soil that is capable of producing disease

purulent
Consisting of or containing pus

reservoir host
Organism that provides a hospitable environment in which pathogens can grow

Rickettsia
Genus of bacteria that are intracellular parasites

sanitize
To remove microorganisms from reusable equipment and surfaces by using chemicals, heat, or ionizing radiation

spores
Bacterial or fungal cells that are resistant to temperature extremes

symptomatic
Having symptoms, such as fever, sore throat, nausea, and vomiting

vector
Carrier, usually an insect, that transmits a disease from an infected person to a noninfected person

virus
Pathogen that can grow and reproduce only after infecting a host cell

Infectious Disease

The health care environment is intended to be a place where people can find help and healing. However, because it brings individuals together, many of whom have infectious diseases or weakened immune systems, it sets the stage for the very real possibility of disease transmission between patients and even health care staff. To prevent such transmission from happening, medical assistants must have an understanding of how disease is transmitted and how to take every reasonable precaution to reduce disease transmission in the medical office.

A **disease** is any condition characterized by subjective complaints (sensations felt by the individual), a specific history, clinical signs, symptoms, and laboratory or radiographic findings. **Infectious diseases**, also called *communicable diseases*, are diseases caused by a microorganism that may be transmitted directly or indirectly between individuals, causing infection.

Microorganisms and Pathogens

Microorganisms are microscopic living organisms, or living organisms too small to be seen with the naked eye. Many different types of microorganisms exist in the environment; however, not all are connected to disease. Those that normally live on and in the human body are known as *normal flora*. A healthy balance of these microorganisms normally exists and provides protection from those that are not part of the body's normal flora. However when this balance is disturbed, a person becomes more vulnerable to illness and disease.

Pathogens are microorganisms that are capable of producing disease. To grow and thrive, most pathogens require nutrients, moisture, warmth, and a suitable (usually neutral) pH environment. Thus, some parts of the human body tend to provide a more hospitable environment for pathogenic growth than others. Some, called *aerobic*, require oxygen; those that must have an oxygen-free environment are called *anaerobic*. There are five main types of pathogens:

- bacteria
- *Rickettsia*
- virus
- fungus
- protozoa.

Bacteria

Bacteria are one-celled organisms that cause such diseases as *Staphylococcus* infection, *Streptococcus* infection (*Strep* throat), gonorrhea, and Lyme disease. There are three types of bacteria:

- cocci (round-shaped)
- bacilli (rod-shaped)
- spirilla (spiral-shaped).

Rickettsia

Rickettsia are a genus of bacteria known as *parasites*, which are organisms that must live inside another living organism in order to survive. *Rickettsia* spread to humans via a **vector**, which is a disease carrier, that transmits a disease from an infected person to a noninfected person. Common vectors are insects, such as ticks, fleas, mites, and lice. Examples of diseases transmitted by rickettsia are typhus and Rocky Mountain spotted fever.

Virus

A **virus** is a pathogen that can grow and reproduce only after infecting a host cell. There are more than 400 types of viruses and they usually act in a parasitic fashion by invading the individual's healthy host cells and taking them over. They then use the host cells' RNA and DNA (genetic material) to reproduce. They are the smallest pathogens and are difficult to treat because the protein in their outer cell membrane prevents antibiotics from affecting them. Viruses cause such diseases as the common cold, hepatitis, chicken pox, and human immunodeficiency virus (HIV).

Fungus

A **fungus** is a simple, single-celled organism, such as yeast, or multicellular colonies, such as mold and mushrooms. Examples of the disease they cause in humans include tinea infections (athlete's foot, ringworm, and so forth) and candidiasis (yeast infections). However, most fungi do not cause disease and are present in the body's normal flora.

Protozoa

Protozoa are disease-causing microorganisms that live mainly in soil. They commonly infect persons with low immunity. Protozoan infections are spread through the fecal-oral route, by ingesting contaminated food or water, or by mosquitoes or other insects carrying the infection. Examples of common protozoan infections are malaria, *Giardia*, and a vaginal infection called *trichomoniasis*. (For more information on pathogenic microorganisms, see Chapter 45, "Microbiology," page 937.)

Chain of Infection

Understanding how microorganisms are spread and persons infected will help the medical assistant more effectively protect herself and her patients. (See *Preventing disease transmission*.) This chain of infection is a series of steps that must occur for disease to spread. Infectious diseases can only spread if all of the links in the chain of infection are active. Therefore, a medical assistant can stop the spread of disease by breaking any link in the chain. The elements of the chain include:

- pathogen
- reservoir host
- means of exit
- mode of transmission
- means of entry
- susceptible host. (See Figure 19-1.)

Pathogen

Pathogens are the first link in the chain of infection. They exist in the everyday environment and usually thrive in warm, moist environments. Those that are present in the blood that can be transmitted through blood or body fluids are called bloodborne pathogens. Examples of common bloodborne pathogens are HIV, hepatitis C, and hepatitis B. Those that are usually harmless but become pathogenic under specific circumstances, such as exposure to an immunocompromised host, are called *opportunistic pathogens.*

Reservoir Host

A **reservoir host** is an organism from which pathogenic organisms such as bacteria or viruses obtain their nourishment.

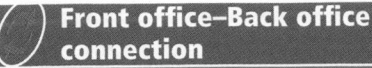

Front office–Back office connection

Preventing Disease Transmission

Microorganisms are introduced into the physician's office on a daily basis by ill patients who speak, cough, sneeze, and touch things with contaminated hands. By doing so, they spread pathogens throughout the reception area and examination rooms. To help break the cycle in the chain of infection, administrative and clinical medical assistants must team up in their efforts to keep the environment as clean as possible. Administrative medical assistants may be responsible for cleaning countertops, windows, and other surfaces in the reception area. Clinical medical assistants may be responsible for cleaning surfaces and equipment in the clinical areas between patients. However, preventing disease transmission is everyone's job, so all members of the team should work together in a cooperative fashion. In addition, they can make sure hand sanitizers and tissues are available to patients in all areas and teach them the importance of hand washing.

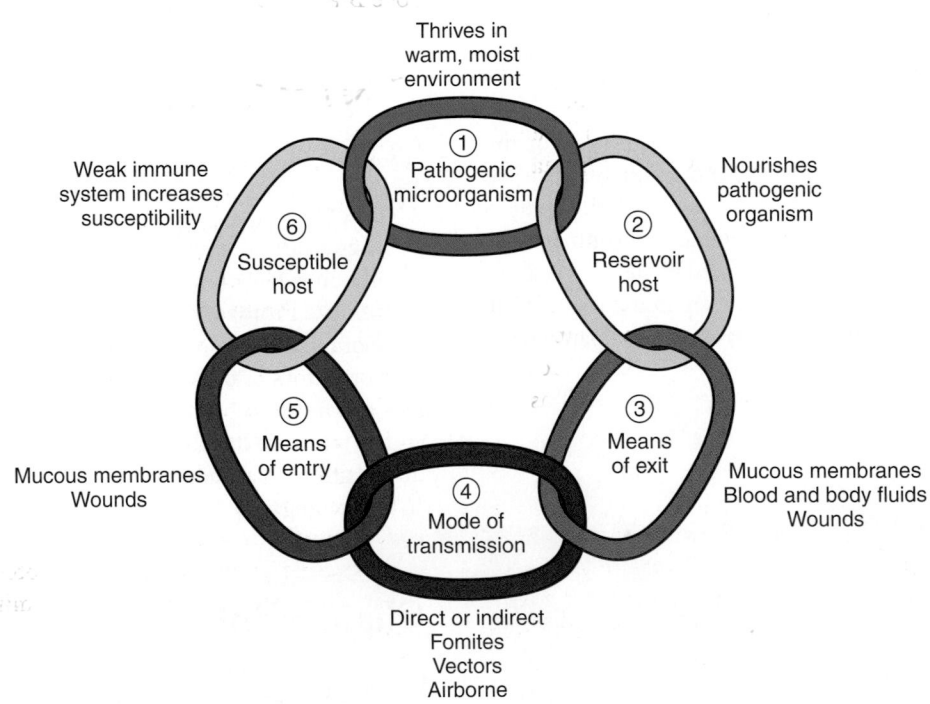

FIG 19-1 Chain of infection.

It provides a hospitable environment in which the pathogen can grow. Living infected hosts may be **symptomatic** (having noticeable signs of disease) or may be asymptomatic (free of symptoms). The reservoir host is considered contagious and can spread the disease to others.

Means of Exit

A common way for pathogens to leave a reservoir host's body is via the mucous membranes. Therefore, any opening of the body that is lined with mucous membranes becomes a potential exit site. Examples include the eyes, nose, mouth, throat, vagina, and rectum. Another exit site might be an interruption in the normal protective structures of the body, such as injury or surgery to the skin and underlying tissues. Pathogens can also exit the body via blood and such body fluids as semen, vaginal secretions, urine, and feces.

Mode of Transmission

A pathogen can be transmitted to another person by direct or indirect contact. Examples of direct contact include skin-to-skin contact such as hand shaking or kissing or the exchange of body fluids such as with needle sharing or sexual contact. Pathogens may also be transmitted via indirect contact with inanimate objects called *fomites*. Virtually any object can be a fomite. Common examples include countertops, hairbrushes, combs, door knobs, drink containers, handles of shopping carts, and pencils. Another type of transmission occurs via vectors, which are usually insects or other arthropods such as fleas, lice, ticks, and vermin that carry pathogens from infected to noninfected individuals.

Airborne transmission, a form of indirect transmission, occurs when an infected individual sprays pathogens into the air by coughing or sneezing. Another individual then inhales the pathogen from the air and becomes infected. Tuberculosis is an example of a disease that is spread by airborne transmission.

Means of Entry

Pathogens gain entry to the body in much the same way as they exit it, usually via contact with mucous membranes or a break in the skin. Therefore, potential entry sites include the eyes, nose, mouth, throat, vagina, and rectum as well as any wounds to the skin.

Susceptible Host

If a host is susceptible, pathogens will grow and multiply, eventually reaching an infectious level. There are a number of conditions that increase host susceptibility and most contribute to a weakened immune system. Common examples include poor hygiene, poor nutrition, stress, other underlying diseases or disorders, some medications, age (very young and very old), and self-destructive behaviors such as tobacco

Patient Education

Breaking the Chain

To help patients avoid infectious disease, the medical assistant should teach these commonsense strategies to help them protect themselves against pathogens:

- Wash your hands frequently throughout the day, especially during cold and flu season, as well as after using the toilet, after blowing your nose, and before eating.
- Teach children how to wash or sanitize their hands.
- Avoid crowds during cold and flu season, if possible.
- Avoid others who are ill.
- Avoid going to work when ill.
- Do not send ill children to school.
- Cover coughs and sneezes with your arm, rather than your hand.
- Avoid sharing drink containers and eating utensils.
- Use hand sanitizer when warm water and soap are not available.
- Avoid unprotected sexual encounters.
- Avoid touching your eyes, nose, and mouth.
- Use hand sanitizers, if available, in medical offices and grocery stores.

use, excessive alcohol intake, and use of illicit drugs. (See *Breaking the chain.*)

Types of Infection

Infections can be categorized according to their general duration and whether they occur only once or recur repeatedly. There are three types of infection:

- *Acute* infections typically have a quick onset and short duration. There may or may not be a clear **prodromal** phase in which symptoms are generally nonspecific. The duration is usually 1 to 3 weeks. An example is the common cold.
- *Chronic* infections last for a long time, sometimes for years or even a lifetime. The patient may be asymptomatic or symptoms may fluctuate. An example of a chronic infection is hepatitis C.
- *Latent* infections are those in which patients experience alternating periods of being symptomatic (relapse) with periods of being symptom-free (remission). The infecting organism, usually a virus, never leaves the body but lies dormant between relapses. A common example is the herpes viruses, which can cause intermittent outbreaks of oral lesions, genital lesions, and shingles.

Stages of Disease

There are several stages in the disease process. The first begins when pathogens first come in contact with and gain access to the body and the last ends when patients are no longer ill and have fully recovered. The duration and severity of the entire process is highly variable. In some cases, it lasts a few short days and in other cases for weeks or even months. Some diseases are so disabling that infected individuals are bedridden, and others are so mild that infected individuals experience few symptoms and continue to carry out their normal daily activities. Stages of disease include:

- incubation
- prodromal
- acute
- declining
- convalescent. (See Figure 19-2.)

Incubation Stage

The **incubation** stage, sometimes called the *latent* period, is the beginning stage of an infectious disease and starts at first contact with the pathogen. During this stage, the patient may be asymptomatic but is commonly considered contagious. The incubation stage is the interval between exposure and the appearance of the first symptoms. Incubation time varies from days to weeks or months, depending on the disease.

Prodromal Stage

The **prodromal** stage marks the interval between the earliest symptoms and the appearance of a rash or elevated

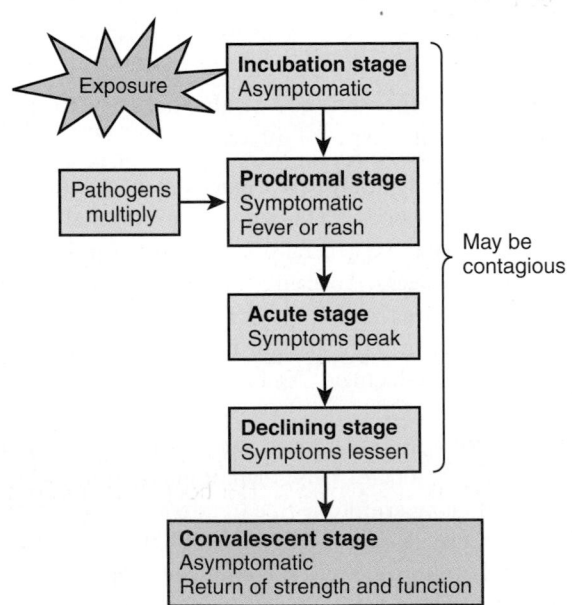

FIG 19-2 The stages of disease.

temperature. Patients who are febrile (have a fever) also commonly complain of such generalized symptoms as malaise (feeling of discomfort), fatigue, weakness, and generally feeling unwell.

Acute Stage

The acute stage is when symptoms peak and the patient feels the worst. He continues to be contagious and should avoid others in order to prevent spreading the disease. He should heed medical advice, which commonly includes taking prescribed medications, resting, and drinking nonalcoholic and noncaffeinated beverages.

Declining Stage

The declining stage begins with the end of the acute stage. It is characterized by a continuation of the disease but a lessening of the symptoms. The patient notices that he is beginning to feel better and may wish to begin resuming normal activities.

Convalescent Stage

The convalescent stage of disease is the recovery period. It begins when disease symptoms disappear and continues until the patient has regained full strength and returns to a normal state of health. The medical assistant should caution patients to avoid overexertion or prematurely discontinuing medical or other therapies during the declining and convalescent stages. Doing so could cause a relapse. (See *Taking medications as prescribed.*)

The Body's Defense Mechanisms

The body's natural protective mechanisms normally work amazingly well to protect human beings from pathogens. There are three main types of defense mechanism:

- mechanical
- chemical
- cellular.

Mechanical Defenses

Mechanical defenses include certain structures and functions of the body. For example, the skin is a structure that protects a person from the external environment. Tiny hairs within the nasal cavity help filter the air by removing debris. The lower airways are lined with special membranes that have cilia (threadlike projections) that move in a wavelike fashion to propel debris upward so that it can be coughed out or swallowed. Protective reflexes, such as coughing and sneezing, are triggered by the presence of foreign debris in the respiratory tract. A cough is a forceful expiratory effort

Patient Education

Taking Medications as Prescribed

Many patients who fail to take their medication as prescribed are labeled "noncompliant" by their health care providers. However, many patients may not understand *why* the medication should be taken a certain way. The medical assistant should strive to explain to patients why they should take medication as prescribed. If they understand, patients are more likely to comply with the treatment plan. Here are some common reasons why patients do not take medications as prescribed:

- **Feeling better.** Some patients think they no longer need the medication when they begin feeling better. In some cases, as with pain medication, this perception is accurate. However, the effectiveness of such medications as antibiotics depends on completion of the full course of treatment. Discontinuing early could cause a relapse and worsening of the illness. Furthermore, discontinuing medication early exposes the pathogens to the medication without fully destroying them. This brief but inadequate exposure is a major contributor to the rise in antibiotic-resistant organisms so prevalent today.

- **Saving some for later.** Some patients discontinue medication early so they will have some left for future use. This practice is dangerous, of course, because the current medication may not be the best choice for whatever future illness arises. Furthermore, having only a small amount of medication like antibiotics may be worse than having none at all, leading to relapse or drug resistance, as discussed.

- **Fitting the schedule.** Some patients change dosing times or frequencies to fit better with their daily schedule. Changing dosing times is sometimes okay, but the medical assistant should encourage the patient to check with the physician before making any changes.

- **Increasing the dose.** Some patients take more than the prescribed dose hoping for an increased effect or a faster response. Doing so puts them at risk for drug toxicity but does not increase the healing benefit.

- **Reducing the effects or cost.** Some patients take less than the prescribed dose, hoping to reduce unpleasant adverse effects, save money, or make the medication last longer. Doing so results in decreased effectiveness of the medication and provides no benefits to the patient. If the patient feels the adverse effects of a drug are unacceptable, the medical assistant should encourage him to consult with the physician regarding possible solutions.

that is difficult, if not impossible, to suppress and can literally be lifesaving. When an individual sneezes, air is expelled forcefully though the nose and mouth by a spasmodic contraction of muscles that normally facilitate respiration. This action helps clear irritating debris and microorganisms from the nasal passages.

Other physical protective mechanisms in the body include the flushing action of certain body fluids. For example, the tear glands of the eyes produce a fluid that continually bathes and cleanses the eyes. Because the eyes are extremely sensitive, when foreign particles enter them the tear glands respond by increasing production of tears to flush the debris away. Flushing action also occurs in the urinary tract where urine is produced in the kidneys and follows a one-way path through the ureters (long, narrow tubes) to the bladder and out of the body via the urethra. This one-way flow of fluid helps prevent pathogens from moving upward through the urethra into the urinary tract, where they might cause infection.

Chemical Defenses

The body has some chemical barriers that help protect it from pathogens. For example, the skin contains sebaceous glands, which are present nearly everywhere except the palms of the hands and soles of the feet. These glands secrete an oily substance that not only helps keep skin supple and healthy but actually kills some types of pathogens. The fluids in the stomach are normally very acidic, which effectively kills most swallowed pathogens. The fluid in tears and the urinary tract is also somewhat acidic, which is generally not conducive to bacterial growth.

In addition, the body produces a group of glycoproteins (compound of carbohydrate and protein), called *interferons*, that have antiviral activity. Some are produced by white blood cells in response to pathogen invasion, especially viruses. They help mark the invading pathogens for destruction. They also inhibit virus production within infected cells. Various types of interferons are used to treat diseases such as hepatitis B and C, Kaposi's sarcoma, and multiple sclerosis.

Also, some enzymes produced by the body protect against pathogens. A great example is lysozyme. This enzyme, which is present in tears, saliva, and other bodily secretions, acts to inhibit the growth of bacteria by damaging their cell walls.

Cellular Defenses

Various cells also act to protect the body from pathogens. These defenses include:

- inflammatory response
- cell-mediated immunity
- antibody-mediated immunity.

Inflammatory Response

The inflammatory response is the body's immediate immuno-logical defense against injury, infection, or allergy. This response protects the body from invasion by foreign pathogens and sets in motion a series of events that repair tissue damage. In the inflammatory response, tissue trauma causes the release of several chemicals that cause inflammation:

- *Histamine* is a chemical that causes a variety of responses, depending on the site of injury. In soft tissue, it causes the dilation of blood vessels, which helps improve circulation to the injured area and increases the arrival of white blood cells to the scene.
- *Prostaglandins* are hormones that are formed rapidly and act in the immediate area of the injury. They produce vasodilation, vascular permeability, and platelet aggregation and stimulate pain receptors.
- *Kinin* is a chemical that increases blood flow and the permeability of small blood capillaries. (See Figure 19-3.)

As a result, localized inflammation occurs, indicated by redness, swelling, heat, pain, and decreased function. Some of these changes indicate that the body is at work healing itself. For example, the increase in circulation and vessel permeability allows specialized white blood cells (phagocytes) to enter the injured area and begin engulfing and desbroying microorganisms, foreign antigens, and cellular debris in a process known as ***phagocytosis***. (See Figure 19-4.) Increased circulation also brings oxygen and nutrients to the area so that repair can occur. However, edema (swelling) can contribute to the patient's discomfort. In addition, the chemicals that set the whole process in motion also cause increased pain perception.

When the body's natural defenses are unsuccessful in eliminating invading organisms, infection may occur. However, inflammation and infection are not the same. Symptoms of localized infection are similar to those of inflammation but may become more pronounced. In infection, such signs of inflammation as redness, swelling, heat, and pain may be present along with fever and generalized malaise. Localized sites of injury may produce **purulent**, or pus-containing, drainage, which is rich in dead white blood cells, bacteria, and cellular debris.

Immunity

Immunity is defined as protection from infectious disease. Immunity is categorized as active or passive. Active and

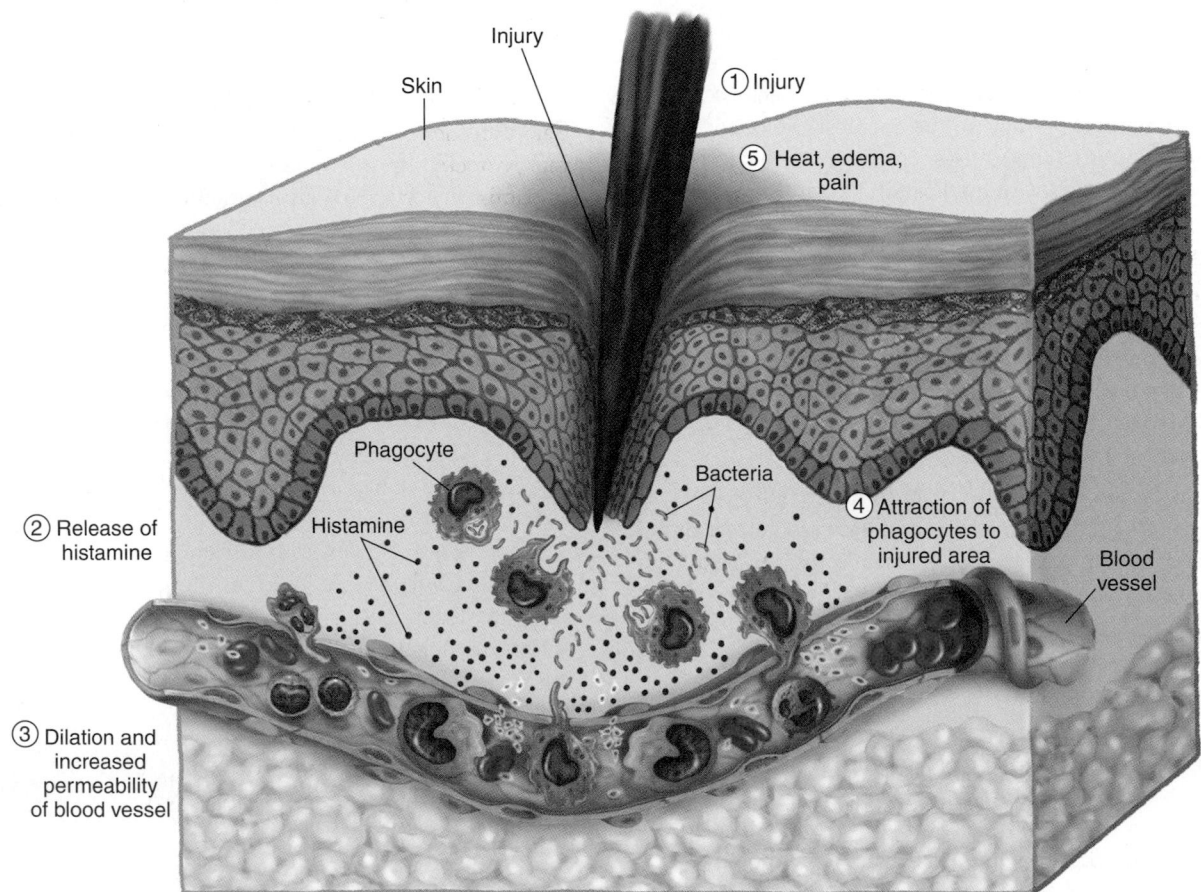

FIG 19-3 Inflammatory response.

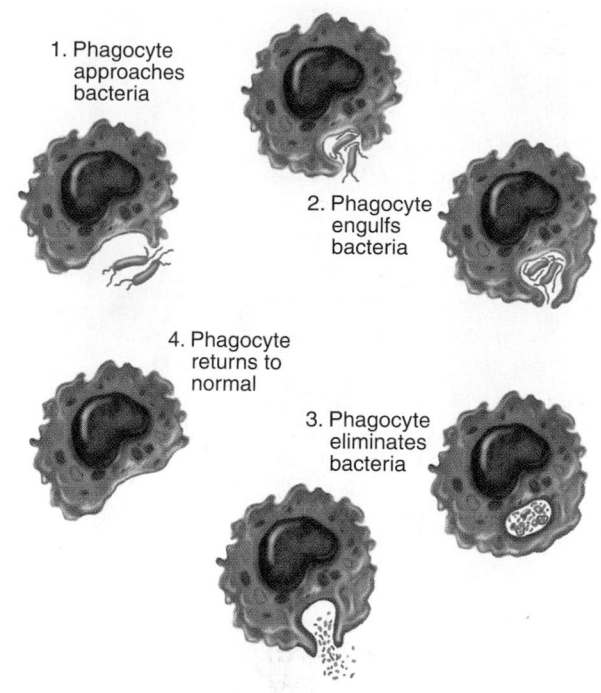

1. Phagocyte approaches bacteria

2. Phagocyte engulfs bacteria

4. Phagocyte returns to normal

3. Phagocyte eliminates bacteria

FIG 19-4 Phagocytosis.

passive immunity are further categorized as acquired naturally or artificially.

Active Natural Immunity

Active natural immunity develops when the body is exposed to a pathogenic microorganism. All microorganisms contain **antigens**, which are markers that identify cells as being part of the body (self) or not part of the body (nonself). Antigens on the body's own cells are called *autoantigens* and all others are *foreign antigens*. During the initial exposure to the pathogen, a person usually develops symptoms of disease. This initial exposure also stimulates white blood cells to develop **antibodies**, which are immunoglobulins specifically tailored to that pathogen's antigen. Those antibodies later combine with that antigen when it presents itself again (during a second exposure) to mark the microorganism for destruction by macrophages, another type of white blood cell.

Active Artificial Immunity

Active artificial immunity develops when an antigen is purposely introduced into a person's body in the form of a vaccine. Examples of vaccines include mumps, measles, and rubella (MMR) or oral poliomyelitis vaccine (OPV). Vaccines generally contain a live, altered (weakened) microorganism or all or part of a dead microorganism. The antigen in the vaccine has been altered in some way so that it will stimulate antibody formation without causing disease.

Passive Natural Immunity

Passive natural immunity develops when already formed antibodies are passed from mother to fetus across the placenta during pregnancy. A pregnant woman has, through the course of her life, been exposed to a variety of pathogenic organisms and developed antibodies against many of them. Some of these antibodies cross the placenta to the fetus. After the infant is born, the antibodies continue to provide protection against disease for several months. In addition, if the woman breastfeeds the infant, additional antibodies are passed to the infant through breast milk. In both cases, the preformed antibodies passed to the infant help to protect him until his body begins developing his own antibodies.

Passive Artificial Immunity

Passive artificial immunity develops when preformed antibodies are developed in an animal or in another human and are then injected into an individual who has experienced a known exposure. This introduction of antiserum provides the individual with temporary passive immunity. Situations in which such an injection might be given include known exposures to rabies, botulism, venomous snakes or spiders, hepatitis, and diphtheria. (See Figure 19-5.)

Standard Precautions

Safety in the medical office is of utmost importance, including protecting staff and patients from injury and disease transmission. Two organizations that play an important role in safety guidelines and regulation in medical offices are the Centers for Disease Control and Prevention (CDC) and the Occupational Safety and Health Administration (OSHA).

In the 1980s, the CDC created a set of guidelines called *universal precautions* to instruct health care providers on how to minimize the risk of disease transmission when providing

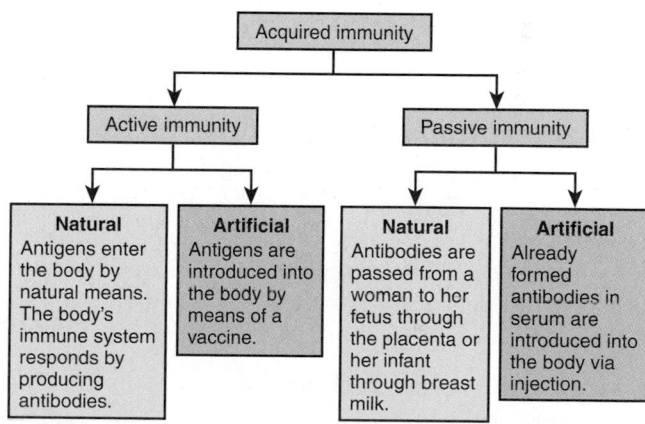

FIG 19-5 Types of immunity.

care. The CDC later revised the guidelines and renamed them *standard precautions.* The revision expanded the guidelines to cover more body fluids and routes of exposure. In general, standard precautions advise health care providers about the handling of any blood or body fluids (except sweat) that might contain blood or infectious organisms. Such body fluids include semen, vaginal secretions, cerebrospinal fluid (CSF), synovial joint fluid, pleural fluid (from the lining of the lungs), peritoneal fluid (from the abdominal cavity), pericardial fluid (from between the heart and its lining), amniotic fluid, and any other body fluid or substance that contains visible blood.

The Occupational Safety and Health Administration (OSHA) is regulated by the U.S. Department of Labor to ensure safe, healthy working conditions for Americans. OSHA guidelines for bloodborne pathogens were developed to decrease the transmission of diseases in the workplace. Upon hire, medical assistants learn about OSHA guidelines relevant to medical office safety and must review them on a regular basis, usually annually. OSHA guidelines dictate that employers provide workers with personal protective equipment (PPE), supplies, and equipment required for the safe disposal of contaminated or dangerous items. Regulations also include mandatory vaccinations against communicable diseases and protocols to follow in the event of an exposure.

Personal Protective Equipment

The practice of standard precautions requires health care providers to wear PPE that is appropriate to each situation, depending on the degree of risk. In the medical office, common PPE includes such items as gloves, masks, eye protection, shoe covers, and gowns to wear during minor office surgeries and procedures when there is a risk of contact with blood or body fluids. The medical assistant and other staff should wear PPE that fits adequately and should replace it if it becomes contaminated or damaged. She should appropriately discard gloves that have become contaminated, punctured, or torn and replace them immediately. Appropriate eye protection includes a face shield or safety glasses that prevent splashing into the eyes. (See Figure 19-6.)

Disposal of Biohazardous Waste

Containers that hold blood or body fluids, such as those used to store or transport specimens, and containers with regulated waste are required to have the biohazard label. (See Figure 19-7.) Red leakproof bags are used for such contaminated supplies as gloves, gauze, bandages, gowns, and linens.

Sharps and Needlestick Safety

The medical assistant must develop careful habits regarding handling materials that are considered "sharps," such as

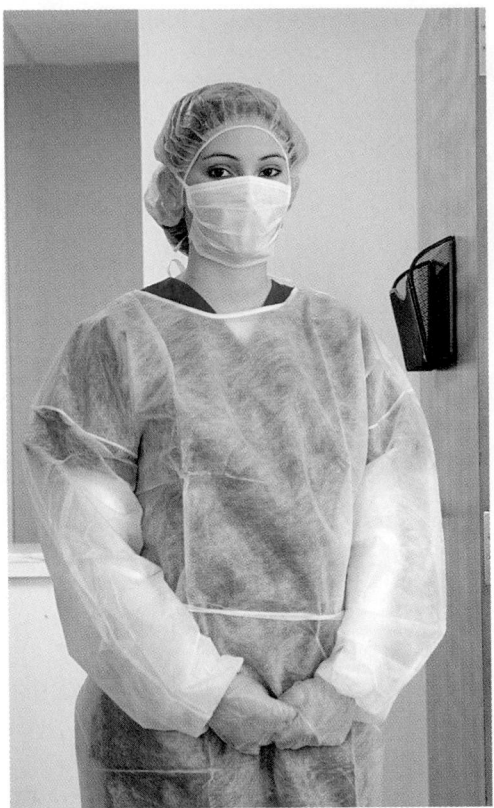

FIG 19-6 Personal protective equipment (PPE).

needles, scalpel blades, capillary tubes, and broken glass or slides. She must dispose of such items in puncture-resistant containers. Furthermore, the medical assistant should never recap an uncapped needle, especially one that is contaminated (used), and should carefully examine trays and work areas for needles or any sharp objects after procedures are completed. She can do so safely by sorting through instruments and supplies with a pair of forceps, rather than by hand. She can then use the forceps to pick up and discard items as needed.

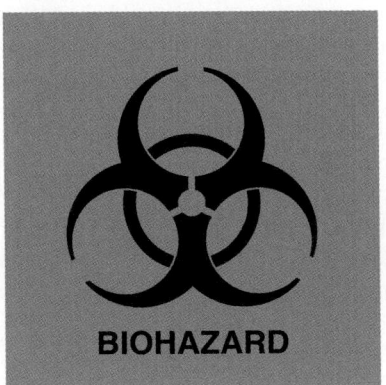

FIG 19-7 Biohazard symbol.

Medical assistants must be in the habit of removing and replacing sharps and biohazard containers before they are full. This reduces risk of injury from trying to place items in a container that is too full. Furthermore, medical assistants must know the policy and procedure for disposal of biohazard waste at the facility in which they work.

In the year 2000, the U.S. Congress signed into law the Needlestick Safety and Prevention Act in an effort to reduce the occupational exposure from sharps injuries. This act was a modification of OSHA's Bloodborne Pathogens Standard and provided more specific directives to employers to identify, evaluate, and implement safer medical devices and to maintain a sharps injury log. (See *Protecting each other.*)

Front office–Back office connection

Protecting Each Other

Accidents involving contaminated substances are common in health care. Many incidents where a health care worker suffers an injury are the result of the sloppy habits of coworkers. Here is a small sample of such events:

- A housekeeper is stuck by a contaminated needle left in a bundle of soiled linens.

- A medical assistant cleaning up after a procedure is stuck in the finger by a suture needle left on the tray.

- As a medical assistant reaches for an overflowing biohazard container placed on an upper shelf in a dirty utility room, it opens and spills its contents over his face.

- A nurse pulls up a nearby chair to sit in while engaged in a conversation with a patient, not noticing the uncapped syringe and needle left there by the laboratory technician, and so sits on the contaminated needle.

- A laboratory technician retrieves a specimen left by a medical assistant. The specimen lid has come loose in transport and contaminated fluid has spilled inside of the specimen bag and soaked the outside of the specimen cup.

- A kitchen worker in a local hospital is poked by a contaminated needle left on a meal tray by a nurse.

What do these events have in common? Members of the health care team were needlessly endangered by the sloppy habits of their coworkers. The safety and well-being of all health care workers depends on each other's good habits.

Vaccinations

In most cases, a medical assistant must provide documentation of all necessary vaccinations prior to employment. Examples include the hepatitis B vaccination and testing for tuberculosis exposure. If the medical assistant has not completed certain vaccinations, the CDC requires the employer to provide them at no cost to the employee within 10 days of becoming employed. The hepatitis B vaccine is administered in a series of three injections; the second injection is administered 6 weeks after the first, and the third injection is administered 6 months after the first. An employee can decline to receive the immunization by completing and signing the proper paperwork, which the office manager will keep in her employee file. If the employee later requests the immunization, the CDC requires the employer to make it available.

Exposure Control

In the event of exposure to a pathogen, the medical assistant must follow the facility policy, which is dictated by several guidelines and requirements set by government agencies. Most exposure control guidelines address exposure to a bloodborne pathogen or a biohazardous material spill.

Bloodborne Pathogen Exposure

If a medical assistant or other staff member is exposed to a bloodborne pathogen, the employee must wash or flush the exposed area and then report the incident to the employer right away. OSHA guidelines require employers to develop exposure control plans and make these plans known to employees. The employee involved must document the event by completing an incident report. The employer is also required to follow up on the exposure incident by documenting the exposure and related circumstances and identifying the source individual and the status of the source individual if he consents to testing for human immunodeficiency virus (HIV) or hepatitis B virus (HBV). The employer must offer the employee the option of having her blood tested for HIV and HBV as well as post-exposure treatment in accordance with the current recommendations from the U.S. Public Health Service. Furthermore, the employer must provide counseling to the employee regarding precautions she must take and what possible illness signs or symptoms to report.

Biohazard Spill

The medical assistant must be familiar with office protocol and CDC recommendations for responding to a biohazard spill. The first priority is protecting herself by applying gloves and other PPE. Next, she should contain the spill with paper towels and then cover the entire spill with 10% bleach solution and let it stand for at least 20 minutes.

When cleaning up the spill, she must use a mechanical device, rather than her hands. She should then place all items in a biohazard container and repeat the bleach application, waiting another 20 minutes. She must document the incident according to office policy.

Asepsis

Asepsis refers to a condition free from pathogens. There are three levels involved in asepsis:

- sanitization
- disinfection
- sterilization.

Sanitization

Sanitization of an object or surface, or the removal of microorganisms using chemicals, heat, or ionizing radiation, is the first line of defense in ensuring asepsis in the health care environment. The single most effective standard precaution practice that breaks the chain of infection and protects everyone is consistent, proper hand hygiene and sanitization. Proper sanitization of equipment and supplies is also essential.

Hand Sanitization

Standard precautions dictate cleaning the hands with soap and warm water or with an antiseptic agent prior to and immediately after any direct contact with patients, after any potential contact with pathogenic organisms, after using the toilet, and any time the hands become visibly soiled. Other times to sanitize the hands include the beginning of each work day, before and after placing patients in examination rooms, before and after cleaning examination rooms, before and after assisting the physician with procedures, before and after cleaning equipment, before putting on gloves, after removing gloves, before and after taking a break, before eating or drinking anything, and at the end of each work day.

When washing her hands, the medical assistant must remember to cover all parts of her hands with soap and water, rub them together to create friction for at least 15 seconds, and then rinse well. (See *Procedure 19-1: Washing hands with soap and water.*)

Alcohol-based hand sanitizers contain 60% to 95% ethanol or isopropyl alcohol. When the medical assistant uses an alcohol-based hand sanitizer, she should follow the manufacturer's directions, which generally include covering all hand surfaces with the sanitizer, including the hands, the fingers, between the fingers, and the wrists. She should then allow her hands to air dry.

There are several advantages to alcohol-based hand sanitizers. They act fast, significantly reduce the number of microorganisms on the skin, and cause minimal skin irritation. They take less time to use than soap and water and require no towel drying. Additionally, allergic responses to these products are rare. (See *Procedure 19-2: Sanitizing hands with an alcohol-based hand sanitizer,* page 300.) The medical assistant must still wash her hands with warm water and soap after several hand sanitizer uses or whenever hands are visibly soiled. In either case, sanitizing the hands in view of the patient sets a good example and assures him that the medical assistant is using proper aseptic technique.

Sanitization of Equipment and the Environment

Sanitization decreases the number of microorganisms from reusable equipment and surfaces. To sanitize an instrument, the medical assistant will usually rinse it under cold water and scrub it with an enzymatic detergent. In some cases, the medical assistant might use an ultrasonic bath where sound waves cause vibrations to loosen debris from instruments. Sanitization allows the heat, gas, or sterilizing chemicals to penetrate all surfaces. It must occur before disinfecting and sterilizing can take place. When performing sanitization, the medical assistant should wear utility or heavy-duty gloves and other PPE, such as goggles, to reduce the risk of exposure to contaminated materials. She must rinse all instruments and equipment under cool running water. For increased efficiency, the medical assistant should try to rinse instruments as soon as possible after use. After rinsing, the medical assistant should clean them by removing debris with a scrub brush. She must carefully scrub all parts of an instrument, including hinges, ratchets, and serrations. At this point, it is also best to check each piece of equipment to ensure it is in proper working order. The medical assistant should try to use detergents that produce no suds or low suds. To prevent self-injury, the medical assistant should point instruments with sharp edges away from her body while cleaning them. She should rinse items with hot water and dry them thoroughly, leaving hinged instruments in the open position. (See *Procedure 19-3: Sanitizing equipment,* page 300.)

In addition to equipment, the medical assistant must sanitize the environment of the medical office, including such surfaces as countertops and examination tables. Such solutions as a combination of 10 parts water to 1 part household bleach are inexpensive, easy to use, and effective. Other commercial sanitizing solutions are available and effective as well. Regardless of the products used, the medical assistant should always take time to read the labels, follow the directions, and note the material safety data sheet (MSDS) information, which provides data about ingredients and measures to take in the event of a spill or exposure. This information is provided by the manufacturer of each substance and is included on the individual package labels. Each medical office must also keep copies of this information on-site.

PROCEDURE 19-1

Washing hands with soap and water

Task
Perform hand washing.

Conditions
- Sink
- Soap
- Timer
- Nail stick or brush
- Paper towels
- Waste container

Standards
In the time specified and within the scoring parameters determined by the instructor, the student will successfully perform hand washing with soap and water.

Performance Standards
1. Remove all rings and jewelry because jewelry harbors microorganisms and push your watchband up to expose your wrists.
2. Stand in front of the sink without touching the sink edge or countertop to prevent water or microorganisms from being transmitted to the front of your uniform.
3. Turn on the water to a comfortable temperature.
4. Apply soap to your hands (approximately 5 ml or 1 tsp) and work it into a lather, being sure to cover all parts of your hands and wrists. Using friction, continue to wash hands and wrists for 15 seconds.
5. Using an orange stick or a fingernail, clean under the edges of all of your fingernails to help remove microorganisms.
6. Pointing your hands and fingers down, rinse your hands under the running water.

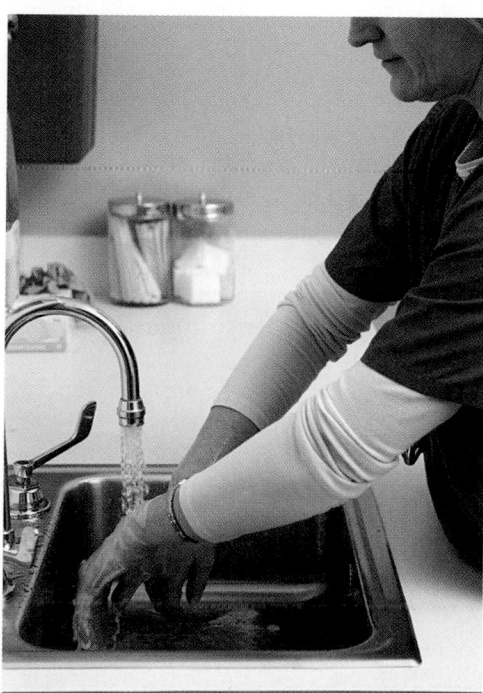

Rinse your hands and fingers while pointing them down.

7. Dry your hands with a disposable towel, then discard the used towel in a waste container.
8. Use a dry, disposable towel to turn off the water to maintain infection control.
9. Dispose of the towel in a waste container.

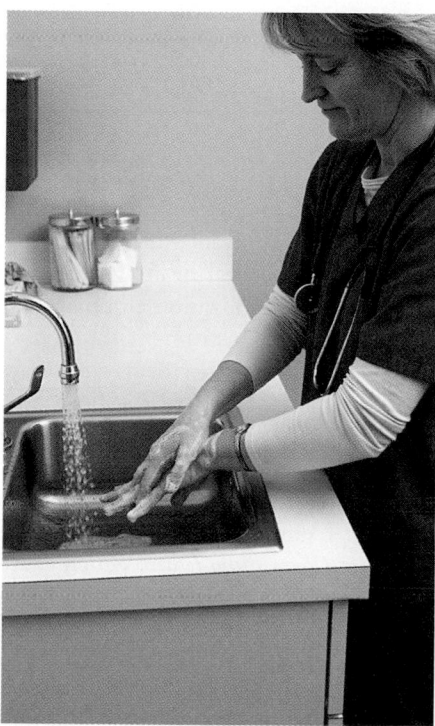

Cover all parts of your hands and wrists.

PROCEDURE 19-2

Sanitizing hands with an alcohol-based hand sanitizer

Task
Sanitize hands using an alcohol-based hand sanitizer.

Conditions
- Alcohol-based hand sanitizer

Standards
In the time specified and within the scoring parameters determined by the instructor, the student will successfully perform hand sanitization using an alcohol-based hand sanitizer.

Performance Standards
1. Remove all rings and jewelry because jewelry harbors microorganisms and push your watchband up to expose your wrists.
2. Read the label of the alcohol-based hand sanitizer and verify that it contains 60% to 95% alcohol.
3. Apply enough sanitizer to cover all the surfaces of your hands and wrists.
4. Rub the sanitizer over the surfaces of your hands, fingers, fingernails, and wrists.
5. Allow your hands to air dry.

PROCEDURE 19-3

Sanitizing equipment

Task
Perform sanitization of equipment.

Conditions
- Sink
- Brush with stiff bristles
- Low-sudsing, chemical disinfectant soap
- Gown or apron with a plastic, leakproof backing
- Utility gloves
- Goggles
- Towels
- Soap

Standards
In the time specified and within the scoring parameters determined by the instructor, the student will successfully sanitize equipment for reuse.

Performance Standards
1. Wash or sanitize your hands to ensure infection control and assemble supplies.
2. Using soap, scrub all instruments with a bristle brush under running water to remove debris.
3. Clean all surfaces of the instruments and open any hinges to allow better exposure of instruments to hot water and air.
4. Rinse the instruments thoroughly with hot water.
5. Place the instruments on a towel for drying.
6. Remove your gloves and wash your hands to ensure infection control.

Disinfection

Although the medical assistant could disinfect instruments used in noninvasive procedures by placing them in boiling water at 212ºF (100ºC) for 15 minutes, doing so is not practical in most medical offices. Thus, **disinfection** typically involves the application of a substance to equipment, surfaces, or other items to kill pathogenic microorganisms.

The medical assistant should be sure to sanitize most instruments and equipment before disinfecting them. Other items a medical assistant should disinfect include surfaces, such as countertops and trays, some types of furniture, and even the skin. Disinfecting agents appropriate for instruments, surfaces, furniture, and equipment include chlorine, iodine, 70% isopropyl alcohol, hydrogen peroxide, or a 1:10 solution of household bleach and water (1 part bleach to 10 equal parts of water). Bleach solution must be prepared daily because it loses potency over time. Agents appropriate for the skin include povidone-iodine (Betadine), if the patient is not allergic to iodine, and 70% isopropyl alcohol. Many other disinfecting agents are too harsh for the skin. Regardless of the agents used, the medical assistant should be sure to read labels and use these agents according to directions. (See *Procedure 19-4: Disinfecting equipment*.)

Sterilization

In surgical asepsis, all instruments and supplies must be sterile. Although sanitization kills most microorganisms, it does not kill **spores** (bacterial or fungal cells resistant to temperature extremes). Sterilization eliminates all microorganisms from a surface or instrument through exposure to chemicals, ionizing radiation, dry heat, gas, or steam. Prior to sterilization, instruments must have been sanitized and disinfected. Some pathogens are easily destroyed; others, such as spores, are very resistant to temperature extremes and are difficult to destroy. However, the process of sterilization kills them. Examples of pathogenic organisms that produce spores are *Clostridium tetani*, which causes tetanus, and *Clostridium botulinum*, which causes food poisoning.

Sterilization should take place in a part of the medical clinic specifically set aside for this purpose. One area should be designated as the receiving area where nonsterile items are placed. Some of the supplies used by the medical assistant in this area include receiving basins, sterilization wrapping

PROCEDURE 19-4

Disinfecting equipment

Task
Perform equipment disinfection.

Conditions
- Sink
- Disinfectant chemical solution
- Container for instruments
- Timer
- Water

Standards
In the time specified and within the scoring parameters determined by the instructor, the student will successfully disinfect equipment.

Performance Standards
1. Wash or sanitize your hands to ensure infection control and assemble supplies.
2. Put on utility gloves.
3. Sanitize all instruments prior to disinfecting.
4. Read the manufacturer's instructions on the label of the disinfectant solution.
5. Prepare the disinfectant as directed.
6. Place the sanitized instruments into a container.
7. Apply the disinfectant to the instruments.
8. Soak the instruments for the required time, according to the manufacturer's instructions.
9. Dry the instruments with towels.
10. Store the instruments appropriately for future use.
11. Remove your gloves and wash your hands to ensure infection control.

paper, sterilization indicator strips, sterilization tape, sterilization pouches, and gloves. When items have been sterilized, the medical assistant should place them in a different area designated as the receiving area for sterile supplies. Types of sterilization techniques include chemical, dry heat, steam, gas, and radiation. One of the most common methods of sterilizing reusable instruments in the medical office is by using an autoclave.

Autoclave

An **autoclave** is a device that sterilizes items using steam pressure at a temperature of 250° to 270°F (120° to 130°C) with 15 lb of pressure for a specific amount of time, depending on the contents to be sterilized. Subjecting items to steam under pressure causes the proteins in microorganisms to coagulate; when the chamber cools, the condensation of the steam causes the explosion of the microorganism cells, ensuring their complete destruction.

Prior to sterilization in the autoclave, the medical assistant should sanitize and, in some cases, disinfect instruments. She must then package or wrap them appropriately. Some packs contain single instruments and others contain a combination of items needed for a specific procedure.

For sterilization to occur efficiently, the surfaces of all objects must be subjected to the moisture, heat, and pressure of the autoclave. Therefore, the medical assistant must follow several guidelines for packaging and preparing items properly. For example, she must leave all hinged instruments open, pack items so they do not touch each other, and pack items loosely into the autoclave so that all parts of the instruments can be fully exposed to the steam and pressure. Many packs include disposable or reusable towels. Muslin cloth, a common reusable material used in sterile packs, is porous, allowing the steam to pass through and enabling the instruments to dry easily as well. Polypropylene autoclave bags are also available. (See *Procedure 19-5: Wrapping a pack for autoclaving,* page 302.)

Surgical packs are commonly wrapped twice using two towels, one inside the other. When a medical assistant includes a large number of items in a pack, she should put them into trays so that the contents can be carefully organized. Regardless of the size or content of the pack, the medical assistant should always place a sterilization indicator strip inside the pack and use special tape to close the pack. These heat-sensitive items change color when sterilized to indicate that the sterilization process is successful. When the medical assistant has wrapped the items, she must identify the contents by labeling the outside of the pack, including the date and her initials.

The medical assistant should always follow the manufacturer's instructions that accompany the autoclave used in her office. However, some general guidelines apply to wrapping instruments and loading, operating, and unloading all autoclaves.

Wrapping Instruments and Loading the Autoclave

When wrapping instruments and loading the autoclave, the medical assistant should be sure to follow these guidelines:

- Make sure all items were previously sanitized.
- Use only material approved for autoclaving to wrap instruments, and examine the wrap for holes or fraying before each use.
- Wrap and arrange all items to allow exposure of all surfaces. (Allow 1" to 3" between the pack and the walls of the autoclave.)
- Wrap hinged instruments open for best exposure.
- Wrap sharp instrument tips with gauze to prevent puncturing the wrap.
- Label packs using permanent marker with the contents, date, and her initials.

PROCEDURE 19-5

Wrapping a pack for autoclaving

Task
Wrap a pack for autoclaving.

Conditions
- Disinfectant chemical solution
- Container for instruments
- Timer
- Water
- Sanitized instruments to be sterilized
- Wrapping towels (2)
- Sterile indicator strips and tape for securing contents
- Marker pen

Standards
In the time specified and within the scoring parameters determined by the instructor, the student will successfully wrap a pack for sterilization.

Performance Standards
1. Wash or sanitize your hands to ensure infection control.
2. Identify the type of pack to be used. Gather the instruments and other equipment.
3. Lay the towels flat in a diamond configuration and place the instruments in the center.
4. Open all hinged instruments. If the hinged instruments can touch, separate them with a 2 × 2 gauze pad to maximize surface exposure of the instruments.
5. Place the sterile indicator strip at the top of the contents to allow the user to verify the sterility of the package contents.
6. Bring the bottom of the diamond up to cover the contents and fold the tip of the corner.

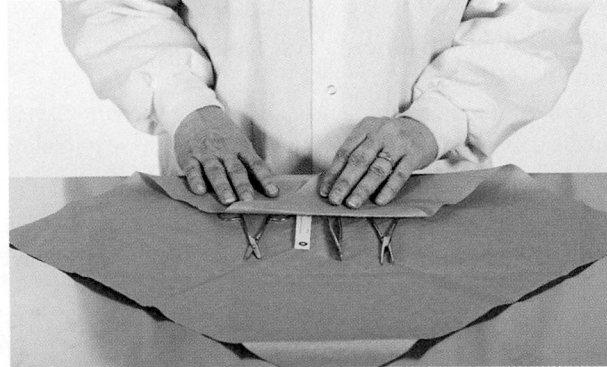

7. Bring one side of the wrap over to cover the contents and fold up the tip of the corner.
8. Bring the other side of the wrap over to cover the contents and fold up the tip of the corner.

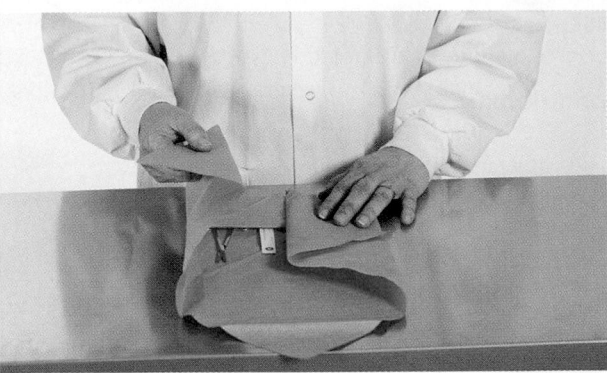

9. Fold the bottom of the wrap over, including the instruments, to align with the top edges of the side folds.

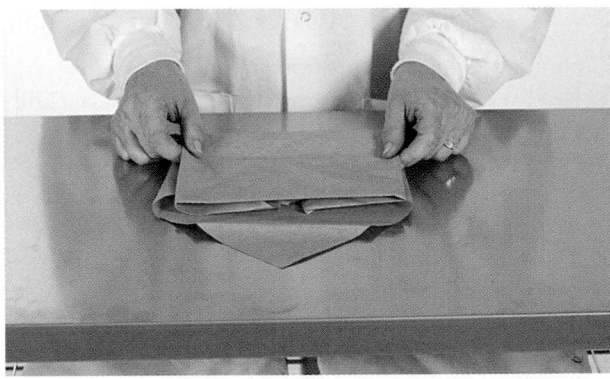

10. For packages that must be double-wrapped, place the package in the center of a second sheet of wrapping material and repeat steps 6 to 9 to facilitate sterile technique when the package is opened.
11. Bring the top of the wrap down and seal the top flap with sterile indicator tape.
12. Label the tape with the contents, the date, and your initials to allow the user to verify the contents and date of sterilization.

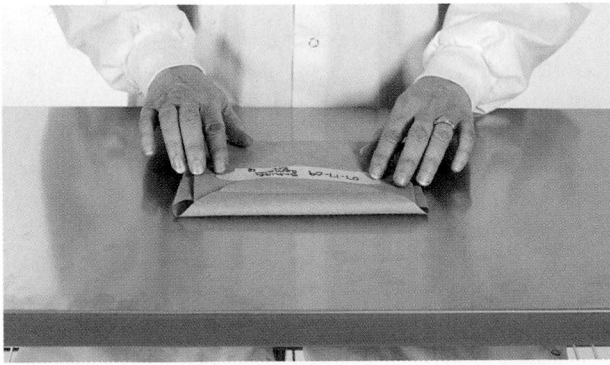

- Arrange containers on their sides and leave the lids ajar.
- Leave instruments unwrapped that do not need to be sterile for use (such as vaginal speculums).

Operating the Autoclave

After wrapping instruments and loading the autoclave, the medical assistant should follow these guidelines for operating the autoclave:

- Use only distilled water to prevent mineral deposits.
- Set the autoclave to at least 250°F (121°C), depending on the item to be sterilized, and 15 lb per square inch (psi) of pressure.
- Begin the processing time after the autoclave reaches the desired operating conditions of temperature and pressure.
- Process unwrapped items for 20 minutes.
- Process small wrapped items for 30 minutes.
- Process large or tightly wrapped items for 40 minutes.

Unloading the Autoclave

When the autoclave sterilization process is complete, the medical assistant should unload the autoclave following these guidelines:

- After completion, open the door slightly and carefully, using heat-resistant gloves, to let steam escape.
- Do not remove wrapped items until they have completely cooled and dried.

Storing Sterilized Items

After sterilization with the autoclave, the medical assistant should store the packs in a dry place. Items sterilized in towels or cloth are considered sterile for 28 to 30 days. Items sterilized in polypropylene autoclave bags are considered sterile for as long as 6 months.

Autoclave Maintenance

The autoclave itself is an important piece of medical equipment and requires careful care and attention to keep it in top operating condition. General guidelines include daily washing of the inner chamber as well as regular draining of the water so that the medical assistant can clean the autoclave with an approved solution. To clean the autoclave, the medical assistant must use distilled water and run two consecutive sterilization cycles. She must also wipe down the inner chamber of the autoclave and remove and scrub the inner shelves. For specific instructions on how to clean the autoclave, the medical assistant should refer to the manufacturer's instructions for the autoclave in her office.

Quality Control

The medical assistant should conduct and document quality-control testing on the autoclave on a regular schedule. Documentation should include a description of the test, the date, and the results. In the event of incomplete or inadequate sterilization, the medical assistant should file a report that describes the problem she encountered and the steps she took to correct it. Additional documentation should reflect satisfactory autoclave performance. (See *Procedure 19-6: Using an autoclave for sterilization,* page 304.)

Chemical Sterilization

Some instruments cannot withstand the high temperatures of the autoclave, such as fiber-optic endoscopes. Therefore, they need sterilization using chemicals. The medical assistant should mix the sterilization solution carefully according to the instructions on the container and mark the solution container with the date of preparation and expiration. She should be sure to use gloves and other PPE for protection if the solution is caustic. Then she should immerse the items in the solution for a specified period of time, commonly 8 or more hours. Upon completion, she must remove the items from the solution with sterile transfer forceps, rinse them with sterile water, dry them with sterile towels, and place them on the sterile field so that they are ready for use.

Types of Asepsis

Within the health care professions, there are two types of asepsis: *medical asepsis* and *surgical asepsis.*

Medical Asepsis

Medical asepsis refers to the destruction of pathogenic organisms after they leave the body. More specifically, medically aseptic technique is a method of performing procedures and providing patient care so that pathogenic organisms are not transmitted from the ill patient to other patients or anyone else. The simplest way to apply medical asepsis is to follow standard precautions consistently. The medical assistant should always consider collected specimens to be contaminated, whether labeled or not. Body fluids that are not considered contaminated are tears, sweat, and saliva. However, medical assistants should always be cautious and wear examination gloves when there is any possibility of contamination.

Surgical Asepsis

Surgical asepsis is the practice of destroying all pathogenic organisms before they enter the body. More specifically, surgical aseptic technique is a method of performing invasive procedures so that patients are protected from pathogenic microorganisms. When performing invasive procedures, the medical assistant must use this technique. Invasive procedures are those in which the patient's normal protective barriers are punctured or disrupted in some manner. Examples of some procedures that require surgical asepsis include injections, urinary catheterization, wound care, and such surgical procedures as tissue biopsy or repair and suturing of lacerations. (See *Medical versus surgical asepsis,* page 305.)

PROCEDURE 19-6

Using an autoclave for sterilization

Task
Perform sterilization.

Conditions
- Packages ready to be sterilized
- Autoclave procedure manual
- Autoclave

Standards
In the time specified and within the scoring parameters determined by the instructor, the student will successfully perform sterilization using an autoclave.

Performance Standards
1. Wash or sanitize your hands to ensure infection control.
2. Load wrapped, labeled packages into the autoclave.

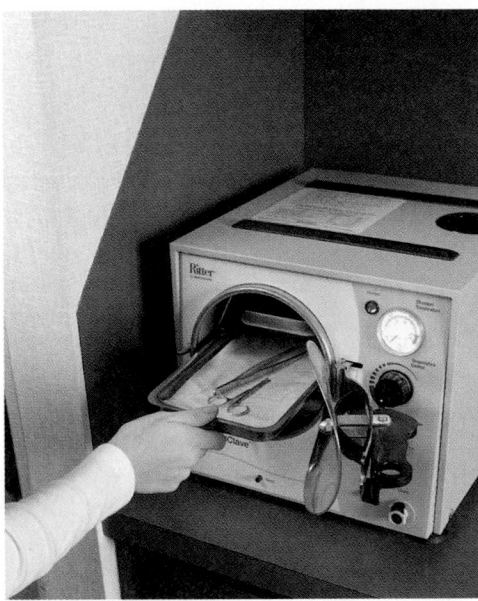

Autoclave loaded with instruments wrapped in a polypropylene autoclave bag

3. Position packages so they are not touching. If sterilizing containers, place containers on their sides so that the steam can circulate around all packages, allowing adequate sterilization to occur.
4. Close the autoclave door and secure it.
5. Following manufacturer's instructions, plug the autoclave's electrical cord into a power outlet and turn on the power.
6. Set the indicator to the contents loaded into the autoclave, such as glass, cloth, or instruments.
7. Set the temperature and pounds of pressure.
8. Set the exposure time.
9. Press the start button.
10. Make sure that the autoclave starts and the door remains secured until the sterilization and drying time are complete.
11. Prior to removing the contents, wash your hands and dry them thoroughly to keep the outside of the packages as clean as possible.
12. Place the sterile packages in a dry storage area.

Medical versus surgical asepsis

In general, medical aseptic technique is used to protect health care providers and others from the patient's pathogenic microorganisms. Surgical aseptic technique is used to protect the patient from any pathogenic organisms external to his body. Here are some examples of procedures that require medical and surgical asepsis.

Medical asepsis

- Taking a patient's temperature
- Removing an old dressing from a patient's wound
- Scrubbing and disinfecting used surgical instruments
- Emptying an emesis basin

Surgical asepsis

- Inserting a urinary catheter
- Administering an intramuscular injection
- Applying a new dressing to a patient's wound
- Opening a sterile package
- Setting up a tray for the physician to perform suturing

Chapter Summary

- Because the health care environment brings individuals together, many of whom have infectious diseases or weakened immune systems, it sets the stage for the very real possibility of disease transmission between patients and even health care staff. To prevent such transmission from happening, medical assistants must have an understanding of how disease is transmitted and how to take every reasonable precaution to reduce disease transmission in the medical office.
- Potentially harmful organisms, such as bacteria, fungi, and protozoa, are found on and in the body. Normally, a healthy balance of these microorganisms exists; however, when this balance is disturbed, the individual becomes more vulnerable to illness and disease.
- Pathogens are microorganisms capable of producing disease. To grow and thrive, most pathogens require nutrients, moisture, warmth, and a suitable pH environment. Therefore, some parts of the human body tend to provide a hospitable environment for pathogenic growth.
- The five main types of pathogens are bacteria, *Rickettsia*, virus, fungus, and protozoa.
- Learning about the chain of infection helps medical assistants understand how microorganisms are transmitted and how people become infected. The elements of the chain consist of the pathogen, reservoir host, means of exit, mode of transmission, and susceptible host.
- Infections can be categorized according to their general duration and whether they occur only once or repeatedly. Types of infection are acute, chronic, and latent.
- There are several stages in the disease process, including incubation, prodromal, acute, declining, and convalescent stages.
- The body's natural protective mechanisms normally protect human beings from pathogens. These mechanisms take on mechanical, chemical, and cellular forms.
- Mechanical defense mechanisms include the skin, mucous membranes, protective reflexes such as coughing and sneezing, and the flushing action of body fluids such as tears and urine.
- Chemical defense mechanisms include secretions of the sebaceous glands, acidic fluids in the stomach, fluids of tears and the urinary tract, and the activity of interferons and certain enzymes.
- When the body's natural defenses are unsuccessful in eliminating invading organisms, infection may occur. Symptoms of localized infection include redness, swelling, heat, pain, fever, and general malaise.
- Immunity is a powerful defense system within the body that responds to the invasion of foreign substances, such as bacteria, viruses, fungi, and parasites. When these substances enter the body, the body's immune system recognizes them as foreign and attacks them.
- There are several types of acquired immunity, including natural active immunity, artificial active immunity, natural passive immunity, and artificial passive immunity.
- The Occupational Safety and Health Administration (OSHA) ensures safe, healthy working conditions for Americans. OSHA guidelines for bloodborne pathogens were developed to decrease the transmission of diseases in the health care setting.
- In the medical office, common personal protective equipment includes such items as gloves, masks, eye protection, shoe covers, and gowns to wear during minor office surgeries and procedures when there is a risk of contact with blood or body fluids.
- Medical assistants must dispose of biohazardous wastes appropriately. Containers that have blood or body fluids are required to have the biohazard label. Red leakproof bags are used for contaminated supplies, such as gloves, gauze, bandages, gowns, and linens.
- In most cases, medical assistants must provide documentation of all necessary vaccinations prior to employment. Examples include the hepatitis B vaccination and testing for tuberculosis exposure. If the medical assistant has not completed certain vaccinations, the employer will provide them at no cost to the employee within 10 days of becoming employed.

- In the event of an exposure, the medical assistant must wash or flush the exposed area and then report the incident to the employer right away. OSHA guidelines require employers to develop exposure control plans and make this plan known to employees. Medical assistants must be familiar with office protocol for responding to a biohazard spill.
- Asepsis is a condition free from pathogens. Within the health care professions, there are two types of asepsis: medical asepsis and surgical asepsis.
- Medical asepsis refers to the destruction of pathogenic organisms after they leave the body. More specifically, medically aseptic technique is a method of performing procedures and providing patient care so that pathogenic organisms are not transmitted from the ill patient to other patients or anyone else.
- The simplest way to apply medical asepsis is to consistently follow standard precautions, that is, guidelines developed by the Centers for Disease Control (CDC) for the protection of all people who come into contact with blood and any other potentially infectious substances that come from the body.
- The most effective standard precaution practice that breaks the chain of infection and protects everyone is consistent, proper hand hygiene.
- Medical assistants must sanitize their hands regularly with soap and warm water or alcohol-based hand sanitizer.
- Sanitization must occur before sterilization can take place and involves the removal of microorganisms from reusable equipment and surfaces by use of chemicals, heat, or ionizing radiation.
- Disinfection is defined as the application of a disinfecting agent to equipment, surfaces, or other items to kill pathogenic microorganisms. However, this process does not always kill all microorganisms and does not kill spores (bacterial or fungal cells resistant to temperature extremes).
- Surgical asepsis is the destruction of all pathogenic organisms before they enter the body. More specifically, surgically aseptic technique is a method of performing invasive procedures so that patients are protected from pathogenic microorganisms.
- When using surgical asepsis, all instruments and supplies must be sterile. Therefore, they must have been previously treated or prepared in a manner that eliminated all microorganisms.
- An autoclave is a device that sterilizes items by steam pressure at temperatures of 250° to 270°F (120° to 130°C) with 15 lb of pressure for a specific amount of time, depending on the contents to be sterilized.

Team Work Exercises

1. Divide into teams of four or five students. Create a plan in writing that designates disinfection duties that each member of the team might perform at the end of each day to be sure that the office is clean and safe for patients the following day. Consider the accidental exposures listed in *Protecting each other* on page 297. Put into writing the strategies that could have been employed by members of the team to prevent these accidents. Share your team's plan with the rest of the class.
2. Divide into teams of three to five students. Select several items that are commonly sterilized by autoclave. Take turns demonstrating for the rest of the class different ways in which items might be properly wrapped and prepared for autoclaving. Use as many variations in packaging and wrapping technique as you can think of, including sterilization wrap, sterilization pouches, and sterile towels.

Cases Studies

1. Your coworker, Elizabeth, is assisting with a minor office surgery when she accidentally punctures her finger (through her glove) with the needle used to inject medication into the patient. She is embarrassed and ashamed that she was careless enough to let this happen. Elizabeth tells you about the incident and asks you not to tell anyone. What should you do?
2. The facility you work for asks you to develop a pamphlet for patients. The pamphlet will be used to inform patients about commonsense, everyday measures they can use to prevent disease transmission and keep healthy during cold and flu season. What data will you include?

Resources

- Centers for Disease Control and Prevention website: *www.cdc.gov*
- Free infection-prevention online course: *www.engenderhealth .org/IP/index.html*
- OSHA website: *www.osha.gov*
- World Health Organization website: *www.who.int/en*

The Patient Interview

Learning Objectives

Upon completion of this chapter, the student will be able to:

- define and spell the key terms in the glossary
- describe the purpose and the key components of the patient interview
- list nine interviewing techniques and the purpose of each
- identify effective strategies for interviewing the talkative patient and the quiet patient
- differentiate among closed questions, open-ended questions, and directive statements and give an example of each
- list five obstacles to effective interviewing and discuss an effective alternative strategy for each
- describe techniques that may be used to help patients feel more comfortable discussing sensitive information
- list at least three examples of age-appropriate interviewing techniques
- list the main components of the medical history
- conduct a patient interview to obtain a medical history
- accurately document the patient's medical information on a history form
- describe three methods of documentation.

CAAHEP Competencies

Clinical Competencies
  Patient Care
    Obtain and record patient history
General Competencies
  Professional Communications
    Recognize and respond to verbal communications
  Legal Concepts
    Establish and maintain the medical record
    Document appropriately

ABHES Competencies

Professionalism
  Be courteous and diplomatic
Communication
  Be attentive, listen, and learn
  Adapt what is said to the recipient's level of comprehension
  Interview effectively
  Receive, organize, prioritize, and transmit information expediently
  Recognize and respond to verbal and nonverbal communication
  Principles of verbal and nonverbal communication
  Adaptation for individualized needs
Administrative Duties
  Prepare and maintain medical records
Clinical Duties
  Interview and record patient history
Legal Concepts
  Document accurately

Procedures

  Interviewing a patient to obtain a medical history

Chapter Outline

  First Impressions
  Interviewing Techniques
    Talkative Patient
    Quiet Patient
  Obstacles to Effective Interviewing
    Offering Opinions and Advice
    Offering False Reassurance
    Using Technical Language
    Talking Too Much
    Asking Judgmental Questions
    Discussing Sensitive Topics
    Age-Appropriate Communication
  Medical History
  Documentation
    Documentation Types
      Source-oriented
      Problem-oriented
  Chapter Summary
  Team Work Exercises
  Case Studies
  Resources

Key Terms

acronym
Word created from the first letters of a series of words

active listening
Nonverbal communication that indicates the listener has heard the message and concerns of the patient

closed question
Question that can be answered with one word

directive statement
Statement that guides the listener in discussing topics as directed

layperson
Nonmedical person

medical jargon
Terminology and abbreviations used in medicine that are not readily understood by laypersons

open-ended question
Question that requires more than a one-word answer

problem-oriented medical record
System of documentation that includes the database, problem list, plan, and progress notes

rapport
Empathetic relationship

redirecting
Guiding the patient back to relevant subject matter

reflecting
Validating the patient's feelings and concerns

restating
Rewording a statement to check for accuracy

silence
Communication strategy that allows the patient time to process information and formulate a response

source-oriented medical record
System of documentation that includes a note for each patient visit, arranged in reverse chronological order

summarizing
Clarifying the patient's key issues

First Impressions

Most patients enter the health care setting because they wish to meet with their health care provider. However, the physician is rarely the first person the patient encounters. After checking in with the receptionist, the patient is usually greeted by a medical assistant. The medical assistant plays an important role in connecting the patient and physician. In addition to weighing the patient, showing him to an examination room, and obtaining vital signs, the medical assistant asks questions about the patient's medical history. This chapter focuses on the role of the medical assistant in the history-taking process and effective interviewing strategies.

The interviewing process generally occurs in three parts:

- *Initiation*—During initiation, the medical assistant introduces herself to the patient and any family members that may be accompanying him. She also seeks clarification regarding the purpose of the visit. Because this part of the conversation may include the patient's personal health care information, it should take place in the private examination room. By using effective communication techniques and body language, the medical assistant conveys respect for the patient.
- *Body*—During the main part, or body, of the interview, the medical assistant uses therapeutic communication techniques to establish trust and rapport. She gathers more detailed information about the nature of the patient's problem as well as his goals and expectations for care. The amount of detailed information the medical assistant obtains depends on the nature of the visit and the office policy.
- *Summary*—The medical assistant closes the interview with a brief summary of the main points of the conversation. This summary allows the patient to make additions, corrections, or clarifications to the information.

Interviewing Techniques

The medical assistant should use several interviewing techniques to ensure that she obtains the most complete, relevant information possible about the patient and his problem in a timely manner. Such techniques can be modified as needed in any situation. For example, a patient may feel reluctant to discuss personal topics or answer questions about his personal habits. On the other hand, a talkative patient might give lengthy answers and get sidetracked with detailed stories that do not provide essential health information. In such situations, the busy medical assistant must use proven interviewing techniques in order to obtain accurate information and complete the interview in a timely fashion. Here are some of the most common interviewing techniques used to respond to these different communication styles:

- A **closed (direct) question** seeks specific information and invites a reply in the form of a one-word answer, such as "yes" or "no," or a number, such as "43." An example of a closed question is "How old are you?"
- An **open-ended question** encourages the patient to answer the question in whatever manner he or she prefers and allows elaboration, such as "What brings you here today?"
- A **directive statement** guides the patient in discussing whatever topic is indicated by the interviewer—for example, "Tell me how you injured your ankle".
- **Restating** checks the listener's understanding and interpretation of the patient's message and invites confirmation or correction.
- **Reflecting** validates the patients' feelings and concerns—for example, "It sounds like you feel upset that the treatment didn't work and you are worried that your condition is worsening."
- **Redirecting** guides the patient back to relevant subject matter, such as "You mentioned earlier that your headaches are getting worse. Please tell me more about that."
- **Summarizing** clarifies key issues for the medical assistant and the patient—for example, "Based on what you've told me your main issues of concern today are…"
- **Active listening** is nonverbal communication that indicates the medical assistant is hearing and attending to the message and the concerns of the patient. She focuses all of her energy on being fully present with the patient and uses body language, such as leaning forward, eye contact, head nodding, and facial expression to convey her attention and concern.
- **Silence** allows the patient ample opportunity to process what has been said and think about what he wants to say next. In allowing him this gift of time, the medical assistant communicates acceptance and caring.

Talkative Patient

A talkative patient can make the medical assistant's job interesting and enjoyable. However, she can also present a challenge. The medical assistant is generally busy and does not have extra time to listen to many of a talkative patient's stories. Therefore, the medical assistant may often find herself in the difficult situation of needing to interrupt the patient to ask questions, give instructions, or even exit the room. Finding ways to do this without appearing rude or insensitive can be challenging. The medical assistant will find it helpful to follow these steps in interviewing such a patient:

1. *Set clear expectations* of the interview. For example, the medical assistant might tell a patient, "Mrs. Singh, I'd like to ask you a few questions about your menstrual history."
2. *Ask closed questions* to gather very specific data, as necessary, by asking questions that typically require a one-word answer. For example, the medical assistant might ask the patient, "How old were you when you first began having menstrual periods?"
3. *Restate the message* in order to verify accurate understanding of key information and allow the patient to confirm or correct it. For example, the medical assistant may say to the patient, "You were 13 years old when you began menstruating."
4. *Redirect* the patient in a kind, yet assertive manner if she wanders too far off the subject. This technique is most effective if followed up by a closed question or a directive statement. For example, the medical assistant might say, "I'd like to hear more about your menstrual pattern. How many days does each menstrual period usually last?" or, "I'd like to hear more about your menstrual discomfort. Please describe the pain you said you typically have."

Quiet Patient

The quiet patient is one who may be withdrawn or shy. Such a patient typically talks very little, providing one- or two-word answers that reveal little detail. When interviewing such a patient, the medical assistant should use these techniques:

- *Use open-ended questions*, which require (or encourage) more elaborate answers.
- *Practice wording questions ahead of time.* Most people find open-ended questions difficult to phrase. Therefore, medical assistants should practice wording open-ended questions ahead of time.
- *Use directive statements*, rather than questions. Such statements allow the medical assistant to direct the conversation to relevant subjects and prompt the patient to disclose information.

All three techniques described may be effective or ineffective, depending on how they are used. Therefore, the medical assistant should become familiar with the advantages and potential disadvantages of each in order to use them most effectively. (See *Using interviewing techniques effectively*, page 310.)

In addition, a patient who is quiet or shy may be much more willing to share questions and concerns in writing. Providing the patient with a self-assessment tool before the patient interview allows him to approach these subjects in a less embarrassing way. The medical assistant or physician can then follow up on the subjects in the interview, as appropriate. (See *Self-assessment questionnaire*, page 310, and *Self-assessment of needs*, page 310.)

Using interviewing techniques effectively

This table lists three common interviewing techniques with advantages and disadvantages of each.

Technique	Example	Advantage	Disadvantage
Closed question	• "Would you mind telling me about your health history?" • "Do you have pain?" • "How are you today?"	• Helps get specific information from overly talkative patients. • Saves time when the medical assistant is extremely busy.	• May be answered with "no," which becomes a barrier to further communication. • May be answered simply with "yes" or another one-word answer, such as "fine" or "terrible," which requires further questioning.
Open-ended question	• "What brings you here today?" • "Why don't you describe your pain?" • "Why are you here today?"	• Discourages patient from providing one-word answers when elaboration is desired. • Allows patient to discuss issues of personal concern.	• May entice the overly talkative patient to tell lengthy stories or get sidetracked. • May not elicit the specific information desired.
Directive statement	• "Tell me about your current problem." • "Describe the pain you are having." • "Tell me how you've been feeling."	• Easier to phrase than open-ended questions. • Allows the interviewer to focus on specific areas of concern. • Discourages one-word answers.	• Can seem like a command unless worded carefully and spoken tactfully.

Front office–Back office connection

Self-Assessment Questionnaire

In some medical offices, the administrative medical assistant will ask a patient to complete a questionnaire while he is waiting in the reception area. Doing so can save the clinical medical assistant some time during the interview process. It may also provide a more comfortable way for patients to discuss personal topics such as sexual function. Questions asked on such questionnaires vary with the medical specialty area; however, here are some common examples:

• What is the main problem that brings you to the clinic?

• What do you think might be causing your current physical problem?

• Where have you traveled in the past 2 years and when?

• Are stress or conflict common in your household?

• Do you fear being harmed in your own home?

• Are you experiencing sexual problems or a change in sex drive?

• Do you enjoy your work?

• Do you frequently feel depressed or anxious?

• Have you seriously thought about suicide?

Patient Education

Self-Assessment of Needs

The medical assistant or office manager should consider adding questions to the self-assessment questionnaire that can help the patient identify his goals for the visit and his own learning needs. Doing so can help the medical assistant and physician understand the patient's expectations and learning needs and how to direct patient education efforts. Having patients answer such questions in writing also gives the medical assistant clues about the patient's reading and writing ability. Such questions might include:

• What do you hope to accomplish on this visit?

• What do you most want the physician to know?

• What do you most wish to know and understand about your condition, disease, or disorder?

• What is your greatest fear regarding your condition, disease, or disorder?

Obstacles to Effective Interviewing

When communicating with patients, the medical assistant must be thoughtful and deliberate in word choice and body language. Doing so requires a degree of focus and concentration not normally used in everyday conversation with family and friends. If she is not careful, the medical assistant may unintentionally lapse into ineffective communication patterns. If she is not always mindful in her communications with patients, the medical assistant could convey the wrong message to the patient and, perhaps worse, break the law. In order to avoid obstacles to good communication with patients, the medical assistant should become familiar with such obstacles and develop skills to avoid them. Common obstacles include:

- offering opinions and advice
- offering false reassurance
- using technical language
- talking too much
- asking judgmental questions.

Offering Opinions and Advice

The medical assistant should always refrain from offering opinions or medical advice. The medical assistant who offers opinions and advice to patients risks acting outside of her scope of practice, putting herself in legal jeopardy. Furthermore, doing so takes the responsibility for decision making away from the patient. Instead, she should try to answer the question with a question, such as asking the patient what he thinks is a reasonable course of action, based on the information provided by the physician. Additionally, she might inquire whether the patient needs more information before making a decision. The medical assistant may also need to refer the patient back to the physician for answers to some questions.

Offering False Reassurance

The desire to provide reassurance is natural, but doing so could convey an inaccurate message that the patient may later resent. As much as patients wish for reassurance, they also need and deserve honesty. Responding in any other manner invalidates and trivializes the patient's concerns. The medical assistant must also remember that only the physician may reveal certain information to patients, such as a diagnosis or prognosis. Instead of offering false reassurance, the medical assistant should use reflection to acknowledge and validate the patient's concerns and feelings. When she feels compelled to provide some reassurance, she should make statements that are honest, yet vague. For example, instead of saying, "I'm sure everything will turn out just fine," the medical assistant might say, "We will do

everything in our power to provide you with the best care possible."

Using Technical Language

Using **medical jargon,** which is technical or specialized language used mainly by medical professionals, tends to add to the patient's confusion and anxiety, especially if he has a perceptual deficit or is not a native English speaker. In such a case, the patient may not understand what has been said but may feel too embarrassed to admit it. When speaking with patients, the medical assistant should keep language and vocabulary professional and appropriate. However, she should also choose terms easily understood by the average **layperson** (nonmedical person). (See *Good interviewing is a team effort,* page 312.)

Talking Too Much

The overly talkative medical assistant risks offending patients and robs them of the opportunity to discuss their concerns. The medical assistant should remember that effective communication happens when she talks little and listens much. In addition, allowing silent pauses encourages the reluctant patient to share concerns.

Asking Judgmental Questions

Questions should be worded as neutrally as possible. Poorly worded questions may imply a negative judgment and discourage the patient from providing a truthful, accurate response. The medical assistant should practice ways to word delicate questions so she can feel more comfortable asking them and convey a message of acceptance. Doing so will encourage patients to be more forthcoming about such information. For example, a judgmental question might be, "You don't drink alcohol do you?" or, "Do you drink alcohol?" A more neutral alternative is, "How much alcohol do you drink during an average week?" Of course, some people do not drink alcohol at all; however, if so, they will simply say so. If the patient does drink alcohol, he will feel more inclined to give an honest, accurate answer if asked in a nonjudgmental way.

Discussing Sensitive Topics

When interviewing a patient to obtain the medical history, the medical assistant must commonly ask questions about personal subjects, such as sexual activity, use of birth control, number of sexual partners, bowel and bladder function, and menstrual pattern. While some patients are not shy about discussing such subjects, many find such conversations uncomfortable or embarrassing. There are several strategies the medical assistant can employ to help ease the patient's discomfort and promote more effective communication:

- *Consider the environment.* Before beginning the interview, the medical assistant must give due consideration to such

Front office–back office connection

Good Interviewing Is a Team Effort

Administrative and clinical medical assistants must work stogether to accomplish the patient interview in an effective manner. Here are some examples of the contribution each person can make.

Administrative medical assistant

- Verify demographic information when the patient checks in, including current address, phone number, employer, and insurance.

- Notice whether the patient has language, perceptual, or sensory deficits or other issues that might hinder the interviewing process. Let the clinical medical assistant know immediately and discreetly to allow her time to plan success strategies.

- Give the patient a self-assessment questionnaire to complete prior to the interview and note whether the patient has difficulty completing it or if anyone else helps with it.

- Check in with the clinical medical assistant discreetly to see if a patient and an accompanying individual might need to be separated for part of the interview and work out a cooperative plan to accomplish doing so.

Clinical medical assistant

- Quickly glance at the updated demographic data gathered by the administrative medical assistant to identify clues to significant changes in the patient's home situation (such as a change of occupation or loss of insurance). Tactfully follow up on these changes during the interview as appropriate.

- Communicate special requests (such as asking the administrative medical assistant to keep parents occupied while you interview their teenage daughter) in a timely, respectful manner.

- Convey appreciation to the administrative medical assistant for any cues or help offered to foster mutual respect and team spirit.

---

environmental issues as privacy and patient comfort. Also, reminding the patient that all information will be kept in strict confidence will reassure the patient.

- *Establish guidelines.* After introducing herself, the medical assistant should establish the guidelines of the interview so that the patient understands the nature and purpose of the questions the medical assistant will ask. If the patient seems hesitant to answer questions, the medical assistant should explain why such information is important in providing a complete health picture.

- *Begin with general questions.* The medical assistant should begin with general questions and save more personal questions for later in the interview when some degree of trust and **rapport** (the development of an empathetic relationship) has been established. If a patient refuses to answer a question, the medical assistant should not press the matter but leave it for the physician to pursue. (See *Looking for clues.*)

Age-Appropriate Communication

In order to interview a patient effectively, the medical assistant must adapt her vocabulary and interviewing strategies to the age of the patient. Techniques for interviewing a toddler will differ from those for interviewing a teenager. Both will differ from techniques for interviewing an elderly person. Age-appropriate interviewing techniques include:

Patient Education

Looking for Clues

A professional medical assistant acts as a sort of health care detective. Throughout the patient interview, she gathers data about the patient's current health practices and concerns. She must get into the habit of noticing clues the patient offers that may signal a potential learning need. The medical assistant can address simple topics right away. For example, if a patient asks what the normal range is for blood pressure measurement, the medical assistant can share that data. However, she may need to refer more complex topics to the physician (or even another provider). The medical assistant should make a special note about the patient's significant learning needs and be sure to bring them to the physician's attention.

- Children
  - Drop to the child's level or sit at eye level in order to make eye contact without looking down on the child.
  - Speak at a normal volume.
  - Use a kind, yet firm tone.

- Provide a simple explanation of procedures before doing them.
- Use simple, age-appropriate language.
- Let the child remain on the parent's lap, if desired.
- Offer limited choices when possible but do not ask the child if he or she wants to do something that is not optional (such as get an injection).
- Offer praise and positive reinforcement whenever possible.
- Include the child in the conversation and direct some simple questions to the child so that she feels included.
- Allow the child to touch some of the equipment, such as a stethoscope, to help to alleviate anxiety about it.
- Save uncomfortable procedures for last.
- Be truthful about uncomfortable procedures (such as injections) but err on the side of understating rather than exaggerating the truth. (Children are unlikely to forgive or forget being lied to.)

- Older children and adolescents
  - Use age-appropriate language and vocabulary.
  - Offer choices whenever possible.
  - Take extra care to provide for privacy, because patients in this age group are acutely self-conscious about their bodies.
  - Explain procedures prior to doing them.
  - Explain findings.
  - Assure the patient of his normalcy.
  - Allow the patient to ask questions and answer them as completely and honestly as possible.
  - Take advantage of opportunities to teach the patient about relevant health and wellness issues as well as disease prevention or management.

- Elderly patients
  - Be aware of and adapt communication techniques for any sensory or perceptual deficits, such as diminished hearing or vision.
  - Allow elderly patients time to process information and formulate responses.
  - Do not assume that all elderly patients are hard of hearing, forgetful, or senile.
  - Convey respect and address the patient by his last name (such as *Mr. Pederson*) unless specifically requested by the patient to do otherwise. (See Figure 20-1.)

Additional strategies for effectively providing care for pediatric and geriatric patients is addressed in depth in Chapter 33, "Pediatrics," on page 641, and Chapter 35, "Geriatrics," on page 707.

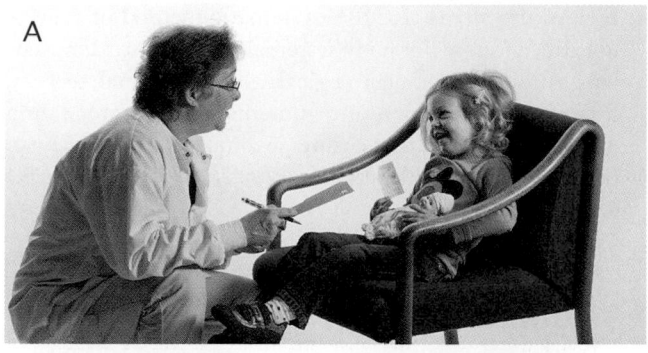

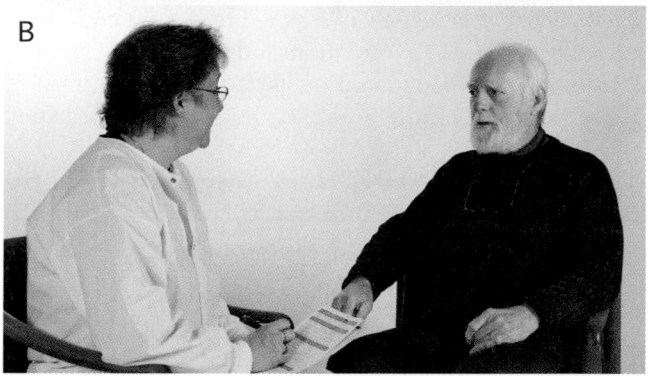

FIG 20-1 Age-appropriate interviewing techniques. (A) Interviewing a child. (B) Interviewing an elderly person.

Medical History

The initial patient interview is usually conducted to obtain a detailed medical history. In some cases, the physician will conduct this entire interview. In other cases, the medical assistant may be responsible for conducting part of it. The standard medical history includes:

- **database**—logistical data, such as the patient's name, address, date of birth (DOB), and insurance coverage; initial physical examination findings; and initial laboratory test results
- **past medical history** (PMH)—immunizations, allergies, prior surgeries (sometimes listed separately as prior surgical history [PSH]), past or current disorders and diseases, and traumatic injuries
- **family history** (FH)—health information about parents, siblings, and children, which may provide clues about the patient's risk factors and emotional support system. (If parents are deceased, the medical assistant should record their ages at time of death and cause of death.)
- **social history** (SH)—patient's occupation, hobbies, lifestyle, education, activity level, sleep habits, sexual activities, dietary practices, and use of tobacco, alcohol, and illicit drugs

- **review of systems** (ROS)—systematic method of collecting data about major body systems, including cardiovascular, gastrointestinal, neurological, musculoskeletal, urinary, reproductive, sensory, integumentary, respiratory, and endocrine systems, that ensures a comprehensive review of the patient's overall health. (See *Procedure 20-1: Obtaining a medical history.*)

Documentation

The patient's chart serves as a record of the patient's medical history as well as a place for recording ongoing care. The chart is also a communication tool because a variety of providers, including the primary care physician, consulting physician specialists, nurses, therapists, and medical assistants, will all read and contribute to parts of it. The patient's chart also serves as a legal document because it is the official record of all care provided as well as the patient's response to such care. Because the patient's chart serves these important purposes, all entries in the chart must be thorough, legible, and professional. (See *Charting do's and don'ts.*)

Documentation Types

There are several methods of documentation commonly used by health care providers. Traditionally, physicians dictate entries that are subsequently typed by a transcriptionist and then entered into the chart. Many health care providers still use this method. However, with the increasing popularity of electronic health records (EHR), more health care

---

PROCEDURE 20-1

Obtaining a medical history

Task
Interview a patient to obtain a medical history.

Conditions
- Patient history form
- Black and red ink pens
- Clipboard
- Private area to conduct the interview

Standards
In the time specified and within the scoring parameters determined by the instructor, the student will successfully conduct a patient interview to obtain the patient's health history.

Performance Standards
1. Wash or sanitize your hands to ensure infection control and assemble supplies.
2. Greet and identify the patient by his last name to convey respect. Use a pleasant, professional manner and introduce yourself to put the patient at ease.
3. Guide the patient to a private, quiet, comfortable area to ensure privacy. Explain the purpose and nature of the interview to help patient understand why certain information is requested.
4. Gather medical information to complete the history form using therapeutic communication techniques to put patient at ease, develop trust and rapport, and facilitate information gathering.
5. Review the self-history section if one was completed to clarify patient responses.
6. Throughout the interview, explain or translate any medical terms the patient does not understand to enhance patient understanding and accuracy of responses.

7. Allow the patient adequate time to answer each question. Some patients need extra time to process questions and formulate responses.
8. Record the patient's allergies in red ink so that this critical safety information is easily visible.
9. Speak in a pleasant, unhurried manner using adequate volume and enunciation to enhance the patient's understanding.
10. Use culturally appropriate body language to convey respect and facilitate communication.
11. Repeat the patient's answers as needed for clarification or confirmation to ensure the accuracy of the communication.
12. Write legibly in black ink, which is less likely to fade and will photocopy better when records must be copied.
13. Document all data accurately and objectively in measurable terms to ensure accuracy and legal defensibility.
14. If more explanation is needed than the space on the form allows, mark it with an asterisk (*) and write an explanation in the "comments" section to allow inclusion of significant details.
15. Thank the patient to convey respect and explain the next step in the examination to help the patient feel less anxious.
16. Invite the patient to use the restroom (and collect a specimen if appropriate) before the examination to promote patient comfort during the examination.

Charting do's and don'ts

All members of the health care team should be aware of these common charting do's and don'ts.

Do

- Identify all documents with patient name and account number.
- Record data on the correct forms.
- Write legibly and spell correctly.
- Use black ink.
- Sign and date all entries.
- Include appropriate credentials after the signature (such as CMA, LPN, RN, and so forth).
- Use only abbreviations and symbols approved by the facility.
- Keep a current list of medications used by the patient (including prescription medications, over-the-counter preparations, and nutritional supplements) in the front of the chart.
- Indicate the patient's own words or statements by using quotation marks.
- Record data in a factual, accurate, nonjudgmental manner. Strategies for doing so include quoting the patient's description of symptoms and quantifying measurable factors by using a pain scale and descriptive adjectives, such as red, pale, warm, cool, and so forth.
- Use correct medical terminology, rather than layman's terms (such as *sutures*, rather than *stitches*).

- Correct errors by drawing one line through the erroneous entry, writing the date and time and a brief explanation, signing the correction, and then writing in the correct entry.

Date	
01/30/09: 9:15 a.m.	~~Pt c/o pain 7/10. in low back described as "sharp & intense."~~ ~~Administered 2 Vicodin per MD order~~ ~~————————————— S. Gonzalez, CMA~~ Wrong chart. ————— S. Gonzalez, CMA. 0915. 01/30/09

- Identify any information added at a later time as a "Late Entry" with the *current* date and time indicated.

Don't

- Do not chart in pencil.
- Do not obliterate errors in any manner (such as erasing or using correction fluid). The erroneous entry must remain legible.
- Do not go back at a later time and add information in a manner that attempts to conceal the fact of the time discrepancy.
- Do not make up new abbreviations or symbols or use any that are not approved by the facility.
- Do not chart subjective assumptions or opinions—for example, "The patient was angry and irrational." Instead, chart the objective data that led to that assumption—for example, "Patient shouted and swore at his wife and left the room before the examination was completed."

---

providers are using computers to enter their own notes directly into the patient's medical record. Regardless of whether a health care provider performs documentation using transcription, handwritten notes, or a computer, a medical practice will usually follow a common documentation system. Two of the most common documentation systems used are:

- source-oriented
- problem-oriented.

Source-oriented

The **source-oriented medical record (SOMR)** is a traditional method of documentation that includes a note for each patient visit. The notes are arranged in reverse chronological order, with the most recent visit first. The advantage of this system is that it tells the patient's "story" in the order in which it occurred. The disadvantage of this system is the

extensive amount of time required to search through the chart and locate specific data.

Problem-oriented

The **problem-oriented medical record (POMR)** is a more efficient system of documentation that organizes data in a logical manner intended to identify, clarify, and resolve problems. The four key parts of the POMR system include:

- *database*—the patient's medical history, laboratory and diagnostic test results, and physical examination findings
- *problem list*—the patient's problems listed individually with an assigned number
- *plan*—current findings with a description of the current treatment plan
- *progress notes*—notes about each identified problem with a summary of the patient's complaints, current condition, and responses to treatment provided

SOAP or SOAPE

In the problem-oriented medical record, progress notes are written using the SOAP or SOAPE method. This **acronym** stands for:

- *s*ubjective
- *o*bjective
- *a*ssessment
- *p*lan of care
- *e*valuation (added for the SOAPE method).

Subjective

The *subjective* part of the SOAP method is information that is known only by the patient and that the patient must share with the health care team for them to be aware of it. Examples of subjective data include description of pain, nausea, and emotional distress. In order to make the subjectivity of such data clear in the written record, the medical assistant should include the patient's own words enclosed within quotation marks or include such words as *the patient reports* or *the patient stated.*

Objective

The *objective* part of the SOAP method is data obtained through the observations of the health care provider. The medical assistant recording such data should record it as accurately as possible using quantitative terms. Examples of objective data include physical examination findings, weight, vital signs, and test results. (See *Subjective versus objective data*)

Assessment

The *assessment* part of SOAP is the physician's conclusion about the patient's condition, or the diagnosis. In some cases, the diagnosis is not yet certain. In such cases, the physician may indicate this by listing the most likely diagnoses. For example, if the physician suspects either angina or gastroesophageal reflux disease (GERD) as the patient's diagnosis, she must document it as *angina vs. GERD.*

When a diagnosis remains unconfirmed, the physician may list the patient's primary symptom with the goal to rule out (R/O) the most life-threatening diagnosis related to that symptom. If that diagnosis is ruled out, then the physician will investigate other possible causes next. To document such an instance, the physician must indicate the symptom and the diagnosis to rule out—for example, for a symptom of chest pain, the physician will first attempt to rule out a myocardial infarction (MI) by documenting *chest pain, R/O MI.*

Plan of care

The *plan of care* section of SOAP is where the physician describes how the patient's health problem will be further evaluated and treated. The plan may include further diagnostic studies, laboratory tests, medications, and treatments as well as surgery or other therapies and patient education.

Evaluation

The added element of *evaluation* creates the SOAPE method. Evaluation describes the patient's understanding of the overall plan as well as his compliance with it. Not all medical practices add the evaluation part.

Chapter Summary

- The medical assistant plays an important role in connecting the patient and physician. In this regard, the medical assistant may help with the patient interview.
- Interview techniques should be modified as needed for the individual situation in order to obtain complete, relevant information in a timely manner.
- Communication techniques include closed questions, restating, redirecting, open-ended questions, and directive statements.
- Establishing guidelines sets clear expectations of the interview.
- Medical assistants must be aware of potential obstacles to effective interviewing, including offering advice, providing false reassurance, using medical jargon, being too talkative, and implying judgment.
- The medical assistant can employ certain strategies to ease a patient's discomfort when discussing sensitive topics, including providing privacy and comfort, explaining the purpose and nature of the interview, and assuring the patient that all information will be kept confidential.
- The medical assistant must adapt vocabulary and interviewing strategies to the age of the patient.
- The patient's medical history typically includes the database, past medical history, family history, social history, and a review of systems.
- The patient's chart serves as a record of the patient's medical history, a communication tool, and a legal document.
- With the increasing popularity of electronic health records (EHR), more health care providers are using computers to enter their own notes directly into the patient's medical record.

Subjective vs. objective data

Here is a handy tip to help you remember the difference between subjective and objective data:
Subjective data is what the patient **s**ays.
Objective data is what you **o**bserve.

- Types of documentation commonly used by health care providers include source-oriented medical records and problem-oriented medical records.
- Progress notes are written using the SOAP or SOAPE method, which includes subjective data, objective data, assessment, plan of care and, sometimes, evaluation.

Team Work Exercises

1. Working in groups of four or five, students should create posters that illustrate the various parts of the medical record and the purpose and nature of each, including the database, past medical history, family history, social history, and review of systems.
2. Working in groups of four or five, students should create posters that illustrate the various parts of SOAPE documentation, listing examples of the type of data contained in each, including subjective data, objective data, assessment, plan of care, and evaluation.

Case Studies

1. Melinda Cross is a 22-year-old patient who has come to the clinic for the first time to establish care. She is quiet and shy and reluctant to disclose personal information. Her current chief complaint is pelvic discomfort and dysuria. The medical assistant must obtain a complete health history, including information about sexual activity, birth control, menstrual pattern, and current symptoms. List and describe strategies the medical assistant might employ to put this patient at ease and obtain the necessary data.
2. Gloria Sherman is a 69-year-old patient visiting the clinic for her annual checkup. She is a friendly, talkative woman who loves to tell stories and gets easily sidetracked. She has multiple medical complaints and is eager to discuss them all at great length. The medical assistant must obtain a complete health history, including information about Mrs. Sherman's current complaints in a time-effective manner. List and describe strategies the medical assistant might employ to keep this patient on track.

Resources

- Miller, W.R., and Rollnick, S.: *Motivational Interviewing: Preparing People for Change,* 2nd ed. New York: Guilford Press, 2002.
- Simulated patient encounters: *medicus.marshall.edu*
- Tips for interviewing children: *www.casanet.org/library/ advocacy/interviewing.htm* and *www.kidscounsel.org/ interviewing child client.pdf*

Vital Signs

Learning Objectives

Upon completion of this chapter, the student will be able to:

- define and spell the key terms in the glossary
- list normal values for temperature, pulse, respiration, blood pressure, and pulse oximetry
- describe variables that might affect temperature, pulse, respiration, blood pressure, and pulse oximeter readings
- discuss potential causes of fever and list common symptoms
- describe the three common fever patterns
- cite four types of thermometers and demonstrate how to measure a patient's temperature with each
- list common factors that can affect pulse rate, rhythm, and strength
- locate and identify the major pulse sites on the human body
- differentiate between internal and external respiration
- discuss the three key characteristics of respiration
- differentiate between systolic and diastolic blood pressure
- list and describe factors that commonly impact blood pressure
- cite risk factors for hypertension and identify which are modifiable
- describe the five types of sounds commonly heard when obtaining a blood pressure measurement and discuss the significance of each
- explain how a pulse oximeter measures blood oxygen levels

- list several factors that might interfere with an accurate pulse oximeter reading
- demonstrate several trouble-shooting techniques when obtaining the arterial oxygen saturation (SpO_2) measurement.

CAAHEP Competencies

Clinical Competencies

Patient Care

Obtain vital signs

ABHES Competencies

Clinical Duties

Take vital signs

Procedures

Measuring oral temperature using a digital thermometer

Measuring axillary temperature using a digital thermometer

Measuring rectal temperature using a digital thermometer

Measuring temperature using a tympanic thermometer

Measuring temperature using a temporal thermometer

Measuring radial pulse and respirations

Measuring apical heart rate

Measuring blood pressure

Measuring oxygen saturation using a pulse oximeter

Chapter Outline

Vital Signs Proficiency
Temperature
  Fever
  Thermometer Types and Uses
    Glass thermometer
    Digital thermometer
    Tympanic thermometer
    Chemical thermometers
    Temporal thermometer
  Disinfecting Thermometers
  Celsius versus Fahrenheit
Pulse
  Pulse Sites
    Temporal
    Carotid
    Brachial
    Radial
    Apical
    Femoral
    Popliteal
    Dorsalis pedis
    Posterior tibialis
Respiration
  Characteristics of Respiration
    Rate
    Rhythm
    Depth
Blood Pressure
  Evaluating Blood Pressure
    Korotkoff sounds
    Postural vital signs
Oxygen Saturation
Chapter Summary
Team Work Exercises
Case Studies
Resources

Key Terms

apnea
Temporary absence of breathing

auscultatory gap
Disappearance of tapping sounds during phase II of a blood pressure measurement

bradypnea
Abnormally slow breathing

core temperature
Temperature within the body's deep internal structures

diastolic pressure
Blood pressure between heart contractions

diurnal rhythm
Normal daily cyclic fluctuation in body temperature

dyspnea
Labored or difficult breathing

expiration
The act of exhaling

external respiration
Movement of air into and out of the lungs

homeostasis
State of equilibrium in the body

hyperventilation
Increased ventilation resulting in a higher blood pH

inspiration
The act of inhaling

Korotkoff sounds
Sounds heard when auscultating blood pressure

point of maximal impulse
Point on the chest wall at which cardiac contractions are best seen or felt

postural vital signs
Vital signs performed to test for orthostatic hypotension

pulse deficit
Difference between the apical pulse and radial pulse

pulse pressure
Difference between systolic and diastolic pressures

sleep apnea
Temporary cessation of breathing during sleep

sphygmomanometer
Blood pressure cuff

systolic pressure
Tension exerted against arterial walls during ventricular contraction and represented by the top number in a blood pressure reading

tachycardia
Abnormally rapid heart rate

tachypnea
Abnormally rapid breathing

Vital Signs Proficiency

Measurement of vital signs (VS) is among the most common procedures medical assistants perform on a daily basis. Such routine, yet very important measurements provide valuable information about a patient's health status. Thus, a medical assistant must become proficient in vital signs measurement. Furthermore, a medical assistant should maintain proficiency, regardless of her chosen specialty, so she can help out whenever needed by obtaining an accurate set of vital signs (See *Stat vital signs.*) Vital signs include temperature, pulse, respiration, blood pressure, and oxygen saturation.

Temperature

Body temperature (T) is an indicator of health and disease. It is regulated by the hypothalamus in the brain and is an important part of **homeostasis**, or the state of dynamic equilibrium in the body. However, a number of physiologic factors can impact temperature. As much as 85% of body heat is lost through the skin. The rest is lost through the lungs and excretions of the bowel and bladder. The body creates heat energy as a by-product of metabolism and exercise. Body temperature also increases temporarily in response to infection, dehydration, hormonal fluctuations, and exposure to a warm environment. Conversely, body temperature decreases slightly with exposure to a cold environment and in elderly patients. It may also be decreased in patients with hypothyroidism or those who have suffered traumatic injury.

Normal body temperature varies with the time of day and the site of measurement. **Core temperature** is the tempera-

 Front office–Back office connection

Stat Vital Signs

Measuring vital signs is one of the most basic yet most important jobs of the medical assistant. Therefore, regardless of whether a medical assistant ends up working in the clinical or administrative setting, she must make the commitment to maintain proficiency in this skill. Doing so will be appreciated by others during times of short staffing or an emergency. During an emergency or urgent situation, the administrative medical assistant will be able to help out by getting a quick set of vital signs, including an oximeter reading. By doing so, she will help to establish critical patient baseline information quickly and free up the clinical medical assistant for more complex clinical tasks, such as performing a stat ECG or administering medications.

ture within the body's deep internal structures, such as the bladder and heart. Core temperature is slightly higher than peripheral body temperature taken in the mouth or axilla. In general, normal body temperature of a healthy individual fluctuates 1° or 2°F between 97.5° and 99.5°F (36.4° to 37.3°C) and averages 98.6°F (37°C). However, some persons, especially elderly persons, may have an average temperature as low as 96.8°F. Body temperature also follows a cyclic fluctuation called the **diurnal rhythm,** which causes body temperature to be lower in the morning and higher in the late afternoon. (See *Factors that affect body temperature.*)

Fever

Fever, sometimes called *pyrexia,* is not an illness itself but is a common symptom of illness caused by bacterial or viral infection. Other causes of fever include tumors, the breakdown of necrotic (decaying) tissue, central nervous system (CNS) damage, and certain diseases. Depending on the cause and severity of a fever, the physician may elect to refrain from treating it because an increase in body temperature is thought to be a natural response designed to inhibit the growth of some bacteria and viruses. Even so, febrile (fever) illness in infants under 3 months of age is evaluated carefully because it may indicate a serious condition.

Onset of fever may be rapid or slow. The patient may exhibit chills and an increased pulse and respiratory rate that continues. The patient feels warm to the touch and may complain of thirst, anorexia (loss of appetite), headache, and malaise (feelings of discomfort, weakness, and fatigue). The fever may subside slowly or suddenly and the patient may experience diaphoresis (profuse sweating). This change is known as the *crisis,* but is commonly described by the layperson as the fever "breaking." During the course of the fever, body temperature fluctuates according to one of three pattern types:

- continuous
- intermittent
- remittent. (See *Fever patterns,* page 322.)

Factors that affect body temperature

A number of factors impact body temperature, including:

- *external environment,* such as heat, humidity, cold, and wind

- *age,* as in elderly persons, who commonly have body temperatures that are 1° to 2°F lower than the average 96.8°F for most persons (due in part to a slower metabolism in elderly persons)

- *infection or illness* (elevated temperature, or *fever*).

Thermometer Types and Uses

Body temperature is measured with a thermometer. There are several different types of thermometers available. (See Figure 21-1.) Each has advantages and disadvantages. Most are available in the medical office and are also available for purchase in most drugstores and some grocery stores. Some electronic versions allow medical assistants the option of measuring in Fahrenheit or Celsius. The best choice of thermometer depends on a number of variables, including the patient's age, condition, level of consciousness, and ability to cooperate, as well as on facility policy. Regardless of the type of thermometer used, the medical assistant must be familiar with the function and care of each type.

Glass Thermometer

Glass thermometers are no longer used in the medical office. However, many patients still keep and use them at home. Because the older mercury thermometers have been deemed unsafe, medical assistants should advise patients to properly dispose of them. (See *Mercury thermometer disposal,* page 323.) There are mercury-free glass thermometers available that function in a similar way to the older types. These thermometers contain a nontoxic silver or red-colored fluid. They do not require a battery and come in oral and rectal versions. Some are available with magnifying optical cases, which make them easier to read. Many also have dual scales, allowing the patient to read the temperature in Fahrenheit or Celsius. Medical assistants should be familiar with the proper use of glass thermometers because some patients may own them and may need instruction in their use.

Digital Thermometer

Digital thermometers are battery operated and portable and can obtain a temperature reading in a minute or less. The temperature is displayed on a light-emitting diode (LED)

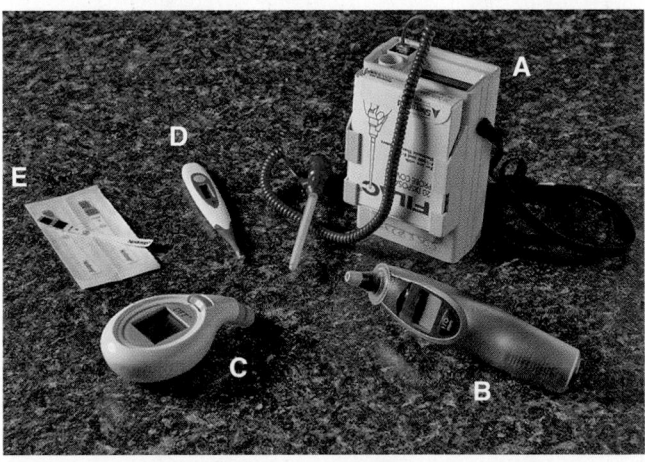

FIG 21-1 Types of thermometers. (A) Oral (or rectal) digital. (B) Tympanic. (C) Temporal. (D) Rectal. (E) Disposable.

Fever patterns

This table lists fever patterns along with a description of each.

Pattern	Description
Continuous	Fever that fluctuates slightly yet remains consistently above normal

Pattern	Description
Intermittent	Fever that fluctuates widely between relatively high levels to normal or even subnormal levels

Pattern	Description
Remittent	Fever that fluctuates widely, yet remains above normal until it finally resolves

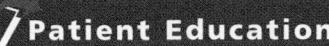

Patient Education

Mercury Thermometer Disposal

Because of the health hazards associated with mercury, thermometers that contain this heavy metal are no longer recommended for use in body temperature measurement. The medical assistant should check with patients regarding the type of thermometer they use at home. If a patient uses a mercury thermometer, the medical assistant should instruct the patient on the proper methods for disposing of this toxic substance, including these guidelines:

- Never throw a mercury thermometer in the garbage because the mercury will eventually make its way into the environment and impact animals and humans.

- Instead, call a household hazardous waste collection facility. Most municipalities conduct periodic collections of household hazardous waste. Contact the local municipal waste disposal organization for more information.

- Mercury poisoning can occur by ingestion, inhalation, or even through skin exposure. It affects the central nervous system, kidneys, and liver and causes alterations in sensation, taste, and movement. It also causes vision disturbances, stupor, and even coma.

- In pregnant women, mercury crosses the placenta and affects fetal development. Children subjected to mercury poisoning show lowered intelligence, poor muscle coordination, and impaired hearing.

- Persons concerned about possible mercury poisoning should contact the regional poison control center; state, county, or local health department; the Agency for Toxic Substances and Disease Registry (ATSDR); or their physician for advice.

---

screen. Some types come with oral and rectal probes. (See *Procedure 21-1: Measuring oral temperature using a digital thermometer*, page 324.) A disposable cover, or sheath, fits over the probe for sanitary use and makes cleaning between patients unnecessary. A digital thermometer may also be used to measure oral, axillary, or rectal temperature. (See *Procedure 21-2: Measuring axillary temperature using a digital thermometer*, page 325.)

The medical assistant should avoid taking the patient's temperature rectally if other reliable means are available. There is potential for rectal trauma if the procedure is not performed carefully, as well as potential embarrassment to the patient. However, rectal temperature readings are considered among the most accurate because the rectum is a highly vascular, closed cavity. The medical assistant may use this route for infants, small children, patients who are unconscious, or those for whom other temperature routes are deemed unreliable. When measuring the patient's temperature rectally, the medical assistant must take measures to ensure privacy and careful positioning. In addition, she must be sure to document that she took the temperature rectally, because rectal temperature readings are generally 1°F higher than those taken by other routes. (See *Procedure 21-3: Measuring rectal temperature using a digital thermometer*, page 326.)

Tympanic Thermometer

A tympanic thermometer, also called an *aural thermometer*, is a small, handheld device with a tympanic probe that fits into the outer part of the ear canal. It is covered with a disposable sheath for sanitary use, which makes cleaning between

patients unnecessary. The tympanic thermometer provides a reading in under 2 seconds. The tympanic thermometer records the temperature of the tympanic membrane, which is protected inside the ear canal. This type of thermometer is used when taking an oral temperature is not possible or practical, such as with a small child or after a patient has just had something hot or cold to drink. However, the medical assistant must take care to use proper technique in order to obtain accurate results, including making sure that the thermometer fits snugly into the ear canal and is pointed slightly forward toward the tympanic membrane. (See *Procedure 21-4: Measuring temperature using a tympanic thermometer*, page 327.)

Chemical Thermometers

Chemical thermometers come in disposable and reusable versions. They contain a heat-sensitive substance that changes color when exposed to body heat. Although not as accurate as other types of thermometers, they are convenient for home use. Disposable, single-use thermometers are placed under the tongue for the designated time (usually 60 seconds) and then read according to the number of small dots that have changed color. Temperature strips may be pressed onto the forehead and read when the colors stop changing (usually 15 seconds). They are especially convenient for the worried parent who wishes to check the fever of a sleeping child.

Temporal Thermometer

The temporal thermometer is a newer type of thermometer. It allows a fast, noninvasive method of taking a temperature

(Text continues on page 328)

PROCEDURE 21-1

Measuring oral temperature using a digital thermometer

Task

Measure oral body temperature using a digital thermometer.

Conditions

- Digital thermometer
- Oral probe
- Probe cover
- Waste container
- Pen
- Patient's medical record

Standards

In the time specified and within the scoring parameters determined by the instructor, the student will successfully measure and record a patient's oral temperature using a digital thermometer.

Performance Standards

1. Wash or sanitize your hands to ensure infection control and assemble supplies.

2. Prepare the oral probe for use according to the manufacturer's directions to prevent errors and ensure accuracy.

3. Greet and identify your patient and introduce yourself. Explain the procedure and ask if the patient has smoked, exercised, or had anything to eat or drink within the past 30 minutes. These activities can affect the accuracy of the temperature measurement.

4. Apply the disposable probe cover, making sure it locks into place to ensure infection control and activate the thermometer.

5. Place the probe under patient's tongue in the pocket on either side of the frenulum linguae to access the warmest part of the mouth.

6. Instruct the patient to close her mouth. Continue holding the end of the probe to keep it in the proper position.

7. Remove the probe after the thermometer beeps and read the number on the digital display screen. Eject the probe cover into the waste container by pressing the ejection button and without touching the probe cover to prevent transfer of microorganisms.

8. Return the probe to its storage position in the thermometer unit to turn off and reset the thermometer and return the thermometer to its base to ensure easy access for future use.

9. Wash or sanitize your hands and disinfect equipment if indicated to ensure infection control.

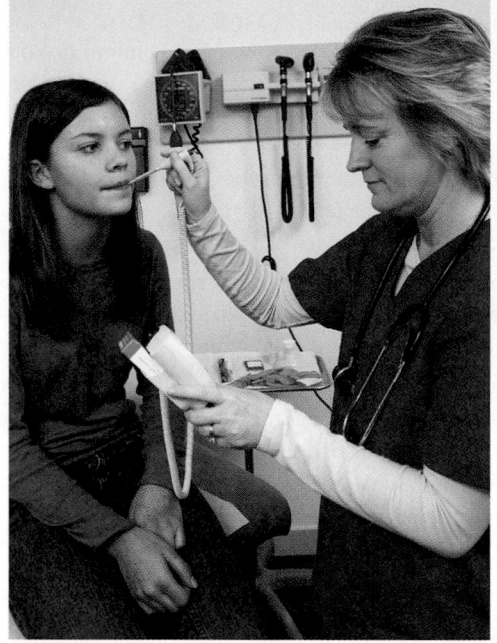

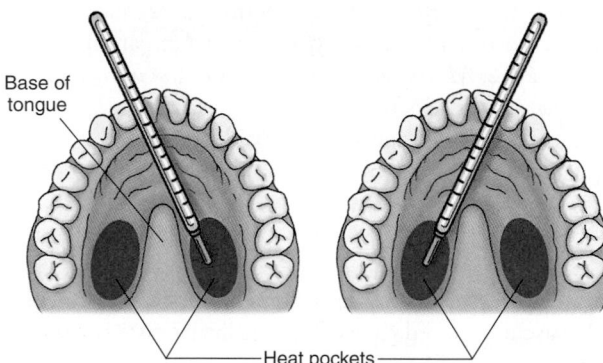

Correct placement of an oral thermometer

10. Record the patient's temperature in the medical record, including the date and time, to ensure accurate documentation and make the information available to the physician.

Date	
05/26/09: 9:45 a.m.	T: 98.4° F. ------------------------------------ S. Lind, CMA

PROCEDURE 21-2

Measuring axillary temperature using a digital thermometer

Task
Measure axillary body temperature using a digital thermometer.

Conditions
- Digital thermometer
- Oral probe
- Probe cover
- Waste container
- Pen
- Patient's medical record

Standards
In the time specified and within the scoring parameters determined by the instructor, the student will successfully measure and record an individual's axillary temperature using a digital thermometer.

Performance Standards
1. Wash or sanitize your hands to ensure infection control and assemble supplies.
2. Greet and identify your patient, introduce yourself, and explain the procedure to ease the patient's anxiety.
3. Prepare the oral probe for use according to the manufacturer's directions to ensure accuracy.
4. Assist the patient in removing or loosening clothing around the shoulder and arm as needed to provide access to the axilla.
5. Pat the axilla dry if needed to ensure accuracy.
6. Apply a disposable probe cover, making sure it locks into place, to activate the thermometer and ensure infection control.
7. Insert the probe into the center of the axilla pointing toward the upper chest. Tell the patient to hold his upper arm snugly against the side of his rib cage and assist him as necessary to ensure accuracy by preventing exposure of the probe to air. Hold the probe in place until you hear the beep sound that indicates the reading is complete.
8. Remove the probe and read the number on the digital display screen. Eject the probe cover into the waste container by pressing the ejection button without touching the probe cover to ensure infection control.
9. Return the probe to its storage position in the thermometer unit to turn off and reset the thermometer and return the thermometer to its base to ensure easy access for future use.

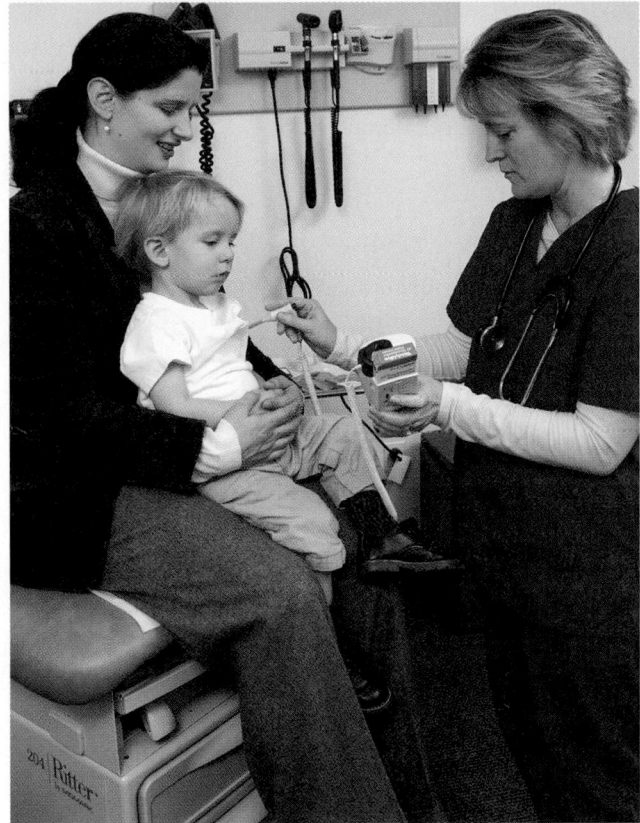

Insert the probe into the center of the axilla pointing toward the upper chest.

10. Wash or sanitize your hands and disinfect equipment if indicated to ensure infection control.
11. Record the patient's temperature in the medical record, including the method of measurement (in this case, axillary), the date, and the time, to ensure accurate documentation and make the information available to the physician.

Date	
06/27/09: 9:56 a.m.	T: 101.2° F (axillary). ------------------------------------S. Lind, CMA

■ **PROCEDURE 21-3**

Measuring rectal temperature using a digital thermometer

Task
Measure rectal body temperature.

Conditions
- Digital rectal thermometer
- Rectal probe
- Probe cover
- Lubricant
- Tissues
- Nonsterile examination gloves
- Waste container
- Pen
- Patient's medical record

Standards
In the time specified and within the scoring parameters determined by the instructor, the student will successfully measure and record the patient's rectal temperature.

Performance Standards
1. Wash or sanitize your hands to ensure infection control and assemble supplies.
2. Greet and identify the patient and introduce yourself to ease patient anxiety.
3. Prepare the rectal probe for use, according to the manufacturer's instructions. Apply a disposable probe cover to ensure infection control, making sure it locks into place to turn the thermometer on.
4. Apply nonsterile examination gloves to ensure infection control.
5. Assist the patient in removing clothing below the waist. Assist the adult or child patient into a Sims or side-lying position. Drape the patient as completely as possible, exposing only the anal area to ensure privacy, warmth, and comfort while providing access to the anal opening. Position the infant patient on his abdomen.

6. Apply lubricant to the tip of the thermometer to ensure easier insertion and minimize patient discomfort. Insert the thermometer into the rectum past the external sphincter. For an infant or small child, take care to insert it no more than 1/2" and no more than 1" for an older child or adult to avoid causing injury. Continue holding the probe end to prevent it from slipping out or further in.
7. Remove the probe after the beeping sound. To prevent transfer of microorganisms, eject the probe cover into the waste container without touching the probe cover and dispose of examination gloves.
8. Read the number on the digital display screen.
9. Offer tissues to the adult or child patient so she can wipe off excess lubricant herself. Wipe excess lubricant from the infant.
10. Return the probe to its storage position in the thermometer unit to turn off and reset the thermometer and return the thermometer to its base to ensure easy access for future use.
11. Wash or sanitize your hands and disinfect equipment if indicated to ensure infection control.
12. Assist the patient with positioning and dressing as needed to put patient at ease.
13. Record the patient's temperature in the medical record, including the method of measurement (in this case, rectal), the date, and the time, to ensure accurate documentation and make the information available to the physician.

Date	
12/10/09; 9:30 a.m.	T: 99.8° F. (rectal) ------------------------------W. Jones, CMA

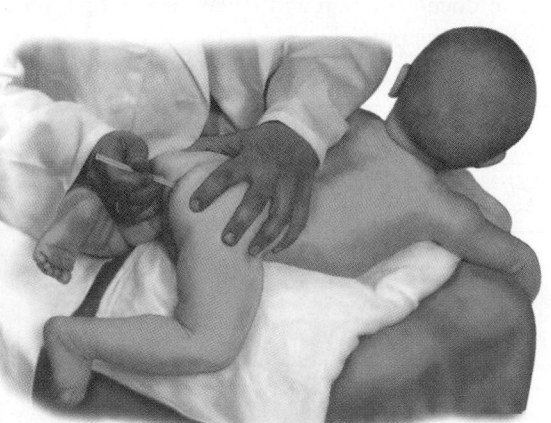

Taking an infant's rectal temperature

PROCEDURE 21-4

Measuring temperature using a tympanic thermometer

Task
Measure body temperature using a tympanic thermometer.

Conditions
- Tympanic thermometer
- Probe cover
- Waste container
- Pen
- Patient's medical record

Standards
In the time specified and within the scoring parameters determined by the instructor, the student will successfully measure and record a patient's body temperature using a tympanic thermometer.

Performance Standards
1. Wash or sanitize your hands to ensure infection control and assemble supplies.
2. Greet and identify your patient, introduce yourself, and explain the procedure to ease the patient's anxiety.
3. Prepare the tympanic thermometer for use according to the manufacturer's directions, making sure that probe lens is clean and the display screen is adjusted for the patient's age to prevent errors and ensure accuracy.
4. Apply the disposable probe cover, making sure that it snaps into place to activate the thermometer and ensure infection control.
5. When the thermometer display reads READY, straighten the patient's ear canal with your other hand by gently pulling the auricle up and backward for patients over age 3 or by gently pulling the pinna down and backward for younger patients to straighten the ear canal.
6. Insert the probe into the patient's ear canal just far enough to seal the opening but without applying pressure to minimize patient discomfort while ensuring accuracy.

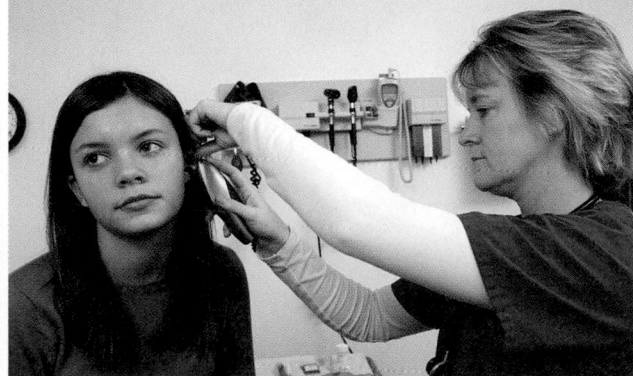

Insert the probe into the patient's ear canal without applying pressure.

7. Press the button and hold it down briefly, as indicated in the manufacturer's instructions. Check the temperature reading that appears on the display screen.
8. Remove the probe and eject the probe cover into a waste receptacle without touching it to ensure infection control.
9. Record the patient's temperature in the medical record, including the method of measurement (in this case, tympanic), along with the ear in which it was measured, the date, and the time, to ensure accurate documentation and make the information available to the physician.

Date	
11/20/09; 1:30 p.m.	T: 99.8° F (tympanic, left ear). -------------------S. Lind, CMA

by scanning the thermometer across the forehead over the temporal artery where it detects infrared readings of blood flow in the temporal artery. Disposable covers may be placed over the probe or it can be cleaned between patients with a disinfectant wipe. Evidence indicates that this method of temperature measurement is as accurate as obtaining a rectal temperature and may be more accurate than the tympanic method. Because it is fast and noninvasive, this method is quickly gaining popularity among patients and health care providers. (See *Procedure 21-5: Measuring temperature using a temporal thermometer.*)

Disinfecting Thermometers

The medical assistant should disinfect reusable thermometers between uses. The World Health Organization (WHO) recommends two methods for disinfecting reusable thermometers: with 70% isopropyl alcohol or a 1:100 bleach solution. To disinfect with 70% isopropyl alcohol, the medical assistant should moisten a clean cloth or gauze pad with alcohol, carefully wipe the thermometer, hold the cloth around it for 30 seconds, and then discard the cloth and let the thermometer air dry. To disinfect with a 1:100 bleach solution, the medical assistant should use a clean cloth or

---

■ PROCEDURE 21-5

Measuring temperature using a temporal thermometer

Task
Measure body temperature using a temporal thermometer.

Conditions
- Temporal thermometer
- Probe cover or disinfectant wipe
- Waste container
- Pen
- Patient's medical record

Standards
In the time specified and within the scoring parameters determined by the instructor, the student will accurately measure and record a patient's temporal temperature.

Performance Standards
1. Wash or sanitize your hands to ensure infection control and assemble supplies.
2. Greet and identify the patient, introduce yourself, and explain the procedure to ease the patient's anxiety.
3. Apply a disposable probe cover, as necessary, to ensure infection control.
4. Scan the probe across the patient's forehead over the temporal artery as indicated in the manufacturer's instructions.

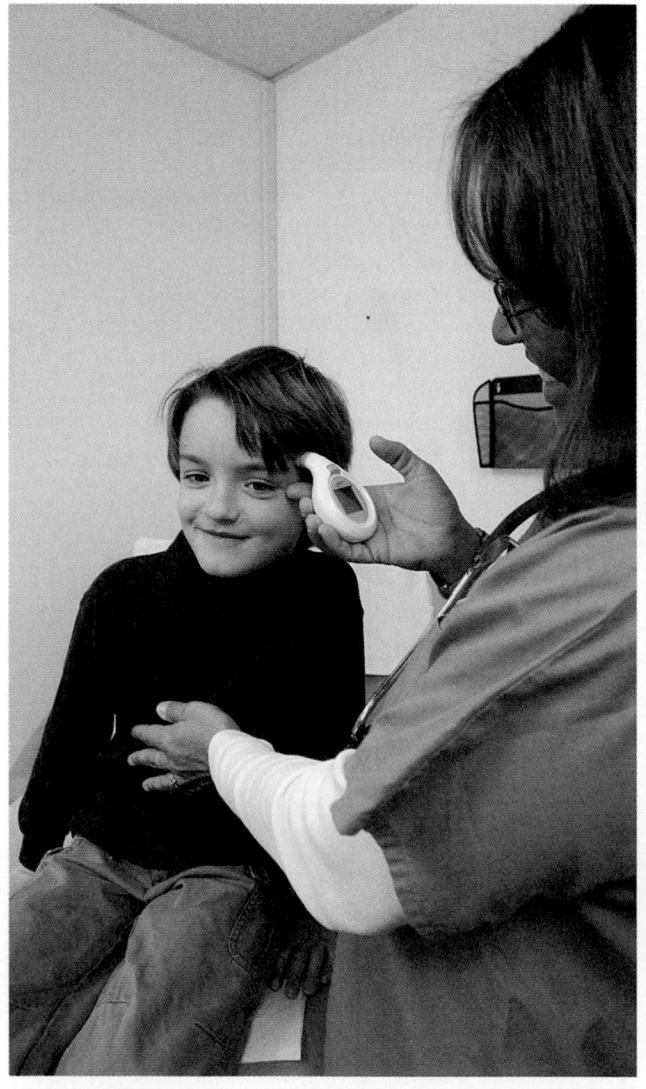

Scan the probe over the temporal artery.

PROCEDURE 21-5—cont'd

5. Read the temperature on the digital display screen.
6. Eject the probe cover into the waste container without touching the probe cover or clean the probe with a disinfectant wipe to ensure infection control.
7. Wash or sanitize your hands to ensure infection control.
8. Record the patient's temperature in the medical record, including the method of measurement (in this case, temporal), the date, and the time, to ensure accurate documentation and make the information available to the physician.

Date	
11/20/09; 9:30 a.m.	T: 99.8° F (temporal). ------------------------------C. Chapin, CMA

gauze pad dipped in the bleach solution to wipe the thermometer. Alternatively, she may soak the thermometer for 10 minutes and then allow it to air dry. Reusable thermometers should be disinfected in this manner or according to office policy any time they have come into contact with body fluids. Tympanic thermometers can be disinfected in a manner similar to other thermometers except that the tip of the probe surface should not get wet, because disinfectant may ruin it. Thus, the medical assistant should be sure to use a probe cover whenever she uses a tympanic thermometer.

Celsius Versus Fahrenheit

Historically, the Fahrenheit scale has been used for temperature measurement in the United States. While many measurements in the United States are still typically nonmetric, metric is the standard scale for measurement within the health care setting. Even so, medical offices may record temperatures using the Fahrenheit or Celsius scale, so the medical assistant should be familiar with both and follow facility policy. In some situations, the medical assistant may need to convert temperature readings from one system to another. (See *Temperature conversions*.)

Pulse

Each time the heart beats, the chambers of the heart contract. This contraction propels blood forward through the circulatory system. As the left ventricle contracts, it forces blood into the aorta, the largest artery in the body. From the aorta, it moves through smaller and smaller arteries throughout the rest of the body. Because the arteries are essentially already full of blood, when the new supply of blood is forced into them by the beating heart, a wavelike pulsation is created as the elastic arteries expand. This pulsation can be felt (palpated) when the medical assistant places the pads of her fingers over a superficial artery. Veins do not pulsate because blood moves through them under much lower pressure. (See *Factors that affect pulse*.)

Temperature conversions

Medical assistants must know how to convert temperatures between Fahrenheit and Celsius. The formulas for conversion are:

$°C = (°F - 32) \times 5/9$

$°F = (9/5 \times °C) + 32$

OR

$°C = (°F - 32) \div 1.8$

$°F = (°C \times 1.8) + 32$

Factors that affect pulse

There are a number of factors that can affect pulse rate, rhythm, and strength. The medical assistant must consider all of these factors when assessing the patient's pulse, including:

- Age—Pulse rate decreases with age. A newborn infant's pulse may be as high as 160 beats/minute and an adult's pulse may be as slow as 60 beats/minute.
- Sex—Women tend to have slightly faster resting pulse rates than men.
- Exercise habits—People who are very athletic may have a normal resting pulse as slow as 40 beats/minute.
- Emotional state—Pulse rate normally increases with exercise and emotional states such as fear, anxiety, anger, and excitement.

Continued

Factors that affect pulse—cont'd

- Pregnancy and other metabolic conditions—Conditions that increase the metabolism, such as pregnancy and hyperthyroidism, will increase the pulse.
- Medication—Some medications may increase or decrease a patient's pulse rate. For example, lanoxin is a cardiac medication that slows the heart rate, and albuterol is a pulmonary medication that opens the air passages but causes **tachycardia** (rapid heart beat) as an adverse effect.
- Fever—Fever increases a patient's pulse rate.
- Arrhythmia—Cardiac arrhythmias (abnormal rhythms) may cause an irregular pulse and may cause some pulsations to be stronger than others.
- Hypertension—A person with hypertension may have a bounding pulse which is very strong and easily palpated.
- Dehydration—A person who is dehydrated may have a weak pulse that is difficult to palpate.

Front office–Back office connection

Using Pulse Points to Control Bleeding

In the event of a bleeding emergency, the administrative medical assistant may be asked to apply pressure to a pulse point while the clinical medical assistant applies direct pressure to the wound with an absorbent dressing. Thus, it is important for an administrative medical assistant to remember where the pulse points are located.

Pulse Sites

There are many pulse points in the body. A pulse point is any area where the pulse can be felt by pressing a superficial artery against a bone. Such areas may be palpated to evaluate circulation in that area or to count heart rate. In cases of hemorrhage, the pulse point can also be compressed to control bleeding. (See *Using pulse points to control bleeding.*) Common pulse points include:

- temporal
- carotid
- brachial
- radial
- apical
- femoral
- popliteal
- dorsalis pedis
- posterior tibialis. (See Figure 21-2.)

Temporal

The temporal pulse is located over the temporal bone, lateral to the eyes. It is rarely used to measure pulse but pressure may be exerted there to control the bleeding of a head wound.

Carotid

The medical assistant can locate the carotid pulse by pressing her fingertips into the groove between the larynx and the sternocleidomastoid muscle on either side of the neck.

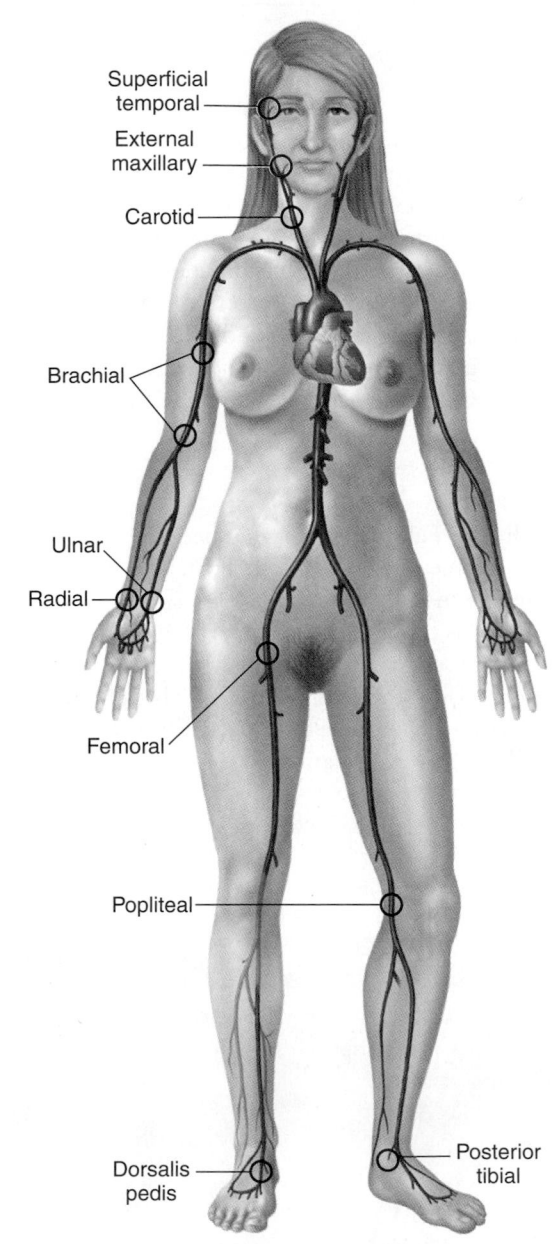

FIG 21-2 Common pulse points.

Because it is one of the strongest pulses in the body and easily accessible, it is used to assess a patient's circulation during cardiopulmonary resuscitation (CPR). A person may also assess his own carotid pulse during exercise. Because it provides the major blood supply to the brain, the medical assistant should use just enough pressure to feel the pulse without occluding blood flow and should only palpate it on one side at a time.

Brachial

The medical assistant can palpate the brachial pulse at the antecubital space in the bend of the arm, anterior to the elbow. This is the site the medical assistant will auscultate when measuring blood pressure. It is also the site for assessing pulse during infant CPR.

Radial

The radial pulse is the most common pulse used for checking the pulse rate. It is located in the distal part of the forearm on the inner aspect of the wrist, just below the base of the thumb. Because the artery lies over the radius (giving this pulse point its name), the medical assistant should be able to feel it easily when pressing the point with the pads of her fingers. (See *Counting radial pulse*.) The most accurate and easiest measurement of pulse and respiration occurs when these measurements are taken together. (See *Procedure 21-6: Measuring radial pulse and respirations*, page 332.)

Apical

The apical pulse is more accurately referred to as the *apical heart rate* because it is usually auscultated with a stethoscope.

It lies over the apex of the heart at the fifth intercostal space at the midclavicular line. It is just below the nipple in men. In a patient who is young and thin, the medical assistant may be able to palpate this pulse easily as the **point of maximal impulse (PMI),** which is where the apex of the heart touches the inner chest wall and pulsations can sometimes be observed and felt. The PMI is typically located in the fourth or fifth intercostal space along the midclavicular line. However, the medical assistant may find it difficult to palpate it in others. Regardless, she can easily auscultate the apical heart rate in nearly everyone. An apical heart rate measurement is helpful if a patient has an irregular heart rhythm or a radial pulse that is difficult to palpate. When listening to the patient's heart, the medical assistant must be sure to note that each heartbeat includes two sounds in quick succession. These sounds are commonly described as a "lubb-dupp" sound. Each lubb-dupp is counted as one heartbeat.

Additionally, the medical assistant may check the patient for a **pulse deficit** by counting the apical heart rate and the radial pulse and noting the difference, if any. In some cases, such as in patients with a common abnormal heart rhythm known as *atrial fibrillation*, the apical heart rate may be higher than the radial pulse. Such a result may happen if some of the heart contractions are weaker than others and do not generate a high enough stroke volume to create a palpable radial pulse. In such a case, the apical heart rate is more accurate, and the medical assistant should record it in the medical record. (See *Procedure 21-7: Measuring apical heart rate*, page 333.)

A medical assistant will commonly use a stethoscope to check a patient's vital signs. Therefore, she should become

---

Patient Education

Counting Radial Pulse

To teach a patient how to take his pulse, the medical assistant should follow these simple steps:

- Tell the patient to position a clock or wristwatch with a second hand within easy view.
- Show the patient how to locate his radial pulse in both wrists.
- Let the patient continue palpating his radial pulse in whichever wrist is easiest for him.
- Palpate his pulse in his other wrist so you are both palpating it at the same time.
- Count for a full minute and then compare numbers. (The numbers may not match exactly but should only vary by one or two beats.)

Some patients may wish to complete the process more quickly by counting for 30 seconds and then multiplying by 2. Although this practice may be acceptable if the pulse is regular, counting for a full minute ensures greater accuracy. Medical assistants typically count for just 30 seconds and multiply by 2 once they become very proficient in obtaining vital signs. However, whenever a patient has an irregular pulse, even the medical assistant should count for 1 full minute. The medical assistant should make sure that this practice is acceptable to the physician before allowing the patient to estimate pulse rate in this way.

PROCEDURE 21-6

Measuring radial pulse and respirations

Task
Measure and record radial pulse and respirations.

Conditions
- Clock or watch
- Pen
- Patient's medical record

Standards
In the time specified and within the scoring parameters determined by the instructor, the student will accurately measure and record radial pulse and respirations.

Performance Standards
1. Wash or sanitize your hands to ensure infection control and assemble supplies.
2. Greet and identify the patient, introduce yourself, and explain the procedure to ease patient anxiety.
3. Assist the patient into a comfortable sitting position with his arm relaxed and slightly flexed to make the pulse easier to palpate and ensure an accurate resting pulse measurement.
4. Grasp the patient's wrist with the pads of your middle three fingers placed over the radial site and apply just enough pressure to distinctly palpate the pulse. Pressing too hard may occlude the pulse. Do not palpate with the thumb, to avoid feeling your own pulse instead of the patient's.

5. Count the pulse for 30 seconds as measured with your watch and multiply by 2 to save time while preserving accuracy.
6. To count respirations, continue holding the patient's wrist while looking at your watch so the patient will not be aware that you are counting respirations and, thus, will continue to breathe normally. Count the patient's respirations for 30 seconds, then multiply by 2. Be sure to note the character of the respirations, including depth and rhythm, to provide information about respiratory function.
7. Record the patient's pulse and respirations in the medical record, including date and time, to ensure accurate documentation and make the information available to the physician.
8. Wash or sanitize your hands to ensure infection control.

Date	
07/16/09: 11:50 a.m.	P: 66, reg, strong. R: 16, reg, nonlabored ----S. Lind, CMA

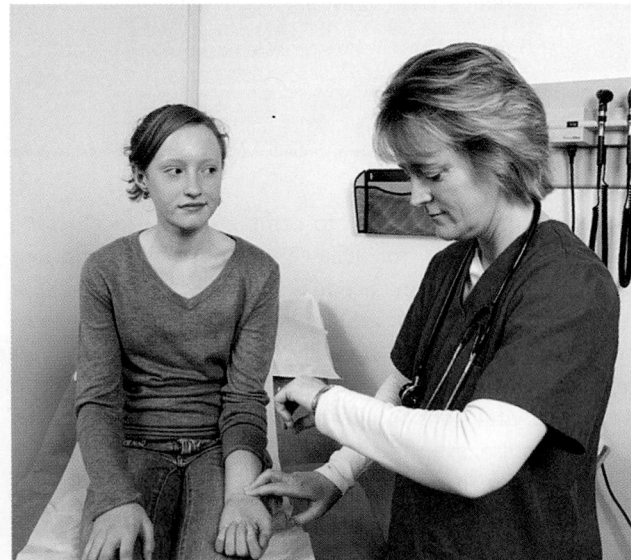
Place the pads of your fingers over the radial site.

PROCEDURE 21-7

Measuring apical heart rate

Task
Measure and record a patient's apical heart rate.

Conditions
- Watch with a second hand
- Stethoscope
- Patient examination gown
- Antiseptic wipe
- Pen
- Patient's medical record

Standards
In the time specified and within the scoring parameters determined by the instructor, the student will accurately measure and record the apical heart rate.

Performance Standards
1. Wash or sanitize your hands to ensure infection control and assemble supplies.
2. Greet and identify the patient, introduce yourself, and explain the procedure to ease patient anxiety.
3. Clean the earpieces and chest piece of the stethoscope with an antiseptic wipe to ensure infection control.
4. Assist the patient in undressing from the waist up and putting on an examination gown, if preferred, with the opening in the front. (Some male patients prefer not to wear a gown. However, the medical assistant should be sure to offer one.) Place the patient in a sitting or reclining position to ensure patient comfort while allowing apical access.
5. Because apical heart sounds are heard best with the bell, place the bell of the stethoscope over the apical area (fifth intercostal space at the midclavicular line), applying just enough pressure to ensure full contact with the skin. Pressing too hard may diminish the sound.

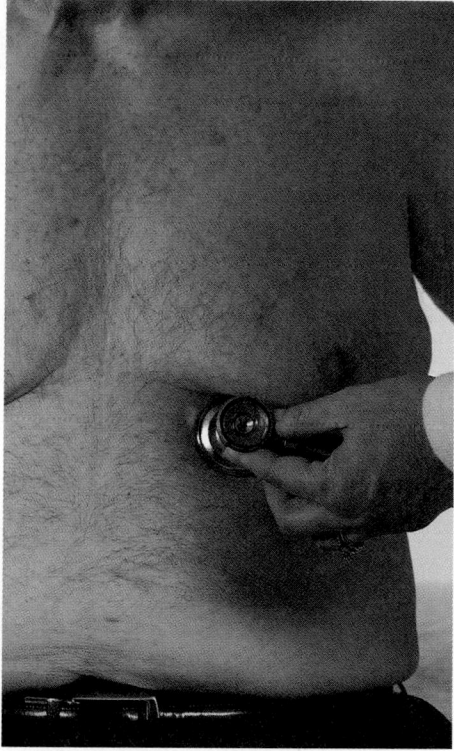

Place the bell of the stethoscope over the apical area.

6. Count the heart beat for a full minute as measured with your watch to ensure accuracy, especially in patients with irregular heart rhythms.
7. Wash or sanitize your hands and sanitize the earpieces and chest piece of the stethoscope to ensure infection control.
8. Record the patient's apical heart rate and rhythm in the medical record, including the date and time, to ensure accurate documentation and make the information available to the physician.

Date	
07/21/09; 3:50 p.m.	AP: 72, reg. ---------------------------------- J. Morgan, CMA

familiar with this important piece of medical equipment. The parts of a stethoscope include the earpieces, called *binaurals,* tubing, and chest piece. (See Figure 21-3.) The chest piece includes a diaphragm, which is a large, round disc, and may also include a bell on the opposite side, which is smaller in diameter and concave in shape. The diaphragm is helpful when listening to high-pitched sounds and the bell is more useful for listening to low-pitched sounds. When using the stethoscope, the medical assistant must make sure the chestpiece is turned in the correct direction or no sound will be heard.

Femoral

The femoral pulse is located where the upper leg bends, in the inguinal area very near the groin. It is most easily palpated by pressing the pads of the fingers firmly downward when the patient is lying supine. This pulse is not commonly

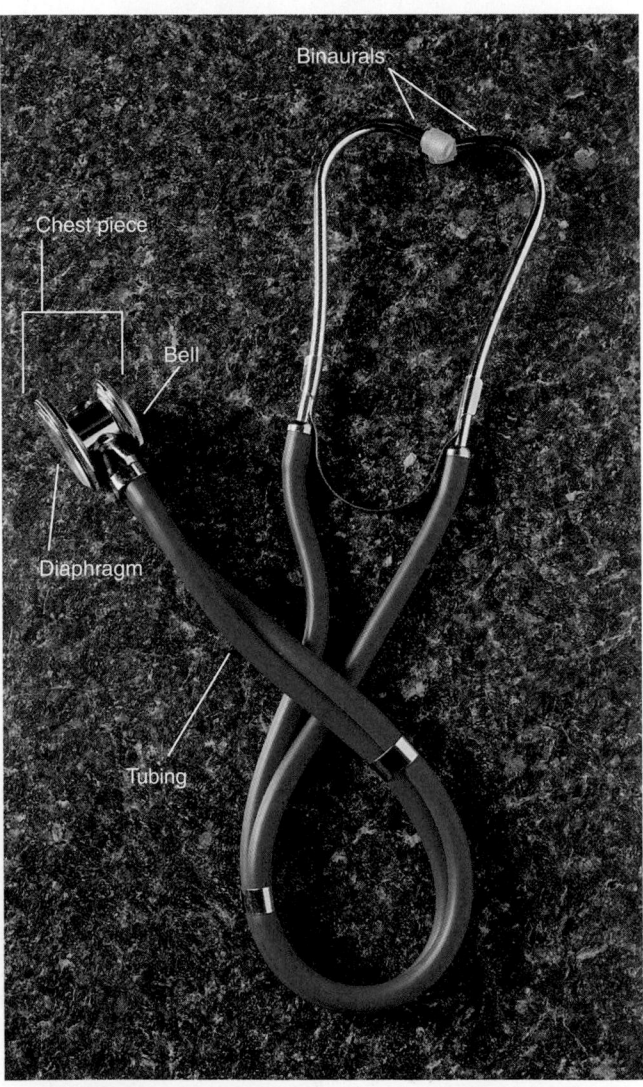

FIG 21-3 Parts of the stethoscope.

used, but may be very useful with patients who are in cardiac arrest or have very weak radial and carotid pulses.

Popliteal

The popliteal pulse is usually difficult to locate and palpate. It is located behind the knee and must be palpated with the leg in a slightly flexed position. This site is sometimes used to assess circulation in the lower leg.

Dorsalis Pedis

The dorsalis pedis pulse is located on the top of the foot near the extensor tendon of the great toe. It is easily palpated in some patients but difficult in others and possibly congenitally absent. It is palpated to assess circulation in the foot.

Posterior Tibialis

The posterior tibialis pulse lies slightly inferior and posterior to the inside ankle bone. It is easy to palpate in some individuals and difficult in others. It is used to assess circulation in the foot.

Respiration

Respiration involves the movement of air into and out of the lungs so that gas exchange can occur in the alveoli, which are the tiny air sacs in the lungs. Even though oxygen is necessary to sustain life, oxygen levels are not the main stimulus for breathing in most people. The real stimulus is the lowered pH level of the blood caused by carbon dioxide (CO_2) buildup. As the pH level drops, a message is sent to the medulla oblongata in the brain, which then sends out a message to the body to increase the rate and depth of respiration. As a result, more CO_2 is blown off and eliminated from the body. Blood pH rises back to a more normal level and homeostasis is maintained. Conversely, when the pH level rises too high, messages to and from the medulla oblongata stimulate a decrease in the rate and depth of respiration, which allows the body to retain more CO_2, thus lowering the pH level to normal.

External respiration involves the movement of air in and out of the lungs. **Inspiration,** or the act of breathing in, occurs when the diaphragm and other muscles contract, pulling the thorax (rib cage) upward and outward. At the same time, the lungs expand, causing air to be pulled in through the mouth and nose. Inspiration is the active phase of breathing and requires the muscles to work. However, **expiration,** or the act of breathing out, is usually passive. The diaphragm and other muscles simply relax, allowing the rib cage to return inward and downward as air is expelled from the lungs.

The medical assistant should be aware of factors that might impact respiration. Some are normal variations in response to physical and emotional stress. Others may be indicators of illness or disease. (See *Factors that affect respiration*.)

Characteristics of Respiration

While a person may exert some voluntary control over respiration, it is generally an automatic or involuntary function controlled by the nervous system. Respirations are most easily and accurately measured when performed simultaneously with pulse measurement. The medical assistant should continue to hold the patient's wrist in a manner that allows for easy observation of her watch as well as the patient's chest. Doing so prevents the patient from being aware that the medical assistant is measuring his respirations, which might cause him to self-consciously alter his breathing pattern. There are three major characteristics of respiration:

- rate
- rhythm
- depth.

Rate

The medical assistant should count the respiratory rate in breaths per minute. One breath includes inspiration and expiration. The normal respiratory rate for adults is 12 to 20 breaths per minute, but the rate varies with age and other factors. (See *Normal respiratory rate by age*.) **Bradypnea** is the term for abnormally slow breathing. While bradypnea is uncommon, it can occur in certain disease states. **Apnea** refers to the absence of breathing. **Sleep apnea** is a condition in which the individual stops breathing for short periods of time while sleeping due to temporary obstruction of the upper airway. This condition is usually associated with severe snoring and can have a profound impact on a person's quality of life. **Tachypnea** is a state of abnormally rapid breathing. It may be caused by many factors, including such respiratory disorders as asthma and emphysema. Tachypnea commonly occurs when an individual is exercising or physically working. Another common cause of tachypnea is **hyperventilation,** which may occur when an individual is feeling anxious or upset. This problem corrects itself as the individual calms down.

Rhythm

The normal respiratory pattern is described as *even* and *regular*. However, normal interruptions in the respiratory pattern may occur when an individual sighs or yawns. Rhythm also varies with speech patterns. Abnormal variations in rhythm may occur with injury or disease. For example, if a person has sustained an injury to the ribs, the breathing pattern may be more rapid and shallow due to pain experienced when the patient takes a deeper breath. Patients with lung disease such as asthma or chronic obstructive pulmonary disease (COPD) may easily develop dyspnea. In a patient with **dyspnea,** respirations may be more rapid and the expiratory phase becomes prolonged because the patient must work harder to breathe out.

Depth

Depth of respiration varies with physical activity and may be described as *normal, deep,* or *shallow.* Respirations become deeper with physical exertion and become more shallow at rest. Depth is also impacted by injury or disease. For example, a patient with a rib injury or one who has undergone recent chest or abdominal surgery may experience increased pain when taking deep breaths. Even so, such patients must

---

Factors that affect respiration

The rate and depth of respirations may increase or decrease in relation to many factors. Some of the most common are listed here.

Increased rate

- severe pain (Depth may be increased or decreased depending on the location and type of pain.)
- fever

Increased rate and depth

- emotions, such as fear, anger, anxiety, or excitement
- physical exertion or exercise
- illness
- condition that causes acidosis, such as severe diabetic coma, exacerbation of chronic obstructive pulmonary disease, asthma, or breathing impairment due to a brain or chest injury

Decreased rate and depth

- illness
- condition that causes alkalosis, such as excessive intake of antacids or severe or prolonged vomiting

---

Normal respiratory rate by age

Normal respiratory rate varies with age. Here are normal ranges for respiratory rates by age group:

- *newborn*—30 to 60 breaths/minute
- *infant (less than 6 months)*—30 to 50 breaths/minute
- *toddler (less than 2 years)*—25 to 32 breaths/minute
- *child*—20 to 30 breaths/minute
- *adolescent*—16 to 19 breaths/minute
- *adult*—12 to 20 breaths/minute.

be instructed and encouraged to take frequent, deep breaths and even cough in order to keep the alveoli open and fully functioning. Occasionally, disease states can impact respiratory depth. An example is the patient in a diabetic coma. Such an individual will involuntarily exhibit a respiratory pattern that is rapid and deep.

Blood Pressure

Blood pressure is one of the most common measurements taken in the medical office. It reflects the pressure exerted against arterial walls by blood and is recorded as a fraction. The **systolic pressure,** the top numbers, indicates the highest pressure, or tension, exerted against arterial walls during ventricular contraction. **Diastolic pressure,** the lower number, represents the lowest pressure exerted against the arterial walls when the heart is at rest between contractions. The difference between the two is the **pulse pressure** and should be 30 to 50 mm Hg. *Hypertension* is defined as sustained blood pressure readings above 140/90 mm Hg. (See *Nonmodifiable risk factors for hypertension.*) However, ideal blood pressure for all adults is below 120/80 mm Hg. (See *Modifying heart rate and blood pressure.*)

Blood pressure normally varies from person to person. Normal diurnal variations also alter blood pressure in the same person during the day. Lower readings are common in the morning when metabolism is slower. Blood pressure rises throughout the day, typically peaking in the late

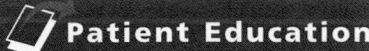

Patient Education

Modifying Heart Rate and Blood Pressure

Measurement of a patient's vital signs commonly creates a great opportunity for teaching because many patients want to know what normal values should be and what their vital sign values are. If the patient's resting heart rate and blood pressure is abnormally high, he may be interested in hearing about what he can do to bring them back to normal. Here is a simple list of commonsense strategies the medical assistant can share with the patient for modifying his heart rate and blood pressure:

- Exercise regularly, including aerobic activity, such as walking briskly, jogging, swimming, or bicycling several times a week for at least 20 to 30 minutes at a time (or as recommended by your physician).

- Stop smoking or other tobacco use.

- Achieve and maintain optimal weight for height.

- Learn and use stress reduction measures, such as meditation and relaxation activities.

- Eat a healthy, well-balanced, low-fat diet.

- Keep alcohol intake to 2 drinks per day or less (or as recommended by your physician).

Nonmodifiable risk factors for hypertension

Although some risk factors for hypertension, such as diet and exercise, are modifiable, there are several nonmodifiable risk factors for hypertension, including:

- age
- gender
- genetics.

Age

Normal values for blood pressure slowly increase with age until individuals reach adulthood. Blood pressure may continue to increase with advancing age as atherosclerosis and other disorders develop. However, as more is learned about the risk that hypertension poses for other disorders, most physicians are taking a more aggressive approach to managing it.

Gender

Blood pressure measurements in boys and girls do not differ significantly, but once they reach adulthood the situation changes. Adult men tend to have higher blood pressures than adult women. However, at more advanced age, the situation reverses and postmenopausal women have higher blood pressures than elderly men.

Genetics

There is some evidence that some of the physical contributors to hypertension and heart disease may be genetic. Therefore, a person whose parents both died of heart disease in their 50s would be at a higher-than-average risk for developing the same disorders. Along the same lines, some ethnic groups have a higher incidence of specific diseases and disorders, including hypertension. For example, African Americans have a higher risk of developing hypertension than other ethnic groups, and those who develop it have a higher risk for such complications as stroke, heart attack, and death.

afternoon or evening. The medical assistant must be aware of the many factors that impact blood pressure. Those that cause a temporary elevation in blood pressure, such as exercise, must be accounted for whenever possible. Therefore, if the patient just climbed a flight of stairs to enter the medical office, the medical assistant should ensure that he sits and rests for 20 to 30 minutes before checking his blood pressure. (See *Factors that affect blood pressure.*) Medications can also impact blood pressure. Therefore, the medical assistant should record all medications in the patient's medical record. Even if altering blood pressure is the desired effect of the medication, the physician must be aware of the medication in order to make an accurate evaluation.

Evaluating Blood Pressure

The medical name for the blood pressure cuff is ***sphygmomanometer***. It includes a cuff with an inner inflatable bladder, a bulb with a control valve, and a gauge. When inflated, the cuff compresses the brachial artery and cuts off blood flow. As it slowly deflates, it measures the pressure exerted by the blood pumping back through the artery and into the arm.

Measuring blood pressure is a very common task for the medical assistant. Therefore, she must be proficient in this skill. However, she may find it a challenge to obtain an accurate blood pressure measurement in some people. When facing such a situation, the medical assistant can use special strategies to increase her chances of obtaining an accurate measurement. (See *Strategies for accurate blood pressure measurement.*)

Factors that affect blood pressure

In addition to the normal diurnal variations in a person's blood pressure, other factors can have a temporary impact on blood pressure.

Temporary increase
- emotions, such as fear, anger, anxiety, and excitement
- severe pain
- exercise or physical exertion

Temporary decrease
- fluid volume deficit, such as from hemorrhage or dehydration
- sudden position change, such as moving from lying down to sitting or standing (most severe if fluid volume deficit is also present)
- some medications, such as general anesthesia or opiate analgesics

---

Korotkoff Sounds

The sounds heard when listening to blood pressure vary. This fact was first noted and reported by Russian neurologist Nikolai Sergeyevich Korotkoff. He divided the sounds, now known as ***Korotkoff sounds***, into five categories. (See Figure 21-4.) These categories, or phases, include:

- *Phase I* is the first sound heard as blood begins to surge back into the constricted artery. This sound is usually a sharp tapping sound that may begin faintly and progressively grow louder. This first tapping sound is the systolic pressure.

- *Phase II* occurs as the tapping sound takes on a swishing or murmuring quality. This sound is more quiet and muffled and, in some cases, disappears completely. When it disappears, it is known as the ***auscultatory gap***. The needle may continue to drop another 30 mm Hg or so before the sound returns. This absence may lead an inexperienced medical assistant to believe she was mistaken about hearing the first sound. However, the experienced medical assistant learns to trust what is heard

---

Strategies for accurate blood pressure measurement

Obtaining an accurate blood pressure reading can be challenging in some patients. Here are some strategies the medical assistant can use to increase her success in this important skill:

- Eliminate room noise, such as talking or music.
- Use a good-quality stethoscope with ear pieces that fit snugly and comfortably.
- Use a cuff that is an appropriate size for the patient's arm.
- Position the patient in a comfortable sitting or lying position.
- Have the patient remove her arm from clothing, rather than rolling up a sleeve tightly.
- Avoid placing the cuff or stethoscope diaphragm over layers of clothing.
- Make sure the cuff is positioned correctly on the patient's arm.
- Make sure the patient's arm is fully extended yet relaxed.
- Place the stethoscope firmly against the patient's arm at the correct spot (identified by palpating the brachial pulse).
- Inflate the bulb to an appropriate level for the patient and deflate it slowly enough to clearly hear the correct systolic sound.

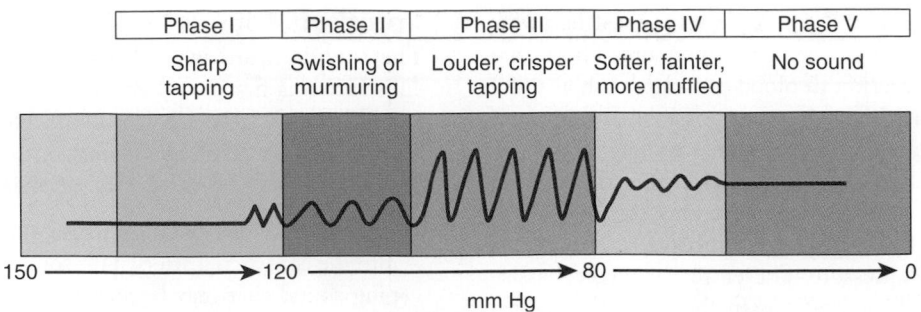

Phase I	Phase II	Phase III	Phase IV	Phase V
Sharp tapping	Swishing or murmuring	Louder, crisper tapping	Softer, fainter, more muffled	No sound

150 ——————→ 120 ——————→ 80 ——————→ 0

mm Hg

FIG 21-4 Korotkoff sounds.

PROCEDURE 21-8

Measuring blood pressure

Task

Measure and record blood pressure.

Conditions

- Sphygmomanometer (blood pressure cuff)
- Antiseptic wipes
- Stethoscope
- Waste container

Standards

In the time specified and within the scoring parameters determined by the instructor, the student will accurately measure and record the patient's blood pressure.

Performance Standards

1. Seat the patient in a quiet room for several minutes prior to checking her blood pressure to ensure an accurate reading.
2. Wash or sanitize your hands to ensure infection control and assemble supplies.
3. Greet and identify the patient, introduce yourself, and explain the procedure to ease patient anxiety.
4. Minimize room noise by turning off music (if playing) and asking the patient to refrain from talking to ensure accuracy in hearing blood pressure.
5. Roll up the patient's sleeve about 5" above the elbow or assist the patient in removing her arm from clothing because a tightly rolled sleeve may interfere with circulation and the accuracy of measurement.
6. Select the proper size cuff for each patient. The cuff bladder should be long enough to wrap around 80% of the patient's arm and wide enough to cover two-thirds of the upper arm. A cuff that is too large or too small will result in a less accurate measurement.
7. Apply the deflated cuff to the patient's upper arm with the arrow over the brachial artery and the lower cuff edge at least 1" above the bend of the elbow to ensure accuracy.

8. Position the gauge so you can easily read it because it is difficult to move the gauge after you begin.
9. Palpate the brachial pulse with one hand and tighten the valve on the inflation bulb with the other hand. Then inflate the cuff and note the reading on the gauge when you are no longer able to palpate the pulse to help identify the approximate systolic blood pressure.
10. Deflate the cuff and apply the stethoscope to the area of the brachial pulse, making sure the earpieces fit snugly and comfortably in your ears and are pointed forward and downward. A correct fit improves the ability to hear blood pressure sounds.
11. Place the stethoscope diaphragm directly on the patient's skin over the site of the brachial artery to ensure accuracy in hearing blood pressure.
12. Make sure the patient's arm is relaxed at heart level. With the patient's arm fully extended, hold the stethoscope over the brachial pulse with your thumb while pressing the back of the elbow with your index and middle finger, which brings the brachial artery closer to the surface and the stethoscope.

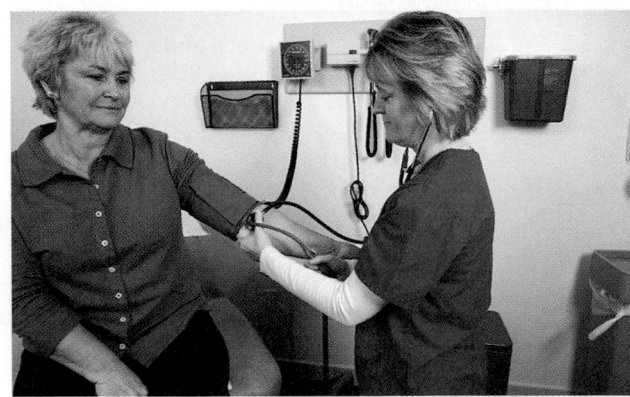

With the patient's arm fully extended, hold your stethoscope over the brachial pulse.

PROCEDURE 21-8—cont'd

13. Position the stethoscope tubing so that it hangs freely without rubbing on anything to eliminate noise interference.

14. Quickly inflate the bulb until the gauge measures approximately 30 mm Hg higher than the palpated reading to ensure that the systolic reading can be heard.

15. Release the pressure at a steady rate of 2 to 3 mm Hg per second. Releasing the pressure too fast or too slow may result in falsely high or low readings.

16. Note when the first sounds are heard (phase I) and record this measurement as the systolic pressure even if the sounds disappear and then return again (auscultatory gap) because the auscultatory gap may be considered a normal finding. (Be sure to note the auscultatory gap in the patient's medical record because, depending on the patient, it could be an abnormal finding.)

17. Note when the sounds completely disappear and record this as the diastolic pressure.

18. Measure and record blood pressure in both arms during an initial patient assessment and whenever the reading is in doubt to ensure accuracy.

19. Wait at least 1 minute between measurements if a repeat blood pressure measurement is required because repeating blood pressure measurement too quickly may result in an inaccurate reading.

20. Because the blood pressure gauge is marked in even numbers, record blood pressure in even numbers and as a fraction (such as *132/72*).

21. Remove the cuff from the patient's arm and return it to the appropriate place. Clean the stethoscope earpieces with alcohol or another antiseptic solution as dictated by office policy and return it to its appropriate place so that it will be clean and available for the next use.

22. Wash or sanitize your hands to ensure infection control.

23. Record the patient's blood pressure measurement in the medical record, including the date and time, to ensure accurate documentation and make the information available to the physician.

Date	
05/26/09; 9:52 a.m.	BP: 132/84. ------------------------------------ S. Lind, CMA

and confidently reports the first sound as the systolic pressure. Because an auscultatory gap is sometimes present with hypertension and some forms of heart disease, it should be noted in the medical record or verbally reported to the physician.

- *Phase III* occurs as the sound reappears (if it disappeared) or becomes louder and more crisp. This sound continues in a rhythmic pattern.
- *Phase IV* begins as the sounds become softer and fainter and take on a more muffled quality. Occasionally, these soft, muffled sounds continue to zero. The point at which the sounds become noticeably softer and fainter should be recorded as the diastolic reading in children. When this change occurs in adults, the physician may want the medical assistant to record three numbers. For example, in the pressure measurement *118/78/62 mm Hg*, the number *118* represents the systolic reading, the number *78* represents phase IV, and the number *62* represents the diastolic reading.
- *Phase V* occurs when the sounds completely disappear. This is recorded as the diastolic sound. (See *Procedure 21-8: Measuring blood pressure.*)

Postural Vital Signs

Occasionally, a physician may ask a medical assistant to check **postural vital signs,** which are vital signs that test for orthostatic hypotension. To measure postural vital signs, the medical assistant must check the patient's pulse and blood pressure in two or three positions (lying supine, sitting, and standing). Throughout the procedure, she must leave the blood pressure cuff in place. Some physicians ask the medical assistant to record pulse and blood pressure immediately after each position change. Others want the medical assistant to wait for 1 to 3 minutes after the position change before measuring vital signs. Therefore, the medical assistant must communicate with the physician to clarify his expectations. The data gathered from checking postural vital signs can help the physician determine if patients are volume depleted or suffering from some other condition that makes them prone to dizziness or syncope (fainting) upon sitting up or standing. Thus, when measuring postural vital signs, the medical assistant should be sure to ask the patient about such symptoms as dizziness, lightheadedness, or vertigo.

Oxygen Saturation

Measurement of arterial oxygen saturation (SpO_2) is becoming more common in acute care and ambulatory care settings. This measurement, done with a pulse oximeter, allows indirect measurement of oxygen bound to hemoglobin on red blood cells. The oximeter includes a probe with an LED and a photodetector. (See Figure 21-5.) The lightwaves from the LED are absorbed differently by hemoglobin, depending on how well it is saturated with oxygen. This difference is sensed by the photodetector and is calculated into the SpO$_2$ reading by the oximeter.

To obtain an accurate SpO$_2$ reading, the medical assistant must select a pulse oximeter probe that is appropriate for the patient. The medical assistant can clip a digit probe onto the patient's finger and an earlobe probe onto the patient's ear. Disposable sensor pads may be used on an adult's nose or an infant's foot.

Normal adult values for the SpO$_2$ are 95% to 100%. However, long-time smokers and those with chronic lung disease tend to run lower baseline values. The medical assistant should consult with the physician to identify a desirable SpO$_2$ goal for such patients. While the oximeter is a valuable tool, the medical assistant should understand its limitations. For example, the accuracy of pulse oximeter readings decreases as arterial oxygen levels drop below 70%. Other variables also impact the accuracy of the oximeter reading. (See *Factors that affect pulse oximeter readings*.) Therefore, the medical assistant must use good judgment in order to obtain

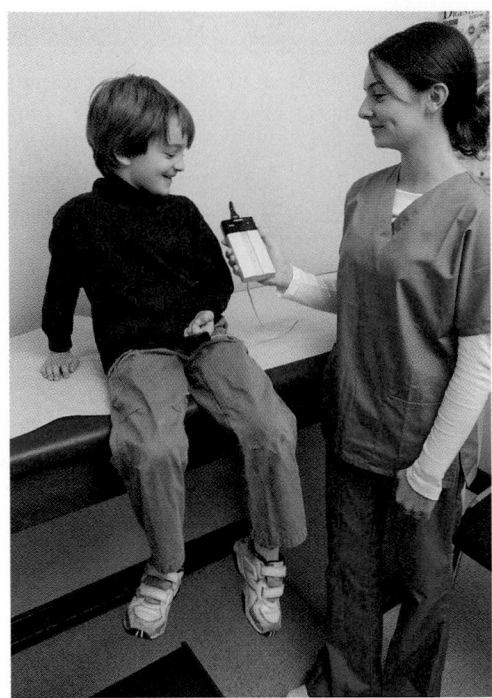

FIG 21-5 Pulse oximeter.

Factors that affect pulse oximeter readings

This table lists the most common factors that interfere with pulse oximeter readings and the corrective measures the medical assistant can take.

Interfering Factors	Corrective Measures
Outside light source	Close blinds or curtains
Carbon monoxide (CO) caused by smoke inhalation or poisoning (artificially elevates SpO$_2$ reading)	Do not use oximeter. Draw blood (per the physician's order) to obtain arterial blood gases.
Motion of patient's hand or finger	Hold the patient's arm and hand to provide support and minimize movement.
Jaundice (yellowish skin color due to liver disease)	Consider obtaining arterial blood gases (per the physician's order).
Intravascular dyes (methylene blue) (artificially lowers SpO$_2$ reading)	Consider using a backup measurement, such as arterial blood gases (per the physician's order).
Pale, cool hand and fingers of patient	Promote circulation by hanging the patient's arm and hand dependently (lower than the heart) for several minutes. Warm the patient's hand and fingers for several minutes with a warm moist towel. Alternatively, take another reading using a probe on the patient's ear or nose.
Edematous hands and fingers of patient	Use a probe on the ear or nose.
Excessively tight probe on patient's finger	Use a probe on the ear or nose or slightly open the finger clip while holding it on the patient's finger.
LED reading of questionable accuracy	Compare with the reading on another finger or on the ear or nose using the appropriate probe. Alternatively, apply the probe to your own finger and see what your reading is. If it is consistent with your baseline, then the oximeter is probably working fine.

PROCEDURE 21-9

Measuring oxygen saturation using a pulse oximeter

Task

Measure and record arterial oxygen saturation using a pulse oximeter.

Conditions

- Pulse oximeter with probe
- Acetone or nail polish remover
- Antiseptic wipe
- Pen
- Patient's medical record

Standards

In the time specified and within the scoring parameters determined by the instructor, the student will successfully measure the patient's oxygen saturation with a pulse oximeter.

Performance Standards

1. Wash or sanitize your hands to ensure infection control and assemble supplies.
2. Greet and identify your patient and introduce yourself to ease patient anxiety.
3. Explain the procedure and reassure the patient that it will not hurt to ease patient anxiety.
4. Clean the probe with an antiseptic wipe to ensure infection control.
5. Identify the patient's baseline reading, if available in the medical record, to provide a basis for comparison.
6. Identify the most appropriate site for the sensor probe and select the appropriate probe to ensure accurate measurement.
7. Position the patient comfortably and instruct him to breathe normally.
8. If a digital sensor is used on the finger, remove any nail polish and support the patient's lower arm because nail polish and movement may interfere with the reading.
9. Apply the probe and activate the oximeter. Wait several seconds and observe the pulse waveform and audible beep. Note the LED reading when it reaches a constant value. If necessary, check the radial pulse to verify accuracy.
10. Remove the probe and clean it with a disinfectant wipe to prevent transmission of pathogens to the next patient.
11. Return the oximeter to its correct location so that it will be available for the next use.
12. Wash or sanitize your hands to ensure infection control.
13. Record the SpO_2 level in the patient's medical record, including the date and time. Include data regarding oxygen use and the presence of fever to ensure accurate documentation and make the information available to the physician.

Date	
09/01/08; 1:50 p.m.	SpO_2 97%, O_2 @ 2 L per NC, Temp 99.8° F ------------------ -- S. Gonzales, CMA

the most accurate reading possible. She should also remember the guideline, "treat the patient, not the machine." Because machines and technology of any kind are tools, they are not foolproof. The medical assistant must always remember to look at the patient. If he looks well and states that he feels well, the medical assistant should double-check the equipment and get another reading. If the patient is symptomatic or if a low reading is still obtained, the medical assistant should consult with a nurse or physician right away. (See *Procedure 21-9: Measuring oxygen saturation using a pulse oximeter.*)

Chapter Summary

- Body temperature is regulated by the hypothalamus and is an important part of homeostasis. A number of factors may affect temperature, including infection, dehydration, exercise, and environment.
- Fever is a common symptom of illness caused by bacterial or viral infection. Depending on the cause and severity of a fever, the physician may elect not to treat it.
- Onset of a fever may be rapid or slow. The course of a fever follows one of three patterns: continuous, intermittent, or remittent.
- There are several types of thermometers, including glass, digital, tympanic, chemical, and temporal.
- The medical assistant should always disinfect nondisposable thermometers any time they have come into contact with body fluids.
- The pulse is generated by the heart each time it contracts to create a heartbeat. Some of the factors that affect pulse rate, rhythm, and strength include age, gender, emotional state, and metabolism.

- Cardiac arrhythmias may cause an irregular pulse and may cause some pulsations to be stronger than others.
- Pulse sites are present where a superficial artery is palpated against a bone. Common locations of pulse sites include the temporal, carotid, brachial, radial, apical, femoral, popliteal, dorsalis pedis, and posterior tibialis pulses.
- External respiration is the process of moving air into and out of the lungs. Inspiration, or the act of breathing in, occurs when the diaphragm and other muscles contract, pulling the thorax upward and outward. Expiration, which is usually passive, occurs when respiratory muscles relax and expel air from the lungs.
- Characteristics of respiration include rate, rhythm, and depth. These characteristics are all impacted by many variables, including age, physical activity, medications, and illness.
- Blood pressure is one of the most common measurements taken in the medical office. It reflects the pressure exerted against the walls of the arteries and is recorded as a fraction, with the systolic pressure represented by the top number and the diastolic pressure represented by the lower number.
- Hypertension is defined as sustained readings above 140/90 mm Hg. However, ideal blood pressure for all adults is below 120/80 mm Hg.
- Blood pressure may vary between persons and fluctuate even within the same day for the same person. Some factors that affect blood pressure include age, gender, and genetics. These factors are also nonmodifiable risk factors for hypertension and heart disease.
- Factors that may temporarily affect blood pressure include emotions, pain, physical exertion, fluid volume, and body position.
- Medications may also affect blood pressure. Such effects may be intentional, as with antihypertensive medication, or simply the adverse effect of a medication, such as an opiate analgesic.
- Measuring blood pressure is one of the most common procedures a medical assistant performs. She can achieve proficiency with practice.
- When listening to the patient's blood pressure, the medical assistant may notice five different types of sounds, known as *Korotkoff sounds.*
- Measurement of the arterial oxygen saturation level (SpO_2) with a pulse oximeter is becoming more common in acute care and ambulatory care settings. This measurement allows indirect measurement of oxygen bound to hemoglobin on red blood cells.
- The pulse oximeter is a useful tool, but good technique must be used to obtain reliable data.

Team Work Exercises

1. Divide into teams determined by your instructor and identify a location within the community to provide free screening of vital signs. Some potential locations include a shopping mall or senior center. Be sure to obtain permission from the owners or managers of the facility. Divide responsibilities among team members so that the following tasks are accomplished:
   a. appropriate and timely contact with facility managers and obtaining permission
   b. making logistical plans (identifying physical location for screening; obtaining tables, chairs, and equipment; and clarifying plans for transport and setup of equipment)
   c. organizing scheduling so that the table is staffed throughout the day (for example, team members may wish to work in pairs in 2-hour blocks of time)
   d. designating who is responsible for clean up at the end of the day and how it will occur
   e. identifying appropriate informational and resource literature and obtaining it to keep on hand
   f. creating a plan for when a client has significantly abnormal vital signs as well as advice that might be offered to the client (clarify the parameters of what constitutes "significant" with your instructor). **Note:** Medical assisting students cannot dispense medical advice. However, they can inform patients that a diagnosis cannot be made based on one isolated reading and that they should follow up with their health care providers if any concerns arise.
   g. keeping a written record of each person's age, gender, and vital signs (to turn in to the instructor per her instructions).
2. Divide into five teams. From cards prepared by the instructor (one card each for temperature, pulse, respiration, blood pressure, and SpO_2), each team must draw one card. Each team will role-play two versions of a scenario in which the medical assistant obtains the vital sign measurement from the patient. In version one, the medical assistant must make every common mistake possible that might affect the accuracy of the measurement. In version two, the team members must demonstrate correct technique that will ensure the accuracy of the measurement and review helpful tips for ensuring accuracy.

Case Studies

1. Miko Ono is a certified medical assistant (CMA) who works in an internal medicine office. One morning, she obtains vital signs and a weight on a new patient. His weight is 212 lb. However, office policy requires her to record patient weight in metrics. How should Miko record this patient's weight? Because the physician suspects this patient may be dehydrated, she asks Miko to obtain a set of postural vital signs. Describe how Miko will obtain these vital signs.

2. Jim Walker is a CMA who works in a family practice clinic. One day, he is helping provide care for an elderly patient who has Parkinson disease as well as diabetes. When attempting to check the patient's oxygen saturation with a pulse oximeter, Jim has difficulty obtaining a reliable reading. Explain some of the physical factors that might be hindering this process. List some troubleshooting strategies that Jim might employ to get a reliable reading.

Resources

- Practical guide to vital signs measurement: *medicine.ucsd.edu/clinicalmed/vital.htm*
- Taking vital signs: *http://healthfieldmedicare.suite101.com/article.cfm/taking_vital_signs__temperature*
- Vital signs information: *www.healthsystem.virginia.edu/uvahealth/adult_cardiac/vital.cfm*

Physical Examination

Learning Objectives

Upon completion of this chapter, the student will be able to:

- define and spell key terms in the Glossary
- describe the purpose of the physical examination
- list and describe six examination techniques commonly used by the physician
- list the supplies and equipment most commonly used in the physical examination and describe the purpose of each item
- discuss the medical assistant's role in preparing the patient examination room
- describe the medical assistant's role in preparing a patient for an examination
- explain how the medical assistant helps the physician and patient during an examination
- demonstrate how to assist a patient into nine different positions for examination
- demonstrate how to measure a patient's height and list at least one reason such a measurement is taken and documented
- demonstrate how to measure a patient's weight and list at least three reasons such a measurement is taken and documented.

CAAHEP Competencies

Clinical Competencies
Fundamental Principles
Practice standard precautions

Patient Care
Prepare and maintain examination and treatment areas
Prepare patients for and assist with routine and specialty examinations
Prepare patients for and assist with procedures, treatments, and minor office surgeries
General Competencies
Legal Concepts
Document appropriately
Patient Instruction
Provide instruction for health maintenance and disease prevention

ABHES Competencies

Clinical Duties
Prepare patients for procedures
Prepare patient for and assist physician with routine and specialty examinations and treatments and minor office surgeries

Procedures

Assisting with physical examination
Assisting the patient to the sitting position
Assisting the patient to the supine and dorsal recumbent positions
Assisting the patient to the Sims position
Assisting the patient to the lithotomy position
Assisting the patient to the semi-Fowler and Fowler positions
Assisting the patient to the Trendelenburg position
Assisting the patient to the knee-chest position
Measuring weight and height

Chapter Outline

Purpose of the Physical Examination

In order to diagnose and treat disorders and diseases, health care providers must gather information about the patient. The information-gathering process involves three phases:

- history taking
- physical examination
- diagnostic testing.

In some cases, the physical examination will be brief and limited in scope—for example, the patient who complains of a simple sore throat. In such a case, the physician may ask a few questions; examine only the patient's respiratory system, including the ears, nose, mouth, throat, and lungs, and be done in as little as 10 minutes. Diagnostic testing may or may not be done. On the other hand, a new patient visiting a primary care physician for the first time to establish regular care will likely undergo an examination that could take up to an hour and cover all body systems. Depending on the patient's age, diagnostics might include blood tests, urinalysis, routine mammography, colonoscopy screening, and other tests. (See *Scheduling the physical examination.*)

Physical Examination Techniques

The medical assistant commonly interacts with the patient before the physician does. Therefore, she must be alert to clues about the patient's concerns. Some characteristics she might note include the patient's general appearance, posture, gait (manner of walking), skin condition, willingness to make eye contact, indicators of pain or difficulty breathing, and issues related to hygiene and grooming. If the medical assistant has significant concerns based on these observations, she should communicate them to the physician. The physician generally conducts a brief interview prior to the examination, which provides an opportunity for the patient and physician to further discuss the patient's concerns. During the physical examination process, the physician generally uses some specific, predictable techniques known as *inspection, palpation, percussion, auscultation, mensuration,* and *manipulation.*

Inspection
Inspection involves gathering information about the patient through observation. The physician notes the patient's general appearance and behaviors, including how she walks, talks, speaks, and makes eye contact; her tone of voice; and other behaviors. In the course of the physical examination, the physician visually examines each body part before and during the hands-on examination.

Palpation

Palpation involves examination of the patient's external body through touch with the hands and pads of the fingers. Light palpation of the skin reveals information about temperature, moisture, and texture. Deep palpation may be used to feel the size, shape, symmetry (similarity in shape and size on both sides of the body), and firmness of organs to detect the presence of masses. A great deal of information can be obtained through direct touch. For example, checking **skin turgor** (resistance of the skin to deformation when grasped between the fingers) provides information about a patient's hydration state. (See Figure 22-1.)

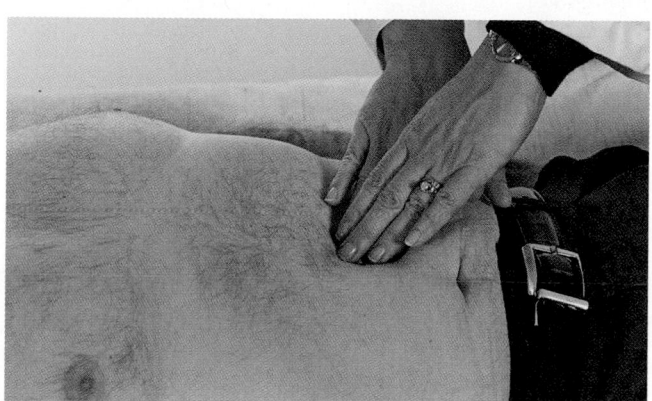

FIG 22-1 Palpating the abdomen.

Percussion

Percussion involves tapping on body structures with the fingers or a small hammer to note the sound elicited. The nature of the sound reveals information about the structures beneath. For example, the abdomen will usually have a more tympanic (high-pitched, vibrating) sound due to greater air content; the area over the liver usually sounds more dull due to its denser, vascular structure. Direct percussion involves tapping directly on the patient's skin. Indirect percussion involves laying the nondominant hand or finger on the patient's skin and then tapping it with the fingers of the dominant hand. (See Figure 22-2.)

Auscultation

Auscultation involves listening to body sounds with a stethoscope. The physician commonly auscultates the patient's lungs to determine whether they sound clear or have abnormal sounds due to narrowed airways or the presence of fluid. He also auscultates the patient's abdomen to assess bowel sounds. Normal sounds include stomach gurgling caused by intestinal peristalsis, the progressive, wavelike, involuntary movement that propels the contents forward. The physician also auscultates heart and vascular sounds, noting the rhythm as well as the presence of such abnormal sounds

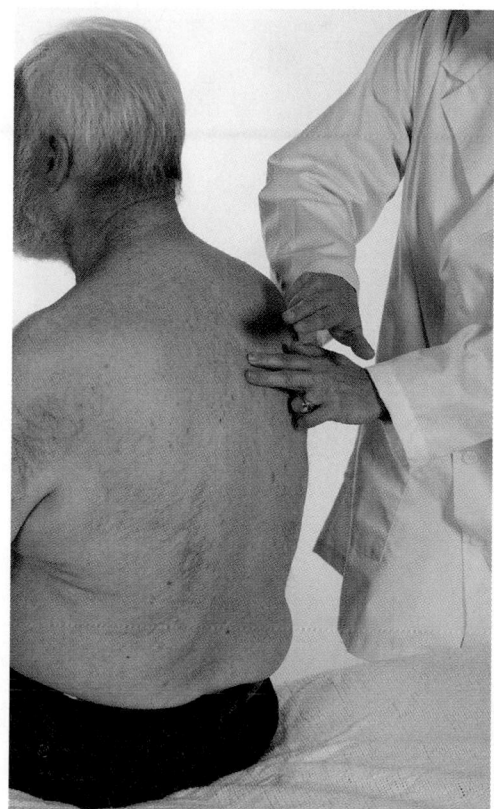

FIG 22-2 Percussing the lungs.

as murmurs (blowing or swishing sound in the heart) and bruits (abnormal arterial or venous swishing sounds heard on auscultation). (See Figure 22-3.)

Mensuration

Mensuration involves various body measurements that may include height or, in the case of an infant, length. The circumference of the head, chest, abdomen, and extremities are sometimes measured as well. Measurements of joint motion may also be taken to determine degree of flexion and extension.

Manipulation

Manipulation involves the application of hands-on techniques to assess joint symmetry and note passive range of motion. It may also be used to employ therapeutic force to increase joint mobility and realign dislocated joints. Manipulation may be done with or without anesthesia or sedation.

Components of a Physical Examination

The medical assistant's presence may not be required for every examination or treatment. However, in cases where

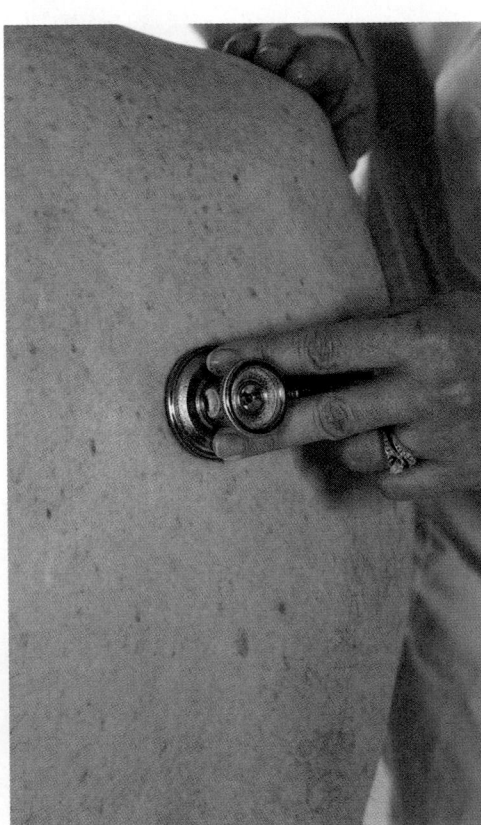

FIG 22-3 Auscultating lung sounds.

the physician and patient are of the opposite gender—especially when the procedure involves areas of the body usually considered private—the medical assistant should remain in the room. The presence of a second professional in the room provides reassurance to the patient and protects the physician from potential lawsuits.

In order to anticipate the patient's and physician's needs, the medical assistant must understand the format of a routine physical examination. The medical assistant can usually predict the sequence that the physician will follow and, thus, predict his needs. The standard physical examination is organized according to body system and, to some extent, follows a head-to-toe order. However, the physician may vary the examination depending on many factors, including the patient's age, chief complaint, and purpose for the visit. After the medical assistant works with a physician for a short time, she will become more adept at developing a system that works smoothly.

The physical examination generally includes components in this order:

- general appearance
- skin
- arms and hands
- head and neck
- eyes
- ears
- nose
- mouth and pharynx
- chest and lungs
- cardiovascular function
- breasts
- abdomen
- genitalia and rectum
- legs and feet
- mental status.

The physician will examine each component for normal and abnormal findings. (See *Common physical examination findings.*)

Preparing for the Physical Examination

The medical assistant helps with the examination process in three key ways. She keeps the examination room ready at all times, prepares the patient for examination, and assists the physician as needed.

Preparing the Examination Room
The medical assistant plays a vital role in helping ensure a smooth, efficient workflow in the medical office. Her

Common physical examination findings

The following table lists common normal and abnormal findings for each component of the physical examination.

Component	Normal Findings	Abnormal Findings
General appearance	• Healthy and well-nourished • Well-groomed • Upright posture and a steady gait	• Malnourished or cachectic (extreme state of malnutrition and muscle wasting) • Morbidly obese • Poor posture or gait
Skin	• Warm, dry, intact, and supple • Appropriate color for ethnicity • Free of lesions • Normal turgor	• Rashes, scales, or lesions • Wounds • Pale, erythematous (reddened), cyanotic (bluish), dusky (poor coloring such as mild cyanosis), or jaundiced (yellowish) • Moist or diaphoretic (profuse sweating) • Taut or edematous (swollen) • Scaly
Arms and hands	• Smooth, supple skin with appropriate color for ethnicity • Absence of rashes or lesions • Present, strong, regular pulses • Full, active range of motion (ROM) with symmetrical and optimal strength and coordination • Smooth, clear nails with convex curve and normal angle of the nail bed to the skin	• Rashes or lesions • Abnormal skin color • Weak, irregular, or absent pulses • Muscle weakness, lack of coordination, or decreased ROM • Absent, brittle, ridged, cracked, yellowed, thickened, or cyanotic nails • Clubbing (enlargement of distal ends of the fingers with no angle from the nail bed to the skin, due to excessive soft tissue growth caused by chronic lung and heart disease)
Head and neck	• Symmetrical head shape • Lustrous or shiny hair that is evenly distributed with a clean scalp that is free of scales or lesions • Supple neck that is free of lumps or tenderness and a nonpalpable thyroid	• Asymmetrical or abnormally sized head • Hair loss • Lumps, scales, lesions, lice, or nits (egg of a louse or any other parasitic insect) on the scalp • Lymphadenopathy (abnormal condition of the lymph glands that causes them to become swollen and tender) in the neck • Enlarged thyroid
Eyes	• Accurate visual acuity and color vision • Intact visual field and extraocular movements (EOM) • Pupils that are equal, round, and reactive to light and accommodation (PERRLA) • White, clear sclera that is free of drainage	• Poor visual acuity, blindness, or color-blindness • Decreased visual field, cloudy lens, or decreased EOM • Pupils that are dilated, constricted, dull, unequal, or slow to react or nonreactive to light or have poor accommodation • Blepharoptosis (drooping of the eyelid) • Sclera that is jaundiced, inflamed, or tearing excessively • Purulent drainage • Exophthalmos (abnormal protrusion of the eyeballs)

Continued

Common physical examination findings—cont'd

Component	Normal Findings	Abnormal Findings
Ears	• Intact hearing • Ears that are symmetrical and normally placed • Pink, patent (wide-open, evident, or accessible) ear canal with minimal cerumen • Pink to pearly gray tympanic membrane that is semitransparent and intact	• Hearing loss or deafness • Ears that are asymmetrical or low-set • Ear canal that is impacted with cerumen or inflamed • Perforated, inflamed, blistered, retracted, or bulging tympanic membrane
Nose	• Straight nose with a midline septum • Patent nares • Pink, moist mucosa • Absent or scant, clear drainage • Intact odor identification	• Deviated septum • Nonpatent nares • Mucous membranes that are inflamed, edematous, boggy, or dry • Purulent drainage • Anosmia (loss of sense of smell) • Polyps (small growths)
Mouth and pharynx	• Structures and membranes that are pink, moist, smooth, and free of lesions • Teeth present with good dental hygiene • Pink, firm gums • Intact gag reflex • Pink tonsils without swelling or exudate (any fluid released from body tissues that has a high concentration of protein cells or solid debris; sometimes containing pus)	• Inflammation, lesions, ulcerations, or dry (tacky) mucous membranes • Dental caries (cavities), loose or absent teeth, loose dentures, or poor oral hygiene • Gingivitis (inflamed gums) • Absent gag reflex • Inflamed, enlarged tonsils with exudate
Chest and lungs	• Symmetrical chest shape with normal anterior-posterior (AP) dimension • Clear lungs • Regular, unlabored respirations	• Asymmetrical, barrel-like chest with increased AP dimension • Decreased lung sounds • Crackles (abnormal sound heard with a stethoscope caused by secretions or sudden opening of tiny collapsed airways) • Rhonchi (low-pitched wheezing, snoring, squeaking, or gurgling sound, caused by mucus or other secretions, heard on auscultation of the lungs with a stethoscope) • Pericardial friction rub (creaking, grating, scratchy, or leathery sound made by inflamed membranes surrounding the heart as they move during the heart beat) • Pleural friction rub (creaking, grating, scratchy, or leathery sound made by inflamed membranes surrounding the lungs as they move during respiration) • Wheezes (continuous musical sound caused by air movement through narrowed respiratory passages) • Irregular or labored respirations

Common physical examination findings—cont'd

Component	Normal Findings	Abnormal Findings
Cardiovascular	• Regular heart rhythm • S_1 and S_2 heart sounds present • Palpable, regular peripheral pulses • Capillary refill (return of normal color in a nail bed or digit after blanching due to pressing on it) less than 3 seconds • Blood pressure within normal range • Normal sinus rhythm (NSR) on electrocardiogram (ECG)	• Irregular heart rhythm • Distant heart sounds, murmur, and S_3 and S_4 heart sounds • Diminished or absent peripheral pulses • Slow or absent capillary refill • Hypertension or hypotension • Abnormal rhythm on ECG
Breasts	• Soft with irregular feel of deep tissue • Symmetrical size, shape, and color of breasts and nipples • Free of lumps, lesions, dimpling, or nipple drainage • Nonpalpable axillary lymph nodes	• Lumps • Abnormal tenderness (although mild tenderness may be normal due to hormonal fluctuations) • Nipple discharge or nipple inversion • Retraction or dimpling of breast tissue or orange-peel appearance • Enlarged axillary lymph nodes
Abdomen	• Soft, nontender, active bowel sounds in all four quadrants • Nonpalpable liver and spleen • Absence of hernias	• Firm, distended, tender abdomen • Hypoactive, hyperactive, or absent bowel sounds • Masses, lesions, or hernias • Hepatomegaly (enlarged liver) or splenomegaly (enlarged spleen)
Genitalia and rectum	• Absence of rashes or lesions • Purulent (forming or containing pus) or foul drainage • Smooth skin • Pink, moist, smooth mucous membranes • Good pelvic floor muscle tone • Smooth, firm, movable testicles • Intact anal sphincter tone • Absence of hemorrhoids or anal fissures (painful linear ulcers on the margin of the anus) • Absence of blood in stool	• Abnormal tenderness • Rashes, lesions, vesicles, or ulcerations • Purulent or foul drainage • Inflamed, edematous, or dry mucous membranes • Weak pelvic floor muscles with prolapse (falling or dropping down) of bladder, rectum, or uterus • Asymmetrical or enlarged testicles • Poor anal sphincter tone • Hemorrhoids or fissures • Positive stool for blood on rectal examination
Legs and feet	• Smooth, supple skin with appropriate color for ethnicity • Absence of rashes, lesions, ulcerations, or edema • Present, strong, regular pulses • Capillary refill less than 3 seconds • Full, active ROM with symmetrical and optimal strength and coordination • Smooth, clear nails • Intact pulses	• Abnormal skin coloring • Rashes, lesions, or edema • Weak, irregular, or absent pulses • Varicosities (condition of having veins that are enlarged and dilated) • Slow capillary refill • Muscle weakness, lack of coordination, or decreased ROM • Nails that are absent, brittle, ridged, cracked, yellowed, or thickened

Continued

Common physical examination findings—cont'd

Component	Normal Findings	Abnormal Findings
Mental status	• Alert and oriented to person, place, and time (A&O × 3) • Appropriate identification of sensory data (such as sharp, dull, soft, and painful) • Intact reflexes	• Confusion or inappropriate verbal responses • Lethargy or agitation • Aphasia (inability to speak) or dysphasia (difficulty speaking) • Short- or long-term memory loss • Diminished or absent reflexes or sensation • Poor coordination • Complaints of vertigo (sensation of moving around in space, or dizziness)

responsibilities include making sure that examination rooms are cleaned, disinfected, and restocked as needed between patients. The medical assistant should check the schedule ahead of time and note the purpose of each patient's visit in order to anticipate the equipment and supplies that will most likely be needed. Having all items ready and close at hand saves time and earns the respect and appreciation of the physician and patient. The patient will also appreciate attention paid to his comfort and privacy needs. The medical assistant must also keep safety and hygiene equipment stocked, including antibacterial soap or cleanser, paper towels, examination gloves, biohazard waste containers, sharps containers, gowns, and masks. The patient who must wait for a few minutes will also appreciate the medical assistant who provides reading material. Such material should include educational pamphlets as well as an assortment of magazines.

Preparing the Patient

The medical assistant should prepare the patient by inquiring about the purpose of the visit, making sure the information in the chart is current, and measuring height, weight, and vital signs. In some cases, she collects urine or blood specimens prior to the examination. If not, the medical assistant should invite the patient to visit the restroom to empty her bladder prior to the examination. Emptying the bladder can help make the examination process more comfortable for the patient—especially when an examination of the abdomen or pelvis will occur. The medical assistant should also provide instructions for undressing and positioning and assist the patient with changing into the examination gown if necessary. (See *Patients with special needs*.)

Front office–Back office connection

Patients with Special Needs

The administrative medical assistant or receptionist should immediately inform the clinical medical assistant of any patients who arrive with special needs (such as a patient who is weak, frail, dizzy, or using such mobility aids as a cane, walker, or wheelchair). Doing so allows everyone to make necessary adjustments to the routine so that extra care and attention can be given to the patient. This small but significant addition to the communication process ensures patient safety, facilitates a smooth work-flow, decreases staff stress, and fosters a spirit of cooperation among health care team members.

Physical Examination Supplies and Equipment

The medical assistant must ensure that examination supplies and equipment are ready, organized, and close at hand and are restocked or disinfected between patients. (See *Physical examination equipment and supplies*.)

Assisting with the Physical Examination

During the examination, the medical assistant acts as a helper to the physician and an advocate for the patient. She helps the physician by handing him needed supplies and

Physical examination equipment and supplies

Here are some of the items usually used during a physical examination, along with a description of their most common uses.

Equipment

- Glass slides—holding specimens that are viewed under a microscope
- Laryngeal and pharyngeal mirrors—examining the pharynx and larynx
- Nasal speculum—examining the nose and nasal mucous membranes
- Otoscope—examining the ear
- Ophthalmoscope—examining the eye
- Penlight—examining the pupils and providing additional light for examination of the throat or other body parts
- Reflex hammer—testing reflexes
- Specimen bottles—holding tissue specimens that will undergo laboratory analysis
- Sphygmomanometer—measuring blood pressure
- Stethoscope—measuring blood pressure and auscultating heart, lungs, and bowel sounds
- Tape measure—measuring the length and circumference of various body parts
- Thermometer—measuring body temperature
- Vaginal speculum—assisting in opening a vagina more fully to facilitate examination

Supplies

- Alcohol pads—cleaning the skin prior to an injection or cleaning some medical equipment
- Cotton balls—applying medication or stopping minor bleeding
- Cotton-tipped applicators—applying medication or collecting a specimen
- Emesis basin—collecting vomitus or sputum from patient
- Gauze pads—dressing a wound, stopping bleeding, or applying medication
- Lubricant—reducing anticipated discomfort from speculum insertion or rectal or vaginal examinations or easing suppository insertion
- Tongue depressor—depressing the tongue for easier examination of the throat

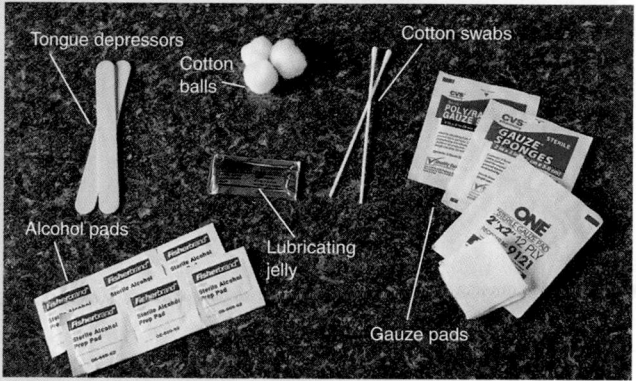

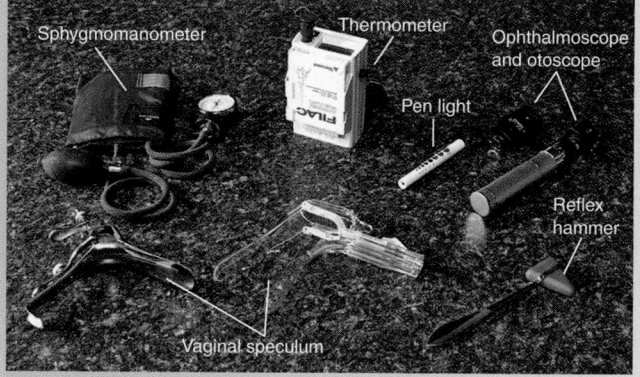

instrumets. (See *Procedure 22-1: Assisting with the physical examination*, pages 354 and 355.) She also pays close attention to the patient and offers reassurance, instruction, and assistance with positioning and draping as needed. After the examination, she may conduct additional diagnostic testing and help schedule the patient for further tests, referrals, or follow-up visits. (See *The teachable moment*, page 355.)

Positioning and Draping

The medical assistant helps with the examination process by instructing and assisting the patient in assuming

PROCEDURE 22-1

Assisting with the physical examination

Task
Assisting the physician with a physical examination.

Conditions
- Examination table
- Specific supplies and equipment for the type of examination being performed
- Drape
- Patient examination gown

Standards
In the time specified and within the scoring parameters determined by the instructor, the student will successfully assist the physician with the physical examination of a patient.

Performance Standards
1. Prepare the examination room, ensuring adequate room temperature and lighting.
2. Wash or sanitize your hands to ensure infection control.
3. Assemble supplies and equipment in the order in which they will be used to ensure a smooth flow to the examination procedure.
4. Obtain the patient's medical record, greet and identify the patient, and introduce yourself to prevent errors and ease patient anxiety.
5. Obtain the patient's weight and height if needed and escort her to the examination room.
6. Review the record with the patient, making sure that the medication list and allergy information are current.
7. Inquire about the purpose of the visit. Record the patient's complaint and symptoms to the degree of detail preferred by the physician.
8. Obtain the patient's vital signs to ensure that important data is current and allow time for the patient to explain and confirm the reason for the visit.
9. Draw blood if needed for laboratory tests. Perform an ECG if ordered.
10. Invite the patient to empty her bladder. If a urine specimen is needed, provide instructions and a specimen container to decrease patient discomfort during the examination and obtain preliminary results of some tests during the patient's visit.
11. Provide the patient with an examination gown and drape. Instruct her to remove all clothing, pointing out where she may hang or lay her clothing. Explain that the gown should be worn with the opening in the front and how the drape should be used.
12. Explain that the patient should sit on the end of the examination table and that the physician will be with her soon to ensure patient understanding.

13. Leave the room so the patient may change in privacy to demonstrate respect for her privacy. However, if she is elderly, weak, or frail or has any symptoms of dizziness, remain in the room to assist her. Help her sit in a regular chair to wait for the physician to prevent falls and ensure the safety of a weak or symptomatic patient.
14. Place the medical record in the designated place for the physician to retrieve and let him know that the patient is ready.
15. Return to the room when directed by the physician to allow time for the physician to interview the patient, if preferred, for a few minutes prior to the examination. (The medical assistant's presence is usually not required for this.)
16. Assist the physician with a general body system examination, including:
    a. Assist the patient into a sitting position on the end of the table if she is not already there. Arrange the drape over her lap.
    b. As the physician examines the patient's upper body (eyes, ears, nose, mouth, throat, and chest), be prepared to hand her items as needed, such as the otoscope, ophthalmoscope, penlight, and tongue depressor.
    c. Dim the lights if directed when the physician examines the patient's eyes to help dilate the patient's pupils.
    d. Throughout the remainder of the examination, continue to hand needed items to the physician and assist the patient in assuming the positions directed by the physician.
    e. Follow standard precautions and take care to handle potentially contaminated items from the physician (such as a tongue depressor, a speculum, and swabs) in a manner that prevents exposure to you.
    f. Dispose of all waste in appropriate containers.
    g. Place specimens in appropriately labeled containers.
17. Upon completion of the examination, assist the patient down from the table and instruct her to get dressed. Leave the room for a few minutes so the patient may change in privacy unless she requires your assistance to show respect for the patient's privacy and protect her safety.
18. Provide the patient with educational information or instructions as directed by the physician and answer questions she may have. Consult the physician or nurse if you are unsure of the answer to a patient's question to ensure that the patient receives the correct information, which is critical.

PROCEDURE 22-1—cont'd

19. Schedule ordered follow-up tests or appointments.

20. Direct the patient back to the reception area. Assist her if needed.

21. Document patient education, instructions, or scheduled tests in the medical record to ensure that the medical record is thorough and accurate.

22. Clean, sanitize, and restock the examination room as needed to prepare the room for the next patient.

Date	
11/01/08: 9:05 a.m.	*Pamphlet titled "Ten ways to Lower Your Cholesterol" given to patient. mammogram scheduled for 11/05/08 ------------------ ----------------------------------- S. Gonzales, CMA*

---

various positions. The purpose of each position is to allow the physician better access to and visibility of the body part being examined. To help promote patient privacy and comfort, the medical assistant should provide careful draping. Here are the 10 examination positions, along with the most common reasons for placing the patient in each:

- The sitting position is commonly used for examination of the upper body, including the head, eyes, ears, nose, throat, neck, chest, lungs, arms, and hands. Common reasons for examining the patient in this position include upper respiratory symptoms (such as a sore throat, sinus pressure, a cough, and an earache) and painful or inflamed joints of the arms, hands, and fingers. (See *Procedure 22-2: Assisting the patient into the sitting position*, page 356.)

- The **supine position,** also called the *horizontal recumbent position,* is commonly used for examination of the breasts, anterior chest, heart, abdomen, and lower extremities. This is a position in which the patient is lying flat, face toward the ceiling. Common reasons for examining the patient in this position include breast cancer screening, heart problems, or pain in the abdomen, lower leg, or foot.

- The **dorsal recumbent position** is sometimes used for rectal and vaginal examinations, particularly if the patient cannot tolerate lying on her back with her feet in stirrups. In the dorsal recumbent position, the patient is lying flat or nearly flat with legs apart, knees bent, and feet near the side edges of the examination table. It may also be used for patients with back or abdominal pain, because bending the knees relieves stress on the lower back and facilitates relaxation of abdominal muscles. It is useful for patients undergoing routine examinations and for those with vaginal or rectal pain, burning, or unusual discharge. It is also useful for those complaining of abdominal, pelvic, or back pain. (See *Procedure 22-3: Assisting the patient into the supine and dorsal positions*, page 357.)

- The **Sims position,** also called the *side-lying* or *lateral position,* is used for anal and rectal examinations, some vaginal examinations, and such procedures as administering rectal suppositories and enemas. In this position, the patient lies on his side with the upper arm forward on the table, lower arm behind, lower leg flexed slightly, and upper leg flexed sharply with his knee resting forward on the examination table. The medical assistant should also consider using this position for a female patient who needs a urinary catheter inserted but cannot tolerate lying supine. In such a case, a second person will be required to support the patient's upper leg. However, the extra effort is worthwhile because the patient with back pain or

Patient Education

The Teachable Moment

Although their time is limited, health care providers, including medical assistants, have many opportunities to provide patient education on a wide range of subjects. To capitalize on what educators refer to as the "teachable moment," the medical assistant must be observant and take notice when a patient expresses interest in a particular subject or concern about an actual or potential health problem. This teachable moment is a time when a patient is especially likely to pay attention to the message shared.

Such opportunities commonly arise when a patient visits for a routine examination. The medical assistant should answer whatever questions she can, consult with the physician on those she cannot, and always try to send the patient home with some type of literature on the subject. Doing so conveys a desire to meet the patient's needs and provides teaching in two different formats: verbal and written. Many brochures also include websites, addresses, and phone numbers where patients can find additional information.

PROCEDURE 22-2

Assisting the patient into the sitting position

Task
Assist the patient into the sitting position.

Conditions
- Examination table
- Table paper
- Examination gown
- Disposable drape or sheet

Standards
In the time specified and within the scoring parameters determined by the instructor, the student will successfully assist the patient into the sitting position.

Performance Standards
1. Greet and identify the patient, introduce yourself, and explain the procedure to prevent errors and ease patient anxiety.
2. Wash or sanitize your hands to ensure infection control.
3. Provide the patient with an examination gown. Describe how fully the patient should undress. Point out where the patient may hang or lay his clothing. Explain that the gown should be worn with the opening in the front.
4. Pull out the footrest of the examination table and explain that he should sit securely on the end of the table with the drape over his lap to ensure patient understanding, proper positioning, and patient safety and comfort.

5. Leave the room for a few minutes so the patient may change in privacy unless he requires your assistance to demonstrate respect for the patient's privacy and safety.
6. Assist the physician as needed with the examination.
7. Upon completion of the examination, assist the patient down from the table and instruct him to get dressed.
8. Return the table footrest to the normal position. Leave the room for a few minutes so the patient may change in privacy unless he requires your assistance to ensure the patient's safety and privacy.
9. Clean, sanitize, and restock the examination room as needed to prepare the room for the next patient.

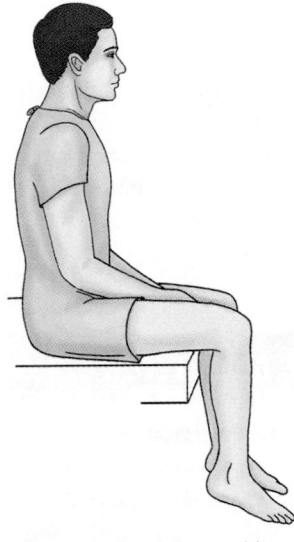

Patient in the sitting position

---

shortness of breath will better tolerate the procedure in this position. Additionally, this position commonly facilitates a better view of the patient's urethral opening. (See *Procedure 22-4: Assisting the patient into the Sims position,* page 358.)

- The **lithotomy position** is primarily used for vaginal examinations and is especially useful when a speculum is required to examine the cervix and collect a specimen for a Papanicolaou (Pap) smear. In this position, the patient reclines face up, with legs apart and feet placed in stirrups. It is used for routine female gynecologic examinations and when women have complaints of pelvic pain or unusual vaginal pain, burning, or discharge. (See

Procedure 22-5: Assisting the patient into the lithotomy position, pages 358 and 359.)

- The **semi-Fowler position** is similar to the Fowler position with the head of the examination table at only 45 degrees. The patient reclines with legs outstretched on the examination table. This position is used for many purposes, including examination of the chest and heart, or for patients who need to rest in a semi-reclining position for comfort reasons.
- The **Fowler position** is similar to the upright sitting position, except that the head of the examination table is elevated as close to 90 degrees as possible to provide support for the patient to lean against and the legs to

PROCEDURE 22-3

Assisting the patient into the supine and dorsal recumbent positions

Task

Assist the patient into the supine and dorsal recumbent positions.

Conditions

- Examination table
- Table paper
- Examination gown
- Pillow
- Disposable drape or sheet

Standards

In the time specified and within the scoring parameters determined by the instructor, the student will successfully assist the patient into the supine and dorsal recumbent positions.

Performance Standards

1. Greet and identify the patient, introduce yourself, and explain the procedure to prevent errors and ease patient anxiety.
2. Wash or sanitize your hands to ensure infection control.
3. Provide the patient with an examination gown. Describe how fully the patient should undress. Point out where the patient may hang or lay her clothing. Explain that the gown should be worn with the opening in the front to ensure patient understanding.
4. Pull out the footrest of the examination table and explain to the patient that she should sit securely on the end of the table with the drape over her lap to ensure patient understanding.
5. Leave the room for a few minutes so the patient can change to ensure patient privacy unless she requires your assistance.
6. When you reenter the room, instruct the patient to lie back and rest her head on the pillow. As she does so, pull out the table extension to support her legs.

7. Ensure that she is lying flat and the drape is positioned properly over her abdomen and legs to ensure proper positioning and the patient's safety, privacy, and comfort.

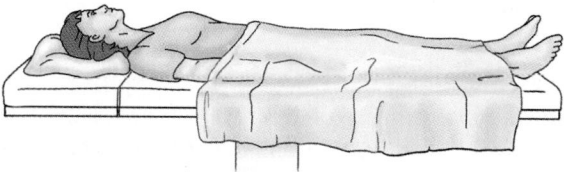

Patient in the supine position

8. To assist the patient into the dorsal recumbent position, instruct her to place the soles of both feet flat on the table with her knees flexed.

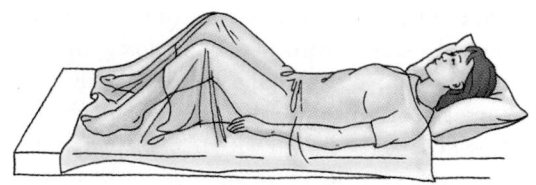

Patient in the dorsal recumbent position

9. Assist the physician as needed with the examination.
10. Upon completion of the examination, assist the patient down from the table and instruct her to get dressed. Return the table footrest to the normal position.
11. Leave the room for a few minutes so the patient may change in privacy unless she requires your assistance to ensure the patient's safety and privacy.
12. Clean, sanitize, and restock the examination room as needed to prepare the room for the next patient.

---

rest outstretched on the examination table. It is used for the same reasons as the sitting position and is particularly useful for patients who are feeling short of breath, because the upright position facilitates maximal lung expansion. (See *Procedure 22-6: Assisting the patient into the semi-Fowler and Fowler positions,* page 360.)

- In the **Trendelenburg position,** the patient lies with her head approximately 30 degrees lower than her outstretched legs and feet. This position is rarely used in the

medical office. It may be useful for patients experiencing shock or dangerously low blood pressure. It is sometimes used for abdominal surgery because gravity causes abdominal contents to shift somewhat toward the chest. Many patients do not tolerate this position well or for long since it makes breathing more difficult. Therefore, the medical assistant should consult with the physician before assisting a patient into this position. (See *Procedure 22-7: Assisting the patient into the Trendelenburg position,* page 361.)

PROCEDURE 22-4

Assisting the patient into the Sims position

Task
Assist the patient into the Sims position.

Conditions
- Examination table
- Table paper
- Examination gown
- Pillow
- Disposable drape or sheet

Standards
In the time specified and within the scoring parameters determined by the instructor, the student will successfully assist the patient into the Sims position.

Performance Standards
1. Greet and identify the patient, introduce yourself, and explain the procedure to prevent errors and ease patient anxiety.
2. Wash or sanitize your hands to control infection.
3. Provide the patient with an examination gown. Describe how fully the patient should undress. Point out where the patient may hang or lay his clothing. Explain that the gown should be worn with the opening in the back.
4. Leave the room for a few minutes so the patient may change in privacy unless he requires your assistance to ensure patient comfort, privacy, and safety.
5. Assist the patient onto the table and into a sitting position. Then instruct him to lie back and rest his head on the pillow. As he does this, pull out the table extension to support his legs.

6. Pull out the footrest and instruct the patient to turn onto his left side. Provide support as needed to ensure that he does not accidentally roll off the table.
7. Position him with his left arm behind his body and his right arm forward with his elbow bent. Instruct him to flex his left leg slightly and his right leg sharply. Place a pillow between his knees.
8. Ensure that the drape is positioned properly to ensure proper positioning and patient safety, privacy, and comfort.

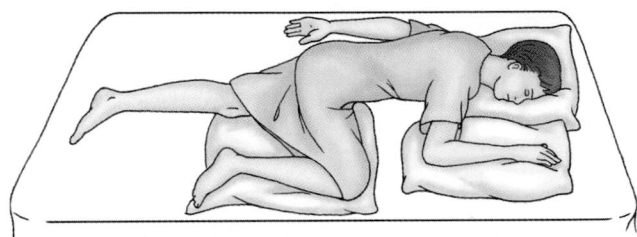

Patient in Sims position

9. Assist the physician as needed with the examination.
10. Upon completion of the examination, assist the patient down from the table and instruct him to get dressed. Return the table footrest to the normal position. Leave the room for a few minutes so the patient may change in privacy unless he requires your assistance.
11. Clean, sanitize, and restock the examination room as needed to prepare the room for the next patient.

PROCEDURE 22-5

Assisting the patient into the lithotomy position

Task
Assist the patient into the lithotomy position.

Conditions
- Examination table
- Table paper
- Examination gown
- Pillow
- Disposable drape or sheet

Standards
In the time specified and within the scoring parameters determined by the instructor, the student will successfully assist the patient into the lithotomy position.

Performance Standards
1. Greet and identify the patient, introduce yourself, and explain the procedure to prevent errors and ease patient anxiety.
2. Wash or sanitize your hands to ensure infection control.
3. Provide the patient with an examination gown. Describe how fully the patient should undress. Point out where the patient may hang or lay her clothing. Explain that the gown should be worn with the opening in the front.
4. Leave the room for a few minutes so the patient may change in privacy unless she requires your assistance.

PROCEDURE 22-5—cont'd

5. Pull out the footrest and assist the patient onto the table into a sitting position. Then instruct her to lie back and rest her head on the pillow. As she does this, pull out the table extension to support her legs. Next, pull out the stirrups and adjust their position to the patient's size. Instruct her to slide down to the bottom of the table and guide her feet into the stirrups.

6. Adjust the drape so that it lies in a diamond formation with one corner draped between the patient's legs to ensure proper positioning and patient safety, privacy, and comfort. (The physician can lift the corner of the drape as needed just prior to the examination.)

7. Assist the physician as needed with the examination.

8. Upon completion of the examination, assist the patient down from the table and instruct her to get dressed. Return the table footrest to the normal position.

9. Leave the room for a few minutes so the patient may change in privacy unless she requires your assistance to ensure patient safety and privacy.

10. Clean, sanitize, and restock the examination room as needed to prepare the room for the next patient.

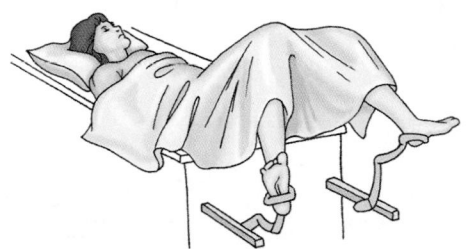

Patient in the lithotomy position

- In the **knee-chest position,** the patient sits on his knees with his chest and face resting forward on a pillow, his arms lying to either side of his head and his buttocks in the air. This position may be awkward, embarrassing, and difficult for many patients to assume. Therefore, the medical assistant must help the patient with positioning and remain with him the entire time to provide stability and emotional support. This position is used for rectal and sigmoid colon examinations and, rarely, for vaginal examinations. (See *Procedure 22-8: Assisting the patient into the knee-chest position,* page 361.)

- The **jack-knife position** requires a special table and is rarely done anywhere but in a urology department. It should be done with the head-up position for patient comfort and ease in breathing. In this position, the patient is in a semi-sitting position with his thighs flexed to 90 degrees. It is useful for male urologic examinations and procedures. (See Figure 22-4.)

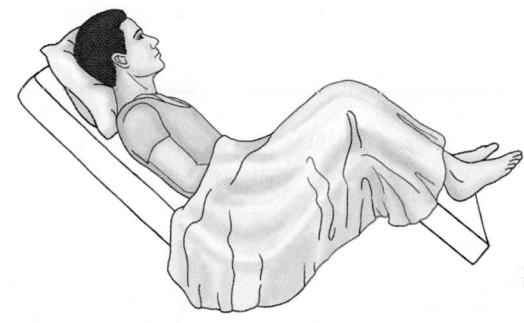

FIG 22-4 Patient in the jack-knife position.

Measurement of Weight and Height

The medical assistant commonly measures a patient's weight and height. The accuracy of this data is important because changes over time may indicate a significant change in a patient's health status.

Measuring Weight

In most acute and long-term care settings patients are weighed in kilograms. In ambulatory care settings, such as medical offices, patients may be weighed in pounds or kilograms, depending on office policy. However, the trend is changing toward using metrics across the board. Therefore, medical assistants must become familiar with the metric system and learn the formulas required for conversion. (See *Weight conversion formulas,* page 362.) In many cases, the patient's weight is

PROCEDURE 22-6

Assisting the patient into the semi-Fowler and Fowler positions

Task
Assist the patient into the semi-Fowler and Fowler positions.

Conditions
- Examination table
- Table paper
- Examination gown
- Pillow
- Disposable drape or sheet

Standards
In the time specified and within the scoring parameters determined by the instructor, the student will successfully assist the patient into the semi-Fowler and Fowler positions.

Performance Standards
1. Greet and identify the patient, introduce yourself, and explain the procedure to prevent errors and ease patient anxiety.
2. Wash or sanitize your hands to control infection.
3. Provide the patient with an examination gown. Describe how fully the patient should undress. Point out where the patient may hang or lay his clothing. Explain that the gown should be worn with the opening in the front.
4. Leave the room for a few minutes so the patient may change in privacy, unless the patient requires your assistance.
5. Pull out the footrest and assist the patient onto the table into a sitting position. Then assist him into the semi-Fowler position by raising the head of the examination table to a 45-degree angle.

6. To assist the patient into the Fowler position, raise the head of the examination table to 90 degrees.
7. Then instruct the patient to lie back and rest his head on the pillow. As he does this, pull out the table extension to support his legs.
8. Ensure that the drape is positioned properly to ensure proper positioning and patient safety, privacy, and comfort.

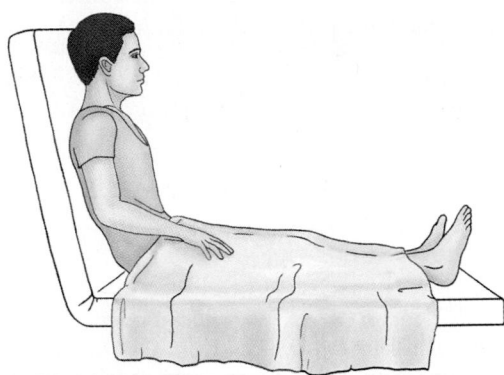

Patient in Fowler position

9. Assist the physician as needed with the examination.
10. Upon completion of the examination, assist the patient down from the table and instruct him to get dressed. Return the table footrest to the normal position.
11. Leave the room for a few minutes so the patient may change in privacy unless he requires your assistance to ensure patient safety and privacy.
12. Clean, sanitize, and restock the examination room as needed to prepare the room for the next patient.

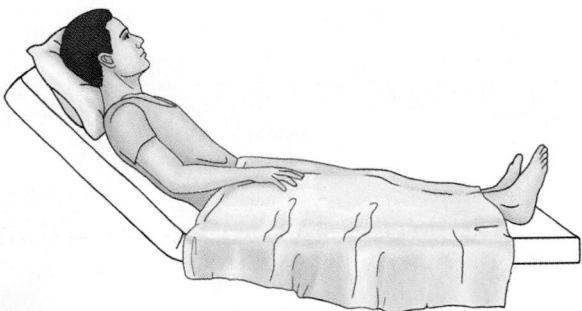

Patient in semi-Fowler position

PROCEDURE 22-7

Assisting the patient into the Trendelenburg position

Task
Assist the patient into the Trendelenburg position.

Conditions
- Examination table
- Table paper
- Examination gown
- Pillow
- Disposable drape or sheet

Standards
In the time specified and within the scoring parameters determined by the instructor, the student will successfully assist the patient into the Trendelenburg position.

Performance Standards
1. Greet and identify the patient, introduce yourself, and explain the procedure to prevent errors and ease patient anxiety.
2. Wash or sanitize your hands to control infection.
3. Provide the patient with an examination gown. Describe how fully the patient should undress. Point out where the patient may hang or lay her clothing. Explain that the gown should be worn with the opening in the front.
4. Pull out the footrest of the examination table and explain that the patient should sit securely on the end of the table with the drape over her lap.
5. Leave the room for a few minutes so the patient may change in privacy unless the patient requires your assistance.

6. Adjust the table so that the head of the table is tilted downward. Ensure that the drape is positioned properly to ensure proper positioning and patient safety, privacy, and comfort. Alternatively, the footrest may be tilted downward so that the knees bend to enhance patient comfort.

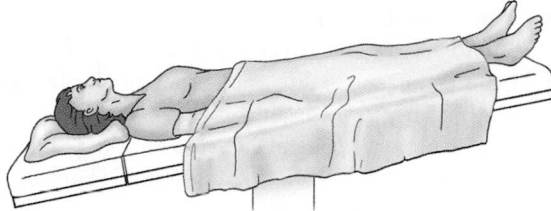

Patient in the Trendelenburg position

7. Assist the physician as needed with the examination.
8. Upon completion of the examination, assist the patient down from the table and instruct her to get dressed. Return the table footrest to the normal position.
9. Leave the room for a few minutes so the patient may change in privacy unless she requires your assistance to ensure patient safety and privacy.
10. Clean, sanitize, and restock the examination room as needed to prepare the room for the next patient.

PROCEDURE 22-8

Assisting the patient into the knee-chest position

Task
Assist the patient into the knee-chest position.

Conditions
- Examination table
- Table paper
- Examination gown
- Disposable drape or sheet

Standards
In the time specified and within the scoring parameters determined by the instructor, the student will successfully assist the patient into the knee-chest position.

Performance Standards
1. Greet and identify the patient, introduce yourself, and explain the procedure to prevent errors and ease patient anxiety.
2. Wash or sanitize your hands to ensure infection control.
3. Provide the patient with an examination gown. Describe how fully the patient should undress. Point out where the patient may hang or lay his clothing. Explain that the gown should be worn with the opening in the back.
4. Leave the room for a few minutes so the patient may change in privacy unless the patient requires your assistance.

Continued

PROCEDURE 22-8—cont'd

5. Pull out the footrest and assist the patient to a sitting position. Then ask him to move back on the table as you pull out the table extension. Assist him into the supine position and then into the prone position by turning onto his side and then onto his stomach. Be sure that he rolls toward you rather than away from you to ensure proper positioning and patient safety, privacy, and comfort.

6. Place a drape over him diagonally with one corner draped over his buttocks and another one over his back to protect patient privacy and modesty and to enable the physician to lift one corner of the drape when ready to begin the examination.

7. Instruct the patient to bend his elbows and rest his arms along side of his head, then to raise his buttocks and chest off the table.

8. Place a pillow beneath his chest for support and instruct him to lower his chest while keeping his buttocks elevated and his back straight.

9. Instruct him to separate his knees and lower legs approximately 12" to ensure proper positioning and provide a wider base of support for safety and comfort.

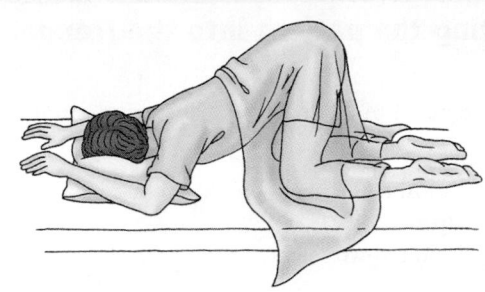

Patient in the knee-chest position

10. Assist the physician as needed with the examination.

11. Upon completion of the examination, assist the patient down from the table and instruct him to get dressed. Return the table footrest to the normal position. Leave the room for a few minutes so the patient may change in privacy unless he requires your assistance to ensure patient safety and privacy.

12. Clean, sanitize, and restock the examination room as needed to prepare the room for the next patient.

Weight conversion formulas

This table lists the formulas for converting a patient's weight from pounds to kilograms and vice versa.

Conversion	Formula	Example
Pounds to kilograms	lb ÷ 2.2 = kg	The patient weighs 220 lb. 220 ÷ 2.2 = 100 kg
Kilograms to pounds	kg × 2.2 = lb	The patient weighs 80 kg. 80 × 2.2 = 176 lb

measured with each office visit. Accuracy in measuring and recording a patient's weight is very important, because medications and procedures are commonly based on a patient's weight. A child's weight is plotted on a growth chart along with his height to identify whether growth patterns are normal. A pregnant woman's weight is carefully noted on each visit as part of the data needed to monitor the pregnancy. A patient on a weight-loss program must also have his weight closely monitored to determine the effectiveness of his weight-loss activities. Any significant change in a patient's weight since his last visit should be brought to the physician's attention because it may indicate a health problem.

Measuring Height

Methods for measuring height vary, depending on the age and size of the patient. Infants and children are measured on each visit so that their growth can be plotted on growth charts. Infants are measured lying down and the measurement is recorded as length in centimeters. When the child reaches toddlerhood and is capable of standing, a standing measurement may be taken. Adult height is typically measured in feet and inches and is done on the first visit and then only as needed—for example, when there is concern about osteoporosis or degenerative changes of the vertebrae. A slight decrease in the height of an elderly patient is not unusual, but may indicate a problem. (See *Procedure 22-9: Measuring weight and height.*)

PROCEDURE 22-9

Measuring weight and height

Task
Measure the patient's weight and height.

Conditions
- Upright balance scale or digital standup scale
- Pen
- Patient's medical record

Standards
In the time specified and within the scoring parameters determined by the instructor, the student will successfully measure the patient's weight and height.

Performance Standards
1. Check the scale to be sure that the pointer floats in the center of the balance frame when all weights are on zero. If the scale is digital, check to make sure it is properly zeroed to ensure that the scale is working properly.
2. Greet and identify the patient, introduce yourself, and explain the procedure to prevent errors and ease patient anxiety.
3. Wash or sanitize your hands to ensure infection control.
4. Instruct the patient to remove her coat or sweater, shoes, and purse (if holding one). Place a paper towel on the scale to provide a clean surface for the patient to stand on and instruct the patient to step onto the scale. Provide assistance as needed to ensure an accurate weight.
5. Instruct the patient to stay still to avoid interfering with the balancing of the scale.
6. Slide the large lower weight to the right to the furthest notched groove that does not cause the pointer to drop to the bottom of the balance frame. Make sure that the weight is securely seated in the groove to avoid incorrect placement of the lower weight, which results in an inaccurate measurement.
7. Slide the smaller upper weight to the right until the pointer is balanced in the center of the balance frame.
8. Add the numbers from the bottom and top together to arrive at the patient's weight to the nearest 1/4 lb. If the scale is digital, note the reading when patient is standing still on the scale.
9. Assist the patient off the scale. Some upright balance scales require that the patient step off so that the calibration rod can be moved upward.
10. Slide the calibration rod up above the patient's approximate height and open the height bar.
11. Assist the patient back onto the scale with her back to it and instruct her to look straight forward to ensure an accurate measurement.
12. Adjust the height bar so that it just touches the top of the patient's head.

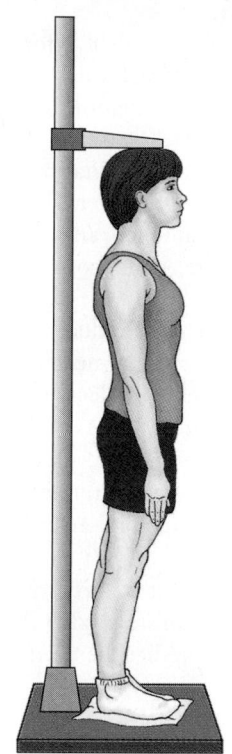

Instruct the patient to stand on the scale with her back to it.

13. Instruct the patient to step off the scale while ensuring that the height bar does not move.
14. Read the measurement where the stationary calibration rod and moveable calibration rods meet to the nearest 1/4".
15. Chart the patient's height and weight in the medical record. Record the weight in pounds or kilograms, depending on office policy to ensure thoroughness and accuracy of the medical record.

Date	
01/15/09: 11:05 a.m.	Wgt 138 $^1/_4$ lb. Hgt: 5' 7 $^1/_4$" ------------- C. Brown, CMA

Chapter Summary

- Health care providers gather information that enables them to diagnose and treat a patient's disorders and diseases. The physical examination is a critical piece of this data-gathering process.
- The standard physical examination is organized according to body system. However, the physician may vary the examination sequence and technique, depending on the patient's age, chief complaint, and purpose of the visit.
- Although the physician conducts the physical examination, the medical assistant must also be alert for clues about potential patient problems and communicate concerns to the physician.
- Physicians use some specific, predictable techniques to examine patients. These techniques are known as inspection, palpation, percussion, auscultation, mensuration, and manipulation.
- The examination format is fairly routine, making it easier for the medical assistant to predict the sequence to be followed and, thus, to predict the needs of the physician and patient.
- The medical assistant helps with the examination process in three key ways. She keeps the examination room ready at all times, prepares the patient, and assists the physician as needed.
- The medical assistant plays a vital role in helping ensure a smooth, efficient workflow, including making sure that examination rooms are cleaned, disinfected, and restocked as needed between patients.
- The medical assistant prepares the patient for the examination and may collect specimens, such as urine and blood.
- The medical assistant must ensure that examination supplies and equipment are ready, organized, and close at hand.
- The medical assistant must become familiar with the equipment most commonly used for physical examinations.
- During the examination, the medical assistant acts as a helper to the physician and as an advocate for the patient. She hands the physician supplies and instruments and pays close attention to the patient and offers reassurance, instruction, and assistance with positioning and draping.
- The medical assistant helps with the examination process by instructing and assisting patients in assuming various positions that allow the physician better access to and visibility of the body part being examined. These positions include the sitting, supine, dorsal recumbent, Sims, lithotomy, semi-Fowler, Fowler, Trendelenburg, knee-chest, and jack-knife positions.
- To help promote patient privacy and comfort, the medical assistant provides careful draping.
- The medical assistant commonly measures the weight and height of patients. Accuracy in obtaining and recording these data is important, because changes over time may indicate a significant change in a patient's health status.

Team Work Exercises

1. Divide into groups of three students. The instructor will write each of the examination positions on a card or small piece of paper and fold it so that it cannot be easily read. Each team will draw one or more cards until all are drawn. After a brief preparation period (as determined by the instructor), each team will present a role-playing scenario in which the medical assistant positions the patient for examination by the physician. Presentations will continue until all positions have been demonstrated.

2. Divide into teams of three or four students. Each team must brainstorm and come up with a plan to deal with the following scenario: You are medical assistants in a busy family practice clinic. An influenza epidemic has hit town and is affecting your patient population as well as the staff at your clinic. You are short-staffed today because your lead nurse, the office manager, and one of the two receptionists are out sick. To make matters worse, you are overbooked because so many of your patients are ill. You each have a strong preference for working in the back office or the front office. However, you are all certified medical assistants and, as such, have been trained to work in both areas. Given the challenges that you all face today, put your heads together and come up with a plan that will help everyone work together effectively to provide good-quality patient care and get the work done. You will have a designated amount of time (as determined by the instructor). Then each of the teams must rejoin the class and share their ideas for coping with this challenging situation.

Case Studies

1. Hachi Macha is a 57-year-old patient who has arrived for his annual health examination. He has been confined to a wheelchair since becoming a double amputee in the Vietnam War. He is a large man who has good use of his arms and hands. The medical assistant needs to measure Mr. Macha's weight and take him to an examination room. What special challenges might be involved in the examination of this patient? Describe some creative solutions to these challenges.

2. Odessa Naia is a 37-year-old woman who is visiting the clinic today for her annual physical examination. She will undergo a pelvic examination and Papanicolaou (Pap)

test. Describe the positions that she might be placed in for this part of her examination and list the advantages and disadvantages of each position.

Resources

- Physical examination overview: *www.en.wikipedia .org/wiki/Physical_examination*
- Physical examination techniques: *http://health.allrefer .com/health/physical-examination-info.html*
- Bickley, L.S., and Szilagyi, P.G.: *Bates' Guide to Physical Examination and History Taking,* 9th ed. Philadelphia: Lippincott Williams & Wilkins, 2007.
- Dillon, P.M.: *Nursing Health Assessment: A Critical Thinking, Case Studies Approach,* 2nd ed. Philadelphia: F.A. Davis Company, 2007.
- Dillon, P.M.: *Nursing Health Assessment: Clinical Pocket Guide,* 2nd ed. Philadelphia: F.A. Davis Company, 2007.
- Jarvis, C.: *Physical Examinations and Health Assessment,* 5th ed. Philadelphia: Saunders, 2007.
- Seidel, H. M., et al.: *Mosby's Physical Examination Handbook,* 6th ed. St. Louis: Mosby, 2006.
- Zator Estes, M.E.: *Health Assessment and Physical Examination,* 3rd ed. Clifton Park, NY: Delmar Cengage Learning, 2006.

Essentials of Medical Terminology

Learning Objectives

Upon completion of this chapter, the student will be able to:

- define and spell key terms listed in the Glossary
- discuss the origins of medical language
- describe medical word elements and how they are combined to create medical terms
- list the three steps used to translate medical terms
- describe seven methods of creating plural word forms
- list seven pronunciation tips and give examples of seven words in the singular and plural forms
- explain the purpose of directional terms and write five statements that use at least one directional term in each.

CAAHEP Competencies

General Competencies

Professional Communications

Respond to and initiate written communications

Recognize and respond to verbal communications

Patient Instruction

Instruct individuals according to their needs

Provide instruction for health maintenance and disease prevention

ABHES Competencies

Communication

Use appropriate medical terminology

Chapter Outline

Origins of Medical Language

Patients sometimes comment that health care providers seem to speak a foreign language. Thus, medical assistants must take care to use language easily understood by the average patient. (See *Be a translator*.) The language of medicine contains many terms that have their origins in a variety of other languages, primarily Greek and Latin. For example, the currently used term *nephro*, which means "kidney," is based on the Greek term *nephros*. The currently used term *oro*, which means "mouth," is based on the Latin term *oris*. The term *hygiene* was derived from the name of the Greek goddess of health, Hygeia. Over time, many other terms have been created as well. Some anatomical terms were named after the person who first identified them, such as the fallopian tubes, which were named after Gabriele Fallopius, a 16th-century Italian student of human anatomy.

Recent advances in medical technology have caused a significant increase in the number of new terms and abbreviations. Some examples include:

- magnetic resonance imaging (MRI), a type of diagnostic radiography that uses a powerful magnetic field to make images of tissues and organs
- percutaneous transluminal coronary angioplasty (PTCA), the surgical repair of a vessel of the heart in which a catheter is inserted into a narrowed vessel and a tiny balloon is inflated to widen it, thereby restoring adequate blood flow to heart muscle.

Regardless of whether a medical assistant is more interested in working in administrative or clinical areas, her effort to learn medical terminology now is a wise investment of her time and energy. Mastering the language of medicine will enable her to communicate fluently with other members of the health care team and record data clearly and accurately in the medical record. Whether she works in a family practice office, pediatrics, sports medicine, or another area of health care, fluency in medical terminology will enhance the medical assistant's effectiveness and her image as a professional.

Medical Word Elements

Understanding medical language begins with learning about common word elements and the categories they fall into. There are five main categories of word elements:

- combining forms
- prefixes
- suffixes
- abbreviations
- pathological terms.

Patient Education

Be a Translator

Because a common complaint of the patient population is that health care providers speak in a language they cannot understand, medical assistants should be prepared to translate the medical language for their patients. There are several ways to help patients understand tricky medical terms, including being prepared to explain terminology and providing other means of learning, including using printed materials.

Sensitivity with skills

The medical assistant's knowledge of medical terminology makes her, in a sense, bilingual. While this knowledge is a great advantage to her professional career, it can become a barrier for patients if she forgets that most of them do not share her language skills. Therefore, as a patient advocate, the medical assistant must be sensitive to the needs of patients and avoid using medical jargon when speaking with them. Additionally, the medical assistant should always offer to translate or explain any terms the patient finds confusing.

Office literature

The medical assistant can use the time that a patient spends waiting in the reception area as an opportunity for patient education. In addition to other literature, the medical assistant can provide cards or pamphlets with translations of terms commonly used in the office. For example, pamphlets placed in a pulmonology department might include such terms as *bronchitis* and *pulmonologist* and abbreviations such as *COPD* for *chronic obstructive pulmonary disease* and *TB* for *tuberculosis*. Pamphlets placed in the cardiac department might include such terms as *tachycardia* and *electrocardiogram* and abbreviations such as *ASHD* for *atherosclerotic heart disease* and *DVT* for *deep venous thrombosis*. Ready access to this type of literature enables patients to begin learning some terminology, increasing their understanding and feelings of empowerment. An added bonus is a decrease in the time the medical assistant must spend translating and explaining medical terms.

Combining Forms

Combining forms are created by joining word roots with combining vowels. A **word root** is the main stem of the word and is the part of the word that conveys the most meaning. For example, in the word *walking*, the root, or main stem, is *walk*. The purpose of a **combining vowel,** which is usually an *o* is to make terms easier to pronounce. The combining vowel has no impact on the meaning of the term and is placed between word parts to link them together. For example, the word root *therm* means "heat." If this word root is joined to an *o*, the result is the combining form *thermo*. A combining vowel should be used when the following word element begins with a consonant, as with the word *thermometer*. However, in cases where the next word element begins with a vowel (a, e, i, o, u), no combining vowel is needed. For example, when the word root *arthr*, which means "joint," is combined with *-itis*, which means "inflammation," no combining vowel is needed because *itis* begins with a vowel. The newly created term *arthritis* means "inflammation of a joint." Note that the key meaning of *joint*, which is inherent in the root *arthr*, remains. However, the newly added *-itis* has modified the meaning. (See *Knowing when to use a combining vowel*.)

Prefixes

Prefixes are word elements located at the beginning of words that modify the word meaning. For example, when the prefix

Knowing when to use a combining vowel

Remembering the purpose of the combining vowel makes it easier to understand when to use one. The combining vowel has no inherent meaning of its own. Its only purpose is to act like the link of a chain to connect other word parts together and make them easier to pronounce. Therefore, if a vowel is already present at the beginning of the next word part, then no additional vowel is needed. On the other hand, if no vowel is present (the next word part begins with a consonant) then a combining vowel is necessary. Here are two examples in which one term uses a combining vowel and the other does not.

micr (small) + **o** (combining vowel) + **scope** (instrument used to view) = **microscope**

appendic (appendix) + **itis** (inflammation) = **appendicitis** (inflammation of the appendix)

diplo ("double" or "twin") is placed before the term *opia* ("vision"), the new word *diplopia* is created, which means "double vision." When the prefix *dys*, which means "bad," "painful," or "difficult," is placed before the term *uria*, which means "urine," the new term *dysuria* is created. The literal translation of this new term is "bad, painful, or difficult urine." However, in common usage it means "painful urination." As this example indicates, the literal translation of terms and their common meanings are sometimes slightly different. (See *Common prefixes*.)

Suffixes

Suffixes are word elements located at the end of a word. Like prefixes, suffixes always modify the meaning of the term in some manner. For example, when the suffix -*dynia* ("pain") is placed after the term *pharyng/o* ("pharynx") the term *pharyngodynia* is created, which means pain in the throat. When the suffix -*dynia* is placed after the combining form *cervic/o* ("neck") the new term *cervicodynia* is created, which means "neck pain." (See *Common suffixes*.)

Common prefixes

The following table lists the most common prefixes used in medical terminology. Some prefixes share the same meaning and are listed together.

Prefix	Meaning	Example
a- an-	without, absence of	**aphasia** (ă-FĀ-zē-ă): absence of speech **anurea** (ăn-Ū-rē-ă): absence of urine
ante-	before, in front of	**antenatal** (ăn-tē-NĀ-tăl): before birth
anti-	against	**antidiarrheal** (ăn-tĭ-dī-ă-RĒ-ăl): against diarrhea (medication)
bi-	two	**bilateral** (bī-LĂT-ĕr-ăl): toward two sides
brady-	slow	**bradypnea** (brăd-ĭp-NĒ-ă): slow breathing
circum-	around	**circumoral** (sĕr-kŭm-Ō-răl): pertaining to around the mouth
dia- trans-	through, across	**diarrhea** (dī-ă-RĒ-ă): flow through **transurethral** (trăns-ū-RĒ-thrăl): through the urethra
diplo-	double, twin	**diploid** (DĬP-loyd): resembling two or twins
dys-	bad, painful, or difficult	**dysmenorrhea** (dĭs-mĕn-ō-RĒ-ă): bad, painful or difficult menstrual flow
endo-	in, within	**endocervical** (ĕn-dō-SĔR-vĭ-kăl): in or within the cervix
epi-	above, upon	**epicardia** (ĕp-ĭ-KĂRD-ē-ă): above or upon the heart
eu-	good, normal	**euthyroid** (ū-THĪ-royd): good or normal thyroid
ex- extra-	away from, external	**exotropia** (ĕks-ō-TRŌ-pē-ă): turning away from **extraocular** (ĕks-tră-ŎK-ū-lăr): external to the eye
hemi-	half	**hemigastrectomy** (hĕm-ē-găs-TRĔK-tō-mē): surgical removal of half of the stomach
hyper- supra-	excessive, above normal	**hyperesthesia** (hī-pĕr-ĕs-THĒ-zē-ă): excessive sensation **supracostal** (soo-pră-KŎS-tăl): pertaining to above the ribs
hypo- sub- infra-	below normal, beneath	**hypocalcemia** (hī-pō-kăl-SĒ-mē-ă): below normal blood calcium **substernal** (sŭb-STĔR-năl): pertaining to beneath the sternum **infrapatellar** (ĭn-fră-pă-TĔL-ăr): pertaining to beneath the patella
inter-	between	**intercellular** (ĭn-tĕr-SĔL-ū-lăr): between cells
macro-	large	**macroplasia** (măk-rō-PLĀ-zē-ă): large formation or growth
micro-	small	**microcardia** (mī-krō-KĂR-dē-ă): small heart

Common prefixes—cont'd

Prefix	Meaning	Example
multi- poly-	many, much	**multigravida** (mŭl-tĭ-GRĂV-ĭ-dă): woman with many pregnancies **polyneuritis** (pŏl-ē-nū-RĪ-tĭs): much nerve inflammation
neo-	new	**neonatology** (nē-ō-nă-TŎL-ō-jē): study of newborns
oligo-	deficient	**oligospermia** (ŏl-ĭ-gō-SPĔR-mē-ă): a condition of deficient sperm
para- peri-	near, beside, or around	**parahepatic** (păr-ă-hē-PĂT-ĭk): pertaining to near, beside, or around the liver **perianal** (pĕr-ē-Ā-năl): pertaining to near, beside, or around the anus
post-	after, following	**postnasal** (pōst-NĀ-zăl): after or following the nose
pre-	before, in front of	**premenstrual** (prē-MĔN-stroo-ăl): before menses
primi-	first	**primigravida** (prī-mĭ-GRĂV-ĭ-dă): woman in her first pregnancy
quadri-	four	**quadriplegia** (kwŏd-rĭ-PLĒ-jē-ă): paralysis of four (extremities)
syn-	union, together, or joined	**syndesis** (sĭn-DĒ-sĭs): binding together
tachy-	rapid	**tachycardia** (tăk-ē-KĂR-dē-ă): rapid heart (beat)
tox-	poison	**toxemia** (tŏk-SĒ-mē-ă): poison blood
uni-	one	**unicellular** (ū-nĭ-SĔL-ū-lăr): pertaining to one cell

Common suffixes

This table lists the most common suffixes used in medical terminology. Some suffixes share the same meaning and are listed together.

Suffix	Meaning	Examples
-al -ac -ar -ary -ic -eal -ous -tic* -tous*	pertaining to	**dermal** (DĔRM-ăl): pertaining to the skin **cardiac** (KĂR-dē-ăk): pertaining to the heart **ocular** (ŎK-ū-lăr): pertaining to the eyes **urinary** (Ū-rĭ-nār-ē): pertaining to urine **gastric** (GĂS-trĭk): pertaining to the stomach **esophageal** (ē-sŏf-ă-JĒ-ăl): pertaining to the esophagus **cutaneous** (kū-TĀ-nē-ŭs): pertaining to the skin **cyanotic** (sī-ăn-ŎT-ĭk): pertaining to blue (color) **edematous** (ē-DĒ-mă-tŭs): pertaining to edema
-asthenia	weakness, debility	**myasthenia** (mī-ăs-THĒ-nē-ă): muscle weakness
-algia -dynia	pain	**arthralgia** (ăr-THRĂL-jē-ă): joint pain **otodynia** (ō-tō-DĬN-ē-ă): ear pain
-arche	beginning	**menarche** (mĕn-ĂR-kē): beginning of menses

*The suffix -tic is a variation of -ic and the suffix -tous is a variation of -ous.

Continued

Common suffixes—cont'd

Suffix	Meaning	Examples
-blast	embryonic cell	**osteoblast** (ŎS-tē-ō-blăst): embryonic bone cell
-cele	hernia	**rectocele** (RĔK-tō-sēl): rectal hernia
-centesis	surgical puncture	**arthrocentesis** (ăr-thrō-sĕn-TĒ-sĭs): surgical puncture of a joint
-cephaly	head	**microcephaly** (mī-krō-SĔF-ă-lē): small head
-cide	kill, destroy	**bacteriocide** (băk-TĔR-ĭ-ō-sīd): destroying bacteria
-clast	to break, surgical fracture	**osteoclast** (ŎS-tē-ō-klăst): breaking a bone
-cyte	cell	**spermatocyte** (spĕr-MĂT-ō-sīt): sperm cell
-derma	skin	**cyanoderma** (sī-ă-nō-DĔR-mă): blue skin
-desis	binding, fixation	**pleurodesis** (ploo-rō-DĒ-sĭs): binding of the pleurae
-dipsia	thirst	**polydipsia** (pŏl-ē-DĬP-sē-ă): much thirst
-ectomy	excision, surgical removal	**appendectomy** (ăp-ĕn-DĔK-tō-mē): excision of the appendix
-edema	swelling	**blepharedema** (blĕf-ăr-ĕ-DĒ-mă): swelling of the eyelids
-emia	condition of the blood	**hypoglycemia** (hī-pō-glī-SĒ-mē-ă): a condition of low blood sugar
-emesis	vomiting	**hyperemesis** (hī-pĕr-ĔM-ĕ-sĭs): excessive vomiting
-esthesia	sensation	**anesthesia** (ăn-ĕs-THĒ-zē-ă): without sensation
-genesis	creating, producing	**hematogenesis** (hē-măt-ō-JĔN-ĕ-sĭs): creating or producing blood
-gram	record	**electrocardiogram** (ē-lĕk-trō-KĂR-dē-ō-grăm): record of heart electricity
-graph	recording instrument	**electroencephalograph** (ē-lĕk-trō-ĕn-SĔF-ă-lō-grăf): instrument for recording brain electricity
-graphy	process of recording	**electromyography** (ē-lĕk-trō-mī-ŎG-ră-fē): process of recording muscle electricity
-gravida	pregnancy	**multigravida** (mŭl-tĭ-GRĂV-ĭ-dă): multiple pregnancies
-ia	condition	**pneumonia** (nū-MŌ-nē-ă): condition of the lungs
-ism		**hypothyroidism** (hī-pō-THĪ-royd-ĭzm): condition of decreased thyroid (function)
-iasis	pathological condition or state, commonly related to the presence of a stone	**cholelithiasis** (kŏl-ō-lĭth-Ĭ-ăs-ĭs): a condition of gall stones
-ist	specialist	**dentist** (DĔN-tĭst): specialist in teeth
-itis	inflammation	**arthritis** (ăr-THRĪ-tĭs): inflammation of a joint
-kinesis	movement	**hyperkinesis** (hī-pĕr-kī-NĒ-sĭs): excessive movement
-kinesia		**hypokinesia** (hī-pō-kī-NĒ-zē-ă): decreased movement
-lith	stone	**nephrolith** (NĔF-rō-lĭth): kidney stone
-logist	specialist in the study of	**cardiologist** (kăr-dē-ŎL-ō-jĭst): specialist in the study of the heart
-logy	study of	**nephrology** (nĕ-FRŎL-ō-jē): study of the kidneys

Common suffixes—cont'd

Suffix	Meaning	Examples
-lysis	destruction of	**hemolysis** (hē-MŎL-ĭ-sĭs): destruction of the blood
-malacia	softening	**chondromalacia** (kŏn-drō-măl-Ā-shē-ă): softening of the cartilage
-megaly	enlargement	**hepatomegaly** (hĕp-ă-tō-MĔG-ă-lē): enlargement of the liver
-meter	instrument for measuring	**arthrometer** (ăr-THRŎM-ĕ-tĕr): instrument for measuring joints
-oid	resembling	**lipoid** (LĬP-oyd): resembling fat
-ole -ule	small	**arteriole** (ăr-TĒ-rē-ōl): small artery **venule** (VĔN-ūl): small vein
-oma	tumor	**lipoma** (lĭ-PŌ-mă): fatty tumor
-opia	vision	**diplopia** (dĭp-LŌ-pē-ă): double vision
-orexia	appetitie	**anorexia** (ăn-ō-RĔK-sē-ă): absence of appetite
-osis	abnormal condition	**vaginosis** (văj-ĭn-ŌS-sĭs): abnormal condition of the vagina
-oxia	oxygen	**hypoxia** (hī-PŎKS-ē-ă): low level of oxygen
-para	to bear offspring	**primipara** (prī-MĬP-ă-ră): first pregnancy
-paresis	slight or partial paralysis	**hemiparesis** (hĕm-ē-par-Ē-sĭs): partial paralysis of half of the body
-pathy	disease	**orchiopathy** (or-kē-ŎP-ăth-ē): disease of the testes
-pause	cessation, stopping	**menopause** (MĔN-ō-pawz): cessation of menses
-penia	deficiency	**erythrocytopenia** (ē-rĭth-rō-sī-tō-PĒ-nē-ă): deficiency of red blood cells
-pepsia	digestion	**dyspepsia** (dĭs-PĔP-sē-ă): bad, painful, or difficult digestion
-pexy	surgical fixation	**mastopexy** (MĂS-tō-pĕks-ē): surgical fixation of the breasts
-phagia	eating, swallowing	**dysphagia** (dĭs-FĀ-jē-ă): bad, painful, or difficult swallowing
-phasia	speech	**aphasia** (ă-FĀ-zē-ă): absence of speech
-phobia	fear	**hemophobia** (hē-mō-FŌ-bē-ă): fear of blood
-phoria	feeling	**euphoria** (ū-FOR-ē-ă): good feeling
-plasm -plasia	formation, growth	**neoplasm** (NĒ-ō-plăzm): new growth **dysplasia** (dĭs-PLĀ-zē-ă): bad, painful, or difficult growth
-plasty	surgical repair	**rhinoplasty** (RĪ-nō-plăs-tē): surgical repair of the nose
-plegia	paralysis	**quadriplegia** (kwŏd-rĭ-PLĒ-jē-ă): paralysis of four extremities
-pnea	breathing	**orthopnea** (or-THŎP-nē-ă): upright breathing
-prandial	meal	**postprandial** (pōst-PRĂN-dē-ăl): after meals
-ptosis	drooping, prolapse	**hysteroptosis** (hĭs-tĕr-ŏp-TŌ-sĭs): prolapse of the uterus
-rrhage -rrhagia	bursting forth	**hemorrhage** (HĔM-ĕ-rĭj): bursting forth of blood **menorrhagia** (mĕn-ō-RĀ-jē-ă): bursting forth of menses

Continued

Common suffixes—cont'd

Suffix	Meaning	Examples
-rrhaphy	suture, suturing	**vasorrhaphy** (văs-OR-ă-fē): suturing of a vessel
-rrhea	flow, discharge	**rhinorrhea** (rī-nō-RĒ-ă): flow from the nose
-salpinx	tube (fallopian or eustachian)	**hemosalpinx** (hē-mō-SĂL-pĭnks): blood in a tube (fallopian or eustachian)
-scope	instrument to view	**laparoscope** (LĂP-ă-rō-skōp): instrument to view the abdomen
-scopy	visual examination	**arthroscopy** (ăr-THRŎS-kō-pē): visual examination of a joint
-spasm	contraction, tension, spasm	**arteriospasm** (ăr-TĒ-rē-ō-spăzm): spasm of an artery
-stenosis	narrowing, stricture	**esophagostenosis** (ē-sŏf-ă-gō-stĕn-Ō-sĭs): stricture of the esophagus
-stomy	mouthlike opening	**tracheostomy** (trā-kē-ŎS-tō-mē): mouthlike opening in the trachea
-therapy	treatment	**hydrotherapy** (hī-drō-THĔR-ă-pē): treatment with water
-tocia	childbirth, labor	**dystocia** (dĭs-TŌ-sē-ă): bad, painful, or difficult labor
-tome	cutting instrument	**crainiotome** (KRĀ-nē-ō-tōm): instrument for cutting the cranium
-tomy	cutting into, incision	**hysterotomy** (hĭs-tĕr-ŎT-ō-mē): incision into the uterus
-tripsy	crushing	**lithotripsy** (LĬTH-ō-trĭp-sē): crushing stones
-trophy	nourishment or growth	**atrophy** (ĀT-rō-fē): absence of growth
-tropia	turning	**exotropia** (ĕks-ō-TRŌ-pē-ă): turning away from
-uria	urine	**hematuria** (hē-mă TŪ-rē-ă): blood in the urine

Abbreviations

Abbreviations are another type of word element used frequently in health care settings because they save time and simplify the speaking and writing of large, difficult-to-pronounce terms. For example, the abbreviation CAD stands for coronary artery disease, which is a narrowing of the lumen of the arteries of the heart. Another example is EGD, which is the abbreviation for the term *esophagogastroduodenoscopy*. (See *Common abbreviations*.) Abbreviations are so numerous in health care that they can cause confusion and even mistakes when not used appropriately. For example, an abbreviation in one specialty area might have a different meaning in another specialty area. Therefore, medical assistants must take care to use only approved abbreviations and should always ask when unsure of what an abbreviation means. (See *Abbreviation miscommunication*, page 376.) Symbols are also often used as a means of reducing the amount of documentation. Examples of commonly used symbols are those for male (♂) and female (♀).

Although many abbreviations are commonly used in health care, there are abbreviations that should no longer be used. Medical assistants must be familiar with these abbreviations in order to correctly interpret past charting as well as to be sure to avoid using them when completing documentation. (See *Discontinued abbreviations*, page 377.)

Pathological Terms

Pathological terms are used extensively in health care and refer to diseases and disorders of various body systems. An example of a pathological term is *multiple sclerosis,* a chronic disease of the central nervous system in which nerves are damaged and may temporarily or permanently lose the ability to transmit messages to muscles and organs. Another example is *impetigo*, which is a highly contagious bacterial infection caused by group A *Streptococcus* or *Staphylococcus aureus* that develops most commonly in young children. Some students struggle to learn pathological terms as well as abbreviations. Learning these terms requires basic memorization, which

Common abbreviations

The following table lists common abbreviations used in most areas of health care along with their corresponding medical terms.

Abbreviation	Term
BM	bowel movement
bid	twice a day
C	Celsius
Ca, CA	calcium, cancer
tid	three times a day
qid	four times a day
c̄	with
s̄	without
c/o	complaint of
Dx	diagnosis
FH	family history
g	gram
gtt	drops
PMH	prior medical history
Hx	history
h, hr	hour
ID	intradermal
IM	intramuscular
INR	International Normalized Ratio
IV	intravenous
K	potassium
Kg, kg	kilogram
L	liter
Mg, mg	magnesium, milligram
ml	milliliter
Na	sodium

Abbreviation	Term
NPC	nonproductive cough
NPO	nothing by mouth
NG	nasogastric
N&V	nausea and vomiting
NPO	nothing by mouth
OTC	over-the-counter
P, p̄	pulse, after
pc	after meals
PO	by mouth
PE	physical examination
PR	per rectum
q	every
qam	every morning
qh	every hour
qhs	every day at bed time (or each evening)
R	respiration
RR	respiratory rate
Rx	prescription
stat	immediately
supp	suppository
Sx	symptom
T	temperature; tablespoon
tab	tablet
Tx	treatment

Front office–back office connection

Abbreviation Miscommunication

Medical assistants become well versed and comfortable with abbreviations used in the area in which they work. However, they may become confused by abbreviations used by providers in other work areas. Thus, the medical assistant must be especially careful with documentation when she floats to an area different from where she normally works. Perhaps she normally works in a family practice department and is asked to float to oncology, neurology, obstetrics, or pediatrics. In addition, a clinical medical assistant might be asked to float to an administrative area or vice versa. Whatever the case, each organization should keep a master list of approved abbreviations for all employees and each department should keep a list of commonly used specialty abbreviations (consistent with the master list) for its employees. When the medical assistant floats to a new area, she should be sure to ask for a copy of these abbreviations to refer to as she completes her documentation duties. Doing so ensures the accuracy of her charting and protects her and her patients from the unpleasant consequences of errors.

This table lists some examples of the many medical abbreviations with multiple meanings.

Abbreviation	Multiple Meanings
BC	bone conduction; birth control
Ca, CA	calcium; cancer
CCU	coronary care unit; critical care unit
ECF	extended care facility; extra-cellular fluid
ED	emergency department; erectile dysfunction
Mg, mg	magnesium; milligram
P, p̄	pulse; after
PA	posteroanterior; pernicious anemia
PI	present illness; previous illness
PND	postnasal drip (drainage); paroxysmal nocturnal dyspnea
RR	respiratory rate; recovery room
RT	radiation therapy; respiratory therapy
T	temperature; tablespoon
TLC	tender loving care; thin layer chromatography; total lung capacity

takes time and effort. However, this effort pays big rewards later in the form of fluency in medical terminology. (See *Memorizing medical terms.*)

Translating Terms

Learning prefixes and suffixes provides significant benefits because it enables students to decipher and translate medical words. There are three simple steps to follow when translating a medical term:

1. identify and translate the *last* word element
2. identify and translate the *first* word element
3. identify and translate the *remaining* word elements in order from left to right.

For example, the term *esophagogastroduodenoscopy* is a large, somewhat intimidating term for most students. However, it can easily be translated using the three steps just described. Beginning students may find it helpful to place slashes between the word elements. After practicing the steps a few times, students will find that it is no longer necessary to use the slashes. To translate esophag / o / gastr / o / duoden / o / scopy, the student should follow the three steps:

1. identify and translate the last term, *-scopy*, which means "visual examination"
2. identify and translate the first term, *esophag/o*, which is a combining form that means "esophagus"
3. identify and translate the remaining terms in order from left to right

   a. first, translate the term *gastr/o*, which is a combining form that means "stomach"

   b. next translate the term *duoden/o*, which is a combining form that means "duodenum" (the first part of the small intestines).

Using the translations in the steps above, the student will determine that the meaning of the medical term *esophagogastroduodenoscopy* is visual examination of the esophagus, stomach, and duodenum.

Discontinued abbreviations

The Joint Commission, formerly called the *Joint Commission on Accreditation of Health Care Organizations (JCAHO),* has identified several abbreviations used in health care as confusing or easily misinterpreted. They have determined that use of these abbreviations could lead to serious errors and possible injury to the patient. Thus, the Joint Commission strongly recommends discontinuing their use in health care practice and documentation. This table lists these abbreviations, along with the reason for their discontinuance and what to use in their place.

Abbreviation	Reason Discontinued	Replacement
U	Mistaken for zero, the number *4* or *cc*	Write out *unit* instead.
IU	Mistaken for *IV* or the number *10*	Write out *international unit* instead.
QD, Q.D, q.d., qd	Mistaken for each other	Write out *daily.*
QOD, qod, Q.O.D., q.o.d.	Period after *Q* and the *o* mistaken for *I*	Write out *every other day.*
Trailing zero (X.0 mg) or lack of leading zero (.X mg)	Decimal point possibly missed	Write *X mg* and *0.X mg*
MS	Can mean *morphine sulfate* or *magnesium sulfate*	Write out *morphine sulfate* or *magnesium sulfate.*
MSO_4, $MgSO_4$	Confused for one another	Write out *morphine sulfate* or *magnesium sulfate.*

Pronunciation and Plural Forms

Most students need a lot of practice before they feel at ease pronouncing medical terms. However, developing good pronunciation habits early can help speed up the process. One step a student can take early on is to memorize the sounds for certain common letter combinations and other rules of pronunciation. (See *Pronunciation guidelines,* page 378.)

Another common obstacle to using correct medical terminology is the rules for changing singular terms to plural terms. Because many terms originate from foreign languages, such as Latin and Greek, the rules for plural terms are not always simple. The student who reviews and understands these rules will achieve a higher level of ease with and understanding of medical terminology. (See *Changing singular to plural,* page 378.)

Directional Terms

Directional terms indicate and describe specific areas on the body. The medical assistant must be able to understand and correctly use **directional terms** in order to accurately communicate descriptive data when speaking with other health care providers and when documenting in the patient's chart. (See *Common directional terms,* page 379.)

Memorizing medical terms

Many medical assisting students find memorizing prefixes, suffixes, combining forms, abbreviations, and pathological conditions requires a great deal of time and effort. To be more effective in the process of memorizing these terms, the student should follow these guidelines:

• Make or purchase ready-made flashcards. Study a few cards each day and keep them handy. Use extra time (when waiting in line at the store or waiting for an appointment) to pull them out and review them.

• Write down several terms and their meanings and give them to friends or family members you see daily. Ask them to quiz you on their "assigned" terms each time they see you.

• Complete the terminology-related student disc activities for this chapter.

• Complete the terminology-related student disc activities for each of the body systems chapters.

• Complete the terminology-related website activities for this chapter and for each of the body systems chapters.

Pronunciation guidelines

This table lists common letter combinations and other pronunciation guidelines to aid in the pronunciation of medical terminology, along with examples.

Letters	Guidelines	Example
ps	Pronounce only the *s*.	**psychology** (sī-KŎL-ō-jē)
pn	Pronounce only the *n*.	**pneumonia** (nū-MŎ-nē-ă)
g and c	Pronounce the soft sound for the letter when used before *e, i,* and *y*.	**gelatin** (JĔL-ă-tĭn) **cycle** (SĪ-kl)
g and c	Pronounce the hard sound for the letter when it is used in front of letters other than *e, i,* and *y*.	**gastric** (GĂS-trĭk) **caffeine** (KĂF-ēn)
ae and oe	Pronounce as a long *e* sound.	**pleurae** (PLOO-rē)
i	When used at the end of a word, pronounce as a long *i* or long *e* sound. (This letter at the end of a word generally indicates a plural.)	**alveoli** (ăl-VĒ-ō-lī)
es	Pronounce as a separate syllable when used at the end of some words.	**nares** (NĀ-rēz)

Changing singular to plural

This table lists singular word endings that are common in medical terminology along with their plural forms, the rule for changing each to plural, and examples.

Singular Form	Plural Form	Rule	Example Singular	Plural
a	*ae*	Retain the *a* and add *e*.	vertebra	vertebrae
ax	*aces*	Drop the *x* and add *ces*.	thorax	thoraces
is	*es*	Drop the *is* and add *es*.	diagnosis	diagnoses
ix, ex	*ices*	Drop the *ix* or *ex* and add *ices*.	appendix	appendices
um	*a*	Drop the *um* and add *a*.	diverticulum	diverticula
us	*i*	Drop the *us* and add *i*.	thrombus	thrombi
y	*ies*	Drop the *y* and add *ies*.	ovary	ovaries

Memorize and Practice

The value to a medical assistant of memorizing medical terms and practicing translating skills is immeasurable. Although such practice requires a fair amount of time and energy up front, it makes so many tasks easier in the long run. Just a few of the benefits enjoyed by those who achieve fluency in medical terminology include:

- increased understanding and enjoyment when reading medical subject manner
- improved test scores because of improved understanding of subject matter and test questions

Common directional terms

This table lists commonly used directional terms along with their combining form or prefix and meaning. Note that most of these terms are listed with their opposites.

Term	Word Element	Meaning
proximal	proxim/o	Nearer to the origin or point of attachment
distal	dist/o	Further from the origin or point of attachment
medial	medi/o	Toward the midline; nearer to the middle
lateral	later/o	Away from the midline; toward the side
superior	super/o	Above or nearer to the head
inferior	infer/o	Beneath or nearer to the feet
anterior	anter/o	Toward or near the front; ventral
posterior	poster/o	Towards or near the back; dorsal
ventral	ventr/o	Front, anterior
dorsal	dors/o	Back; posterior
abduction	ab-	From, away from
adduction	ad-	Toward

- more accurate verbal communication with other health care professionals
- more accurate medical documentation
- increased level of professionalism.

This chapter introduced some combining forms and the many prefixes and suffixes the medical assistant needs to know. Additional combining forms, as well as abbreviations and pathological terms, are introduced in each of the chapters that review body systems and their medical specialties. (See Chapters 25 through 36.) Selected prefixes and suffixes are reviewed in those chapters as well.

Chapter Summary

- Patients sometimes comment that health care providers seem to speak a foreign language. This observation is essentially true because the language of medicine contains many terms that have their origins in a variety of other languages, primarily Greek and Latin. Additionally, recent advances in medical technology have caused a significant increase in the number of new terms and abbreviations.
- Understanding medical language begins with learning about the common word elements, including combining forms, prefixes, suffixes, abbreviations, and pathological terms.
- A combining form is created by joining a word root, which is the part of the word that conveys the most meaning, with a combining vowel, which make the term easier to pronounce.
- A prefix is a word element located at the beginning of a word that modifies the word's meaning.
- A suffix is a word element located at the end of a word that also modifies the word's meaning.
- Abbreviations are used frequently in health care to save time and simplify the speaking and writing of large, difficult-to-pronounce terms.
- Pathological terms refer to diseases and disorders of various body systems.
- There are three simple steps in the process of translating medical terms. The first step is to identify and translate the *last* word element. The second step is to identify and translate the *first* word element. The third step is to identify and translate the *remaining* word elements in order from left to right.
- Developing good pronunciation habits early can help enhance a medical assistant's ease in using medical terms. In addition, understanding the rules regarding converting singular medical terms to plural will help her achieve a higher level of ease with and understanding of those terms.
- Directional terms indicate and describe specific areas on the body.
- The value to a medical assistant of memorizing medical terms and practicing translating skills is immeasurable. Although such practice requires a fair amount of time and energy up front, it increases the medical assistant's understanding of medical literature and helps her with test taking and, most importantly, accuracy, effectiveness, and professionalism on the job.

● This chapter provides an introduction to medical terminology. To become more fluent in the language of medicine, students must study the medical terminology sections of Chapters 25 through 36.

Team Work Exercises

1. Divide into small teams of three or four students for a friendly competition. The instructor will give each team a list of 10 medical terms. The first team to accurately translate or define all 10 of the terms wins the competition.
2. Divide into small teams of three or four students for a friendly competition. The instructor will give each team a list of 10 singular terms. The first team to accurately convert all 10 of the terms to their correct plural forms wins the competition.

Case Studies

1. Alicia Mendoza is a clinical medical assistant who works in a sports medicine clinic. She has noticed on several occasions that another medical assistant frequently uses abbreviations that Alicia does not recognize. When she asked her coworker about it, his reply was "Well, sometimes I make up my own because I just don't have time for all of this documentation we have to do." Alicia is concerned about this response and wants to discuss the subject further. Make a list of all the reasons why making up abbreviations might be a bad idea. Describe how Alicia might approach her coworker to discuss this issue without offending him.
2. The following paragraph contains 29 abbreviations that you must define. Some are located in this chapter and others are located in other clinical chapters. On a separate piece of paper, write each of the abbreviations in the order in which they appear in the story and then write the meaning next to them.

Anatoly Fedor is a 71-year-old ♂. His PMH includes HTN, BPH, and ASHD. He also has a recent Hx of a MI two months ago. After five days in the hospital, he was discharged home and underwent several weeks of PT. Today he came to the clinic c̄ c/o of SOB, frequent NPC, and occasional PND. The medical assistant checked Mr. Fedor's VS and noted that his BP was 166/94, his T was 37°C, his RR was 28, and his weight was 76 Kg, up 3 Kg from his last visit. After a thorough PE and tests, which included a CXR, CBC, and lytes, the physician diagnosed Mr. Fedor with heart failure. The physician ordered an RT Tx for him before he leaves today and also wrote an Rx for furosemide and K supplement to be taken bid PO.

Resources

● Free online medical terminology course: *www.free-ed .net/free-ed/HealthCare/MedTerm-v02.asp*
● Online medical dictionary: *www.medterms.com/script/ main/hp.asp*
● Medical terminology online course: *davisplus.fadavis .com/MTO.cfm*
● Chabner, D.: *Medical Terminology: A Short Course,* 4th ed. New York: W.B. Saunders, 2005.
● Collins, C.: *A Short Course in Medical Terminology.* Philadelphia: Lippincott, Williams & Wilkins, 2007.
● Eagle, S.: *Medical Terminology in a Flash!* Philadelphia: F.A. Davis Company, 2006.
● Gylys, B.A., and Masters, R. M.: *Medical Terminology Simplified: A Programmed Learning Approach by Body Systems,* 3rd ed. Philadelphia: F.A. Davis Company, 2005.
● Hutton, A.: *Pocket Medical Terminology.* New York: Churchill Livingstone, 2004.
● Venes, D., ed.: *Taber's Cyclopedic Medical Dictionary,* 20th ed. Philadelphia: F.A. Davis Company, 2005.

Surgical Asepsis and Assisting with Minor Surgery

Learning Objectives

Upon completion of this chapter, the student will be able to:

- define and spell terms related to surgical asepsis and minor surgery
- describe the role of the medical assistant when assisting with minor surgical procedures
- describe categories of surgical instruments and give examples of instruments in each category
- list common features of surgical instruments
- describe common features of surgical scissors and list at least three types
- describe common types of grasping-clamping instruments
- discuss common features of grasping-clamping instruments
- describe common types of dilating-probing instruments
- list at least three types of specialty instruments
- discuss eleven principles of sterile technique.

CAAHEP Competencies

Clinical Competencies
Patient Care
Prepare patients for and assist with procedures, treatments, and minor office surgeries

ABHES Competencies

Clinical Duties
Apply principles of aseptic technique and infection control
Prepare patient for and assist physician with routine and specialty examinations and treatments and minor office surgeries

Procedures

Performing a surgical scrub
Setting up a sterile field
Applying sterile gloves
Assisting with minor surgery
Performing suture removal
Removing a dressing and applying a new sterile dressing

Chapter Outline

Surgical Role of a Medical Assistant
Surgical Instruments
  Cutting Instruments
    Scissors
    Scalpels
  Grasping-Clamping Instruments
  Probing and Dilating Instruments
    Specula
    Scopes
    Probes, retractors, and dilators
  Specialty Instruments
Biopsy Equipment

Principles of Surgical Asepsis
  Sterile Technique
    Surgical scrub
    Sterile field
    Sterile gloving
Minor Surgical Procedures
  Cryosurgery
  Microsurgery
  Laser Surgery
  Electrosurgery
  Endoscopy
  The Medical Assistant's Role in Minor Surgery
  Patient Preparation and Postoperative Care
  Wound Care
    Sutures
    Staples
  Wound Care Supplies
    Dressings
    Bandages
    Creams, ointments, and solutions
    Anesthetics
Chapter Summary
Team Work Exercises
Case Studies
Resources

Key Terms

anesthesia
Absence of sensation

approximation
Bringing wound edges together closely and evenly

bandage
Nonsterile material applied over the top of dressings to secure them

cryosurgery
Technique that destroys tissue by subjecting it to very cold temperatures; also called *cryotherapy*

dressing
Material placed in or on a wound

electrosurgery
Use of high-frequency electric current to cut, remove, or destroy tissue; also called *electrocautery*

endoscopy
Use of a specialized scope to visually examine a structure

laser surgery
Treatment of tissue by means of colored light beams

microsurgery
Any procedure completed with the use of a special operating microscope

sterile technique
Method that involves performing invasive procedures in a manner that protects patients from pathogens

sterile toss
Technique for placing sterile items on the sterile field without contaminating either one

surgical asepsis
Destruction of all pathogenic organisms before they enter the body

suture
Material used to sew wound edges together or the act of sewing wound edges together

swage
To fuse a suture to a needle

Surgical Role of a Medical Assistant

A medical assistant will commonly assist with minor surgical procedures. These procedures usually take place in a procedure room, rather than a typical examination room. Such rooms are generally more spacious, allowing for easy movement of personnel and equipment, and stocked with surgical supplies and equipment. The medical assistant's role involves preparing the room for procedures, assisting the physician during procedures, providing postprocedure care to patients, and tidying and sanitizing the room after procedures. To be able to fulfill these duties effectively, the medical assistant must be familiar with commonly used supplies and instruments, the principles of surgical asepsis, and the procedures commonly performed in the medical office.

Surgical Instruments

The medical assistant should become familiar with the surgical instruments used in the office in which she works. There are more than 30,000 different types of surgical instruments designed to serve a variety of purposes. Most can be categorized as:

- cutting instruments, such as scalpels and scissors
- grasping-clamping instruments, such as needle holders, clamps, hemostats, and forceps
- probing and dilating instruments, such as dilators, specula, probes, scopes, and retractors
- specialty instruments, including those that do not fit into the other categories and those designed for specific procedures. (See *Identifying surgical instruments*.)

> **Front office–Back office connection**
>
> ## Identifying Surgical Instruments
>
> A medical assisting student who plans to work as an administrative medical assistant might think that identifying surgical instruments is not relevant to her. However, she should strive to learn and remember as much as she can about surgical equipment, instruments, and procedures. Doing so will not only make her a more knowledgeable, versatile, and valuable member of the team, it will also allow her to respond professionally and appropriately if she is one day asked to:
>
> • help out by calling for or retrieving certain instruments from storage

Cutting Instruments

The two most common types of cutting instruments are scissors and scalpels.

Scissors

Scissors come in many sizes and shapes. Surgical scissor types include those with straight or curved blades that are both sharp (s/s), both blunt (b/b), or one sharp and one blunt (s/b). (See Figure 24-1.) Mayo dissecting scissors may be straight or curved with tips that have a beveled edge and slightly rounded points. (See Figure 24-2.) Bandage scissors, also called *dressing scissors*, have one rounded tip and one blunt tip so they can be inserted beneath a patient's bandage without risk of skin injury. Suture scissors, sometimes called *stitch scissors*, have a notch at the end of the blade that is inserted under the suture before cutting. Iris scissors have small, sharp, straight or curved blades that were originally designed for eye surgery but are now used for various procedures. (See Figure 24-3.)

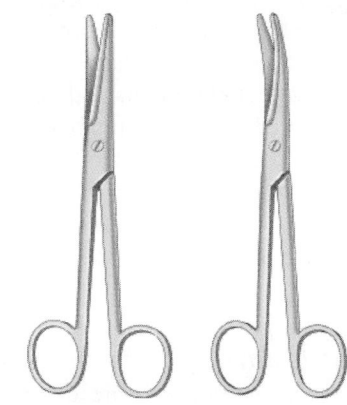

FIG 24-2 Mayo scissors.

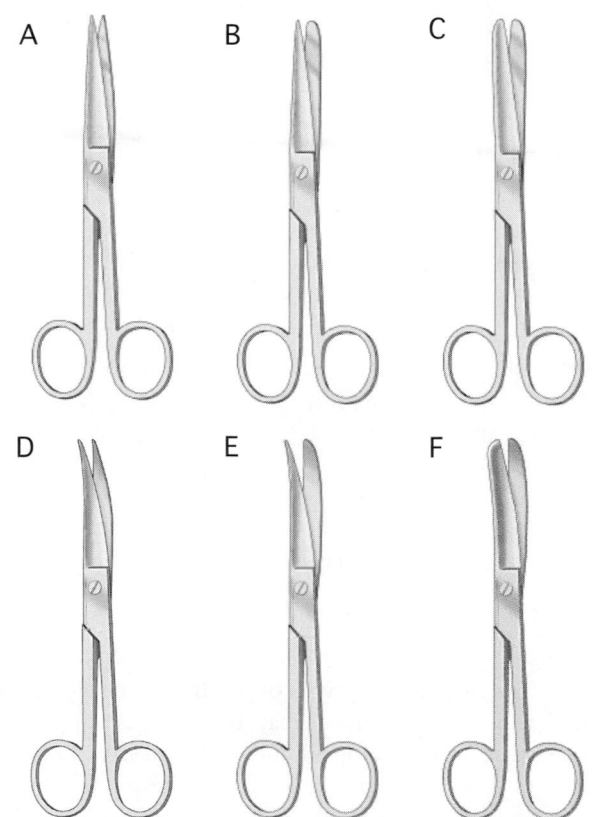

FIG 24-1 Surgical scissors. (A) Straight s/s. (B) Straight s/b. (C) Straight b/b. (D) Curved s/s. (E) Curved s/b. (F) Curved b/b.

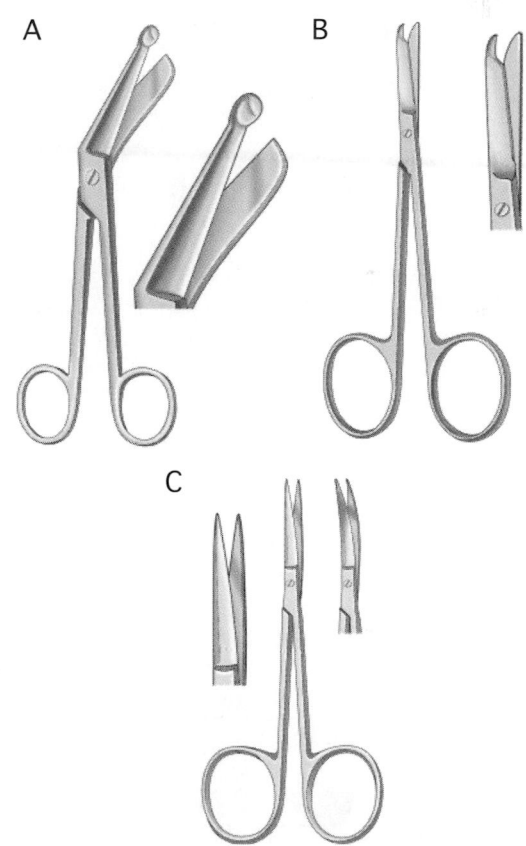

FIG 24-3 Bandage scissors (A). Suture scissors (B). Iris scissors (C).

Scalpels

Scalpels are cutting instruments commonly used to create surgical incisions. A scalpel includes a very sharp blade attached to a handle. They are available as single-use disposable or as handles to which blades may be attached. Both scalpels and handles come in a variety of sizes and shapes. (See Figure 24-4.)

Grasping–Clamping Instruments

The large category of grasping-clamping instruments includes a wide variety of forceps, hemostats, needle holders, and clamps. Forceps are used to grasp tissue during procedures. (See Figure 24-5.) Hemostats and hemostatic forceps are used in surgical procedures to clamp blood vessels in order to stop bleeding. Needle holders are similar to hemostats with a slight variation in design that allows them to securely hold a needle without crushing it. (See Figure 24-6.) Towel clamps are used to fasten sterile towels and drapes in place to secure the sterile field.

Probing and Dilating Instruments

Probing and dilating instruments are designed for procedures in which the physician examines body cavities. Such

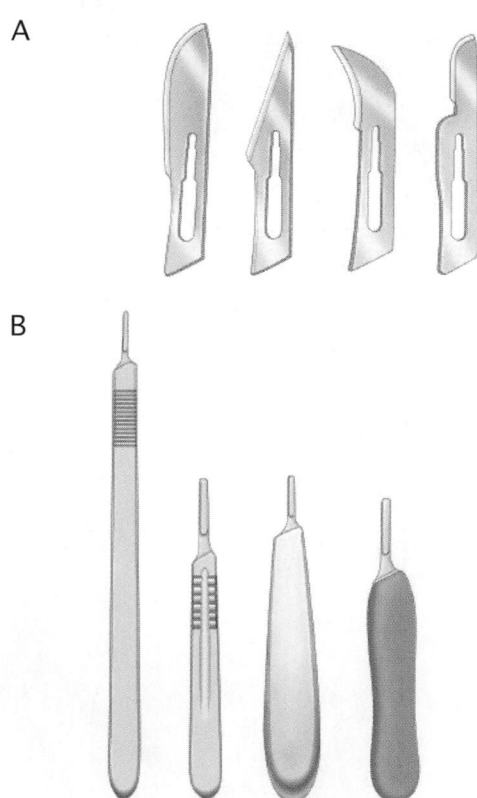

FIG 24-4 Scalpels. (A) Disposable. (B) Handles.

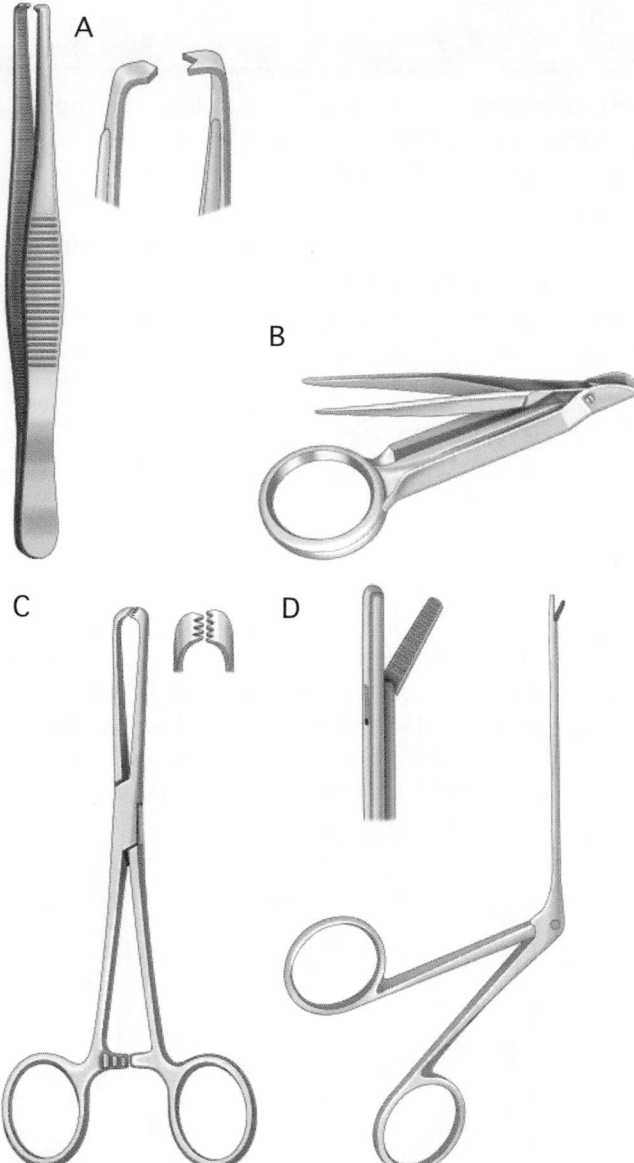

FIG 24-5 Forceps. (A) Tissue forceps. (B) Splinter forceps. (C) Allis tissue forceps. (D) Alligator forceps.

instruments include specula, scopes, probes, retractors, and dilators.

Specula

Two of the most common types of speculum are vaginal and nasal. The vaginal speculum may be made of disposable, clear plastic or reusable metal and is designed to hold the collapsible walls of the vagina apart so the physician may examine the uterine cervix. A nasal speculum is designed to open the nares (nasal openings) wider to aid the physician in examination of the nasal passages. (See Figure 24-7.)

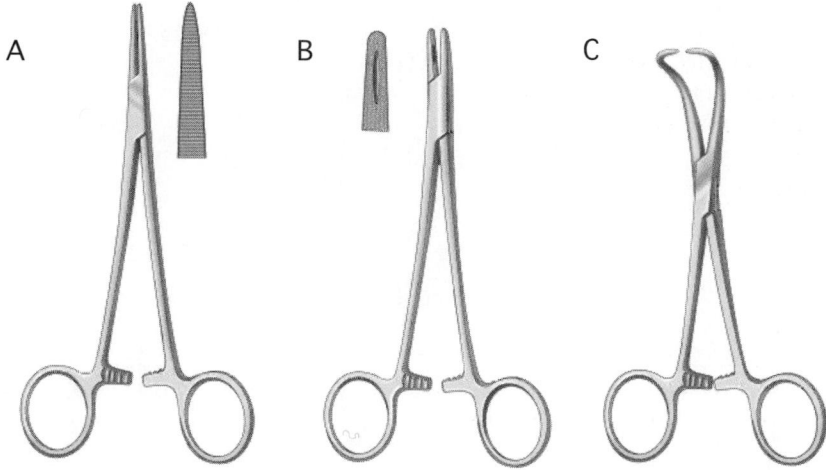

FIG 24-6 Grasping-clamping instruments. (A) Hemostats. (B) Needle holders. (C) Towel clamp.

Scopes

Scopes are lighted instruments designed to aid in the visualization of body cavities, such as the ear, esophagus, stomach, rectum, colon, abdomen, or even the inside of joints. They are generally named for the body part they are designed to examine. For example, the *otoscope* is used to examine the ear, the *arthroscope* is used to examine the inside of joints, and the *anoscope* is used to examine the inside of the anus and the rectum. (See Figure 24-8.)

Probes, Retractors, and Dilators

As their name implies, probes are used to probe deep into wounds or body cavities. Sounds are instruments similar to probes but may be longer and are used to investigate an area for size and shape as well as for the presence of foreign bodies.

Retractors are used to pull wound edges back to allow the physician a better view of and access to the area. They come in a variety of sizes and shapes, depending on their intended use.

Dilators are metal rods with smooth rounded tips on either end. They come in a range of sizes. Smaller to larger sizes may be used to slowly enlarge an opening, such as the uterine cervix. (See Figure 24-9.)

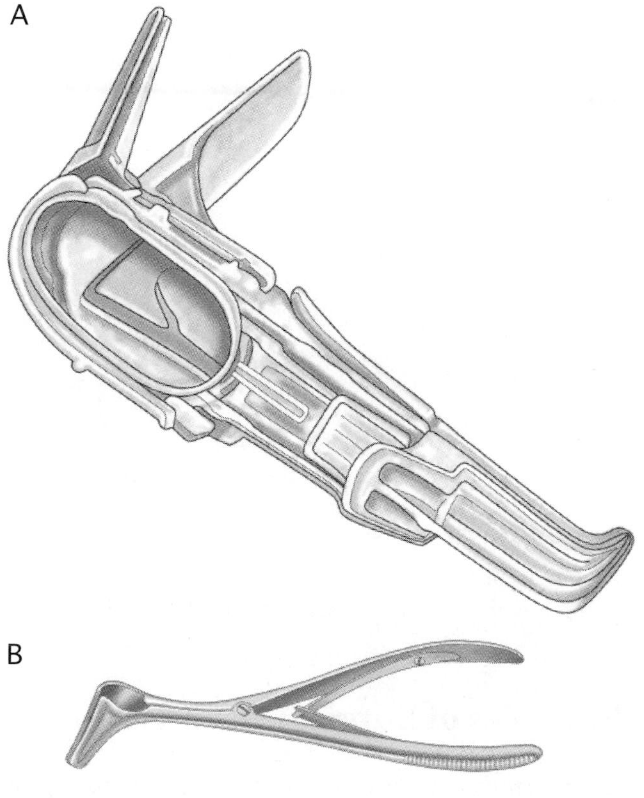

A

B

FIG 24-7 Specula. (A) Vaginal speculum. (B) Nasal speculum.

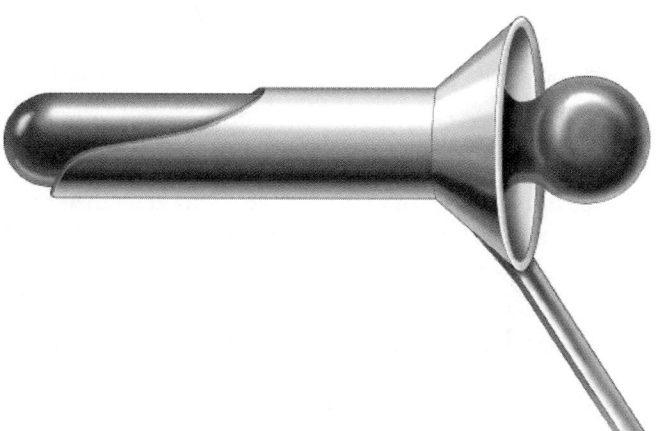

FIG 24-8 Anoscope.

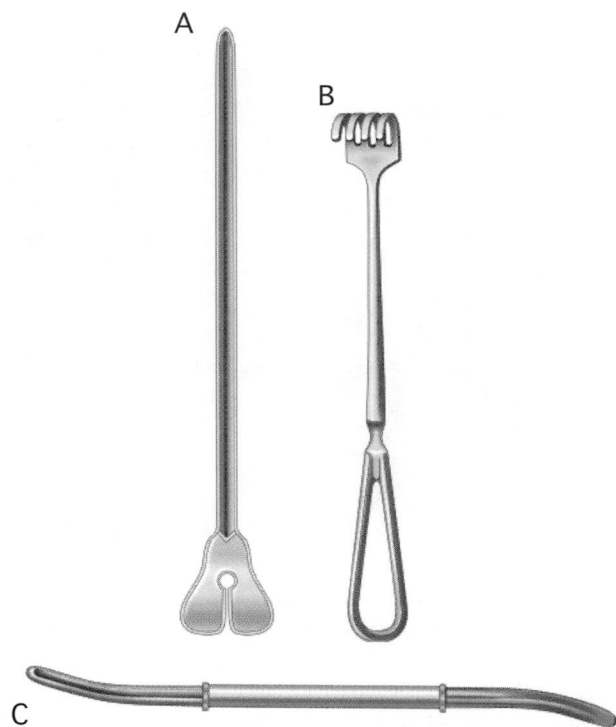

FIG 24-9 Probe, retractor, and dilator. (A) Grooved director probe. (B) Volkmann retractor. (C) Uterine dilator.

Specialty Instruments

A variety of specialty equipment is designed for specialty examinations and procedures. For example, some instruments are designed specifically for gynecological examinations and procedures. The speculum is used to open the walls of the vagina so that the vagina and cervix may be examined. Foerster sponge forceps are used to hold gauze pads to sponge the surgical site and absorb blood or other fluid. A curette is used to scrape the inner walls of the uterus to remove the endometrial lining and abnormal growths. A uterine sound is used to examine the inside of the uterus for size and shape as well as the presence of foreign bodies. A uterine tenaculum is used to grasp and position the cervix for better examination, tissue removal, or other procedures. (See Figure 24-10.) Other specialty equipment includes items designed for eye and ear examinations and procedures. For example, the laryngeal mirror allows the physician to inspect the larynx and other structures deep in the throat. (See Figure 24-11.)

Biopsy Equipment

A biopsy is a procedure in which a physician collects a tissue specimen from a patient to test for cancer or other abnormalities. The most common method for obtaining such a specimen is excision (cutting) with a scalpel or biopsy punch.

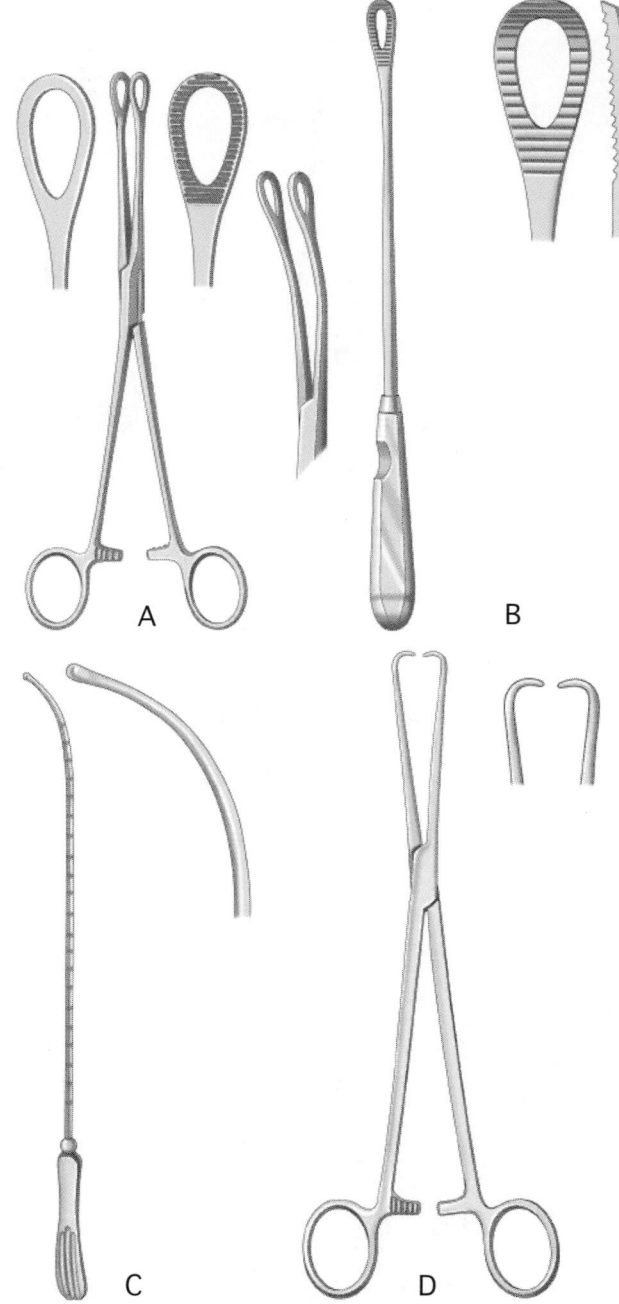

FIG 24-10 Specialty instruments. (A) Foerster sponge forceps. (B) Curette. (C) Uterine sound. (D) Tenaculum.

The physician will commonly collect a fluid specimen by aspiration with a needle and syringe. (See Figure 24-12.)

Principles of Surgical Asepsis

Surgical asepsis is the practice of destroying all pathogenic organisms before they enter the body. More specifically, surgical asepsis refers to the protection of patients from pathogenic

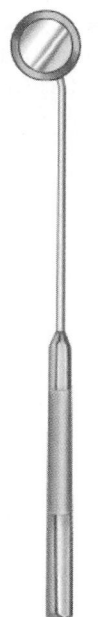

FIG 24-11 Laryngeal mirror.

microorganisms during invasive procedures. Invasive procedures are those in which the patient's normal protective barriers are punctured or disrupted in some manner. Examples of some procedures that require surgical asepsis include injections, urinary catheterization, wound care, and such surgical procedures as tissue biopsy or repair and suturing of lacerations. Surgical asepsis differs from *medical* asepsis, which refers to methods of performing procedures and providing patient care to prevent transmission of pathogenic organisms from the ill patient to other patients or anyone else. Adherence to medical asepsis involves the use of standard precautions. (For more information about medical asepsis, see Chapter 19, "Infection Control and Medical Asepsis," page 287)

Sterile Technique

To adhere to the principles of surgical asepsis, the health care team must understand and follow sterile technique. **Sterile technique,** also called *aseptic technique,* is a manner of performing specific tasks and procedures that protects patients from pathogenic organisms to the fullest extent possible. When a medical assistant first learns sterile technique, she

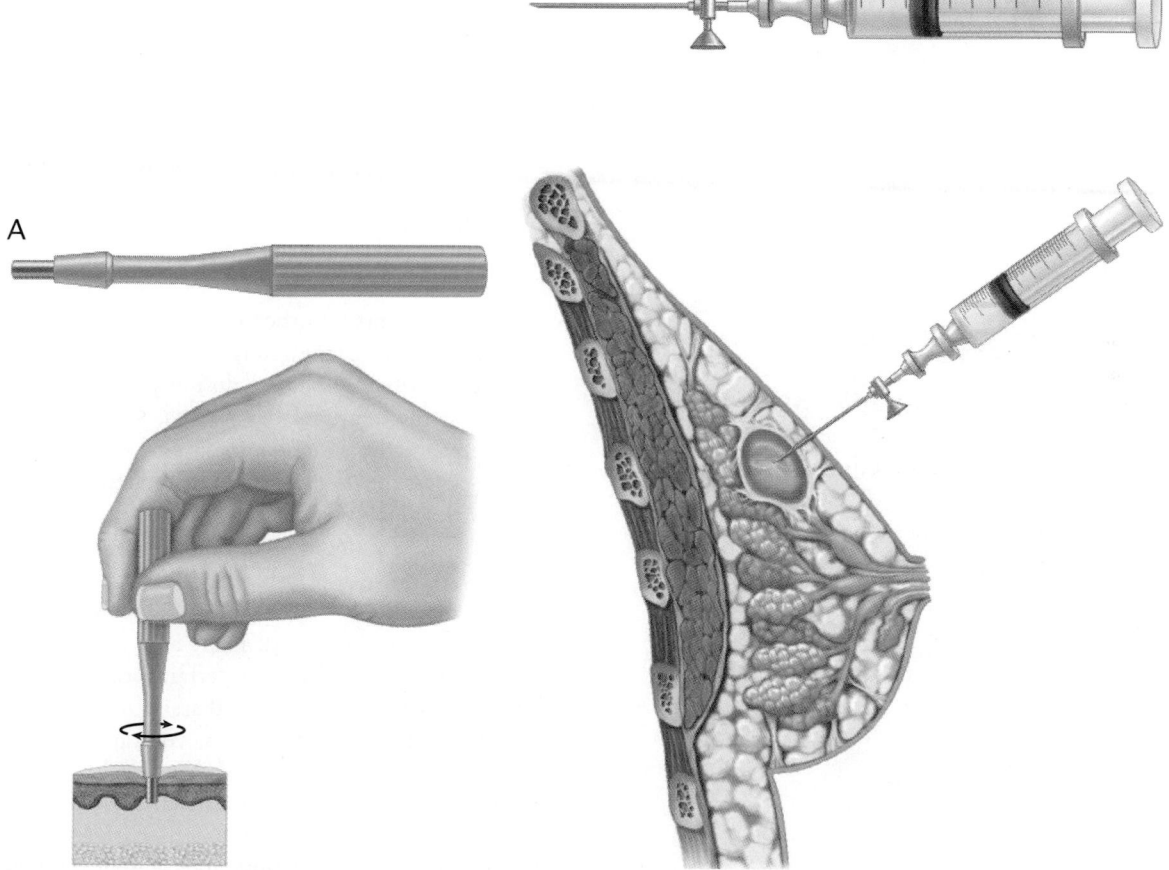

FIG 24-12 Biopsy equipment. (A) Biopsy punch for obtaining a tissue specimen. (B) Syringe and large gauge needle for aspirating a fluid specimen.

may find the many rules confusing and difficult to remember. The most important rule to remember is that *sterile may only touch sterile and nonsterile may only touch nonsterile*. Thus, the medical assistant must know which surfaces are sterile and nonsterile and be sure to protect the sterile field from pathogenic microorganisms. (See Figure 24-13.) Whenever sterile

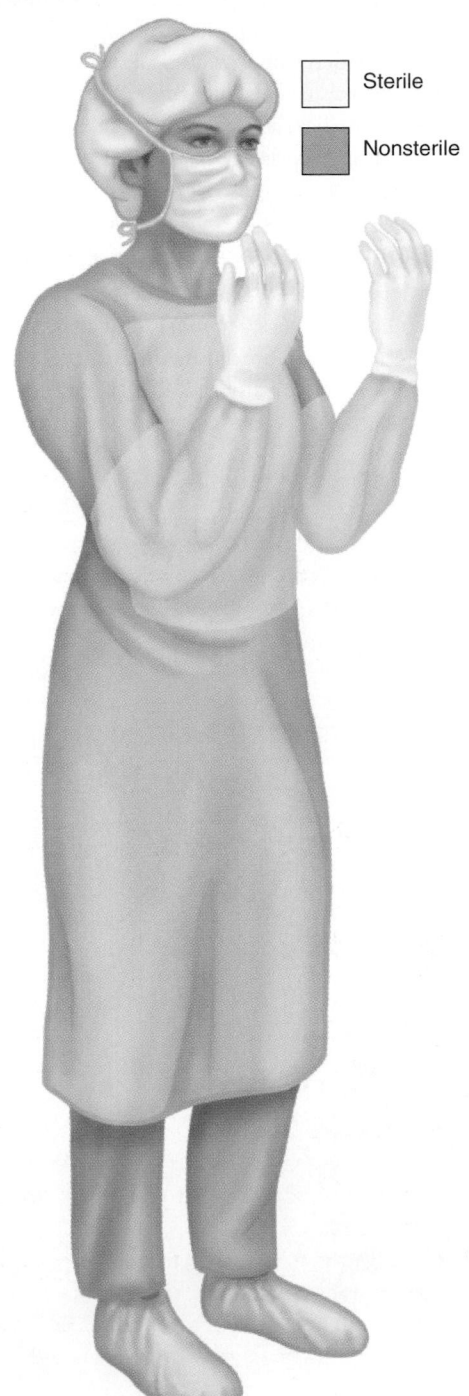

Sterile

Nonsterile

FIG 24-13 The sterile field and nonsterile areas.

and nonsterile items touch one another, contamination occurs, and the team must take corrective steps before the procedure can continue. (See *General rules of sterile technique*.)

Surgical Scrub

Prior to assisting with certain surgical procedures, the medical assistant may need to perform a surgical scrub. This procedure is a type of hand washing that is much more thorough than regular hand washing and follows specific steps. Although the human skin can never be fully sterilized, the surgical scrub is designed to reduce the number of pathogenic microorganisms on the hands and forearms to the greatest extent possible. Ideally, this scrub should take place at a large, deep surgical sink that allows the medical assistant to lean forward and hold both arms upright within the scrub area. Such sinks have automatic controls or ones that can be powered by the feet or knees. This allows the medical assistant to complete the scrub without touching any part of the sink. However, most medical assistants work in offices that have standard sinks, rather than deep surgical sinks. In such a case, the medical assistant must use the best technique possible under the circumstances. (See *Procedure 24-1: Performing a surgical scrub*.)

Sterile Field

Any member of the health care team involved in a sterile procedure must ensure that the supplies or instruments used in an invasive manner during the sterile procedure remain sterile. The first step in ensuring that such instruments are sterile is to understand how to properly sterilize and package such items in advance. (For more information on proper sterilization and packaging procedures, see Chapter 19, "Infection Control and Medical Asepsis.") In addition, when medical assistants or other health care providers open and handle such items, they must adhere to the rules of sterile technique so that the items do not come into contact with any nonsterile items.

After hand washing, the next step in preparing for any sterile procedure is always the arrangement of the sterile field with all necessary supplies and equipment. Medical assistants are commonly required to set up sterile fields—for their use or the use of other health care providers. A sterile field is created to form a sterile work area when a sterile procedure must be performed. There are many variations of the sterile field but they all have certain principles in common. In the medical office, a medical assistant will commonly use a portable device, such as a mayo stand or other mobile stand, for the work surface. The medical assistant must lay down some form of a sterile barrier to create a sterile work surface. In the operating room, a much larger sterile field is created with the use of numerous drapes or towels. When the medical assistant establishes the sterile field, she must

General rules of sterile technique

This table lists some of the most common rules of sterile technique along with their rationales.

Principle	Rationale
The health care provider should never turn his back on the sterile field.	Contamination to the field might occur without the health care provider's knowledge.
Hair should be tied back and not allowed to fall forward.	Hair contains microorganisms that will fall onto the field if hair hangs over it.
Members of a sterile team should always face each other when working, but if they must pass one another in close quarters then they should do so back-to-back or front-to-front.	Facing one another keeps the sterile field in everyone's view. Passing back-to-back or front-to-front prevents touching of sterile to nonsterile body surfaces.
The outer 1'' border of sterile drapes and any sterile wrap must be considered contaminated.	The edge of the drapes are in contact with nonsterile surfaces and are, therefore, contaminated. A 1'' border creates a safety margin.
Any item below waist level must be considered contaminated.	Areas below waist level are commonly out of view and may, therefore, become contaminated without the health care provider's knowledge.
Sterile surfaces that become wet must be considered contaminated unless they include a waterproof layer.	Microorganisms from the surface below can move up through a wet layer of paper or cloth and contaminate the field.
The longer a sterile surface is exposed to the air, the more contamination occurs.	Microorganisms in the air will begin to settle onto the sterile field.
Reaching over the field should be avoided whenever possible.	Microorganisms from the arm or clothing may fall onto the sterile field.
Contaminated items should not be passed over the sterile field.	Contaminated debris and microorganisms may fall onto the sterile field.
Coughing, sneezing, and even talking over the sterile field should be avoided.	Airborne microorganisms from the individual's mouth may fall onto the sterile field.
When pouring sterile solutions into other sterile containers, the bottle should be held high enough to avoid touching any other surface, yet low enough to avoid splashing onto the sterile field.	The outer rim of the bottle is contaminated and will contaminate any surface it touches. Areas of the field that get wet will draw microorganisms into it unless it has a waterproof layer.

PROCEDURE 24-1

Performing a surgical scrub

Task
Perform a surgical scrub.

Conditions
- Deep sink or a surgical sink with foot, knee, or arm controls (if available)
- Surgical soap
- Nail file or fingernail stick
- Surgical scrub brush
- Clean or sterile towels

Standards
In the time specified and within the scoring parameters determined by the instructor, the student will successfully perform a surgical scrub.

Performance Standards
1. Remove all jewelry on hands and arms because jewelry harbors pathogens.
2. Roll long sleeves up above elbows to prevent clothing from getting wet and expose hands and arms for scrubbing.
3. Examine hands and fingernails for breaks or rough areas, because jagged nails can puncture surgical gloves and breaks in the skin put you at risk for exposure to pathogens.
4. Turn on the water to a warm temperature, because warm water more effectively kills pathogens than cold water. Avoid touching your body to the sink's edge to prevent water and microorganisms on the sink's edge from touching your clothes.

Continued

PROCEDURE 24-1—cont'd

5. Wet your hands under the water while holding them upright above waist level so that pathogens will rinse off in a one-way direction.

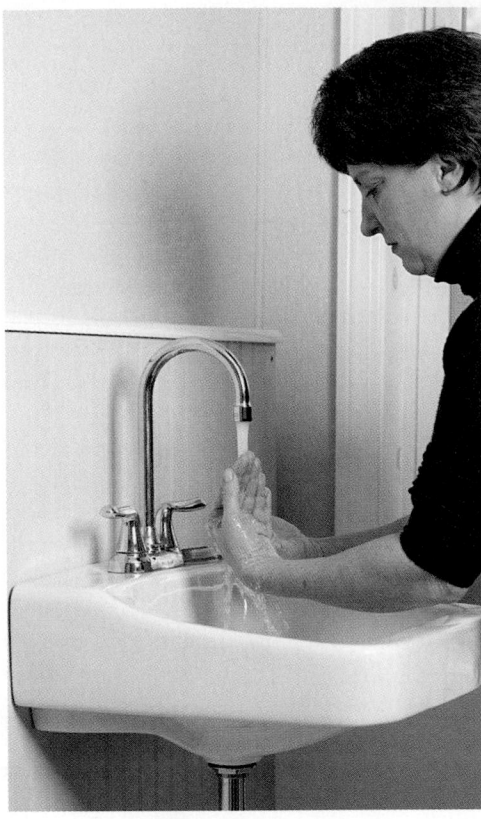

Wet your hands while holding them upright.

6. Clean under all fingernails with a nail file, fingernail stick, or the nail attachment of the scrub brush, if provided.

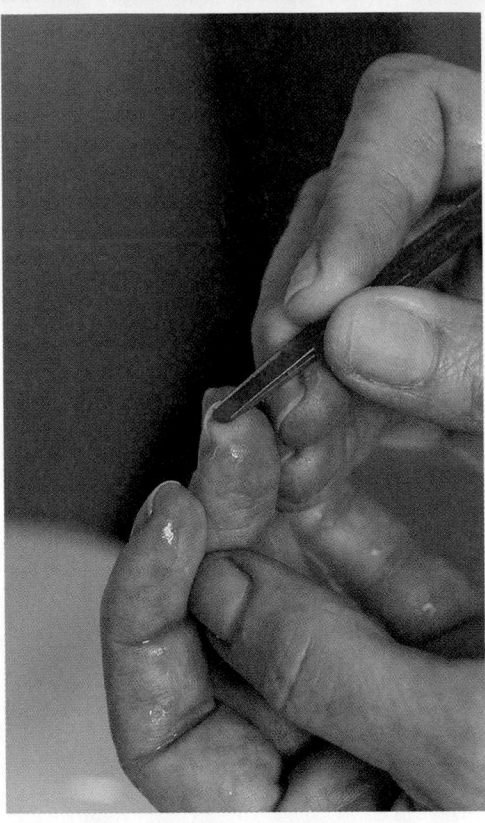

Clean under all fingernails with a fingernail stick.

7. Discard the file or stick without lowering your hands to prevent reintroducing pathogenic microorganisms to your fingernails.

8. Rinse nails by continuing to hold hands upright, allowing water to run over your hands from nails downward and off of your elbows.

9. Apply surgical soap or use a disposable brush impregnated with surgical soap and scrub the palms of your hands in a circular motion.

10. While continuing to hold your hands and fingers upward, follow a set pattern as you scrub the thumbs and each finger, taking care to scrub the base, along each side, and across the nails to ensure thoroughness.

11. Scrub the back of each hand in a circular motion. Total scrub time for each hand should be a minimum of 5 minutes to ensure thoroughness.

PROCEDURE 24-1—cont'd

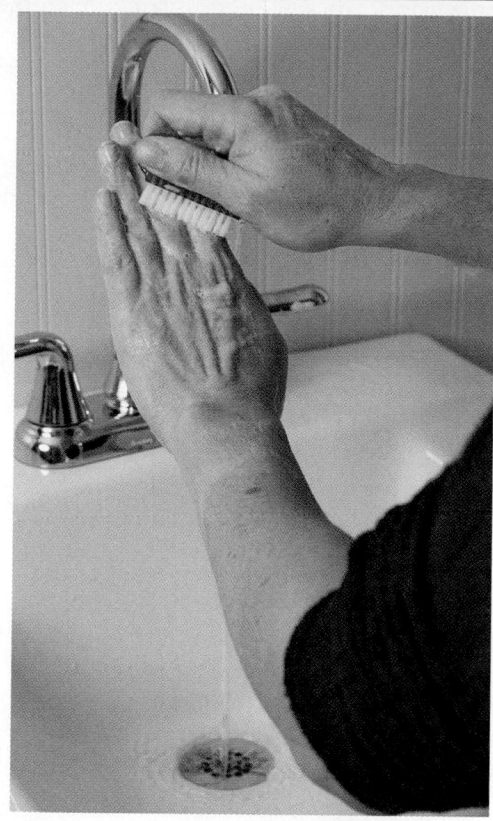

Scrub the back of each hand in a circular motion.

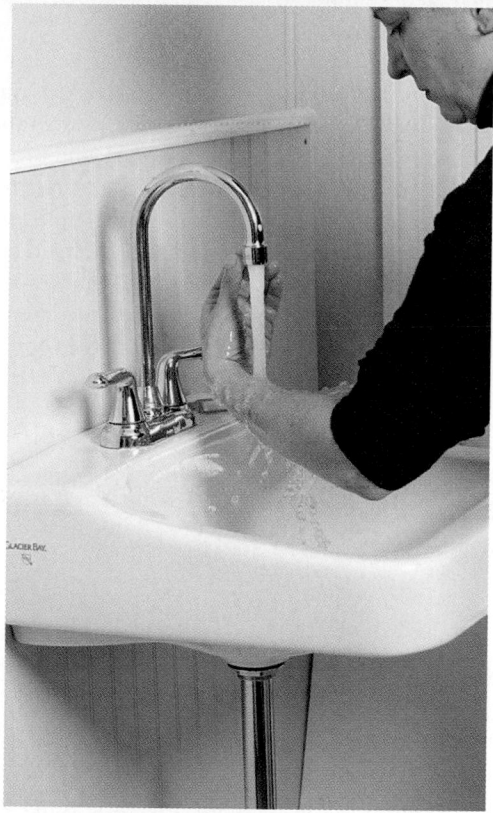

Allow the water to run downward and off of your elbows.

12. Scrub the wrists and the forearms from the distal to the proximal side, which scrubs pathogens from the more clean to the less clean area.

13. Rinse each arm separately by continuing to hold hands upright, allowing the water to run downward and off of your elbows.

14. Discard the scrub brush.

15. Turn off the water using a clean paper towel (or the foot or knee lever on a surgical sink) to maintain cleanliness of the hands.

16. Continue to hold your hands upright and dry one hand and arm with a towel, moving from the distal to the proximal side. If sterile gowning and closed gloving are required, be sure to use a sterile towel for drying to prevent reintroduction of pathogens to the hands and arms.

17. Using the other end of the towel, repeat the drying process on the other hand and arm because the unused end of the towel is cleaner.

18. Avoid touching anything by keeping your hands above your waist to prevent introducing pathogens before gloving.

open all needed supplies and add them to the field, arranged in an organized manner that facilitates effective performance of the procedure.

Next, she must create a sterile barrier using sterile disposable drapes, sterile towels, or even the sterile wrap that encloses some types of supplies. When she creates the barrier, she must open other needed sterile items and drop them onto the field using a technique called the *sterile toss.* To perform this technique, the medical assistant must open the sterile wrapped item or packet away from the field without touching the contents. Then she must hold the wrapper just near enough to the field to carefully toss the items onto it. In this way, sterile items are placed on the sterile field

without contaminating either one and without the need to wear sterile gloves. After all needed items are on the field, the medical assistant or other health care provider may put on sterile gloves and organize items on the field as desired in preparation for the procedure.

Commonly, the medical assistant will use the wrap that encloses an item as the underlying sterile barrier. When opening this or any other sterile wrapped item, the medical assistant should always open the wrap away from the body first, then to each side, and, lastly, toward the body.(See *Procedure 24-2: Setting up a sterile field.*) Following these rules of sterile technique prevents unnecessary reaching over the sterile field. (See *Patients and the sterile field,* page 394.)

PROCEDURE 24-2

Setting up a sterile field

Task
Setting up a sterile field.

Conditions
- Mayo stand or other small table on wheels
- Sterile drape
- Waste receptacle
- Other supplies, as needed for the procedure, such as (used in this example):
  - Sterile solution, such as saline or povidone-iodine (Betadine)
  - Sterile transfer forceps
  - Small sterile cup or basin
  - Two sterile, wrapped 4" × 4" sponges

Standards
In the time specified and within the scoring parameters determined by the instructor, the student will successfully set up a sterile field, add items to the field by sterile toss, use sterile transfer forceps to add an item to the field, and pour a sterile solution.

Performance Standards
1. Select a clean, dry surface above waist level, such as a mayo stand. Items below the waist are considered nonsterile.
2. Assemble the necessary supplies and check the expiration dates on the packages. After the expiration date, a package is considered nonsterile. Also check the label on each one to ensure the package contains the needed items.
3. Place the waste receptacle within easy reach of the work area.
4. Wash or sanitize your hands to ensure infection control.

5. Lay a sterile wrapped drape on the surface in front of you with the top flap pointing toward you; position facilitates correct opening of the package.
6. Grasp and remove the sterilization seal or tape.
7. Grasp the top flap of the wrap by the outer surface near the tip. Then lift and open it away from you.

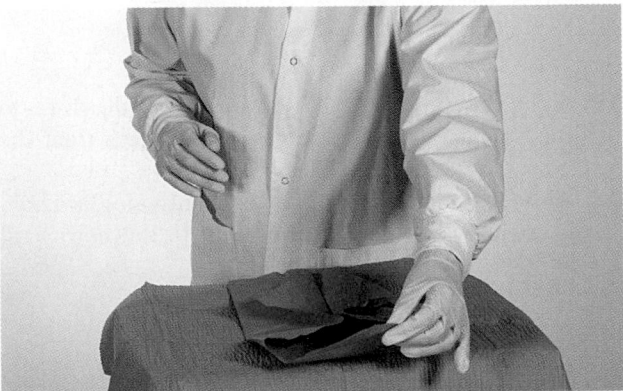

Open the top flap of the wrap away from you.

8. Grasp the side flap by the outer surface near the tip. Then lift and open it to the side.
9. Grasp the other side flap by the outer surface near the tip. Lift and open it to the side, taking care not to touch any of the sterile contents with your fingers. Following the sequence (top, side, side) avoids the need to extend the arm over the sterile field.

PROCEDURE 24-2—cont'd

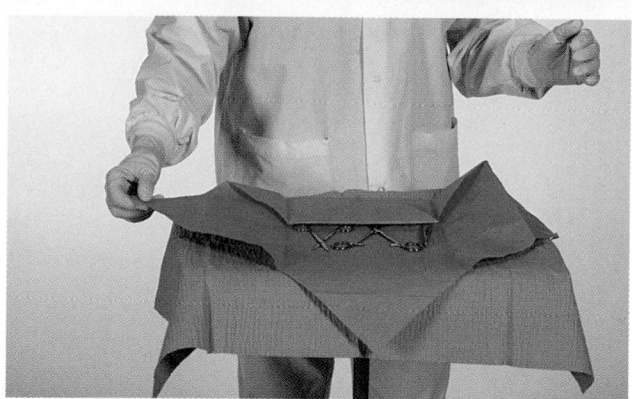

Lift the side flap, taking care not to touch the sterile contents.

10. Carefully pick up top edge of remaining corner of the folded drape. The outer 1" is considered nonsterile, so you may touch it as necessary.

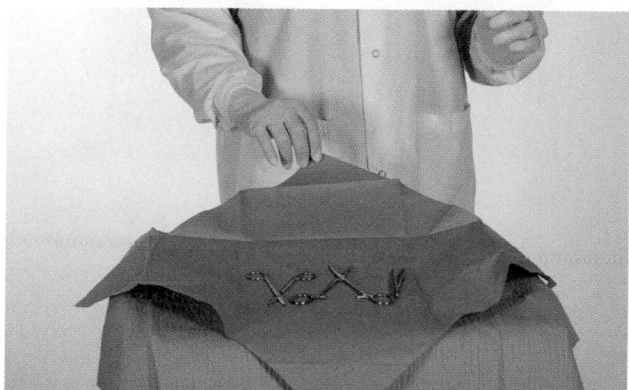

Carefully pick up the top edge of the remaining corner of the folded drape.

11. Lift the drape and let it unfold itself by gravity, rather than shaking it, and make sure that it does not touch anything to avoid contamination.
12. Holding the drape by the outer top corners, lay it over the work surface.
13. If using sterile 4" × 4" gauze pads, take a wrapped pad and grasp each flap of the wrapper between your thumbs and fingers and open the package outward, taking care not to touch the inner contents with non-sterile fingers to prevent contamination.

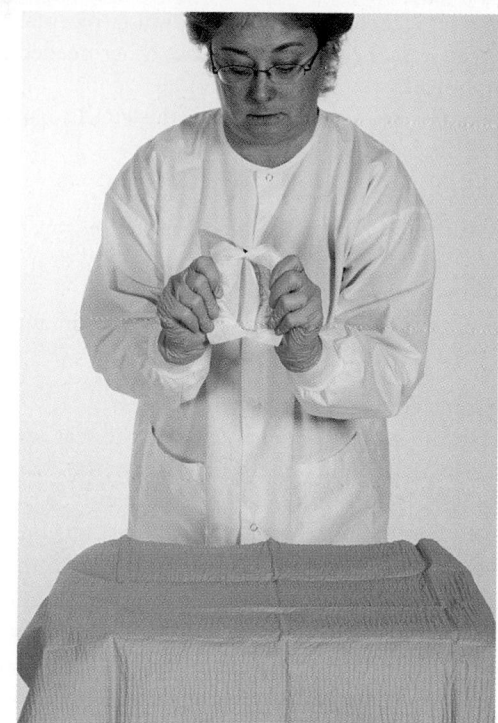

Open the package outward, taking care not to touch the contents.

14. When you have opened the package approximately three-quarters of the way, move over the sterile field and gently toss or drop the item onto the field, taking care not to touch any nonsterile item to the field.

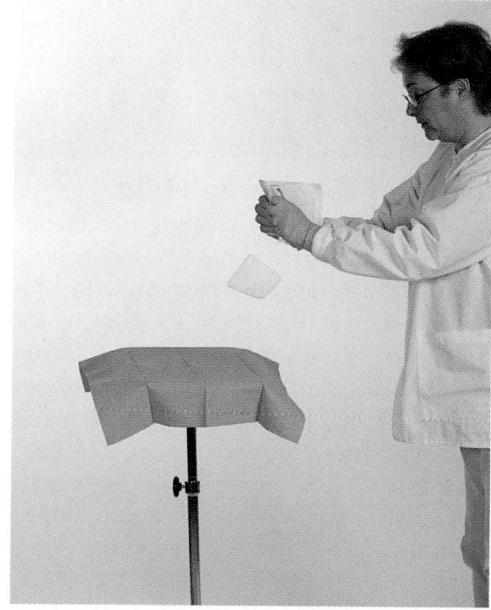

Gently toss or drop the item onto the sterile field.

Continued

PROCEDURE 24-2—cont'd

15. Dispose of the outer wrap in the waste receptacle.
16. Repeat steps 12 to 14 to add any other needed items to the field.
17. Open the package containing the sterile basin but leave the basin on its sterile wrapper.

Using sterile transfer forceps
18. Open the package containing the sterile transfer forceps and grasp them by the handles only to maintain sterility of the tips.
19. Using sterile forceps, grasp the sterile basin and place it in the sterile field where desired.

Pouring a sterile solution onto the sterile field
20. Grasp the sterile container, remove the seal, and then remove the cap. Hold the cap with the open side downward in your nondominant hand or place it nearby (but not on the sterile field) with the open side up to minimize the risk of contamination to the cap.
21. Carefully pour in the required amount of solution, holding the bottle between 1" and 4" above the basin to minimize the risk of contamination from touching the bottle to the basin, while also minimizing the risk of splashing.

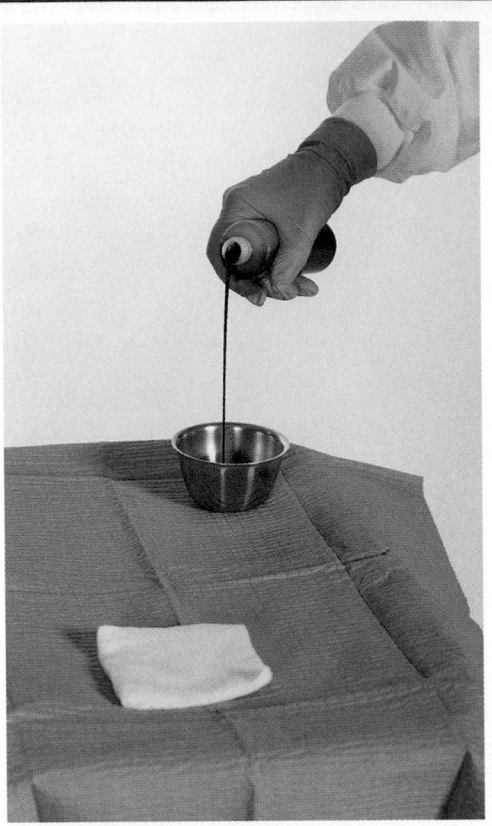

Hold the bottle 1" to 4" above the basin.

22. Recap the sterile bottle and set it aside but not on the sterile field.

Patients and the Sterile Field

Well-meaning patients may unwittingly contaminate a sterile field by touching items out of curiosity or a desire to be helpful. Therefore, the medical assistant should tactfully request that the patient keep his hands away from the sterile drapes and instruments. The medical assistant can explain to the patient that all items have been carefully sterilized with the goal of sparing the patient the unpleasant complications an infection might cause. If the patient is unpredictable (such as a small child), the medical assistant must be aware of the child's movements in order to intervene if necessary. A parent or guardian might also be enlisted to hold the child's hands during the procedure.

Sterile Gloving

Application of sterile gloves is one of the most common sterile procedures that medical assistants perform. Therefore, it is extremely important for the medical assistant to learn how to apply sterile gloves properly and maintain good technique. Regardless of what happens during a procedure, if the medical assistant begins a procedure with contaminated gloves, she contaminates everything she touches and puts the patient in jeopardy. (See *Procedure 24-3: Applying sterile gloves.*)

Minor Surgical Procedures

Many minor surgical procedures are done in the medical office. Common procedures include suturing, suture removal, incision and drainage (I&D) of infections, and removal of

PROCEDURE 24-3

Applying sterile gloves

Task
Apply sterile gloves.

Conditions
- Package of sterile gloves in the appropriate size
- Clean, dry surface such as the top of a mayo stand

Standards
In the time specified and within the scoring parameters determined by the instructor, the student will successfully apply sterile gloves.

Performance Standards
1. Wash your hands with warm water and soap. Dry thoroughly to ensure infection control.
2. Open the outer wrapper, remove the inner pack, and lay the inner pack on the table in front of you, slightly above waist level. Items below waist level are considered contaminated.
3. Grasp paper fold in each hand and open outward without disturbing the gloves inside.

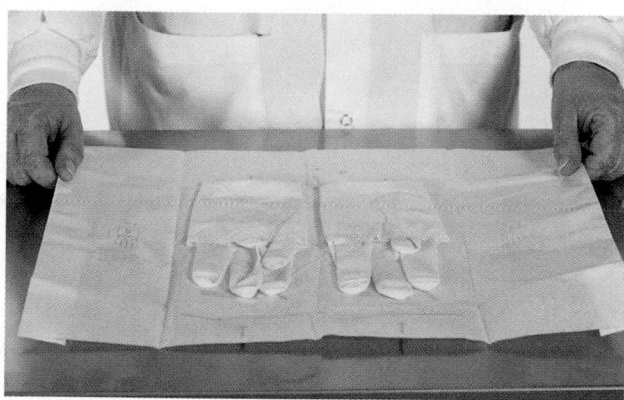

Open the paper outward without disturbing the gloves.

4. Identify the right and left glove.
5. With the first two fingers and thumb of your nondominant hand, grasp the cuff of the dominant hand glove by touching only the inside surface to keep the outside of glove sterile.

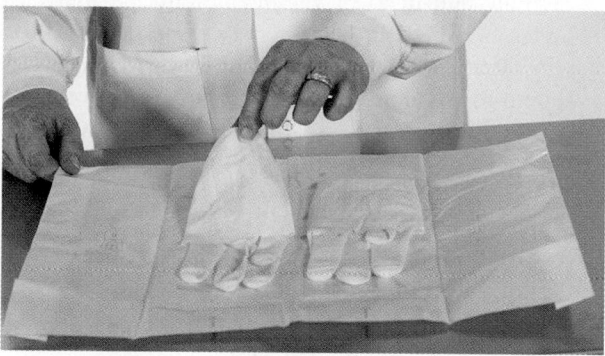

Grasp the cuff of the glove by touching only the inside surface.

6. Insert your dominant hand into the glove while carefully pulling it on with your nondominant hand.

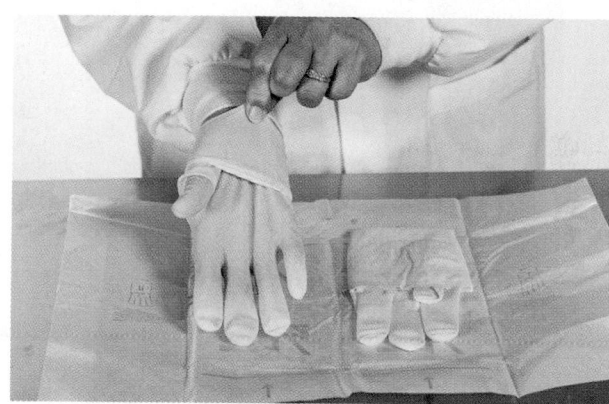

Insert your dominant hand.

7. With your sterile-gloved, dominant hand, slip your fingers under the cuff of the other glove, touching only the sterile side, because only sterile may touch sterile, and lift it off the table.

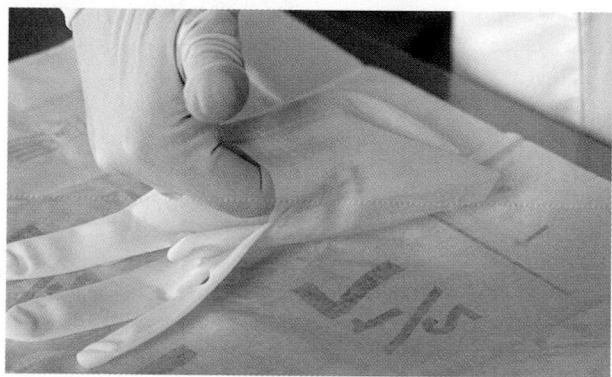

Slip your fingers under the cuff, touching only the sterile side.

Continued

PROCEDURE 24-3—cont'd

8. Insert your nondominant hand into the glove and carefully pull it on by pulling upward and outward under its cuff with the fingers of the other hand. Be very careful not to touch your sterile-gloved fingers or thumb to any nonsterile surface to prevent contamination. Keep your gloved thumb abducted so it does not touch the other arm.

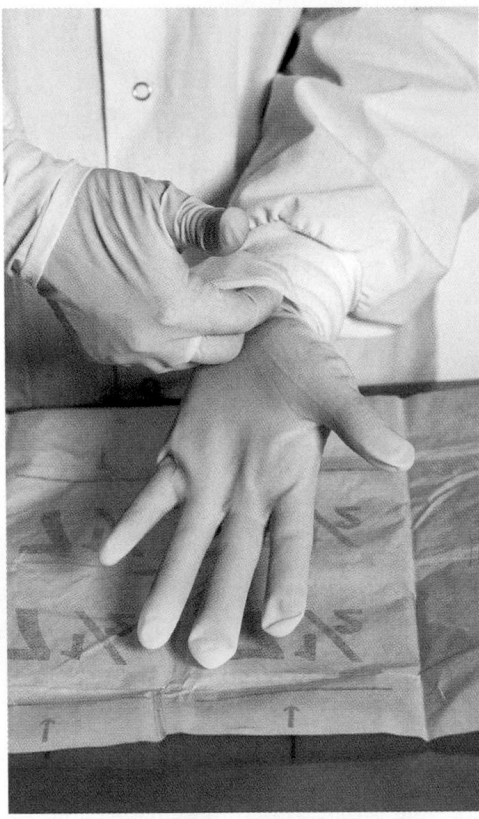

Pull upward and outward under the cuff and keep your thumb abducted.

9. If you are wearing long sleeves, continue pulling the cuff upward in the manner described above until the cuff encircles your sleeve cuff to prevent sleeves from falling too low over the glove and contaminating the wrist area.

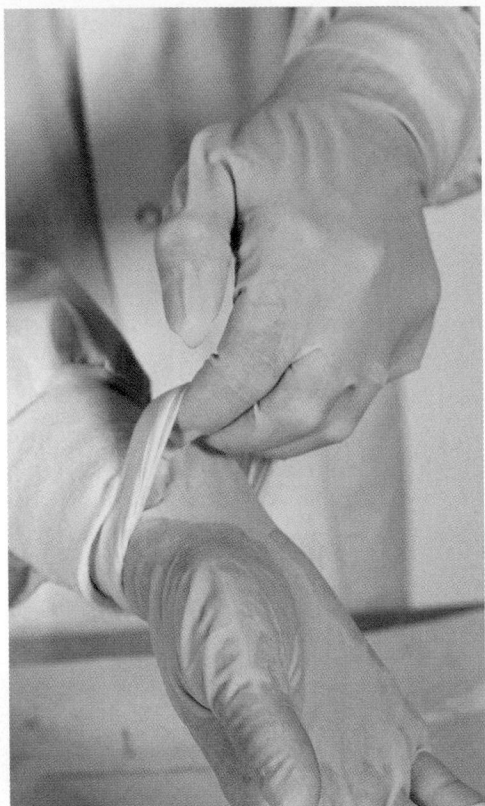

Pull the cuff upward until it encircles your sleeve cuff.

10. After you have applied the second glove, interlock your hands and adjust the fingers of the gloves if necessary to ensure a smooth fit.

Removing gloves
11. Grasp the outer cuff of one glove with the other hand. Do not touch your wrist with the fingers of the contaminated glove to avoid spreading pathogens to your bare skin.

PROCEDURE 24-3—cont'd

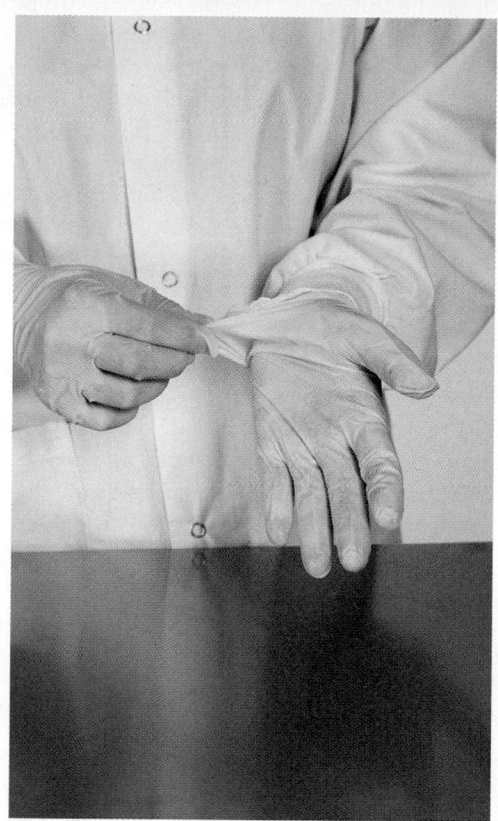

Grasp the outer cuff of one glove without touching your wrist.

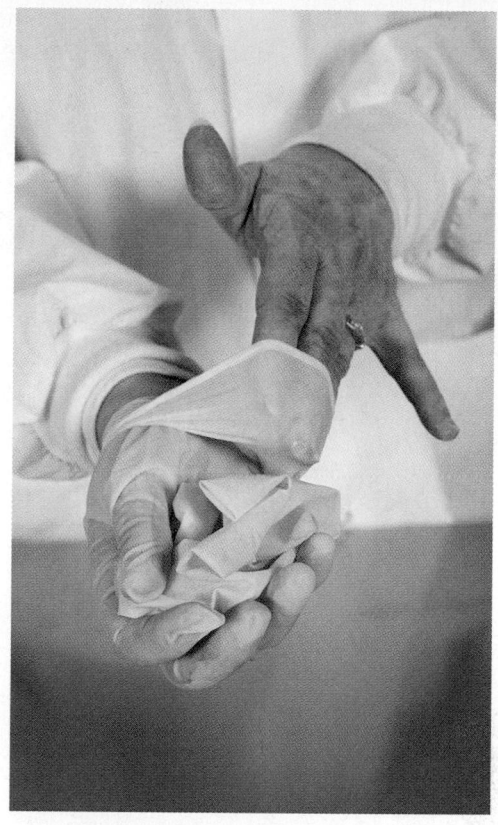

Place your fingers under the cuff next to the skin and pull the glove off.

12. Pull the glove off, turning it inside out, and wad it up in the other gloved hand.

13. Place the fingers of your ungloved hand under the cuff of the gloved hand (next to the skin) and pull the glove off, turning it inside out while enclosing the other glove in the process.

14. Discard in waste receptacle.

ingrown toenails or sebaceous cysts. (See Figure 24-14.) There are some procedures the medical assistant may perform herself if the physician has given the order to do so, including suture or staple removal and application of dressings.

There are many types of surgical procedures that medical assistants may be asked to assist with. Those that involve the use of extreme cold are sometimes called *cryosurgery.* Those performed with the use of specialized microscopes are called *microsurgery.* Those that involve cutting or destroying tissue by the application of electricity are called *electrosurgery.*

Cryosurgery

Cryosurgery, also called *cryotherapy,* is a technique that destroys tissue by subjecting it to very cold temperatures, usually −20°C (−4°F), using a probe that has liquid nitrogen

circulating through it. This procedure is commonly used in ambulatory settings for a wide range of needs, including treating cancer and precancerous conditions. Cryosurgery may be used internally on liver, prostate, bone, or cervical cancer or externally to remove skin lesions. This treatment has fewer adverse effects than many other forms of treatment and usually has a shorter recovery time.

Microsurgery

Microsurgery is a general term that refers to any procedure completed with the use of a special operating microscope. It is useful for delicate procedures on the eyes, nose, sinuses, larynx, genitourinary tract, and any structures with tiny blood vessels and nerves. It is especially useful in the reattachment of severed body parts and organ and tissue transplantation.

A

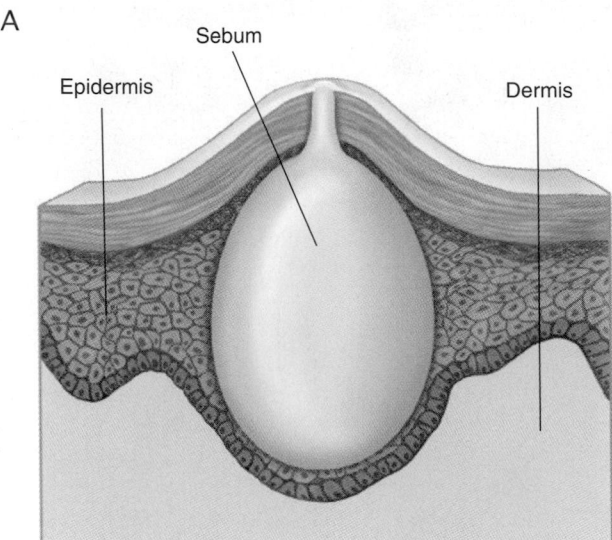

Epidermis   Sebum   Dermis

B

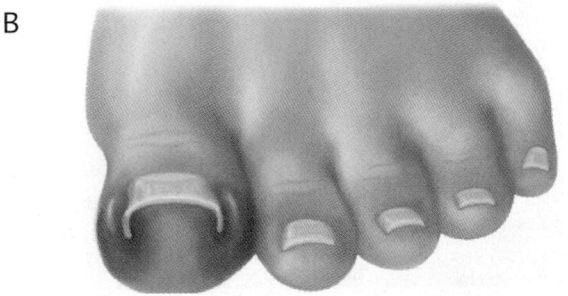

FIG 24-14 Sebaceous cyst (A) and ingrown toenail (B).

Plastic surgeons use microsurgery to perform repair and reconstructive surgeries.

The microscope allows the surgeon to operate on structures that would otherwise be difficult to see by magnifying them up to 40 times their normal size. There are many types of microscopes that can be mounted on the floor or ceiling. All have a set of lenses with zoom functions, a high-intensity light source, and a video camera that displays images on a screen. The physician can operate the microscope using foot or mouth controls.

The physician must also use special microsurgical instruments that allow manipulation of delicate structures. Some of these instruments include specialized forceps, scissors, needle holders, clamps, irrigators, and vessel dilators. Specialized suture material is also used with suture thread as small as 12-0 (0.001 mm). Suture needles for microsurgery also come in many sizes and with different points. Sizes are generally less than 0.15 mm in diameter.

Laser Surgery

Laser surgery is the treatment of tissue by means of a laser. The term *laser* is an acronym for light amplified by stimulated emission of radiation. The laser's beams are so precise that they enable the surgeon to target structures with little injury to surrounding tissues, resulting in minimal scar formation. Lasers were initially most common in the treatment of eye disorders but have become a popular tool for various procedures. Lasers are particularly useful for cosmetic surgery, including the removal of vessels, moles, warts, and other lesions. Improper operation or handling of laser equipment could result in injury. Therefore, medical assistants should undergo special training before assisting with laser surgery or handling laser equipment.

Electrosurgery

Electrosurgery, also called *electrocautery,* involves the use of an electrosurgical unit (ESU) or high-frequency electric current to cut, remove, or destroy tissue. It is a popular method of removing skin tags (small noncancerous growths), tumors, and warts in dermatology and is commonly preferred over laser surgery or cryosurgery. The ESU has a small, electrified probe that burns or vaporizes tissue with minimal bleeding. The device also includes disposable tips for the probe, a grounding cable, and a pad.

Endoscopy

Endoscopy is becoming a popular method of performing internal examinations and procedures. It involves the use of a specialized scope containing a tiny camera and light source to visually examine a structure, such as the upper gastrointestinal (GI) system (esophagus, stomach, duodenum), lower GI system (rectum, colon), respiratory system (trachea, larynx, bronchi), urinary system (urethra, bladder, ureters), inside of the abdomen, and inside of various joints. During such procedures, physicians carefully examine structures, obtain tissue for study, and perform surgical interventions. Just a few examples of common endoscopic procedures include tubal ligation (female sterilization), cholecystectomy (gallbladder removal), and colonoscopy. Scopes may be rigid, semirigid, or flexible. The scopes and associated equipment are expensive and delicate and, thus, require special handling and care. Therefore, medical assistants should be properly trained before handling them or assisting with endoscopic procedures.

The Medical Assistant's Role in Minor Surgery

The medical assistant performs many duties when assisting with minor surgery. She must always examine the room to be sure it has been properly cleaned and prepared. She must familiarize herself with the physicians she works with and note their preferences for room arrangement and supplies. She must be familiar with the procedures to be performed in order to do these tasks. (See *Procedure "recipe" cards.*) She must set up the sterile field for the physician so that, once begun, the procedure can be completed smoothly and efficiently. The medical assistant should make sure that she does not leave opened sterile materials exposed to the air or unattended because contamination may occur. Therefore, she should set up the sterile field just prior to the procedure. However, in some offices it is acceptable to set up trays up to 1 hour ahead of time and cover them with a sterile drape until the procedure begins.

When the procedure begins, the medical assistant plays two key roles:

1. Assist the physician by:
   a. handing him needed supplies or instruments (See *Safe instrument exchange*.)
   b. observing the field and the procedure for any breaks in sterility and notifying the physician if it occurs.
2. Attend to the patient by:
   a. providing instruction about positioning
   b. explaining what is happening
   c. offering reassurance. (See *Procedure 24-4: Assisting with minor surgery*, page 400 to 402.)

Patient Preparation and Postoperative Care

Prior to any surgical procedure, the medical assistant must make sure that the patient has been properly informed and prepared. To do so, the medical assistant must make sure the patient understands the procedure, the physician has satisfactorily answered all of the patient's questions, all preoperative laboratory work has been completed, and the patient has signed an informed consent form. It is the physician's legal responsibility to inform the patient about the procedure and obtain the patient's signature. If this step has not been completed, the medical assistant must alert the physician.

After completion of the surgical procedure the patient may need time to rest, especially if a sedating medication is administered. The medical assistant should make sure the patient is positioned comfortably and safely while resting. She should also ensure that there is a person with the patient to supervise him carefully when he gets up, dresses, and travels home to prevent injury. (See *Preoperative and postoperative education*, page 402.)

Safe instrument exchange

To hand the physician sharp instruments, such as scissors, hold them by their tips and extend the handles toward the physician so that he can securely grasp them in his palm or fingers. Doing so protects the physician from injury and enables him to grasp them securely, reducing the risk of dropping them.

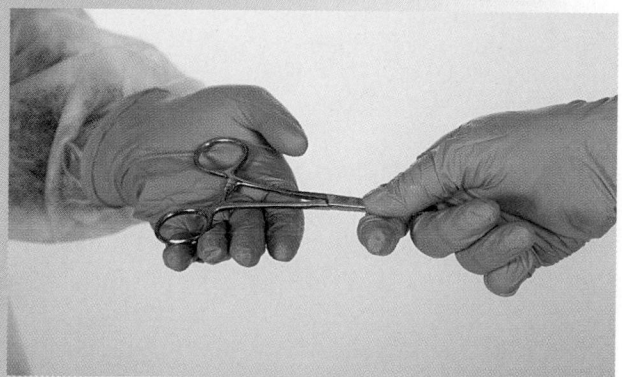

Hold on to the tip of the instrument and extend the handle toward the physician.

Front office–Back office connection

Procedure "Recipe" Cards

Most medical assistants who have moved or temporarily floated to a new department have stories of frustration about trying to locate items and understand physician preferences. Such situations are especially frustrating when a medical assistant is attempting to set up and assist with a procedure. Clinical medical assistants can make the back office "float-friendly" for others by creating (and keeping up-to-date) a "recipe" book of all of the procedures commonly done in the office. Using a three-ring binder makes it easy to remove, replace, and update information. Be sure all information in the book is consistent with office policy.

A list of physician's glove sizes should be located in the front of the book. Each procedure listed in the book should include step-by-step instructions for procedures commonly performed by medical assistants, along with the following information:

- location within the office of commonly needed items
- physician preferences regarding instruments or procedure kits
- physician preferences for room arrangement and patient positioning
- physician preferences for whether the medical assistant is to remain in the room to assist or wants to complete the procedure on her own
- typical postprocedure patient education
- length of time usually required for the procedure.

PROCEDURE 24-4

Assisting with minor surgery

Task

Prepare patient for and assist physician with minor surgery, including application of sterile gloves, setup of the sterile field, and surgical skin preparation.

Conditions

Mayo stand

- Needles and syringes for anesthesia
- Betadine solution and preparation bowls or cups (at least 2)
- Sterile saline solution
- Sterile gauze sponges
- Scalpel and blade
- Operating scissors
- Fenestrated drape
- Hemostats, curved and blunt
- Thumb dressing forceps
- Thumb tissue forceps
- Needle holder
- Suture pack
- Transfer forceps

Side table

- Package of sterile gloves
- Labeled biopsy containers (with formalin)
- Laboratory requisition
- Anesthesia vial
- Alcohol wipes
- Dressing materials, including tape, bandages, and 4" × 4" gauze pads
- Biohazard container
- Betadine solution

Standards

In the time specified and within the scoring parameters determined by the instructor, the student will successfully assist with a minor surgical procedure.

Performance Standards

1. Select a clean, dry surface above waist level, such as a mayo stand, because items below the waist are considered nonsterile.
2. Check the room for cleanliness to ensure infection control.
3. Assemble the supplies for the procedure, inspecting each item for expiration date or contamination to ensure infection control.
4. Wash your hands to ensure infection control.
5. Set up a side table with nonsterile items to avoid contaminating sterile items with nonsterile items.
6. Set up a sterile field on a clean, dry surface.

7. Add sterile items to the sterile field as needed.
8. Apply sterile gloves.
9. Arrange the sterile instruments according to order of use to avoid needing to pass dirty instruments over sterile ones during the procedure.
10. Cover the sterile field with a sterile towel if not used immediately to prevent dust and other airborne microorganisms from settling on the sterile field.
11. Identify the patient and explain the procedure to ease patient anxiety, prevent misidentification of the patient, and facilitate patient compliance.

Surgical skin preparation

12. Prepare the patient's skin according to office procedure or following these steps:
    a. Apply clean examination gloves.
    b. Remove hair from the operative site by carefully shaving, holding the skin taut and shaving in the direction of hair growth to reduce the risk of cutting the skin or by clipping hair short, because shaving can cause small abrasions, increasing risk of infection.

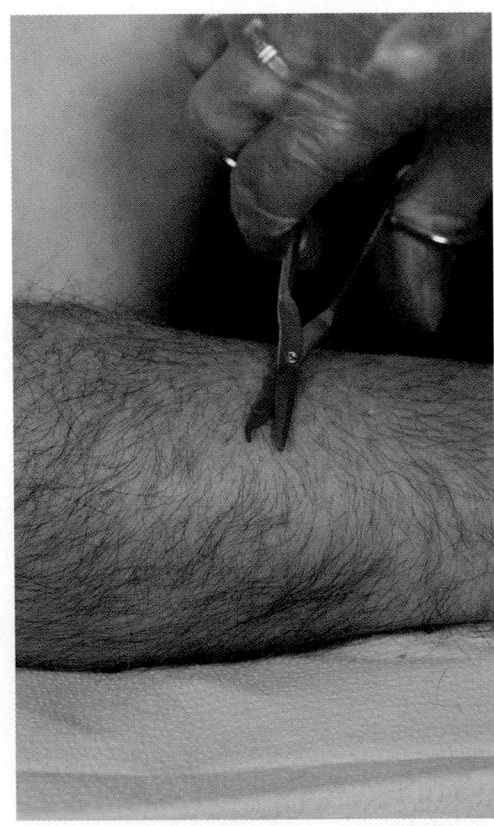

Remove hair from the operative site by shaving or clipping it short.

PROCEDURE 24-4—cont'd

c. Rinse the area with sterile saline solution and pat it dry.

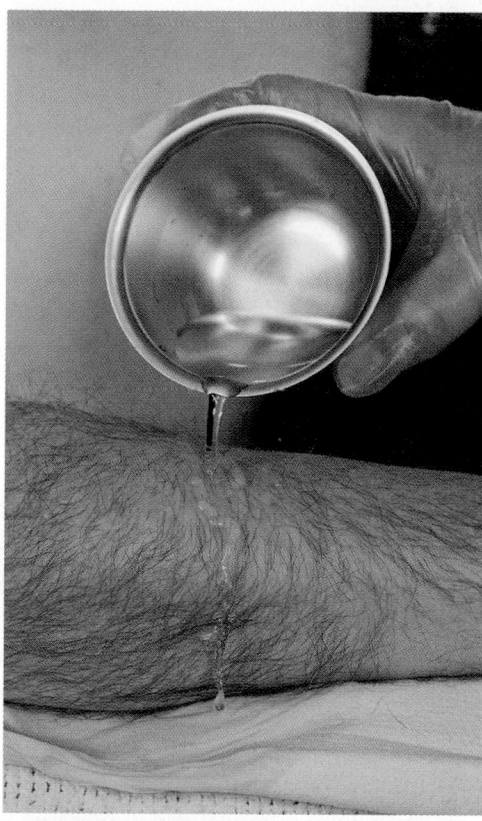

Rinse the area with sterile saline solution.

d. Cleanse the area with an antiseptic solution and a surgical scrub brush by scrubbing gently in a circular motion moving from inward to outward. Do not retrace over the previously scrubbed area.

e. Rinse the area with sterile saline saturated gauze pads and blot it dry.

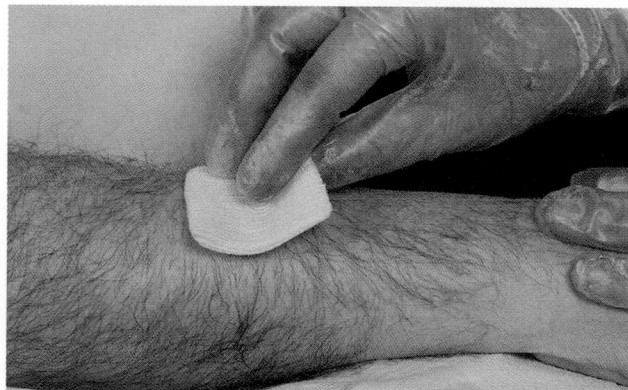

Rinse the area and blot it dry.

f. Clean the area with antiseptic povidone-iodine (Betadine) or alcohol swabs.

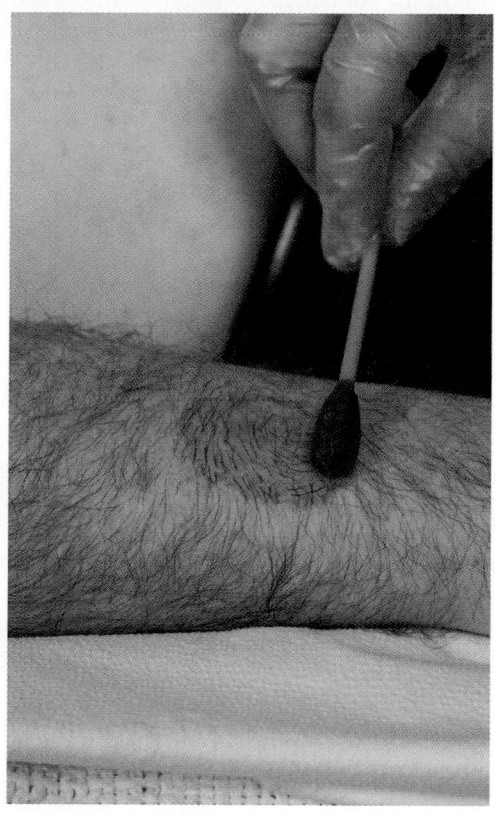

Clean the area with antiseptic povidone-iodine swabs.

g. Allow the area to air dry.
h. Remove your gloves.
i. Sanitize your hands.

13. Remove the sterile towel from the sterile field as the physician applies sterile gloves.

14. Assist the physician with the procedure, according to her requests. Communication throughout the procedure is critical to a good outcome.

15. Throughout the procedure:
   a. Ensure that the physician has the necessary equipment and supplies.
   b. Ensure that the lighting is adequate for the physician to view the surgical field.
   c. Comfort the patient (if awake) during the procedure.
   d. Hand instruments to the physician as requested.
   e. Hold the biopsy container for the physician to place the tissue specimen into, if necessary.
   f. Ensure the biopsy containers or other specimens are properly labeled, tightly covered, and sent to the laboratory with an appropriately completed laboratory requisition form.

Continued

PROCEDURE 24-4—cont'd

16. When the physician completes the procedure, assist her as needed with the application of a dressing.

17. Dispose of contaminated supplies and sharps in an appropriate biohazard sharps container to ensure infection control.

18. Rinse used surgical instruments and soak, sanitize, and sterilize them for reuse.

19. Remove and appropriately dispose of your gloves, gown, and other PPE and wash your hands to ensure infection control.

21. Apply clean gloves and other PPE as needed.

22. Disinfect the treatment area per office protocol.

20. Wash your hands to ensure infection control.

21. Be sure to provide the patient's medical record to the physician for timely documentation of the procedure.

 Patient Education

Preoperative and Postoperative Education

Before a patient undergoes a surgical procedure, the medical assistant must ensure that the patient understands what will happen before and after the procedure. Although patient education for specific procedures will vary, below are general guidelines for preoperative and postoperative patient education.

Preoperative

• Check to be sure that the patient or legal representative has signed the necessary consent forms.

• Give the patient instructions for home preparation that must be completed before the procedure, such as bathing, diet, and medications.

• Call the patient the day before surgery to confirm and remind the patient of such special instructions.

• Remind the patient to leave valuables at home.

• Make sure the patient has someone who can drive him home after the procedure.

Postoperative

• Make sure the patient has recovered sufficiently to be able to travel safely.

• Obtain postprocedure vital signs according to office policy (which may or may not be required for various procedures).

• Inform the patient about residual effects of local or systemic medications used during the procedure.

• Educate the patient about postoperative medications he must take.

• Make sure the patient has made a follow-up appointment if appropriate.

• Discuss wound care or dressing changes with the patient as appropriate. (The most reliable way to verify patient understanding is to have him perform wound care or a dressing change while you observe.) Be sure to include these points:
  • Mild inflammation is normal and is indicated by slight redness, slight edema, mild warmth, and some tenderness.
  • Observe for signs of infection and call the physician if any appear (increased redness, increased pain, increased heat, and foul drainage as well as fever and decreased function).
  • Keep the wound clean and dry.
  • Wash hands with warm water and soap prior to changing dressings.
  • Perform dressing changes daily or as instructed by the physician.
  • Do not apply creams, ointments, or solutions to the wound except as instructed by the physician.
  • Return for suture or staple removal as directed by the physician.
  • Complete antibiotics or other prescribed medication as directed by the physician.

• Discuss other signs or symptoms for which the patient should contact the physician.

• Ask the patient if he has any questions or concerns and answer them or refer them to the physician.

Wound Care

When closing a wound, the physician's goals are to promote timely healing and reduce scar formation. These goals are accomplished through the use of aseptic technique and careful **approximation** of the wound edges (bringing them together closely and evenly). The physician most commonly does this by using sutures or staples.

Sutures

The word *suture* may be used as a noun or a verb. When used as a noun, it refers to a specific type of material used to sew wound edges together. When used as a verb, it refers to the action of sewing the wound edges together. Although suture material and needles may be packaged separately, they are most commonly packaged together with the suture already **swaged** (fused) to the needle. Needles are usually curved and are categorized by curve radius, size, shape, and type of point (round taper, blunt, or cutting). (See Figure 24-15.) Swaged needle-suture sets come packaged in a variety of sizes and shapes as well as a variety of suture gauges (sizes) and lengths. Suture sizes range from the smallest gauge (6-0) to the largest gauge (4). Packages are labeled for easy identification. However, the numbers reflecting size may be listed as *2-0* or *00*, *3-0* or *000*, and so on.

The physician's selection of a suture type and size depends on the tissue type being sutured. For example, smaller suture material is appropriate for delicate tissue where appearance is important, such as on the face. Manmade synthetic absorbable suture, such as Vicryl or PDS II, is used for internal sutures where later removal is not possible or practical. The older variety of surgical gut suture made from a sheep's intestinal tissue is seldom used. Nonabsorbable sutures made of Dacron, cotton, nylon, silk, or even stainless steel are used for external suturing where they can be easily removed. When the patient's wound has healed, suture removal is usually easily accomplished with suture scissors and forceps. The physician will commonly delegate this task to the medical assistant. (See *Procedure 24-5: Performing suture removal*, page 404.)

Staples

In recent years, staples have become a popular choice for wound closure because they are effective, safe, and enable quick, easy wound closure. (See Figure 24-16.) This may be especially true when the patient is particularly anxious, fearful of needles, and has difficulty holding still. However staples are not appropriate in every case and may only be used for external wound closure. Once the wound has healed the staples are easy to remove with a sterile prepackaged staple remover. The medical assistant places the tips of the staple remover under the staple and squeezes the handle, which lifts the staples out.

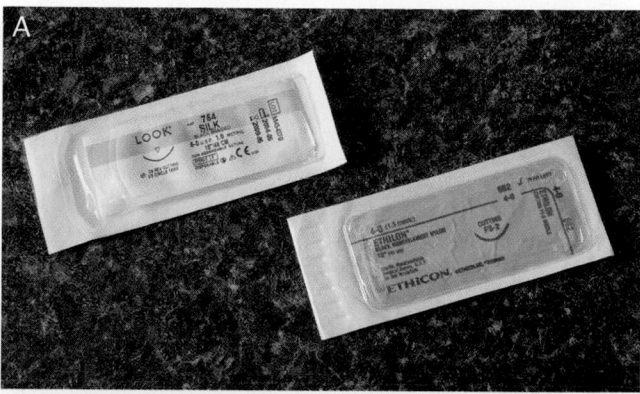

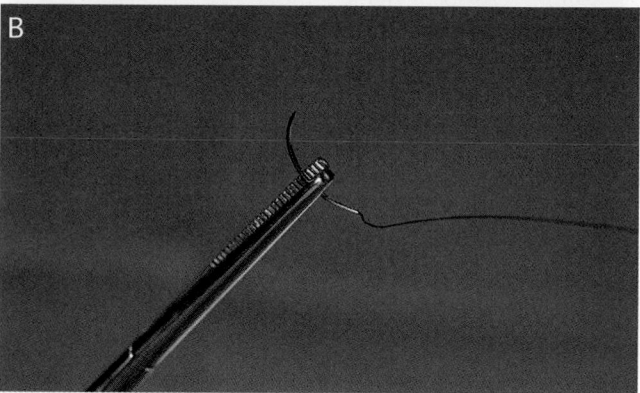

FIG 24-15 Suturing equipment. (A) Suture packs. (B) Swaged needle.

Wound Care Supplies

Every medical facility stocks the most commonly used supplies and equipment used for surgery and wound care for its patient population. Many of these items are disposable and intended for one-time use only. The medical assistant may be required to sanitize and sterilize other items for reuse.

Dressings

Dressings are materials placed in or on a wound and are usually made of gauze. They must be sterile and completely cover the wound. In some cases, a specific type of dressing material, called a *surgical wick* or a *wound packing strip*, such as Iodoform, is used to promote drainage of fluid from an infected wound. Such material may be packaged individually or in a long, narrow strip of sterile material packaged in a bottle. When using this type of material, the medical assistant must take special care to maintain the sterility of the wick that remains in the bottle.

Other common types of dressings include gauze pads or sponges of various sizes. The most common sizes of gauze pads are 4" × 4" (4" square) and 2" × 2" (2" square), although other sizes are available. (See Figure 24-17.) They may be packaged individually in peel-apart sterile packages

PROCEDURE 24-5

Performing suture removal

Task
Perform removal of skin sutures.

Conditions
- Gauze sponges
- Bandage scissors
- Biohazard waste container
- Tape
- Sponge forceps
- Suture scissors or staple remover
- Thumb forceps
- 4" × 4" gauze pads
- Sterile gloves
- Betadine solution or wash

Standards
In the time specified and within the scoring parameters determined by the instructor, the student will successfully remove sutures from a wound.

Performance Standards
1. Wash or sanitize your hands to ensure infection control.
2. Identify the patient and explain the procedure to ease patient anxiety.
3. Open the suture removal kit.

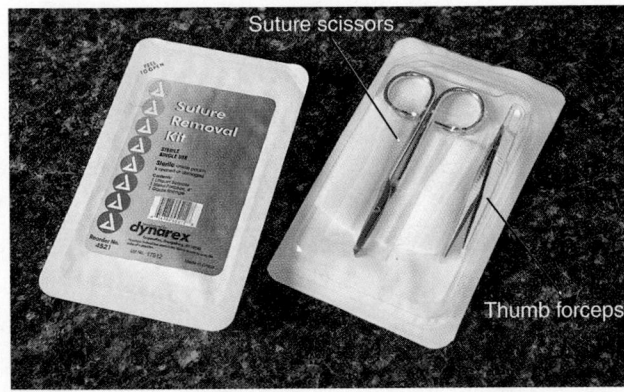

Suture removal kit

4. Apply sterile gloves.
5. Using thumb forceps, gently pick up one knot of a suture.
6. Gently pull upward toward the suture line to avoid cutting the patient's skin with the scissors.
7. Insert the curved notch of the suture removal scissors beneath the suture and cut one side of the suture as close to the skin as possible.

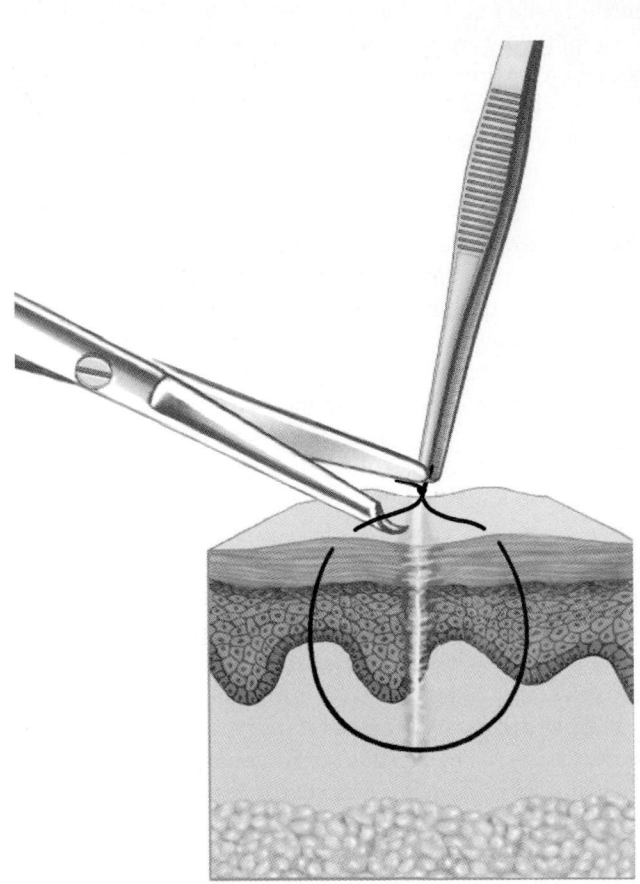

Sutured incision

8. Pull the suture through the skin, being careful to avoid contaminating the wound with the suture tip to prevent infection.
9. Remove all sutures in the same manner.
10. Place each suture on a sterile gauze sponge to avoid contaminating the thumb forceps and enable an accurate count of sutures.
11. Examine the wound to be sure that you have removed all of the sutures. Leaving a suture in the wound may lead to infection.
12. Apply povidone-iodine solution to the area unless the patient is allergic to iodine to inhibit bacterial growth.
13. Apply a sterile dressing if directed to reduce the risk of infection.
14. Remove your gloves and dispose of them in a biohazardous waste container to ensure infection control.
15. Dispose of all used items per OSHA regulations.
16. Wash your hands to ensure infection control.

PROCEDURE 24-5—cont'd

17. Explain wound care to the patient, providing written and verbal instructions to promote patient understanding and timely wound healing.
18. Document the procedure to ensure a complete, accurate medical record.

Date	
09/01/08: 1:30 p.m.	*11 sutures removed from Ⓡ forearm incision ----------------* --*S. Gonzales, CMA*

of two or may be packaged in bulk (one hundred). Some sponges have other material such as cotton or rayon embedded to provide for greater absorption. These are useful when excessive bleeding or fluid drainage is an issue.

The physician will commonly delegate the application or changing of a dressing to the medical assistant. Occasionally, the physician will give specific instructions but usually lets the medical assistant use her judgment in selecting the most appropriate dressing material. In making her decision, she should consider the wound location, size, amount of drainage, and the patient's physical activity level. The dressing must be snug enough to be secure but should be as comfortable as possible and not impede circulation. (See *Procedure 24-6: Removing a dressing and applying a new sterile dressing,* page 406.)

Bandages

Bandages are nonsterile material applied over the top of dressings to secure them. They may be made of gauze in the form of an elastic wrap or a roll that can be wrapped around a dressing. (See Figure 24-18.) Tubular gauze is a popular form of bandage material for distal extremities such as fingers, toes, arms, and legs. Its unique shape makes it easy

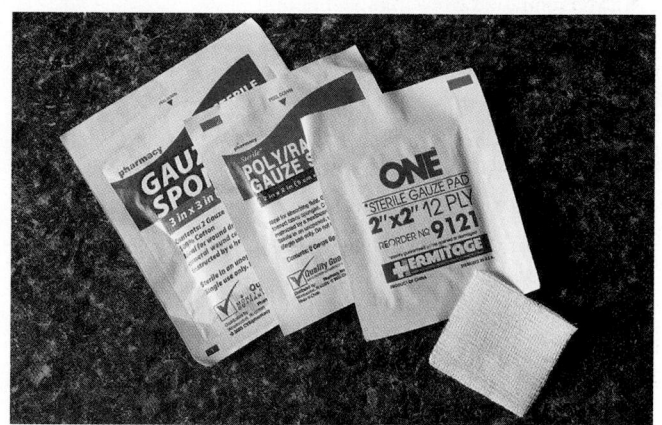

FIG 24-17 Sterile gauze pads.

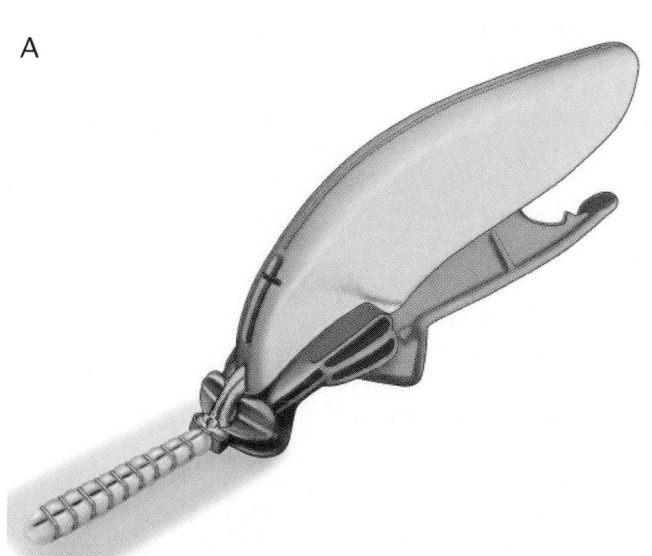

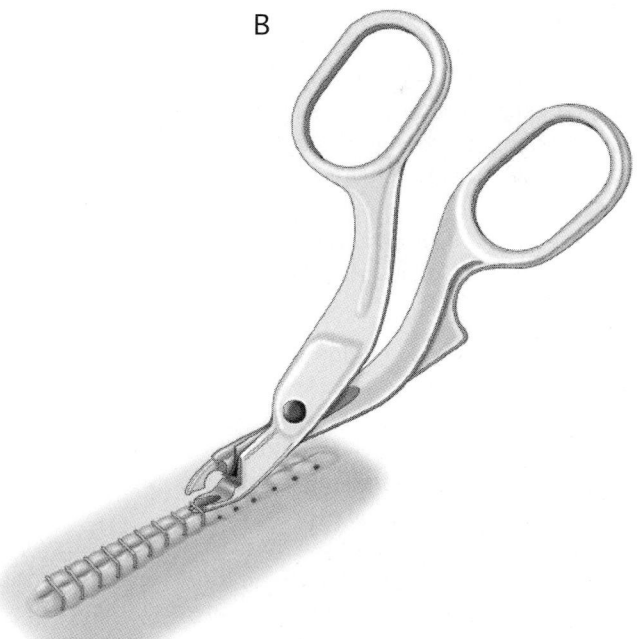

FIG 24-16 Skin stapler (A). Staple remover (B).

PROCEDURE 24-6

Removing a dressing and applying a new sterile dressing

Task

Demonstrate the removal and application of a sterile dressing.

Conditions

- Sterile gloves
- Sterile gauze dressings as needed
- Examination gloves
- Tape
- Waste receptacle
- Sterile saline solution
- Tape, roller gauze, or elastic net as desired

Standards

In the time specified and within the scoring parameters determined by the instructor, the student will successfully remove an old dressing and apply a new, dry, sterile dressing.

Performance Standards

1. Wash or sanitize your hands to ensure infection control.
2. Introduce yourself to the patient and explain the procedure to ease patient anxiety.
3. Note the location, size, and depth of the wound as well as the current dressing material used to determine the amount and type of dressing material needed.
4. Review the physician's order for wound care and dressing change to dress the wound according to the physician's instruction.
5. Gather the needed supplies.
6. Evaluate the patient's current degree of discomfort and whether pain medication is needed to ease the patient's discomfort during the dressing change.
7. Take measures to ensure privacy for the patient.
8. Position the patient on the examination table in a manner that maximizes patient comfort and provides optimal access to the wound.
9. Wash or sanitize your hands to ensure infection control.
10. Set up a sterile field and needed supplies.

Removing the old dressing

11. Apply clean examination gloves and remove the old dressing by following these steps:
    a. Stabilize the old dressing with one hand while carefully pulling the tape off toward the wound to minimize patient discomfort.
    b. Gently remove the dressing in layers.
    c. Before disposing of the dressing, note the amount and character of drainage on the dressing material because such information is important in determining the status of the wound and the amount of new dressing material to apply.
    d. Remove your contaminated gloves and dispose of them in the biohazard waste container to ensure infection control.
12. Wash or sanitize your hands to ensure infection control.

Applying the new dressing

13. Apply sterile gloves.
14. Note the wound's appearance, including size, depth, and any signs of infection.
15. Clean the wound, as ordered. Use sterile saline-moistened gauze to clean from the most to least contaminated area (from wound outward) and from wound margins outward. Alternatively, irrigate the wound with sterile saline, flushing in one direction.
16. Pat the area dry with dry sterile gauze.
17. Apply a sterile dry dressing material as needed over the wound.
18. Secure the dressing in place with tape or another bandage material, such as roller gauze or elastic net.
19. Document the procedure and any patient education about wound care or signs of infection to ensure a complete, accurate medical record.

Date	
06/27/08; 10:56 a.m.	(R) forearm dressing changed. Old dressing with moderate amount of serous drainage. No Sx infection noted. Two sterile 4x4s applied and secured with elastic net. Pt. tolerated procedure well, c/o "slight" pain ———————————— ————————————————————————————S. Gonzales, CMA

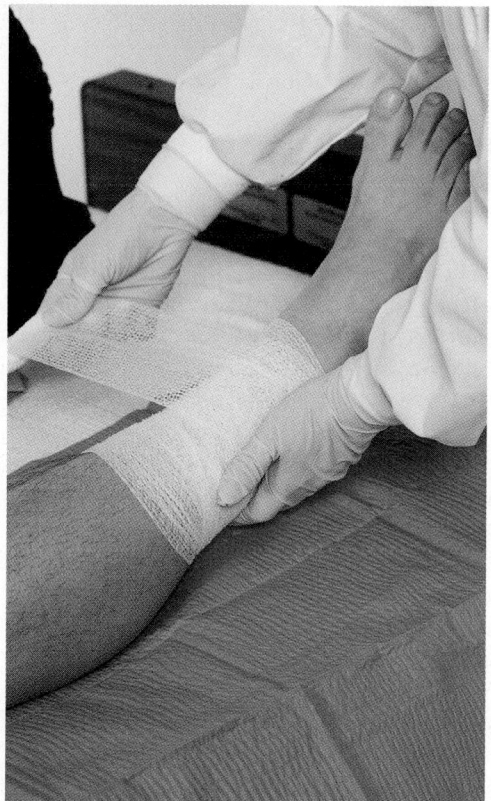

FIG 24-18 Roll bandage applied over a dressing.

to apply. Furthermore, it creates bandages that conform securely and comfortably to these body parts.

Creams, Ointments, and Solutions

In some cases, the physician may instruct the medical assistant to clean or treat a wound with a specific type of cream, ointment, or solution. By far the most popular choice of solution for cleaning the inside of a wound is sterile saline. It is safe, gentle on tissues, and hypoallergenic. Another common solution used is povidone-iodine (Betadine). This comes in the form of an antiseptic solution, a surgical soap, a topical solution (skin preparation or paint), and even an ointment. However, because some patients are allergic to iodine, the medical assistant should only use povidone-iodine and other solutions containing iodine when instructed to do so by the physician and after asking the patient about allergies. An alternative to povidone-iodine is chlorhexidine gluconate (commonly known by its brand name, Hibiclens), which does not stain and contains no iodine. Other antiseptic solutions include isopropyl alcohol and hydrogen peroxide. These solutions are generally reserved for external use (not inside the wound) because alcohol has limited effectiveness as an antiseptic and is painful to wounds. Hydrogen peroxide has a harsh, abrasive action on tissues. In some cases, the physician

will use hydrogen peroxide mixed with equal parts of sterile saline solution. (See Figure 24-19.)

The physician may occasionally order the use of antibacterial creams or ointments. Creams are easier to remove than ointments if the wound is to be cleaned between dressing changes. Silvadene®, an antibacterial cream available by prescription, is often used for burns. It must be applied with a sterile tongue depressor so that the cream in the jar (or tube) maintains its sterility.

Anesthetics

The term *anesthesia* means "absence of sensation." Prior to cleaning or suturing a wound, an anesthetic may be applied to numb the area and reduce patient discomfort. Anesthetics most commonly used in ambulatory care come in topical and injectable forms. Topical anesthetics such as ethyl chloride may be sprayed on or applied with a sponge, cotton ball, or cotton-tipped swab as with EMLA cream. Injectable anesthetics, such as lidocaine (Xylocaine) and procaine (Novocain), are useful for numbing an area before making an incision or suturing. Some products are available with epinephrine, which causes vasoconstriction and is used to reduce bleeding. However, products containing epinephrine should not be used on such body parts as the fingers, toes, nose, earlobes, and other areas with limited circulation. (See Figure 24-20.)

Depending on the procedure and the physician's preference, the medical assistant may be asked to draw up the anesthetic and place it near, but not on, the sterile field. The physician will then administer it before applying sterile gloves. In other cases, the medical assistant may need to place the syringe onto the sterile field using sterile technique and then hold the anesthetic vial for the sterile gloved physician as he draws anesthetic from it. In either case, the vial must be kept on hand so the physician can verify that the correct type of anesthetic is being used.

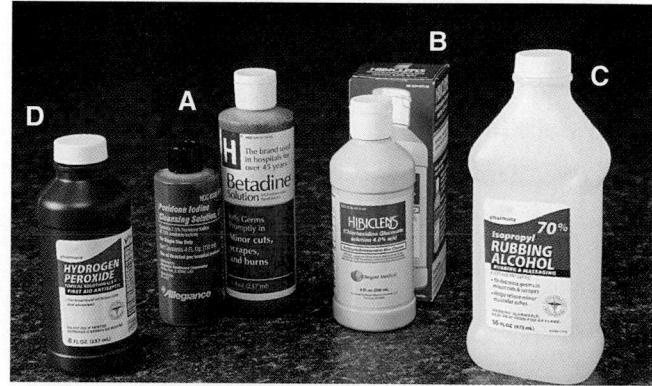

FIG 24-19 Antiseptic solutions. (A) Povidone-iodine. (B) Chlorhexidine gluconate (Hibiclens). (C) Isopropyl alcohol. (D) Hydrogen peroxide.

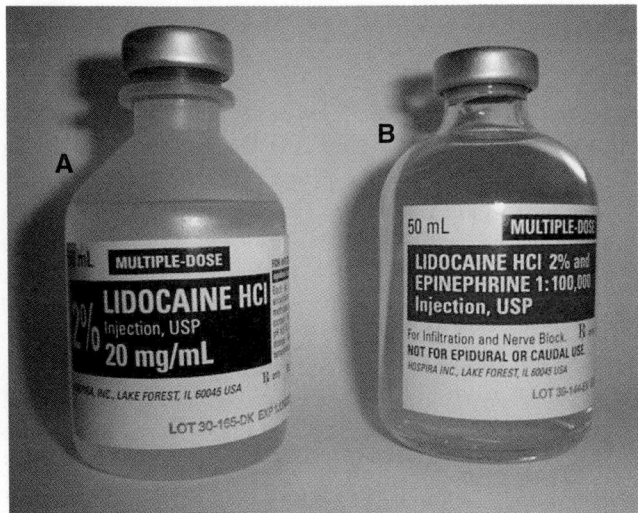

FIG 24-20 Anesthetics. (A) Lidocaine without epinephrine. (B) Lidocaine with epinephrine.

Chapter Summary

- Medical assistants commonly assist with minor surgical procedures. Their role involves preparing the room for procedures, assisting the physician during procedures, providing postprocedure care to patients, and tidying and sanitizing the room after procedures.
- Medical assistants should become familiar with the surgical instruments used in the offices in which they work. Most surgical instruments fall into one of four categories: cutting instruments, grasping-clamping instruments, probing and dilating instruments, or specialty instruments.
- Design features common to certain categories of instruments include finger ring handles or spring handles, box-lock hinges, closing mechanisms, jaws, serrations, ratchets, and teeth.
- Scissors are one of the most common cutting instruments and come in many sizes and shapes. Examples include surgical scissors, mayo dissecting scissors, bandage scissors, suture scissors, and iris scissors. Scalpels are also commonly used cutting instruments.
- The large category of grasping-clamping instruments includes forceps, hemostats, needle holders, and clamps.
- Probing and dilating instruments include specula, such as a vaginal or nasal speculum; scopes, such as an otoscope or anoscope; probes, such as a grooved director probe; retractors, such as a Volkmann retractor; and dilators, such as a uterine dilator.

- Examples of specialty instruments are obstetrical instruments like the vaginal speculum, Foerster sponge forceps, a curette, and a uterine tenaculum.
- To adhere to the principles of surgical asepsis, the health care team must understand and follow the sterile technique, which is a manner of performing specific tasks and procedures that protects patients from pathogenic organisms to the fullest extent possible.
- Surgical asepsis and the use of sterile technique are necessary when performing such invasive procedures as injections, urinary catheterization, and wound care and such surgical procedures as tissue biopsy or repair and suturing of lacerations.
- Prior to assisting with certain surgical procedures, medical assistants may be required to perform a surgical scrub, which is a type of hand washing that is much more thorough than regular hand washing.
- Medical assistants are commonly required to set up sterile fields for their use or for other health care providers. In doing so, they lay down a sterile barrier and then add all needed supplies to the field.
- Application of sterile gloves is one of the most common sterile procedures that medical assistants perform. Therefore, it is extremely important for the medical assistant to learn how to apply sterile gloves properly and maintain good technique.
- Many minor surgical procedures are done in the medical office. Common procedures include suturing, suture removal, incision and drainage (I&D) of infections, and removal of ingrown toenails or sebaceous cysts.
- There are some procedures the medical assistant may perform herself if the physician has given the order to do so, including suture or staple removal and application of dressings.
- There are many types of surgical procedures. Those that involve the use of extreme cold are sometimes called *cryosurgery*. Those performed with the use of specialized microscopes are called *microsurgery*. Those that involve cutting or destroying tissue by the application of electricity are called *electrosurgery*.
- The medical assistant performs many duties when assisting with minor surgery, including preparation of the examination the room, noting physician's preferences for room arrangement and supplies, setting up the sterile field for the physician, assisting the physician, and attending to the patient's needs.
- Prior to any surgical procedure, the medical assistant must make sure that the patient has been properly informed and prepared.
- After completion of the surgical procedure, the medical assistant should make sure the patient is positioned comfortably and safely while resting. To prevent injury, she should also ensure that there is a person with the patient

to supervise him carefully when he gets up, dresses, and travels home.

- When closing a wound, the physician's goals are to promote timely healing and reduce scar formation. These goals are accomplished through the use of sterile technique and careful approximation of the wound edges by suturing or stapling them.

- Suture needles may have the suture material swaged to them. Suture sizes range from the smallest gauge (6-0) to the largest gauge (4). Packages are labeled for easy identification.

- In recent years, staples have become a popular choice for wound closure because they are effective, safe, and enable quick, easy wound closure.

- Dressings are materials, such as gauze pads, that are placed in or on wounds. They are usually made of sterile gauze and are useful for protecting wounds and absorbing drainage.

- Bandages are nonsterile material applied over the top of dressings to secure them. They are commonly made of gauze in the form of rolls that can be wrapped around a dressing or elastic wrap.

- In some cases, the physician may instruct the medical assistant to clean or treat a wound with a specific type of cream, ointment, or solution. Some commonly used solutions are sterile saline, povidone-iodine, Hibiclens, isopropyl alcohol, and hydrogen peroxide.

- Before cleaning or suturing a wound, an anesthetic may be applied to numb the area and reduce discomfort. Anesthetics most commonly used in ambulatory care are topical forms, such as EMLA cream, and injectable anesthetics, such as lidocaine (Xylocaine) and procaine (Novocaine).

Team Work Exercises

1. Divide into small teams. Each team should select and complete a different assignment from this list:
   a. Collect examples of medical instruments that possess some or all of the following characteristics: ratchets, ring-handles, spring handle, box lock, jaws, serrations, and teeth. Create a poster to accompany these instruments that illustrates and defines each feature. Present your poster and example tools to the class and then place them on a table and invite the students to take a close look at each instrument.
   b. Collect examples of cutting instruments and create a poster to accompany these instruments that illustrates and names each of them. Present your poster and instruments to the class and then place them on a table and invite the students to take a close look at each instrument. (Take care to make sure that any sharp points or blades are covered so that no one is injured.)
   c. Collect examples of grasping-clamping instruments and create a poster to accompany these instruments

that illustrates and names each of them. Present your poster and instruments to the class and then place them on a table and invite the students to take a close look at each instrument. (Take care to make sure that any sharp points are covered so that no one is injured.)
   d. Collect examples of probing and dilating instruments and create a poster to accompany these instruments that illustrates and names each of them. Present your poster and instruments to the class and then place them on a table and invite the students to take a close look at each instrument.
   e. Collect examples of specialty instruments and create a poster to accompany these instruments that illustrates and names each of them. Present your poster and instruments to the class and then place them on a table and invite the students to take a close look at each instrument. (Take care to make sure that any sharp points or blades are covered so that no one is injured.)
   f. Collect examples of biopsy tools and create a poster to accompany these instruments that illustrates and names each of them. Present your poster and instruments to the class and then place them on a table and invite the students to take a close look at each instrument. (Take care to make sure that any sharp points or blades are covered so that no one is injured.)

2. Divide into teams to create presentations that illustrate and emphasize the general rules of sterile technique, listed in the table on page 389. Each team will choose a different type of presentation, including:
   a. A poster presentation. Be sure to use color, illustrations, or photos and other creative visuals to make it interesting.
   b. A fun role-playing scenario in which one or more of you create a "sterile" field. In the process, you will break as many of the rules of sterile technique as possible. The class will watch and identify as many things as possible that you did wrong.
   c. The proper way to set up a sterile field, open a sterile pack, add items to the sterile field, and pour a solution into a container on the sterile field.
   d. An audiovisual presentation, such as a slide presentation or video, that describes the guidelines listed in the table.

Case Studies

1. Anthony is a CMA in a family practice office. He has noticed that one of his coworkers, who is also a CMA, checks the physician's schedule for the day to identify any procedures that might be done. He then sets up the procedure trays and puts them in a row in the back room until they are needed. Anthony appreciates his coworker's efforts to get organized for the day but is not sure that preparing all procedure trays for the entire day in the morning is a good idea. List the pros and cons of such a

practice. Describe how this coworker's routine might be modified to make it better.

2. Ernesto is a patient who came to the urgent care center with a deep laceration on his thumb. He says that he accidentally cut himself with his hunting knife while sharpening it. What supplies and equipment will the medical assistant need to gather for this patient? List everything you can think of. Will the physician want to use lidocaine with or without epinephrine? Why? Betadine should be avoided for this patient if he has what allergy? After the physician has sutured Ernesto's laceration, he asks you to apply a dressing. What materials will you use and why? What instructions will you give to Ernesto before he leaves?

Resources

- Encyclopedia of Surgery: *www.surgeryencyclopedia.com/index.html*
- Free online course on infection prevention: *www.engenderhealth.org/IP/index.html*
- National Cancer Institute: *www.cancer.gov/cancertopics/factsheet/Therapy/cryosurgery*

Dermatology

Learning Objectives

Upon completion of this chapter, the student will be able to:

- define and spell terms related to dermatology
- identify key structures of the integumentary system
- discuss the roles of protection and temperature regulation played by the integumentary system
- describe the role of the medical assistant in the dermatology office
- identify common skin diseases and disorders
- differentiate skin lesions
- list commonly used word elements related to the integumentary system
- give at least 10 examples of how new dermatology-related terms may be created by combining prefixes, suffixes, and combining forms
- describe the medical assistant's role in assisting with a tissue biopsy
- list the seven warning signs of cancer
- identify the characteristics of malignant melanoma
- describe physical examination techniques used to evaluate the integumentary system
- list and describe four types of allergy testing
- discuss the purpose of culture and sensitivity testing in the treatment of infection
- describe five types of image enhancement procedures.

CAAHEP Competencies

Administrative Competencies
Process Insurance Claims
Perform diagnostic coding

Clinical Competencies
Diagnostic Testing
Perform immunology testing
Patient Care
Prepare patients for and assist with routine and specialty examination
Prepare patients for and assist with procedures, treatments, and minor office surgery
General Competencies
Patient Instruction
Instruct individuals according to their needs
Provide instruction for health maintenance and disease prevention

ABHES Competencies

Administrative Duties
Perform diagnostic coding
Communication
Use appropriate medical terminology
Clinical Duties
Prepare patients for procedures
Prepare patient for and assist physician with routine and specialty examinations and treatments and minor office surgeries
Collect and process specimens
Perform immunology testing
Instruction
Teach patients methods of health promotion and disease prevention

Procedures
Performing allergy skin testing

Chapter Outline

Structures and Functions of the Integumentary System
Structures of the Skin
Functions of the Skin
Protection
Temperature regulation
Medical Terminology Related to the Integumentary System

Common Integumentary System Diseases and Disorders
Bacterial Skin Infections
Impetigo
Acne
Cellulitis
Folliculitis
Viral Skin Infections
Warts
Herpes viruses
Herpes zoster
Fungal Skin Disorders
Tinea
Candidiasis
Parasitic Infestations
Pediculosis
Scabies
Hypersensitivity and Inflammatory Reactions
Eczema
Psoriasis
Systemic lupus erythematosus
Neoplasms
Basal cell carcinoma
Squamous cell carcinoma
Malignant melanoma
Dermatology Procedures
Assisting with Examination
Allergy Skin Testing
Scratch test
Intradermal test
Patch test
Radioallergosorbent test
Culture and Sensitivity Testing
Image Enhancement Procedures
Dermabrasion and dermaplaning
Microdermabrasion
Chemical peel
Laser resurfacing
Botox™
Chapter Summary
Team Work Exercises
Case Studies
Resources

Key Terms

allergen
Substance that produces a hypersensitivity reaction

atopic
Type of allergic reaction for which there is a genetic predisposition

biopsy
Procedure in which a representative sample of tissue is obtained for microscopic examination

chemical peel
Destruction of superficial layers of the skin using a chemical application in order to remove scars, tattoos, or abnormal pigmentation

cryosurgery
Surgery with cold probes to destroy cancerous tissue

dermabrasion
Procedure in which outer layers of the skin are removed by abrasion with a wire brush or other device

dermaplaning
Procedure in which a dermatome is used to skim off surface layers of the skin to remove scars, tattoos, and fine wrinkles

dermatome
Band or region of skin supplied by a single sensory nerve

diascopy
Procedure in which a glass plate is held against the skin to observe changes related to pressure application

electrodesiccation
Destructive drying of cells by applying electrical energy

erythema
Redness of the skin

laser resurfacing
Use of short pulses of light to treat some skin conditions

melanocyte
Melanin-forming skin cell

microdermabrasion
Gentle abrasion of the skin to reduce fine lines, age spots, and acne scars and stimulate growth of new skin cells and collagen

patch test
Skin test in which a low concentration of a presumed allergen is applied to the skin beneath an occlusive dressing to see if a reaction occurs

pruritus
Feeling of itchiness

radioallergosorbent test
Blood test for allergy that measures small quantities of immunoglobulin E in blood

scratch test
Test in which a dilution of a potential allergen is placed in a lightly scratched area of the skin

Structures and Functions of the Integumentary System

The integumentary system is made up of the skin and related structures, such as hair follicles, tiny blood vessels, fatty tissue, and specialized nerves for detecting heat, cold, pain, and pressure. The integumentary system protects vital organs and helps carry out many essential body functions.

Structures of the Skin

The skin is made up of three layers: the epidermis, the dermis, and the subcutaneous layer. (See Figure 25-1.) The top layer is the epidermis, which is a thin outer layer mostly constructed of nonliving keratinized cells. It is waterproof and provides protection for the deeper layers. The epidermis is thickest on the soles of the hands and feet. The base of this layer, aptly named the *basement membrane,* is where new skin cells are produced. These cells are pushed upward as even newer cells form beneath them. Eventually, they rise near enough to the top that they die, leaving dry, keratinized (hardened) tissue that becomes a part of the epidermal layer.

The dermis lies just beneath the epidermis and is much thicker. It contains a number of structures, including hair follicles, nerves, blood vessels, and some glands. Beneath the dermis is the subcutaneous layer. This layer contains fat tissue as well as the deeper blood vessels, nerves, and hair follicles. It also contains elastin, which provides elasticity, and collagen, which provides strength. The subcutaneous layer provides insulation for deeper structures.

Accessory structures of the skin include the sudoriferous (sweat) glands, sebaceous (oil) glands, hair, and nails. Sebaceous glands are found at the base of hair follicles all over the body and secrete an oily substance called *sebum.* Sudoriferous glands are located throughout the body but are more concentrated in some areas, such as the soles of the feet and palms of the hands.

Functions of the Skin

The skin and accessory structures serve several important functions in the body. Its major functions are protection and temperature regulation.

Protection

The skin protects the body from bacteria and other microorganisms, damaging light from the ultraviolet rays of the sun, and extreme temperatures. Because the outer layer of the skin is waterproof, it prevents organisms from entering even when it gets wet, unless there is a break in the skin. Sebaceous glands secrete an oily substance that inhibits bacterial growth and lubricates the skin to keep it soft and supple. If microorganisms gain entry through breaks in the skin, such

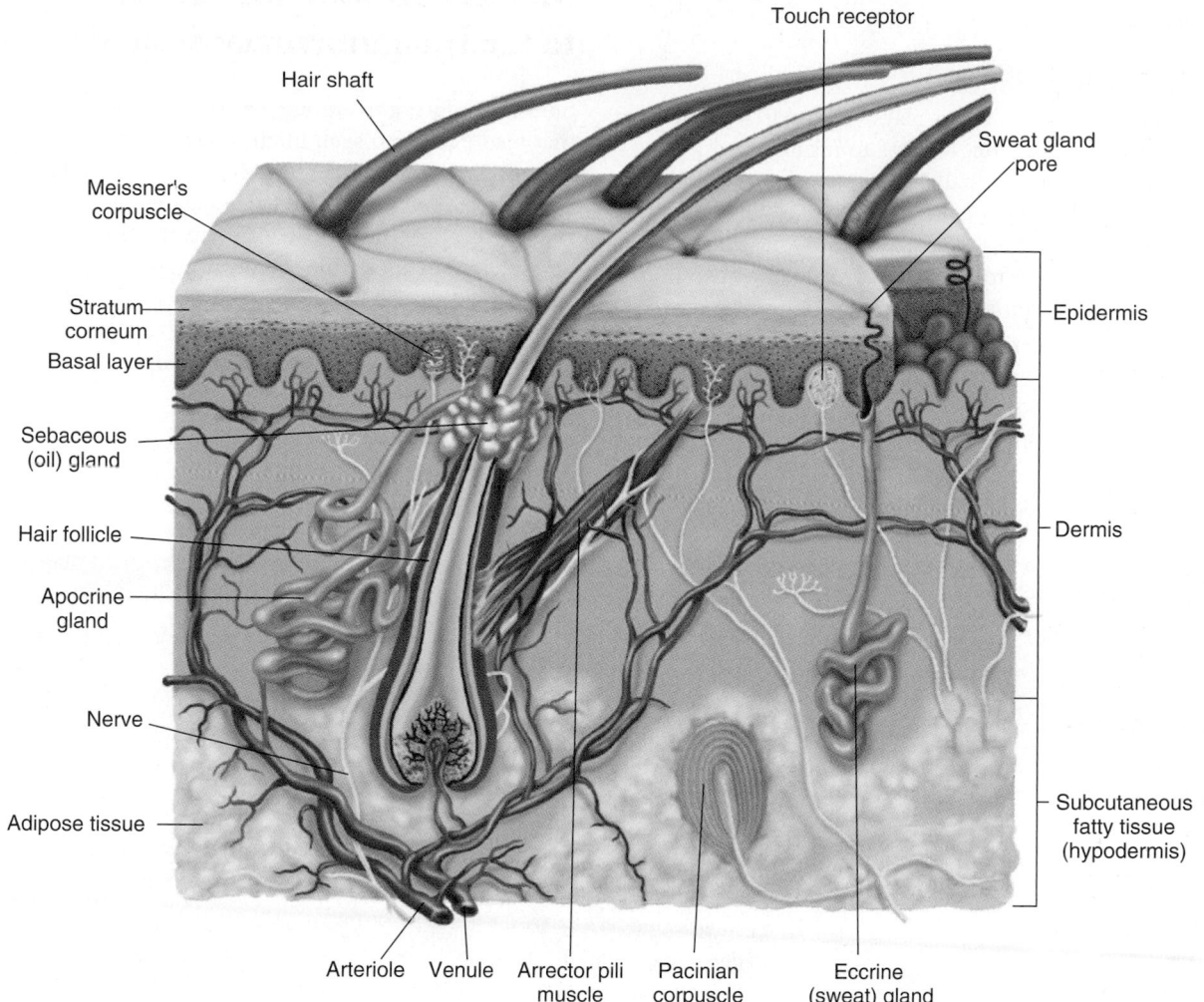

FIG 25-1 Layers and structures of the skin.

as a laceration (a cut or tear in the flesh) or an abrasion (an area where skin or mucous membranes are scraped away), an infection may occur. However as the tissue becomes irritated, a natural inflammatory response occurs. This response triggers increased circulation in the injured area, which is responsible for the appearance of such signs as edema, or swelling, and **erythema,** which is redness that may indicate inflammation or injury. Increased numbers of leukocytes (white blood cells) arrive to fight off the invaders and act to engulf the bacteria. The increased circulation also helps speed the process of healing as debris is cleared away and healthy new cells along with scar tissue fill in the injured area.

The skin also contains **melanocytes,** which are melanin-forming skin cells. In response to ultraviolet light from the sun, melanocytes secrete melanin, a brown pigment that helps filter ultraviolet light and protect the skin from further damage. These cells are responsible for the browning of the

skin known as a *suntan.* The amount of melanin in the skin varies depending on the individual's heredity and ethnicity.

Because the skin contains a number of different specialized nerves and sensory receptors, it plays a vital role in the ability to perceive cold and heat as well as pressure and pain. These messages signal the individual to take measures to increase physical comfort, such as putting on a coat for warmth. In addition, they also provide an important protective function. If the person accidentally touches a hot surface, the heat and pain receptors immediately send a message to the central nervous system (CNS) and the person responds by pulling her hand away. Such a response is a protective reflex, which happens quickly and without conscious thought.

Two accessory structures of the integumentary system play a role in protecting the body. The hair of the head, eyebrows, eyelashes, nose, and ears protects the body by filtering out dust and debris from the air. Nails help protect the ends of the fingers and toes.

Temperature Regulation

The integumentary system also plays an important role in body temperature regulation. It helps to insulate and maintain warmth when the external environment is too cold. As the environment becomes colder, the hands and fingers become pale in color because the blood vessels near the skin's surface constrict in order to give off less heat and conserve it for deeper organs. When the environment is too hot, these same blood vessels dilate (expand) in order to give off more heat. This response causes a flushed appearance. In addition, the sweat glands secrete sweat, which evaporates on the skin's surface and provides even more cooling.

Medical Terminology Related to the Integumentary System

Skin disorders are among the most common problems that lead people to seek medical care. Whether they work in family practice offices, urgent care centers, dermatology clinics, or other areas, medical assistants play an important role in the provision of health care to these patients. To be effective in their role, medical assistants must become well versed in the language and vocabulary that pertain to the integumentary system. The following tables list common medical terminology related to the integumentary system.

Table 25.1 | Word elements

This table contains combining forms, prefixes, and suffixes related to the integumentary system, along with examples of terms that use the word element, a pronunciation guide, and a definition for each.

Combining Form	Meaning	Example	Meaning
adip/o	fat	adipoid (ĂD-ĭ-poyd)	resembling fat
lip/o		lipoma (lĭ-PŌ-mă)	tumor of fat
albin/o	white	albinism (ĂL-bĭn-ĭzm)	condition of (being) white
leuk/o		leukorrhea (loo-kō-RĒ-ă)	white flow or discharge
cutane/o	skin	cutaneous (kū-TĀ-nē-ŭs)	pertaining to the skin
dermat/o		dermatologist (dĕr-mă-TŎL-ō-jĭst)	specialist in the study of skin
derm/o		dermoplasty (dĕr-mō-plăs-tē)	surgical repair of the skin
cyan/o	blue	cyanosis (sī-ă-NŌ-sĭs)	abnormal condition of blue (color)
cyt/o	cell	cytology (sī-TŎL-ō-jē)	study of cells
erythem/o	red	erythematous (ĕr-ĭ-THĒ-mă-tĭs)	pertaining to red
erythr/o		erythrocyte (ĕ-RĬTH-rō-sīt)	red (blood) cell
melan/o	black	melanoma (mĕl-ă-NŌ-mă)	tumor that is black in appearance
myc/o	fungus	mycosis (mī-KŌ-sĭs)	abnormal condition of fungus
necr/o	dead	necrosis (nĕ-KRŌ-sĭs)	abnormal condition of dead (tissue)
onych/o	nail	onychomalacia (ŏn-ĭ-kō-mă-LĀ-sē-ă)	softening of the nail
pil/o	hair	pilophobia (pī-lō-FŌ-bē-ă)	fear of hair
trich/o		trichopathy (trĭk-ŎP-ă-thē)	disease of the hair
scler/o	hardening; sclera	sclerosis (sklĕ-RŌ-sĭs)	abnormal condition of hardening
xer/o	dry	xeroderma (zē-rō-DĔR-mă)	dry skin
xanth/o	yellow	xanthoderma (zăn-thō-DĔR-mă)	yellow skin

Table 25.1 | Word elements—cont'd

Combining Form	Meaning	Example	Meaning
Prefixes			
epi-	above, upon	**epidermis** (ĕp-ĭ-DĚR-mĭs)	above the dermis
sub-	below, beneath	**subcutaneous** (sŭb-kū-TĂ-nē-ŭs)	pertaining to beneath the skin
neo-	new	**neoplasm** (NĔ-ō-plăzm)	new growth
Suffixes			
-cyte	cell	**adipocyte** (ĂD-ĭ-pō-sīt)	fat cell
-derma	skin	**cyanoderma** (sī-ă-nō-DĚR-mă)	blue skin
-oma	tumor	**lipoma** (ăd-ĭ-PŌ-mă)	fatty tumor
-plasia	formation; growth	**dysplasia** (dĭs-PLĂ-zē-ă)	bad (abnormal) growth
-plasty	surgical repair	**dermoplasty** (DĚR-mō-plăs-tē)	surgical repair of the skin
-ist	specialist	**dermatologist** (dĕr-mă-TŎL-ō-jĭst)	specialist in the diagnosis and treatment of skin disorders

Table 25.2 | Pathologic Terms

This table lists some of the most common pathologic terms related to the integumentary system, along with a pronunciation guide and a brief definition for each.

Term	Definition
abrasion ă-BRĂ-zhŭn	Scraping away of skin or mucus membranes
acne ĂK-nē	Inflammatory skin disease of sebaceous follicles common in adolescence that is marked by comedones, papules, and pustules
actinic keratosis ăk-TĬN-ĭk kĕr-ă-TŌ-sĭs	Rough, precancerous macule or papule caused by excessive exposure to ultraviolet light
albinism ĂL-bĭn-ĭzm	Genetic partial or total absence of pigment in the skin, hair, and eyes
alopecia ăl-ō-PĒ-shē-ă	Absence or loss of hair, particularly on the head
basal cell carcinoma BĂ-săl SĔL kăr-sĭ-NŌ-mă	Most common type of skin cancer, which usually begins as a small, shiny papule and eventually enlarges to form a whitish border around a central depression or ulcer that may bleed
carbuncle KĂR-bŭng-k'l	Skin abscess created by the merger of two or more furuncles (boils)
cellulitis sĕl-ū-LĬ-tĭs	Spreading bacterial infection of the skin and subcutaneous tissue
comedo KŎM-ē-dō	Small skin lesions of acne vulgaris, commonly called blackhead or whitehead, depending on the color
corn KORN	Thickening of keratinized skin caused by pressure or friction

Continued

Table 25.2 | Pathologic Terms—cont'd

Term	Definition
cyst SĬST	Closed sack or pouch on or under the skin that contains fluid, solid, or semisolid material
dysplasia dĭs-PLĀ-zē-ă	Area of abnormal tissue growth
ecchymosis ĕk-ĭ-MŌ-sĭs	Discoloration of the skin; also called bruise or contusion
eczema ĔK-zĕ-mă	General term for pruritic, red rash that that weeps and may become crusted, thickened, or scaly; also called dermatitis
edema ĕ-DĒ-mă	When localized or generalized tissue contains excessive fluid
folliculitis fō-lĭk-ū-LĬ-tĭs	Inflammation (and sometimes infection) of hair follicles
furuncle FŪ-rŭng-k'l	Skin abscess; also called boil
hemangioma hē-măn-jē-Ō-mă	A dull red, benign lesion present from birth or appearing within 2 or 3 months; sometimes called a *strawberry nevus*
herpes simplex virus type 1 HĔR-pēz SĬM-plĕx VĪ-rŭs	Virus that causes a lesion on the lips
herpes simplex virus type 2 HĔR-pēz SĬM-plĕx VĪ-rŭs	Virus that commonly causes lesions on the genitals
herpes zoster HĔR-pēz ZŌS-tĕr	Reactivation of the varicella virus, years after an initial infection with chickenpox, that is marked by a painful, vesicular rash along the associated dermatome; also called shingles
impetigo ĭm-pē-TĪ-gō	Contagious bacterial infection of the skin caused by streptococci or staphylococci that is marked by yellow to red weeping lesions that are crusted or pustular
laceration lăs-ĕ-RĀ-shŭn	Cut or tear in the flesh
lentigo lĕn-TĪ-gō	Flat brown spot on the skin related to sun exposure, more common in elderly individuals; commonly called *liver spots* although they are not caused by liver disease
malignant melanoma mă-LĬG-nănt mĕl-ă-NŌ-mă	Cancerous tumor of darkly pigmented skin cells that spreads aggressively and has a high mortality rate
neoplasm NĒ-ō-plăzm	New, abnormal formation of tissue, such as a tumor
nevus NĒ-vŭs	Hyperpigmented area of the skin, such as a mole or birthmark
pediculosis pē-dĭk-ū-LŌ-sĭs	Infestation with lice
petechia pē-TĒ-kē-ă	Tiny red or purple hemorrhagic spot on the skin
postherpetic neuralgia pōst-hĕr-PĔT-ĭk nū-RĂL-jē-ă	Persistent nerve pain from herpes infection that lasts for months after lesions disappear

Table 25.2 | Pathologic Terms—cont'd

Term	Definition
psoriasis sō-RĬ-ă-sĭs	Noncontagious chronic skin disorder in which red scaly plaques with sharply defined borders appear on the body's surface
scabies SKĀ-bēz	Contagious infestation of the skin with the itch mite
seborrheic keratosis sĕb-ō-RĒ-ĭk kĕr-ă-TŌ-sĭs	Benign, scaly skin growth that is yellow, gray, or brown and common in older adults
squamous cell carcinoma SKWĀ-mŭs SĔL kăr-sĭ-NŌ-mă	Form of skin cancer that develops in squamous tissue and grows more rapidly and spreads more easily than basal cell carcinoma
tinea TĬN-ē-ă	Fungal skin infection
verruca plantaris vĕr-ROO-kă plăn-TĂR-ĭs	Wart that grows on the soles of the feet
verruca vulgaris vĕr-ROO-kă vŭl-GĀ-rĭs	Common wart
vitiligo vĭt-ĭl-Ī-gō	Disorder that causes a patchy loss of skin pigmentation

Common Integumentary System Diseases and Disorders

There are innumerable diseases and disorders of the integumentary system. Some of the most common include bacterial infections, viral infections, fungal diseases, parasitic infestations, hypersensitivity and inflammatory reactions, and neoplasms. Many disorders are identified by the type of lesion they produce on the skin. (See *Common skin lesions*, page 418.)

Bacterial Skin Infections

Some of the most common bacterial infections of the skin include impetigo, acne, cellulitis, and folliculitis. Here is a summary of each, along with its corresponding ICD-9-CM code.

Impetigo
ICD-9-CM code: 684

Impetigo is a highly contagious bacterial infection caused by group A *Streptococcus* or *Staphylococcus aureus*. It is most common in young children and accounts for 10% of all cases of children with skin problems who are brought to medical clinics. Areas of the skin that are scraped or scratched are most vulnerable to infection. Lesions may appear anywhere on the body but are most common on the face and extremities. Impetigo appears as tiny vesicles (blisters), which

Table 25.3 | Abbreviations

In dermatology, as with other areas of health care, abbreviations are commonly used. Abbreviations such as the ones listed here save time and effort in documentation and written communications.

Abbreviation	Term
Bx	biopsy
HSV-1	herpes simplex virus type 1
HSV-2	herpes simplex virus type 2
ID	intradermal (injection)
I&D	incision & drainage
RAST	radioallergosorbent test
SLE	systemic lupus erythematosus
SubQ, subcu, or subq	subcutaneous
T	temperature
ung	ointment

Common skin lesions

This table lists some of the most common types of skin lesions, along with a pronunciation guide, a definition, and an illustration for each.

Lesion	Definition	Example
macule MĂK-ūl	Flat, discolored spot on the skin (such as a freckle)	
papule PĂP-ūl	Small, raised spot or bump on the skin (such as a mole)	
nodule NŌD-ūl	Small node	
bulla BŬL-lă	Large blister or skin vesicle filled with fluid	

Common skin lesions—cont'd

Lesion	Definition	Example
vesicle VĔS-ĭ-kl	Clear, fluid-filled blister	
scales Skālz	Areas of skin that are excessively dry and flaky	
fissure FĬSH-ūr	Small, crack-like break in the skin	
ulcer ŬL-sĕr	Lesion of the skin or mucus membranes marked by inflammation, necrosis, and sloughing of damaged tissues	

Continued

Common skin lesions—cont'd

Lesion	Definition	Example
wheal HWĒL	Rounded, temporary elevation in the skin that is white in the center with a red-pink periphery and accompanied by itching	
pustule PŬS-tūl	Small, pus-filled blister	

develop into weeping, **pruritic** (itching, tingling, or faint burning sensation) sores with honey-colored, crusty edges. (See Figure 25-2.) Diagnosis is usually based on medical history and physical examination findings. Occasionally, culture (propagation of microorganisms in a special growth media) and sensitivity (determining susceptibility of bacteria to antibiotics) testing and a Gram stain may be done.

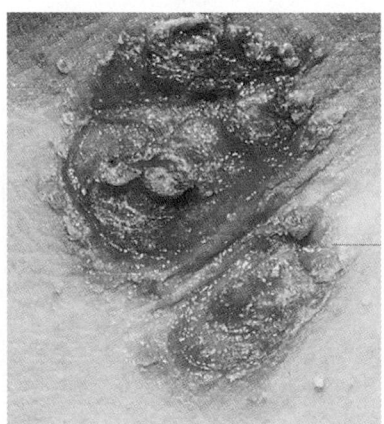

FIG 25-2 Impetigo.

Treatment includes topical antibiotic ointment for small areas and systemic antibiotics for widespread infection. The lesions should be gently scrubbed daily with an antiseptic soap and covered lightly with a dressing. To help prevent the spread of impetigo, the patient's fingernails should be short and clean. Patient education includes discussion of hygiene and avoiding the sharing of linens and towels. In addition, the patient should call the physician if lesions do not begin to heal within 3 days; the skin around the lesions becomes red, warm, and tender; or fever develops. (See *Patient with an unidentified rash*.)

Acne

ICD-9-CM code: 706.1

Acne is the term used to describe a skin disease of the pilosebaceous units (PSUs) in the skin. PSUs include sebaceous (oil) glands and hair follicles. The exact cause of acne is unclear; however, the PSUs apparently become plugged and develop into comedones, which are small skin lesions of acne that include whiteheads and blackheads. Contributing factors include hormonal influences, genetics, and use of some medications or oily cosmetics. Exacerbations may be related to hormonal factors, exposure to oily environments, pollution,

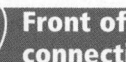

Front office–Back office connection

Patient with an Unidentified Rash

When a patient enters the medical office with a rash of unknown cause, the administrative medical assistant must consider the cause to be potentially contagious. This rule is especially true if the patient is febrile, the rash is weepy, or the rash was potentially caused by a parasitic infestation. The medical assistant should take measures to keep the patient separate from other patients. Doing so can be especially challenging when the patient is a child. If necessary, the administrative and clinical medical assistants should consult with one another about placing the patient directly into an examination room. Isolating potentially infectious patients helps minimize exposure to other patients and health care staff.

humidity, and stress. As infection sets in, the comedones become pustules that can further develop into nodules and cysts. (See Figure 25-3.) Acne is most common among teenagers of all races and ethnicities but may affect adults as well. Acne occurs most commonly where large numbers of sebaceous glands are located, such as on the face, back, and chest. Over 40% of acne sufferers develop skin problems severe enough to seek medical care. In severe cases, it can be disfiguring and cause permanent scarring.

Diagnosis is based on clinical presentation and symptoms. Over-the-counter (OTC) topical preparations such as benzoyl peroxide provide effective treatment in most cases. However, prescription medication may be needed for more severe cases. Such medications include antibiotics and vitamin A derivatives. Some medications such as isotretinoin (Accutane) are known teratogens (substances known to cause abnormal fetal development), so pregnant women should avoid their use. Oral contraceptives or low-dose corticosteroids may be effective for women whose acne is caused by excess androgen (male) hormones. Patients must be encouraged to have realistic expectations of treatment, as people respond differently and it commonly takes 6 to 8 weeks for a full response. Acne

scars may be removed or minimized by **dermabrasion,** which is a process in which a plastic surgeon or dermatologist scrapes away the outermost layer of skin using a wire brush or burr impregnated with diamond particles.

Cellulitis
ICD-9-CM code: 682.9

Cellulitis is a bacterial infection of the dermis and subcutaneous tissues. It is usually caused when group A streptococci and *Staphylococcus aureus* organisms invade the skin through local injury, such as a scrape or cut. It is a common type of skin infection occurring among all races. Facial cellulitis is more common among adults over age 50 and children ages 6 months to 3 years. Perianal cellulitis is more common among children. People at increased risk include those with a weakened immune system, diabetes or other systemic illness, or impaired peripheral circulation and those using corticosteroid medication. Symptoms of cellulitis include localized pain, erythema, edema, warmth, and fever. (See Figure 25-4.) Red streaks may indicate spreading infection.

Diagnosis is usually based on physical examination findings. In more complex cases, laboratory tests may include a complete blood count and blood cultures. In addition, wound secretions may be collected for Gram stain and culture. In severe cases, radiographic studies may reveal gas in the tissues that indicates fasciitis or gangrene, which are surgical emergencies. Treatment includes the administration of antibiotics and, for severe cases, surgical resection. Complications may include loss of localized tissue and septicemia. However, with early diagnosis and appropriate treatment, most people recover fully.

Folliculitis
ICD-9-CM code: 704.8

Folliculitis is the inflammation of hair follicles. It is very common and occurs anywhere on the skin, especially on the face and scalp. Folliculitis develops secondary to irritation caused by the friction of clothing rubbing on the skin or shaving as well as from the blockage of follicles. Infection with *Staphylococcus aureus* may follow. Symptoms include a rash with comedones, pustules, and itching.

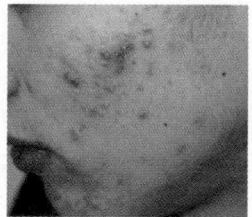

FIG 25-3 Acne. (From Barankin, Freiman, *Derm Notes*. FA Davis, Philadelphia, 2006, p. 53, with permission.)

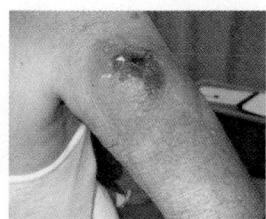

FIG 25-4 Cellulitis. (From Barankin, Freiman, *Derm Notes*. FA Davis, Philadelphia, 2006, p. 74, with permission.)

Diagnosis is based on physical examination findings and symptoms. Occasionally, a culture may be done to identify the infecting organism. Folliculitis can be prevented or minimized by reducing friction from clothing, avoiding shaving if possible, and keeping the skin clean and dry. Treatment includes application of warm, moist compresses; topical or oral antibiotics; or antifungal medications. Folliculitis generally responds well to treatment but has a tendency to recur. A potential complication is the spread of infection.

Viral Skin Infections

Some of the most common viral skin infections include warts, herpes virus, and herpes zoster. Here is a summary of each, along with its corresponding ICD-9-CM code.

Warts

ICD-9-CM code: 078.10 (general code for common warts), 078.11 (genital)

Warts are small, benign skin tumors that are caused by the human papilloma virus (HPV). They are contagious and spread via direct contact. There are many variations of warts, including verruca vulgaris (common warts), commonly found on the hands; venereal (genital) warts, which are sexually transmitted; and verruca plantaris (plantar warts), which grow on the soles of the feet. (See Figure 25-5.) Children and young adults are the populations that commonly get warts. Especially vulnerable are those with weakened immune systems, such as people with acquired immune deficiency syndrome (AIDS) and cancer or those taking chemotherapy or other immunosuppressive medications. Experts estimate that genital HPV infection is the most common type of sexually transmitted disease, with 5.5 million new cases reported yearly and at least 20 million people already infected.

Physical appearance of warts varies depending on the specific type of virus (there are over 100 different types) and the location involved. Warts may be tiny to medium-sized bumps or may have a cauliflower-type appearance. Genital warts, which develop on the genitalia, may be obvious and extensive or subtle and only perceptible using a Papanicolaou (Pap) test, also called a *Pap smear.*

Diagnosis is based on physical examination findings. Treatment options include over-the-counter (OTC) topical medications such as salicylic acid and numerous others. If home treatment does not produce satisfactory results, patients may seek treatment from their health care provider. A common treatment choice is **cryotherapy,** which involves the application of liquid nitrogen to freeze the wart and kill it. Repeated treatments may be needed. Other forms of treatment include application of lactic acid or trichloroacetic acid (TCA). Warts usually disappear without treatment; however, it may take weeks, months, or even years for them to do so. Genital warts in women may cause tissue changes that result in the development of cervical cancer. This development most likely accounts for the growing incidence of cervical cancer among young women. Therefore, the medical assistant should caution patients to use condoms to prevent transmission. Furthermore, women who are sexually active should have regular examinations and Pap tests.

Herpes Viruses

ICD-9-CM code: 054.10 (genital herpes simplex), 054.9 (oral herpes simplex)

There are many variations of the herpes virus. Herpes simplex virus type 1 (HSV-1), also known as *herpes labialis,* most commonly causes lesions on the lips, usually referred to as *cold sores* or *fever blisters.* Herpes simplex virus type 2 (HSV-2) most commonly causes lesions on the genitals. (See Figure 25-6.) In either case, the virus causes repeated eruptions of acutely painful vesicles and then spreads along nerve pathways where it lays dormant between outbreaks. Other variations of herpetic outbreaks include herpes corneae (affecting the cornea), herpes facialis (affecting the face), and herpes menstrualis (appearing during menses). HSV-2 is considered a sexually transmitted disease, with an estimated 90 million people infected worldwide. All forms of herpes are contagious and spread via direct contact with secretions. Triggers that may precipitate repeated outbreaks include stress, illness, immunosuppressive medications, and sun or wind (oral herpes).

Symptoms commonly include sensations of pain, itching, tingling, and burning prior to an outbreak of vesicles. When the rash appears, it includes a red base with small clusters of painful vesicles and pustules that also itch and burn. Systemic symptoms may include fever and malaise, which is a feeling of discomfort, weakness, fatigue, or feeling generally unwell. Diagnosis is based on medical history, including sexual activity and physical examination findings. Treatment usually includes antiviral medications, such as acyclovir or penciclovir, which reduce viral shedding and shorten outbreaks. Analgesics may help reduce pain and tenderness

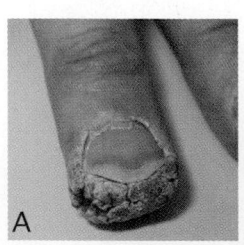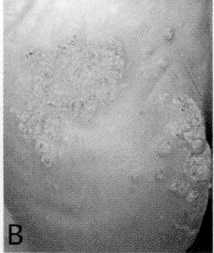

FIG 25-5 Common warts. (A) Plantar warts. (B) (From Barankin, Freiman, *Derm Notes.* FA Davis, Philadelphia, 2006, p. 171, with permission.)

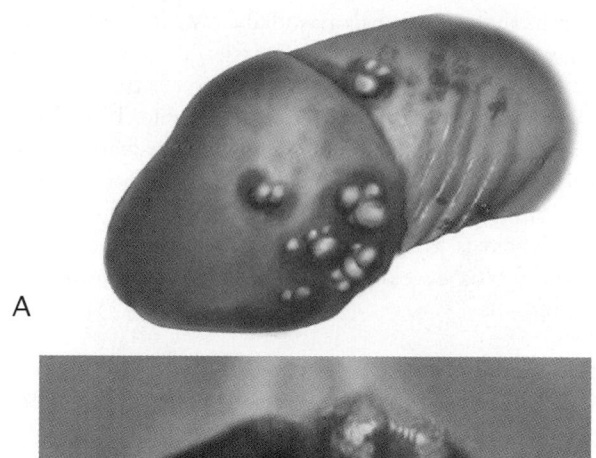

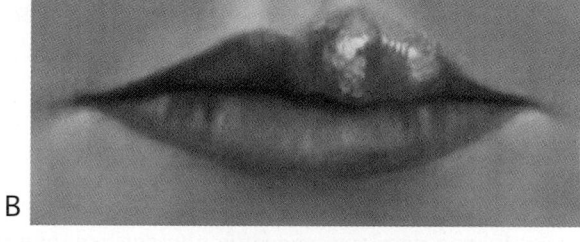

FIG 25-6 Herpes virus. (A) HSV 2— Genital herpes. (From Barankin, Freiman, *Derm Notes*. FA Davis, Philadelphia, 2006, p. 98, with permission.) (B) HSV 1— Herpes labialis.

caused by the lesions. The medical assistant should counsel patients with genital herpes regarding safe sexual practices to reduce the risk of transmission.

There is no cure for herpes and, once acquired, the virus lies dormant in the body until something triggers another outbreak. Individuals should learn to identify their most common triggers and avoid them if possible. They should also take precautions to avoid transmission of the virus to others. Women who are pregnant or are considering becoming pregnant should inform their health care provider if they have genital herpes because transmission during childbirth can result in serious complications for the newborn. (See *Patient with a herpetic rash.*)

Front office–Back office connection

Patient with a Herpetic Rash

There are many types of lesions caused by different herpes viruses. However, the general public associates the term *herpes* with genital herpes. Such misinformation can cause confusion and great embarrassment to the patient. Therefore, administrative and clinical medical assistants must be especially careful when checking in and caring for a patient with a herpetic rash. In addition, such sensitivity is one more important reason to keep communications confidential, especially at the reception desk, where others might overhear what is said.

Herpes Zoster
ICD-9-M code: 053.9

Outbreaks of herpes zoster, also called *shingles*, are caused by a reactivation of the varicella virus. After an initial outbreak of varicella (chickenpox), the varicella zoster virus incorporates itself into nerve cells and lies dormant after patients recover from the initial infection until it is reactivated years later. Between 600,000 and 1 million people develop shingles each year. About 50% of people who live to age 80 will have an outbreak at some time in their life. Persons at increased risk are those taking immunosuppressive medications and those with weakened immune systems, including elderly patients and those with AIDS, Hodgkin disease, or diabetes.

Symptoms of herpes zoster include unilateral distribution of herpetic vesicles along the affected **dermatome** (nerve pathway) of a few segments of spinal or cranial peripheral nerves. (See Figure 25-7.) These vesicles usually develop on the trunk or, sometimes, the face or head. Lesions are described as acutely painful and may burn or itch as well. Other symptoms may include fever, chills, headache, and malaise, depending on the dermatomes involved.

Diagnosis is based on characteristic appearance. Diagnosis may be confirmed by a culture of secretions or, more rarely, by the presence of antibodies in the blood.

Treatment for herpes zoster includes antiviral drugs, such as acyclovir, which reduce viral shedding and the severity and duration of the outbreak if administered within 3 days of onset. Other medications may include corticosteroids, analgesics, and antipruritics.

The duration of outbreaks may last from 10 days to 5 weeks. A potential complication of herpes zoster is postherpetic neuralgia, which is persistent nerve pain that lasts for months after lesions disappear. Fortunately, repeated outbreaks of shingles are uncommon.

Fungal Skin Disorders
Fungal skin disorders are a common complaint. Two of the most common types include the family of tinea infections, which are named for the various parts of the body affected, and candidiasis.

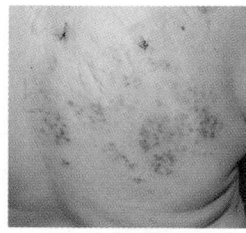

FIG 25-7 Herpes zoster. (From Barankin, Freiman, *Derm Notes*. FA Davis, Philadelphia, 2006, p. 100, with permission.)

Tinea

ICD-9-M code: 110.9 (tinea corporis), 110.0 (tinea capitis), 110.1 (tinea unguium), 110.4 (tinea pedis), 110.3 (tinea cruris)

Tinea infection, also called *dermatophytoses* or *ringworm*, is any fungal skin infection on the body. Various forms include *tinea capitis* (scalp), *tinea corporis* (trunk), *tinea cruris* (genital area, also called *jock itch*), *tinea nodosa* (mustache and beard), *tinea pedis* (feet, also called *athletes foot*), and *tinea unguium* (nails). These types of infections are common. Tinea cruris is most common in adult men and tinea corporis is especially common in children.

Tinea is caused by a fungus and is, therefore, contagious. It is transmitted via direct contact or by touching infected items, such as shoes, combs, clothing, and shower or pool surfaces. It may also be contracted from pets; cats are common carriers. Tinea thrives in warm, moist areas, and skin with a minor injury (such as a scratch or scrape) is more vulnerable.

Symptoms of tinea infection vary, depending on the type and location. Most forms include red, raised, scaly, itchy lesions. (See Figure 25-8.) Patchy hair loss may be evident on the head or, in men, the face. The rash of tinea corporis has circular lesions. Tinea pedis causes the skin of the feet and especially between the toes, to crack, peel, flake, and redden. Patients may complain of itching, burning, and stinging. There may be blisters that break and ooze and become crusty. Affected nails become discolored, thickened, and softened and sometimes crumble.

Diagnosis is based on the appearance of lesions and the patient's description of symptoms. Diagnosis is confirmed by a skin culture or **biopsy,** a procedure in which a representative sample of tissue is obtained for microscopic examination via surgery, syringe and needle, endoscopy, punch technique, or other means. Also, examination of the scraping under a blue light (Wood's lamp) in a dark room can confirm the diagnosis.

Treatment usually includes over-the-counter (OTC) antifungal creams and powders such as miconazole (Monistat, Micatin). Patients should be instructed to continue use for 2 weeks after symptoms have resolved to keep the tinea infection from recurring. They must also keep the affected skin clean and dry, wear clean cotton socks (for tinea pedis),

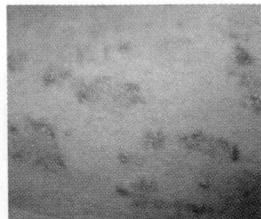

FIG 25-8 Tinea corporis. (From Barankin, Freiman, *Derm Notes.* FA Davis, Philadelphia, 2006, p. 160, with permission.)

and wash sheets and pajamas daily. What's more, they should seek treatment for infected pets.

Tinea infections usually respond well to treatment within 3 to 5 weeks, although recurrence is possible. If infection does not respond to OTC medications, evaluation by a health care provider is recommended. Prescription-strength medication may be needed and includes antifungal creams or pills. There is a risk of a secondary bacterial infection such as cellulitis developing due to skin breakdown from scratching.

Candidiasis

ICD-9-CM code: 112.3 (skin and nails), 112.0 (oral thrush), 112.1 (vaginal yeast)

Candidiasis, commonly called *yeast infection,* is an infection of the mucous membranes or skin caused by *Candida albicans,* which is part of the body's normal flora. It causes an infection when an overgrowth of the organism develops in warm, moist areas, such as the mouth, vagina, nails, and skin folds. Candidiasis develops when the composition of the body's normal flora is disrupted, usually due to antibiotic therapy, or when the normal immune defenses are weakened, commonly due to corticosteroid therapy, chemotherapy, or an immune system disorder such as AIDS. Risk factors for candidiasis include diabetes mellitus and pregnancy.

Symptoms vary depending on the location of the infection. Oral candidiasis, commonly called *thrush,* causes raised, white patches on the oral mucous membranes and tongue with an underlying inflammation. Candidiasis within skin folds causes a reddened, pruritic rash. Vaginal infections cause a thick cheesy discharge and pruritis, a feeling of itchiness. Diagnosis of candidiasis is based on physical examination findings, the patient's description of symptoms and, occasionally, microscopic examination of skin scrapings or vaginal discharge.

Most forms of candidiasis respond to systemic antifungal medication such as oral fluconazole (Diflucan). Oral infections may also be treated with clotrimazole lozenges (Mycelex) or a nystatin solution (Mycostatin, Nilstat) that is swished in the mouth and then swallowed. Antifungal creams or ointments are sometimes applied topically to affected skin folds, and vaginal suppositories may be used for vaginal infections.

Prognosis for most forms of candidiasis is good. Immunocompromised individuals who develop systemic fungal infections may be vulnerable to septicemia, which can be life-threatening if septic shock develops.

Parasitic Infestations

Parasitic infestations include pediculosis (lice) and scabies. Some confusion exists between scabies and lice. Both are skin conditions caused by infestation. Both are very contagious and both cause itching.

Pediculosis

ICD-9-CM code: 132 (general code; see diagnosis for specific code)

Pediculosis is the term used to refer to infestation with a species of louse. There are three species of louse: the head louse, body louse, and pubic louse. Head lice and body lice are very similar in appearance but differ primarily in habitat. Head lice are currently considered the most common human parasitic infestation in the United States and Europe. (See Figure 25-9.) Nits (eggs) are tiny, yellow-white, and oval in shape. They are firmly attached to the side of the hair shaft near the scalp. They are laid by live lice and cannot be transmitted to others. It takes 7 to 10 days for the eggs to hatch and then another 7 to 10 days for the new females to mature and begin laying their own eggs. Adult lice are about the size of sesame seeds and are reddish-brown, wingless, crawling insects that cannot jump or fly. They are rarely found on pets. They feed on human blood and usually live for about 30 days but can only live for 1 to 2 days away from the host.

Head lice are common and primarily affect the scalp and, infrequently, the eyebrows and eyelashes. They are transmitted via direct contact with the infected person's head or with personal items such as scarves, hats, coats, brushes, combs, and towels. Personal hygiene and cleanliness in the home is not a factor. Body lice are found on the body and attach their eggs to the inside of clothing, usually along seam lines. Crab lice are found primarily in the pubic and perianal area.

Symptoms of pediculosis include itching and sores on the scalp from scratching as well as the sensation of something crawling on the skin. Diagnosis is made by careful examination of the hair and scalp for nits or lice. Treatment includes manually ridding the body of parasites, controlling itching, and disinfecting the home environment. Medication and treatment recommendations are modified frequently. The latest recommendations can be found at *http://www .headlice.org.*

Scabies

ICD-9-CM code: 133.0

Scabies is a common, contagious condition in which the skin has been infested with microscopic mites. It is found worldwide and crosses all social classes and races. It spreads quickly in crowded conditions where people have close contact, such as in health care institutions. It is transmitted via direct contact with an infected person or by sharing personal items, such as clothing and bed linens. The scabies rash is intensely pruritic and made up of scaly papules, insect burrows, and secondary infected lesions. (Figure 25-10.) It is most prevalent in skin folds at the wrists, elbows, between fingers, under the arms, in the groin, and under the beltline. The scalp, palms of the hands, and soles of the feet may also be affected. Itching is usually worse at night.

Diagnosis includes differentiating scabies from other skin conditions, such as folliculitis, dermatitis, and impetigo. It is sometimes identified by the characteristic rash. The most common diagnostic test involves scraping the lesion and examining the tissue microscopically for the presence of mites or eggs. An ink test may also be used in which blue or black ink is applied after which the skin is cleaned. Some of the ink absorbs into the mite burrows thus revealing the lesions.

Traditional treatment of scabies involves the application of products containing lindane. However, its use is not advised due to potentially serious adverse effects. A safer alternative is products containing topical 5% permethrin cream (Elimite, Acticin). Application should be repeated in 7 to 10 days when the nits hatch. Other individuals who live in the same household should be treated as well. The home environment should be disinfected as extensively as possible by washing or vacuuming surfaces and washing linens, towels, and clothing in hot water. Pesticide sprays should not be used.

Prognosis is good with adequate treatment. Itching may persist for several weeks after treatment. Reinfestation is possible if the home and personal belongings are not cleaned adequately.

Hypersensitivity and Inflammatory Reactions

Hypersensitivity skin disorders are common, especially in people who suffer from other forms of allergies. Among the most common are eczema and psoriasis. In addition, lupus is a serious inflammatory disorder that may affect the skin or other body systems.

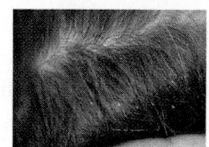

FIG 25-9 Pediculosis capitis. (From Barankin, Freiman, *Derm Notes.* FA Davis, Philadelphia, 2006, p. 127, with permission.)

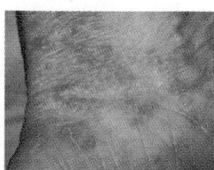

FIG 25-10 Scabies. (From Barankin, Freiman, *Derm Notes.* FA Davis, Philadelphia, 2006, p. 142, with permission.)

Eczema

ICD-9-CM code: 690 (general code for seborrheic dermatitis), 691 (general code for atopic dermatitis), 692 (general code for contact dermatitis); refer to diagnosis for specific code

Eczema, also known as *dermatitis,* is a general term for a group of conditions that affect people of all ages. The most common type is **atopic** eczema, meaning that there is a genetic predisposition for it. It is associated with asthma and hayfever and runs in families.

Eczema is fairly common, affecting 10% to 20% of the general population. It is more common among infants and children and may be acute or chronic. Causes are numerous and include allergies, response to chemicals, scratching the skin, emotional stress, illness, or sun exposure. Eczema is not contagious. Rash appearance and symptoms vary with the severity and type of eczema and the causative agent. The skin may be hot, dry, and pruritic. In more severe forms, the skin may be red, swollen, cracked, weeping, scaly, and itchy and may even bleed.

There is no specific diagnostic test. Diagnosis is based on medical history, patient symptoms, and physical examination findings. At present there is no cure for eczema. However, many children will be free of symptoms by the time they are in their teens. There are a number of treatment options, including application of aluminum acetate astringents (Burow's solution), which is used in dermatology as a drying agent, for weeping skin lesions. Other medications include corticosteroids, emollients, antihistamines, or injections. Known **allergens,** which are any substance that causes a hypersensitivity reaction or abnormal immune response, should be avoided. Clothing made from soft-textured cotton is recommended and should be laundered in mild detergent. Keeping room temperatures below 72°F (22.2°C) and use of room humidifiers may help. Sensitivity to specific allergens may never disappear entirely. However flare-ups can be minimized and symptoms controlled.

Psoriasis

ICD-9-CM code: 696 (general code; refer to diagnosis for specific code)

Psoriasis is a chronic, inflammatory skin disorder characterized by the development of red, scaly plaques. Appearance varies with the specific type. Psoriasis affects 1% to 3% of the world's population and approximately 4.5 million people in the United States. It affects men and women equally but is more common in Caucasians. The specific cause of psoriasis is unknown, although it may be autoimmune in nature. Contributing factors include stress, family history, skin trauma, cold weather, infections, and some medications. It is not contagious.

The typical presentation of psoriasis includes silvery-white scaly plaques or patches with reddened skin beneath and sharply defined borders. (See Figure 25-11.) Lesions may

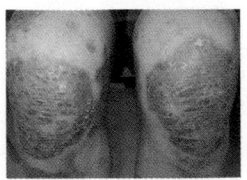

FIG 25-11 Psoriasis. (From Barankin, Freiman, *Derm Notes.* FA Davis, Philadelphia, 2006, p. 133, with permission.)

crack and bleed. They are commonly found on the knees, shins, elbows, buttocks, lower back, ears, and along the hairline; however, the total body surface may be involved in some cases. Age of onset is usually between 15 and 35 years, although it can develop at any age. There is a pattern of exacerbations and remissions but flare-ups can last for years. Many patients report that psoriasis has a significant impact on their quality of life and affects clothing choice (to cover lesions), quality of sleep, and self-esteem. Symptoms include itching and pain.

Diagnosis of psoriasis is based on history, physical examination findings and the patient's description of symptoms. Biopsy may be done when typical lesions and scales are not obvious. There are a number of treatments for psoriasis, including topical corticosteroids, vitamin D, coal tar derivatives, retinoids, and ultraviolet light exposure. Relatively new drugs on the market, known as *biologics,* have been approved for the treatment of psoriasis. The term *biologics* refers to a variety of medicinal products derived from natural sources or produced by biotechnology. Drugs created to treat psoriasis include alefacept (Amevive), efalizumab (Raptiva), and etanercept (Enbrel). Other drugs are still undergoing research. In addition to using prescribed medications, patients are encouraged to maintain self-care, which includes preventing skin trauma and avoiding known triggers. There is no cure for psoriasis. However the disorder can be managed by avoiding triggers and using approved treatments and medications. Approximately 10% to 30% of individuals develop a related form of arthritis known as psoriatic arthritis.

Systemic Lupus Erythematosus

ICD-9-CM code: 710.0

Systemic lupus erythematosus (SLE) is a chronic autoimmune disorder, meaning that the body produces antibodies that targets "self" tissues. These antibodies cause inflammation and degeneration of various connective tissues in the body. The exact cause of the autoimmune response is not fully understood. There is some thought that genetics, viruses, some drugs, female hormones, stress, and ultraviolet light in the form of sunlight, fluorescent lights, and tanning beds may play a role. Lupus that affects only the skin is called *discoid lupus.* However SLE is considered systemic because it can target any number of tissues or organs within the body, including the skin, lungs, heart, joints, kidneys, blood, and nervous system.

SLE affects up to 1.5 million Americans and is eight times more common in women than men. It can occur at any age but is most common in women of childbearing age between the ages of 15 and 45. It is also more common in African Americans, Latinos, Native Americans, and those of Japanese and Chinese descent.

Lupus is marked by exacerbations (periods of illness) and remission (periods of wellness). One of the most prominent features of discoid lupus and SLE is the skin rash that may develop anywhere on the body but is most obvious on the face and scalp. It is generally red and flat but may have raised borders and is painless and does not itch. Other symptoms of SLE depend on the body system affected. General, whole-body symptoms include mild fever, fatigue, anorexia, and weight loss. Other symptoms include myalgias (muscle aches); arthralgias (aching joints); photosensitivity; splenomegaly (spleen enlargement); enlarged, tender lymph nodes; and Raynaud's phenomenon (a circulatory disorder of the fingers and toes). Arthritic changes develop in 90% of those with SLE and cause symptoms of joint pain, stiffness, edema, and possible joint deformity.

There is no single test that definitively diagnoses SLE. Instead, 11 criteria are used to confirm diagnosis. Identification of four or more suggests a diagnosis of SLE. These criteria include:

1. classic "butterfly" rash across the cheeks and nose
2. discoid skin rash
3. photosensitivity
4. ulcerations in the mouth, nose or throat
5. arthritis
6. pleuritis (inflammation in the lining of the lungs) or pericarditis (inflammation in the lining of the heart)
7. kidney abnormalities
8. brain irritation
9. abnormal blood count
10. positive antinuclear antibody (ANA) test
11. immunologic disorder characterized by abnormal immune tests, including anti-DNA or anti-Sm (Smith) antibodies, false-positive blood test for syphilis, anticardiolipin antibodies, lupus anticoagulant, or elevated lipoprotein electrophoresis test.

Other testing that may be helpful includes the erythrocyte sedimentation rate (ESR), blood chemistry testing, tissue biopsies, and fluid specimen analysis.

There is no cure for SLE. Treatment goals aim to relieve symptoms and prevent or minimize complications. A variety of medications may be used to prevent or treat inflammation, including nonsteroidal anti-inflammatory drugs (NSAIDs), such as ibuprofen (Motrin), aspirin, naproxen (Aleve), and sulindac. Severe exacerbations may be treated with corticosteroids. Hydroxychloroquine is helpful for treating SLE patients suffering from skin and joint disease

and fatigue. Those with severe kidney or brain disease may benefit from plasmapheresis, which is a procedure used to remove autoantibodies from the blood. Other immunosuppressive medications may be used as well. General recommendations also include rest and regular, moderate exercise.

Complications from SLE include some forms of cancer, pleuritis, pericarditis, cardiovascular disease, heart attack, kidney failure, stroke, Raynaud's phenomenon, and brain involvement. Some patients go into remission for up to a year and require no treatment during that time. Survival and longevity is variable, depending on how many of the 11 diagnostic criteria are present and which organs are affected. Those with SLE limited to skin and joints have the best prognosis. Those with CNS or kidney disease have a poor prognosis.

Neoplasms

An area of abnormal tissue growth may be identified as a *neoplasm* or *dysplasia*. Such tissue must be evaluated by a pathologist to determine whether it is malignant (cancerous) or benign (noncancerous). The most common way to determine if a neoplasm is cancerous is to surgically remove a piece of the tissue via biopsy and examine it under a microscope. If the tissue is malignant, the next step is to determine whether it is carcinoma in situ (confined to the original site), has spread regionally, or has metastasized (spread to distant sites). Detection of cancer in regional lymph nodes indicates that it has spread into the lymphatic system and may have spread to other, more distant sites.

Cancer is classified according to a system of grading and staging in order to determine the patient's overall prognosis and treatment plan. *Grading* refers to a standardized process of describing cancer cell differentiation, from stage I to stage IV, where stage IV has the least resemblance to normal tissue. *Staging* refers to the extent of dissemination of the cancer, including tumor size as well as regional and distant metastasis.

Treatment of cancer is determined by an oncologist and depends on the type, stage, and grade of the cancer. Treatment options usually include surgery, chemotherapy, radiation therapy, hormone therapy, **cryosurgery** (surgery with cold probes to destroy cancerous tissue), **electrodesiccation** (destructive drying of cells by application of electrical energy), application of chemotherapeutic agents, and administration of medications to boost the immune system. These treatments may be used alone or in combination.

Benign neoplasms of the skin are common and include birthmarks, such as strawberry hemangiomas and nevi (moles). Cancerous neoplasms of the skin are classified as *basal cell carcinoma, squamous cell carcinoma,* and *malignant melanoma.* Together, they make up the most common form of cancer. Areas of the body most commonly affected are those frequently exposed to the sun, such as the face and ears.

Basal Cell Carcinoma
ICD-9-CM code: M8090/3 ("/3" means "malignant, primary site")
Basal cell carcinoma is the most common type of skin cancer and, fortunately, grows slowly and rarely metastasizes. It usually begins as a small, shiny papule and eventually enlarges to form a whitish border around a central depression or ulcer that may bleed.

Squamous Cell Carcinoma
ICD-9-CM code: M8070/3 ("/3" means "malignant, primary site")
Squamous cell carcinoma grows more rapidly than basal cell carcinoma and spreads more easily. It develops in squamous tissue found on the skin or in the mouth, esophagus, bronchi, lungs, or cervix. It may appear as a firm, red nodule, have a scaly appearance, and ulcerate. (See *Seven warning signs of cancer*.)

Malignant Melanoma
ICD-9-CM code: 172 (use 4th digit for specific site)
Malignant melanoma commonly arises from a brown or black mole and has a tendency to spread aggressively to distant sites, making it the most lethal form of skin cancer. Risk factors include sunlight exposure, especially the number of childhood sunburns, as well as fair skin color, red hair, and family history. The initial appearance of malignant melanoma lesions is variable but includes pigmented color (tan, brown, blue, red, black, or white), asymmetry, and irregular borders. Lesions are generally larger than 6 mm in size, often metastasize, and can recur. Therefore, patients should be reevaluated on a regular basis after the malignant

tissue has been surgically removed. (See *Warning signs of malignant melanoma: The ABCD system.*)

Dermatology Procedures

Dermatology is a medical specialty that focuses on the study and treatment of disorders of the integumentary system. While many physicians, including pediatricians and family practice specialists, diagnose and treat minor skin disorders, those who specialize in this area of medicine are *dermatologists*.

The dermatologist is responsible for identifying skin changes and their possible significance. Some skin changes occur as a natural part of the aging process, including loss of elasticity (causing lines and wrinkles on the skin), increased numbers of benign growths and lesions (such as age spots and moles), and scars and other changes due to sun exposure and minor trauma. Other skin changes may reflect poor nutritional status, circulatory problems, or systemic disease.

Some disorders treated by the dermatologist, such as acne, aren't considered serious medical disorders. However, because they have an impact on self-image, these disorders deserve as much attention as more serious medical disorders such as cancer.

Assisting with Examination
To reach an accurate diagnosis, the physician must obtain a medical history, including a description of symptoms. A physical examination of the skin and skin structures is also important. A thorough examination includes the entire body, from head to toes, including the genital area. While performing inspection, the dermatologist must have good lighting and a magnifying lens in order to closely examine any suspicious lesions or growths. He'll pay attention to changes in skin color as well as the presence of any lesions, ulcers, bruises, or rashes. When performing palpation, the dermatologist notes changes in elasticity and texture as well

---

📝 Patient Education

Seven Warning Signs of Cancer
Skin cancer is among the most common forms of cancer, is one of the most preventable, and can be one of the most deadly. Teach your patients about the seven warning signs of cancer so they can detect changes early. The seven warning signs of cancer are:

• Change in bowel or bladder habits

• A sore throat that does not heal

• Unusual bleeding or discharge

• Thickening or a lump in the breast or other area

• Indigestion or difficulty swallowing

• Obvious change in a mole or wart

• Nagging cough or hoarseness.

Warning signs of malignant melanoma: The ABCD system

A helpful way to remember and identify the warning signs of malignant melanoma is the ABCD system:

• **A**ssymetry—One half of the mole does not match the other half.

• **B**order—The edges of the mole are irregular or blurred.

• **C**olor—Varying shades of color throughout include tan, brown, black, blue, red, or white.

• **D**iameter—The mole is larger than 6 mm.

as the presence of lumps, masses, or areas of firmness. The dermatologist may conduct **diascopy,** which is a procedure that allows the dermatologist to observe changes in response to pressure. In some cases, the dermatologist may obtain tissue samples via biopsy for microscopic analysis.

In an examination, the medical assistant must prepare the patient by checking vital signs and obtaining health history, which should include data regarding outdoor activities, family history of skin problems, and use of sunscreen. She should then assist him as needed with undressing and positioning. She must also assist the dermatologist as needed with any procedures. For example, if the dermatologist notices a lesion, he may ask the medical assistant to apply a dressing or obtain a drainage specimen for culture.

Allergy Skin Testing

Allergy skin testing is done to identify what substance or allergen is responsible for triggering an allergic response in a person. This testing evaluates the person's sensitivity to numerous substances, including those common in trees, shrubs, weeds, and grasses; fungus; dust and dust mites; feathers; pet dander; foods; medications; and insect venom. Symptoms of allergies include sneezing; runny nose; and itchy, watery eyes. Allergies can also trigger asthma attacks. When allergies are identified, individuals may be able to avoid or minimize exposure to the offensive substance or take allergy shots to decrease the severity of their reaction.

Allergies are diagnosed through skin or blood testing. Both testing methods expose a person to suspected allergens to see if a reaction occurs. Skin tests are generally preferable due to their reliability, quick results, and low expense.

Scratch Test

A **scratch test,** also called a *skin prick test,* is done by placing a drop of a solution containing a potential allergen on the skin and then pricking the skin with a needle to expose it to the allergen. (See Figure 25-12.) Any smooth surface of the body may be used, including the back, which is a popular site. The locations of scratch tests are documented in some form of a pattern so that any positive reactions can be associated with the correct allergen. A multiheaded testing device is commonly used to allow application of multiple allergen solutions at once. (See Figure 25-13.) They are commonly placed in rows 1 1/2" to 2" apart with as many as 50 tests done at once. A positive reaction is indicated by the development of a wheal, which is a rounded temporary elevation in the skin that is white in the center with a pale red periphery and is accompanied by itching, commonly seen with insect bites and allergic reactions. Wheals usually develop within 30 minutes and indicate that the person is allergic to that allergen. More severe reactions may include itching. Positive reactions are graded on a scale from 2 (least severe) to 4 (most severe). In cases of severe reactions, the solution should be wiped off. (See *Procedure 25-1: Performing allergy skin testing,* page 430.)

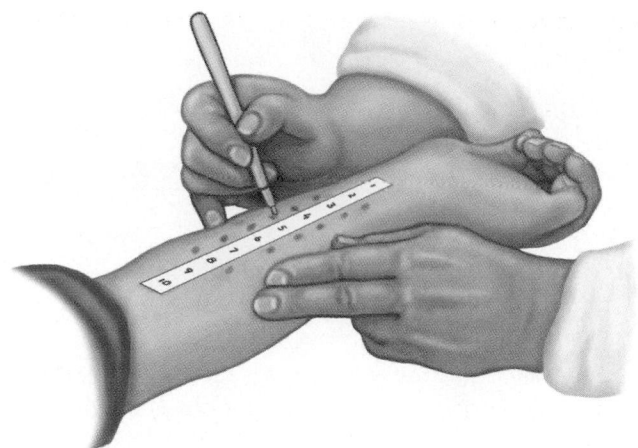

FIG 25-12 Scratch test.

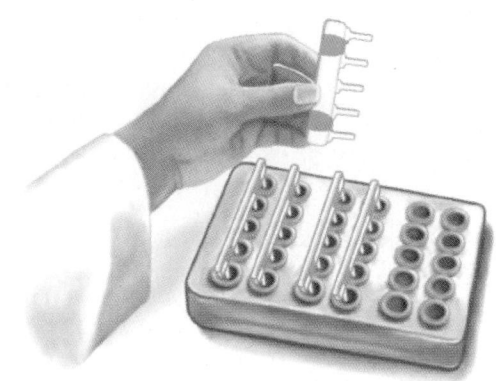

FIG 25-13 Multiheaded testing device.

Intradermal Test

The intradermal test involves the injection of a tiny dose (0.1 to 0.2 ml) of an allergen solution deeper into the skin. As many as 15 different allergens may be tested on each arm. This test may be done when there is no reaction to the scratch test, yet there is still reason to suspect the individual may be allergic. This test is more sensitive than the scratch test and provides more consistent and reliable results. However, a positive reaction to it does not necessarily confirm the allergen is a severe problem for the individual, but does indicate the presence of antibodies. Other information, including the person's history and description of symptoms, is required to determine whether treatment is needed. (See Figure 25-14.)

Patch Test

A **patch test** is used to detect contact dermatitis, a form of skin allergy. In this test a pad soaked in an allergen solution is placed on the skin, covered with cellophane, and left in place for up to 2 days. (See Figure 25-15.) As many as 30 such tests may be done at one time and the reaction is checked within 4 days. (See *Skin testing guidelines,* page 432.)

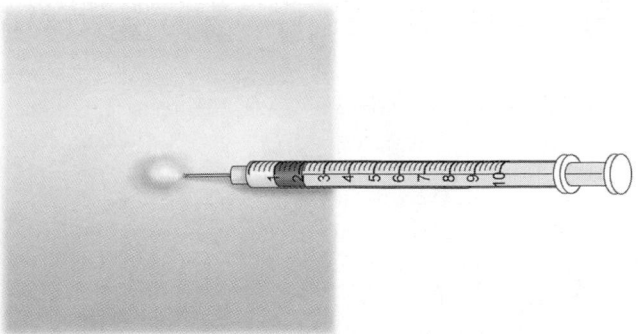

FIG 25-14 Intradermal test with injection of 0.1 to 0.2 ml of solution containing an allergen.

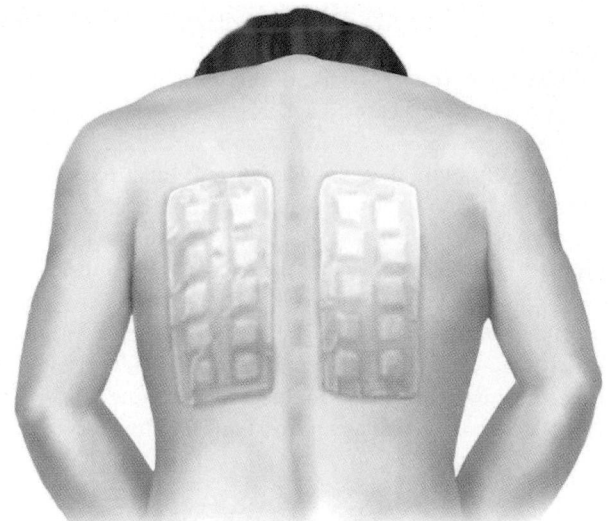

FIG 25-15 Patch test pad soaked in an allergen solution and placed on the skin.

PROCEDURE 25-1

Performing allergy skin testing

Task
Perform an allergy skin prick test.

Conditions
- Allergen solution
- Control solution
- Multiheaded skin-testing device
- Biohazard container
- Marking pen
- Ruler or measuring device
- Tissues
- Nonsterile examination gloves
- Medical record or chart
- Waste container

Standards
In the time specified and within the scoring parameters determined by the instructor, the student will successfully perform an allergy skin prick test.

Performance Standards
1. Wash or sanitize your hands to ensure infection control and assemble supplies.
2. Greet and identify your patient and introduce yourself. Explain the procedure and ask the patient if he has taken any medications in the past 2 weeks that might interfere with the test. Also ask if the patient has applied any creams, ointments, or moisturizers to his skin today. Substances applied to the skin may cause solution from one test site to run onto another test site.
3. Assist the patient onto the examination table into a position that is comfortable for the patient and convenient for testing. (The test site will be the surface of the inner forearm, the outer upper arm, or the back, depending on the number of test sites needed.)
4. Clean the skin site with water or alcohol (per office protocol).
5. Hold the multiheaded skin-testing device next to the patient's skin. Use the marking pen to mark the patient's skin next to each testing site, according to office protocol, to ensure an accurate reading of results.

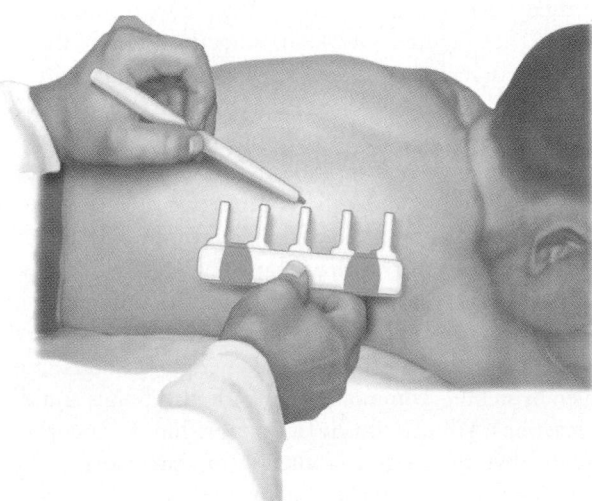

Mark the patient's skin while holding the testing device next to it.

PROCEDURE 25-1—cont'd

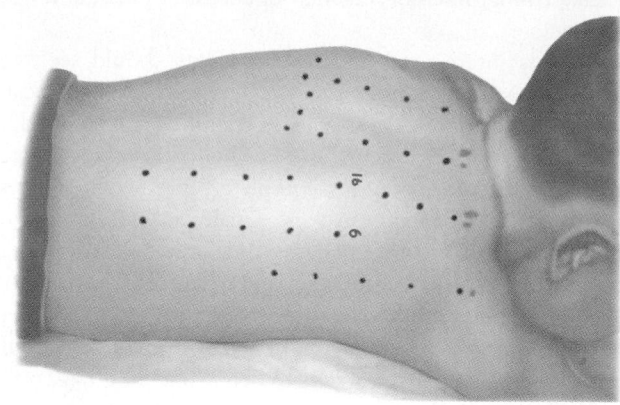

Patient's skin with marks

6. Press the testing device gently against the patient's skin so that the allergen solution enters the top layer of skin.

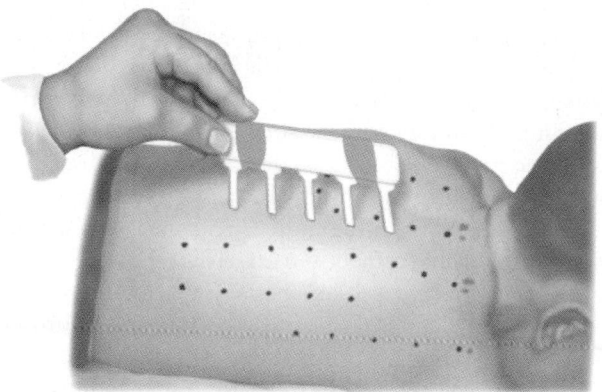

Press the testing device gently against the patient's skin.

7. Repeat steps 6 and 7 with different prepared testing devices until all tests have been completed.

8. Carefully blot (do not wipe) any excess solution with tissue to prevent solution from running between test sites.

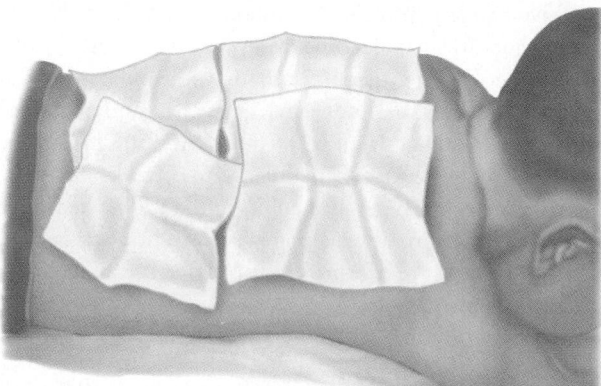

Apply tissue to the patient's skin, without wiping, to blot excess solution.

9. Set the timer for 15 minutes. Give the patient some reading material if desired to help the patient pass the time and provide a distraction from skin discomfort or itching.

10. Note the results and measure any positive reactions in millimeters. If wheals are not round in shape, measure the diameter in both directions and record the average of the two (or according to office policy) to ensure the most accurate measurement.

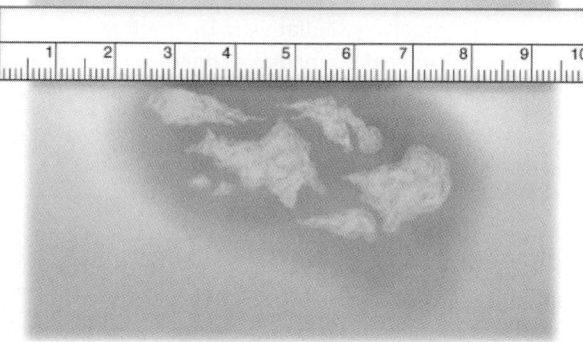

Measure positive reactions in millimeters.

11. Remove markings from the skin with an alcohol solution or water.

12. Reassure the patient that any itching should resolve within 20 minutes or so. Apply a cool compress or cortisone cream for itching (per office protocol) to increase patient comfort.

13. Instruct the patient with positive reactions to remain in the office for at least 20 minutes after completion of the test to provide time for the physician to counsel the patient regarding the test results and to observe the patient for asthma or anaphylaxis.

14. Document results in the medical record according to office policy to ensure accuracy of the medical record.

Date	
07/23/08; 3:12 p.m.	Allergy skin testing completed; Pt. tolerated procedure well; results reviewed by Dr. Lee. ---------------- S. Gonzales, CMA

Skin testing guidelines

Below are the most common guidelines for allergy skin testing. Medical assistants who assist with allergy testing should be familiar with these guidelines as well as any other related policies established by the medical office:

- Antihistamines or allergy medications should be discontinued a minimum of 3 days prior to testing.
- Recommended testing sites include the anterior forearm and the back.
- Sites must be carefully labeled and spaced 1 1/2" to 2" apart.
- Notify the physician immediately if the patient demonstrates signs of anaphylaxis (hives, edema, redness, difficulty breathing, nausea, vomiting, anxiety).
- Keep emergency supplies on hand, such as epinephrine and diphenhydramine hydrochloride (Benadryl).

Radioallergosorbent Test

The **radioallergosorbent test** (RAST) checks blood for the presence of specific allergy antibodies. It may be done instead of or in addition to skin testing and is useful for people who are on medications that suppress the results of skin tests and for those who cannot discontinue antihistamine medication. It is also more specific than skin testing and is helpful in the diagnosis of asthma, allergies, and other lung disorders.

Culture and Sensitivity Testing

A wound culture involves obtaining secretions from the wound using a sterile, cotton-tipped applicator and securing it in a transport medium. It is then transported to the laboratory for microscopic examination and culturing. Culturing is a process in which the sample is applied to a growth medium and placed in a supportive environment to grow for 24 to 72 hours. Aerobic cultures identify organisms that grow and thrive in environments with oxygen. Such organisms are usually found on or near the surface of wounds. Anaerobic cultures identify organisms that grow and thrive in environments with little or no oxygen. Such organisms are usually found in the deeper layers of wounds and ulcers. When the organisms are identified, a sensitivity test exposes the microorganisms to various anti-infective agents to determine which one is most effective in killing them. This testing helps the dermatologist determine the best antimicrobial agent to prescribe for the patient.

Image Enhancement Procedures

Procedures to repair disfigurement and enhance appearance are becoming more and more popular, due in part to medical advances that are making such procedures more affordable and less risky. Common procedures include dermabrasion and dermaplaning, microdermabrasion, chemical peels, and laser resurfacing.

Patients interested in these procedures should seek the care of a qualified dermatologist. The physician should caution patients that results vary, depending on individual anatomy, physical reactions, and healing abilities and, therefore, the outcome is never completely predictable. These treatments may be expensive and usually are not covered by medical insurance. In some cases, they may be used for scar modification or the removal of precancerous skin growths. Such conditions might meet the criteria of "medical necessity" required by insurance companies. Individuals should contact their insurance carriers to determine whether coverage will apply in their individual case.

Dermabrasion and Dermaplaning

Dermabrasion is a process in which a surgeon scrapes away the outermost layer of skin using a wire brush or burr impregnated with diamond particles. **Dermaplaning** is a procedure in which the surgeon uses an instrument called a *dermatome*, which resembles an electric razor, to skim off surface layers of the skin. Both procedures refinish the top layers of the skin and can remove acne scars, scars from previous surgery or accidents, nevi (moles), tattoos, or fine wrinkles and leave a smoother surface. Both procedures can be performed on small areas of skin or the entire face and may be used alone or with other enhancement procedures. Both procedures are usually done under local anesthesia, which numbs the area being treated. Medication may also be administered to help patients feel relaxed yet still awake. In severe cases, general anesthesia may be used. Dermabrasion and dermaplaning usually last from a few minutes up to 90 minutes, depending on the area of skin involved. Cases involving deep scarring may require multiple treatments. Potential complications include infection, skin pigment changes, and scarring.

Microdermabrasion

Microdermabrasion is similar to dermabrasion but is less aggressive and less invasive. It stimulates growth of skin cells and collagen and has become a popular nonsurgical procedure. It involves gentle abrasion or "polishing," which is useful in reducing fine lines, nevi, age spots, and acne scars. Each treatment takes 30 to 60 minutes. About 5 to 12 treatments are recommended, scheduled 2 to 3 weeks apart. It is effective on all skin types and colors and does not require an anesthetic. It may be used along with a light chemical peel for increased effect. Periodic repeat treatments are needed to maintain the effect.

Chemical Peel

A **chemical peel,** also called *chemabrasion* or *chemexfoliation,* is an alternative to dermabrasion. In this procedure, a chemical solution is applied to the skin to improve appearance by removing blemishes, fine wrinkles, and uneven pigmentation. It may also be used to treat scars and tattoos. A chemical peel involves the use of different chemical solutions, depending on the extent of the peel desired; thus, the terms *light, medium,* and *deep* are used to describe the level of chemical peel. Most peels may be safely done in the medical office or outpatient surgical center. The procedure usually doesn't require anesthesia because the chemical solution acts as an anesthetic. (See *Aftercare for the patient undergoing a chemical peel.*)

Laser Resurfacing

Laser resurfacing, also called *photothermolysis,* involves the use of short pulses of light to treat skin conditions. Sometimes called a *laser peel,* this fairly new procedure involves using a carbon dioxide laser to remove fine lines and damaged skin around the eyes and mouth. It is also used to minimize scars and even out areas of uneven pigmentation. During the procedure, a laser is carefully passed over the skin until the appropriate depth is affected to achieve the desired results. This treatment may be done on specific areas or the whole face and takes anywhere from a few minutes to 90 minutes. Recovery includes application of a dressing for several days. Skin crusts may form temporarily but should not be picked off, as scarring may result. Redness is common and may last for several weeks. Repeated treatments may be necessary to achieve desired results. Final results may not be fully apparent for several months.

Botox™

Botox™ treatments have gained increasing popularity in recent years. Botox™ comes from the botulinim toxin and was approved by the FDA over 10 years ago for the treatment of certain problems with eye muscles. Physicians and patients noticed that it also improved the appearance of wrinkles around the eyes. It has since been approved for use in lessening the appearance of wrinkles between the eyebrows. It acts by interfering with contraction of the treated muscles, thereby reducing the appearance of wrinkles. In this procedure, the dermatologist injects a small amount of Botox™. Results occur within 7 days and may last up to 4 months. Common adverse effects are flulike symptoms of headache, upset stomach, and temporary eyelid droop. Cases of botulism are extremely rare but have been reported. (See *Teaching about Botox.*)

Patient Education

Aftercare for the Patient Undergoing a Chemical Peel

The medical assistant should provide these guidelines to the patient undergoing a chemical peel:

- You may experience some temporary flaking, scaling, redness, or dryness.
- You may experience some swelling.
- The physician may prescribe a mild analgesic to relieve discomfort.
- Arrange to have someone help you out at home for a day or two so that you can rest.
- Avoid sun exposure.
- Follow any other instructions given to you by the physician.

Patient Education

Teaching About Botox™

Patients are becoming more curious about Botox™ treatments as a means to temporarily reduce fine lines and wrinkles, and unregulated Botox™ "parties" are even becoming popular. However, there are potential risks and adverse effects associated with this medical treatment. Therefore, be sure your patients are well informed by providing them with the following information:

- Botox™ is only approved to treat wrinkles between the eyebrows.
- Botox™ is only approved for those between the ages of 18 and 65.
- Consult with your physician for appropriate evaluation and treatment.
- Seek treatment only from qualified medical providers in a physician's office or medical clinic.
- Avoid "Botox™ parties" because the person administering the injection may be unlicensed and not properly trained.
- Never share Botox™ solution or needles with others.
- Avoid Botox™ use if your are pregnant or breastfeeding.
- Tell the physician if you are taking antibiotics.
- Tell the physician about nervous or muscular disorders you have.

Chapter Summary

- The integumentary system includes the skin, which is the largest organ of the body. It is made up of the epidermis, the dermis, the subcutaneous layer, and other structures. It plays vital roles in protection, temperature regulation, and insulation.
- Medical assistants must be well versed in language and vocabulary that pertains to the integumentary system. In addition to knowing common combining forms, they should be familiar with common abbreviations and pathological terms.
- Some of the most common disorders of the integumentary system include impetigo, acne, cellulitis, folliculitis, warts, herpes simplex types 1 and 2, herpes zoster, fungal infections, pediculosis, scabies, eczema, psoriasis, SLE, and neoplasms.
- Dermatology is a medical specialty that focuses on the study and treatment of diseases and disorders of the integumentary system.
- To reach an accurate diagnosis, the dermatologist must complete a physical examination of the skin and skin structures. Examination techniques employed include inspection and palpation. Diascopy may also be used.
- The medical assistant prepares the patient by assisting him as needed with undressing and positioning. She also assists the physician with examinations and procedures.
- Allergy skin testing is done to identify a substance or allergen that is responsible for triggering an allergic response in a person. Tests include the scratch (skin prick) test, intradermal test, patch test, and RAST.
- Culture and sensitivity testing may be used to determine what organisms are growing in a wound and the antimicrobial agents that will be most effective in killing them.
- Procedures to repair disfigurement and enhance appearance are becoming more and more popular. Common procedures include dermabrasion and dermaplaning, microdermabrasion, chemical peel, laser resurfacing, and Botox™.

Team Work Exercises

1. Create poster illustrations or three-dimensional models of the skin, including the epidermis, dermis, and subcutaneous layers and key structures. Include appropriate labels. Classmates or the instructor may evaluate creations and choose a winner based on accuracy, use of humor, creativity, or other criteria.

2. Using medical word elements in Tables 23-1, 23-2, and 25-1, create as many terms related to dermatology as you can think of. List the definition of each term next to it. The team with the most terms wins.

Case Studies

1. Shirley Washington is a 54-year-old woman who has come to the dermatology clinic seeking information about image enhancement. She has a history of acne as a teenager that left some scarring. In recent years, she has developed fine lines and wrinkles around her eyes and mouth. She doesn't want to undergo invasive plastic surgery, but is interested in finding out what other options might be available to her. What will you tell her?

2. Wendy and Angela, two high school girls, visit the dermatology clinic together. They tell you that they are gathering information for a school health project about cancer. They are interested in learning about risk factors for cancer and especially want to know about the various types of skin cancer. What will you tell them?

Resources

- About.Com's Dermatology Site: *http://www.dermatology.about.com*
- American Society of Plastic Surgeons (wide variety of information about plastic surgery and image enhancement): *http://www.plasticsurgery.org*
- Centers for Disease Control and Prevention: *http://www.cdc.gov*
- E-medicine: *http://www.emedicine.com/derm/index.shtml*
- Headlice.org from the National Pediculosis Association: *http://www.headlice.org*
- Medline Plus: *http://www.nlm.nih.gov/medlineplus/skinhairandnails.html*
- National Eczema Society: *http://www.eczema.org*.
- National Institute of Arthritis and Musculoskeletal and Skin Diseases (NIAMS): *http://www.niams.nih.gov*
- National Psoriasis Foundation: *http://www.psoriasis.org*
- Nemours Foundation—Kids Health: *http://www.kidshealth.org*
- Skin Care Physicians.com: *http://www.skincarephysicians.com*

Neurology

Learning Objectives

Upon completion of this chapter, the student will be able to:

- define and spell terms related to neurology
- identify key structures of the neurological system
- discuss the roles played by the neurological system
- describe the role of the medical assistant in the neurologist's office
- identify common neurological diseases and disorders
- list commonly used word elements related to the neurological system
- give at least 10 examples of how new neurological related terms may be created by combining prefixes, suffixes, and combining forms
- describe the medical assistant's role in assisting with neurological procedures
- describe physical examination techniques used to evaluate the neurological system.

CAAHEP Competencies

Clinical Competencies

Patient Care

Prepare patients for and assist with routine and specialty examination

Prepare patients for and assist with procedures, treatments, and minor office surgery

General Competencies

Legal Concepts

Document appropriately

Patient Instruction

Instruct individuals according to their needs

ABHES Competencies

Communication

Use appropriate medical terminology

Administrative Duties

Perform diagnostic coding

Clinical Duties

Prepare patients for procedures

Prepare patient for and assist physician with routine and specialty examinations and treatments and minor office surgeries

Collect and process specimens

Instruction

Teach patients methods of health promotion and disease prevention

Procedures

Assisting with a neurological examination

Assisting with lumbar puncture

Chapter Outline

Structures and Functions of the Nervous System

Structures of the Nervous System

Neuron

Central nervous system

Peripheral nervous system

Functions of the Nervous System

Neuron

Central nervous system

Peripheral nervous system

Medical Terminology Related to the Neurological System

Common Nervous System Diseases and Disorders

Disorders of the Central Nervous System

Stroke

Transient ischemic attack

Migraine headache

Epilepsy

Encephalitis

Meningitis

Traumatic brain injury

Spinal cord injury

Parkinson disease

Multiple sclerosis

Brain tumor

Disorders of the peripheral Nervous System

Amyotrophic lateral sclerosis

Bell palsy

Peripheral neuropathy

Carpal tunnel syndrome

Spinal stenosis

Neurology Procedures

Assisting with Examination

Nervous System Tests

Electroencephalography

Lumbar puncture

Computed tomography

Magnetic resonance imaging

Chapter Summary

Team Work Exercises

Case Studies

Resources

Key Terms

affect
Emotional state or *mood*

aura
Subjective sensation that occurs prior to and signals the onset of a migraine headache or a seizure

bradykinesia
Extreme slowness in movement

Brudzinski sign
Patient response in which neck flexion causes flexion of the hips when the patient is lying in a supine position

central nervous system
Nerve tissue that comprises the brain and spinal cord

cerebral concussion
Brief loss of consciousness or brief episode of disorientation or confusion following a head injury

cerebral contusion
Injury involving bruising of brain tissue

contrecoup
Rapid acceleration-deceleration injury of the brain that bruises the front and back of the brain

corpuscallosotomy
Surgical procedure in which the central part of the brain is partially divided in two

embolic
Caused by a moving mass in a blood vessel (embolus)

fasciculation
Visible involuntary muscle twitching

fibrillation
Spontaneous muscle contraction or quivering

homeostasis
State of equilibrium in the body

Kernig sign
Reflexive hamstring contraction and pain when attempting to extend the leg after flexing the hip

motor nerves
Nerves involved in movement

myelin
Layer of phospholipids and protein that forms the myelin sheath of neurons and acts as electrical insulation

neuron
Nerve cell

neurotransmitter
Chemical that plays an important role in nerve impulse transmission

nuchal rigidity
Condition that involves pain and stiffness of the neck and a resulting reluctance to flex the head forward

paresthesia
Abnormal sensation

peripheral nervous system
Portion of the nervous system outside the central nervous system that conveys sensory and motor impulses

sensory nerves
Nerves that convey sensory information

spinal fusion
Surgical immobilization of adjacent vertebrae

thrombotic
Caused by a blood clot

transection
Cutting

Structures and Functions of the Nervous System

The nervous system plays a key role in maintaining **homeostasis**, the state of dynamic equilibrium in the internal environment of the body. More complex than the most advanced computer, the nervous system is capable of storing vast amounts of data as well as receiving and sending thousands of messages throughout the body instantly and simultaneously.

Structures of the Nervous System

An understanding of the nervous system must begin with its most essential element, the neuron. While the nervous system functions as an integrated system, it is more easily understood when divided into its two major parts: the central nervous system (CNS) and the peripheral nervous system (PNS).

Neuron

A **neuron** includes a cell body, dendrites, and axons. The cell body houses the nucleus and organelles, which are a variety of specialized structures within the cell. Dendrites resemble branches coming off of the cell body, much like the branches of a tree. The axons of a neuron are as short as a few millimeters or as long as a meter. They are cordlike projections that are sometimes covered in a myelin sheath made up of a specialized layer of cells. (See Figure 26-1.) Neuron cell bodies grouped together form gray matter. Axons bundled together form white matter, named for the whitish hue of

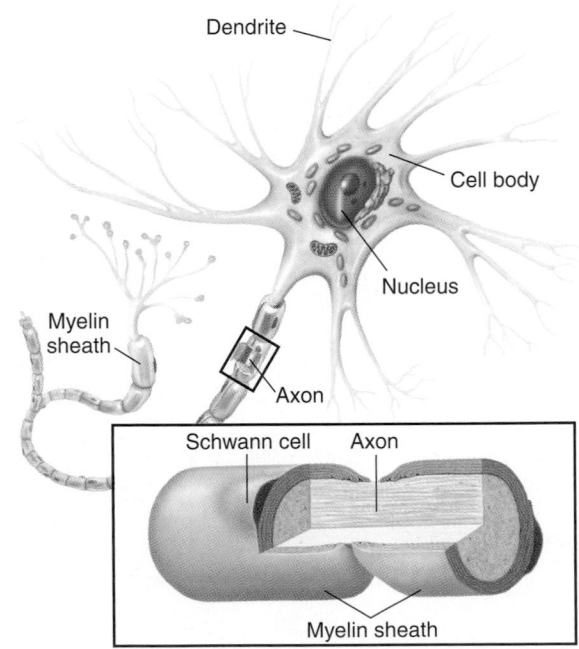

FIG 26-1 Neuron.

the myelin sheaths. Within the PNS, bundles of axons are called *nerves.*

Central Nervous System

The **Central nervous system** (CNS) includes the brain and spinal cord. The brain weighs about 3 lb (1.4 kg) and is made up of three major divisions: the cerebrum, cerebellum, and brainstem. The cerebrum is the largest portion of the brain and lies within the forebrain. Its surface, called the *cortex,* is made up of gray matter and is characterized by deep folds and shallow grooves, which increase its surface area. The cerebral cortex, along with other areas of gray matter, is full of neurons as well as specialized support cells called *glia.* The cerebrum also contains white matter, which makes up the bulk of the tissue of the cerebral hemispheres. This white matter is made up of the axons of the neuron. Buried in the white matter are special nuclei, called *basal ganglia.* The cerebrum is divided into two hemispheres, which are mostly separated by a deep, longitudinal fissure but are joined by the corpus callosum.

The cerebellum is located in the inferior posterior portion of the head. It is about the size of a fist and shaped like a walnut. It is sometimes called the "little brain," and, like the cerebrum, has convolutions (although smaller), an outer cortex, inner white matter, and nuclei below the white matter.

The brainstem runs from the forebrain to the spinal cord. It includes the medulla oblongata, pons, and midbrain. The brain is enclosed and protected by the hard bones of the skull, known as the *cranium.*

The spinal cord extends from the base of the brain down to the second lumbar vertebra and is surrounded by the vertebral column. It is divided into sections that correspond to the vertebra and paired spinal nerves. A cross-section of the spinal cord reveals a butterfly-shaped inner core of gray matter, which contains nerve cell bodies. The gray matter is surrounded by white matter that forms ascending and descending pathways called *spinal tracts.*

The brain and the spinal cord are covered by three membranes called the *meninges,* which continue beyond the end of the spinal cord to the distal end of the sacrum. Cerebrospinal fluid is contained between layers of the meninges and circulates around the brain and spinal cord. It is a colorless, clear fluid similar to blood plasma. (See Figure 26-2.)

Peripheral Nervous System

The **Peripheral nervous system** (PNS) includes 31 pairs of spinal nerves, 12 cranial nerves, and nerves in the arms and

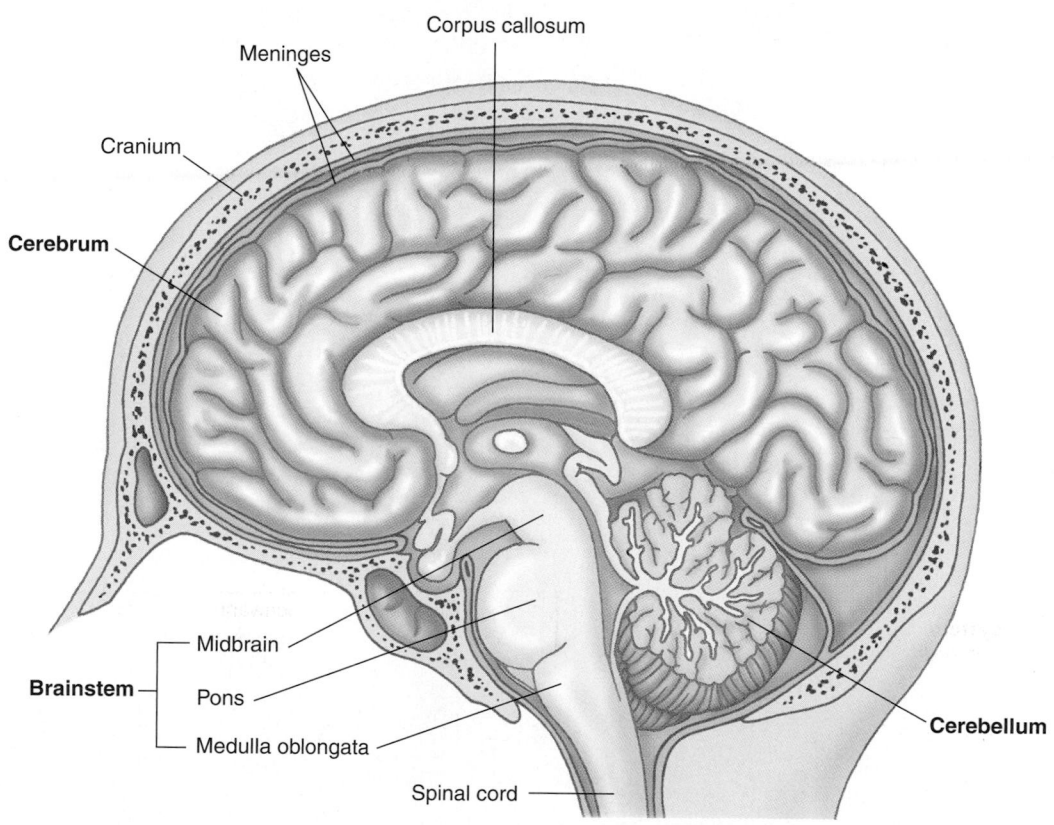

FIG 26-2 Brain.

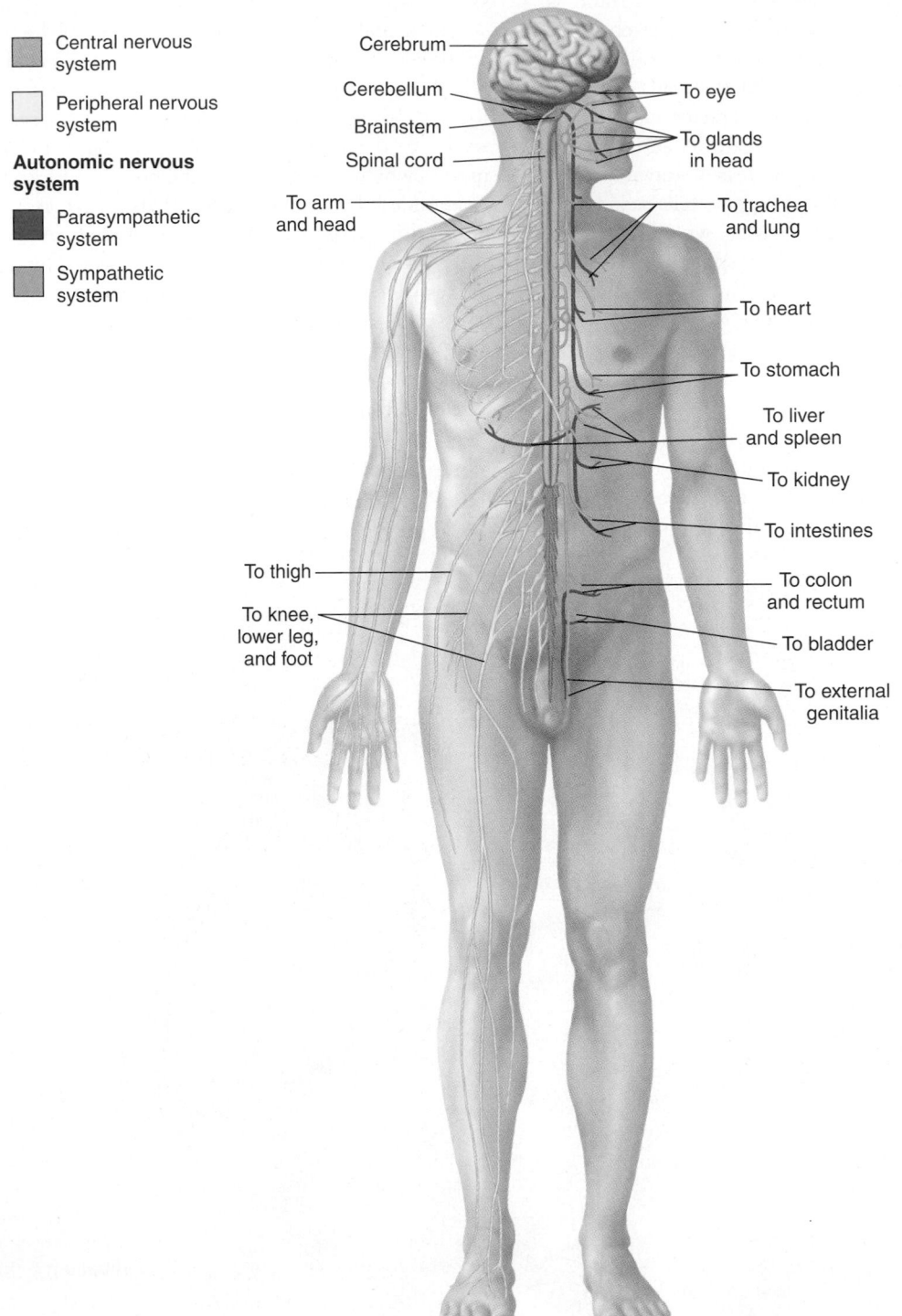

Central nervous system

Peripheral nervous system

Autonomic nervous system

Parasympathetic system

Sympathetic system

Cerebrum

Cerebellum

Brainstem

Spinal cord

To eye

To glands in head

To arm and head

To trachea and lung

To heart

To stomach

To liver and spleen

To kidney

To intestines

To thigh

To colon and rectum

To knee, lower leg, and foot

To bladder

To external genitalia

FIG 26-3 Central and peripheral nervous systems, along with the autonomic nervous system.

legs. The cranial nerves are considered peripheral nerves. Most are called *mixed* nerves because they are made up of sensory and motor neurons. However, some are only sensory or motor. The spinal nerves branch off from either side of the spinal cord between the vertebra. Each spinal nerve is named for and corresponds to the vertebra above it. Spinal nerves are all mixed nerves.

An important part of the PNS is the autonomic nervous system (ANS), which controls involuntary functions. It consists of motor nerves to smooth muscle, cardiac muscle, glands such as sweat glands, and salivary glands. It is further divided into the sympathetic and parasympathetic nervous systems. (See Figure 26-3.)

Functions of the Nervous System

The brain is a complex organ that allows humans to think, reason, express personality, and learn. It is an amazing organ capable of an incredible amount of multitasking. In simple terms, it stores a vast amount of data, processes a wealth of information, controls conscious thought, and keeps all autonomic (automatic) functions working—all at the same time. The spinal cord acts as a messenger, sending information to the brain from the body and from the brain to the body. The functions of the nervous system are organized according to their location in the CNS or the PNS.

Neuron

A neuron works alone or in groups to sense internal and external environmental changes, transmit messages between the brain and body, initiate responses to help maintain the body's state of equilibrium, and facilitate voluntary movement. Dendrites of the neuron, which resemble tree branches, are actually extensions of the cell body and act to sense changes in the body's internal environment by receiving information from other neurons or from sensory receptors and send impulses to the main cell body. Axons are long, cordlike structures that transmit nerve impulses away from the cell body to other neurons, target organs, or muscles. The myelin sheath wrapped around each axon is composed of specialized cells made of a largely lipid substance that provides insulation to the axon, similar to the rubber covering on an electrical cord. The myelin sheath and the interspersed junctions, called *nodes of Ranvier*, allow the axon to function efficiently so that it can conduct impulses at an amazingly rapid rate.

Central Nervous System

The corpus collosum of the cerebrum serves to coordinate activity between the two hemispheres of the cerebrum. The convolutions of the cerebrum increase the surface area where nerve cell bodies are located, thus maximizing their function. The cerebral cortex, or gray matter, of the cerebrum is involved in sensory perception, emotions, and muscle control. The basal ganglia in the white matter of the cerebrum organize motor function. The cerebellum is responsible for posture, balance, and coordination. The brainstem is an essential pathway that conducts impulses between the brain and spinal cord. The cranium provides a strong, hard enclosure that protects the brain from injury.

The spinal cord is the pathway for sensory impulses to the brain from the rest of the body and motor impulses from the brain to the rest of the body. It also mediates stretch reflexes and the defecation and urination reflexes. The vertebral column provides a bony structure to surround and protect the spinal cord. In conjunction with surrounding muscles, it also allows movement of the torso and provides an upright framework for the rest of the skeleton.

The meninges provide a supportive structure for many small blood vessels on the brain's surface. They also provide protection to the brain and spinal cord by housing the cerebrospinal fluid, which continuously circulates and provides a cushion to protect against injury from impact and sudden movement.

Peripheral Nervous System

In the PNS, the 12 cranial nerves originate in the brain and brainstem and innervate such structures as the eyes, ears, nose, face, tongue, and some muscles in the throat and neck. (See Figure 26-4.)

A key function of the 31 pairs of spinal nerves is the innervation of the skin and muscles of the limbs. Specific areas of the skin associated with specific spinal nerves are called *dermatomes*. (See Figure 26-5.) In some disorders, pain or other sensations caused by spinal nerve injury are felt along the associated dermatome, rather than the actual site of injury. Thus, a patient suffering from spinal nerve root compression sometimes feels pain or other symptoms in his arms or legs, rather than his back.

The autonomic nervous system (ANS) within the PNS controls involuntary functions. Its motor nerves control smooth muscle, cardiac muscle, and glands such as sweat glands and salivary glands. Within the ANS, the sympathetic nervous system is responsible for the survival response known as the *fight or flight response*. This response prepares a person for action, whether it is to run from danger or to respond in some other way. The corresponding physical changes within the body include increased heart rate and force, increased blood pressure, increased blood glucose levels, bronchodilation, and decreased peristalsis. These changes provide the body with increased energy and oxygen while slowing some functions (such as digestion) that are less important at the time. The parasympathetic nervous system essentially creates an opposite response and dominates during nonstressful times. Some of its effects include decreased heart rate, bronchoconstriction, and increased peristalsis.

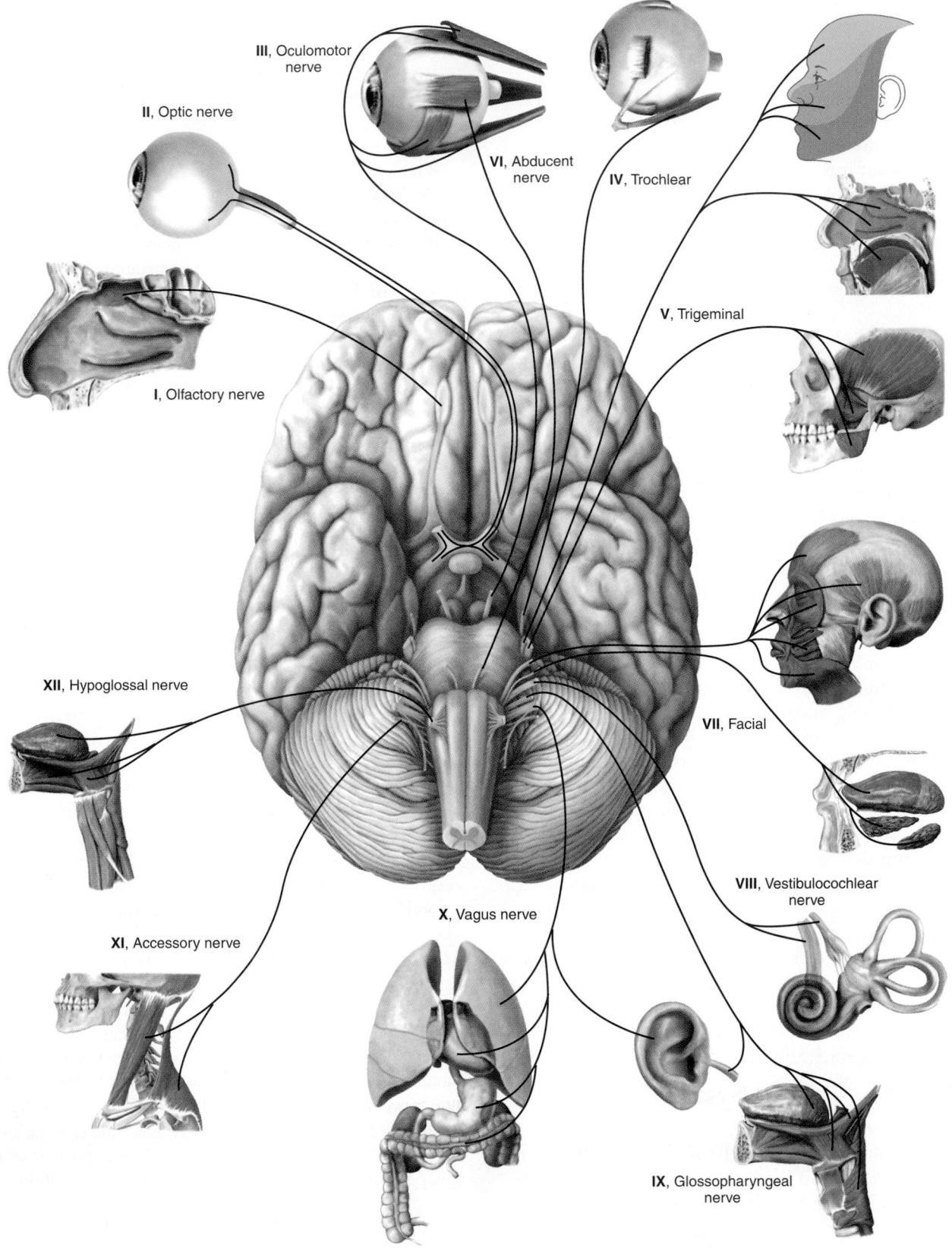

III, Oculomotor nerve

II, Optic nerve

VI, Abducent nerve

IV, Trochlear

V, Trigeminal

I, Olfactory nerve

XII, Hypoglossal nerve

VII, Facial

VIII, Vestibulocochlear nerve

XI, Accessory nerve

X, Vagus nerve

IX, Glossopharyngeal nerve

FIG 26-4 Cranial nerve locations and functions.

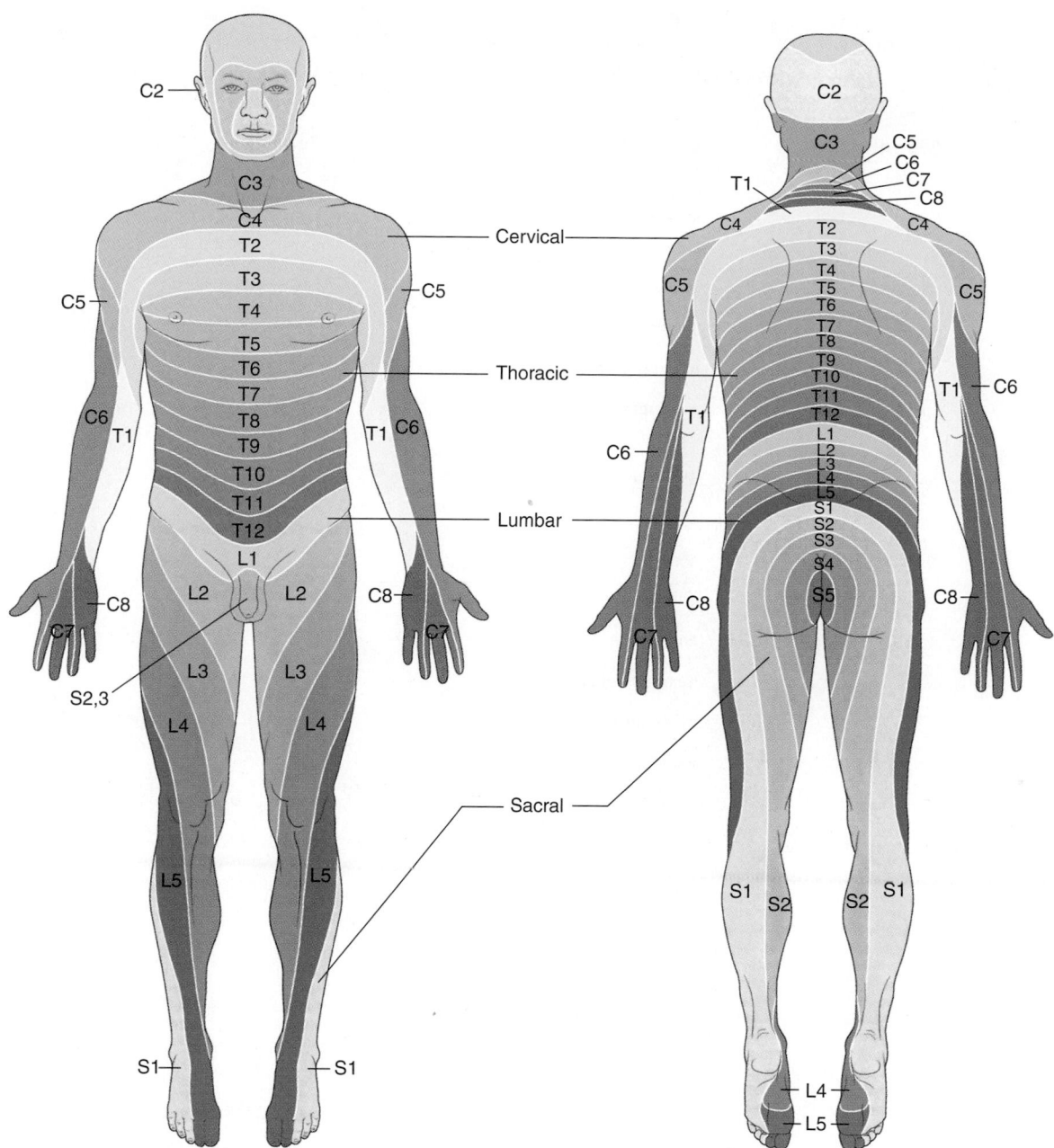

FIG 26-5 Dermatomes.

Medical Terminology Related to the Neurological System

Neurological disorders cause symptoms that are distressing and uncomfortable to the individuals experiencing them, thus leading them to seek help from their health care providers. Whether medical assistants work in family practice offices, urgent care centers, neurology departments, or other areas, they play an important role in the provision of health care to these patients. To be effective in their role, medical assistants must become well versed in the language and vocabulary that pertain to the nervous system. The following tables list common medical terminology related to the nervous system.

Common Nervous System Diseases and Disorders

There are many diseases and disorders affecting the nervous system. Here are some of the most common with

Table 26.1 | **Word Elements**

This table contains combining forms, prefixes, and suffixes that pertain to the nervous system, along with their meanings, and examples with a pronunciation guide and definition.

Word Element	Meaning	Example	Meaning
Combining Forms			
cerebr/o	brain	cerebrovascular (sĕr-ē-brō-VĂS-kū-lăr)	pertaining to the brain and vessels
encephal/o		encephalocele (ĕn-SĔF-ă-lō-sēl)	herniation of the brain
gli/o	glue or gluelike	glioma (glī-Ō-mă)	gluelike tumor
mening/o	meninges	meningitis (mĕn-ĭn-JĪ-tĭs)	inflammation of the meninges
meningi/o		meningioma (mĕn-ĭn-jē-Ō-mă)	tumor of the meninges
myel/o	spinal cord; bone marrow	myelography (mī-ĕ-LŎG-ră-fē)	process of recording activity in the spinal cord or bone marrow
neur/o	nerve	neurocytoma (nū-rō-sī-TŌ-mă)	tumor of nerve cells
spin/o	spine	spinal (SPĪ-năl)	pertaining to the spine
Prefixes			
a-	without, absence of	aphasia (ă-FĀ-zē-ă)	absence of speech
an-	without, absence of	anesthesia (ăn-ĕs-THĒ-zē-ă)	absence of sensation
dys-	painful or difficult	dysphagia (dĭs-FĀ-jē-ă)	painful or difficult swallowing
hemi-	half	hemiplegia (hĕm-ē-PLĒ-jē-ă)	paralysis of half (of the body)
micro-	small	microcephaly (mī-krō-SĔF-ă-lē)	small head
poly-	much, many	polyneuritis (pŏl-ē-nū-RĪ-tĭs)	inflammation of many nerves
para-	beside or near; two	paraplegia (păr-ă-PLĒ-jē-ă)	paralysis of two (legs)
quadri-	four	quadriplegia (kwŏd-rĭ-PLĒ-jē-ă)	paralysis of four (extremities)
Suffixes			
-al	pertaining to	spinal (SPĪ-năl)	pertaining to the spine
-algia	pain	neuralgia (nū-RĂL-jē-ă)	nerve pain
-cele	hernia	meningomyelocele (mĕ-nĭng-gō-MĪ-ĕ-lō-sēl)	herniation of the meninges and spinal cord (spina bifida)
-eal	pertaining to	meningeal (mĕn-ĬN-jē-ăl)	pertaining to the meninges
-esthesia	sensation	hyperesthesia (hī-pĕr-ĕs-THĒ-zē-ă)	increased sensation
-logist	specialist in the study of	neurologist (nū-RŎL-ō-jĭst)	specialist in the study of nerves (nervous system disorders)
-logy	study of	neurology (nū-RŎL-ō-jē)	study of nerves (nervous system disorders)
-paresis	slight or partial paralysis	hemiparesis (hĕm-ē-păr-Ē-sĭs)	slight or partial paralysis of half (of the body)
-pathy	disease	neuropathy (nū-RŎP-ă-thē)	disease of the nerves
-phagia	swallowing	dysphagia (dĭs-FĀ-jē-ă)	painful or difficult swallowing
-phasia	speech	dysphasia (dĭs-FĀ-zē-ă)	difficult speech
-plegia	paralysis	blepharoplegia (blĕf-ă-rō-PLĒ-jē-ă)	paralysis of the eye or eyes
-ptosis	drooping	blepharoptosis (blĕf-ă-rō-TŌ-sĭs)	drooping of the eyelid
-trophy	nourishment or growth	atrophy (ĂT-rō-fē)	absence of growth

Table 26.2 | **Pathologic Terms**

This table lists some of the most common pathologic terms related to the nervous system with a pronunciation guide and brief definition for each.

Term	Definition
amyotrophic lateral sclerosis ă-mī-ō-TRŌ-fĭk LĂT-ĕr-ăl sklĕ-RŌ-sĭs	Chronically progressive, degenerative neuromuscular disorder that destroys motor neurons of the body; also called *Lou Gehrig disease*
Bell palsy BĔL PAWL-zē	Disorder of the seventh cranial nerve that causes temporary weakness or paralysis of one side of the face
carpal tunnel syndrome KĂR-păl TŬN-ĕl SĬN-drōm	Syndrome that is characterized by pain or numbness of the median nerve in the hand and forearm and caused by nerve compression and inflammation due to cumulative trauma from repetitive motion
encephalitis ĕn-sĕf-ă-LĪ-tĭs	Disorder that involves inflammation of the brain
encephalomeningitis ĕn-sĕf-ă-lō-mĕn-ĭn-JĪ-tĭs	Disorder that is a combination of encephalitis and meningitis
epilepsy ĔP-ĭ-lĕp-sē	Chronic disorder of the brain marked by recurrent seizures, which are repetitive, abnormal electrical discharges within the brain
Huntington chorea kō-RĔ-ă	Hereditary nervous disorder that leads to bizarre, involuntary movements and dementia
meningitis mĕn-ĭn-JĪ-tĭs	Infection of the meninges, the spinal cord, and the cerebrospinal fluid, usually caused by an infectious illness
migraine headache MĪ-grān HĔD-āk	Familial disorder marked by episodes of throbbing, severe headache that is commonly unilateral and, sometimes, disabling
multiple sclerosis MŬL-tĭ-pl sklĕ-RŌ-sĭs	Chronic autoimmune disease that affects the central nervous system, causing inflammation and degeneration of the myelin sheath that protects nerve fibers
Parkinson disease PĂR-kĭn-sŏn dĭ-ZĔZ	Chronic, degenerative disease of the central nervous system that results in movement disorders and changes in cognition and mood
peripheral neuropathy pĕr-ĬF-ĕr-ăl nū-RŎP-ă-thē	Dysfunction of nerves that transmit information to and from the central nervous system with resulting pain, altered sensation, and muscle weakness
poliomyelitis pōl-ē-ō-mī-ĕl-Ī-tĭs	Inflammation of the spinal cord caused by a virus, possibly resulting in spinal and muscle deformity and paralysis
sciatica sī-ĂT-ĭ-kă	Severe pain of the sciatic nerve that radiates from the buttocks to the feet
shingles SHĬNG-lz	Unilateral, painful vesicles that appear on the upper body and are caused by the herpes zoster virus
spinal stenosis SPĪ-năl stĕ-NŌ-sĭs	Disorder that involves narrowing of an area of the spine that puts pressure on the spinal cord and nerve roots
stroke STRŌK	Sudden loss of neurological function due to vascular injury to the brain; also called *cerebrovascular accident (CVA)* and *brain attack*
transient ischemic attack TRĂNS-ē-ĕnt ĭs-KĒ-mĭk ă-TĂK	Temporary impairment of neurological functioning due to a brief interruption in blood supply to a part of the brain

Table 26.3 | **Abbreviations**

In neurology, as with other areas of health care, abbreviations are commonly used. Abbreviations such as the ones listed below save time and effort in documentation and written communications.

Abbreviation	Term
ALS	amyotrophic lateral sclerosis, also called *Lou Gehrig's disease*
CNS	central nervous system
CSF	cerebrospinal fluid
CT	computed tomography
CVA	cerebrovascular accident; also called *stroke* or *brain attack*
EEG	electroencephalography
EMG	electromyogram
ICP	intracranial pressure
LP	lumbar puncture
MRI	magnetic resonance imaging
MS	multiple sclerosis
PNS	peripheral nervous system
TIA	transient ischemic attack

a summary of each, along with its corresponding ICD-9 code.

Disorders of the Central Nervous System

Some of the most common diseases and disorders of the central nervous system include stroke, transient ischemic attack, migraine headache, epilepsy, encephalitis, meningitis, traumatic brain injury, spinal cord injury, Parkinson disease, multiple sclerosis, and tumors.

Stroke

ICD-9-CM code: 436

Stroke, also called *cerebrovascular accident (CVA)* and *brain attack,* is the sudden loss of neurological function due to vascular injury to the brain. More than 700,000 individuals suffer from strokes annually in the United States. At greatest risk are those over age 65 with a family history of cerebrovascular disease. Cerebrovascular disease is caused by **atherosclerosis** of cerebral arteries, which is the narrowing and loss of elasticity of vessels due to accumulation of fatty cholesterol deposits.

Strokes are classified as *hemorrhagic* or *ischemic.* Hemorrhagic strokes occur when a vessel in the brain ruptures and bleeds. Risk factors for hemorrhagic strokes include hypertension and the presence of aneurysms, which are weak, bulging areas in a vessel, or arteriovenous malformations (AVMs), which are abnormal clusters of tiny veins connected directly to tiny arteries without a capillary bed between. The cause of ischemic strokes is **thrombotic**, meaning caused by a blood clot, or **embolic**, meaning caused by an embolus, which is a substance in the bloodstream that becomes lodged in a small vessel. (See Figure 26-6.) Risk factors for ischemic stroke include cerebrovascular disease, atrial fibrillation (a type of heart irregularity), tobacco use, alcohol abuse, and clotting disorders.

Signs and symptoms of stroke are highly variable depending on the extent of injury and the specific part of the brain affected. The patient usually exhibits symptoms on the opposite side of the body from the side of the brain injured. A left-sided stroke may cause right-sided paralysis or weakness and a right-sided stroke may cause left-sided symptoms. Other symptoms are usually sudden in onset and may include **paresthesia** (altered sensation, such as numbness, stinging, or burning, that results from injury to nerves) and weakness on one side of the body, vision loss or changes, dysphasia (difficulty speaking or understanding speech), dysphagia (difficulty swallowing), severe headache, dizziness, confusion, altered consciousness, and difficulty with gait (manner of walking) and balance.

Diagnosis is usually based on signs and symptoms. Radiological studies, such as computed tomography (CT), magnetic resonance imaging (MRI), and magnetic resonance angiography (MRA), are used to confirm the diagnosis and differentiate hemorrhagic from ischemic strokes. In the case

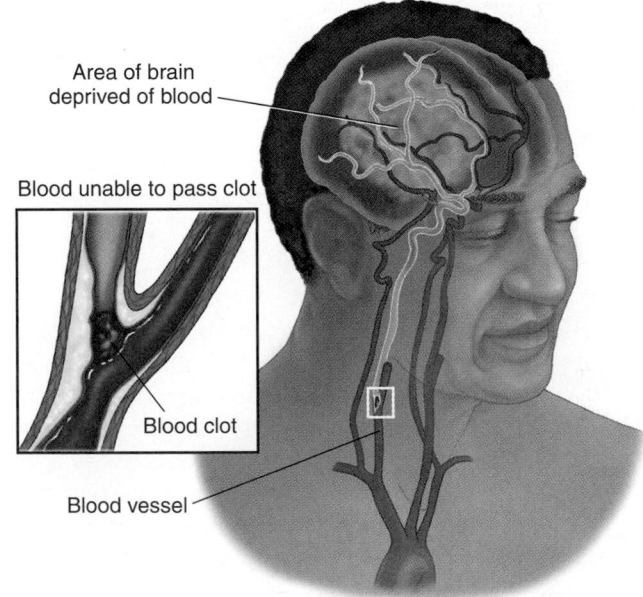

Area of brain deprived of blood

Blood unable to pass clot

Blood clot

Blood vessel

FIG 26-6 Thrombotic stroke.

of a hemorrhagic stroke, lumbar puncture (LP) may reveal the presence of blood in the CSF.

Treatment of ischemic strokes involves the administration of thrombolytic and anticoagulant medications. Thrombolytics are powerful drugs that dissolve blood clots. Anticoagulants are medications that delay or prevent blood clot formation. Criteria for the use of thrombolytic agents are very strict. The drug must be started within a specific time frame, usually 3 hours or less from the onset of symptoms, and cannot be given to anyone at risk for hemorrhage. Anticoagulant medication protects the individual from another stroke while the body heals itself. Treatment of hemorrhagic stroke includes surgery to remove blood clots from the brain and repair identified aneurysms. Other treatment is highly individualized and depends on the type and severity of the stroke and personal factors, such as age and baseline health status. Extended hospitalization may be required. As the patient recovers and enters the rehabilitation phase, emphasis is placed on reestablishing an optimal level of independence in all activities of daily living (ADLs), such as eating, bathing, toileting, dressing, and mobility. The rehabilitation period commonly takes months.

Stroke is the third leading cause of death in the United States. It commonly produces long-term or permanent disability in those who survive. Common deficits include impairment of movement, mobility, and speech. However, many individuals are able to recover significant function with the help of physical, occupational, and speech therapies. (See *Caring for stroke victims*.)

Transient Ischemic Attack

ICD-9-CM code: 435 (use 4th digit to code specific site)
Transient ischemic attack (TIA) is the temporary impairment of neurological functioning due to a brief interruption in blood supply to a part of the brain. Unlike stroke, the impairment is temporary in nature and neurological function is fully restored within minutes or hours. An estimated quarter of a million Americans experience a TIA each year. Rates are higher in Hispanic and African American populations.

TIAs are commonly caused by tiny particles of atherosclerotic plaque or tiny blood clots that dislodge from a heart valve or artery wall and travel in the bloodstream to the brain. Because of their tiny size, they are quickly dissolved by the body's protective mechanisms before permanent damage results. Vascular spasm can also cause TIAs. Risk factors for TIA include cerebrovascular disease, tobacco use, alcohol abuse, hypertension, and clotting disorders.

Signs and symptoms of TIA are variable and temporary. They include one-sided weakness, paresthesias, visual changes or vision loss, dysphasia, dysphagia, dizziness, confusion, altered consciousness, and difficulty with gait and balance. Deficits usually resolve within minutes or hours and signs and symptoms may resolve by the time the patient is evaluated. Therefore, a careful history and description from the patient and any witnesses is essential. Because a TIA is viewed as a possible warning sign of a future stroke, it must be taken seriously.

Diagnostic testing is done to try to determine the cause and may include MRI and CT scans to examine cerebral arteries. Carotid Doppler studies may identify carotid artery narrowing. Treatment of the TIA is not necessary. However, measures to prevent stroke are critical and may include anticoagulant medication, management of hypertension, and surgery to remove carotid artery plaque. Patients are advised to reduce or eliminate modifiable risk factors, such as tobacco and alcohol abuse, as well as lose weight and include regular exercise in their daily routine.

Migraine Headache

ICD-9-CM code: 346.9 (unspecified)
Migraine headaches are a familial disorder marked by episodes of severe throbbing headache that is commonly unilateral and sometimes disabling. They affect more than 28 million Americans and are three times more common in women than in men.

The cause of migraine headaches is not fully understood, although they tend to run in families, are worse early in life, and generally improve in later years. Current theories about causes include involvement of the trigeminal nerve, imbalances in such chemicals as serotonin, and vascular dilation and inflammation. Many risk factors and potential triggers have also been identified, including hormonal changes and such foods as red wine, beer, aged cheese, chocolate, aspartame, and monosodium glutamate. Other triggers include stress, bright lights, fumes, perfumes, smoke, exertion, fatigue, environmental changes, and some medications.

Front office–Back office connection

Caring for Stroke Victims

Patients who suffer from stroke and other neurological injuries receive their early care in the hospital. However, those who recover will return to the medical office for follow-up care. Many of them may be struggling with some residual neurological deficit that impacts their ability to move, process information, respond, and speak. Therefore, medical assistants must remember to be patient, speak clearly, and allow such patients ample time to respond.

Some individuals experience an **aura**, which is a type of sensory warning prior to the onset of the migraine. Auras may include flashes of light, visual changes, or tingling in the arms or legs. Signs and symptoms of migraine headache vary somewhat with the individual but commonly include throbbing pain on one or both sides of the head, nausea with or without vomiting, photophobia (sensitivity to light), and phonophobia (sensitivity to sound). Untreated migraines usually last between 4 and 72 hours. They may occur once a year or as often as every week.

Diagnosis is nearly always based on the patient's description of symptoms and a physical examination. However, if the headaches have a sudden, severe onset or have changed significantly in frequency or character, a more thorough neurological evaluation and diagnostic testing may be warranted. Such tests might include a CT or MRI scan and an LP so that cerebrospinal fluid can be evaluated.

Treatment of migraine headaches has improved dramatically in recent years and numerous medications are now available, including ibuprofen (Motrin), a nonsteroidal anti-inflammatory drug (NSAID), and acetaminophen (Tylenol) and other analgesics. In addition, one of the newer triptans, rizatriptan (Maxalt), helps abort the headache. People who experience more than two migraines per month commonly benefit from preventive medications, such as the antihypertensive lisinopril (Zestril), the antidepressant nortriptyline (Pamelor), and the antiseizure medication valproic acid (Depakote).

In most cases, migraines cannot be totally eliminated. However, the prognosis for most individuals is good. Effective management for each person depends on identifying and eliminating or minimizing exposure to triggers and determining the most effective medication regimen. (See *Caring for patients with migraine*.)

Epilepsy

ICD-9-CM code: 345.90 (unspecified)

Epilepsy is a chronic disorder of the brain marked by recurrent seizures, which are repetitive abnormal electrical discharges within the brain. Epilepsy seizure types have been categorized as *partial, generalized,* or *unclassified.* With generalized seizures, the excessive nervous activity affects both sides of the brain. With partial seizures, also called *focal* or *local* seizures, activity begins in one part of the brain but may occasionally evolve into a generalized seizure.

As many as 2% to 3% or 2.3 million Americans have epilepsy and 125,000 new cases are diagnosed each year. Those most commonly affected are children and those over age 70. The cause of epilepsy is not clear but is thought to result from congenital or acquired brain disease. Various types of stimuli may trigger a seizure, including withdrawal from antiseizure medication, head trauma, illness, emotional or physical stress, fatigue, specific foods and chemicals, and flickering or flashing lights.

Signs and symptoms of epilepsy depend on the type of seizures involved. (See *Types of seizures.*) Diagnosis is based on a history and description of symptoms and a description of the seizure activity. A thorough neurological evaluation is required. A number of diagnostic studies may be done, including electroencephalogram (EEG), CT scan, MRI scan, and LP.

Treatment of epilepsy is aimed at reducing the number and severity of seizures. A variety of medications are available, including phenytoin (Dilantin), phenobarbital (Luminal), carbamazepine (Tegretol), valproic acid (Depakene), and gabapentin (Neurontin). For patients whose epilepsy does not respond to medication, surgical options may be considered, including implanting a vagal nerve stimulator, excision of the brain tissue responsible for triggering the seizures, and **corpuscallosotomy**, in which the central part of the brain, the corpus callosum, is partially divided in two. These surgical procedures effectively reduce the severity and frequency of seizure activity and make the individual more responsive to antiseizure medication. Treatment during an actual seizure should focus on protecting the individual from injury by removing nearby objects and providing privacy (when possible). Nothing should be inserted in the individual's mouth.

The prognosis for epilepsy is generally good depending on the severity of the disorder and how responsive the patient is to treatment. In some cases, the seizures cannot be totally eliminated. However, in most cases, the severity and frequency can be reduced, resulting in an improved quality

---

Front office–Back office connection

Caring for Patients with Migraine

The misery of migraine headaches is difficult to describe and is generally incomprehensible to those who have never had them. A sensitive response by administrative and clinical medical assistants will be greatly appreciated by such patients. Simple but thoughtful measures include:

- quickly escorting the patient to an examination room if one is available
- dimming the lights in the examination room
- offering an ice pack
- keeping noise to a minimum
- asking about nausea
- offering an emesis basin and a cool, wet washcloth.

Types of seizures

The following table lists the most common types of seizures and the defining characteristics of each.

Seizure Type	Characteristics
GENERALIZED SEIZURES	
tonic-clonic (formerly called *grand mal***)**	• Duration: 2 to 5 minutes • Intense muscle tension followed by jerking movements • Loss of consciousness • Bowel and bladder incontinence • Postictal state for up to an hour, characterized by fatigue, lethargy, and confusion
tonic	• Duration: 30 seconds to several minutes • Intense muscle tension • Loss of consciousness
clonic	• Duration: several minutes • Muscle contraction alternating with relaxation
absence (formerly called *petit mal***)**	• Duration: several seconds • Patient appearing to be conscious but is not • No postictal state • More common in children • Familial tendency
myoclonic	• Duration: several seconds • Brief jerking or stiffening of extremities
atonic	• Sudden loss of muscle tone that may cause the patient to fall • Postictal state characterized by confusion
PARTIAL SEIZURES	
complex partial (also called *psychomotor* **or** *temporal lobe***)**	• Duration: 1 to 3 minutes • Loss of consciousness that involves odd behaviors, such as lip smacking, patting, and picking at clothing or other items • No recollection of the event by the patient
simple partial	• Patient remaining conscious • Patient possibly experiencing an aura prior to the seizure, which might include a feeling of déjà vu, an offensive smell, or a painful sensation • Unilateral extremity movement • Unusual sensations • Autonomic symptoms that may include a change in heart rate, flushing, and epigastric discomfort

of life for the patient. A life-threatening complication of epilepsy is status epilepticus, which is characterized by continuous or recurrent seizure activity.

Encephalitis

ICD-9-CM code: 323.9 (unspecified)

Encephalitis is inflammation of the brain and is usually associated with meningitis, which is the inflammation of the meninges. The two combined are known as *encephalomeningitis*. Encephalitis, which affects approximately 20,000 Americans each year, is usually caused by a virus. Those most commonly involved viruses are the arboviruses (group of viruses carried by insects, such as mosquitoes and ticks), herpes virus, AIDS, influenza, measles, chickenpox, and rabies. Some types of fungi and protozoa may also be involved.

Patients with encephalitis may exhibit a wide variety of neurological symptoms, including seizures, fever, abnormal reflexes, muscle weakness, paralysis, and confusion. The individual may eventually lapse into a comatose state. Diagnosis is based on a history and description of signs and symptoms. Cerebrospinal fluid (CSF) is obtained via LP and examined to determine the causative organism. Other diagnostic tests include CT and MRI scans.

Treatment of encephalitis is aimed at the underlying cause. Acyclovir is given for herpesvirus infections and rabies is treated with rabies immune globulin and vaccine. In all cases, treatment is supportive and focuses on managing increased intracranial pressure (ICP) with diuretics and corticosteroids.

The prognosis for encephalitis depends on the timeliness of diagnosis and treatment. In many cases, rehabilitation and therapy is needed for the treatment of residual neurological deficits.

Meningitis

ICD-9-CM code: 322.9 (unspecified)

Meningitis is an infection of the meninges, the spinal cord, and CSF and is usually caused by an infectious illness. The incidence worldwide ranges from 0.5 to 5 per 100,000 individuals. Those at greatest risk include infants and children and those in the military or living in dormitories. Other risk factors include a history of splenectomy, exposure to active and passive tobacco smoke, and exposure to those who are ill with meningitis.

The cause of meningitis is usually viral or bacterial, although fungi, amoebas, or chemical irritation may also be causative factors. The most common infecting organisms include *Streptococcus pneumoniae* and *Niesseria meningitides*. Fortunately, the practice of including the Hib vaccine with childhood immunizations has drastically reduced the incidence of the *Haemophilus influenzae* meningitis. Some types of bacterial and viral meningitis are contagious and may be transmitted through exposure to large-droplet respiratory or oral secretions by coughing or kissing. Those at greatest risk are those who live in the same household or have close physical contact with infected persons.

Common signs and symptoms of meningitis include headache; high fever; stiff, painful neck; nausea; vomiting; photophobia; confusion and fatigue; and seizures. Many of these symptoms may not be obvious in infants, who may exhibit loss of appetite, vomiting, irritability, or lethargy.

Definitive diagnosis is based on examination of CSF, which may appear slightly cloudy due to increased white blood cells, protein, glucose, and bacteria. Most importantly, it will reveal the causative organism in the case of bacterial meningitis. Physical examination findings may include **nuchal rigidity**, which is pain and stiffness of the neck with a resulting reluctance to flex the head forward, a positive **Kernig sign**, which is the reflex contraction and pain in the hamstring muscles when attempting to extend the leg after flexing the hip, and **Brudzinski sign**, in which neck flexion causes flexion of the hips when the patient is lying in a supine position. Deep tendon reflexes are also increased.

Treatment for meningitis must be aggressive to reduce the risk of death and disability. Differentiating bacterial from viral meningitis is important to determine the appropriate treatment and prevent transmission. Furthermore, identifying the specific causative organism in cases of bacterial meningitis is crucial in determining the appropriate antibiotic. Intravenous steroids reduce the risk of death and disability. Other medications may be given to reduce pain, fever, and seizure activity. The patient's room should be kept dark and quiet to reduce environmental stimuli. In the case of bacterial meningitis, family members and those with close direct contact may be treated with antibiotics as a preventive measure.

Viral meningitis is usually less severe than bacterial meningitis with a better prognosis. Bacterial meningitis has a greater risk of causing brain damage, disability, or even death. Mortality rates are between 10% and 40%, with the highest rates in the elderly. Between 11% and 19% of those who survive meningitis will suffer permanent deficits, such as hearing loss, mental retardation, and limb loss.

Traumatic Brain Injury

Cerebral concussion—ICD-9-CM code: 850.9 (unspecified)
Cerebral contusion—ICD-9-CM code: 851

More than 1.5 million Americans suffer from traumatic brain injury each year. Fortunately, approximately 75% of these cases involve only mild concussion. The incidence of head injury is greatest in adolescents, elderly patients, men, and African Americans.

Cerebral concussion is a vague term that refers to a brief loss of consciousness or brief episode of disorientation or confusion following a head injury. ***Cerebral contusion*** refers to bruising of brain tissue and is, therefore, the more severe of the two injuries. The most common cause of cerebral concussion and contusion is a blow to the head, or a ***contrecoup*** type of injury, in which there is a rapid acceleration followed by deceleration that throws the brain forward and backward within the skull. As a result, delicate brain tissue and small vessels may be torn by the force or cut by sharp protrusions within the bony cranium. (See Figure 26-7.)

Cerebral concussion usually results in a brief episode of loss of consciousness, confusion, or disorientation. Other temporary symptoms may include headache, drowsiness,

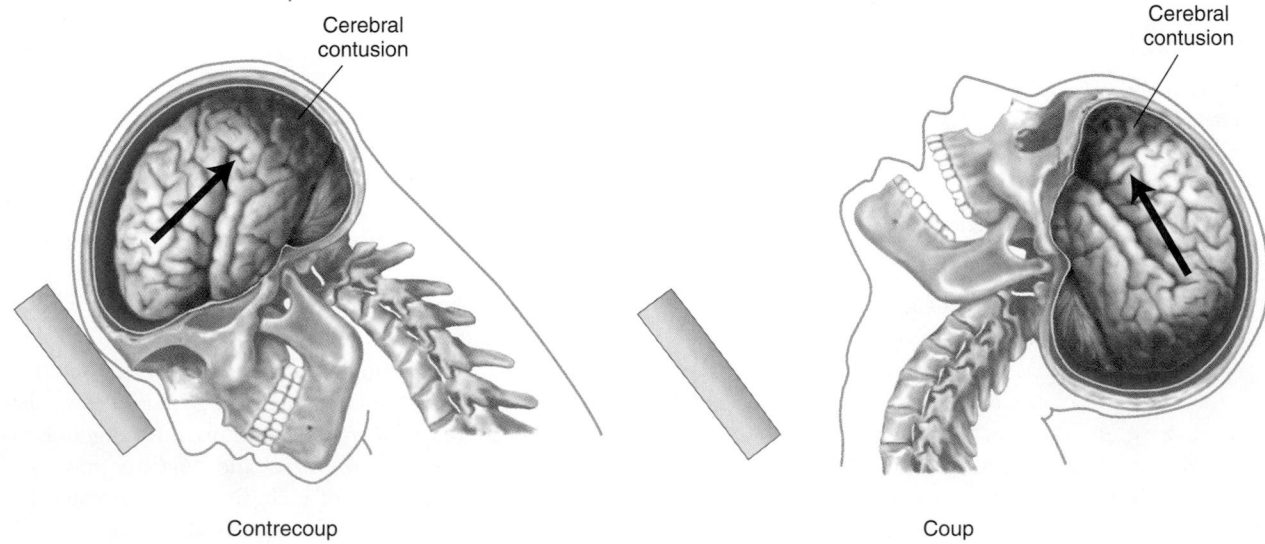

Cerebral contusion

Cerebral contusion

Contrecoup

Coup

FIG 26-7 Brain injury. (A) Contrecoup. (B) Coup.

and visual changes. The symptoms of contusion are generally more severe due to tiny cerebral hemorrhages and edema and include more prolonged loss of consciousness, memory problems, and vomiting.

Diagnosis is based on neurological evaluation as well patient signs and symptoms. A CT scan is recommended for those with loss of consciousness lasting more than 1 minute or those with deteriorating neurological status. A CT scan revealing a "salt and pepper" appearance caused by tiny hemorrhages confirms the diagnosis of cerebral contusion. Spinal films should also be done to rule out spinal injury.

Treatment of mild concussion is conservative and usually involves rest and analgesics. Treatment of severe concussion and cerebral contusions is more aggressive and hospitalization is usually required. The focus of care is on reducing and managing intracranial pressure (ICP), which can contribute to further brain injury if it rises too high.

Prognosis is good with mild concussion. Those with more severe concussion may develop post-concussion syndrome, which includes memory problems, depression, and dizziness. The prognosis for cerebral contusion is more guarded, with a risk of escalating ICP and microhemorrhages progressing to hematoma. In either case, compression of the brain increases the risk of further injury with a higher likelihood of permanent neurological deficit.

Spinal Cord Injury

ICD-9-CM code: 344.1 (paraplegia), 344.0 (quadriplegia)
Spinal cord injury involves traumatic bruising, crushing, or tearing of the spinal cord. **Transection** (cutting) of the spinal cord may be partial or complete, depending on the mechanism of injury (means by which injury occurred). Approximately 14,000 individuals in the United States suffer from acute spinal cord injury each year and another 300,000 to 400,000 are living with some degree of chronic disability as a result of spinal cord injury. More than 80% of acute spinal cord injury patients are young adult white males. Alcohol or mood altering drugs are a factor in more than half of all spinal cord injuries.

The cause of spinal cord injury is some type of traumatic force, most commonly a motor vehicle accident. Other causes include violence in the form of shootings and stabbings, falls, and injuries from sports, such as diving and football.

Initial signs and symptoms of spinal cord injury include loss of function, sensation, and reflexes below the site of the injury. However, with time and medical care, some return of function may occur. The degree of permanent deficit is widely variable and depends on the location, extent, and nature of the injury. Some individuals with relatively minor injury may regain full function, while others may be left permanently paralyzed from the neck down.

Diagnosis of spinal cord injury is based on a thorough neurological evaluation and radiological studies, including x-rays of the spine, CT scan, and MRI. Treatment involves stabilization of the patient in the emergency department, followed by transfer to the critical care unit. The spinal cord and vertebrae may be stabilized by application of Gardener-Wells tongs and traction. (See Figure 26-8.) This stabilization protects the spinal cord from further damage until the patient is deemed stable enough for surgery. During surgery, bone fragments and hematomas are removed and the spine is stabilized through **spinal fusion**, which is the surgical immobilization of adjacent vertebrae by grafting bone or insertion of hardware. Subsequently, application of a halo traction brace may enable increased mobility. (See Figure 26-9.)

Victims of spinal cord injury suffer from profound, life-altering injury as well as severe emotional trauma. The long-term prognosis varies and depends on the location, type, and severity of injury. In general, the higher the injury occurs on the spinal cord, the more severe the consequences and the more grim the prognosis. As the patient moves into the rehabilitation phase, emphasis is placed on restoration of optimal function and independence. Rehabilitation takes many months. Many patients require special medical care and must pay careful attention to self-care for the remainder of their lives in order to avoid such complications as pressure ulcers and autonomic dysreflexia. The eventual causes of death for those who survive the initial injury include pneumonia, pulmonary embolism, and kidney failure. (See *Autonomic dysreflexia*, page 450.)

Parkinson Disease

ICD-9-CM code: 32.0
Parkinson disease is a chronic degenerative disease of the central nervous system that results in movement disorders

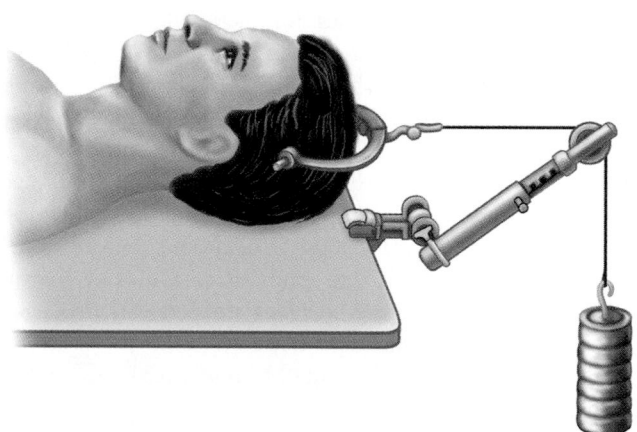

FIG 26-8 Patient with Gardener-Wells tongs and traction.

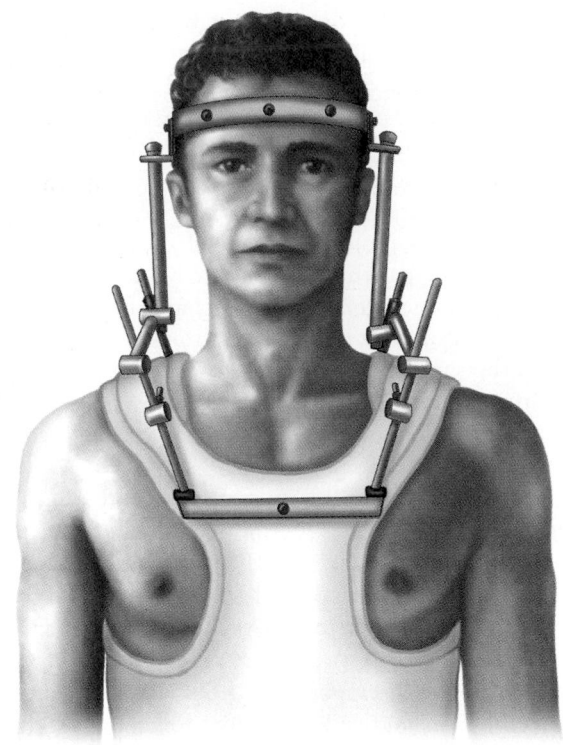

FIG 26-9 Patient with halo brace.

and changes in cognition and mood. It affects 1.5 million Americans, is most common in patients over age 65, and is more common in men than women.

The cause of Parkinson disease is not fully understood; however, it does tend to cluster in families. The symptoms are caused by a deficiency of dopamine. Dopamine is a type of **neurotransmitter**, which is a chemical released by an axon terminal to inhibit or excite a target cell. Neurotransmitters play an important role in nerve impulse transmission. With a deficiency in these neurotransmitters, nerve impulse transmission becomes dysfunctional.

Early symptoms of Parkinson disease include gradual onset of aching and fatigue in the extremities followed by resting hand tremor. Muscle rigidity develops and the classic, pill-rolling tremor of the hands becomes prominent. The face develops a masklike, nonexpressive appearance and the voice becomes softer and quieter. **Bradykinesia**, a slow, hesitating pattern of movement, develops. In addition, the individual develops a shuffling gait that tends to speed out of control with walking. The posture becomes stooped with the neck bent forward. The individual develops difficulty initiating movements, such as standing up or turning over in bed. Swallowing difficulty is common and difficulty in managing oral secretions may eventually cause drooling. In some cases, mental slowing also occurs.

Autonomic dysreflexia

Autonomic dysreflexia is a potentially life-threatening complication for patients with spinal cord injury. The most common triggers are bowel distention, caused by constipation, or bladder distention, caused by urinary retention. The effects of autonomic dysreflexia are immediate and profound. Unless the patient gets immediate attention, autonomic dysreflexia may progress to a stroke. The best way for individuals to avoid this life-threatening complication is to maintain regular and effective bowel and bladder elimination patterns.

The most common symptoms of autonomic dysreflexia are:

- hypertension
- profuse sweating above the spinal cord lesion
- severe, throbbing headache
- blurred vision
- apprehension
- nausea.

Diagnosis is based on presenting signs and symptoms and a thorough neurological evaluation. Dopamine levels in urine may be decreased. There is no known cure for Parkinson disease. Medical treatment includes levodopa-carbidopa (Sinemet) and other dopamine agonists. Other medications may be given to reduce oral secretions, tremor, and muscle rigidity. A multidisciplinary team approach is required to help the patient and family cope with this disabling disease.

Because Parkinson disease is a progressive, degenerative disorder with no known cure, the outlook may be disheartening for those affected. Average life expectancy from the time of diagnosis is 10 years. However, many individuals live much longer and, with supportive care, are able to maintain a good quality of life.

Multiple Sclerosis
ICD-9-CM code: 340

Multiple sclerosis (MS) is thought to be a chronic autoimmune disease. Autoimmune diseases occur when the body's immune system loses the ability to distinguish its own "self" cells from foreign or "non-self" cells. As a result, the immune system attacks the cells and tissues that it has misidentified. In the case of multiple sclerosis, the autoimmune disorder affects the central nervous system and causes inflammation and degeneration of the myelin sheath that protects nerve fibers. Attacks are usually episodic, resulting in repetitive episodes of disrupted nerve impulse conduction. There are several different types of MS; however, the most common is the relapsing-remitting type, which affects 85% of patients with MS. It is characterized by increasingly frequent attacks in which the individual experiences worsening symptoms alternating with periods of remission.

Approximately 500,000 people in the United States have been diagnosed with MS. It is twice as common in women than men, with typical onset between the ages of 20 and 40. It is also more common in cold climates.

The cause of MS is not fully understood, although it is thought to have an autoimmune basis. The immune system mistakenly recognizes the myelin sheath of nerve fibers as foreign and attacks it. Degeneration and malfunction occurs as a result. Triggers for MS include infections, viruses, and pregnancy. There is a familial component; children of patients with MS are 15 times more likely to develop MS than the average person.

Symptoms of MS vary widely and may include weakness, fatigue, muscle spasms, altered gait, tremors, bowel and bladder dysfunction, sexual dysfunction, vertigo, tinnitus (ringing, buzzing, tinkling, or hissing sound in the ear), hearing loss, visual changes, altered sensation, dysphasia, dysphagia, anxiety, mood fluctuations, short-term memory deficits, inattentiveness, and impaired judgment.

Diagnosing MS commonly takes time because the symptoms are intermittent and variable and other disorders must be ruled out. This process can be frustrating to patients. Diagnostic studies include MRI and CT scans, which indicate the presence of MS plaques.

There is currently no cure for MS. Acute exacerbations may be treated with corticosteroids. Some medications may reduce the frequency and severity of relapses for some types of MS. However, they are expensive and not effective in every case. Therefore, therapy must be individualized. Patients with MS must develop a plan of self-care in which the focus is protection of the immune system. Regular, moderate exercise; good nutrition; adequate rest; and minimizing stress are all key components of such a plan.

Prognosis for patients with MS varies and depends on the type of MS involved. In general, life expectancy is less than that of the general population.

Brain Tumor
ICD-9-CM code: 239.6

Tumor is a vague term used to describe any type of abnormal mass or growth of tissue that is different from neighboring tissue. A brain tumor is any type of abnormal mass growing within the cranium.

Approximately 190,000 Americans are diagnosed with brain tumors each year. They are more common among populations of industrialized countries and among Whites.

The composition of brain tumors varies with the type and there are more than 120 different types. Examples include cysts, abscesses, and a variety of benign and cancerous growths. Most are named for the tissue from which they originate and approximately half result from cancer that has spread from another site in the body. The specific cause of many types of brain tumors is unknown.

Signs and symptoms of brain tumors are usually related to the pressure exerted on surrounding structures and increased ICP. Such signs and symptoms include headaches, seizures, nausea, vomiting, loss of consciousness, memory problems, personality changes, muscle weakness, sensory loss, aphasia, alterations in gait and balance, and visual disturbances.

Diagnosis of brain tumor is based on a description of signs and symptoms, a thorough neurological evaluation, a medical history, and results of an MRI or CT scan. Examination of CSF may reveal cancerous cells, indicating spread of the cancer to the spinal cord. Edema of the optic nerve may be apparent on ophthalmic examination. Study of tissues obtained through surgery or biopsy determine whether the growth is cancerous or benign.

Treatment for brain tumors depends on the type and location of the tumor. When possible, a tumor may be surgically removed. In any case, measures are taken to relieve ICP and associated symptoms. Antiseizure medication is given to treat or prevent seizures and corticosteroids may be given to decrease inflammation, thereby decreasing ICP. When the tumor is cancerous, surgery is usually followed with chemotherapy or radiation therapy.

Prognosis depends on the type and location of the tumor. The general 5-year survival rate is just over 30%. However, the outcome is generally more favorable for younger patients, those with small tumor size, those with absence of mental changes at the time of diagnosis, and those in which the entire tumor is successfully removed. Survival rate is nearly 70% in children; however, many of them live with some degree of permanent neurological deficit caused by the tumor or adverse effects of treatment.

Disorders of the Peripheral Nervous System

Some of the most common diseases and disorders of the peripheral nervous system include amyotrophic lateral sclerosis, Bell palsy, peripheral neuropathy, carpal tunnel syndrome, and spinal stenosis.

Amyotrophic Lateral Sclerosis
ICD-9-CM code: 335.20

Amyotrophic lateral sclerosis (ALS), also called *Lou Gehrig's disease,* is a chronic, progressive, degenerative neuromuscular disorder that destroys motor neurons of the body. It affects approximately 30,000 Americans with 5,600 new cases diagnosed each year. Men are affected more than women, and Whites are more commonly affected. Typical onset is between the ages of 40 and 70. The cause of ALS is unclear, although one form that affects approximately 10% of ALS patients is hereditary.

ALS affects the motor nerves of the body and usually leaves sensory nerves and cognitive function intact. The typical course involves muscle weakness and fatigue that begins in the extremities and progresses to the trunk and head. It eventually affects respiratory muscles and muscles of the head, neck, and face. As a result, individuals become progressively paralyzed and eventually experience difficulty with breathing, speech, and swallowing. Life expectancy is only about 5 years from the time of diagnosis. Death is usually due to respiratory complications.

There is no specific diagnostic test for ALS. Therefore, the diagnosis is achieved by ruling out other disorders. A thorough neurological evaluation and medical history are required. EMG and nerve conduction velocity (NCV) may reveal muscle **fasciculations** (visible, involuntary twitching of muscle fibers) and **fibrillations** (quivering or spontaneous contraction of muscle fibers). Muscle biopsy reveals atrophy.

There is currently no cure for ALS. Survival time may be extended by use of riluzole (Rilutek), a medication approved for the treatment of ALS. The focus of care is on supportive, palliative care with the goal of helping the individual to maintain an optimal level of independent function. Palliative care is care that attempts to relieve pain and suffering but does not provide a cure. Priority must be given to protecting respiratory function. Medications may be used to decrease muscle spasticity and pain and to reduce oral secretions. A multidisciplinary approach to care is essential and should involve the patient, patient's family, physician, nurses, medical assistants, therapists, case managers, and hospice workers. The patient and family should be given information about community resources, support groups, and advance directives.

Bell Palsy
ICD-9-CM code: 351.0
Bell palsy is a disorder of the seventh cranial nerve that causes temporary weakness or paralysis of one side of the face. It usually comes on suddenly and takes months to resolve. It affects approximately 40,000 individuals each year in the United States. It is equally common in men and women and is most common between the ages of 15 and 60. It is more common among pregnant women and patients with diabetes or upper respiratory infections.

Bell palsy occurs when the seventh cranial nerve becomes inflamed, swollen, and compressed. The underlying cause is unknown; however, it is believed that a virus may serve as the triggering event.

Symptoms of Bell palsy vary somewhat. In most cases, there is some degree of paralysis that causes drooping of the facial features on the affected side. (See Figure 26-10.) Other symptoms may include twitching, weakness, drooling, eye dryness, impaired taste, excessive tearing, headache, ringing in the ears, and difficulty eating or drinking.

Diagnosis is based on the patient's signs and symptoms. A neurological examination is required. An EMG test will detect nerve damage. CT scan, MRI, and skull x-rays may be done to rule out other disorders.

There is no cure for Bell palsy. However corticosteroids may be given to decrease inflammation and swelling. Antiviral medications may be given if a viral cause is suspected. Analgesics and warm, moist compresses may help relieve pain. Because the individual may be unable to effectively blink or close the eye, measures must be taken to protect the eye and keep it moist, including use of artificial tears and an eye patch.

The prognosis for those with Bell palsy is very good. Recovery is complete in most cases but may take as long as 6 months. In some cases, the symptoms may never fully resolve and, in a very small number of cases, the paralysis may be permanent. Recurrences are rare.

Peripheral Neuropathy
ICD-9-CM code: 356.9
Peripheral neuropathy is a dysfunction of nerves that transmit information to and from the brain and spinal cord.

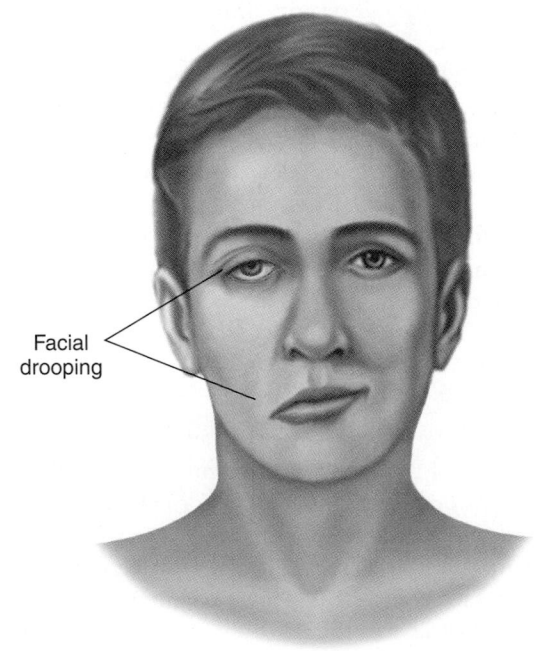

Facial drooping

FIG 26-10 Bell palsy.

The disorder is characterized by pain, altered sensation, and muscle weakness. It may affect a single nerve or nerve group or may affect multiple nerves. Experts do not agree about the definition of peripheral neuropathy, which makes its incidence difficult to estimate. However, they all agree that it is extremely common.

The cause of peripheral neuropathy is not clear. However, a number of disorders are associated with it, including diabetes, alcoholism, AIDS, rheumatoid arthritis, systemic lupus erythematosus (SLE), ingestion of toxic substances and some drugs, and nerve injury from prolonged immobility or compression.

The symptoms of peripheral neuropathy may be motor, sensory, or both and vary widely depending on the nerve or nerves affected. The most common sensory symptoms are nerve pain and numbness. Motor symptoms include weakness, muscle twitching, atrophy, muscle cramps, loss of movement, and loss of coordination. Damage to autonomic nerves that impact involuntary or semivoluntary functions may result in such signs and symptoms as blurred vision, dizziness, diarrhea, constipation, urinary incontinence, and impotence, among others.

Diagnosis is based on a detailed history and neurological examination. Tests may include an EMG, nerve conduction tests, and nerve biopsy. Blood tests may be done to identify or rule out underlying medical disorders, such as diabetes or nutritional deficits.

Therapy is individualized depending on the symptoms. Goals include treating underlying disorders or nutritional deficiencies. Physical and occupational therapy may help build muscle strength and coordination. Braces, splints, or mobility aids may improve independence. Emphasis is placed on safety with a goal of preventing falls or injuries to extremities with decreased sensation. Such medications as analgesics, anticonvulsants, and antidepressants may help alleviate pain.

The prognosis for peripheral neuropathy is variable, depending on the specific cause. In cases where an underlying disorder can be cured or treated, the outlook is positive. However, in some cases, nerve damage is permanent.

Carpal Tunnel Syndrome

ICD-9-CM code: 354.0

Carpal tunnel syndrome is a common type of entrapment neuropathy that occurs when the median nerve in the forearm and hand becomes compressed or irritated as a result of inflammation. It is three times more common in women than men. Also at risk are persons with diabetes or other metabolic disorders that affect the peripheral nerves.

Carpal tunnel syndrome occurs as a result of increased pressure on the median nerve, which runs down the forearm into the wrist. (See Figure 26-11.) In some cases, the problem has a congenital cause, meaning the carpal tunnel,

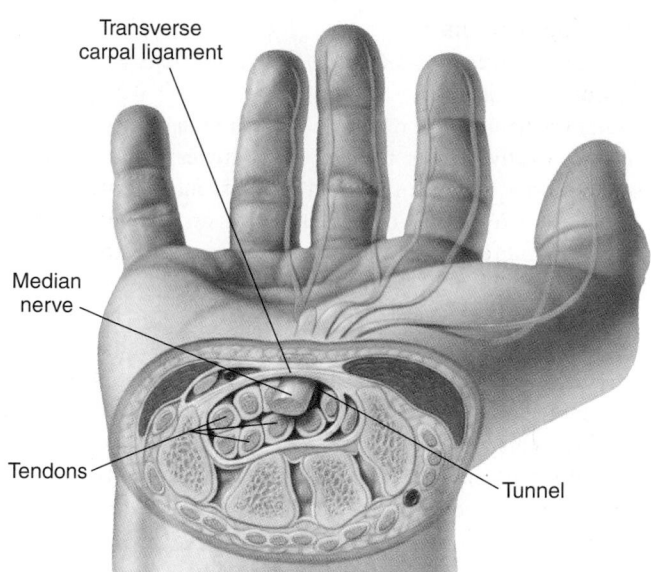

FIG 26-11 Carpal tunnel syndrome.

through which the median nerve travels, is smaller in some people. Contributing factors include injury to the wrist, rheumatoid arthritis, and work stress in which the wrist is subjected to vibrations or repetitive movements. Carpal tunnel syndrome is especially common in individuals who perform assembly-line work, such as sewing, manufacturing, cleaning, or packing meat.

Symptoms of carpal tunnel syndrome begin gradually, increase over time, and are commonly worse at night. They include tingling, itching, weakness, numbness, and pain that radiates up the arm.

Diagnosis is usually based on signs and symptoms and physical examination. The wrist may be tender, warm, red, and swollen. Diagnosis can be confirmed with a nerve conduction study and ultrasound.

Treatment for carpal tunnel syndrome begins with treating an underlying cause such as arthritis. Initial treatment is usually conservative and includes resting the wrist by splinting or avoidance of exacerbating activities. In addition, cool packs and NSAIDs may help relieve inflammation and pain. Corticosteroids may be taken orally or injected directly into the wrist to relieve inflammation. Some individuals find that chiropractic and acupuncture treatments are helpful. Yoga has been found useful in decreasing pain and increasing grip strength. The carpal tunnel release surgical procedure is recommended for those whose symptoms last longer than 6 months and who have not found relief with other measures. The surgery does not require hospitalization and can be done under local anesthesia. Recovery is usually complete but can take several months. Recurrence is uncommon.

Spinal Stenosis

ICD-9-CM code: 956.0 (sciatic nerve injury), 724.00 (spinal stenosis)

Spinal stenosis is the narrowing of an area of the spine. It most typically affects the upper or lower back and puts pressure on the spinal cord and spinal nerve roots. (See Figure 26-12.) It currently affects an estimated half a million Americans and is most common in those over age 50.

In some cases, patients are born with spinal stenosis. However, it usually develops later in life, secondary to degenerative changes associated with aging. Primary contributors include osteoarthritis, disk herniation, ligament changes, misalignment of the vertebra, spinal tumors, traumatic injuries, and disorders of bone tissue formation. Any of these conditions can result in compression of spinal cord or spinal nerve roots, causing the associated symptoms.

Signs and symptoms of spinal stenosis vary, depending on the severity and the specific location. Patients commonly experience pain, numbness, or cramping in the legs, back, neck, shoulders, or arms. Patients may also complain of decreased sensation in the extremities, balance problems, and bowel and bladder dysfunction.

Diagnosis of spinal stenosis is based on medical history, description of signs and symptoms, and a thorough examination of the spine. Radiologic studies help confirm the diagnosis and may include spinal x-rays, MRI, CT scan, CT myelogram, and bone scan.

Nonsurgical interventions for spinal stenosis include NSAIDs (such as ibuprofen) and analgesics (such as acetaminophen) for pain as well as rest; moderate exercise; physical therapy; wearing a back brace or corset; epidural steroid injection; and an anesthetic injection known as *nerve block*. Surgical options, which usually provide long-term relief, include decompressive laminectomy, laminotomy, and spinal fusion.

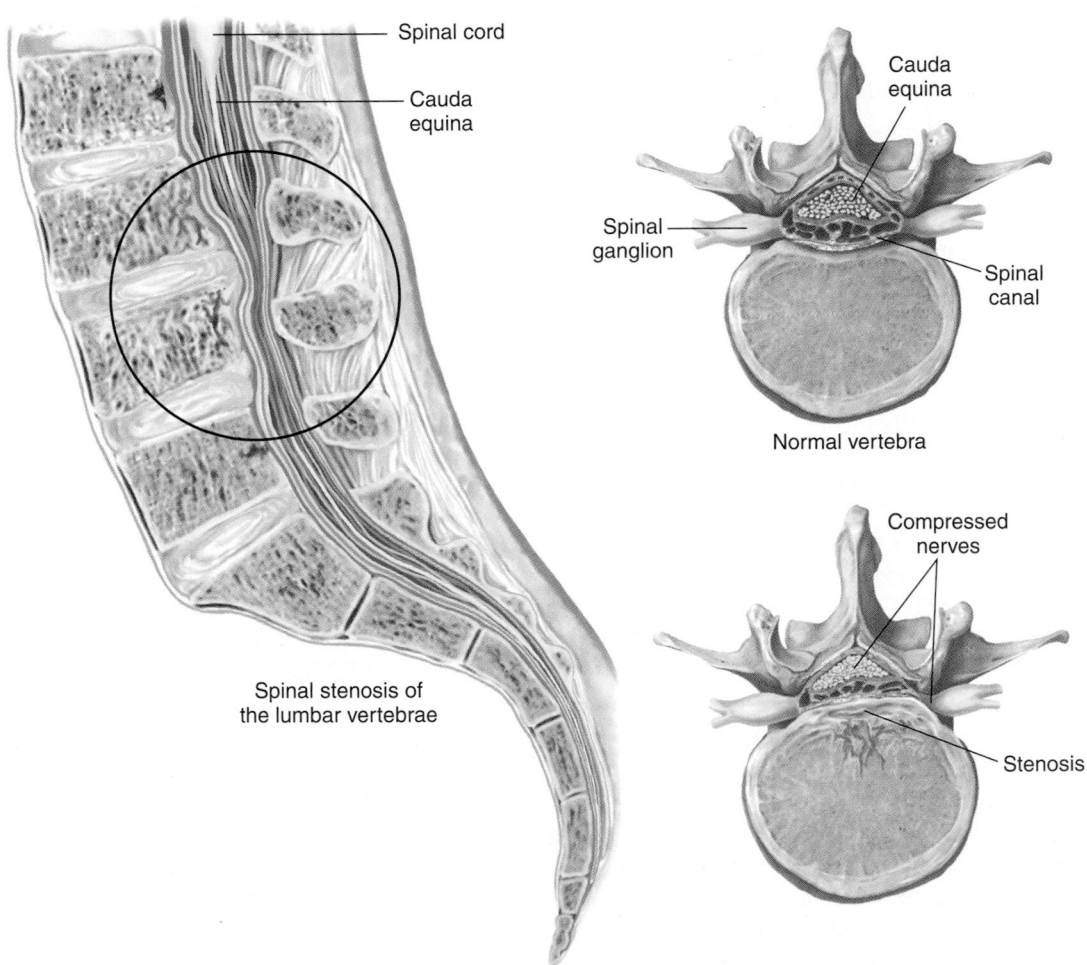

FIG 26-12 Spinal stenosis.

Neurology Procedures

Neurology is a medical specialty that focuses on the study and treatment of diseases and disorders of the nervous system. A physician who specializes in this area of medicine is a neurologist.

Assisting with Examination

The medical assistant must prepare the patient for neurological evaluation by first checking vital signs and updating health history, including data regarding medications, allergies, family history, and recent symptoms of concern to the patient. In addition, the medical assistant should pay special attention to subtle clues about neurological functioning and possible deficits. While it is the neurologist's role to conduct a thorough neurological evaluation, any significant observations made by the medical assistant might help the physician identify issues of special concern. Thus, the medical assistant should note the patient's general appearance, hygiene, dress, and **affect**, which is the emotional reaction associated with an experience (also called *mood*). She should note whether the patient understands and responds appropriately to questions and commands, as well as any difficulty with short-term memory and disturbances in gait, movement, strength, coordination, or speech. She should then assist the patient as needed with undressing and positioning and also assist the neurologist as needed with the examination and any procedures. (See *Procedure 26-1: Assisting with a neurological examination,* page 456.)

Nervous System Tests

The medical assistant working in the neurology department may help with patient evaluations by conducting or assisting with a variety of diagnostic procedures. Each of these procedures helps to evaluate the patient's condition and to gather data necessary for the diagnosing and treatment of neurological disorders.

Electroencephalography

Electroencephalography is the process of amplifying, recording, and analyzing the electrical activity of the brain. The printed record obtained is called an electroencephalogram (EEG). A variety of electrodes are placed at specific locations on the patient's scalp. (See Figure 26-13.) The machine then records the electrical activity at each site and measures the difference in activity between various sites. In resting adults the most common waveform is called the *alpha rhythm* and it includes $8^{1}/_{2}$ to 12 waves per second. Characteristic waveform changes occur depending on whether the individual is sleeping, awake and restful, or concentrating. In some cases, neurological diseases may

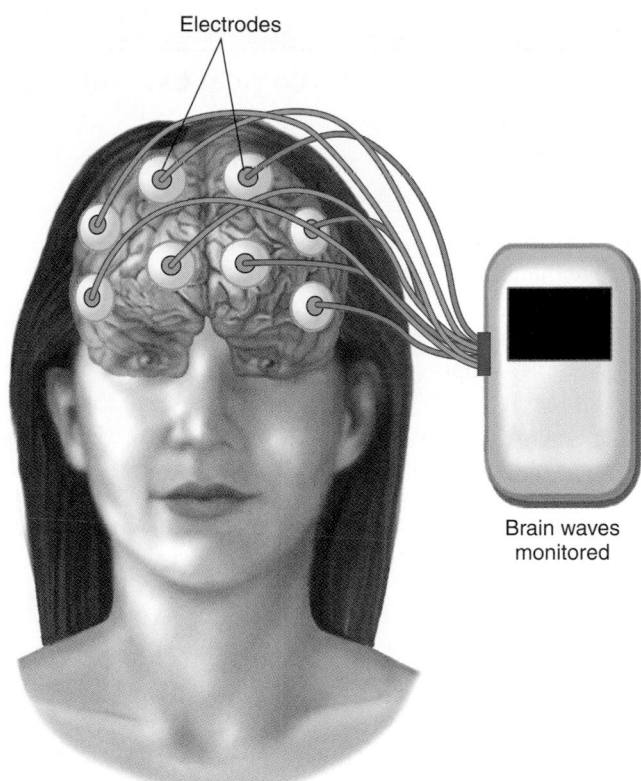

FIG 26-13 Patient undergoing EEG testing.

cause waveform changes. For example, *delta waves* are slow, irregular waves normally found only in infants, small children, and sleeping adults. They are an abnormal finding in wakeful adults. *Theta waves* are slow, regular waves that indicate a decline in brain function. A *flatline* EEG indicates an absence of brain activity and is part of the criteria for determining brain death. (See Figure 26-14.) EEG has

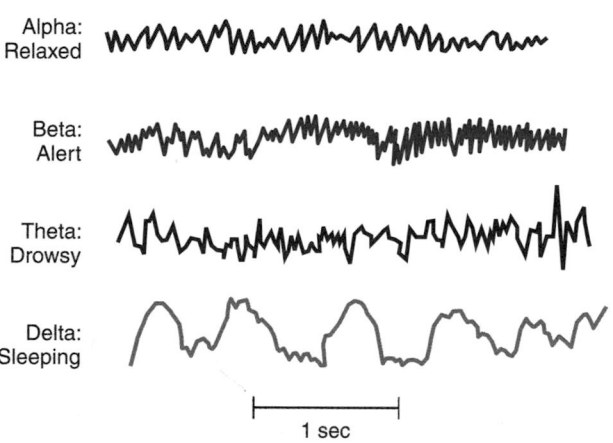

FIG 26-14 EEG wave patterns.

PROCEDURE 26-1

Assisting with a neurological examination

Task
Prepare the patient for and assist the physician with a complete neurological examination.

Conditions
- Examination table
- Drape
- Patient examination gown
- Specific supplies and equipment including but not limited to:
  - neurology reflex hammer
  - safety pin
  - otoscope
  - ophthalmoscope
  - penlight
  - tongue blade
  - tuning fork
  - pinwheel
  - cotton ball
  - items for testing heat and cold sensation per physician's instructions
  - small containers of sweet and salty solutions per physician's instructions
  - items for odor identification per physician's instructions.

Standards
In the time specified and within the scoring parameters determined by the instructor, the student will successfully assist with a neurological examination.

Performance Standards

1. Complete preliminary steps as for any general physical examination. Assist the patient into positions as instructed by the physician. Arrange the drape for warmth and privacy.
2. As the physician examines the patient, be prepared to hand him items as needed, such as the otoscope, ophthalmoscope, penlight, and tongue depressor.

3. Dim the lights if directed when the physician examines the patients' eyes to help the patients' eyes dilate.
4. Throughout the remainder of the examination, continue to assist the patient in assuming the positions directed by the physician and continue to hand needed items to the physician.
5. Follow standard precautions and take care when receiving any potentially contaminated items from the physician (such as the tongue depressor, speculum, or swabs) and handle them in a manner that prevents exposure to you.
6. Dispose of all waste in appropriate containers.
7. Place any obtained specimens in appropriately labeled containers.
8. Upon completion of the examination, assist the patient down from the table and instruct her to get dressed. Leave the room for a few minutes so the patient may change in privacy unless she requires your assistance to protect and respect the patient's safety and privacy.
9. Schedule any ordered follow-up tests or appointments.
10. Direct the patient back to the reception area. Assist her if needed.
11. Document patient education, instructions, or scheduled tests in the medical record to ensure that the medical record is thorough and accurate.
12. Clean, sanitize, and restock the examination room as needed so that the room will be ready for the next patient.

Date	
04/23/09; 11:55 a.m.	*Neurological examination completed by Dr. Lee. EEG scheduled for 4/24/09 at 8:10 a.m. ------------------------------------- S. Gonzales. CMA*

been especially useful in the evaluation of seizure disorders and locating lesions within the brain.

Lumbar Puncture
Lumbar puncture (LP) is a procedure in which a hollow needle is inserted into the subarachnoid space below the end of the spinal cord, usually at the L3 to L4 intervertebral space. (See Figure 26-15.) The needle is used to withdraw CSF for analysis, inject dye, or drain fluid in order to relieve

pressure. Presence of blood in the CSF might indicate a stroke. Presence of bacteria might indicate bacterial meningitis. Elevated levels of protein or other substances might indicate a variety of other neuromuscular disorders.

Lumbar punctures are performed on hospitalized patients at the bedside, in surgical centers, and in clinics in special procedure rooms. Therefore, the medical assistant must be prepared to assist with this procedure and to monitor the patient afterward. (See *Procedure 26-2: Assisting with lumbar*

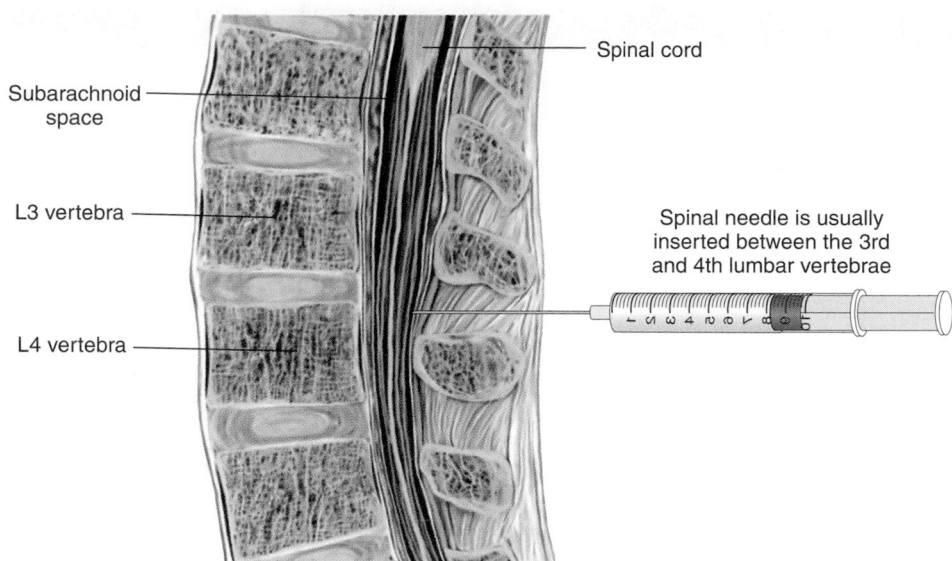

Subarachnoid space

Spinal cord

L3 vertebra

L4 vertebra

Spinal needle is usually inserted between the 3rd and 4th lumbar vertebrae

FIG 26-15 Lumbar puncture.

puncture, page 458.) Facility policy must be followed regarding observing the patient for adverse effects, treating discomfort, and monitoring fluid intake and vital signs. (See *Teaching about lumbar puncture,* page 459.)

Computed Tomography

Computed tomography (CT) scanning is a radiographic technique that uses a computer to create a clear x-ray image of selected sections of anatomy. The images can be created in "slices" as thin as 1 mm. The procedure may be done with or without a contrast medium, which is injected before the scan. When used, the contrast medium enhances the images of certain structures. (See Figure 26-16.)

Magnetic Resonance Imaging

Magnetic resonance imaging (MRI) is a type of diagnostic radiography that uses powerful magnetic fields to create images of soft tissues and organ structures in the body. MRI is especially useful for imaging structures in the musculoskeletal and central nervous systems. The precise location of tumors or lesions within the brain can be detected, allowing a surgeon a clear three-dimensional picture of what might be encountered before performing surgery. (See Figure 26-17.) While contrast agents may be used with MRI, they are not required to create clear images of most structures. This type of procedure should not be used on a patient who has a cardiac pacemaker or other type of metal in the body. (See *Teaching about MRI,* page 459.)

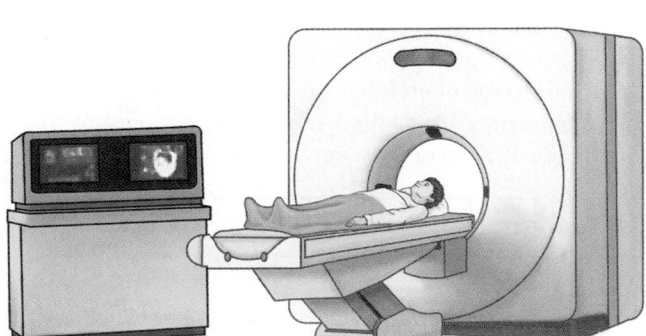

FIG 26-16 Patient undergoing a CT scan.

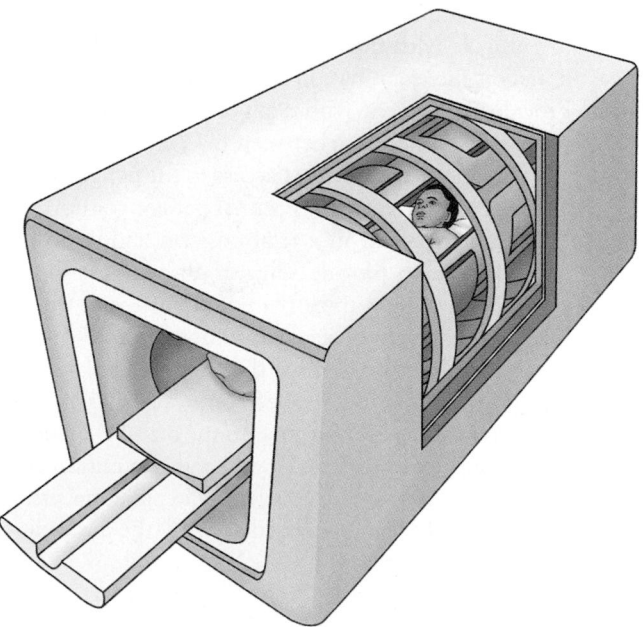

FIG 26-17 Patient undergoing an MRI scan.

Assisting with lumbar puncture

Task

Prepare an individual for and assist with lumbar puncture to collect a specimen for CSF analysis.

Conditions

- Local anesthetic
- Disposable lumbar puncture tray
- Mayo-type of supply stand
- Marker to label specimen tubes
- Sterile gloves
- Syringe and needle
- Patient examination gown
- Drape

Standards

In the time specified and within the scoring parameters determined by the instructor, the student will successfully assist with lumbar puncture.

Performance Standards

1. Greet and identify your patient and introduce yourself to prevent errors and ease patient anxiety.
2. Review the nature of the procedure and determine whether the patient has any questions.
3. Check to make sure a consent form has been signed to ensure that the patient understands the procedure and possible effects and to reinforce information already given by the physician.
4. Instruct the patient to empty his bladder to increase patient comfort during the procedure.
5. Give the patient an examination gown. Instruct him to put it on with the opening in the back and then lie down on the examination table on his left side.
6. Provide the patient with a pillow for his head and a second pillow to place between his knees if desired to allow the physician the best access to the patient's lumbar spine, while ensuring optimal patient comfort.
7. Position the patient in a fetal position and cover him with a drape to provide warmth and privacy for the patient and to maximize the spread of the L4-to-L5 space, making correct needle insertion easier and safer.
8. Wash your hands, assemble the supplies, and set up a sterile field, including needed sterile supplies.
9. Perform sterile skin preparation on the patient's lumbar area to decrease microorganisms in critical areas and reduce the risk of infection at the puncture site.
10. Assist the physician as needed with the procedure, including:

   a. Hold the anesthetic vial upside down at an angle so the physician can aspirate fluid from it or pour it into a sterile cup on the sterile field.
   b. Provide reassurance to the patient and assist him in holding still in the fetal position to make the procedure easier for the physician and reduce the risk of injury to the patient.
   c. Hold the top of the manometer if requested by the physician.
   d. If pressure readings are taken, instruct the patient to refrain from talking or holding his breath.
   e. If directed by the physician, assist the patient in straightening his legs to increase the accuracy of the pressure readings.
   f. Mark the specimens sequentially according to the order in which they are collected (for example, "#1," "#2," and "#3").
   g. Complete the laboratory requisition form and package the specimens for transport to ensure that results are accurately reported and accurately documented.

11. After the physician has completed the procedure and applied an adhesive bandage to the site, position the patient in a prone or supine position as directed by the physician.
12. Instruct the patient to lie flat for the required number of hours because lying flat, especially in the prone position, reduces likelihood of CSF leakage at the puncture site. It also reduces the risk of postprocedure headache for the patient.
13. Measure and record the patient's vital signs, provide liquids, and evaluate the patient for discomfort according to facility policy. Through careful monitoring, the medical assistant becomes aware of any changes in the patient's status. Promoting fluid intake helps the body replace the lost CSF fluid, reducing risk of headache.
14. Dispose of supplies, taking care to place sharps and contaminated items in appropriate biohazard waste containers.
15. Clean the room per facility protocol and sanitize your hands to maintain infection control.
16. Document data in the patient's chart to ensure that the medical record is complete and accurate.

Date	
02/19/09: 11:15 a.m.	*LP performed by Dr. Greer. Specimen sent to lab. Pt lying prone. denies pain. VSS ————————————————* *———————————————— S. Gonzales, CMA*

Patient Education

Teaching About Lumbar Puncture

The medical assistant may share the following information with the patient preparing to undergo a lumbar puncture:

- The physician will explain the exact nature and purpose of the procedure.

- You will be asked to read and sign an informed consent form. This is your opportunity to ask the physician any questions you may have.

- Proper positioning is very important. You will be asked to lay on your left side or sit on the side of the examination table and lean forward on a pillow. In either case, you will flex your thighs and bend your head and chest as far forward as possible to assume the fetal position.

- Holding very still is extremely important. Someone will help you to do so.

- The physician will give you a local anesthetic to numb the area.

- The most common adverse effect is headache. You can minimize this and other potential complications by drinking fluids and laying down after the procedure as instructed.

Patient Education

Teaching About MRI

The medical assistant may share the following information with the patient preparing to undergo a magnetic resonance imaging (MRI) scan:

- You must remove any metal objects from your body, such as earrings, body jewelry, and watches.

- You should not undergo this procedure if you have metal inside your body—for example, a pacemaker or metal clip, pin, or rod.

- You will be asked to lay very still on a flat surface for the duration of the procedure, which usually takes between 30 and 90 minutes.

- The test itself is not painful.

- You may hear sounds coming from the pulsing of the magnetic field; this sound is normal.

- You will be able to talk with staff by microphone during the procedure.

- Please let the technicians know ahead of time if you suffer from claustrophobia.

Chapter Summary

- The nervous system is made up of the central and peripheral nervous systems. It plays a key role in maintaining homeostasis in the body and is capable of storing and processing vast amounts of data.

- Medical assistants must be well versed in the language and vocabulary that pertain to the nervous system. In addition to knowing common combining forms, prefixes, and suffixes, they should be familiar with common abbreviations and pathological terms.

- Some of the most common disorders of the neurological system include stroke, transient ischemic attack, migraine headaches, epilepsy, encephalitis, meningitis, cerebral concussion, cerebral contusion, spinal cord injury, Parkinson disease, multiple sclerosis, brain tumor, amyotrophic lateral sclerosis, Bell palsy, peripheral neuropathy, carpal tunnel syndrome, and spinal stenosis.

- Neurology is a medical specialty that focuses on the study and treatment of diseases and disorders of the nervous system.

- To reach an accurate diagnosis, the neurologist must complete a thorough evaluation of the nervous system.

- The medical assistant prepares the patient by assisting him as needed with undressing and positioning. She also assists the physician with examinations and procedures.

- Procedures commonly used to diagnose neurological disorders include electroencephalogram, lumbar puncture, computed tomography, and magnetic resonance imaging.

Team Work Exercises

1. Teams will select or be assigned one of the following assignments.

   - Research about the Mini Mental State Examination. Return to class with the following information prepared:
     a. purpose of the tool
     b. type of clients most commonly evaluated with this tool
     c. how the results are scored
     d. implications of low scores
     e. a role-play scenario in which the medical assistant evaluates the patient using the tool.

   - Research about the Glasgow Coma Scale. Return to class with the following information prepared:
     a. purpose of the tool
     b. type of clients most commonly evaluated with this tool
     c. how the results are scored

d. implications of low scores

e. a role-play scenario in which the medical assistant evaluates the patient using the tool.

- A chart or poster that reflects the following information:

a. name and function of each of the 12 cranial nerves

b. method that might be used by the physician to evaluate each of the nerves

c. a role-play scenario where the "physician" evaluates at least 4 of the cranial nerves

- A chart, illustration, or poster that reflects the following information:

a. dermatomes of the body

b. description of how the information in this chart might be useful in understanding a patient's sensory symptoms

c. a list and description of some of the tools that might be used to evaluate sensory function in a client without causing harm (heat, cold, sharp, dull, etc.).

2. Using medical word elements in the tables in this chapter, create as many terms related to neurology as you can think of. List the definition of each term next to it. The team with the most terms wins.

Case Studies

1. Mr. and Mrs. Sommersby have an appointment today. Mr. Sommersby recently suffered from a stroke and now walks with the aid of a walker. They both convey their concerns about his risks of falling and injuring himself. What are some of the questions that the medical assistant might ask to learn more about the Sommersbys' home environment? What are some suggestions that the medical assistant might offer to help reduce Mr. Sommersby's risk of injury in and around the home?

2. Hector Gonzalez is a 49-year-old Hispanic patient who woke up this morning and found the left side of his face paralyzed and drooping. He was extremely upset when he arrived and was sure that he had suffered from a stroke. He shares that his father died of a stroke and he is afraid this means he is going to die. He has a wife and several children depending upon him for support and he is worried about them. After a neurological evaluation, Mr. Gonzalez was diagnosed with Bell palsy. After the examination, the physician asked the medical assistant to provide more information about Bell palsy to Mr. Gonzalez. What information will you share?

Resources

- ALS Association: *www.alsa.org*
- Centers for Disease Control and Prevention: *www.cdc.gov*
- E-medicine: *www.emedicine.com*
- Hyman-Newman Institute for Neurology and Neurosurgery: *www.nyneurosurgery.org*
- Mayo Clinic: General—*www.mayoclinic.org;* Tools for Healthier Lives—*www.mayoclinic.com*
- Medline Plus: *www.nlm.nih.gov/medlineplus*
- The Michael J. Fox Foundation for Parkinson's Research: *www.michaeljfox.org*
- National Brain Tumor Foundation: *www.braintumor.org*
- National Institute of Neurological Disorders and Stroke: *www.ninds.nih.gov*
- National Parkinson Foundation: *www.parkinson.org/NETCOMMUNITY/Page.aspx?&pid=201&srcid=-2*

Cardiology and Lymphatics

Learning Objectives

Upon completion of this chapter, the student will be able to:

- define and spell terms related to the cardiovascular and lymphatic systems
- identify key structures of the cardiovascular and lymphatic systems
- describe the electrical conduction system of the heart
- discuss the roles played by the cardiovascular and lymphatic systems
- describe the role of the medical assistant in the cardiology office
- identify common cardiovascular and lymphatic disorders
- list commonly used word elements related to the cardiovascular and lymphatic systems
- give at least 10 examples of how new cardiology-related terms may be created by combining prefixes, suffixes, and combining forms
- describe physical examination techniques used to evaluate the cardiovascular and lymphatic systems
- list and describe types of cardiovascular testing done in or out of the cardiology office
- demonstrate the performance of an electrocardiogram (ECG).

CAAHEP Competencies

Clinical Competencies
Diagnostic Testing
Perform electrocardiography
Patient Care
Prepare and maintain examination and treatment areas
Prepare patients for and assist with routine and specialty examinations

General Competencies
Patient Instruction
Instruct individuals according to their needs
Provide instruction for health maintenance and disease prevention

ABHES Competencies

Clinical Duties
Prepare patients for procedures
Prepare patient for and assist physician with routine and specialty examinations, treatments, and minor office surgeries
Perform electrocardiograms
Instruction
Teach patients methods of health promotion and disease prevention

Procedure
Performing a 12-lead ECG

Chapter Outline

Structures and Functions of the Cardiovascular System
Structures of the Cardiovascular System
Heart
Circulatory system
Functions of the Cardiovascular System
Heart
Circulatory system
Structures and Functions of the Lymphatic System
Structures of the Lymphatic System
Thymus
Spleen
Functions of the Lymphatic System
Thymus
Spleen
Medical Terminology Related to the Cardiovascular and Lymphatic Systems

Common Cardiovascular and Lymphatic System Diseases and Disorders
Cardiovascular System
Hypertension
Coronary artery disease
Myocardial infarction
Heart failure
Aneurysm
Atrial fibrillation
Varicose veins
Deep vein thrombosis
Shock
Anemia
Leukemia
Lymphatic System
Hodgkin disease
Non-Hodgkin lymphoma
Acquired immune deficiency syndrome
Cardiology and Lymphatics Procedures
Assisting with Examination
Electrocardiography
Preparing the electrocardiograph machine
Electrocardiograph paper
Standardization
Leads and electrodes
Preparing the patient
Recording the ECG
Rhythm interpretation
Artifacts
Artificial Cardiac Pacemaker
Implantable Cardioverter Defibrillator
Cardiac Stress Test
Holter Monitoring
Event Recorder
Chapter Summary
Team Work Exercises
Case Studies
Resources

461

Structures and Functions of the Cardiovascular System

The cardiovascular system is made up of the heart and the circulatory system, including arteries, veins, and capillaries. The cardiovascular system provides oxygen and nutrients to the entire body.

Structures of the Cardiovascular System

The structures of the cardiovascular system include the heart, located in the center of the chest, and the complex system of arteries, veins, and capillaries that are distributed throughout the entire body.

Heart

The heart is a muscular organ about the size of a closed fist. (See Figure 27-1.) It is located in the center of the chest and slightly to the left in an area called the *mediastinum*. The heart has three layers: the outer lining, called the *epicardium*, the middle muscular layer, called the *myocardium*, and the inner lining, called the *endocardium*. The heart is enclosed in a fibrous membrane called the *pericardium* or *pericardial sac*, which also contains a small amount of fluid called *pericardial fluid*.

The heart has two upper chambers, the right and left atria, and two larger, lower chambers, the right and left ventricles. The left ventricle is larger and more muscular than the right because of its greater workload. The right and left sides of the heart are divided by a thick layer of muscle tissue called the *septum*.

There are four valves in the heart. The tricuspid valve exits the right atrium into the right ventricle, and the mitral, or *bicuspid*, valve exits the left atrium into the left ventricle. The pulmonary valve exits the right ventricle into the pulmonary artery, and the aortic valve exits the left ventricle into the aorta.

The largest part of the heart, the lower left, is known as the *apex*. This site is best for auscultating sounds from the mitral valve and is where the **apical pulse** is best heard. Auscultating the apical pulse for one full minute is considered the most accurate method of measuring heart rate and is the preferred method in situations where accuracy is critically important.

Circulatory System

The circulatory system is composed of all the vessels of the body. (See Figure 27-2.) Major vessels entering and exiting the heart include the aorta, which is the largest artery in the body; right and left pulmonary arteries, which connect the right ventricle to the lungs; the superior and inferior vena cava, which are the largest veins in the body; and the right and left pulmonary veins, which connect the lungs to the left

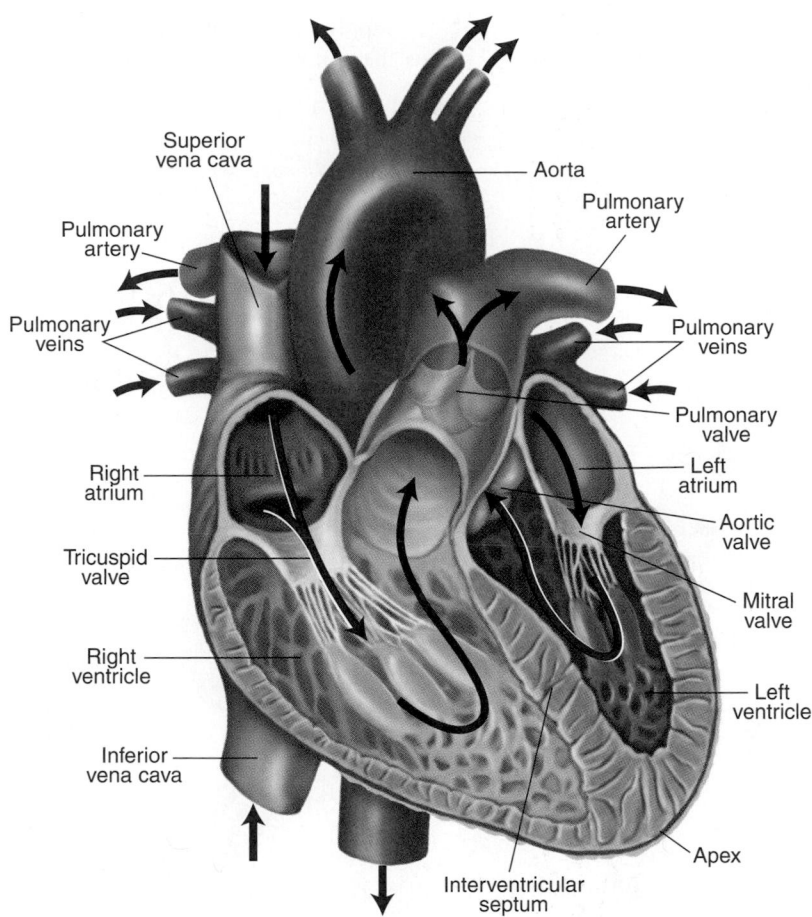

Superior
vena cava

Aorta

Pulmonary
artery

Pulmonary
artery

Pulmonary
veins

Pulmonary
veins

Pulmonary
valve

Right
atrium

Left
atrium

Aortic
valve

Tricuspid
valve

Mitral
valve

Right
ventricle

Left
ventricle

Inferior
vena cava

Apex

Interventricular
septum

FIG 27-1 Structures of the heart.

atrium. Blood flows from the heart to the body through smaller and smaller arteries, eventually ending in capillary beds. Capillaries are the tiniest blood vessels in the body. Capillaries also connect arteries and veins. Blood leaves capillary beds and is returned to the heart by way of larger and larger veins.

Functions of the Cardiovascular System

The heart serves as a pump that propels blood throughout the entire circulatory system. The heart and the circulatory system deliver much-needed oxygen and nutrients to all parts of the body.

Heart

The heart is a hollow, muscular organ that generates its own contractions approximately 60 to 100 times per minute throughout a person's entire life span. At an average rate of 72 beats per minute, the heart beats 104,000 times per day, and 38,000,000 times per year. The heart is enclosed within the pericardial sac, which contains a very small amount of pericardial fluid. This fluid acts as a type of lubricant and serves to reduce friction as the heart repeatedly contracts and relaxes.

Blood flows through both sides of the heart simultaneously and each side pumps blood to different parts of the body. (See Figure 27-3.) Blood that is low in oxygen but high in carbon dioxide (CO_2) returns from the body to the right atrium via the inferior and superior vena cava. The atria are smaller than the ventricles and do approximately 30% of the workload of the heart, while the larger, more muscular ventricles do the other 70% of the work. Both atria contract at the same time, each pumping blood to a different area. As the right atrium contracts, blood is forced downward through the tricuspid valve into the right ventricle. As the right ventricle contracts, it forces blood up and out through the pulmonary valve into pulmonary arteries. The pulmonary arteries lead to the lungs, where CO_2 is exchanged for oxygen (O_2). The pulmonary arteries are the only arteries in the body that transport deoxygenated blood.

Oxygen-enriched blood then returns through the pulmonary veins to the left atrium. The pulmonary veins are the only veins in the body that transport oxygenated blood. As the left atrium contracts, it forces blood downward through the mitral valve into the left ventricle. As the left ventricle contracts, it forces blood upward and out through the aortic valve into the aorta and out to various parts of the body. Branching off the base of the aorta are the right and left coronary arteries, which provide the heart with its own blood supply and ensure that the heart always receives a generous share of richly oxygenated blood.

Conduction System

A cluster of specialized cells in the right atrium called the *sinoatrial (SA) node* serves as a natural pacemaker for the heart and initiates an electrical impulse about 60 to 100 times

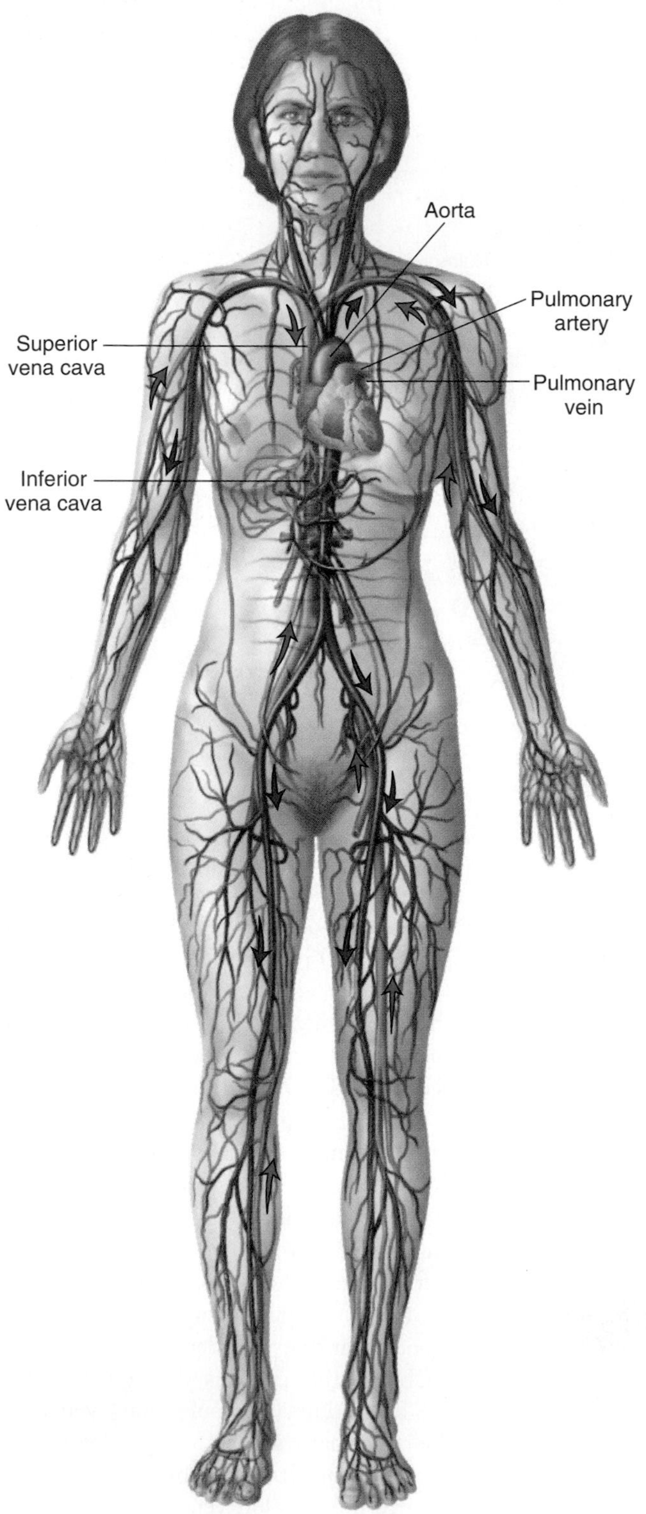

FIG 27-2 Structures of the circulatory system.

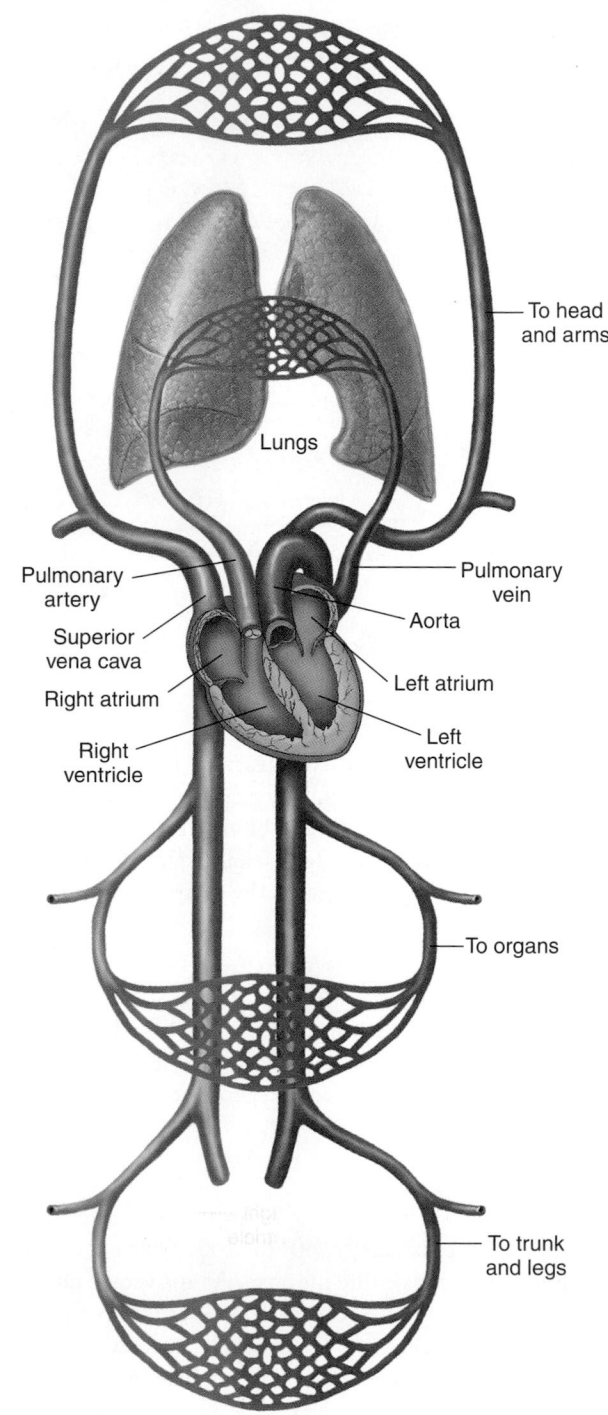

FIG 27-3 Cardiopulmonary circulation.

per minute. Each of these impulses is transmitted throughout all muscle cells of the heart, resulting in electrical **depolarization**. Depolarization is an electrical change in cardiac muscle cells in which the inside of the cells become positive in relation to the outside. This depolarization causes individual cardiac muscle cells in the atria to contract in unison.

Within the floor of the right atrium is a backup pacemaker, the atrioventricular (AV) node. It receives the impulse from the SA node and transmits it onward to both ventricles via the bundle of His, located within the septum and the Purkinje fibers, distributed through the septum and throughout the ventricles. As the electrical impulse is transmitted throughout the ventricles, all ventricular muscle fibers contract in unison. This contraction occurs just slightly after the contraction of the atria and the combination of the two results in one complete heartbeat. This entire process is repeated with each heartbeat. (See Figure 27-4.)

Cardiac Cycle

The contraction and relaxation of the four heart chambers creates each heartbeat and is known as the *cardiac cycle*. Each cardiac cycle takes approximately 0.8 second. The

pressure created by pumping blood, known as **blood pressure**, is written as two numbers, one written over the other, such as 120/80. The upper number, called the **systolic pressure,** is a measurement of the highest pressure exerted against artery walls during ventricular contraction, or **systole**. The lower number, called the **diastolic pressure**, measures the lowest pressure exerted against artery walls during ventricular relaxation, or **diastole**.

Large arteries in the body that have a strong pulse and are easily palpated are known as **pulse points**. These points, sometimes called *pressure points,* may be compressed to slow bleeding in the case of hemorrhage. (Common pulse points are illustrated in Chapter 21, "Vital Signs," on page 319.)

Circulatory System

The aorta, the largest artery of the body, delivers oxygen-rich blood from the heart to various parts of the body via **systemic circulation**. As blood leaves the aorta, it moves through smaller and smaller arteries, all of which have thick, muscular walls because they carry blood under high pressure. The tiniest arteries, called *arterioles,* terminate in capillary beds. Capillaries are the tiniest blood vessels in the body and

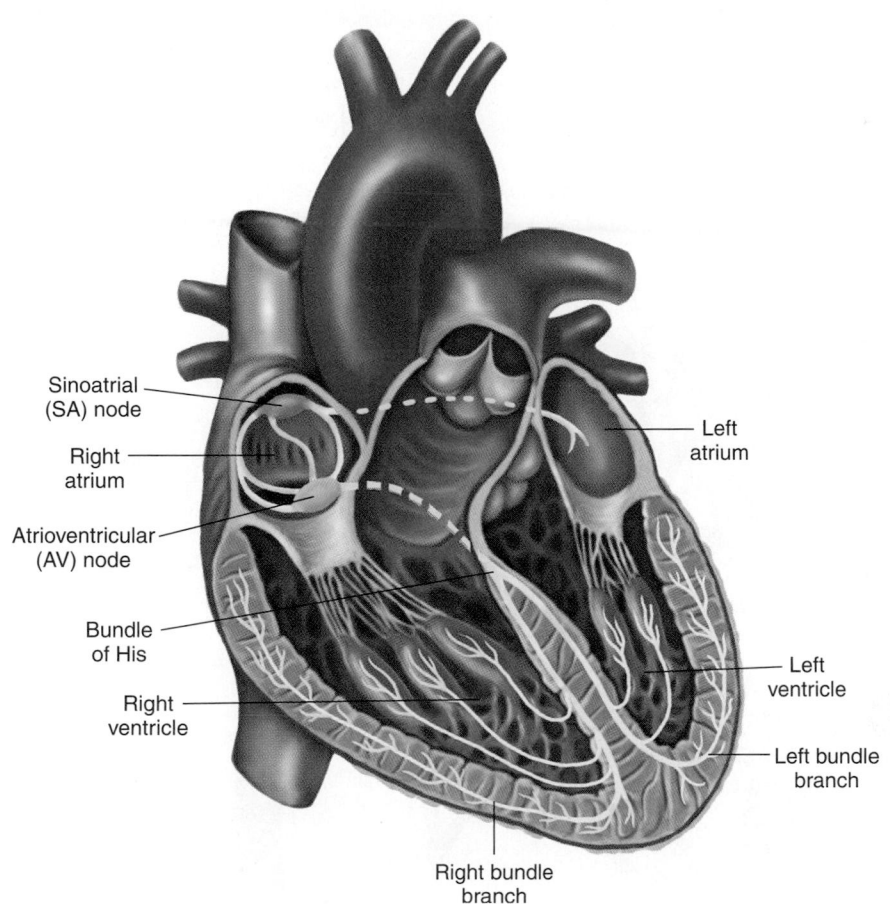

Sinoatrial (SA) node

Right atrium

Atrioventricular (AV) node

Bundle of His

Right ventricle

Left atrium

Left ventricle

Left bundle branch

Right bundle branch

FIG 27-4 Electrical conduction system of the heart.

are where the exchange of gases and nutrients occurs. Capillaries have walls that are only one cell thick, making them semipermeable. This permeability facilitates the delivery of oxygen and nutrients to tissue cells and the retrieval of carbon dioxide. Blood that is low in oxygen and high in carbon dioxide leaves the capillaries and enters tiny veins called *venules*. Venous blood continues flowing through larger and larger veins until it returns to the heart via the superior and inferior vena cava. It then returns to the lungs, which facilitate the release of carbon dioxide.

Venous blood travels under much less pressure than arterial blood. Because of this lack of pressure, venous blood cannot easily flow against gravity to ascend the legs and return to the heart. Fortunately, veins contain one-way valves that facilitate circulation by preventing the backflow of blood. The pumping action created by the contraction and relaxation of leg muscles also helps to propel the blood forward.

Structures and Functions of the Lymphatic System

Lymph is tissue fluid that has entered lymph capillaries and made its way into larger lymph vessels. It is a clear, colorless, alkaline fluid made up mostly of water along with some protein, salts, urea, fats, and white blood cells. Lymphatic vessels are found throughout the body alongside arteries,

veins, and capillaries. While blood vessels rely on the pumping action of the heart, there is no pump for the lymphatic vessels. Instead, lymph flow is facilitated by the pumping action of skeletal muscle contraction. The lymphatic system includes lymph nodes, commonly called *glands*, which serve as filters to clean debris from lymph and also to produce some white blood cells. Because of these functions, the lymphatic system is also considered part of the immune system.

Structures of the Lymphatic System

Lymph is excess fluid from tissues that is eventually returned to the circulatory system via lymphatic vessels. While located in tissue spaces, it is called *interstitial fluid* or *intercellular fluid*. When located within lymphatic vessels, it is called *lymph*. Lymphatic vessels are located throughout the body and are connected to the superior vena cava, which is where lymph enters the circulatory system and is combined with blood. Lymph nodes are distributed along lymphatic vessels, with higher concentrations in the neck, axilla, groin, and the mesentery of the abdomen. (See Figure 27-5.) There are two sets of lymph nodes in the oropharynx, commonly known as the tonsils and adenoids. These nodes can become tender and swollen when the individual has a cold or sore throat. This occurs when lymph nodes that have been working to filter bacteria, virus, or other substances from lymph become overwhelmed and inflamed. An inflamed gland may be referred

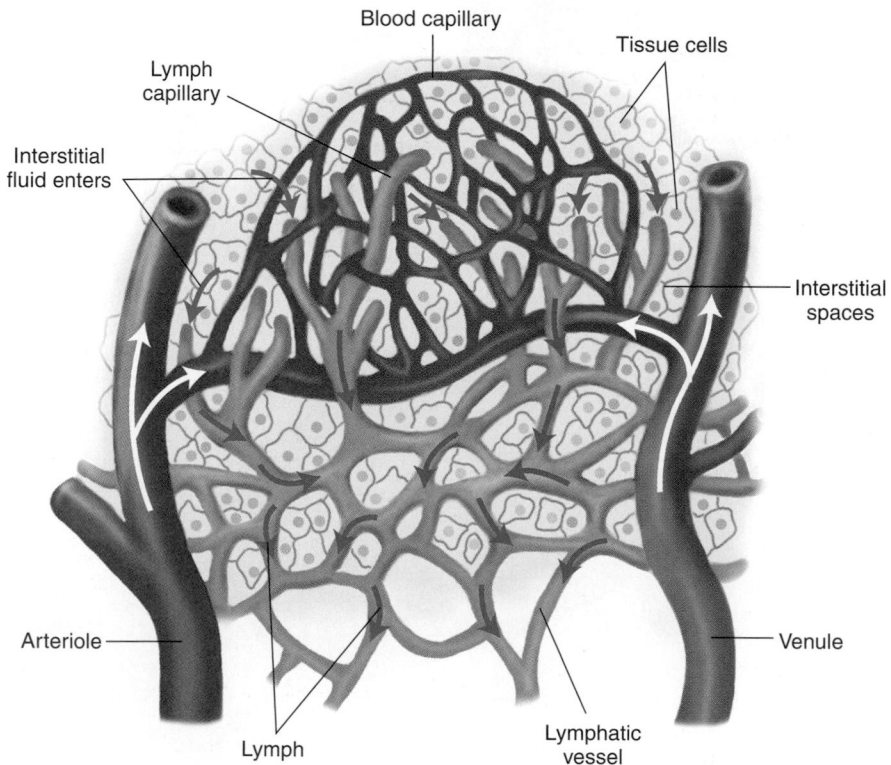

FIG 27-5 Lymphatic vessels.

to as *adenitis* or adenopathy. Other organs of the lymphatic system include the thymus gland and spleen.

Thymus

The thymus gland is located in the mediastinum above the heart. It consists of two fused lobes and is divided into an outer cortex mostly composed of immature T lymphocytes (a type of white blood cell) and an inner medulla. The thymus grows until puberty and then gradually shrinks in size as individuals age.

Spleen

The spleen is a dark red, oval-shaped, lymphoid organ located in the left upper quadrant of the abdomen just under the ribs. It is surrounded by an outer capsule of connective tissue and is divided into compartments. (See Figure 27-6.)

Functions of the Lymphatic System

The lymphatic system includes an intricate network of lymph vessels that collect and filter excess tissue fluid and return it to circulation. This system plays a major role in the immune system because lymph nodes are rich in white blood cells (WBCs), which engulf bacteria and cellular debris through a process known as **phagocytosis**. The body responds to infection and inflammation by increasing production of phagocytes.

Thymus

The thymus is most active during the prenatal period and early years of life. It plays a role in cellular immunity and is believed to play a role in protecting the body against cancer. T-lymphocytes, also known as *killer T cells,* mature in the thymus and then circulate to the spleen, lymph nodes, and other lymphoid tissue, where they are involved in cell-mediated immune responses.

Spleen

The spleen contains a supply of 100 to 300 ml of blood and 30% of the body's total platelets, most of which can be returned to circulation in the event of hemorrhage. Because of its location and rich blood supply, the spleen may be injured if the individual sustains a blow to the abdomen. Such an injury may require a splenectomy (surgical removal of the spleen) to stop internal bleeding. Fortunately, most people can survive without their spleen, although their immune system will be slightly weakened, leaving them more vulnerable to infection.

During prenatal development, the spleen forms red and white blood cells. After birth, RBCs are produced by the spleen only in cases of severe need. However, the spleen continues creating WBCs as well as antibodies as part of its role in the immune system. Phagocytosis occurs to remove microorganisms, cell debris, and blood cells that are damaged, old, abnormal, or marked by antibodies.

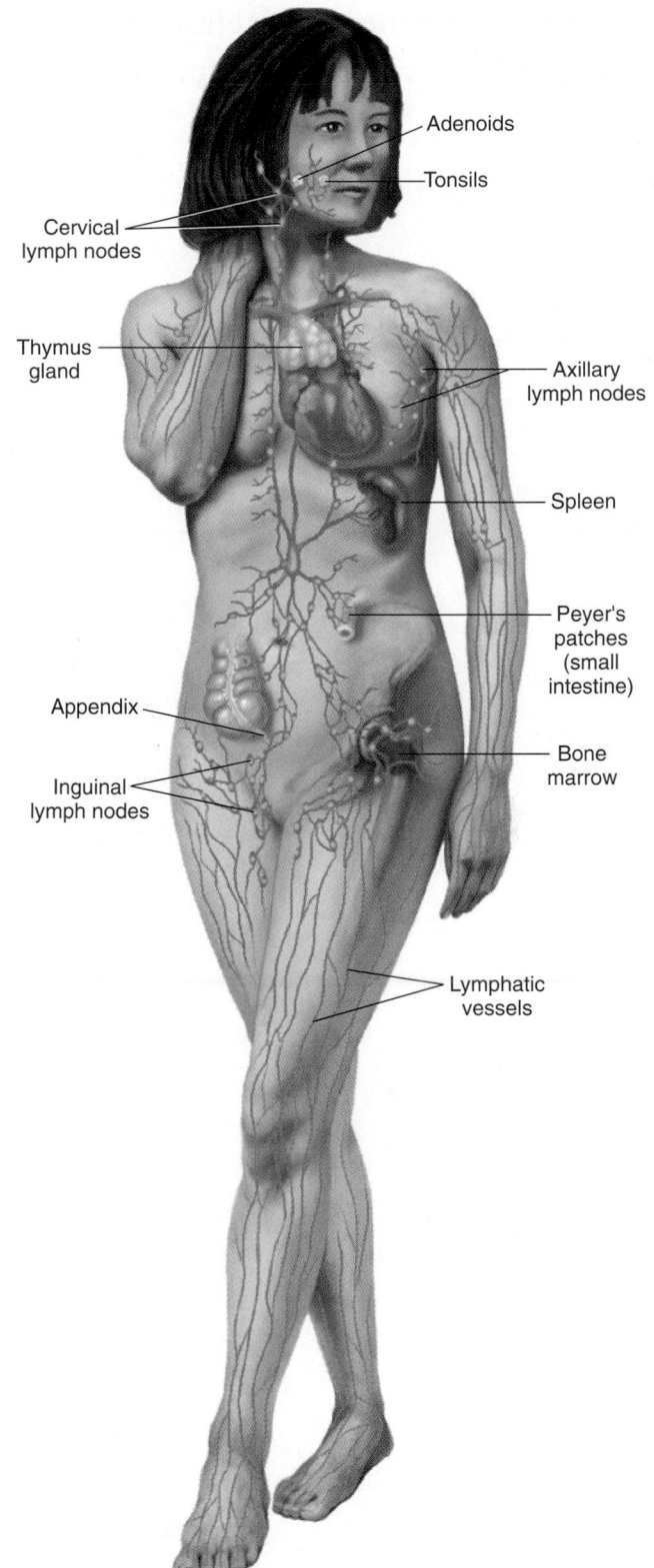

FIG 27-6 Lymphatic system.

Medical Terminology Related to the Cardiovascular and Lymphatic Systems

Cardiovascular disorders are among some of the most common and most serious problems treated in health care today. Lymphatic disorders, though slightly less common, can be equally devastating to those affected by them. Medical assistants who work in family practice offices, urgent care centers, cardiology clinics, or other areas play an important role in the provision of health care to these patients. To be effective in this role, the medical assistant must become well versed in the language and vocabulary that pertain to these body systems. The following tables list common medical terminology related to the cardiovascular and lymphatic systems.

Table 27.1 | Word Elements

This table contains combining forms, prefixes, and suffixes related to the cardiovascular and lymphatic systems along with examples of terms that use the word element and a pronunciation guide.

Word Element	Meaning	Example	Meaning
Combining Forms			
aden/o	gland	**adenoma** (ăd-ĕ-NŌ-mă)	tumor of a gland
angi/o	vessel	**angioedema** (ăn-jē-ō-ĕ-DĒ-mă)	swelling of a vessel
vas/o		**vasorrhaphy** (văs-OR-ă-fē)	suture of a vessel
aort/o	aorta	**aortostenosis** (ā-or-tō-stĕ-NŌ-sĭs)	narrowing or stricture of the aorta
arteri/o	artery	**arteriosclerosis** (ăr-tē-rē-ō-sklĕ-RŌ-sĭs)	hardening of the artery
ather/o	thick, fatty	**atheroma** (ăth-ĕr-Ō-mă)	thick, fatty tumor
atri/o	atria	**atrioventricular** (ā-trē-ō-vĕn-TRĬK-ū-lăr)	pertaining to the atria and the ventricles
cardi/o	heart	**tachycardia** (tăk-ē-KĂR-dē-ă)	condition of a rapid heart (beat)
electr/o	electric	**electrocardiogram** (ē-lĕk-trō-KĂR-dē-ō-grăm)	electrical recording of the heart
hem/o	blood	**hemolytic** (hē-mō-LĬT-ĭk)	pertaining to destruction of the blood
hemat/o		**hematemesis** (hĕm-ăt-ĔM-ĕ-sĭs)	vomiting of blood
lymph/o	lymph	**lymphoma** (lĭm-FŌ-mă)	lymph tumor
phleb/o	vein	**phleborrhexis** (flĕb-ō-RĔK-sĭs)	rupture of a vein
ven/o		**venostasis** (vē-nō-STĀ-sĭs)	stopping of a vein (refers to slowed blood flow)
splen/o	spleen	**splenomegaly** (splē-nō-MĔG-ă-lē)	enlargement of the spleen
thromb/o	thrombus (clot)	**thrombophlebitis** (thrŏm-bō-flĕ-BĪ-tĭs)	inflammation of a vein in the presence of a clot
ventricul/o	ventricle	**ventriculostomy** (vĕn-trĭk-ū-LŎS-tō-mē)	mouthlike opening in the ventricle
Prefixes			
brady-	slow	**bradycardia** (brād-ē-KĂR-dē-ă)	condition of a slow heart (beat)
micro-	small	**microcardia** (mī-krō-KĂR-dē-ă)	condition of a small heart
supra-	above	**supraventricular** (soo-pră-vĕn-TRĬK-ū-lăr)	pertaining to above the ventricles
tachy-	rapid	**tachycardia** (tăk-ē-KĂR-dē-ă)	condition of a rapid heart (beat)
Suffixes			
-cyte	cell	**thrombocyte** (THRŎM-bō-sīt)	clotting cell (term sometimes used for platelets)
-centesis	surgical puncture	**phlebocentesis** (flĕb-ō-sĕn-TĒ-sĭs)	surgical puncture of a vein (more commonly, but less accurately, called *phlebotomy*)

Table 27.1 | **Word Elements—cont'd**

Word Element	Meaning	Example	Meaning
-edema	swelling	lymphedema (lĭmf-ĕ-DĒ-mă)	swelling caused by lymph fluid
-emia	condition of the blood	leukemia (loo-KĒ-mē-ă)	a condition of white blood cells (refers to malignancy of the blood)
-genesis	creating, producing	hemogenesis (hēm-ō-JĔN-ĕ-sĭs)	creating or producing blood
-gram	record	electrocardiogram (ē-lĕk-trō-KĂR-dē-ō-grăm)	record of heart electricity (cardiac rhythm)
-graphy	process of recording	angiography (ăn-jē-ŎG-ră-fē)	recording of a vessel (radiological picture)
-logist	specialist in the study of	hematologist (hēm-ă-TŎL-ō-jĭst)	specialist in the study of blood
-lysis	destruction	hemolysis (hē-MŎL-ĭ-sĭs)	destruction of blood
-megaly	enlargement	cardiomegaly (kăr-dē-ō-MĔG-ă-lē)	enlargement of the heart
-ole -ule	small	arteriole (ăr-TĒ-rē-ōl) venule (VĔN-ūl)	small artery small vein
-pathy	disease	adenopathy (ăd-ĕ-NŎP-ă-thē)	diseased gland
-penia	deficiency	erythrocytopenia (ĕ-rĭth-rō-sī-tō-PĒ-nē-ă)	deficiency of red blood cells
-rrhage	bursting forth	hemorrhage (HĔM-ĕ-rĭj)	bursting forth of blood (severe bleeding)
-rrhexis	rupture	phleborrhexis (flĕb-ō-RĔK-sĭs)	rupture of a vein
-rrhaphy	suture, suturing	vasorrhaphy (văs-OR-ă-fē)	suturing of a vessel
-stenosis	narrowing, stricture	aortostenosis (ā-or-tō-stĕ-NŌ-sĭs)	narrowing or stricture of the aorta

Table 27.2 | **Pathologic Terms**

This table lists some of the most common pathologic terms related to the cardiovascular and lymphatic systems with a brief definition of each.

Term	Definition
Cardiovascular	
anemia ă-NĒ-mē-ă	Reduction in the mass of circulating red blood cells
aneurysm ĂN-ū-rĭzm	Dilation in the wall of a blood vessel due to weakness or a congenital defect
angina ăn-JĬ-nă	Chest pain or pressure caused by insufficient oxygen supply to the heart muscle
arrhythmia ă-RĬTH-mē-ă	Irregular heart rhythm
arterial occlusion ăr-TĒ-rē-ăl ō-KLOO-zhŭn	Blockage of blood flow through an artery
arteriosclerosis ăr-tē-rē-ō-sklĕ-RŌ-sĭs	Thickening and loss of elasticity and contractility in artery walls

Continued

Table 27.2 | Pathologic Terms—cont'd

Term	Definition
atherosclerosis ăth-ēr-ō-sklē-RŌ-sĭs	Condition in which fatty plaque deposits accumulate on the inner walls of arteries
bruit brwē	Abnormal arterial or venous swishing sound heard on auscultation
cardiomyopathy kăr-dē-ō-mī-ŎP-ă-thē	Any of several diseases that affects the heart muscle
crackles KRĂ-kĕls	Abnormal lung sound heard on auscultation that is produced by air passing over retained airway secretions or the sudden opening of collapsed alveoli
deep vein thrombosis DĒP VĀN thrŏm-BŌ-sĭs	Blood clot within a vein deep in the legs
embolus ĔM-bō-lŭs	Mass of undissolved solid, liquid, or gaseous matter floating in the blood
endocarditis ĕn-dō-kăr-DĪ-tĭs	Infection or inflammation of the valves and inner lining of the heart
heart failure HĂRT FĂL-yĕr	Inability of the heart to circulate blood effectively enough to meet the body's needs
hypertension hī-pĕr-TĔN-shŭn	Condition in which blood pressure is higher than 140/90 on three separate readings that are several weeks apart
ischemia ĭs-KĒ-mē-ă	Temporary reduction in blood supply to a localized area of tissue
leukemia loo-KĒ-mē-ă	Malignancy of the blood in which immature blood cells multiply at the expense of other cells
murmur MŬR-mŭr	Blowing or swishing sound in the heart due to turbulent blood flow or backflow through a leaky valve
myocardial infarction mī-ō-KĂR-dē-ăl ĭn-FĂRK-shŭn	Loss of living heart muscle as a result of coronary artery occlusion; also called a *heart attack*
orthopnea or-THŎP-nē-ă	Labored breathing that occurs when lying flat and is relieved by sitting upright
paroxysmal nocturnal dyspnea păr-ŏk-SĬZ-măl nŏk-TŪR-năl DĬSP-nē-ă	Episodic dyspnea at night that occurs repeatedly and without warning
petechiae pē-TĒ-kē-ē	Small, purplish, hemorrhagic spots on the skin that appear in patients with platelet deficiencies and in many febrile illnesses
postphlebitic syndrome pŏst-flĕ-BĬ-tĭc SĬN-drŏm	Condition sometimes following deep vein thrombosis in which the individual experiences chronic edema and aching
prehypertension prē-hī-pĕr-TĔN-shŭn	Condition in which systolic blood pressure measures between 120 and 140, diastolic blood pressure measures between 80 and 90, or both
premature atrial contraction prē-mă-CHŬR Ā-trē-ăl kŏn-TRĂK-shŭn	Heartbeat stimulated by a group of irritable cells in the atria other than the SA node
premature ventricular contraction prē-mă-CHŬR vĕn-TRĬK-ū-lăr kŏn-TRĂK-shŭn	Heartbeat stimulated by a group of irritable cells in the ventricles

Table 27.2 | Pathologic Terms—cont'd

Term	Definition
primary hypertension PRĬ-mă-rē hī-pĕr-TĔN-shŭn	Hypertension that has no identifiable cause; also called *essential hypertension*
pulmonary edema PŬL-mŏ-nĕ-rē ĕ-DĒ-mă	Accumulation of fluid in the interstitium and alveoli of the lungs
pulmonary embolism PŬL-mŏ-nĕ-rē ĔM-bō-lĭzm	Obstruction of a pulmonary artery from an embolus
rhonchi RŎNG-kī	Low-pitched snoring, squeaking, or gurgling sound heard during auscultation of the lungs and caused by partial airway obstruction from mucus
secondary hypertension SĔ-kŭn-dăr-ē hī-pĕr-TĔN-shŭn	Hypertension caused by an identifiable factor
shock SHŎK	Syndrome marked by inadequate perfusion and oxygenation of cells, tissues, and organs due to low blood pressure
venous stasis VĒ-nŭs STĀ-sĭs	Sluggish blood flow caused by venous congestion
varicose vein VĂR-ĭ-kōs VĀN	Enlarged, dilated vein
Lymphatic	
acquired immunedeficiency syndrome ă-KWĪRD ĭm-ūn dē-FĬSH-ĕn-sē SĬN-drōm	Late-stage infection with the human immunodeficiency virus
Hodgkin disease HŎJ-kĭn dĭ-ZĒZ	Malignant lymphoma characterized by giant Reed-Sternberg cells
lymphadenopathy lĭm-făd-ĕ-NŎP-ă-thē	Enlargement and tenderness of lymph nodes due to local or regional infection or tumor growth
lymphosarcoma lĭm-fō-săr-KŌ-mă	Cancer of the lymphatic tissue not related to Hodgkin disease
mononucleosis mŏn-ō-nū-klē-Ō-sĭs	Acute infection with the Epstein-Barr virus, which causes sore throat, fever, fatigue, and enlarged lymph nodes
non-Hodgkin lymphoma nŏn-HŎJ-kĭn lĭm-FŌ-mă	Group of malignant tumors of B or T lymphocytes

Table 27.3 | Abbreviations

In cardiology and lymphatics, as in other areas of health care, abbreviations are commonly used. Abbreviations such as the ones listed below save time and effort in documentation and written communications.

Abbreviation	Term	Abbreviation	Term
Cardiovascular System		*Cardiovascular System*	
AIDS	acquired immune deficiency syndrome	BP	blood pressure
ASHD	arteriosclerotic heart disease	CABG	coronary artery bypass graft

Continued

Table 27.3 | **Abbreviations—cont'd**

Abbreviation	Term	Abbreviation	Term
DVT	deep vein thrombosis	PVC	premature ventricular contraction
HTN	hypertension (high blood pressure)	RBC	red blood cell
INR	International Normalized Ratio	PTT	partial thromboplastin time
LA	left atrium	RA	right atrium
LV	left ventricle	RV	right ventricle
MI	myocardial infarction	WBC	white blood cell
PAC	premature atrial contraction	*Lymphatic System*	
PND	paroxysmal nocturnal dyspnea	AIDS	acquired immune deficiency syndrome
PTCA	percutaneous transluminal coronary angioplasty	HIV	human immunodeficiency virus
PT	prothrombin time	PCP	*Pneumocystis* pneumonia

Common Cardiovascular and Lymphatic System Diseases and Disorders

There are innumerable diseases and disorders of the cardiovascular and lymphatic systems. Some of the most common include hypertension, coronary artery disease (CAD), myocardial infarction (MI), heart failure, and acquired immune deficiency syndrome (AIDS).

Cardiovascular System

Disorders of the cardiovascular system include hypertension, coronary artery disease, myocardial infarction, heart failure, aneurysm, atrial fibrillation, varicose veins, deep vein thrombosis, shock, anemia, and leukemia.

Hypertension
ICD-9-CM code: 401

Hypertension, commonly known as *high blood pressure*, is a condition in which three separate blood pressure readings over several weeks' time measure the systolic pressure above 140, the diastolic pressure above 90, or both. It is further categorized as stage 1 (systolic of 140 to 159 or diastolic of 90 to 99) and stage 2 (systolic 160 or above or diastolic 100 or above). With the goal of identifying and treating hypertension earlier, experts have now defined prehypertension as systolic readings between 120 and 140 and/or diastolic readings between 80 and 90. One-third of American adults over age 35 have hypertension and a third of those do not know it. Incidence of hypertension increases with age

and is higher in the African American population than other ethnic groups.

Hypertension is classified as secondary, which means that it is caused by an underlying disorder, or primary (also called *essential*), which means that the specific cause is unclear. Secondary hypertension makes up 5% to 10% of all cases, and primary hypertension makes up the other 90% to 95% of cases. Causes of secondary hypertension include kidney disease, congenital abnormalities of the aorta, and narrowing of certain arteries. Risk factors for primary hypertension include pregnancy, obesity, tobacco use, a family history of hypertension, and endocrine disorders such as diabetes.

Hypertension is known as a silent killer because most people are asymptomatic until complications arise due to advanced disease. In some cases, individuals may complain of headache. However, unless high blood pressure is noted through the course of routine health screening or when individuals seek care for other problems, the first indicator may be a complication such as stroke or heart attack. Diagnosis is easily made based on repeated high blood pressure readings over several weeks' time.

Treatment of hypertension depends on the severity. In most cases, health care providers try to employ conservative measures first. Such measures include modification of identified risk factors, such as weight loss, elimination of tobacco use, dietary changes, alcohol intake restriction (1 to 2 drinks per day), and regular aerobic exercise. If these measures fail to achieve the desired result or the hypertension is extreme, the provider will prescribe medication. The most commonly used medications include diuretics and antihypertensives. Because of the large list of medications to choose from and the variation in individual response, the provider must personalize each treatment plan for the individual patient.

Hypertension is a major contributor to the development of several serious conditions, including coronary artery disease, heart failure, heart attack, kidney failure, stroke, and vision loss. Therefore, health care providers should take the condition seriously and treat it aggressively whether the patient is symptomatic or not.

Coronary Artery Disease
ICD-9-CM code: 414.0

Coronary artery disease (CAD) is defined as a narrowing of the **lumen** (the space within a vessel or other tubelike structure) of the arteries of the heart due to atherosclerosis, which is a condition marked by cholesterol-lipid-calcium deposits on the inner walls of arteries. It is the most common type of heart disease and is the leading cause of death of men and women in industrialized nations. Approximately 13 million Americans currently suffer from CAD and nearly half a million people die from the disease each year.

CAD results from the development of atherosclerosis and arteriosclerosis (changes in arterial walls caused by thickening, hardening, and loss of elasticity), which impedes blood flow to heart muscle. (See Figure 27-7.) Risk factors include hypertension, tobacco use, sedentary lifestyle, obesity, diabetes, advanced age, and family history of CAD.

Individuals with CAD are asymptomatic until the disease has advanced enough to cause angina (chest pain or pressure caused by insufficient blood flow and oxygen delivery to heart muscle) or heart attack. Symptoms of angina include chest pain and pressure or burning that may radiate to the neck, jaw, back, shoulders, or arms. Other symptoms of angina include nausea, vomiting, and diaphoresis (profuse sweating). Symptoms are brought on by physical exertion, emotional stress, eating large meals, or being in a cold environment. Symptoms of angina are temporary (usually lasting less than 30 minutes) and relieved by rest and nitroglycerine.

Diagnosis of CAD is based on presenting signs and symptoms (if any) and the results of diagnostic tests. Tests may include a 12-lead electrocardiogram (ECG), cardiac catheterization, echocardiogram, chest x-ray, cardiac stress test, and blood lipid studies.

Treatment of CAD depends on the severity of the disease and whether or not symptoms are present. In most cases, health care providers will employ conservative measures first. These measures include lifestyle modification, such as weight loss, elimination of tobacco use, low-fat diet, alcohol restriction, and regular aerobic exercise. If these measures fail to achieve desired results or lipid levels are extreme, the provider will prescribe medication to reduce cholesterol and triglyceride levels. If the disease is limited to one or two areas within cardiac arteries, the patient may undergo

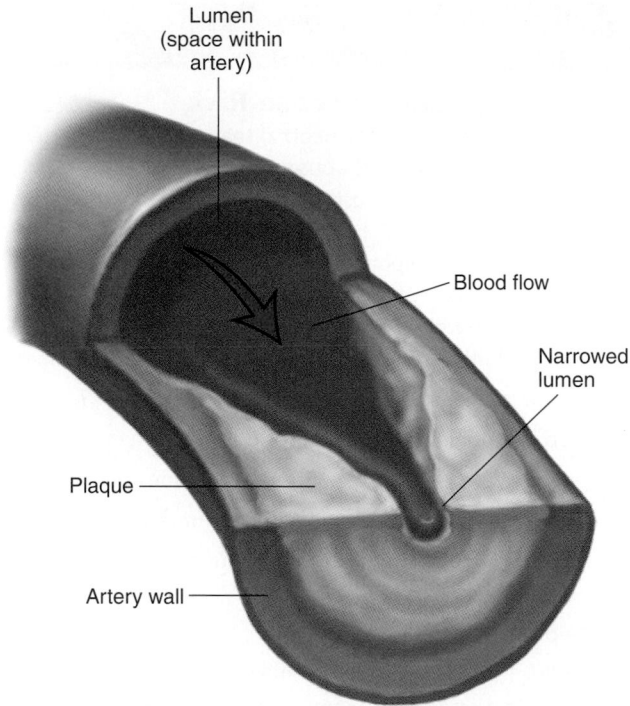

Lumen (space within artery)

Blood flow

Narrowed lumen

Plaque

Artery wall

FIG 27-7 Coronary artery disease.

coronary **angioplasty**. In this procedure, the surgeon will place a stent or inflate a tiny balloon to open narrowed vessels. When disease is more extensive, the patient may undergo open heart surgery to place coronary artery bypass grafts (CABGs) to divert blood around areas of narrowing or blockage.

Prognosis for CAD varies, depending on the extent and severity of disease and the individuals' underlying health status. Health care providers must take the condition seriously, because disease progression increases the risk of death from heart attack or other complications. However, early diagnosis and aggressive management usually results in significantly increased length and quality of life. (See *Reducing heart disease risk*, page 474.)

Myocardial Infarction
ICD-9-CM code: 427.5

Myocardial infarction (MI), commonly called *heart attack*, is defined as the death of heart muscle related to coronary artery occlusion (blockage), which cuts off the supply of oxygen and nutrients. Over 1 million individuals in the United States suffer from an MI each year and about half of them die. Risk factors for MI are the same as for CAD and include atherosclerosis and arteriosclerosis, hypertension, tobacco use, sedentary lifestyle, obesity, diabetes, advanced age, and family history of heart disease. Symptoms of MI include pain, pressure, fullness, heaviness or squeezing sensation in the chest, arms, neck, jaw, back or epigastric

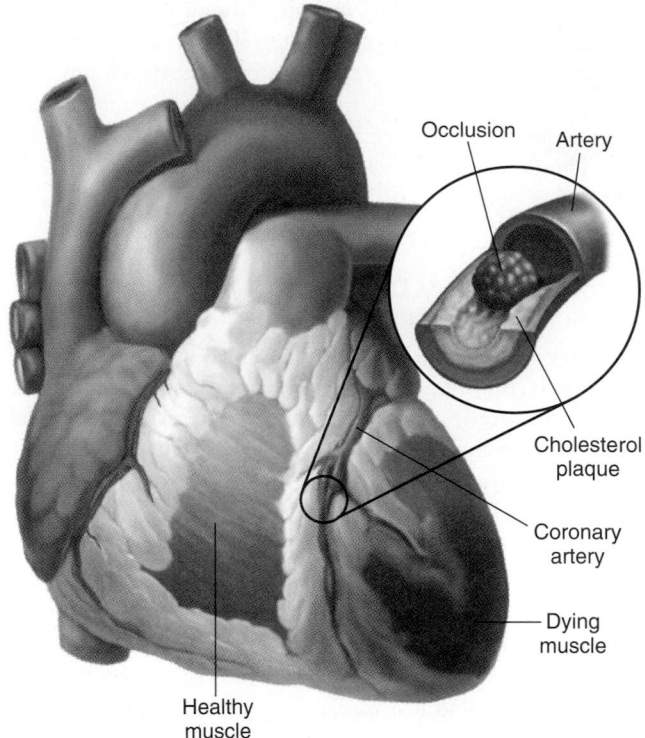

FIG 27-8 Myocardial infarction.

area; dyspnea; nausea; diaphoresis; and lightheadedness. MI commonly causes heart arrhythmias (irregularity or loss of rhythm of the heartbeat, also called *dysrhythmias*). Half of those who suffer from an MI die within the first hour of symptom onset. (See Figure 27-8.)

Diagnosis of MI is based on presenting signs and symptoms and results of diagnostic testing. Immediate tests include a 12-lead ECG and blood tests to check cardiac enzymes. The blood test that is considered most reliable is the **troponin** level, which determines how much heart muscle damage has occurred. When the patient's condition is stable, testing may be done to determine the extent of CAD and whether surgical intervention is needed. Such tests may include a nuclear heart scan, cardiac catheterization, and coronary angiography. These tests allow close inspection of heart chambers, valves, and coronary arteries.

A MI is a life-threatening emergency and the effectiveness of treatment depends on early, aggressive treatment. Unfortunately, many individuals delay seeking medical attention for 2 to 12 hours. (See *MI warning signs*.) Initial medications include aspirin, nitroglycerine, thrombolytics, beta-blockers, and morphine. These drugs are usually followed by anticoagulants and, if needed, medication to manage hypertension and lower triglycerides and cholesterol levels. Other supportive care includes treatment of arrhythmias, administration of

IV fluids, and respiratory support. In some cases, emergency angioplasty is done to treat severely narrowed coronary arteries. Rehabilitation focuses on two areas: exercise and education. Each patient follows an individualized exercise plan that supports him in gaining strength and endurance. The plan is designed around the patient's abilities, energy level, and personal interests. Education addresses risk reduction through lifestyle modification and newly prescribed medications.

A MI is a significant event that destroys some heart muscle. For those who survive the first post-MI hour and receive timely diagnosis and treatment, prognosis is good, with a 95% survival rate. Recovery and rehabilitation may take several weeks or months. (See *Patient with chest pain*.)

Heart Failure

ICD-9-CM code: 427.5

Heart failure, formerly called *congestive heart failure*, is the inability of the heart to pump enough blood to meet the needs of the body. The left ventricle is the part of the heart most affected in this condition. When the left ventricle is affected, the condition is referred to as *left-sided heart failure* and results in decreased effectiveness in pumping oxygen-rich blood to all parts of the body. Failure of the right ventricle, called *right-sided heart failure*, is less common. This condition impedes effective pumping of blood that returns

Patient Education

MI Warning Signs

Unlike in the movies, the fact that someone is having a heart attack is not always immediately apparent. Consequently, a person sometimes waits too long to summon help. The medical assistant should provide the following guidelines to patients at risk for a myocardial infarction (MI).

Major signs of MI

Major signs of an MI include:

- mild or severe chest pain, pressure, fullness, heaviness, or squeezing that is constant and lasts for more than a few minutes or goes away and then returns
- discomfort in other areas of the upper body, such as one or both arms or the back, neck, jaw, or upper stomach
- shortness of breath with or without chest discomfort
- nausea
- breaking out in a cold sweat
- dizziness or lightheadedness.

Different in women

A woman's symptoms may vary from the major symptoms above and may include:

- nausea
- shortness of breath
- back or jaw pain
- chest discomfort (not as common).

What to do?

If you suspect that you or a companion may be experiencing an MI, take these measures:

- Call 911.
- If you are the person experiencing symptoms, do NOT drive yourself to the hospital.
- While waiting for an ambulance, rest in a position of comfort to decrease oxygen demands on your heart.
- Take one aspirin.
- Take nitroglycerine if it has been prescribed.

Front office–Back office connection

Patient with Chest Pain

When a patient enters the medical office with complaints of pain, pressure, heaviness, or a squeezing sensation in the chest that may be accompanied by dyspnea, he must be treated as if he could be having a myocardial infarction (MI). An immediate and cooperative effort from administrative and clinical medical assistants and other staff is required to:

- Notify the physician.
- Assist the patient to an examination room and onto an examination table.
- Bring the code cart or supply cart that contains cardiac monitoring equipment, emergency cardiac medications, intubation equipment, and oxygen delivery equipment.
- Prepare for a STAT electrocardiogram (ECG).
- Prepare to draw blood for STAT laboratory tests.
- Prepare to start an IV.
- Call 911 if directed by the physician so the patient can be transported to a hospital.

Minutes saved can mean lives saved. Therefore, the office staff should develop and follow a clear protocol for such situations and all members of the health care team should be familiar with their roles so that everything is handled efficiently without duplication of effort.

to the lungs via the right side of the heart. Even so, as heart failure progresses, both sides of the heart become affected.

Approximately 5 million Americans suffer from heart failure, and the incidence is increasing. More than half a million individuals are newly diagnosed each year, and about 300,000 people die annually from heart-failure-related causes. Those at greatest risk for developing heart failure include African Americans and the elderly.

Heart failure is caused by ineffective pumping of the ventricles. The ventricles may lose effectiveness after heart muscle is lost due to MI or the heart is weakened by cardiomyopathy or other disorders, such as diseased heart valves, congenital heart defects, heart arrhythmias, CAD, diabetes, and hypertension. Damage from disorders such as kidney failure, sepsis (systemic response to massive infection), and other illnesses also contributes to heart failure.

Because left-sided heart failure results in fluid buildup in the lungs, the most common signs and symptoms are related to respiratory problems. Individuals commonly complain of shortness of breath, especially with exertion, and general fatigue. Some individuals may experience orthopnea (dyspnea when lying flat that is relieved by sitting up) or paroxysmal nocturnal dyspnea (PND) (episodes of dyspnea at night that occur repeatedly and without warning). Other symptoms include lower extremity edema, decreased oxygen saturation, and the presence of crackles (fluid in alveoli) heard on auscultation.

Diagnosis of heart failure is based on signs and symptoms, medical history, and diagnostic testing. An echocardiogram, which creates a moving picture of the heart using sound waves, is one of the most useful tests. It reveals data about the heart's size, shape, and valve function. It also reveals areas of poor blood flow and whether all parts of the heart are contracting normally. Chest x-ray reveals pulmonary edema (fluid in the interstitium and alveoli of the lungs) and cardiomegaly (enlarged heart). A blood test of B-type natriuretic peptide (BNP) will be elevated.

Treatment of heart failure includes the administration of diuretics, antihypertensives, and digoxin (Lanoxin). Diuretics stimulate filtration and excretion of urine. Excretion of urine reduces intravascular fluid and allows fluid to shift from the lungs back into blood vessels, thereby relieving dyspnea. Antihypertensives decrease the workload of the heart. Digoxin increases cardiac muscle contractility, thereby strengthening the pumping force of the heart. In cases of valvular disease, heart valve replacement may be considered. Heart transplantation is considered only in extreme cases.

Of those with heart failure, approximately 10% to 20% die each year. However, early diagnosis and medical management can prolong life and increase its quality for most people.

Aneurysm
ICD-9-CM code: 442.9

An aneurysm is an abnormal dilation in the wall of a blood vessel (usually an artery) by more than 50% due to weakness in the vessel wall. Brain aneurysm is the most common type, and abdominal aortic aneurysm (AAA) is the second most common type. (See Figure 27-9.)

One in fifteen Americans has a brain aneurysm, although most will not realize it unless they become symptomatic. Every year, approximately 30,000 will suffer from bleeding. Brain aneurysms are most common in adult women between the ages of 35 and 60. However, AAA is most common among White males over the age of 60, and approximately 15,000 Americans die from a ruptured AAA each year.

Atherosclerosis and weakness in the vessel wall is the cause of AAA. Brain aneurysms are usually congenital. General risk factors that compound vessel injury and increase aneurysm expansion and risk of rupture include diabetes, hypertension, tobacco use, alcohol abuse, and insomnia.

A patient with a brain aneurysm or an AAA is usually asymptomatic unless the aneurysm ruptures. Rupture of a brain aneurysm causes sudden severe headache and hemorrhagic stroke. Rupture of an AAA causes pain in the abdomen or back that may radiate into the groin or flank. The patient may also complain of a feeling of fullness. Without immediate medical attention, severe hypotension, shock, and death quickly follow.

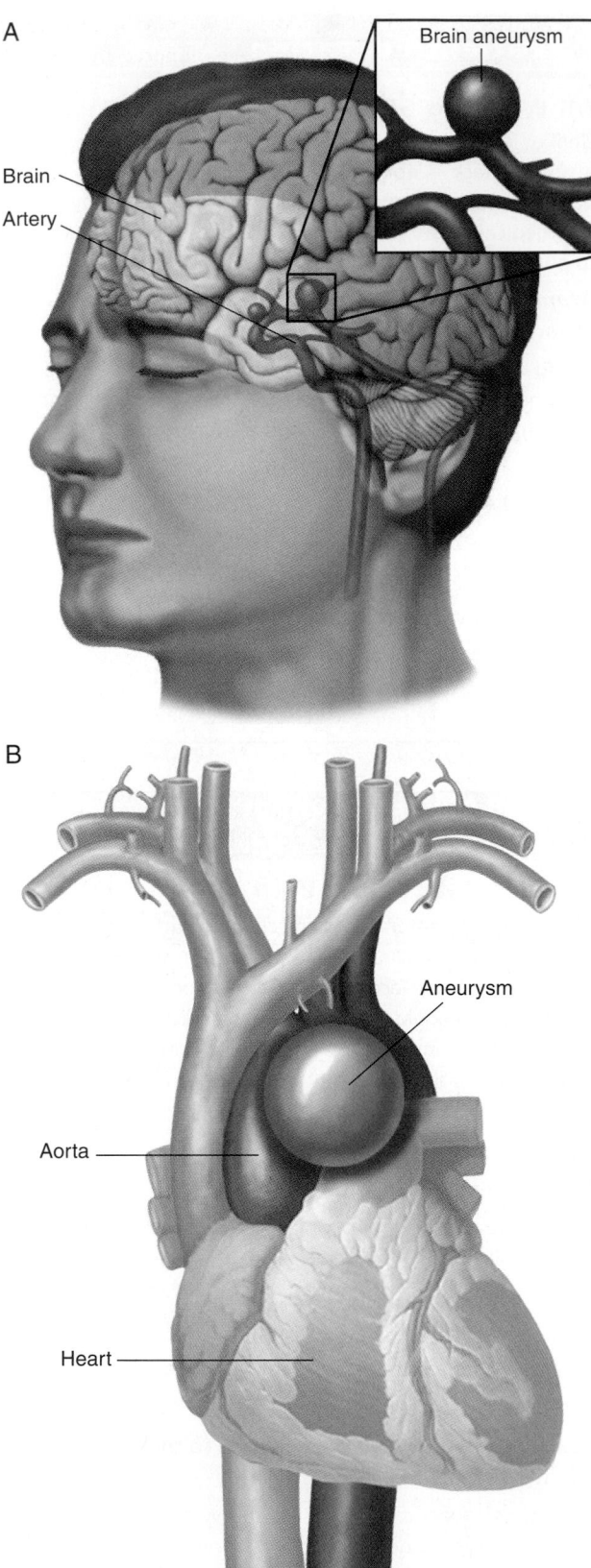

FIG 27-9 Aneurysm. (A) Brain aneurysm. (B) Aortic aneurysm.

Diagnosis of an abdominal aneurysm may be discovered on examination when a pulsating mass is noted in the mid-abdomen. A bruit (abnormal swishing sound) may be heard upon auscultation. Radiological studies, such as MRI, CT scan, and ultrasound, confirm the diagnosis for all types of aneurysms. In some cases, aneurysm is noted when patients undergo examination or radiological testing for other purposes.

When an aneurysm is found, it is usually examined repeatedly over time to determine whether it is increasing in size. This approach is sometimes called "watchful waiting." Traditional treatment of unstable aneurysms includes surgery to insert a graft or clip to stabilize the area. In the late 1990s, a treatment method known as *coil embolization* was developed to treat brain aneurysms. In this procedure, a microcatheter is inserted through a large vessel near the groin and threaded to the aneurysm. Coils are inserted into the aneurysm, filling it from within and thus plugging it and preventing blood from entering. When a patient is identified as having a dissecting (tearing) or ruptured aneurysm, emergency measures are initiated, including surgery, blood and fluid replacement, and respiratory support.

Prognosis depends on the type and location of the aneurysm and whether or not it is identified prior to rupture. When intervention occurs prior to rupture, chances of survival are good. However, once an aneurysm ruptures, the survival rate is low. Among those who suffer a ruptured brain aneurysm, 10% to 15% will die before reaching a hospital. Of those who survive the initial event, 50% will die within 30 days. Of those who survive long-term, approximately 50% will have some type of permanent neurological deficit.

Atrial Fibrillation
ICD-9-CM code: 427

There are many types of heart arrhythmias. By far, the most common is atrial fibrillation. It occurs when irritable myocardial cells in the atrium, other than the SA node, fire chaotically. As a result, the atria quiver uncontrollably rather than contracting normally. The ventricles, in turn, contract irregularly at a faster rate than normal, which results in a rapid, irregular heartbeat. Because of their chaotic quivering, the atria are ineffective in emptying and some blood may pool there and form a clot.

Atrial fibrillation affects as many as 10% of all individuals over the age of 70, or about 2.2 million Americans. The underlying cause of atrial fibrillation is not always clear. Known triggers are many and include stress, exercise, alcohol withdrawal, cardiac surgery, cocaine intoxication, hypoxia, MI, pulmonary embolism (PE), and others. Chronic atrial fibrillation also occurs in those with chronic forms of heart disease.

Individuals with atrial fibrillation are sometimes asymptomatic. However, most experience rapid, irregular heart beat; hypotension; and chest **palpitations** (sensation of rapid or irregular beating of the heart). Other symptoms include shortness of breath, dizziness, and exercise intolerance.

Atrial fibrillation is diagnosed using a 12-lead ECG. However, atrial fibrillation is sometimes intermittent in nature and may be missed by an ECG, which only detects arrhythmias occurring at the moment the ECG is performed. Therefore, accurate diagnosis may require the patient to wear a Holter monitor or an event recorder. These devices allow the detection of abnormal heart beats as the individual goes about her daily routine. Other diagnostic techniques may include echocardiography and trans-esophageal echocardiography.

Conservative treatment of atrial fibrillation includes medication, such as digoxin, that slows the heart rate and may restore normal sinus rhythm (NSR). If medication is not successful, the patient will undergo **cardioversion**, which is a synchronized shock of electrical current delivered to the chest wall while the patient is under sedation and analgesia. If these measures are unsuccessful, the patient may undergo **ablation** (destruction of electrical conduction pathways) of the AV node. Subsequent placement of a pacemaker may prevent the chaotic atrial impulses from affecting the ventricles and ensure a stable heart rate.

Prognosis for those with atrial fibrillation is good with accurate diagnosis and treatment. Even when restoration of NRS is not achieved, people commonly lead productive lives for many years with atrial fibrillation at a controlled rate. Potential complications include blood clot formation in the atria that may embolize to the brain and other vital organs and cause life-threatening complications, such as stroke or pulmonary embolism.

Varicose Veins
ICD-9-CM code: 454

Varicose veins are enlarged, dilated superficial veins that most commonly develop in the legs. An estimated 12 million Americans suffer from varicose veins. Women suffer from varicose veins more than men, with over 40% of all women over age 50 affected.

Varicosities develop in veins rather than arteries because venous blood travels under low pressure and must fight against gravity to return to the heart. Blood flow is helped along by the presence of one-way valves in veins as well as the pumping action of surrounding leg muscles. However, when valves become incompetent and fail to close properly, blood movement becomes sluggish. This sluggishness results in vein engorgement, which further exacerbates valvular incompetence. It is unclear why this problem develops in some individuals and not in others; however, family history of varicose veins is a known risk factor. Others risk factors include obesity, pregnancy, and prolonged sitting or standing.

Signs and symptoms of varicose veins include the appearance of distended, knotted-appearing superficial veins of the legs and feelings in the legs of pain, aching, and fatigue. Symptoms worsen with prolonged standing and are temporarily relieved by elevating the legs.

Diagnosis is based on appearance of the veins and a description of symptoms from the patient. Conservative treatment aims at relieving symptoms and promoting venous blood return to the heart. It includes rest periods during which legs are elevated above the heart, wearing support hose, and ambulation or leg exercises every hour throughout the day. Patients should avoid activities that impede circulation, including wearing hose with tight leg bands, wearing girdles, crossing the legs, and sitting or standing for a prolonged time. Weight loss is encouraged if obesity is a factor. More aggressive treatment includes **ligation** and stripping (surgical procedures to remove the affected veins) or injection of a sclerosing solution that causes the vein to collapse, harden, and, eventually, atrophy.

In most cases, varicose veins pose no significant health risk other than discomfort and embarrassment related to their appearance. However, severe varicose veins do contribute to the development of deep vein thrombosis, which can be serious.

Deep Vein Thrombosis
ICD-9-CM code: 451
Deep vein thrombosis (DVT), also known as *thrombophlebitis*, occurs when a blood clot develops in a deep vein, usually in the legs. The condition most commonly develops in adults over the age of 60 and those with impaired mobility, such as those with paralysis.

DVT usually occurs secondary to vessel injury and blood stasis (sluggish blood flow) caused by poor circulation and immobility. Platelets begin to gather and fibrin formation occurs in areas of injury, creating a blood clot, and then inflammation ensues. Other contributing factors include clotting disorders, heart failure, estrogen use, malignancy, obesity, and pregnancy.

Common symptoms of DVT include a dull ache in the area of the clot, a feeling of heaviness, and localized edema, redness, and heat. A tentative diagnosis is based on physical examination findings, description of symptoms, and tenderness on palpation. Diagnosis is confirmed with compression ultrasonography, which reveals the failure of a vein to compress where a clot is located. Radiographic venography may also help confirm the diagnosis.

Treatment of DVT includes administration of an anticoagulant medication, such as heparin or enoxaprin (Lovenox), followed by warfarin (Coumadin). The patient should rest and refrain from exercise until the condition resolves. The

health care provider may also advise the patient to elevate the limb and apply warm compresses.

A potential complication of DVT is embolization of the clot to the lungs, resulting in pulmonary embolism (blood clot in the lungs), which may be a life-threatening event. However, with timely diagnosis and intervention, most individuals recover without incident. In some cases, postphlebitic syndrome, a chronic condition marked by edema and aching, may develop.

Shock
ICD-9-CM code: 785.50 (unspecified; failure of peripheral circulation), 785.51 (cardiogenic), 785.59 (other)
Shock is a syndrome of inadequate perfusion and oxygenation of cells, tissues, and organs as a result of low blood pressure. It is classified according to the underlying cause. Types of shock include cardiogenic (cardiac failure), hemorrhagic (blood loss), septic (massive infection), and anaphylactic (allergic). Incidence varies with the type of shock involved. Regardless of the cause, all forms of shock, if severe enough, ultimately lead to severe hypotension. As a result, vital organs of the body are not adequately **perfused**, resulting in organ system dysfunction and possible death.

Early symptoms of shock are variable, depending on the underlying cause; however, they always include anxiety and a decreased level of consciousness. Late signs of shock include tachycardia, profound hypotension, diaphoresis, confusion, pallor, a dramatic drop in oxygen saturation levels, a dramatic decrease in urinary output, and, eventually, death.

Diagnosis is based on recent medical history, the patient's presenting signs and symptoms, and physical examination findings. Because shock may be life-threatening, timely diagnosis is important, as is aggressive treatment tailored to the specific cause. Hypotension is treated by blood transfusion or administration of IV fluids and vasoactive medications. The patient may be admitted to an intensive care unit, placed on cardiac monitors, and provided with respiratory support.

Prognosis for the individual experiencing shock depends on the underlying cause and how quickly diagnosis and treatment begin. The outcome for a patient suffering from mild shock is good if appropriate treatment is initiated. However, survival for those suffering from severe, late-stage shock is poor.

Anemia
ICD-9-CM code:280 to 289 (depends on specific type)
Anemia is not a disease, but rather a symptom of disease. It is defined as a reduction in the mass of circulating red blood cells. An individual is considered anemic when her hemoglobin level drops below a specified point. However, normal

values vary depending on gender, pregnancy status, age, the altitude at which a person lives, and race.

Approximately 3.4 million Americans suffer from some form of anemia. Those most commonly affected include women and those with chronic disease. Some of the numerous causes of anemia include blood loss, vitamin or mineral deficiencies, drop in red blood cell production as a result of kidney or bone marrow failure, or disorders that cause excessive red blood cell destruction.

Signs and symptoms of acute anemia include weakness, fatigue, light-headedness, tachycardia, tachypnea, dyspnea, heart palpitations, angina, and headache. Chronic anemia may cause pallor and fissures at the corners of the mouth.

In general, an individual has symptomatic anemia when the hemoglobin content of the blood is less than that required to meet the oxygen-carrying demands of the body. Diagnosis of a specific type of anemia is usually done by examining red blood cells (RBCs) and other blood components under the microscope to determine their shape, size, and color characteristics.

Treatment of anemia depends on the underlying cause. For example, iron deficiency anemia is treated with iron and vitamin C supplements. Pernicious anemia is treated with vitamin B_{12} supplements, and sickle cell anemia is treated with supplemental iron and blood transfusions. Prognosis for individuals suffering from anemia depends on the specific type, the underlying cause, and the individual's response to therapy.

Leukemia
ICD-9-CM code: 204.0, 204.1, 205.0, 205.1 (depends on specific type)

Leukemia is a malignancy of the blood and blood-forming tissues, including the bone marrow, spleen, and lymph nodes. There are a number of different types of leukemia, including acute and chronic forms. The chronic forms have a relatively slow course that averages 4 years, while the acute forms are fatal within months or even weeks.

In the United States, approximately 29,000 adults and 2,000 children are diagnosed with some form of leukemia each year. Acute lymphocytic leukemia (ALL) is the most common type of leukemia to affect children. The other three types—acute myelogenous leukemia (AML), chronic lymphocytic leukemia (CLL), and chronic myelogenous leukemia (CML)—may occasionally affect children but develop mostly in older adults.

In all types of leukemia, abnormally rapid proliferation of one type of white blood cell (WBC) results in reduced production of other types of WBCs, RBCs, and platelets. The underlying cause is not always fully understood. Suspected triggers or contributors are thought to include viruses, tobacco use, chemical exposure, some drugs, previous radiation treatment, other types of cancer, and genetic factors.

Signs and symptoms of leukemia include fatigue, fever, frequent infections, pallor, petechiae (tiny purple-red hemorrhagic spots under the skin), and easy bruising or bleeding. Individuals may also experience hepatomegaly, splenomegaly, enlarged axillary or cervical lymph nodes, tenderness over bony areas, headache, weight loss, and bone and joint pain.

Diagnosis is based on signs and symptoms, physical examination findings, and examination of the blood and bone marrow. CBC with differential may reveal anemia as well as an abnormal count of the different types of WBCs, platelets, and RBCs. A lumbar puncture may be done to obtain spinal fluid for examination. Treatment of leukemia varies with the specific type and usually involves chemotherapy, bone marrow transplantation, or both.

Prognosis for individuals suffering from leukemia depends on the specific type and timeliness of diagnosis and treatment as well as other factors, such as whether a suitable bone marrow donor is identified. Survival rates vary dramatically, from 20% to 75%, depending on the type of leukemia and other factors.

Lymphatic System
Hodgkin Disease
ICD-9-CM code: 201.90

Hodgkin disease, also known as *lymphoma,* is a malignancy of the lymph system. It initially affects lymph nodes and eventually spreads throughout the lymphatic system, involving the spleen, liver, and bone marrow.

About 7900 new cases of Hodgkin disease are diagnosed each year in the United States. Those most commonly affected include young adults between the ages of 15 and 40 and those over age 55.

The cause of Hodgkin disease is not fully understood. However, the Epstein-Barr virus has been found in approximately 50% of those with the disease. Therefore, a link between the two is suspected. Other risk factors include a weakened immune system from chemotherapy or radiation, from human immunodeficiency virus or AIDS, or from immunosuppressive therapy related to organ transplantation. A family history of Hodgkin disease is also a risk factor.

In the early stages of Hodgkin disease, patients may be asymptomatic except for a painless lump in the axilla or neck. Other signs and symptoms are similar to influenza and include fever, anorexia, weight loss, fatigue, itching, and night sweats. Eventually, tumors develop.

Diagnosis of Hodgkin disease is confirmed upon finding the giant Reed-Sternberg cells in biopsied lymph node tissue. Staging is done to determine how advanced the disease is and to determine the best course of treatment. There are five stages, with stage I being early disease involving a single lymph structure through stage V, which involves widespread disease. Chest, abdomen, and pelvic CT scans may be done to determine the extent of disease.

Treatment for Hodgkin disease includes chemotherapy alone or in combination with radiation therapy. Combinations of agents known by such acronyms as BEACOPP and others are common. Bone marrow transplantation may also be done.

Approximately 1300 Americans die from this disease each year, a 60% drop in mortality since the 1970s. Prognosis depends on the stage of metastasis at the time of diagnosis. Early disease is confined to one or a few nodes, while advanced disease has spread to both sides of the diaphragm or throughout the body. Those with early disease have a 5-year survival rate as high as 90%.

Non-Hodgkin Lymphoma
ICD-9-CM code: 202.8

Non-Hodgkin lymphoma is a group of more than 30 types of malignancies of B or T lymphocytes. These malignancies affect approximately 54,000 Americans each year. The disease is more common in men than women. The cause of non-Hodgkin lymphoma is unclear. However, those who have received previous treatment with immunosuppressive therapies have a risk 100 times greater than others. Other risk factors include infection with AIDS and Epstein-Barr viruses, the *Helicobacter pylori* bacteria, and exposure to some chemicals used to kill weeds and insects.

Early symptoms of non-Hodgkin lymphoma are similar to Hodgkin disease and include painless lymphadenopathy and, sometimes, fever, night sweats, fatigue, abdominal pain or swelling, and weight loss.

Diagnosis is determined by identifying malignant cells via lymph node biopsy and bone marrow examination. CT scans and MRI are done to help determine the extent of spread. Treatment of non-Hodgkin lymphoma includes radiation therapy, chemotherapy, and bone marrow transplantation.

Prognosis depends on the specific type of non-Hodgkin lymphoma involved and the timeliness of diagnosis and treatment. Some types spread slowly and respond well to treatment; others spread quickly, respond to treatment poorly, and are rapidly fatal.

Acquired Immune Deficiency Syndrome
ICD-9-CM code: 042

Acquired immune deficiency syndrome (AIDS) is a late-stage infection of the human immunodeficiency virus (HIV), which progressively weakens the immune system. This disease was first reported in the United States in 1981 and has since become a worldwide epidemic. Two human immunodeficiency viruses have been identified: HIV-1 and HIV-2. Most HIV infections in West Africa are caused by HIV-2. Most other cases in the world are caused by HIV-1. HIV is a retrovirus, which means that it cannot survive on its own but invades human CD-4 lymphocytes and uses them as its host cell. As the virus proliferates and destroys CD-4 lymphocytes, it leaves the body vulnerable to infection. Diagnostic criteria for diagnosis of AIDS includes HIV infection with a CD-4 helper T-cell count of less than 200, the presence of an opportunistic infection, the presence of an AIDS-defining malignancy, or a combination of these criteria.

AIDS is the fourth most common cause of death worldwide and is the leading cause of death in Africa. While anyone can be infected with the AIDS virus, the most common victims have limited access to health care and are poor, heterosexual, and between the ages of 15 and 44. Approximately 1 million cases of AIDS have been reported in the United States and about half of those individuals have died. It is estimated that only about 10% of those infected with AIDS have been diagnosed. Approximately 40,000 Americans are newly infected each year and more than 40 million individuals are infected with AIDS worldwide.

HIV is acquired through direct contact with infected bodily fluids, such as blood, blood products, semen, and vaginal secretions of another person. The most common means of AIDS transmission includes unprotected sexual intercourse, injection drug use, and children born to infected mothers. It is not spread through casual contact, such as shaking hands and hugging. Health care workers may contract the disease through needlestick injuries and major exposure to mucus membranes, such as splashing of blood or body fluids into the eyes and nose. However, the practice of standard precautions significantly minimizes this risk.

About 1 to 2 weeks after exposure to HIV, individuals commonly experience flulike symptoms of fever, body aches, and sore throat. However, few people recognize this as a warning that they have contracted HIV. For the most part, individuals are asymptomatic in the early stages and may unwittingly transmit the virus to others. As the disease progresses and the immune system weakens, opportunistic infections are frequent. Common examples of opportunistic infection include *Pneumocystis* pneumonia (PCP), cytomegalovirus, infections with *Candida albicans,* and malignancies. These infections cause anorexia, weight loss, fatigue, fevers, chills, sweats, breathlessness, pneumonia, diarrhea, lymphadeonopathy (tender, enlarged lymph nodes), and skin rashes. In some cases, dementia develops.

Confirmation of HIV infection is based on the detection of HIV antibodies in the blood by the enzyme-linked immunosorbent assay (ELISA) and Western blot test. If the ELISA test is positive, the test is repeated. Confirmation of diagnosis is done with the Western blot test. Trained clinic personnel can employ newer testing methods, which produce results within 60 minutes and involve testing the blood or swabbing the inside of the mouth around the gums. A home test is also available. The test includes instructions for obtaining a drop of blood by pricking the finger and applying it to the enclosed card, which must be mailed to a laboratory for testing. Because the individual uses an identification number, this system ensures privacy and confidentiality. As with other HIV testing, the patient must confirm positive results by undergoing a Western blot test. Disease progression is monitored by checking CD-4 lymphocyte counts and viral load. As the disease progresses and the immune system weakens, the CD-4 count decreases and viral load increases.

There is currently no cure for HIV or AIDS. Treatment includes the use of highly active antiretroviral therapies (HAART), which include a drug that inhibits HIV-1 protease and drugs that block viral reverse transcriptase. General measures that protect the immune system and protect against other infections are advised. These measures include getting immunized, use of anti-infective medications as needed, avoidance of high-risk behaviors, good nutrition, adequate sleep, moderate exercise as tolerated, and avoidance of others with communicable diseases or infections.

AIDS is ultimately a fatal disease. However, individuals with AIDS are living much longer, healthier lives than in the past, due to advances in treatment. Current life expectancy is approximately 10 years from the time of diagnosis. Even so, the prognosis varies widely, depending on the individual's self-care practices and access to health care resources. (See *Immunocompromised patients*.)

Front office–Back office connection

Immunocompromised Patients

Patients with diseases like leukemia and AIDS are commonly immunocompromised, which means they are especially vulnerable to acquiring other infectious diseases within the medical office. Clinical and administrative medical assistants should collaborate with the other health care providers in the office to identify steps they can take to ensure the welfare of such patients. Such measures may include:

- establishing a plan for immunocompromised patients to enter the office through a lesser-used entrance

- immediately escorting the patient to an examination room

- providing the patient with a mask to wear while in the medical office

- providing a supply of masks for the patient to keep at home for their next trip to the clinic

- remembering to carefully practice standard precautions

- ensuring that health care personnel with infectious conditions (such as the common cold) do not come in contact with the patient.

Cardiology and Lymphatics Procedures

Cardiology is a medical specialty that focuses on the study and treatment of disorders of the cardiovascular system. While many physicians diagnose and treat cardiac disorders, those who specialize in this area of medicine are called *cardiologists*.

Assisting with Examination

To reach an accurate diagnosis, the physician must obtain a medical history, including a description of symptoms, and perform a comprehensive physical examination. The physician inspects the skin for discoloration that might indicate poor circulation as well as distended neck veins or lower-extremity edema that might indicate fluid overload related to heart failure. The physician carefully auscultates the heart to detect abnormal sounds. He also auscultates the lungs for abnormal sounds, such as crackles or rhonchi (low-pitched snoring, squeaking, or gurgling sounds), that indicate the presence of fluid.

The medical assistant must prepare the patient by checking vital signs and obtaining a health history, which may include family history, risk factors for CAD, and new or unusual symptoms the patient has experienced. She should then assist the patient as needed with undressing and positioning and assist the physician as needed with the examination and procedures.

Electrocardiography

Electrocardiography is a common, painless, noninvasive procedure that can be done in the physician's office during a routine physical examination. The **electrocardiogram** (ECG) is the written record that is produced from this procedure and is created by use of an **electrocardiograph** machine. The electrocardiograph machine is connected to the patient with wires and electrodes that are sensitive to the electrical impulses generated by the patient's heart. This electrical activity is represented on electrocardiograph paper through specific waveforms, which are then reviewed and analyzed by the physician. The information obtained aids in the diagnosis and treatment of cardiac problems. ECGs are also commonly done prior to major surgical procedures to establish baseline health information about a patient and to identify potential cardiac disorders. Because this data is so important, the medical assistant must have a good understanding of how to obtain an accurate ECG.

Preparing the Electrocardiograph Machine

To obtain accurate ECG tracings, the medical assistant must be familiar with the ECG machine and equipment in the medical office and become proficient in its use. (See Figure 27-10.)

Electrocardiograph Paper

The paper used in ECG machines is pressure- and heat-sensitive. The ECG machine includes a stylus that becomes hot when the machine is turned on. The stylus marks the ECG paper as it moves horizontally past at a specific rate. The paper is also a type of graph paper, with vertical and horizontal lines at 1-mm intervals and bold horizontal and vertical lines at 5-mm intervals. The space between each vertical line represents 0.04 second of time, and the space between bold vertical lines (5 tiny boxes) represents 0.2 second of time. The space between horizontal lines represents amplitude or voltage. When the machine is properly calibrated, 10 mm of amplitude (10 tiny boxes or 2 large boxes) equals 1 millivolt (mV) of electrical activity. (See Figure 27-11.)

Standardization

All ECG machines are standardized in the same way so that an ECG can be interpreted in the same manner, regardless what part of the world a patient is in. To ensure this consistency, the medical assistant must check for standardization,

or *calibration,* of the ECG machine each time she conducts an ECG. To check for standardization, the medical assistant must first make sure that the machine is set at 1 STD. Then she must verify that 1 mV of electricity causes the stylus to move 10 mm vertically by quickly pushing the STANDARDI-ZATION button. The machine should respond by creating a deflection that is 10 mm (10 tiny boxes) high vertically and 2 mm (2 tiny boxes) wide horizontally. (See Figure 27-12.) The manufacturer's manual explains the exact method for adjusting the machine to create perfect standardization.

Leads and Electrodes

The medical assistant must place electrodes on the patient's arms, legs, and chest to sense cardiac electrical activity. Each of the electrodes is connected to color-coded leadwires (commonly called *leads*) by a metal clip. The leadwires transmit data about cardiac electrical activity to the ECG machine. The ECG machine amplifies the electrical activity and represents it on the ECG paper by characteristic waveforms created by deflection of the stylus. Older ECG machines use metal disks, rubber bands, and suction cups to attach the electrodes and keep them in place. Such equipment is cumbersome and difficult to use, especially when time is of the essence. Therefore, most medical offices now use disposable,

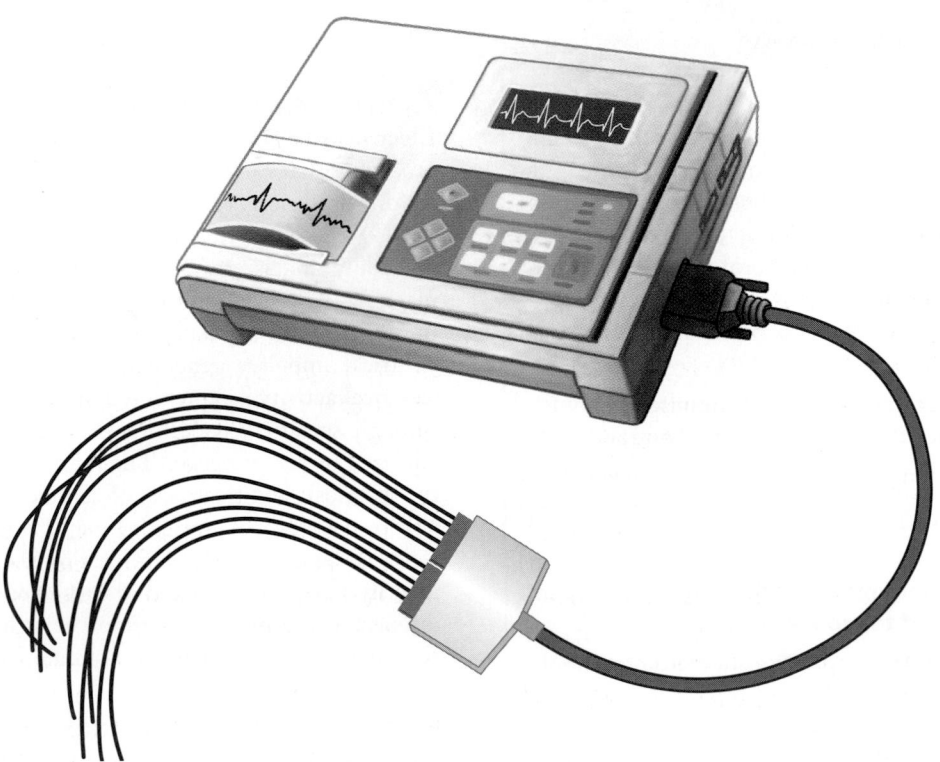

FIG 27-10 ECG machine.

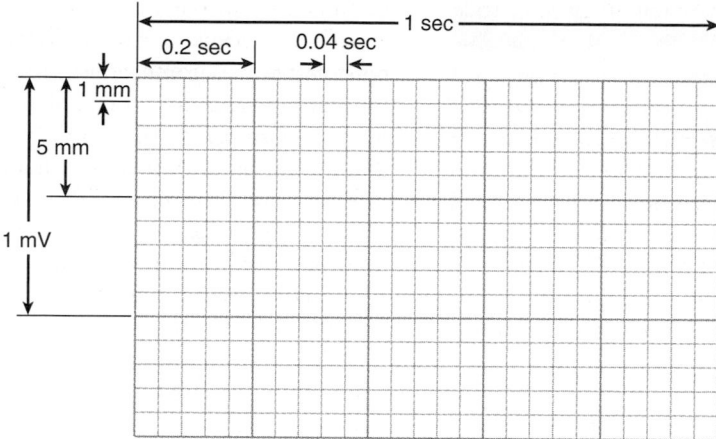

FIG 27-11 ECG paper.

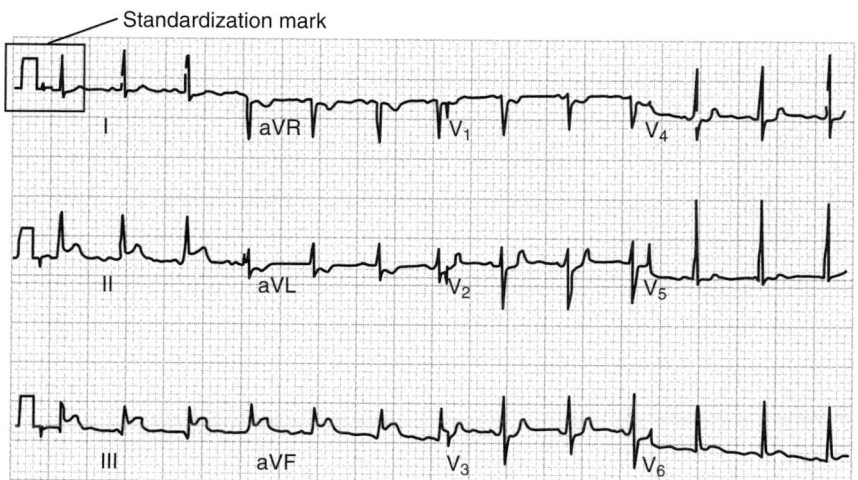

FIG 27-12 Standardization mark.

self-adhesive electrodes that are impregnated with the optimal amount of electrolyte gel.

Correct leadwire placement enables the ECG machine to record electrical activity of the heart from different viewpoints. Frontal leads include leads I, II, III, aV_R, aV_L, and aV_F. Other leads are on the horizontal plane. These leads include the six precordial leads, or *chest leads*. Each lead records electrical activity between positive and negative electrodes. When depolarization of heart muscle occurs toward a positive electrode, it creates a positive, or upright, deflection. If it occurs toward a negative electrode, it creates a negative, or downward, deflection. (See *Lead placement,* page 484.)

Color coding and labels make accurate attachment of leadwires to electrodes easy. The RA lead is attached to the right arm lead, the LA lead is attached to the left arm lead, and so on. In the case of a patient who has had a limb amputated, the medical assistant should place the limb electrodes above the amputation, making sure to place the electrodes directly across from each other. She should not place electrodes on scars, skin growths, or open wounds. If the patient has excessive hair, the medical assistant may need to clip the hair on the area before placing the electrodes. Shaving should be avoided because shaving commonly causes small nicks in the skin that can put the patient at risk for infection.

Preparing the Patient

Medical assistants and other health care providers who routinely perform ECGs sometimes forget that the procedure does not feel routine to a patient, who may be anxious, embarrassed, confused, or in pain. Therefore, the medical assistant must be sensitive and take care to properly prepare the patient so that an accurate tracing can be obtained and the patient is as comfortable as possible. Although the patient must disrobe above the waist, he should be offered a gown (with the opening in the front). The medical assistant

Lead placement

Although there are 10 electrodes, heart activity is recorded from 12 different angles, thus the term *12-lead electrocardiogram (ECG)*. Electrodes are applied to the patient in these specific locations:

- V_1—fourth intercostal space at the right sternal border
- V_2—fourth intercostal space at the left sternal border
- V_3—midway between V_2 and V_4
- V_4—fifth intercostal space, in the left midclavicular line
- V_5—lateral to V_4, in the left anterior axillary line
- V_6—lateral to V_5, in the left midaxillary line
- RA and LA—anterior surface of the upper arms near the shoulder
- RL and LL—clean, dry, fleshy areas of the lower legs.

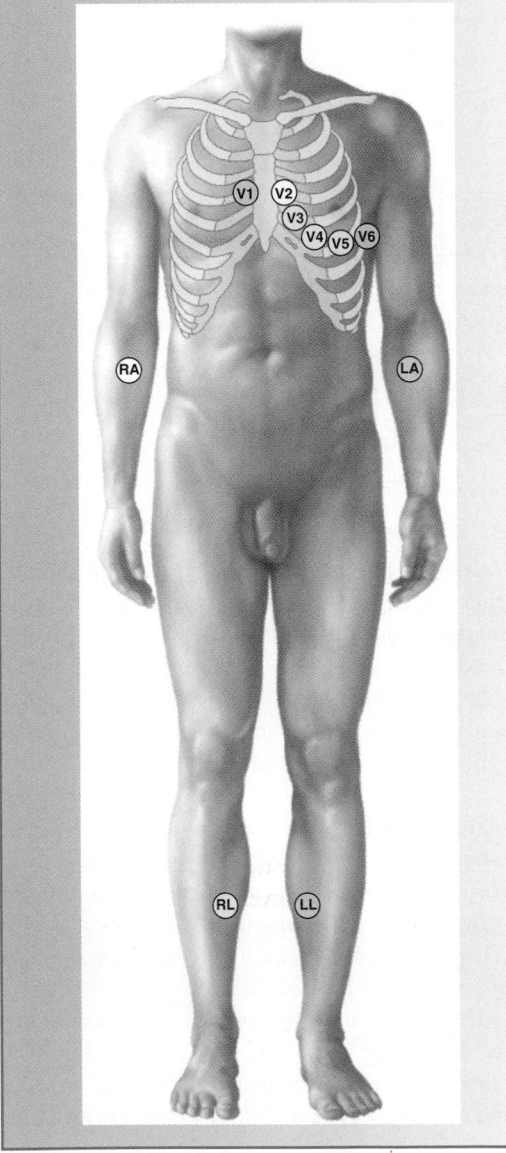

should carefully drape a female patient, in particular, during the procedure to protect her privacy to the greatest extent possible without compromising the accuracy of the ECG tracing. The medical assistant should position the patient in a supine position or semi-Fowler position if short of breath. The patient should not cross or dangle his legs. The medical assistant should record in the patient's chart his current medications and vital signs. Alternatively, some machines allow the medical assistant to program these details into the machine, which will print them on the ECG tracing. The medical assistant should reassure the patient that the procedure will be painless and should remind him to lie still and breathe normally.

Recording the ECG

There are a variety of ECG machines, so the medical assistant should become familiar with the ECG machine used in her office. Most types currently in use perform labeling and standardization automatically. However, the medical assistant may need to enter information about the patient's gender, age, and medications. Six-channel ECG machines print and label all 12 leads and include a strip across the bottom of the paper in lead II. This type of machine completes a recording quickly. When the recording is complete, the medical assistant must review it for clarity, the presence of electrical interference, or other problems. If the recording appears satisfactory, the medical assistant must give it to the physician for review and analysis. She should then help the patient get off the examination table and dress, as needed.

Rhythm Interpretation

To be able to accurately examine the ECG waveforms, the medical assistant must understand what each one represents. The first waveform occurs when the muscle cells of the atria depolarize. This electrical activity causes the stylus to deflect upward, creating the P wave. It is usually a slight upward, rounded wave. After a brief pause, the ventricles depolarize. This depolarization generates a greater amount of electrical activity, causing a larger deflection of the stylus, creating the Q, R, and S waves, more commonly known as the *QRS complex*. This complex is followed by a brief period with no electrical activity, causing the ST segment, where the stylus remains at the baseline. Next, ventricular repolarization occurs, creating the T wave. (See Figure 27-13.)

The physician is responsible for analyzing and interpreting the ECG tracing. However, because the medical assistant routinely performs ECGs, she must be familiar with the most common rhythms—especially those that may be life-threatening. Basic rhythm interpretation involves several simple steps, including:

- calculation of the ventricular rate
- calculation of the atrial rate
- measurement and examination of the waveforms.

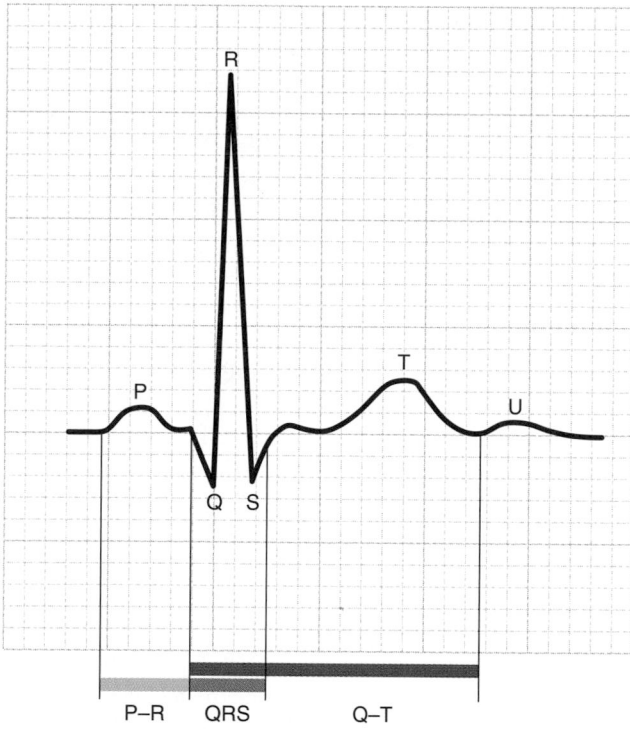

FIG 27-13 ECG waveforms.

Calculation of the Ventricular Rate

The simplest way to calculate the ventricular rate is to count the number of R waves in a 6-second strip (30 large squares) and multiply by 10, or count the number of R waves in a 3-second strip (15 large squares) and multiply by 20. Three-second segments are generally easy to identify on rhythm strips by small marks across the top of the strip. This system is fairly accurate as long as the rhythm is regular. For grossly irregular rhythms, this system is less reliable. The normal adult heart rate is between 60 and 100 beats/minute.

Calculation of the Atrial Rate

Calculation of the atrial rate is similar to calculating the ventricular rate except that P waves are counted instead of R waves. This step may seem redundant and unnecessary. However, in some abnormal rhythms, the atria and ventricles function out of sync with one another and may have different rates. Counting P waves allows the examiner to identify this abnormality. Isolated QRS complexes that occur earlier than expected are called *premature atrial contractions* (PACs). In a PAC, the electrical impulse originates somewhere in the atria other than the SA node. Occasional PACs are generally not of concern. However, patients experiencing frequent PACs accompanied by symptoms of chest pain, shortness

of breath, or dizziness must receive evaluation and treatment.

Examination of the P Waves

When examining the P waves, the medical assistant should note whether there is consistently a P wave in front of every QRS complex. She should also note whether P waves are upright and rounded and whether all P waves have the same appearance.

Measurement of the PR Interval

The PR interval represents the time required for the electrical impulse to spread from the SA node through the atrial muscle cells and the AV node. The PR interval should be measured from the beginning of the P wave (where it leaves the baseline) to the beginning of the QRS complex. All PR intervals should be of the same length and should measure between 0.12 and 0.20 second (3 to 5 tiny boxes).

Measurement of the QRS Complex

The QRS complex represents the time required for the electrical impulse to spread through the right and left ventricles. The QRS complex is measured from the beginning of the Q wave to the end of the S wave and should be less than 0.12 second in length. All QRS complexes should be of consistent shape and size. Isolated QRS complexes that occur earlier than expected and are wide and oddly shaped represent **premature ventricular contractions** (PVCs). In PVC, the electrical impulse originates somewhere within the ventricles. Occasional PVCs are generally not of concern. However, patients experiencing frequent PVCs accompanied by symptoms of chest pain, shortness of breath, or dizziness must receive evaluation and treatment.

Examination of the ST Segment

The ST segment should be *iso-electric,* which means that it should be at the baseline. However, some patient factors may cause variations in the ST segment. For example, ST segment elevation or depression may suggest myocardial ischemia or even myocardial infarction and should be examined by the physician immediately, particularly if the patient is symptomatic.

Examination of the T Wave

The T wave may be curved upward with a rounded top, more sharply peaked, or even inverted, depending on a number of patient factors. For example, patients with hyperkalemia (elevated blood potassium) usually exhibit tall, peaked T waves.

Examination of the QT Interval

The QT interval is measured from the beginning of the QRS complex to the end of the T wave. It represents the time required for the impulse to spread through the muscle cells of the ventricles and for repolarization to occur. The normal QT interval length is between 0.32 and 0.44 second long. (See *Common ECG rhythms*.)

Artifacts

Because electrocardiograph machines are sensitive to electrical activity, they sometimes record electrical activity from sources other than the patient's heart. Examples include electricity from nearby equipment or even the patient's own noncardiac muscle movement. When the ECG stylus moves in response to this interfering electrical activity, it records markings on the ECG strip known as **artifacts**, which are distracting and irrelevant. (See *Common types of artifact*, page 490.) The medical assistant must review the ECG tracing for the presence of artifacts or other errors that may require her to perform the test again. (See *Procedure 27-1: Performing a 12-lead ECG*, page 492.)

Artificial Cardiac Pacemaker

An artificial pacemaker is a device that delivers electrical impulses to the heart to stimulate a heartbeat. The purpose is to maintain an adequate heart rate in individuals whose natural heart rate is too slow or irregular due to a malfunction of the SA node or a block in the electrical conduction system. The pacemaker is implanted under a patient's skin, usually on the left anterior chest wall, and has electrodes that are implanted into the heart muscle. There are numerous makes and models of pacemakers and each can be programmed specifically for the needs of the patient. Pacemakers may be programmed to stimulate atrial contraction, ventricular contraction, or both (dual channel). The physician can set the pacemaker to pace the heart all of the time or only as needed when the patient's SA node fires below a specified rate. Pacemaker spikes may or may not show up on the ECG tracing, depending on the type and setting of pacemaker. If present, pacemaker spikes appear as small vertical lines just before the P wave (if pacing the atria) or just before the QRS complex (if pacing the ventricles) or both. A rate-responsive pacemaker senses the patient's physical activity and responds by increasing or decreasing the rate.

Implantable Cardioverter Defibrillator

An implantable cardioverter defibrillator (ICD), also called an *automated implantable cardioverter defibrillator* (AICD), is a small device slightly larger than a pacemaker that is implanted in patients at risk for life-threatening arrhythmias, such as ventricular fibrillation and ventricular tachycardia. Some devices are actually a combination of a pacemaker and a defibrillator. ICDs continually monitor the individual's heart rate and rhythm. If a patient develops a potentially life-threatening arrhythmia, the ICD delivers an electrical shock to the heart with the goal of restoring normal sinus rhythm.

Cardiac Stress Test

A cardiac stress test is a test performed to evaluate the heart's response to physical exercise. This test has a number of other names, including *exercise stress test, exercise treadmill test, exercise tolerance test, stress test, exercise ECG test,* and, if radioactive isotopes are used, *nuclear stress test*. This test may be useful for patients who experience angina caused by stenosis of 75% or more of a coronary artery. In the test, the patient walks on a treadmill or is given IV medication that causes a response similar to the body's response to exercise. During the procedure, the medical assistant monitors the patient's heart rate, blood pressure, and any symptoms. The American Heart Association recommends a cardiac stress test for patients with a medium risk of coronary artery disease based on the risk factors of smoking, hypertension, family history of heart disease, high cholesterol, and diabetes. However, patients who have had an MI within the previous 48 hours and those with unstable angina, uncontrolled arrhythmias, or certain other unstable conditions should not undergo stress testing. Because the cardiac stress test does subject the patient to physical stress, close monitoring is important. Members of the testing team must be familiar with emergency protocols and should be prepared to respond if the patient develops arrhythmias, dyspnea, chest pain, or an actual MI. The medical assistant or other staff member should keep emergency cardiac medications and equipment on hand, and the testing team must be familiar with their use.

Holter Monitoring

The Holter monitor is a portable device that records the patient's cardiac rhythm over a 24- or 48-hour period. This type of testing, also known as *ambulatory electrocardiography*, is useful when the patient complains of an irregular heartbeat or other symptoms that are intermittent and therefore difficult to obtain on a 12-lead ECG in the medical office. The medical assistant should apply the Holter monitor electrodes to the patient and show him how to carry the monitor in a small pouch with a shoulder strap. She should instruct him to wear the device while participating in normal daily activities and to record in a journal when he feels any symptoms, such as heart palpitations and dizziness, or if he engages in heavy physical activity. After wearing the monitor for the designated period of time, the patient returns it to the medical office, where the data is downloaded. A cardiologist then reviews and interprets it and discusses the results with the patient.

The medical assistant may be responsible for applying and removing the monitor as well as providing the patient with instructions. The patient may not shower or bathe while wearing the Holter monitor, but may take a sponge bath. The medical assistant may need to clip chest hair to ensure good electrode adhesion. The patient keeps the

Common ECG rhythms

This table describes the features of some of the most common electrocardiograph (ECG) rhythms. Some are considered normal while others may be life-threatening.

Rhythm	Characteristics	Signs and Symptoms	Required Response
Sinus Rhythms			
Normal sinus rhythm (NSR) (From Jones, *ECG Success: Exercises in ECG Interpretation*. FA Davis, Philadelphia, 2008, p. 20, with permission.)	• Rate: 60 to 100 beats/minute • Rhythm: regular • PR interval: 0.12 to 0.20 second • QRS complex: <0.12 second	• None	No special action is required.
Sinus bradycardia (From Jones, *ECG Success: Exercises in ECG Interpretation*. FA Davis, Philadelphia, 2008, p. 21, with permission.)	• Rate: <60 beats/ minute • Rhythm: regular • PR interval: 0.12 to 0.20 second • QRS complex: <0.12 second	• Usually none	Notify the physician if the patient is symptomatic.
Sinus tachycardia (From Jones, *ECG Success: Exercises in ECG Interpretation*. FA Davis, Philadelphia, 2008, p. 21, with permission.)	• Rate: >100 beats/minute • Rhythm: regular • PR interval: 0.12 to 0.20 second • QRS complex: <0.12 second	• Usually none	Notify the physician if the patient is symptomatic.
Sinus arrhythmia (From Jones, *ECG Success: Exercises in ECG Interpretation*. FA Davis, Philadelphia, 2008, p. 22, with permission.)	• Rate: fluctuates with respiratory pattern • Rhythm: regular • PR interval: 0.12 to 0.20 second • QRS complex: <0.12 second	• None	No special action is required.

Continued

Common ECG rhythms—cont'd

Rhythm	Characteristics	Signs and Symptoms	Required Response
Atrial Arrhythmias			
Sinus rhythm with premature atrial contractions (PACs) (From Jones, *ECG Success: Exercises in ECG Interpretation*. FA Davis, Philadelphia, 2008, p. 29, with permission.)	• Rate: 60 to 100 beats/minute • Rhythm: regular, except when PACs occur • PR interval: 0.12 to 0.20 second; may vary in the PACs • QRS complex: <0.12 second	• Usually none • Possible palpitations	No special action is required.
Atrial fibrillation (From Jones, *ECG Success: Exercises in ECG Interpretation*. FA Davis, Philadelphia, 2008, p. 32, with permission.)	• Rate: possibly rapid • Rhythm: irregular • P waves: none • PR interval: none • QRS complex: <0.12 second	• Palpitations, dyspnea, and dizziness possible with rapid, uncontrolled rate • Possibly no symptoms with controlled rate	Notify the physician if the patient is symptomatic.
Atrial flutter (From Jones, *ECG Success: Exercises in ECG Interpretation*. FA Davis, Philadelphia, 2008, p. 31, with permission.)	• Rate: atrial, rapid (250 to 350 beats/minute); ventricular, variable (125 to 175 beats/minute) • Rhythm: usually regular • P waves: none identifiable; instead, "saw-tooth" patterned flutter waves • QRS complex: <0.12 second	• Possible palpitations, shortness of breath, and dizziness	Notify the physician immediately.

Common ECG rhythms—cont'd

Rhythm	Characteristics	Signs and Symptoms	Required Response
Ventricular Arrhythmias			
Sinus rhythm with premature ventricular contractions (PVCs) (From Jones, *ECG Success: Exercises in ECG Interpretation*. FA Davis, Philadelphia, 2008, p. 46, with permission.)	• Rate: 60 to 100 beats/minute • Rhythm: regular except when PVCs occur • PR interval: 0.12 to 0.20 second, none when PVCs occur • QRS complex: <0.12 second, except PVCs, which show up as bizarrely shaped, wide QRS complexes with no preceding P wave.	• Usually none unless PVCs are frequent • Possible palpitations	No special action is required unless the patient is symptomatic.
Ventricular tachycardia (From Jones, *ECG Success: Exercises in ECG Interpretation*. FA Davis, Philadelphia, 2008, p. 54, with permission.)	• Rate: rapid, usually 100 to 220 beats/minute • Rhythm: usually regular • P waves: none • QRS complex: wide, oddly shaped, and >0.12 second	• Dramatic hypotension • Loss of consciousness	This is a life-threatening emergency that requires you to contact the physician immediately. If the patient is pulseless and breathless, initiate cardiopulmonary resuscitation (CPR).
Ventricular fibrillation (From Jones, *ECG Success: Exercises in ECG Interpretation*. FA Davis, Philadelphia, 2008, p. 57, with permission.)	• Rate: rapid (350 to 450 beats/minute) • Rhythm: irregular; chaotic • P waves: none • QRS complex: none	• Loss of consciousness • Loss of pulse • Imminent death	This is a life-threatening emergency that requires you to contact the physician immediately. If the patient is pulseless and breathless, initiate cardiopulmonary resuscitation (CPR).

Continued

Common ECG rhythms—cont'd

Rhythm	Characteristics	Signs and Symptoms	Required Response
Asystole 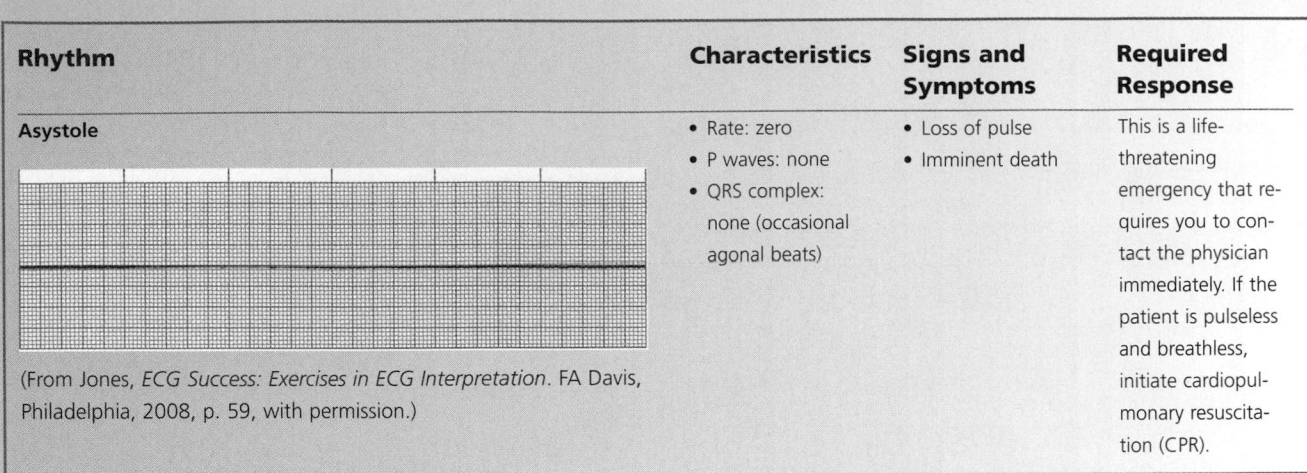 (From Jones, *ECG Success: Exercises in ECG Interpretation*. FA Davis, Philadelphia, 2008, p. 59, with permission.)	• Rate: zero • P waves: none • QRS complex: none (occasional agonal beats)	• Loss of pulse • Imminent death	This is a life-threatening emergency that requires you to contact the physician immediately. If the patient is pulseless and breathless, initiate cardiopulmonary resuscitation (CPR).

Common types of artifact

It is important for the medical assistant to become familiar with common types of artifact so she can minimize interference when obtaining electrocardiograms (ECGs). The patient and physician depend on the medical assistant to provide accurate ECGs to aid in accurate diagnosis and create an effective treatment plan.

The following table lists the types of artifacts that commonly interfere with accurate ECG recording, along with a description and sample tracing, typical causes, and solutions.

Artifact	Cause	Solution
Somatic tremor—causes small, irregular, jagged peaks and may give the tracing a fuzzy appearance 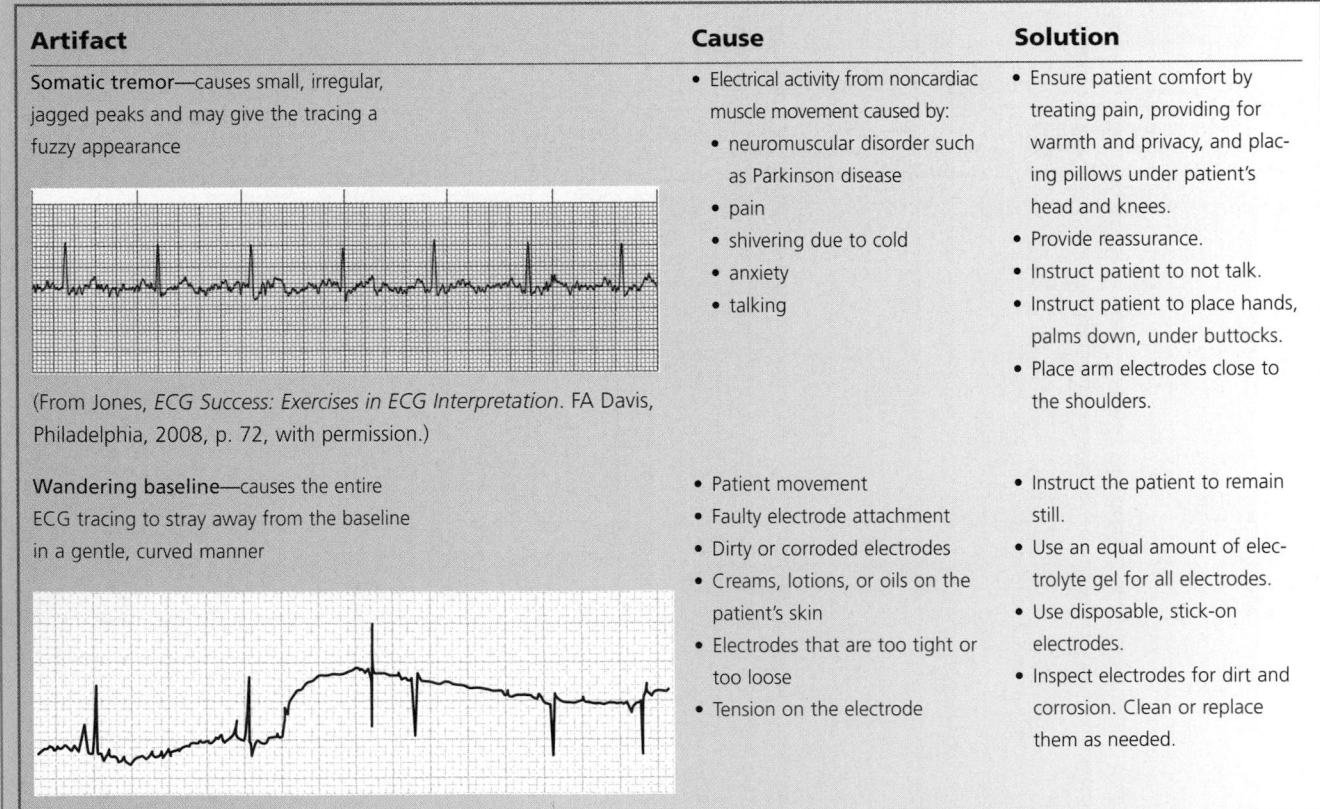 (From Jones, *ECG Success: Exercises in ECG Interpretation*. FA Davis, Philadelphia, 2008, p. 72, with permission.)	• Electrical activity from noncardiac muscle movement caused by: • neuromuscular disorder such as Parkinson disease • pain • shivering due to cold • anxiety • talking	• Ensure patient comfort by treating pain, providing for warmth and privacy, and placing pillows under patient's head and knees. • Provide reassurance. • Instruct patient to not talk. • Instruct patient to place hands, palms down, under buttocks. • Place arm electrodes close to the shoulders.
Wandering baseline—causes the entire ECG tracing to stray away from the baseline in a gentle, curved manner	• Patient movement • Faulty electrode attachment • Dirty or corroded electrodes • Creams, lotions, or oils on the patient's skin • Electrodes that are too tight or too loose • Tension on the electrode	• Instruct the patient to remain still. • Use an equal amount of electrolyte gel for all electrodes. • Use disposable, stick-on electrodes. • Inspect electrodes for dirt and corrosion. Clean or replace them as needed.

Common types of artifact—cont'd

Artifact	Cause	Solution
		• Clean the patient's skin with alcohol. • Clip (do not shave) chest hair if necessary. • Tape leadwire 1" to 2" below the clip.
Alternating current (AC) interference—causes a series of short spikes (From Geiter, *E-Z ECG: Basic Step-by-Step Interpretation*. FA Davis, Philadelphia, 2007, p. 301, with permission.)	• Electrical currents from nearby equipment or wires	• Plug ECG machine into 3-prong, grounded outlet. • Avoid crossing leadwires. • Unplug nearby electrical equipment. • Move the examination table away from the wall. • Turn off the overhead fluorescent lights. • Perform ECGs in the room furthest away from other electrical equipment.
Interrupted baseline—appears as large, irregular fluctuations in which the stylus moves to the margins of the ECG paper (From Jones, *ECG Success: Exercises in ECG Interpretation*. FA Davis, Philadelphia, 2008, p. 71, with permission.)	• Interruption of electrical connection caused by patient movement • Broken leadwires • Loose cable tips	• Instruct the patient to remain still. • Replace the leadwires. • Attach the cable tips firmly to the electrodes.

monitor in a pouch that is attached to a belt or slung over the shoulder. (See Figure 27-14.)

Event Recorder

An event recorder, sometimes called a *King of Hearts monitor*, is a small portable monitor that the patient can wear around the neck like a pendant or place in a shirt pocket. It is attached to two electrodes on the patient's chest that may be activated by the patient when he feels such symptoms as chest pain, dizziness, and palpitations. The data is then sent to the cardiology clinic via the telephone for analysis. This type of device is ideal for patients whose symptoms are intermittent and unpredictable and, therefore, unlikely to manifest during an ECG test. Event recorders may be worn for as long as 30 days to capture events likely to be missed by an ECG or even a Holter monitor. Most event recorders allow telephone transmission of recordings, so the medical assistant should also provide the patient with instructions about how to do this. Lastly, the medical assistant should give the patient contact information in case he has questions or concerns. (See *Wearing an event recorder*, page 492.)

PROCEDURE 27-1

Performing a 12-lead ECG

Task
Obtain an accurate 12-lead ECG recording.

Conditions
- ECG machine with cable and paper
- 10 disposable, self-adhesive electrodes
- Examination gown
- Drape

Standards
In the time specified and within the scoring parameters determined by the instructor, the student will successfully obtain an accurate 12-lead ECG recording.

Performance Standards

1. Wash or sanitize your hands to ensure proper infection control and assemble supplies.
2. Greet and identify your patient, introduce yourself, and explain the procedure to prevent errors and ease patient anxiety.
3. Instruct the patient to remove socks or pantyhose as well as clothing above the waist, including undergarments to facilitate the placement of electrodes. Assist the patient as necessary.
4. Position the patient on the examination table in the supine position. Drape her for warmth and privacy.
5. Turn on the machine. Enter the patient's name, date, time, and patient's current cardiac medications into the machine or write the information on the tracing paper to ensure proper identification of the tracing and provide relevant data.
6. Clean the patient's skin with alcohol at each site where an electrode will be placed and clip hair if

necessary to remove skin oils or hair that would interfere with secure sensor adhesion.

7. Apply self-adhesive electrodes to a dry, clean, intact, fleshy area on the extremities across from one another and to the cleaned areas on the chest.
8. Connect the leadwires to the electrodes using the alligator clips. Make sure the correct leads are connected to the correct electrodes. Do not cross leadwires to help prevent artifact.
9. Press the AUTO button on the ECG machine. The machine runs automatically once the AUTO button is pressed. Watch for artifacts and make corrections as needed to get an acceptable tracing.
10. Disconnect the leadwires from the electrodes and then remove the electrodes from the patient.
11. Assist the patient off the examination table and with dressing as needed.
12. Clean and return the ECG machine to storage so it will be ready for the next use.
13. Mount the ECG tracing in the patient's chart or give it to the physician as directed.
14. Document the procedure in the patient's chart to ensure a complete, accurate medical record.
15. Wash or sanitize your hands.

Date	
11/22/08; 9:30 a.m.	ECG recording obtained and given to physician for review. ———————————————— S. Gonzales, CMA

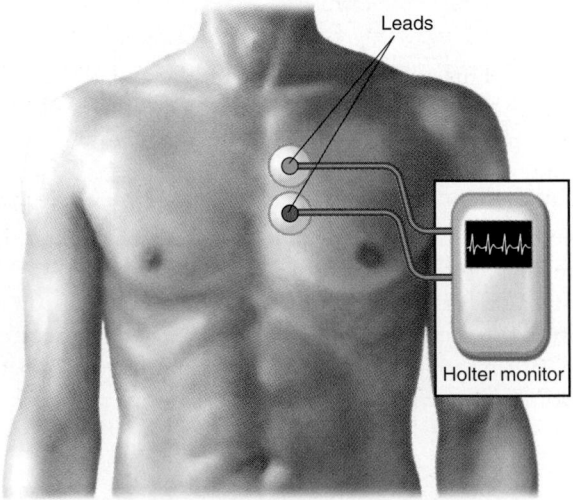

FIG 27-14 Holter monitor.

Leads

Holter monitor

Patient Education

Wearing an Event Recorder
The medical assistant should be sure to give the patient who is to wear an event recorder the following instructions:

- Trigger the event recorder any time you feel symptoms, such as shortness of breath, palpitations, weakness, and dizziness.
- Remove the event recorder before bathing and reapply it immediately afterward.
- Keep a diary of your daily activities and any symptoms you experience.
- Change the electrodes and batteries daily as instructed.

Patient Education—cont'd

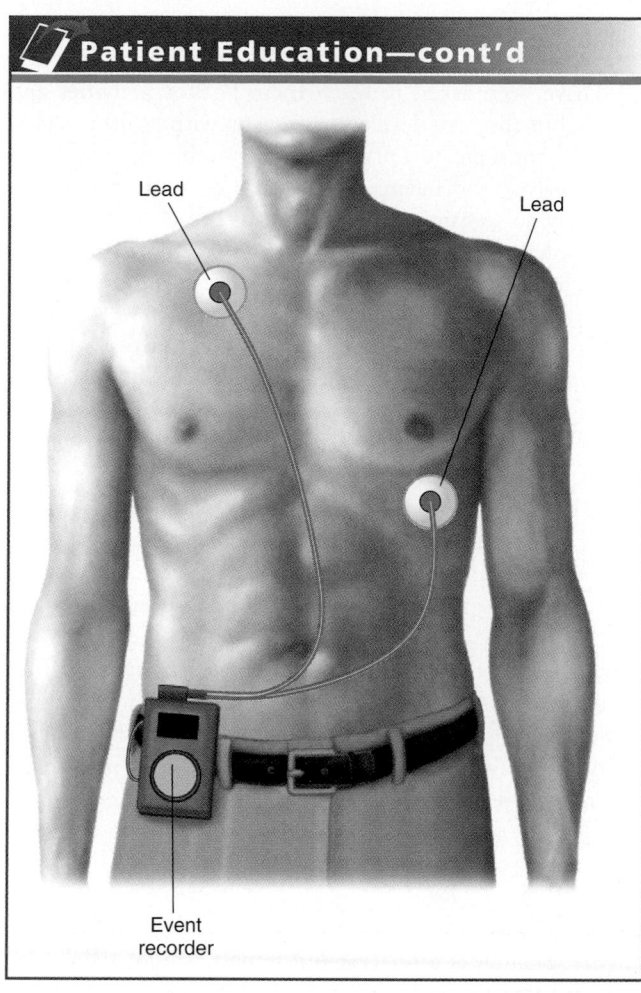

Lead

Lead

Event
recorder

Chapter Summary

- The heart is a muscular organ located in the center of the chest that beats an average of 60 to 100 times per minute and pumps blood throughout the circulatory system.
- Blood flows from the heart to all parts of the body and, eventually, into capillary beds (where oxygen and carbon dioxide are exchanged in the tissues) and then returns to the heart by way of the veins.
- The heart contains its own specialized electrical conduction system, which includes the SA node, the AV node, the bundle of His, and the Purkinje fibers.
- The cardiac cycle includes systole, the phase of heart chamber contraction, and diastole, the phase of heart chamber relaxation.
- Lymphatic vessels are found throughout the body and carry lymph fluid from the tissues back into vascular circulation. Lymph nodes are rich in WBCs and help clean bacteria and cell debris from lymph fluid.

- The thymus, located in the mediastinum above the heart, plays a major role in the immune system. It grows until puberty and then gradually shrinks in size as a person ages.
- The spleen, located in the left upper quadrant of the abdomen, creates WBCs as well as antibodies as part of its role in the immune system. It also contains a supply of RBCs that can be made available to the cardiovascular system in the event of hemorrhage.
- Medical assistants must become well versed in the language and vocabulary that pertain to the cardiology and lymphatic systems so they can communicate effectively with other members of the health care team.
- Medical assistants should become familiar with the more common diseases and disorders of the cardiovascular system, including hypertension, coronary artery disease (CAD), myocardial infarction (MI), heart failure, aneurysm, atrial fibrillation, varicose veins, deep vein thrombosis (DVT), shock, anemia, leukemia, Hodgkin disease, non-Hodgkin lymphoma, and acquired immune deficiency syndrome (AIDS).
- Cardiology is a medical specialty that focuses on the study and treatment of disorders of the cardiovascular system. Medical assistants help with the provision of care to patients in the cardiology office by helping with examinations, procedures, and testing.
- Medical assistants commonly perform 12-lead ECGs. To effectively carry out their duties, they must understand how to prepare the ECG machine, read the paper, assess for standardization, apply the leads and electrodes, prepare the patient, and record the ECG.
- The physician is responsible for interpreting the ECG rhythm and diagnosing the patient. However, because medical assistants routinely perform ECGs, they must be familiar with common rhythms, including those that indicate a life-threatening condition.
- Steps to rhythm interpretation involve calculation of the atrial and ventricular rates and measurement and examination of the waveforms.
- To obtain accurate and useful ECGs, medical assistants must be familiar with common forms of artifact, including somatic tremor, wandering baseline, AC interference, and interrupted baseline, and take measures to prevent them.
- Artificial pacemakers are devices that deliver electrical impulses to the heart to stimulate a heartbeat and maintain an adequate heart rate in individuals whose natural heart rate is too slow or irregular.
- An ICD is a small device that is implanted in patients at risk for life-threatening arrhythmias, such as ventricular fibrillation and ventricular tachycardia. Some devices are actually a combination of a pacemaker and a defibrillator.

- Cardiac stress testing is done to evaluate the heart's response to physical exercise.
- The Holter monitor is a portable device that records the patient's cardiac rhythm over a 24- or 48-hour period. This type of testing is useful when the patient complains of an irregular heartbeat or other symptoms that are intermittent and therefore difficult to obtain on a 12-lead ECG in the medical office.
- An event recorder is a small portable monitor that is attached to two electrodes on the patient's chest and may be activated by the patient when he feels such symptoms as chest pain, dizziness, and palpitations. It may be worn for as long as 30 days to capture events likely to be missed by an ECG or even a Holter monitor.

Team Work Exercises

1. Divide into teams of 4 to 6 students each. Select one of the scenarios below and create a role-playing presentation for the rest of the class in which you fulfill all criteria of the scenario. Provide handouts for the class that summarize the key points of your presentation. List on the handout all the resources you accessed for your presentation.
   a. Mrs. Dough walks into the office complaining of nausea and pain in her left arm and jaw. She is feeling slightly short of breath. She does not lose consciousness or experience a cardiac arrest. Your team must demonstrate, through role-playing, how this situation ought to be handled up to—but not including—the point where Mrs. Dough is transferred to the hospital by ambulance. To each member of the team, you must assign roles, such as patient, patient's spouse, administrative medical assistant, clinical medical assistant, nurse, physician, laboratory technician, and so forth.
   b. Mrs. Dough recently experienced a small MI, was treated at the hospital, and is in the office for her first post-discharge visit. The physician has asked you to:
      - review with her measures she can take to reduce her risk of a repeat MI, hypertension, and CAD
      - teach her about her new medications, which include metoprolol, aspirin, and nitroglycerine.
   c. Your office team has been asked to visit a nearby elementary school for their Healthy Heart day. You have been asked to teach them about the anatomy of the heart and how the blood flows through the body. You must create a plan that gets the children physically involved and having fun while they are learning. You may do so using such methods as games, skits, puppet shows, or anything that is interactive, colorful, and fun. The students in the class will be the "children" (ages 6 to 11) in your audience.
   d. Your office team has been asked to visit a nearby elementary school for their Healthy Heart day. You have been asked to teach them healthy activities and habits they can develop to grow up with healthy hearts. You must create a plan that gets the children physically involved and having fun while they are learning. You may do so using such methods as games, skits, puppet shows, or anything that is interactive, colorful, and fun. The students in the class will be the "children" (ages 6 to 11) in your audience.
   e. Your team is to create a story that utilizes as many cardiac and lymphatic medical terms and abbreviations as you can. The story may be serious or humorous. However, all medical terms must be accurately spelled and their use must fit within the context of the story. After you have created your story, read it to the class. Each time a medical term or abbreviation is used, the story's reader must pause and allow another member of the team to translate the term or abbreviation for the listeners.
2. Divide into teams of 4 to 6 students each. Your instructor will provide each team with one or more cardiac rhythm strips. Analyze the strips to the best of your ability. When you have agreed on what the strip represents, you must present your findings to the rest of the class and explain your rationale for the conclusions you have reached.

Case Studies

1. Mrs. Schultz is a 66-year-old female patient who complains that her heart is "racing" or "skipping" a beat and she sometimes feels dizzy. She does not know if it is worth "bothering anyone about" or if she should just go home and not worry about it. What will you say to her? What type of response would you anticipate the physician making?
2. Mrs. Smith has her 5-year-old son in the pediatrician's office, stating that he has a sore throat and slight fever. The mother has noticed that the glands in his neck are swollen but that he also has lumps under his arms. What is the likely cause of the lumps under his arms?

Resources

- Latest AIDS information, news, and research: *www.aids.org*
- American Heart Association: *www.americanheart.org*
- Auscultation Assistant: *www. med.ucla.edu/ wilkes/inex.htm*
- ECG Library: *www.ecglibrary.com/*
- Heart Institute for Children: *www.thic.com*
- Leukemia and Lymphoma Society: *www.leukemia.org/hm_lls*

Pulmonology

Learning Objectives

Upon completion of this chapter, the student will be able to:

- define and spell terms related to pulmonology
- identify key structures of the pulmonary system
- discuss the roles played by the pulmonary system
- describe the role of the medical assistant in the pulmonologist's office
- identify common pulmonary diseases and disorders
- list commonly used word elements related to the pulmonary system and give at least 10 examples of how new pulmonary-related terms may be created by combining prefixes, suffixes, and combining forms
- describe the medical assistant's role in assisting with pulmonary procedures
- describe physical examination techniques used to evaluate the pulmonary system.

CAAHEP Competencies

Administrative Competencies
Process Insurance Claims
  Perform diagnostic coding
Clinical Competencies
Diagnostic Testing
  Perform respiratory testing
Patient Care
  Prepare patients for and assist with routine and specialty examinations
  Prepare patients for and assist with procedures, treatments, and minor office surgeries

General Competencies

Patient Instruction
  Instruct individuals according to their needs
  Provide instruction for health maintenance and disease prevention

ABHES Competencies

Clinical Duties
  Prepare patients for procedures
  Prepare patient for and assist physician with routine and specialty examinations and treatments and minor office surgeries
  Perform respiratory testing

Procedures

Performing respiratory testing
Teaching a patient to use an MDI
Administering oxygen via nasal cannula

Chapter Outline

Structures and Functions of the Pulmonary System
  Structures of the Pulmonary System
    Upper airway
    Lower airway
    Lungs
  Functions of the Pulmonary System
    Upper airway
    Lower airway
    Lungs
Medical Terminology Related to the Pulmonary System
Common Pulmonary System Diseases and Disorders
  Common Upper Respiratory System Diseases and Disorders
    Allergic rhinitis
    Upper respiratory infection
    Sinusitis
    Pharyngitis
  Common Lower Respiratory System Diseases and Disorders
    Pneumonia
    Influenza
    Chronic obstructive pulmonary disease
    Bronchitis
    Asthma
    Emphysema
    Pulmonary tuberculosis
    Epstein-Barr virus
    Lung cancer
Pulmonology Procedures
  Assisting with Examination
  Diagnostic Testing
    Pulmonary function tests
    Bronchoscopy
    Mantoux test
    Peak-flow measurement
  Treatments
    Metered-dose inhaler
    Nebulizer treatments
    Incentive spirometry
    Oxygen therapy
Chapter Summary
Team Work Exercises
Case Studies
Resources

Key Terms

antitussive
Medication that suppresses the cough reflex

aspiration
Unintentional inhalation of any substance other than air

bronchoscopy
Examination of the bronchi through a specialized instrument called a *bronchoscope*

chest physiotherapy
Type of therapy that includes percussion (clapping) over the thorax or vibration and positioning to facilitate loosening and removal of respiratory secretions

circumoral cyanosis
Blue coloring around the mouth due to inadequate oxygenation

corticosteroids
Medications that suppress the immune response and decrease inflammation

crackles
Abnormal crackly lung sound heard with a stethoscope

dyspnea
Painful or difficult breathing

exhalation
Act of breathing out; also called *expiration*

expectorant
Medication that liquefies and loosens respiratory secretions to aid in expelling them

febrile
Fever causing

hemoptysis
Coughing up blood

hypoxia
Deficient level of oxygen

hypoxic drive
Backup system of respiration that stimulates breathing in a patient who is retaining carbon dioxide

incentive spirometer
Handheld device used by the patient to inhale a maximal breath to keep lungs expanded and functional

inhalation
Act of breathing in; also called *inspiration*

lobectomy
Surgical removal of a lobe of a lung

lymphadenopathy
Swollen, tender cervical lymph nodes

Mantoux test
Test to identify tuberculosis exposure

metered dose inhaler
Handheld device used to inhale medication into the lungs

nasal cannula
Oxygen tubing designed to deliver oxygen into a patient's nose

nebulizer
Device that produces a fine spray or mist to deliver medication to the air passages and lungs

peak-flow meter
Handheld device used to measure an individual's lung capacity

pH scale
Scale used to measure acidity or alkalinity of a substance

pleural membranes
Double membranes that cover the lungs and line the thoracic cavity

pulmonology
Field of medicine that studies and treats respiratory disorders

pulmonologist
Physician who specializes in the diagnosis and treatment of respiratory disorders

pneumonectomy
Surgical removal of an entire lung

pulmonary function test
Measurement of air flow and lung volumes; also called *spirometry*

purulent
Consisting of or containing pus

rhonchi
Coarse gurgling sound heard on auscultation that is caused by secretions in the air passages

wedge resection
Surgical removal of a small part of a lung

wheeze
Somewhat musical sound heard in the lungs, usually with a stethoscope, that is caused by partial airway obstruction

Structures and Functions of the Pulmonary System

The pulmonary system, also called the *respiratory system,* is made up of the upper airways, lower airways, and the lungs. The pulmonary system facilitates breathing and the exchange of gases like oxygen and carbon dioxide that is so vital to life and health.

Structures of the Pulmonary System

The pulmonary system is divided into the upper and lower airways and the lungs. (See Figure 28-1.)

Upper Airway

The main structures of the upper airway consist of the mouth, nose, sinuses, and pharynx (throat). The pharynx is further divided into the nasopharynx (back of the nose) and oropharynx (back of the mouth). The nose begins with the nares (nostrils) and extends back to the nasopharynx. The nasal passages are divided into right and left sides by the nasal septum. The hard palate divides the nasal cavity from the mouth, which sits beneath it. The sinus cavities are air-filled spaces named for the facial bones within which they are located. They include the maxillary, frontal, ethmoidal, and sphenoidal sinuses. Many of the upper airway structures are shared by the gastrointestinal and sensory systems.

Lower Airway

The lower airways consist of the epiglottis, trachea, bronchial tubes, and lungs. The trachea (sometimes called the *windpipe*) begins superiorly with the larynx (sometimes called the *voice box*) and extends inferiorly to the middle of the chest. It is approximately 5" long and gets its shape and strength from numerous rings of cartilage. In the center of the chest, the trachea divides into the two primary bronchi, each of which leads to smaller and smaller bronchi and, eventually, to tiny bronchioles. The structure of bronchi changes to less cartilage and more smooth muscle as they become smaller. The bronchioles end at the alveoli, which are microscopic air sacs within the lungs. There are approximately 300 million alveoli in each lung. They are covered with a delicate capillary bed (microscopic blood vessels), which provide them with a rich blood supply.

Lungs

The lungs are divided into lobes; the right lung has three and the left lung has two. The lungs are covered with two thin membranes known as the **pleura**. The visceral pleura lies directly on the lungs. The parietal pleura lines the inner wall of the thorax. A small amount of pleural fluid lies in the space between the two membranes. This space is sometimes

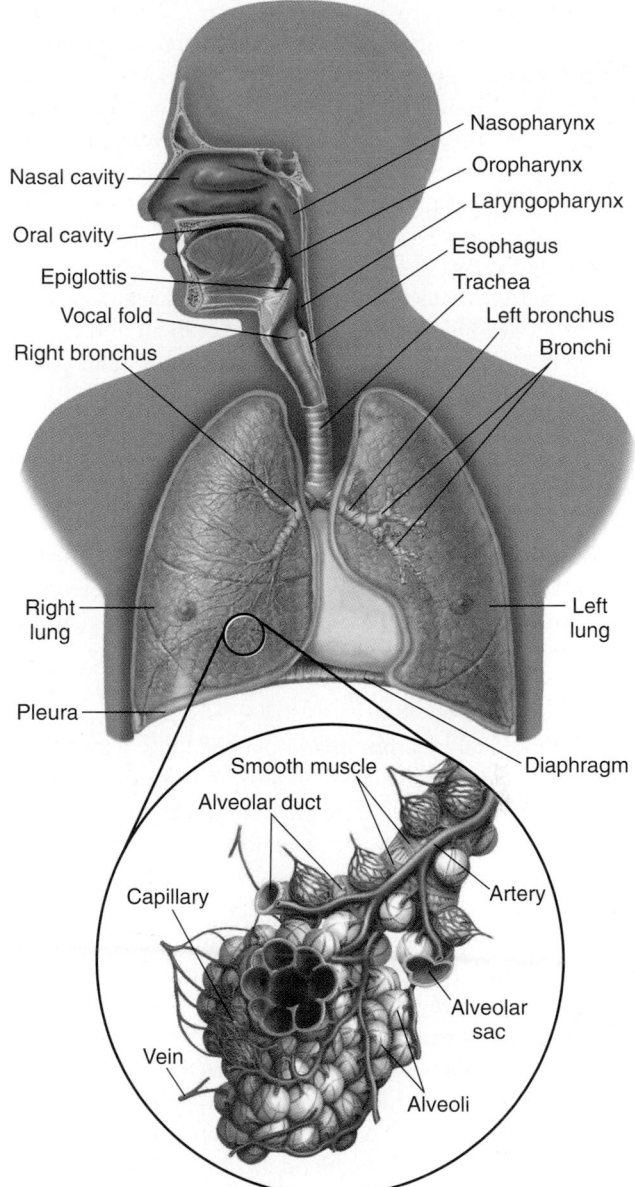

FIG 28-1 Respiratory system.

referred to as a *potential* space because there is nothing there other than a small amount of this fluid.

Functions of the Pulmonary System

The functions of the pulmonary system can be further broken down to those of the upper and lower airways and the lungs.

Upper Airway

The structures of the upper airway act to cleanse, moisten, and warm inhaled air before it continues its journey to the lungs. Mucous membranes that line these structures contribute moisture to humidify the air. Cilia (tiny hairs) within the nasal cavity help filter the air by removing debris. The rich blood supply of all of these structures warms the air as it passes through. Sinus cavities serve to decrease the weight of the skull, provide resonance for the voice, and produce mucus, which helps eliminate microorganisms as it drains into the nasal cavities.

Lower Airway

The epiglottis acts as a doorway to the trachea and serves a vital protective function by opening to let in air and closing to keep out food and fluid. The larynx vibrates as air passes through it, creating vocal sounds. The numerous C-shaped cartilage rings of the trachea provide strength and keep it open. The trachea and bronchi have ciliated mucous membrane linings, which serve to further moisten air and secrete mucus to trap foreign debris that has been inhaled. The cilia move in a wavelike fashion to propel debris upward. The trachea and bronchi are extremely sensitive and the presence of foreign particles stimulates a powerful cough reflex that further helps to expel foreign debris.

Lungs

As the individual breathes in and out the lungs expand and contract. The elastic quality that allows the lungs to do this is sometimes called *recoil*. The pleural fluid between the visceral and parietal pleura acts as a sort of lubricant, which helps the process along as the lungs continually expand and contract.

A person takes oxygen (O_2) into the lungs through the act of **inhalation**, or breathing in, which is usually an unconscious act. However, a person may exert conscious control to take extra large breaths or even hold his breath for a short time. At some point, however, he will have an overwhelming urge to breathe, which is triggered by a buildup of carbon dioxide (CO_2) when a person stops breathing in oxygen. This buildup of CO_2 in the blood causes it to become more acidic. To be healthy, a person's blood must remain slightly alkaline—within the narrow range of 7.35 to 7.45 on the **pH scale**, which is a tool for measuring the acidity or alkalinity of the blood. As the blood becomes more acidic, the pH level drops, triggering the urge to breathe. The act of inhalation brings fresh, oxygen-rich air into the person's lungs so it can be absorbed into his blood. The act of **exhalation**, or breathing out, allows the body to eliminate excess CO_2, thus restoring a normal blood pH level. Contrary to what most people think, the stimulus to breathe is not lower oxygen levels in the blood, but the lowered pH level caused by CO_2 buildup.

Gas exchange, so vital to life, takes place within the millions of tiny alveoli contained within each lung. They expand somewhat like tiny balloons during inhalation as air enters and fills them. They contract and partially deflate during exhalation as much of the air moves out of the lungs. Because the walls of the alveoli and the capillary beds are each just one cell thick, gases move easily back and forth. Excess CO_2 leaves the capillaries and moves into the air space in the alveoli and is then exhaled. Oxygen moves from the air space in the alveoli into the capillary blood and is then distributed to various parts of the body via the circulatory system.

Medical Terminology Related to the Pulmonary System

Pulmonary disorders are common and affect every segment of the population at some time, leading them to seek medical care in both acute and ambulatory settings. To be effective in their role, medical assistants must become well versed in the language and vocabulary that pertain to the pulmonary system. The following tables list common medical terminology related to the pulmonary system.

Table 28.1 | Word elements

This table contains word elements that pertain to the pulmonary system, along with examples of terms that use the combining form and a pronunciation guide.

Element	Meaning	Example	Meaning
Combining Forms			
aer/o	air	**aerophagia** (ĕr-ō-FĀ-jē-ă)	swallowing air
bronch/o	bronchus	**bronchitis** (brŏng-KĪ-tĭs)	inflammation of the bronchus
bronchi/o		**bronchiectasis** (brŏng-kē-ĔK-tă-sĭs)	dilation or expansion of the bronchus
chondr/o	cartilage	**chrondroplasty** (KŎN-drō-plăs-tē)	surgical repair of the cartilage

Table 28.1 | **Word elements—cont'd**

Element	Meaning	Example	Meaning
Combining Forms			
epiglott/o	epiglottis	**epiglottal** (ĕp-ĭ-GLŎT-ăl)	pertaining to the epiglottis
laryng/o	larynx	**laryngitis** (lăr-ĭn-JĪ-tĭs)	inflammation of the larynx
nas/o	nose	**nasogastric** (nā-zō-GĂS-trĭk)	pertaining to the nose and stomach
rhin/o		**rhinitis** (rī-NĪ-tĭs)	inflammation of the nose (runny nose)
muc/o	mucus	**mucoid** (MŪ-koyd)	resembling mucus
or/o	mouth	**oral** (Ō-răl)	pertaining to the mouth
stomat/o		**stomatitis** (stō-mă-TĪ-tĭs)	inflammation of the mouth
orth/o	straight	**orthopnea** (or-THŎP-nē-ă)	breathing in the straight (upright) position
ox/o	oxygen	**anoxia** (ăn-ŌK-sē-ă)	condition of no oxygen
pharyng/o	pharynx	**pharyngeal** (făr-ĬN-jē-ăl)	pertaining to the pharynx
pleur/o	pleura	**pleurodynia** (ploo-rō-DĬN-ē-ă)	pain in the pleura
pneum/o	lung, air	**pneumonia** (nū-MŌ-nē-ă)	condition of the lung
pneumon/o		**pneumonectomy** (nū-mŏn-ĔK-tō-mē)	surgical excision of the lung
pulmon/o	lung	**pulmonary** (PŬL-mō-nĕ-rē)	pertaining to the lung
sinus/o	sinus	**sinusoid** (SĪ-nŭs-oyd)	resembling a sinus
thorac/o	thorax	**thoracentesis** (thō-ră-sĕn-TĒ-sĭs)	surgical puncture of the thorax
tonsill/o	tonsils	**tonsillitis** (tŏn-sĭl-Ī-tĭs)	inflammation of the tonsils
trache/o	trachea	**tracheotomy** (trā-kē-ŌT-ō-mē)	surgical incision into the trachea
Prefixes			
circum-	around	**circumoral** (sĕr-kŭm-Ō-răl)	pertaining to around the mouth
hypo-	below, beneath	**hypoxia** (hī-PŎKS-ē-ă)	condition of low oxygen
intra-	within	**intrathoracic** (ĭn-tră-thō-RĂS-ĭk)	pertaining to within the thorax
para-	beside, near	**paranasal** (păr-ă-NĀ-săl)	pertaining to beside or near the nose
peri-	beside, near	**peritonsillar** (pĕr-ĭ-TŎN-sĭ-lăr)	pertaining to beside or near the tonsils
post-	after, following	**postnasal** (pōst-NĀ-zăl)	pertaining to the posterior portion of the nose
Suffixes			
-ary	pertaining to	**pulmonary** (PŬL-mō-nĕ-rē)	pertaining to the lungs
-algia	pain	**stomatalgia** (stō-mă-TĂL-jē-ă)	mouth pain
-centesis	surgical puncture	**pleurocentesis** (ploo-rō-sĕn-TĒ-sĭs)	surgical puncture of the pleura
-cyte	cell	**chondrocyte** (KŎN-drō-sīt)	cartilage cell
-desis	binding	**pleurodesis** (ploo-rō-DĒ-sĭs)	binding the pleura

Continued

Table 28.1 | Word elements—cont'd

Element	Meaning	Example	Meaning
Suffixes			
-ectomy	excision, surgical removal	**laryngectomy** (lăr-ĭn-JĔK-tō-mē)	surgical removal of the larynx
-logist	specialist in the study of	**pulmonologist** (pŭl-mŏn-ŎL-ō-jĭst)	specialist in the study and treatment of lung disorders
-ole	small	**bronchiole** (BRŎNG-kē-ōl)	small bronchus
-plasty	surgical repair	**rhinoplasty** (RĪ-nō-plăs-tē)	surgical repair of the nose
-plegia	paralysis	**laryngoplegia** (lă-rĭng-gō-PLĒ-jē-ă)	paralyzed larynx
-scope	instrument used to view	**laryngoscope** (lăr-ĪN-gō-skōp)	instrument used to view the larynx
-scopy	visual examination	**bronchoscopy** (brŏng-KŎS-kō-pē)	visual examination of the bronchi
-stomy	mouthlike opening	**tracheostomy** (trā-kē-ŎS-tō-mē)	mouthlike opening in the trachea

Table 28.2 | Pathologic Terms

This table lists some of the most common pathologic terms related to the pulmonary system with a brief definition for each.

Term	Definition
acute respiratory distress syndrome	Hypoxemia and respiratory failure due to severe inflammatory damage to the lungs after severe infection or trauma
allergic rhinitis (ă-LĔR-jĭk rī-NĪ-tĭs)	Inflammation of the nasal membranes due to allergies; also called *hay fever*
asthma (ĂZ-mă)	Disorder in which airways overreact to certain triggers with inflammation, resulting in narrowing, mucus production, and dyspnea; also called *reactive airway disease*
atelectasis (ăt-ĕ-LĔK-tă-sĭs)	Partial collapse of lung tissues, such as alveoli and bronchioles
bronchitis (brŏng-KĪ-tĭs)	Infection of the bronchial passages, usually by a virus but possibly by bacteria
chronic obstructive pulmonary disease	Group of chronic lung disorders that includes emphysema, chronic bronchitis, and asthma and creates obstructive changes in the bronchi and alveoli; also called *chronic obstructive lung disease (COLD)*
croup (KROOP)	Acute viral disease, usually in children, marked by a barking, "seal-like" cough and respiratory distress
cystic fibrosis (SĬS-tĭk fī-BRŌ-sĭs)	Fatal genetic disease that causes frequent respiratory infections, increased airway secretions, and chronic obstructive pulmonary disease in children
emphysema (ĕm-fī-SĒ-mă)	Common chronic obstructive respiratory disorder that causes permanent, destructive changes to respiratory structures
empyema (ĕm-pī-Ē-mă)	Collection of infected fluid (pus) in a body cavity, usually between the pleura
epistaxis (ĕp-ĭ-STĂK-sĭs)	Nosebleed
Epstein-Barr virus (ĔP-stēn BĂR)	Infection caused by the Epstein-Barr virus (EBV), which is a member of the herpesvirus family; also known as *mononucleosis* or *glandular fever*
glomerulonephritis (glŏ-mĕr-ū-lō-nĕ-FRĪ-tĭs)	Type of kidney infection

Table 28.2 | Pathologic Terms—cont'd

Term	Definition
hemothorax (hē-mō-THŎ-răks)	Condition in which blood has collected between the pleural linings of the lungs
hypercapnia (hī-pĕr-KĂP-nē-ă)	Chronic retention of carbon dioxide in the blood
influenza (ĭn-floo-ĔN-ză)	Group of viral respiratory illnesses marked by fever, headache, muscle aches, rhinitis, fatigue, sore throat, dry cough, and gastrointestinal symptoms
lung cancer	Group of several different types of cancer, including small cell, non–small cell, squamous cell, adenocarcinoma, and large cell lung cancer
orthopnea (or-THŎP-nē-ă)	Need to remain upright in order to breathe effectively
pharyngitis (făr-ĭn-JĪ-tĭs)	Sore throat
pleural effusion (PLOO-răl ĕ-FŪ-zhŭn)	Collection of fluid in the pleural space
pneumonia (nū-MŌ-nē-ă)	Viral or bacterial infection of the lungs
pneumothorax (nū-mō-THŎ-răks)	Condition in which air has collected between the pleural linings of the lungs
pulmonary tuberculosis (PŬL-mō-nĕ-rē tū-bĕr-kū-LŌ-sĭs)	Contagious lung infection caused by the *Mycobacterium tuberculosis* organism
sinusitis (sī-nŭs-Ī-tĭs)	Inflammation of the lining of the sinus cavities
upper respiratory infection	Acute inflammation of the mucous membranes of the nasal passages and throat caused by a virus; also called *the common cold* or *coryza*
severe acute respiratory syndrome	Viral respiratory illness marked by head and body aches, fever, and cough that may lead to severe pneumonia
stridor (STRĪ-dor)	Medical emergency marked by a high-pitched upper airway sound (heard without a stethoscope) that indicates airway obstruction

Table 28.3 | Abbreviations

In pulmonology, as with other areas of health care, abbreviations are commonly used. Abbreviations such as the ones listed here save time and effort in documentation and written communications.

Abbreviation	Term	Abbreviation	Term
ABGs	arterial blood gases	**RT**	respiratory therapy
ARDS	acute respiratory distress syndrome	**SARS**	sudden acute respiratory syndrome
COPD	chronic obstructive pulmonary disease	**SOB**	shortness of breath
CPR	cardiopulmonary resuscitation	**Stat**	immediately
CO₂	carbon dioxide	**TB**	tuberculosis
O₂	oxygen	**URI**	upper respiratory infection
PND	paroxysmal nocturnal dyspnea	**VC**	vital capacity

Common Pulmonary System Diseases and Disorders

There are many disorders affecting the pulmonary system. Here are some of the most common ones with a summary of each, along with its corresponding ICD-9-CM code.

Common Upper Respiratory System Diseases and Disorders

Common upper respiratory system diseases and disorders include allergic rhinitis, upper respiratory infection, sinusitis, and pharyngitis.

Allergic Rhinitis

ICD-9-CM code: 477 (base code), 477.0 (due to pollen), 477.1 (due to food), 477.2 (due to animal hair), 477.8 (due to other allergen)

The term *rhinitis* means inflammation of the nasal membranes. When rhinitis is caused by allergies it is sometimes also called *hay fever* because the most common cause is allergy to seasonal plant pollens. It affects nearly 40 million people, or approximately 20% of the U.S. population. Costs associated with treating allergic rhinitis and its complications are over $5 billion per year.

The primary risk factor for allergic rhinitis is a genetic predisposition. Susceptible people develop sensitivity to certain allergens and then experience reactions when subsequently reexposed to those allergens. Triggers are numerous. The most common triggers include pollen, dust, mold, and pet dander. Signs and symptoms of allergic rhinitis include sneezing, nasal congestion, itching, redness, postnasal drip, runny nose, and sinus congestion. Systemic symptoms may include malaise, fatigue, and sleepiness. Symptoms may last for hours or days.

Diagnosis is based on the patient's description of symptoms and physical examination findings. Treatment includes the use of antihistamines, decongestants, and nasal steroids. Patients should be counseled to avoid allergens when possible and to consider the use of filters in their home. Desensitization may be accomplished through injections. Allergies are generally chronic but can usually be managed reasonably well with medications. Potential complications include otitis media, acute and chronic sinusitis, and eustachian tube dysfunction.

Upper Respiratory Infection

ICD-9-CM code: 460

Upper respiratory infection (URI), also called *coryza*, is more commonly known as the *common cold* because it is so common. In fact, it is the reason most frequently given for missed school and work, with an estimated 1 billion cases in the United States each year. Children experience an average of three to eight colds each year.

More than 200 viruses are known to cause the common cold, which is very contagious. Virus particles are contained within nasal secretions and are easily spread when individuals wipe their nose and then touch other people or objects. The virus can also be spread via tiny airborne droplets when someone sneezes. The most contagious time is within the first 2 to 3 days of a cold.

Symptoms vary with the specific virus but generally include runny nose, nasal congestion, sneezing, sore throat, cough, headache, malaise, pharyngitis (sore throat), muscle aches, headache, and decreased appetite. Very young children may run a fever as high as 102°F, but older children and adults are usually afebrile. Symptoms occur within 2 to 3 days from exposure and usually last 7 to 10 days.

Diagnosis is based on a description of symptoms and physical examination findings. Treatment includes fluids and rest. Over-the-counter medications including analgesics may lessen the severity of symptoms. Antibiotics are not appropriate because they have no effect on viruses. Most people recover fully from URIs but complications may include secondary otitis media, sinus infection, bronchitis, pneumonia, and an exacerbation of asthma in those with asthma.

Sinusitis

ICD-9-CM code: 461.9 (acute, unspecified), 473.9 (chronic, unspecified)

Sinusitis is a condition in which the lining of the sinus cavities becomes inflamed. An estimated 30 million people in the United States suffer from sinus disease and over $65 billion is spent each year on medical care and surgical treatments. Sinusitis is caused when the sinus cavities become blocked due to swelling or growth of polyps. Primary contributors include bacterial and viral infections. Other contributors include overuse of decongestant nasal sprays and smoking.

A common sign of acute sinusitis is when a URI seems to improve and then worsens again. Pressure or pain is commonly felt in the face, including the cheeks, forehead, between the eyes, or even the teeth. Other symptoms may include nasal congestion, fever, malaise, and a cough and pharyngitis (due to postnasal drainage) that are worse in the mornings.

Diagnosis is usually based on a description of symptoms and physical examination findings. In some cases, x-rays, computed tomography (CT) scan, or magnetic resonance imaging (MRI) of the sinuses reveal thickening of the mucosa and presence of increased fluid. The physician may prescribe antibiotics for 10 to 14 days. The medical assistant should be sure to tell the patient to take the medication for the entire period, even though symptoms may begin to improve after a few days. The physician may also prescribe decongestants. Other treatment includes rest, fluids, moist heat compresses, humidifiers, and hot showers (to breathe the warm, humidified air). Most people recover fully with appropriate diagnosis and treatment. Potential complications include chronic sinusitis, osteomyelitis, and orbital cellulitis.

Pharyngitis
ICD-9-CM code: 462

Pharyngitis is the inflammation of the pharynx. In the United States, children have an average of five episodes and adults have an average of two episodes of pharyngitis per year. The usual cause of pharyngitis is a viral URI and seasonal allergies, which cause postnasal drainage that irritates the throat. Organisms that may be responsible for bacterial pharyngitis include *Streptococcus, Mycoplasma pneumoniae, Chlamydia pneumoniae,* and *Neisseria gonorrhoeae.* Infection is spread from person to person by direct contact and contact with oral secretions. Other causes of pharyngitis include sinus infection, diphtheria, and mononucleosis caused by the Epstein-Barr virus. Risk factors that make people more vulnerable to pharyngitis include inhaling pollutants, smoking, and secondhand smoke.

Patients with pharyngitis describe the throat as scratchy and sore. Swallowing is painful and may be difficult. Upon examination, the pharynx appears red and edematous and the tonsils may be swollen and have white spots of **purulent** (pus) exudate. Other symptoms may include fever and cough. Cervical lymph nodes are usually tender and swollen.

Diagnosis is based on a description of symptoms and physical examination findings. A throat culture may be used to differentiate viral from bacterial pharyngitis. A quick in-office test, called the *rapid Strep test,* provides results in about 15 minutes. However, negative results must be confirmed by a culture because the test is not 100% accurate. Viral pharyngitis usually resolves without medication and responds well to conservative treatment, including analgesics and warm saline gargles. Antibiotics are prescribed for bacterial pharyngitis. Most people recover fully with conservative treatment. However, potential complications include rheumatic fever, scarlet fever (with streptococcal infections), tonsillary abscess, and glomerulonephritis (a type of kidney infection). Those who suffer from chronic infections may benefit from a tonsillectomy.

Common Lower Respiratory System Diseases and Disorders

Common lower respiratory diseases and disorders include pneumonia, influenza, chronic obstructive pulmonary disease, bronchitis, asthma, emphysema, tuberculosis, Epstein-Barr virus, and lung cancer.

Pneumonia
ICD-9-CM code: 486

Pneumonia is a viral or bacterial infection of the lungs that may be mild or severe and, in some cases, is life-threatening.

In past years, a third of those infected died from pneumonia. However, since the advent of antimicrobial medications, most people with access to medical care recover. More than 3 million people in the United States develop pneumonia each year and more than a half million of them are hospitalized.

Pneumonia may be caused by bacteria, viruses, or chemical irritants. In some cases, the infecting organisms become airborne when the ill person coughs or sneezes. If another person inhales the infectious organisms and the organisms grow in that person's lungs, pneumonia develops. Another common cause of pneumonia is **aspiration** (inhalation) of chemical irritants such as stomach fluids, food, or drink, which might occur during cardiopulmonary resuscitation (CPR) or a choking episode. Those at greatest risk for developing pneumonia include those with weakened immune systems, chronic lung disease, heart disease, alcoholism, seizure disorders, and swallowing disorders.

Symptoms of pneumonia include coldlike symptoms followed by fever, productive cough, shaking chills, shortness of breath, chest pain with deep breaths, muscle aches, and malaise. Diagnosis is based on a description of symptoms, physical examination findings, and a chest x-ray, which may reveal whitened areas (opacities) that indicate consolidation (solidification due to engorgement). Lung sounds heard on auscultation usually include **wheezes** and **crackles** caused by inflammation of the airways and fluid accumulation. The physician may order a sputum sample to identify the causative microorganism. A culture and sensitivity test determine the most appropriate antimicrobial agent to use for treatment. Examination of a blood sample may reveal increased WBCs.

Treatment is based on the cause. Bacterial pneumonia is treated with antibiotics. Patients with other forms of pneumonia are usually treated with supportive care, including oxygen, fluids, and respiratory support. Prognosis and survival is generally good. However, there is a 5% mortality rate, usually affecting patients in a weakened state. Complications include pleural effusion and empyema.

Influenza
ICD-9-CM code: 487

Influenza, commonly called the *flu,* is a common, contagious, acute viral respiratory illness. Outbreaks can occur as often as every year and affect approximately 20% of the U.S. population each year. Of those affected, over 200,000 are hospitalized and more than 35,000 die. Those at greatest risk are the very young, very old, and those with chronic health disorders.

There are a number of flu viruses, commonly categorized as types A, B, and C. They are most commonly spread from person to person through respiratory droplets and secretions from coughing, sneezing, and kissing. They are also spread through a person's contact with contaminated surfaces (such as a door knob) and then touching the mouth or nose. A person may be infectious up to 1 day before symptom development and up to 5 days after. (See *Virus transmission reduction.*)

Common signs and symptoms of the flu include fever as high as 104°F (40°C), headache, muscle aches, nasal congestion or rhinitis, fatigue, sore throat, dry cough, and such GI symptoms as nausea, vomiting, and diarrhea. Diagnosis of influenza is usually based on physical examination findings and a description of symptoms. A positive throat culture confirms the diagnosis. If secondary bacterial pneumonia is suspected, the physician may order a sputum specimen for analysis.

Treatment of influenza usually includes supportive care, such as fluids, rest, analgesics, and antipyretics. Sore throat may also be soothed by warm saltwater gargles and throat lozenges. Amantadine, an antiviral agent, may be helpful in some cases. In severe cases, hospitalization may be needed. Antibiotics are not effective against the flu virus but may be appropriate for secondary bacterial infections. Aspirin should not be given to children because of the risk of Reye syndrome.

Patient education should be aimed at prevention through flu vaccination and standard precautions such as hand washing. Most individuals can also benefit from a yearly flu vaccination, which is generally available each fall. (See *Influenza vaccination.*) Prognosis is generally good and most people recover

---

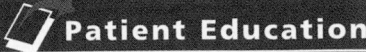

Patient Education

Influenza Vaccination

Medical assistants commonly administer influenza vaccinations. The following general information will help you answer questions your patients may have.

- Vaccination is recommended for health care providers and vulnerable individuals, such as the elderly, residents of long-term-care facilities, those with cancer and lung disease, those with weakened immune systems, infants between ages 6 and 23 months, and children on long-term aspirin therapy.

- Individuals should consult with their physician prior to being vaccinated.

- Influenza vaccination should NOT be given to individuals:
  - with allergies to chicken or to eggs
  - who have experienced a previous severe reaction to flu vaccine
  - with a history of Guillain-Barré syndrome in the past 6 weeks
  - under age 6 months
  - who are currently ill with a **febrile** (fever-causing) illness (should wait until they are well to receive the vaccination).

Front office–Back office connection

Virus Transmission Reduction

Following are measures that front and back office staff can take to reduce transmission of cold and influenza viruses:

- Keep tissue and a dispenser of antimicrobial lotion at the reception desk. Encourage patients to use both.

- Keep antimicrobial lotion at each nurse's station and at strategic locations in the facility and encourage employee use.

- If toys or books are kept in the reception area for children, select those that are nontoxic, easy to disinfect, and unlikely to harbor microorganisms.

- Avoid coming to work if you have a communicable illness.

- Obtain an annual influenza vaccination.

- Practice good self-care to keep your immune system strong.

- Remind patients, family, and friends about the value of good hand washing.

---

fully. However, complications many include dehydration, bacterial pneumonia, bronchitis, and sinus or ear infections.

Chronic Obstructive Pulmonary Disease
ICD-9-CM code: 490

Chronic obstructive pulmonary disease (COPD) includes a variety of lung disorders that create obstructive changes in the air passages and alveoli. These disorders include chronic bronchitis, asthma, emphysema, bronchiectasis, cystic fibrosis, and pneumoconiosis. COPD affects 11% of the U.S. population.

The greatest risk factor for COPD is smoking. Others include exposure to air pollution, dust, and chemicals and repeated lower respiratory infections. Although the pathophysiology is different in each disease, the result of all is impaired air exchange. As chronic air trapping occurs, the patient's chest changes dimension, becoming more barrel-like. The lungs also flatten on the bottom, robbing the diaphragm of its effectiveness. Cilia, tiny hairlike structures in the airway, normally move foreign debris upward to be coughed out. However, in smokers, the cilia become clogged with tar and lose effectiveness. As a result of these and other physical changes, a patient with COPD will eventually begin to experience some or all of the following symptoms:

- Orthopnea is the need to remain upright in order to breathe effectively. Physicians commonly quantify the severity of orthopnea by the number of pillows a patient uses while sleeping (for example, *three-pillow orthopnea*).

- Hypercapnia is the chronic retention of CO_2. In some cases, this changes the way a person's body determines when to breathe and he begins to function according to a **hypoxic drive**, which means he feels the urge to breathe when his O_2 level gets too low instead of when his CO_2 level gets too high. This change poses a risk when the patient needs supplemental O_2 because, if his blood oxygen levels rise too high, he may lose the urge to breathe, leading to respiratory arrest. Hypercapnia can also cause mental cloudiness and lethargy.

- Chronic **hypoxia** is a chronic lack of oxygen. As gas exchange becomes less effective, breathing becomes more and more difficult. Eventually, the individual becomes O_2-dependent. Yet, in the last stages of the disease, supplemental O_2 is of little help. The person feels chronically short of breath and suffers from severe **dyspnea** (painful or difficult breathing) with the slightest exertion. (See Figure 28-2.)

Bronchitis

ICD-9-CM code: 466 (acute), 491 (chronic)

Bronchitis is an infection of the bronchial passages that is usually caused by a virus. It can occur in acute and chronic forms. Both forms have the same characteristics except that chronic bronchitis persists for weeks, months, or even years and causes permanent destructive changes in the lungs. The infectious microorganisms are spread through respiratory secretions by coughing, sneezing, or direct contact. Those most vulnerable to bronchitis are those who smoke and those with chronic respiratory conditions.

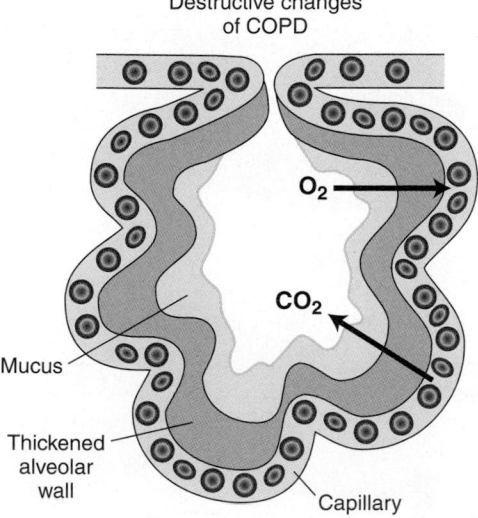

Destructive changes of COPD

O_2

CO_2

Mucus

Thickened alveolar wall

Capillary

FIG 28-2 Destructive changes in COPD.

The most common symptom of bronchitis is a persistent cough that typically produces thick sputum. Other symptoms include wheezing, shortness of breath, and mild fever. Acute bronchitis usually lasts for around 1 week but the cough may continue for several weeks. Lungs are usually clear to auscultation but occasionally scattered wheezes and crackles may be heard. The primary symptom of chronic bronchitis is a chronic cough that is generally worse in the mornings. Symptoms are exacerbated by other respiratory infections.

Diagnosis is usually based on history and symptoms. Testing may be done to rule out other disorders and may include chest x-ray, blood and sputum analysis, and arterial blood gases analysis. In addition, **pulmonary function tests**, also called *spirometry*, are used to evaluate the respiratory system. These tests, commonly conducted in a pulmonology clinic, provide more detailed information about the patient's lung capacity.

Because the cause of bronchitis is usually viral, antibiotics are of little help. Treatment is generally conservative and includes fluids, rest, air humidifiers, and cough medication. A cough that produces thick secretions may be treated with **expectorant** medication, which helps loosen and liquefy secretions so they are more easily expelled. Coughs that are nonproductive may be treated with **antitussive** medication, which suppresses the cough reflex. In some cases, bronchodilator medication may be used to help open narrowed airways. **Corticosteroids**, which suppress the immune response, may be used to decrease inflammation. Patients with chronic bronchitis may eventually need oxygen therapy and more aggressive pulmonary care, including **chest physiotherapy**, which involves percussion (clapping) over the thorax or vibration and positioning to facilitate loosening and removal of respiratory secretions. Smoking cessation is encouraged. If a secondary bacterial infection is suspected, antibiotics may be prescribed.

Patients with acute bronchitis usually recover completely, although the cough may linger for several weeks. The prognosis for those with chronic bronchitis is more guarded because of the cumulative damage, which results in obstructive changes.

Asthma

ICD-9-CM code: 493.90 (acute), 493.20 (chronic)

Asthma is a disorder in which the airways overreact to certain triggers with inflammation that results in narrowing and production of thick mucus, causing breathing difficulty. Asthma usually affects individuals who also suffer from allergies.

Asthma affects approximately 20 million Americans and costs an estimated $18 billion dollars each year in direct and indirect costs. It is estimated that each day 30,000 people suffer an asthma attack, 40,000 miss school or work, several thousand visit the emergency room, 1,000 are admitted to the hospital, and 14 people die. Asthma is the most common chronic disease suffered by children. It accounts for 25% of emergency room visits and 10 million outpatient visits. Even more alarming is the fact that asthma-related deaths have increased by more than 50% among all age groups and by 80% among children since 1980. Ethnic groups such as African Americans and Latino populations suffer higher rates of illness and death. These differences appear to be correlated with poverty, poor air quality, indoor allergens, and lack of access to adequate education and medical care.

There are two types of asthma: allergic and nonallergic. Allergic asthma is caused by allergens such as pollen, dust mites, pet dander, or other irritants that are inhaled into the lungs and air passages, causing inflammation. Nonallergic asthma is triggered by such factors as exercise, cold air, stress, anxiety, smoke, and viruses. Risk factors for asthma include genetics, poor air quality, and poverty.

Signs and symptoms of both forms of asthma include coughing, wheezing, shortness of breath, and chest tightness. Increased respiratory effort and dyspnea commonly result in anxiety, tachycardia, and pallor. The individual prefers to sit upright for maximal lung expansion and may have difficulty speaking in complete sentences. Auscultation of the lungs reveals "tight"-sounding lungs with wheezing and decreased breath sounds.

In an emergent situation, diagnosis is usually based on the patient's description of symptoms, physical examination findings, oxygen saturation readings, and peak-flow measurement. A peak-flow meter is a handheld device the patient can use to measure the volume of air that he is able to inhale and exhale. The physician may order pulmonary function tests but usually defers them for the critical patient. Chest x-ray reveals changes related to hyperinflation of the lungs and mucus plugs. Allergy testing may also be done.

Acute asthmatic episodes are treated with such medications as albuterol and epinephrine. Both medications cause relaxation of the smooth muscle in the airways, allowing them to open. Depending on the severity of the attack, corticosteroids may also be used because of their potent anti-inflammatory effect and their ability to decrease airway reactivity. Long-term management includes identification of allergens, desensitization therapy, preventive medications such as steroid inhalers, and avoidance of known triggers.

Prognosis is variable and depends on the type and severity of the asthma and the patient's access to health care resources.

Emphysema
ICD-9-CM code: 492.8

Emphysema is a common chronic obstructive respiratory disorder that involves permanent damage to the alveoli and flattening of the diaphragm, leading to COPD. Emphysema affects as many as 30 million Americans and causes over 100,000 deaths each year.

There are a number of contributors to the development of emphysema, including industrial exposure and repeated or chronic respiratory infections. However, the main risk factor is cigarette smoking. As the lungs are repeatedly subjected to the irritants and toxins in cigarette smoke, the delicate alveoli lose their elasticity and become permanently distended like tiny balloons that have been inflated too many times. They also erode and thicken, thereby functioning less effectively. Loss of elasticity results in air trapping and the thorax begins to develop the barrel-like shape characteristic of COPD. The diaphragm also flattens, losing much of its effectiveness.

Most patients are asymptomatic until they lose over half of their lung function. This lack of symptoms leads many into a false sense of security, believing they still have time to quit smoking before any real damage is done. Initial signs of emphysema include dyspnea with exertion, which gradually worsens, and the development of a chronic productive cough. Weight loss occurs and as heart failure develops, lower-leg edema also develops. Fingernail clubbing develops due to microvascular changes. (See Figure 28-3.) The patient experiences progressively worse orthopnea and chronic hypoxia, which causes **circumoral cyanosis** (blue color around the mouth) during acute episodes. Other symptoms include tachycardia and hypertension.

Diagnosis is based on history and physical examination findings, chest x-ray, and pulmonary function tests. Tidal volume and residual volume are increased while vital capacity and expiratory volume are decreased. Radiologic studies reveal a flattened diaphragm and cardiomegaly. On good days, the lungs may sound clear; however, auscultation with a stethoscope will reveal decreased breath sounds. On bad days, the lungs will sound wheezy with scattered crackles and **rhonchi**, which are coarse, gurgling sounds heard

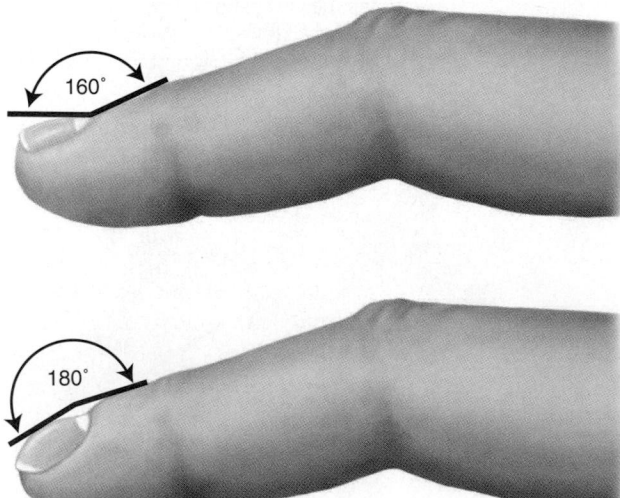

FIG 28-3 Fingernail clubbing.

on auscultation caused by secretions in the air passages. Arterial blood gas (ABG) analysis may reveal chronically low oxygen saturation and carbon dioxide retention.

Treatment for emphysema includes various medications to manage the disease and treat acute exacerbations. Some may be delivered via inhalation therapy with a metered-dose inhaler (MDI) or a **nebulizer**, which is a device that produces a fine spray or mist to deliver medication to the deep air passages of the lungs. For acute exacerbations, the physician may prescribe IV or oral corticosteroids. Expectorants may help make a productive cough more effective and antibiotics are appropriate if a secondary bacterial infection is suspected. Nutrition becomes an issue as patients lose their appetite and the ability to complete a meal without dyspnea. Eventually, supplemental oxygen is needed. However, patients must carefully follow physician recommendations because too much oxygen can sometimes cause complications. During the last few years of life, the patient with emphysema has great difficulty performing basic self-care tasks due to extremely poor activity tolerance.

Emphysema causes permanent destructive changes to respiratory structures and has significant impact on quality of life and longevity. Prognosis is poor and depends largely upon how early the patient receives diagnosis and treatment and whether further exposure to irritants is eliminated. Death from emphysema and other forms of COPD is common in the United States. (See *Teaching about COPD*.)

Pulmonary Tuberculosis

ICD-9-CM code: 011.90

Pulmonary tuberculosis is a contagious lung infection that can also spread to and affect other organ systems. An estimated 30,000 Americans are affected by TB. Populations that suffer from poverty, crowding, unsanitary conditions, malnutrition, and poor access to health care suffer higher rates than others. Pulmonary TB is acquired most commonly by individuals who have weakened immune systems that do not isolate the primary infection, including very young and very old patients and those who are immunocompromised, such as patients with AIDS or those on antirejection or chemotherapeutic medication.

TB is caused by infection with the organism *Mycobacterium tuberculosis*. Primary infection with *M. tuberculosis* usually begins in the lungs after inhalation of the bacterium shed by the cough or sneeze of a contagious individual. In most cases, the lungs successfully encapsulate the infection and the individual recovers without further complications. Pulmonary TB may develop several weeks after the primary infection or may develop or recur after lying dormant for a number of years. Those who are immunocompromised are more likely to experience such a reactivation at a later time.

Up to 20% of individuals with pulmonary tuberculosis may be asymptomatic. Others have a productive cough,

---

Patient Education

Teaching About COPD

The medical assistant should be sure to include these points when teaching a patient about chronic obstructive pulmonary disease (COPD):

- Stop or reduce smoking. Information on smoking cessation programs is available.
- Avoid secondhand smoke and other pollutants.
- Avoid exposure to others with contagious respiratory disorders.
- Obtain an annual influenza vaccination.
- Plan small, nutritious meals with between-meal snacks.
- Consider drinking high-energy, nutritious supplements such as Ensure.
- Take a daily multiple vitamin.
- Take medication as prescribed.
- Keep emergency medication (such as an inhaler) handy.
- Pace activity with frequent rest periods.
- Use purse-lipped breathing when you feel severely short of breath.
- Do not smoke or use flames around oxygen.
- Keep well hydrated to help thin respiratory secretions.

---

hemoptysis (coughing up blood), fever, night sweats, weight loss, anorexia, fatigue, chest pain, and dyspnea.

Diagnosis is based on history, symptoms, and physical examination findings. Auscultation of the lungs may reveal crackles. Other findings include cervical lymph node enlargement and tenderness. The tuberculin skin test (PPD) is a first-line test; a positive reaction to the test indicates exposure to tuberculosis but does not confirm the presence of active disease. In addition, when an individual has tested positive, the TB skin test will always test positive and is of no further use. Other diagnostic testing includes chest x-ray, which reveals multiple opacities (light areas) that may coalesce (run together) and tubercle lesions and cavities, and bronchoscopy (visual examination of the large air passages of the lungs) with collection of sputum (lung secretions) for culturing, which detects the presence of the tubercle bacillus, confirming the diagnosis.

The course of treatment usually lasts 6 months or longer and includes administration of multiple medications, including rifampin (Rifadin), isoniazid (Nydrazid), and others. Because all antitubercular drugs have some toxicity, the medical assistant and physician must conduct thorough patient education and careful monitoring. The medical assistant should also emphasize the importance of completing treatment to prevent relapse and reduce the risk of antibiotic resistance.

Symptoms generally resolve within 3 weeks, although chest x-ray will not reveal improvement until later. Prognosis is excellent if the disease is diagnosed and treated early. Delayed treatment can result in permanent lung damage. Incomplete treatment contributes to the emergence of drug-resistant strains.

Epstein-Barr Virus
ICD-9-CM code: 075

The Epstein-Barr virus (EBV), also called *infectious mononucleosis,* is an infection marked by fever and fatigue. EBV has infected an estimated 95% of adults under age 40. When the virus infects a person during his teen or young adult years, it causes infectious mononucleosis between 35% and 50% of the time. Younger children are commonly asymptomatic or have such a mild case that it is indistinguishable from other mild viruses. Adults older than age 35 rarely have an active infection.

EBV is a member of the herpesvirus family and is transmitted by intimate contact with saliva of an infected person, giving it the name "kissing disease" among young people. It is not usually transmitted via air as cold viruses are or via blood. Because many healthy people have the virus and don't know it, most are not at significant risk for acquiring an active infection from anyone else. Therefore, no special precautions are recommended.

Symptoms include fever, pharyngitis, **lymphadenopathy** (swollen and tender cervical lymph nodes), headaches, fatigue, and anorexia. Splenomegaly or hepatomegaly may also develop. If symptoms last longer than 4 months, chronic EBV infection may be present.

Diagnosis is based on history, description of symptoms, and diagnostic tests. Common tests include the monospot test, antinuclear antibody (ANA) test, and CBC test, which may reveal elevated WBC count and elevation in a specific type of WBCs called *lymphocytes.* The Paul-Bunnell heterophile antibody test may be used to confirm the diagnosis.

There is no cure for EBV and treatment aims to relieve symptoms, including bed rest, fluids, and analgesics. Corticosteroids may help relieve pharyngitis and lymphadenopathy. The physician may recommend the avoidance of sports and demanding physical activities. Aspirin should not be given to young people. Because EBV is a virus, it does not respond to antibiotics.

Symptoms usually resolve within 4 weeks and complete recovery occurs within 3 to 4 months. Once a person is infected, the virus commonly remains dormant in the body. In most cases, it causes no further problems for the individual. However, in rare cases it can play a role in the development of Burkitt's lymphoma and nasopharyngeal carcinoma. A rare but serious complication is splenic rupture, which can cause life-threatening hemorrhage.

Lung Cancer
ICD-9-CM code: 162.9

Lung cancer involves the proliferation of cancer cells in lung tissues. There are two general types of lung cancer: small cell and non-small cell. Lung cancer causes 90% of all cancer-related deaths in the United States. Small cell lung cancer accounts for 20% of all lung cancer and develops almost exclusively in smokers. Non-small cell lung cancer comprises over approximately 80% of lung cancer cases. Squamous cell carcinoma, a type of non-small cell lung cancer, comprises approximately 30% of all lung cancer cases and is most common in men. Adenocarcinoma, another type of non-small lung cell cancer, comprises approximately 40% of all lung cancer cases and is most common in women and nonsmokers. A third type of non-small cell lung cancer, known as *large cell carcinoma,* comprises the other 10% of all lung cancer cases. African Americans have a higher risk of lung cancer, develop it at an earlier age, and are less likely to survive. The higher risk in this group is thought to be related to less access to health care, rather than genetics.

The cause of each type of lung cancer is still not fully understood. However, research has proven that the single largest contributor to the disease is the use of tobacco, which is known to contain over 3500 chemicals—many of them carcinogens—as well as toxic metals and radioactive compounds. Other contributors to lung cancer include second-hand smoke, asbestos, air pollution, and radon, which is an odorless gas released from the breakdown of uranium in water and soil. As tissue cells are damaged by these substances, they change and, in some cases, become cancerous.

Patients with lung cancer are commonly asymptomatic until the disease is far advanced. The most common first symptom is an unexplained cough or a chronic "smoker's cough" that worsens or changes in character. Other signs and symptoms include hemoptysis, dyspnea, chest pain, new onset of wheezing, prolonged hoarseness, fatigue, anorexia, weight loss, bone pain, headache, and repetitive episodes of bronchitis or pneumonia.

Screening for lung cancer is controversial and is not currently recommended by the American Cancer Society. Chest x-rays and CT scans check for abnormal lesions or masses. However, the definitive diagnostic test for any form of cancer is analysis of a biopsied tissue specimen. Such specimens may be obtained through a sputum specimen, bronchoscopy, mediastinoscopy, transthoracic needle biopsy, thoracentesis, or video thoracoscopy. If cancer is detected, the physician stages it according to a system that classifies it based on the extent of spread. Tests used to determine staging include MRI and PET scans. Staging is important in determining the most appropriate treatment plan.

Treatment for the individual patient depends on a number of factors, including the type and stage of the cancer and the patient's underlying health status. The physician may perform surgery to remove cancerous lesions if the cancer remains localized. Procedures include **wedge resection** (removal of only the affected part of the lung), **lobectomy** (removal of an entire lobe), or **pneumonectomy** (removal of an entire lung). Also, lymph node biopsy identifies whether the cancer has spread into the lymphatic system.

Chemotherapy, radiation therapy, or both are common treatments for lung cancer. Chemotherapy involves the use of medications to kill cancer cells, shrink them, or slow their growth, thereby making the patient more comfortable and prolonging life. Radiation therapy uses targeted x-rays to kill cancer cells or shrink tumors. The mode of delivery depends on the type and stage of the cancer.

The prognosis for individuals with lung cancer is generally poor but varies somewhat, depending on the type of cancer and how early it is detected. Small cell cancer grows and spreads rapidly with a very poor prognosis. All forms of lung cancer that respond well to initial treatment commonly reappear months or years later and are less responsive to treatment at that time. The 5-year survival rate for all types of lung cancer is only 15%.

Pulmonology Procedures

Pulmonology is a medical specialty that focuses on the study and treatment of diseases and disorders of the respiratory system. However, all primary care providers evaluate and treat patients with common respiratory disorders. Patients with more severe or complex respiratory illness are usually referred to the **pulmonologist**, a specialist in the diagnosis and treatment of respiratory disorders.

Some disorders treated by the pulmonologist, such as URI, aren't considered serious medical disorders. However, because of their potential for adverse complications in compromised individuals, these disorders deserve as much attention as more serious medical disorders such as lung cancer. (See *Front office breathing emergency*.)

Assisting with Examination

To reach an accurate diagnosis, the pulmonologist must assess the patient's medical history, including a description of symptoms, as well as perform a physical examination of upper and lower airways. In an examination, the medical assistant must prepare the patient by checking vital signs and obtaining the health history, which should include data regarding allergies, new respiratory symptoms, and medications.

Front office–Back office connection

Front Office Breathing Emergency

The administrative medical assistant should never make a patient who complains of shortness of breath wait in the reception area. She should act quickly to:

- notify the physician, nurse, or clinical medical assistant immediately
- assist the patient to a chair and send someone for a wheelchair
- make sure the patient is wheeled to an examination room right away
- obtain emergency contact information for a patient who arrives alone
- assist the clinical staff, if requested, by ordering emergency tests or consultations.

She should then assist the patient as needed with undressing and positioning. Patients should undress above the waist, put on the examination gown with the opening in the front, and sit upright on the examination table. Doing so allows the physician easy access to the patient's thorax in order to perform inspection, palpation, percussion, and auscultation anteriorly, posteriorly, and laterally. The medical assistant should provide the patient as much privacy as possible, assist the physician as needed with the examination, and perform ordered diagnostic tests. She must also assist the pulmonologist as needed with any procedures.

Diagnostic Testing

Respiratory disorders are extremely common. Therefore, regardless of what type of setting they work in, most medical assistants help provide care for patients with some form of respiratory illness or disorder. Diagnostic tests commonly done in a pulmonology office include pulmonary function tests and bronchoscopy. Simple tests that might be done in any medical office include the Mantoux test and peak-flow measurement.

Pulmonary Function Tests

Pulmonary function tests (PFTs), also called *spirometry,* are a group of tests used to evaluate the respiratory system and determine the degree of airway obstruction caused by obstructive disorders. The test measures various aspects of expiratory flow and lung volume.

- *Total lung capacity* is the total volume of air in the lungs after a maximal inhalation. It is reduced in patients with restrictive lung disease and increased in those with obstructive lung disease.

- *Tidal volume* is the volume of air typically inhaled and exhaled with each normal breath. It is reduced in elderly patients and those with restrictive lung disease.
- *Vital capacity* is the volume of air that can be exhaled from the lungs after a maximal inspiration. It is reduced in elderly patients and those with atelectasis and pulmonary edema.
- *Residual volume* is the amount of air remaining in the lungs after a forced maximal exhalation. It is increased in elderly patients and those with COPD.
- *Functional residual capacity* is the amount of air remaining in the lungs after a normal exhalation. It is increased in elderly patients and those with COPD. (See Figure 28-4.)
- *Forced expiratory volume (FEV)* is the amount of air that can be quickly exhaled.
- *FEV1* is the volume of air that can be forcibly exhaled in 1 second.
- *Forced vital capacity (FVC)*, also called *FEV6*, is the amount of air that can be completely and forcibly exhaled after a maximal inhalation. (See *Procedure 28-1: Performing respiratory testing*.)

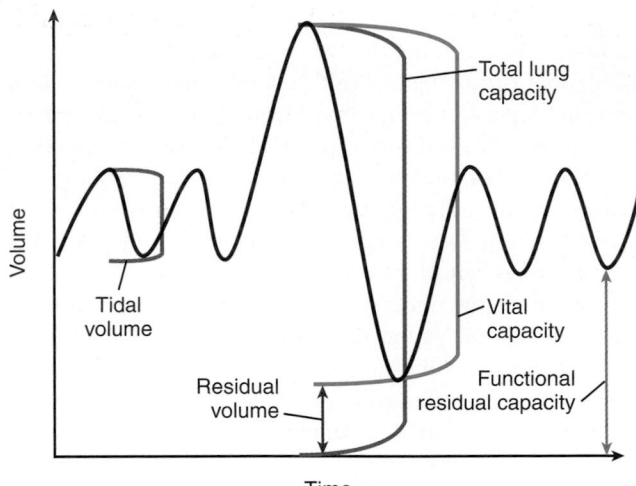

FIG 28-4 Pulmonary function test.

Performing respiratory testing

Task
Assist a patient in the use of a spirometer for respiratory testing.

Conditions
- Spirometer with recording paper
- Disposable tubing
- Disposable mouthpiece
- Disposable nose clips
- Biohazardous waste container
- Patient's medical record

Standards
In the time specified and within the scoring parameters determined by the instructor, the student will successfully assist a patient in the use of a spirometer to complete respiratory testing.

Performance Standards
1. Greet and identify your patient to prevent errors. Introduce yourself and explain the procedure to ease patient anxiety.
2. Wash or sanitize your hands to ensure infection control.
3. Assemble supplies and equipment. Apply new disposable tubing and mouthpiece.
4. Obtain the patient's height and weight to accurately calculate predicted values.
5. Enter the patient's age, gender, height, and weight into the computer to ensure accurate calculation of predicted values.
6. Ask the patient to loosen tight clothing and sit upright near the machine to increase the patient's ease when performing breathing maneuvers.
7. Describe and demonstrate the breathing maneuver to the patient to help him understand how to perform the procedure and feel less self-conscious about doing it himself.
8. Gently apply the nose clips to his nose to keep air from escaping out of his nose and coach him in performing the maneuver to help him complete the procedure successfully, using these instructions:
   a. Take in as deep a breath as you possibly can.
   b. Put the mouthpiece in your mouth with your lips snugly around it.
   c. Blow out forcefully as hard as you can for as long as you can until your lungs feel completely empty.

PROCEDURE 28-1—cont'd

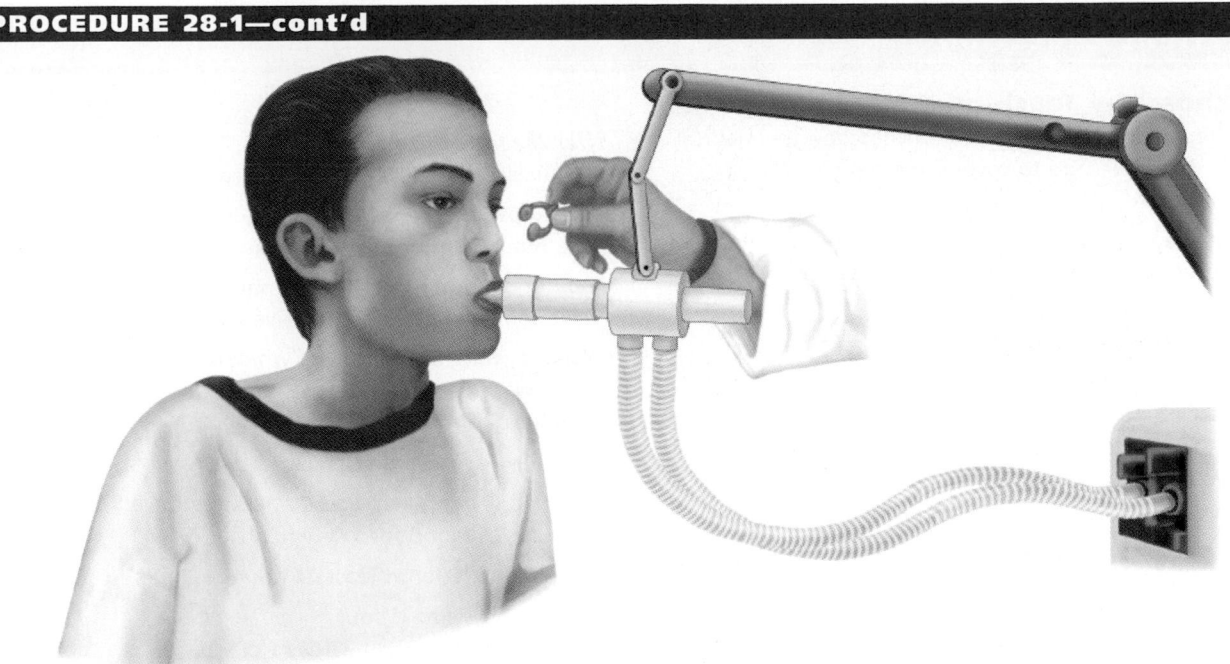

Apply nose clips to patient's nose and coach him through the steps of the maneuver.

9. Repeat the maneuver until three optimal readings have been obtained to ensure accurate results.
10. Remove the nose clips, disposable mouthpiece, and tubing. Discard them all in the biohazardous waste container. Allow the patient to rest for a few minutes because the patient may feel slightly dizzy from the deep breathing.
11. Sanitize your hands, print the report, and enter all data in the patient's medical record, including his name, the date, the time, the name of the test, and your signature to ensure the accuracy and completeness of the medical record.

Date	
07/07/08; 10:21 a.m.	Spirometric testing completed. See report for details. ——————————————————————S. Gonzales, CMA

12. Clean the spirometer according to the manufacturer's instructions and put away all equipment to ensure infection control and prepare the equipment for the next use.

Bronchoscopy

Bronchoscopy is a procedure in which the physician views a patient's airways using a bronchoscope in order to examine them, remove foreign objects or a growth, or collect tissue for biopsy. The physician may use a rigid or flexible bronchoscope, depending on the purpose. Flexible bronchoscopes are more useful for viewing small airways and removing small tissue specimens and usually do not require general anesthesia. Rigid bronchoscopes are more useful for treating bleeding and removing foreign objects or large tissue samples and usually require general anesthesia. The physician performs a bronchoscopy in a hospital setting or the procedure room of a medical clinic. The medical assistant should be sure to explain the procedure to the patient as well as provide patient education on how to prepare for the test. (See *Bronchoscopy teaching*, page 512.)

A large x-ray machine called a *fluoroscope* may be used to transmit a picture to a monitor, which provides an enlarged picture and the ability to record a video of the procedure.

Mantoux Test

The **Mantoux test**, also called the *purified protein derivative (PPD) test*, detects tuberculosis infection. The test involves the intradermal injection of purified protein derivative just beneath the top layer of the skin on the inner aspect of the forearm. The nurse or medical assistant evaluates the site between 48 and 72 hours later for evidence of induration

Patient Education

Bronchoscopy Teaching

When preparing a patient for a bronchoscopy, the medical assistant should be sure to cover these topics.

First steps

- You will be able to discuss the procedure with the physician beforehand, so you can get answers to all of your questions.
- The physician will ask you to sign a consent form.
- The physician or medical assistant will ask some questions, including:
  - What medications are you taking?
  - Do you bleed easily?
  - Are you or could you be pregnant?

Prior to the procedure

- You may undergo a chest x-ray to help the physician identify the area to look at during the procedure.
- Eat and drink nothing within 8 to 10 hours of the procedure.
- Empty your bladder just before the procedure.
- You may be asked to remove:
  - dentures
  - eyeglasses or contacts
  - hearing aids
  - jewelry
  - wigs
  - makeup
  - all or most of your clothing (you will be given a gown to wear).
- You may be given medication, such as:
  - topical anesthetic spray
  - medication to relax you
  - medication to dry up oral secretions.

After the procedure

- You will rest for 2 to 3 hours afterward.
- If a biopsy was done you may undergo a chest x-ray to rule out pneumothorax (air leakage).
- Do not operate a car or other equipment. Be sure to have someone available to drive you home.
- You may have a sore throat, which you can relieve by using warm saltwater gargles or sucking on throat lozenges.
- You may have a hoarse voice.
- If a biopsy was taken, you may cough up very small amounts of blood for a few hours.
- Do not smoke for at least 24 hours.
- Call the physician if you:
  - cough up more than 2 Tbs of blood
  - have difficulty breathing
  - run a fever greater than 100°F (38°C).

General information

- The procedure will not interfere with your ability to breathe.
- You may receive oxygen through your nose.
- The staff will monitor your heart rate, blood pressure, and oxygen levels throughout the procedure.
- The procedure usually takes 1 hour or less.
- Results of a biopsy or culture are usually available 2 to 7 days after the procedure.

(hardening). An area of induration larger than 10 mm is considered positive, which means the patient has a current or prior tuberculosis infection.

Peak-Flow Measurement

A **peak-flow meter** is a handheld device used to measure a patient's lung capacity. It provides less detailed information than pulmonary function tests but has the advantage of being portable and easy to use. Therefore, patients may obtain an objective measurement of lung capacity at home, work, school, or elsewhere whenever they feel short of breath. The patient can compare these measurements with her normal baseline values to determine whether to take medication or call the medical office. To use the peak-flow meter, the patient takes a deep breath and blows into the meter as quickly and forcefully as possible. Keeping a peak-flow diary helps the patient determine what her normal baseline values are and allows comparison and objective measurement during times of illness or exacerbation of an underlying respiratory disorder. It is especially useful for patients with asthma. (See Figure 28-5.)

Treatments

Treatments for respiratory disorders include use of a metered-dose inhaler, a nebulizer, incentive spirometry, and oxygen therapy.

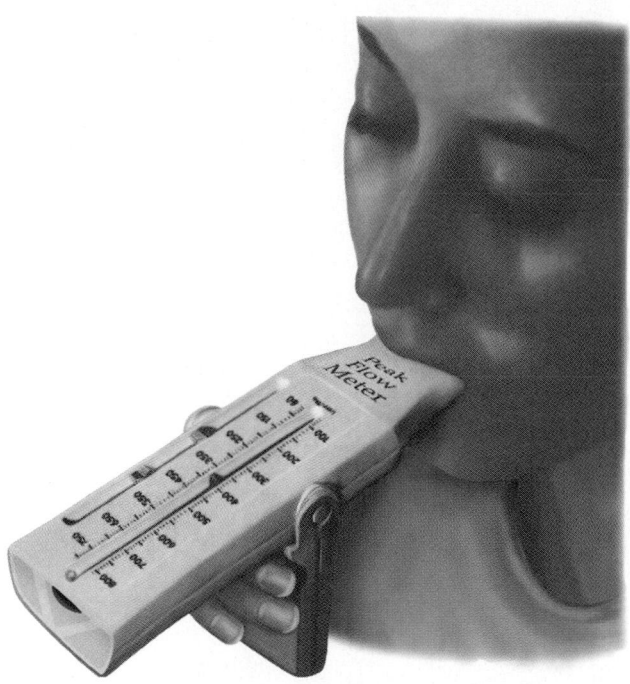

FIG 28-5 Peak-flow meter.

Metered-Dose Inhaler

Patients with respiratory disorders such as asthma and emphysema are commonly given a prescription for a **metered-dose inhaler** (MDI), which allows the patient to deliver medication directly into his air passages and lungs. MDIs with spacers are also available for patients who have trouble using MDIs. (See *Using a spacer*.) Inhalers may be prescribed for use on a regular schedule or on an as-needed (prn) basis. However, in instances when use of an inhaler does not provide adequate relief of symptoms, the patient may administer medication using a nebulizer. (See Figure 28-6.) The medical assistant may teach the patient to use an **incentive spirometer** for postoperative or home use. The patient uses this handheld device several times throughout the day to inhale a maximal breath to keep lungs expanded and functional. The patient may also receive oxygen administration in the medical office on a temporary basis or may need instruction for home oxygen use. (See *Procedure 28-2: Teaching a patient to use an MDI*, page 515.)

Nebulizer Treatments

A nebulizer is a device that produces a fine spray or mist to deliver medication to the air passages and lungs. It creates the mist by rapidly passing air through a liquid or by vibrating a liquid at a high frequency so that the particles produced are extremely small and become aerosolized. For example, albuterol (Proventil, Accuneb), which relaxes muscles in the airways, is delivered in this manner. This muscle relaxation allows air passages to open more fully, enabling

the patient to breathe better. Such an effect is especially useful for patients experiencing an exacerbation of a disorder such as asthma or emphysema.

As a general rule, doctors prefer to prescribe inhalers, rather than nebulizers, because they are cheaper, more portable, and deliver less medication, which means less risk of adverse effects. However, nebulizers work especially well for infants and very small children who are unable to use MDIs effectively. Although physicians prefer MDIs for use by older individuals, a nebulizer may be prescribed for an individual with serious respiratory disease or severe asthma attacks. In selected cases, the physician will also prescribe nebulizers for home use. However, nebulizer use is most common in clinics and hospitals. If the physician prescribes a home-use nebulizer for a patient, the medical assistant should be sure to provide adequate education to ensure the maximal therapeutic benefit. (See *Using a home nebulizer*, page 516.)

Incentive Spirometry

An incentive spirometer is a handheld device used by a patient to fully expand the lungs by inhaling as deeply as possible to keep lungs clear. Patients who use this device are commonly postoperative patients and those at risk for developing atelectasis (partial lung tissue collapse). There are many styles of incentive spirometers; however, all have similar components, including a mouthpiece, tube, and ball or piston. The patient inserts the mouthpiece into his mouth and then must breathe in slowly and as deeply as he can. As he does so, a small ball or piston rises in the tube, which has

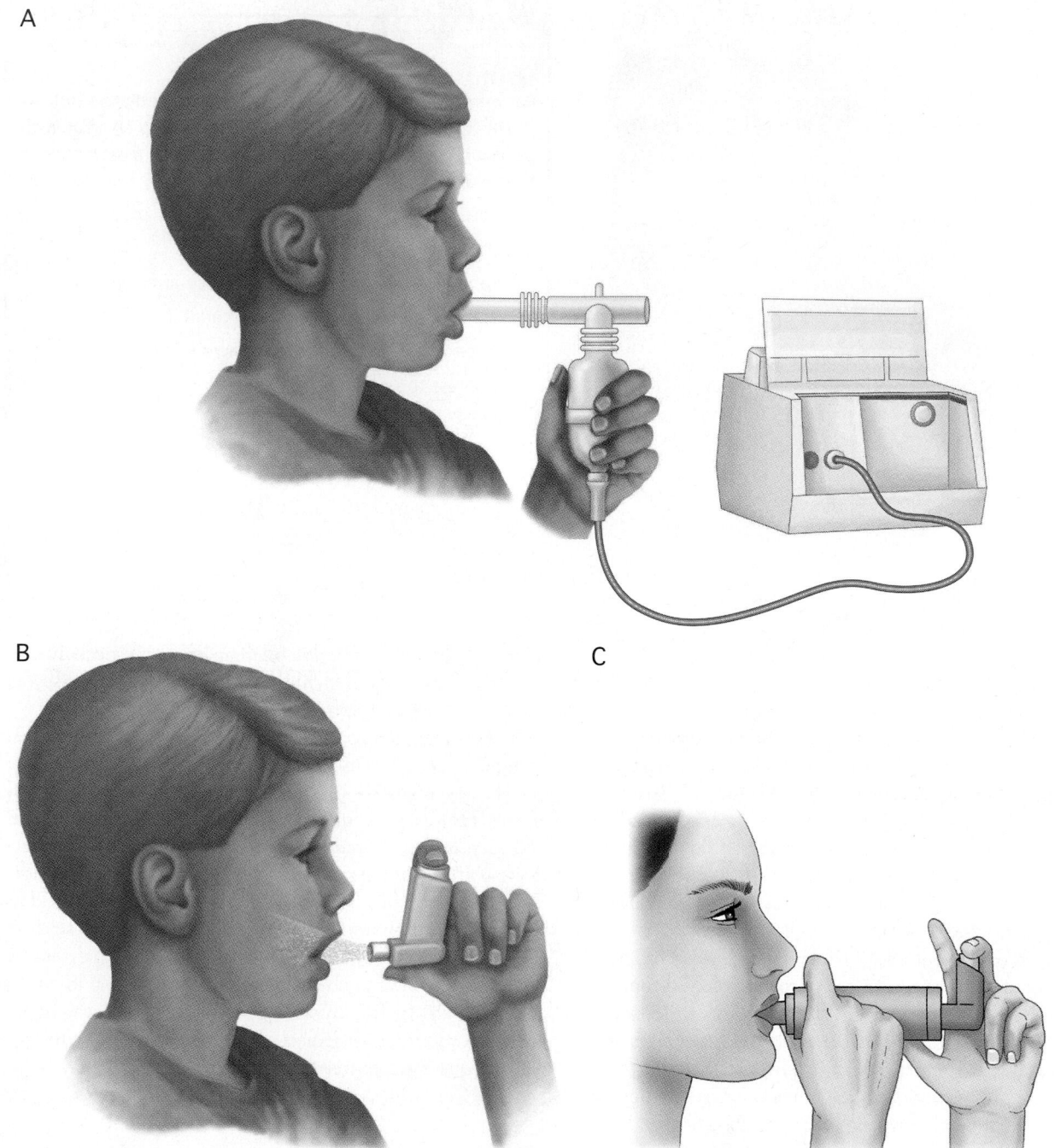

FIG 28-6 (A) Nebulizer. (B) MDI. (C) MDI with spacer.

markings on it. The patient should hold his breath for as long as possible and then breathe out. After resting for a few seconds, the patient should repeat the process. Postoperative patients should complete a set of 10 breaths every hour or two while awake. In most cases, the patient can stop using the incentive spirometer when they return home from the hospital. However, patients who are prone to respiratory infections or are sedentary may be instructed to use an incentive spirometer at home. These individuals should follow the instructions of their physician.

Oxygen Therapy

Patients who suffer from acute or chronic respiratory disorders sometimes need supplemental oxygen therapy. In most

PROCEDURE 28-2

Teaching a patient to use an MDI

Task
Teach a patient how to use a metered-dose inhaler (MDI).

Conditions
- Metered-dose inhaler
- Patient's medical record

Standards
In the time specified and within the scoring parameters determined by the instructor, the student will successfully teach a patient to use an MDI.

Performance Standards

1. Greet and identify your patient to prevent errors. Introduce yourself and explain the procedure to ease patient anxiety.
2. If possible, ask the patient to watch an MDI demonstration video to introduce the patient to the proper use of an MDI.
3. Wash or sanitize your hands to ensure infection control.
4. Using a placebo MDI or one prescribed for the patient, point out the mouthpiece and cover and the medication canister. Indicate how the canister is depressed to initiate a puff of medication to familiarize the patient with the parts and function of the device.
5. Instruct the patient to use purse-lipped breathing to slow and control his breathing rate. Remove the cap from the mouthpiece and shake the MDI for 5 to 10 seconds to mix the medication, preparing the MDI for use.

6. Hand the MDI to the patient and instruct him to hold it upside down 1" to $1^1/_2$" in front of his open mouth to enable him to inhale more of the aerosolized medication into his lungs, rather than depositing it on the back of his mouth.
7. Instruct the patient to exhale and then, just after beginning to inhale, to depress the canister. The patient should continue to inhale slowly for 5 to 6 seconds to help move more of the aerosolized medication into the deeper airways and leave less on the back of the throat.
8. Instruct the patient to hold his breath for 8 to 10 seconds, if possible, and then to exhale through pursed lips to facilitate the deposit of the medication into his lungs before exhalation.
9. If more than one puff is prescribed, instruct the patient to wait for several minutes before repeating the procedure to allow the patient to rest and provide time for the initial dose to work, which (with medications such as bronchodilators) will enable more effective inhalation of the second dose.
10. Document the session in the patient's medical record to reflect the teaching that occurred and ensure a complete, accurate medical record.

Date	
11/03/08: 9:55 a.m.	Instructed Pt in use of MDI. Return demonstration performed ----------------------------------S. Gonzales, CMA

---

cases, the need is temporary. However, in the case of some chronic disorders such as COPD, patients may become chronically oxygen-dependent. The goal of oxygen therapy is to relieve or prevent hypoxemia (low blood oxygen levels). Regardless of the need, oxygen administration, as with any drug, is dependent on a physician's order. In some cases, improper administration of oxygen can cause adverse effects. In addition, some patients with COPD, who chronically retain carbon dioxide (CO_2), can actually lose their drive to breathe if too much oxygen is administered. The standard flow rate for such patients is usually 1 to 2 L per minute.

Home-delivery vendors deliver the oxygen and related equipment to the patient as well as set it up and instruct the patient on its proper use. However, the physician and medical assistant must closely monitor the patient on oxygen therapy and provide comprehensive education for safe, effective home use, including fire hazards around oxygen. Although it will not burn spontaneously, oxygen can help to ignite and fuel a fire if a spark or flame is present.

Different devices deliver different percentages of oxygen, referred to as *fraction of inspired oxygen* (FIO_2). The most common device for oxygen delivery in the clinic or home setting is disposable tubing with a **nasal cannula**, sometimes referred to as *nasal prongs*, which are attached to an oxygen tank or a wall outlet. The prongs of the cannula are usually curved in shape and fit most comfortably in the patient's nose with the prongs pointed downward toward the base of the patient's nose. (See Figure 28-7.) The nasal cannula is for low-flow oxygen only. The most common setting is 2 L/minute, although anywhere between 1 and 6 L may be administered. However, a flow rate greater than 4 L will quickly dry the nasal mucosa and a humidifier should be attached for prolonged use. For flow rates above 5 or 6 L, the patient should use a mask. (See *Procedure 28-3: Administering oxygen via nasal cannula,* page 516.)

Patient Education

Using a Home Nebulizer

The medical assistant teaching a patient how to use a home nebulizer should be sure to include these steps:

• Breathe normally most of the time, but take an occasional deep breath and hold it for 5 to 10 seconds to help distribute the medication into the deep air passages.

• If administering a nebulizer to an infant or small child, use a mask. If the child will not tolerate wearing a mask, hold the mask in front of her face as she breathes.

• Sit upright to ensure maximal lung expansion.

• Clean the nebulizer and equipment after each use according to the manufacturer's instructions to avoid the growth of microorganisms.

• Bronchodilators provide immediate relief but commonly cause the temporary adverse effects of nervousness, tremors, heart palpitations, and increased blood pressure.

• Steroids can cause oral thrush and sore throat, so be sure to rinse the mouth after use.

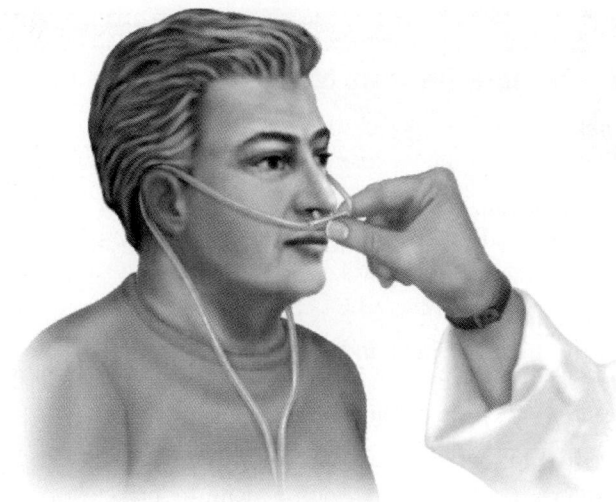

FIG 28-7 Oxygen therapy using a nasal cannula.

PROCEDURE 28-3

Administering oxygen via nasal cannula

Task

Administer oxygen to a patient using a nasal cannula.

Conditions

- Nasal cannula
- Oxygen tubing
- Oxygen source
- Oxygen flow meter
- Appropriate room signs
- Patient's medical record

Standards

In the time specified and within the scoring parameters determined by the instructor, the student will successfully administer oxygen to a patient using a nasal cannula.

Performance Standards

1. Greet and identify your patient to prevent errors. Introduce yourself and explain the procedure to ease patient anxiety.
2. Wash or sanitize your hands to ensure infection control.
3. Connect the nasal cannula to the oxygen tubing (unless tubing is packaged preconnected). Attach the tubing to the oxygen source and set it at the prescribed level to avoid having to adjust the oxygen flow when administering it to the patient. Check for oxygen flow out of the nasal cannula to ensure patency of the tubing.
4. Place the tips of the cannula into the patient's nares with the curved prongs pointing downward to ensure that the oxygen will flow into the nasal passages, rather than against the roof of the nose.
5. Place the tubing on either side of patient's head and wrap it behind the patient's ears (similar to the ear pieces on a pair of glasses) so that the tubing then lies forward on his chest. Adjust the plastic slide so that the tubing is comfortably snug under the patient's chin to ensure that the tubing is secure during movement but the patient is comfortable.
6. Document the procedure in the patient's medical record to ensure a complete, accurate medical record.

Date	
08/07/08; 8:55 a.m.	O₂ applied at 2 L per NC.------------------S. Gonzales, CMA

Chapter Summary

- Oxygen is essential for human life. The pulmonary system allows the human body to exchange oxygen for carbon dioxide through inspiration and expiration.
- Key structures of the pulmonary system include the mouth, nose, sinuses, nasopharynx, oropharynx, trachea, bronchi, and lungs. Gas exchange occurs in the tiny alveoli, which are microscopic air sacs.
- Medical assistants must be well versed in the language and vocabulary that pertain to the pulmonary system. In addition to knowing common word elements, they should be familiar with common pathological terms and abbreviations.
- Some of the most common disorders of the pulmonary system include allergic rhinitis, URI, sinusitis, pharyngitis, pneumonia, influenza, tuberculosis, mononucleosis, lung cancer, and obstructive disorders such as bronchitis, asthma, and emphysema.
- Pulmonology is a medical specialty that focuses on the study and treatment of diseases and disorders of the respiratory system. Medical assistants assist physicians in pulmonology as well as in other settings with patient examinations, diagnostic testing, and procedures.
- Pulmonary function tests (PFTs) are a group of tests used to evaluate the respiratory system and are used to determine the degree of airway obstruction that exists with obstructive disorders.
- The physician performs a bronchoscopy using a bronchoscope to examine the patient's airways, remove a foreign object or growth, or collect tissue for biopsy.
- The Mantoux test identifies whether an individual has been exposed to tuberculosis.
- A peak-flow meter is a handheld device that may be used to measure a patient's lung capacity. It provides less detailed information than pulmonary function tests but has the advantage of being portable and easy to use.
- A metered-dose inhaler (MDI) is a handheld device that delivers medication directly into the air passages and lungs. Physicians prescribe inhalers for use on a regular schedule or on an as-needed basis.
- An incentive spirometer is a handheld device used by a patient to fully expand the lungs by inhaling as deeply as possible. Postoperative patients and those at risk for developing atelectasis commonly use this device.
- Patients who suffer from acute or chronic respiratory disorders sometimes need supplemental oxygen therapy. The goal of oxygen therapy is to relieve or prevent hypoxemia.

Oxygen should be administered by physician order only. Consistent monitoring and comprehensive education on oxygen home use is essential.

Team Work Exercises

1. Divide into groups of three or four students. Each group must role-play one of the following scenarios (as determined by the instructor) for the rest of the class:
   a. An 8-year-old child is diagnosed with asthma. The physician prescribes an albuterol inhaler. The medical assistant must teach the child and parent(s) how to use it with and without a spacer.
   b. A 72-year-old man with COPD is taking a nebulizer home so that he can have home treatments three times per day, as needed. He is extremely hard of hearing and somewhat forgetful. Therefore, the medical assistant must teach the patient and his wife how to use the nebulizer.
   c. Mrs. Vargas is a 38-year-old woman who will be undergoing a bronchoscopy. She speaks and understands very little English. The medical assistant must provide Mrs. Vargas and her teenage daughter with instructions regarding what to expect before and after the procedure. An interpreter will be used.
2. Divide into groups of three to four students. Each team must compose a story. In writing the story, the team must use as many medical terms, pathological terms, and abbreviations included in this chapter as possible. The stories may be serious, funny, or silly. However, the terms must be used accurately within the context of the story. The instructor will determine a time limit for writing the story. At the end of the time period, a representative of each team must read the story aloud to the rest of the class.

Case Studies

1. Albert Washington is a 67-year-old patient with COPD. He comes to the clinic complaining of feeling worse than usual with a frequent cough that produces "thick green stuff." The physician asks the medical assistant to collect a sputum specimen from Mr. Washington. Describe what the medical assistant should do.
2. Mr. Washington (see previous case study) states that he sometimes turns his home oxygen up when he feels especially short of breath. His wife is concerned and states that she doesn't believe he should be doing this. They cannot agree on this issue and have asked the medical assistant to settle their argument. What should the medical assistant tell them?

Resources

- American Cancer Society information on lung cancer: *www.cancer.org*
- American Lung Association: *www.lungusa.org*
- CDC influenza guidelines: *www.cdc.gov/flu*
- Information on asthma and allergies: *www.aaaai.org* and *www.aafa.org*
- Information on lung diseases: *www.nlm.nih.gov/medlineplus/lungdiseases.html*
- Information on pneumonia: *www.medicinenet.com/pneumonia*
- Information on pulmonary disorders and conditions:*www.pulmonologychannel.com*
- National Emphysema Foundation: *www.emphysemafoundation.org*

Endocrinology

Learning Objectives

Upon completion of this chapter, the student will be able to:

- define and spell terms related to endocrinology
- identify key structures of the endocrine system
- describe the functions of the endocrine system
- describe the role of the medical assistant in endocrinology
- identify common endocrine diseases and disorders
- list the major hormones of the endocrine system
- list the major glands of the endocrine system
- differentiate between type I and II diabetes mellitus
- identify complications of diabetes mellitus
- identify patient education regarding endocrine system diseases and disorders
- list commonly used word elements related to the endocrine system and give at least 10 examples of how new endocrine related terms may be created by combining prefixes, suffixes, and combining forms
- describe the medical assistant's role in assisting with endocrinology procedures
- list common tests for endocrine system diseases and disorders.

CAAHEP Competencies

Administrative Competencies
Process Insurance Claims
  Perform diagnostic coding

Clinical Competencies
Patient Care
  Prepare patients for and assist with routine and specialty examinations
  Prepare patients for and assist with procedures, treatments, and minor office surgeries
General Competencies
Patient Instruction
  Instruct individuals according to their needs
  Provide instruction for health maintenance and disease prevention

ABHES Competencies
Administrative Duties
  Perform diagnostic coding
Clinical Duties
  Prepare patients for procedures
  Prepare patient for and assist physician with routine and specialty examinations and treatments and minor office surgeries
Instruction
  Teach patients methods of health promotion and disease prevention

Procedures
  Teaching a patient to provide foot care

Chapter Outline
Structures and Functions of the Endocrine System
  Structures of the Endocrine System
  Functions of the Endocrine System
    Pineal gland
    Pituitary gland
    Thyroid gland
    Adrenal glands
    Pancreas
    Thymus gland
    Ovaries
    Testes
    Negative feedback system
Medical Terminology Related to the Endocrine System
Common Endocrine System Diseases and Disorders
  Types of Diabetes
    Type 1 diabetes
    Type 2 diabetes
    Gestational diabetes
  Thyroid Disorders
    Hypothyroidism
    Hyperthyroidism
Endocrinology Procedures
  Assisting with Examination
  Endocrine System Tests
    Fasting blood glucose
    Glucose tolerance test
    Glycosylated hemoglobin
    Urine glucose test
    Glucometer testing
    Thyroid tests
    Thyroid scan
    Radioactive iodine uptake
Chapter Summary
Team Work Exercises
Case Studies
Resources

Key Terms

endocrinologist
Medical doctor who specializes in the diagnosis and treatment of endocrine diseases and disorders

endocrinology
Study of the structures and functions of the endocrine system

exophthalmos
Symptom of protruding eyeballs, usually caused by a severe form of hyperthyroidism called *Graves disease*

fasting
Practice of denying the body all food or nutrition, usually for a specified period of time before laboratory tests or surgical procedures

glucometer
Instrument used to measure glucose levels in the blood

glucosuria
Presence of glucose in the urine

goiter
Enlarged thyroid gland

growth hormone
Hormone secreted by the pituitary gland to stimulate growth of bones and tissues; also called *somatotropin*

hyperglycemia
Abnormally high blood glucose level

hyperthyroidism
Condition of having excessive levels of thyroid hormone in the body

hypertrophy
Excessive growth of tissue

hypoglycemia
Abnormally low blood glucose levels

hypoglycemic
Drug that lowers blood glucose levels

hypothyroidism
Condition of inadequate levels of thyroid hormone in the body

negative feedback system
Control system in which an increase or decrease in a substance stimulates an opposite response by a hormone

peripheral
Away from the trunk of the body; in the extremities

polydipsia
Increased thirst

polyphagia
Increased appetite

polyuria
Increased urination

venous
Pertaining to the veins or the blood in the veins

Structures and Functions of the Endocrine System

The endocrine system is made up of all the major glands of the body. It regulates many body functions through the action of various hormones. (See Figure 29-1.)

Structures of the Endocrine System

The pituitary gland is a small, round, pea-sized structure attached to the lower surface of the hypothalamus in the brain. The pituitary gland is divided into an anterior lobe and a posterior lobe.

The thyroid gland, one of the largest endocrine glands, is highly vascular and is located in the base of the neck. It is shaped similar to the letter H and has two lobes located on each side of the trachea, which are connected by a narrow band. Four tiny parathyroid glands lie on the posterior surface of the thyroid gland within its connective tissue.

The two adrenal glands are triangular in shape and located on top of each kidney within the retroperitoneal cavity (in the back of the abdomen). They are made up of an outer layer called the *adrenal cortex* and an inner part called the *adrenal medulla*.

The pancreas is a long, somewhat flat organ that is located in the upper left quadrant of the abdomen. The endocrine portion of the pancreas includes the pancreatic islets, also called the *islets of Langerhans*.

The pineal gland, sometimes referred to as the *pineal body*, is shaped like a pine cone and located in the brain above and behind the thalamus.

The thymus gland consists of two symmetrical lobes located in the mediastinum (midchest area). It is proportionately larger in infants and children and shrinks in size as people age.

The reproductive glands, sometimes called the *gonads*, are the ovaries and testes. The ovaries are flat, oval-shaped structures located on each side of the uterus in the lower abdominal cavity, attached to the broad ligament. The ovaries contain the graafian follicles, in which are the immature ova, or eggs. The testes are egg-shaped glands located in the scrotum of the male reproductive tract.

Functions of the Endocrine System

The endocrine system is a complex network of glands that regulate and secrete hormones that act directly on target organs or stimulate other glands to secrete different hormones. Hormone levels in the blood vary according to bodily functions. Glands sense the varying levels and work to increase or decrease the level of glandular secretion to maintain a balance. In most cases, hormones work in pairs to maintain the appropriate balance, with one hormone acting

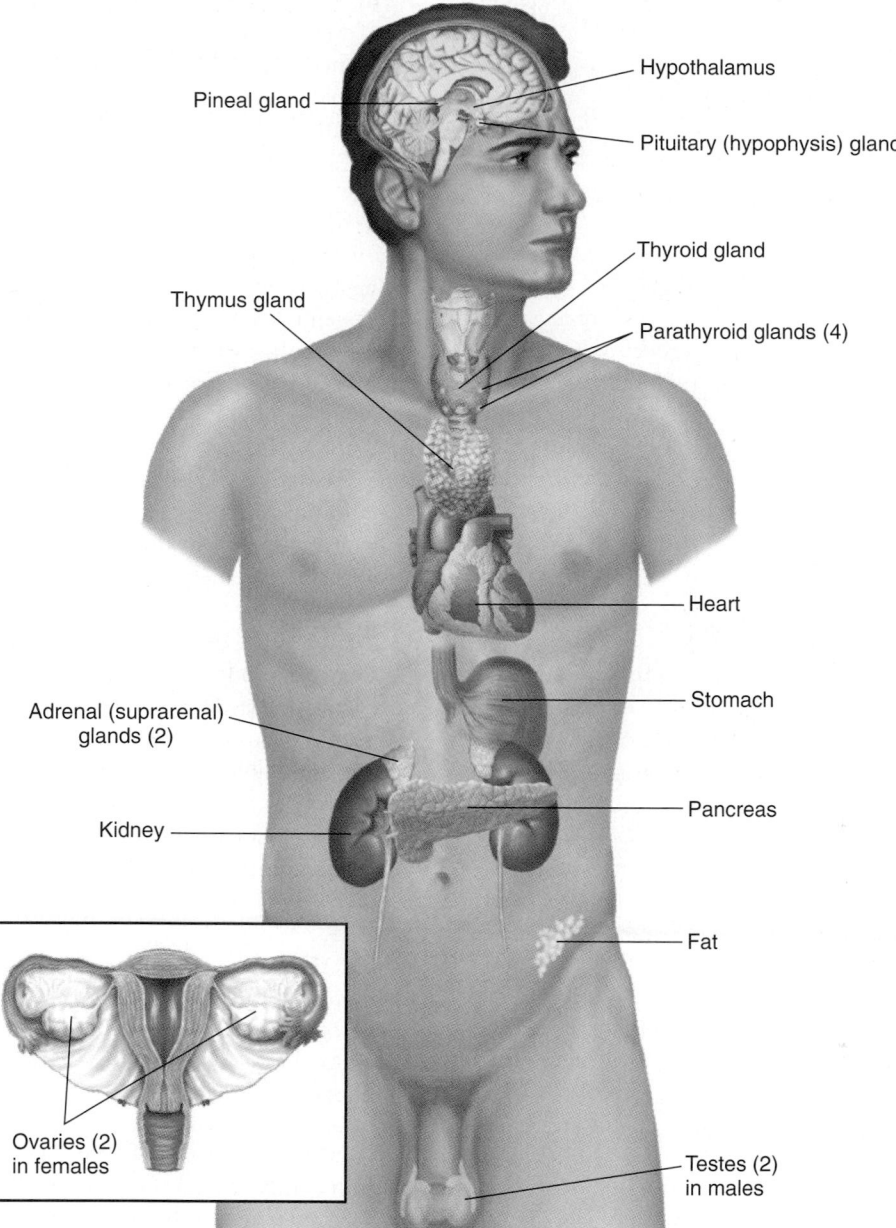

FIG 29-1 Endocrine system.

to raise levels of other substances when needed and the other acting to lower levels when needed. For example, the hormones calcitonin and parathyroid hormone function in an opposite, yet complementary, fashion to maintain an optimal level of calcium in the blood. Endocrine glands are also responsible for the development and maturation of individuals from children to adolescents and, eventually, to adults capable of reproduction. Endocrine glands also play a role in the body's ability to metabolize food and store energy.

Pineal Gland

The pineal gland produces the hormone melatonin, which influences the body's natural circadian rhythm, or sleep-wake cycle.

Pituitary Gland

The pituitary gland is commonly called the *master gland* because it controls all of the other glands in the body. Even so, it is actually controlled by the hypothalamus. The anterior and posterior lobes of the pituitary gland produce many different hormones.

Anterior Lobe

The anterior lobe is responsible for secreting six different hormones:

- **growth hormone** (GH), which promotes the growth of body structures, such as bones
- thyroid stimulating hormone (TSH), which affects the growth and functioning of the thyroid gland
- follicle-stimulating hormone (FSH) and luteinizing hormone (LH), which are referred to as *gonadotropins* because they act on the gonads—the ovaries in the female to produce an ovum and the testes in the male to produce sperm
- prolactin, which acts on mammary glands to produce milk
- adrenocorticotropic hormone (ACTH), which acts on the adrenal glands to secrete glucocorticoids, including cortisol.

Posterior Lobe

The posterior lobe secretes two hormones:

- oxytocin, which acts on the uterus to promote contractions during labor and delivery of a baby
- antidiuretic hormone (ADH), which acts on the kidneys to increase the absorption of water. (See Figure 29-2.)

Thyroid Gland

The thyroid gland produces the two thyroid hormones, triiodothyronine (T_3) and thyroxine (T_4), which are responsible for growth throughout childhood and regulation of body metabolism. For the thyroid gland to function properly, iodine must be obtained in the diet. The thyroid gland also secretes the hormone calcitonin, which is responsible for regulating calcium and phosphorus levels in the blood. The parathyroid glands on the surface of the thyroid gland secrete parathormone (PTH), which also helps regulate calcium and phosphorus levels in the blood.

Adrenal Glands

The adrenal glands secrete several hormones:

- Epinephrine, also known as *adrenalin,* is released during the "fight-or-flight" response to increase the body's ability to cope with stress or trauma. Epinephrine enables the body to respond to stressful situations by converting stored glucose into energy, dilating the pupils, opening the airways, and decreasing peristalsis.
- Aldosterone plays a role in regulating and maintaining the body's balance of water as well as sodium and other electrolytes.
- Cortisol is the body's natural steroid and works to decrease inflammation.
- Androgens are responsible for the secondary sexual characteristics in females and males.

Pancreas

In addition to its important role in the digestive process, the pancreas secretes insulin and glucagon. The beta cells of the pancreas secrete insulin after food is eaten to metabolize carbohydrates and break them down into glucose. Insulin stimulates cells to take up glucose from the blood so that it can be used for energy. As a result, blood glucose levels decrease. The alpha cells of the pancreas secrete glucagon to increase glucose levels in the blood by stimulating the liver to release stored glucose, called *glycogen.* Glycogen is also stored in the muscles and can convert into glucose during times of need, such as during exercise or prolonged periods without meals.

Thymus Gland

The main function of the thymus gland is to produce T-lymphocytes that are necessary for the immune system. It plays an active role in the immune system in childhood but shrinks and becomes less active as a person ages.

Ovaries

The ovaries produce an ovum during each menstrual cycle and secrete estrogen and progesterone. Estrogen helps develop sexual characteristics in the female, including breasts and pubic hair. It also plays a vital role in the menstrual cycle and is important in the prevention of osteoporosis in postmenopausal women. Progesterone is necessary to prepare and maintain the uterus for a fertilized ovum.

Testes

The testes secrete testosterone, which is responsible for the development of male characteristics during puberty, such as deepening of the voice, growth of facial and pubic hair, and increased muscle development. It is also necessary in the production of sperm.

Negative Feedback System

Within the endocrine system, glands and hormones work together to maintain homeostasis in the body by utilizing a **negative feedback system.** The system is considered *negative* because it works in opposites to maintain an optimal level of certain substances in the body. Each gland produces a hormone that serves to oppose another substance. The gland may increase or decrease production of the hormone to stimulate a corresponding decrease or increase of the other substance. Thus, this system works much like a thermostat functions, activating the production of heat in response to falling temperatures (a decrease in the normal level) or decreasing heat production in response to achieving the optimal heat level or a level that is too high.

Almost all endocrine glands operate in a negative feedback system. For example, the parathyroid glands secrete parathyroid hormone, which regulates blood calcium levels. A decrease in calcium levels in the blood (below the

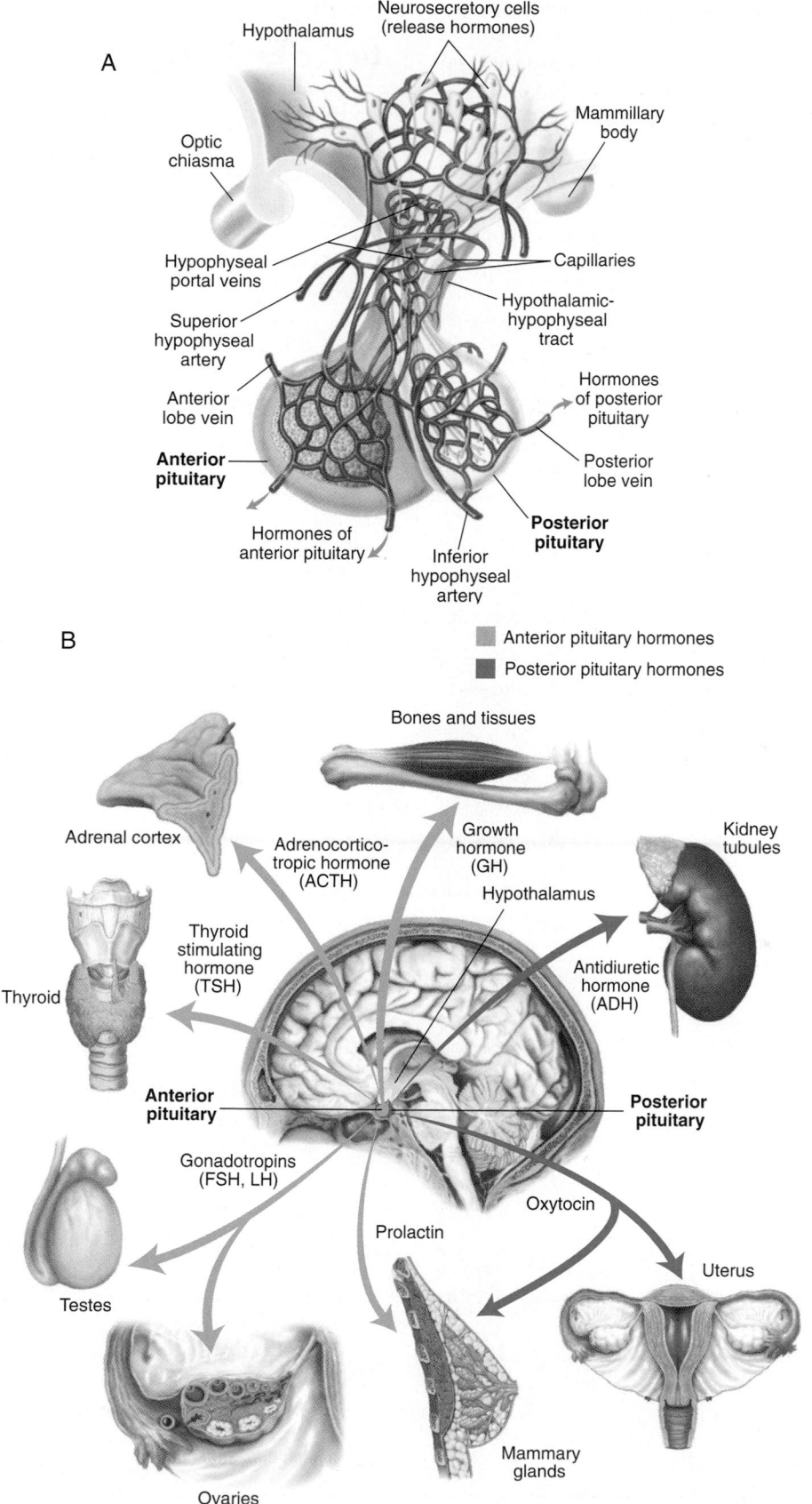

FIG 29-2 Pituitary gland. (A) Anterior and posteroir view. (B) Hormones and target glands.

normal level) stimulates the parathyroid glands to secrete more parathyroid hormone. Parathyroid hormone stimulates the bones to release more calcium. It also facilitates calcium uptake from the kidneys into the bloodstream. Thus, blood calcium levels increase back to the normal level. In addition, if blood calcium levels increase (above the normal level), the parathyroid glands decrease production of parathyroid hormone. Either way, the response of the parathyroid glands is a negative (opposite) response to the stimulus of a decrease or increase in blood calcium levels.

Medical Terminology Related to the Endocrine System

Endocrine disorders are common and affect every segment of the population at some time, leading them to seek medical care in acute and ambulatory care settings. To be effective in their role, medical assistants must become well versed in the language and vocabulary that pertain to the endocrine system. The following tables list common medical terminology related to the endocrine system.

Table 29.1 | **Word Elements**

This table contains combining forms, prefixes, and suffixes related to the endocrine system, along with examples of terms that use the word element, a pronunciation guide, and a definition for each.

Combining Form	Meaning	Example	Meaning
Combining Forms			
aden/o	gland	**adenopathy** (ăd-ĕ-NŎP-ă-thē)	Disease of a gland
adrenal/o	adrenal	**adrenalectomy** (ăd-rē-năl-ĔK-tō-mē)	Surgical removal of the adrenal gland
adren/o	gland	**adrenal** (ăd-RĒ-năl)	Pertaining to the adrenal gland
calc/o	calcium	**hypercalcemia** (hī-pĕr-kăl-SĒ-mē-ă)	Excessive calcium in the blood
gluc/o	sugar	**glucogenesis** (gloo-kō-JĔN-ĕ-sĭs)	Creating glucose
glyc/o	glucose	**glycosuria** (glī-kō-SŪ-rē-ă)	Sugar in the urine
hydr/o	water	**hydrolysis** (hī-DRŎL-ĭ-sĭs)	Destruction of water
oophor/o	ovary	**oophorectomy** (ō-ŏf-ō-RĔK-tō-mē)	Surgical removal of the ovaries
ovari/o		**ovarioptosis** (ō-vă-rē-ŏp-TŌ-sĭs)	Prolapse of the ovary
orch/o	testes	**orchopathy** (ōr-KŎP-ă-thē)	Disease of the testes
orchi/o		**orchiectomy** (ōr-kē-ĔK-tō-mē)	Surgical removal of the testes
orchid/o		**orchidopexy** (ōr-kĭ-dō-PĔK-sē)	Surgical fixation of the testes
test/o		**testomegaly** (tĕs-tō-MĔG-ă-lē)	Enlargement of the testes
pancreat/o	pancreas	**pancreatography** (păn-krē-ă-TŎG-ră-fē)	Process of recording the pancreas
parathyroid	parathyroid	**parathyroidectomy** (păr-ă-thī-royd-ĔK-tō-mē)	Surgical removal of the parathyroid gland
thym/o	thymus	**thymoma** (thī-MŌ-mă)	Tumor of the thymus
thyroid/o	thyroid	**thyroiditis** (thī-royd-Ī-tĭs)	Inflammation of the thyroid
toxic/o	toxin, poison	**toxicologist** (tŏks-ĭ-KŎL-ō-jĭst)	Specialist in the study of toxins
Prefixes			
an-	without, absence of	**anorchidism** (ăn-OR-kĭ-dĭzm)	Absence of testes
anti-	against	**antiglycemic** (an-tī-glī-SĒ-mĭk)	Pertaining to against sugar (refers to a medication that lowers the blood glucose level)

Table 29.1 | Word Elements—cont'd

Combining Form	Meaning	Example	Meaning
Prefixes			
eu-	good, normal	**euthyroid** (ū-THĬ-royd)	Good or normal thyroid
hyper-	excessive, above	**hyperglycemia** (hī-pĕr-glī-SĒ-mē-ă)	Excessive blood sugar
hypo-	below, beneath	**hypocalcemia** (hī-pō-kăl-SĒ-mē-ă)	Below (low) blood calcium
Suffixes			
-algia	pain	**orchialgia** (or-kē-ĂL-jē-ă)	Pain in the testes
-cele	hernia	**ovariocele** (ō-VĀ-rē-ō-sēl)	Herniation of the ovary
-ectomy	surgical removal	**orchiectomy** (or-kē-ĔK-tō-mē)	Surgical removal of a testicle
-ic	pertaining to	**pancreatic** (păn-krē-ĂT-ĭk)	Pertaining to the pancreas
-lith	stone	**pancreatolith** (păn-krē-ĂT-ō-lĭth)	Pancreatic stone
-logist	specialist in the study of	**toxicologist** (tŏks-ĭ-KŌL-ō-jĭst)	Specialist in the study of poisons
-megaly	enlargement	**thyroidomegaly** (thī-royd-ō-MĔG-ă-lē)	Enlargement of the thyroid
-oma	tumor	**thymoma** (thī-MŌ-mă)	Tumor of the thymus
-osis	abnormal	**toxicosis** (tŏks-ĭ-KŌ-sĭs)	Abnormal condition of toxin or poisoning
-otomy	incision	**thyroidotomy** (thī-royd-ŌT-ō-mē)	Incision into the thyroid
-pexy	surgical fixation	**orchidopexy** (OR-kĭd-ō524-sē)	Surgical fixation of a testicle
-rrhexis	rupture	**ovariorrhexis** (ō-vă-rē-ō-RĔK-sĭs)	Rupture of an ovary

Table 29.2 | Pathologic Terms

This table lists some of the most common pathologic terms related to the endocrine system, along with a pronunciation guide and a brief definition for each.

Term	Definition
acromegaly ăk-rō-MĔG-ă-lē	Rare disorder in which the pituitary gland becomes overactive after the individual has reached adulthood, secreting excessive amounts of human growth hormone (hGH), which affects the bones and tissues of the face and extremities causing them to become disproportionately enlarged compared with the rest of the body
Addison disease ĂD-ĭ-sŭn dĭ-ZĔZ	Disorder involving adrenal gland failure, which results in a chronic metabolic disorder that requires steroid hormone replacement therapy
congenital hypothyroidism kŏn-JĔN-ĭ-tăl hī-pō-THĬ-royd-ĭzm	Type of hypothyroidism present at birth that results in arrested physical and mental development; formerly called *cretinism*
Cushing syndrome KOOSH-ĭng SĬN-drōm	Rare disorder caused by prolonged, excessive secretion of glucocorticoids by the adrenal glands, resulting in altered fat distribution and muscle weakness; also called *hypercortisolism*
diabetic ketoacidosis dī-ă-BĔT-ĭk kē-tō-ăs-ĭ-DŌ-sĭs	Abnormal condition that occurs in uncontrolled diabetes and results in the accumulation of ketone bodies secondary to the oxidation of fats; also called *diabetic coma*

Table 29.2 | Pathologic Terms—cont'd

Term	Definition
diabetes insipidus dī-ă-BĒ-tēz ĭn-SĬ-pĭ-dŭs	Disorder caused by lack of vasopressin and marked by output of abnormally large amounts of dilute urine, which results in increased thirst and the need for a dramatic increase in fluid intake
diabetes mellitus dī-ă-BĒ-tēz mĕl-Ĭ-tĭs	Chronic metabolic disorder in which the pancreas secretes insufficient amounts of insulin or the body is insulin resistant
dystocia dĭs-TŌ-sē-ă	Difficult labor caused by a small pelvic outlet or a large baby, commonly related to macrosomia
eclampsia ē-KLĂMP-sē-ă	Condition caused by pregnancy-induced hypertension in which the woman experiences severe hypertension, convulsions, and coma
gestational diabetes jĕs-TĀ-shŭn-ăl dī-ă-BĒ-tēz	Diabetes that begins during pregnancy secondary to insulin resistance and altered glucose metabolism
gigantism JĬ-găn-tĭzm	Disorder in which the pituitary gland secretes excessive amounts of hGH during childhood, resulting in an abnormally large adult
goiter GOY-tĕr	Enlarged thyroid gland
Graves disease GRĀVZ dĭ-ZĒZ	Form of hyperthyroidism caused by an autoimmune response that may cause exophthalmos
hyperpituitarism hī-pĕr-pĭ-TŪ-ĭ-tăr-ĭsm	Disorder in which the pituitary gland secretes excessive amounts of hGH
hyperthyroidism hī-pĕr-THĬ-royd-ĭzm	Condition of having excessive levels of thyroid hormone in the body
hypopituitarism hī-pō-pĭ-TŪ-ĭ-tă-rĭzm	Condition that involves diminished secretion of pituitary hormones as a result of dysfunction of the anterior lobe of the pituitary gland; also called *underactive pituitary gland*
hypothyroidism hī-pō-THĬ-royd-ĭzm	Condition of having inadequate levels of thyroid hormone in the body
insulin shock ĬN-sŭ-lĭn SHŎK	Condition caused by too much insulin, in which the blood glucose level is too low; usually below 40 mg/dl; also called *hypoglycemia*
macrosomia măk-rō-SŌ-mĭ-ă	Condition of an abnormally large neonate caused when glucose crosses the placenta from a diabetic mother, causing the infant's pancreas to make more insulin and storage of excess glucose in the baby's body in the form of fat
myxedema mĭks-ē-DĒ-mă	Life-threatening condition of severe hypothyroidism, including such symptoms as fatigue; dry, brittle hair; cold intolerance; weight gain; constipation; mental apathy; physical sluggishness; muscle aches; and skin changes due to infiltration by mucopolysaccharides, which gives it a waxy, coarsened appearance with nonpitting edema
nephropathy nĕ-FRŎP-ă-thē	Disease of the kidneys commonly caused by poorly controlled diabetes
neuropathy nū-RŎP-ă-thē	Disease of the nerves with many causes, including diabetes
panhypopituitarism păn-hī-pō-pĭ-TŪ-ĭ-tăr-ĭzm	Condition resulting from diminished secretion of all hormones secreted by the anterior pituitary gland

Table 29.2 | Pathologic Terms—cont'd

Term	Definition
pituitary dwarfism pĭ-TŪ-ĭ-tār-ē DWĂR-fizm	Form of hypopituitarism that results from the deficiency of hGH during childhood, resulting in stunted growth
pregnancy-induced hypertension PRĔG-năn-sē ĭn-DOOST hī-pĕr-TĔN-shŭn	Complication of pregnancy marked by increasing blood pressure, urine protein, and edema
retinopathy rĕt-ĭn-ŌP-ă-thē	Disease of the retina, commonly caused by diabetes
thyrotoxicosis thī-rō-tŏks-ĭ-KŌ-sĭs	Sudden, life-threatening episode of worsening of hyperthyroidism symptoms
type 1 diabetes dī-ă-BĒ-tēz	Chronic metabolic disorder characterized by an absence of insulin production, resulting in hyperglycemia; also called *juvenile onset diabetes* and *insulin-dependent diabetes mellitus (IDDM)*
type 2 diabetes dī-ă-BĒ-tēz	Metabolic disorder caused by decreased insulin production and decreased sensitivity of the body to the insulin that is produced, which results in hyperglycemia; also called *adult onset diabetes* and *non-insulin-dependent diabetes mellitus (NIDDM)*

Table 29.3 | Abbreviations

In endocrinology, as in other areas of health care, abbreviations are commonly used. Abbreviations such as the ones listed here save time and effort in documentation and written communications.

Abbreviation	Definition	Abbreviation	Definition
ADH	antidiuretic hormone	GH	growth hormone
ACTH	adrenocorticotropic hormone	IDDM	insulin-dependent diabetes mellitus; also called *type 1 diabetes*
BG	blood glucose; also called *blood sugar*		
BS	blood sugar; also known as *blood glucose*	K	potassium
Ca	calcium	LH	leuteinizing hormone
CA	cancer	Na	sodium
DM	diabetes mellitus	NIDDM	non-insulin-dependent diabetes mellitus; also called *type 2 diabetes*
FBG	fasting blood glucose; also called *fasting blood sugar*	PTH	parathormone; also called *parathyroid hormone*
FBS	fasting blood sugar; also called *fasting blood glucose*	T_3	triiodothyronine
fsbs	finger stick blood sugar	T_4	thyroxine
FSH	follicle-stimulating hormone	TSH	thyroid-stimulating hormone

Common Endocrine System Diseases and Disorders

There are many disorders affecting the endocrine system. Some of the most common include type I and type II diabetes mellitus, gestational diabetes, hypothyroidism, and hyperthyroidism.

Types of Diabetes

Diabetes may occur in three forms, including type 1, type 2, and gestational diabetes.

Type I Diabetes

ICD-9-CM code: 250.90 (fifth digit modifier required)
Diabetes mellitus is a chronic metabolic disorder characterized by **hyperglycemia** (abnormally high blood glucose level). Type I diabetes is commonly referred to as *insulin-dependent diabetes mellitus* (IDDM) and is sometimes also called *juvenile onset diabetes*. However, people can develop type 1 diabetes into early adulthood. An estimated 0.3% to 0.4% of the population has type I diabetes. Onset usually begins in childhood. High-risk groups include Native Americans, African Americans, Pacific Islanders, and Mexican Americans. Incidence may be as high as 20% in these groups.

Type I diabetes is caused by autoimmune destruction of the beta cells in the pancreas, which are responsible for producing insulin, a hormone that makes glucose available to the cells of the body for energy. This lack of insulin causes blood glucose levels to rise out of control while the cells of the body are starved for glucose.

Onset of type I diabetes is commonly acute. A person usually experiences **polydipsia** (increased thirst), **polyphagia** (increased appetite), **polyuria** (increased urination), and weight loss. The physician commonly makes an initial diagnosis after the person is hospitalized with diabetic ketoacidosis (DKA), which occurs from continued, severe hyperglycemia. DKA commonly has a gradual onset, preceded by infection or illness. Symptoms include abdominal pain, cramps, nausea, vomiting, headache, irritability, tachycardia, hypotension, fruity breath odor, and flushed, dry skin. Many of these symptoms are related to the severe dehydration that occurs. The condition will deteriorate into a diabetic coma and can be fatal if not treated.

Diagnosis of diabetes mellitus is based on medical history, signs and symptoms, and results of diagnostic testing. Diagnostic tests include a random blood glucose level, fasting blood glucose level, glycosylated hemoglobin level, and a glucose tolerance test. Presence of the classic symptoms and two separate fasting blood glucose levels of more than 126 mg/dl or a random glucose level over 200 mg/dl confirms the diagnosis.

Treatment for type I diabetes includes dietary modification, regular exercise, careful foot and eye care, and supplemental insulin. Because gastric juices (stomach acid) will break down insulin, it must be injected, rather than administered orally. Therapy must be individualized. Some people do well with one or two injections per day of long-acting insulin, but others may require several injections per day of shorter-acting insulin. Another option is a continuous infusion of short-acting insulin using an insulin pump. This device is attached to a catheter that is inserted into the abdomen, releasing a steady amount of insulin into subcutaneous tissue. This manner of administration closely mimics the body's natural way of infusing insulin from the pancreas. The management goal is to maintain a balanced blood glucose level without great fluctuations.

In years past, the prognosis for those with type I diabetes was grim and few lived beyond childhood. As treatment options have improved, life expectancy has increased significantly. However, many patients still continue to suffer from devastating long-term consequences, including blindness caused by retinopathy, limb loss caused by peripheral neuropathy, peripheral vascular disease, and eventual kidney failure caused by nephropathy. Fortunately, diabetes is better understood today and treatment options are more effective. Risk of these disabling long-term complications, while still real, has lessened considerably. In fact, research indicates that those who develop good self-care habits and maintain tight control over blood glucose levels on a daily basis can now lead long, productive, reasonably healthy lives. (See *Diabetic self-care.*)

Type II Diabetes

ICD-9-CM code: 250.90 (fifh digit modifier required)
Type II diabetes is an endocrine disorder marked by decreased insulin production and decreased sensitivity to insulin. It is also referred to as *non-insulin-dependent diabetes mellitus* (NIDDM) and *adult-onset diabetes*. It usually appears after the age of 40 but can occur at any age. It is estimated that 6.6% of the population has type II diabetes. However, it is probable that many people remain undiagnosed because they are usually asymptomatic in the early years. Those at greatest risk are obese middle-aged people with sedentary lifestyles. The incidence of type II diabetes is rapidly growing in this country due to childhood and adult obesity.

Type II diabetes is caused by decreased insulin production and decreased sensitivity of the body to the insulin that is produced. As a result, individuals develop hyperglycemia. The cause of type II diabetes is linked to family history, obesity, and a sedentary lifestyle. In the early stages, most patients with type II diabetes are asymptomatic and may, therefore, be unaware that they have diabetes. As hyperglycemia worsens, signs and symptoms are similar to those for type I diabetes, including polydipsia, polyphagia, and polyuria. In addition, the patient may notice weight gain and delayed wound healing. Onset of symptoms with type II diabetes is more gradual and the development of DKA is less likely.

Diagnosis for type II diabetes is similar to type I and is based on medical history, signs and symptoms, and results of

Patient Education

Diabetic Self-Care

In teaching the diabetic patient proper self-care measures, the medical assistant should be sure to include the following information:

- Eat frequent, small, well-balanced meals throughout the day, rather than three large meals.
- Monitor intake of carbohydrates and calories, according to the plan recommended by your physician or dietitian.
- Engage in moderate, regular physical exercise according to the recommendations of your physician.
- Check your blood glucose levels routinely, according to the recommendations of your physician.
- There are many types of glucometers on the market; find and use the one that best fits your lifestyle and personal needs.
- Consider using a system of mapping your injection sites to prevent overuse of any one site.
- Consult with a dietitian to determine dietary guidelines that best meet your needs.
- Develop a habit of regularly inspecting and caring for your skin and feet.
- Keep a list of resources handy for when you have questions or concerns.

diagnostic testing. Diagnostic tests include a random blood glucose level, fasting blood glucose level, glycosylated hemoglobin level, and a glucose tolerance test. Presence of the classic symptoms and two separate fasting blood glucose levels of more than 126 mg/dl or a random glucose level over 200 mg/dl confirms the diagnosis.

Some patients with type II diabetes can control their blood glucose level with diet and regular exercise, whereas others may need to take oral hypoglycemic medications that stimulate the pancreas to produce insulin or make the body more responsive to insulin. (See *Hypoglycemia versus hyperglycemia,* page 530.) As a result, glucose becomes available to the cells of the body and blood glucose level normalizes. In some patients, the pancreas eventually stops producing insulin. When this happens, they must begin injecting insulin to manage glucose levels. (Regardless of whether insulin production ceases altogether, the diabetes type remains type II; it does not change to type I.)

Diabetes is a chronic disease for which there is no identified cure. However, with proper diagnosis and management most diabetics can lead long, healthy lives. The key is daily management that prevents the destructive changes that occur gradually over time. Complications include retinopathy leading to blindness, nephropathy leading to kidney failure, and neuropathy and peripheral vascular disease, leading to delayed wound healing, tissue necrosis, and limb loss. (See *Foot and skin care,* page 531.) Diabetics are also at increased risk for heart disease, which puts them at risk for heart attack.

Gestational Diabetes
ICD-9-CM code: 648.80

Gestational diabetes is diabetes that begins during pregnancy due to insulin resistance and altered glucose metabolism. Gestational diabetes affects approximately 4% of all pregnant women, or around 135,000 American women each year. Those at greatest risk include women over age 25, those with a history of gestational diabetes during a previous pregnancy, those with a family history of diabetes, and those who are overweight at the start of pregnancy. Additional risk factors include African American, Native American, or Hispanic ethnicity and having had a previous stillbirth or a baby weighing more than 9 lb at birth.

The cause of gestational diabetes is not fully understood. It is known that placental hormones, which help the baby grow, cause insulin resistance in the mother's body. Subsequently, the mother develops hyperglycemia as glucose levels rise in her blood. Gestational diabetes usually subsides after delivery. However, such women have a 50% chance of developing type II diabetes later in life.

Gestational diabetes usually doesn't begin until the 24th to 28th week of pregnancy (5th or 6th month) and most women are asymptomatic. Those who do experience symptoms usually exhibit polydipsia, polyphagia, and polyuria.

Screening for gestational diabetes is just one of the many reasons women should seek health care before and during pregnancy. Measuring blood glucose level and screening for diabetes is part of routine perinatal care. Diagnosis of diabetes is similar to other types of diabetes. Many physicians recommend a glucose challenge test between 24 and 28 weeks' gestation. Management of gestational diabetes is similar to that for other forms of diabetes and includes careful attention to diet; regular, moderate exercise; monitoring glucose levels; and supplemental insulin as needed.

With careful management, the woman can experience a normal, healthy pregnancy and delivery. However, there are potential complications that can arise, especially when maternal hyperglycemia is poorly controlled. The most life-threatening of these is pregnancy-induced hypertension (PIH), which can cause eclampsia, in which the woman experiences severe hypertension, convulsions, and coma. Another complication is the need for a caesarean section (c-section) delivery due to macrosomia, which is an abnormally large baby at birth. Macrosomia is caused by the transfer of maternal glucose across the placenta, giving the baby hyperglycemia. In response, the baby's pancreas makes more insulin, which then causes the excess glucose to be stored in

Hypoglycemia versus hyperglycemia

This table lists the laboratory values for hypoglycemia and hyperglycemia, along with the onset, most common signs and symptoms, cause, and most common treatment for each.

	Onset	Signs and Symptoms	Cause	Treatment
Hypoglycemia (glucose < 40 mg/dl)	Acute	• Fatigue, tremor • Hunger • Restlessness, dizziness, confusion • Irritability, combativeness • Heart palpitations • Moist, clammy skin • Eventual loss of consciousness	• Too much insulin • Not enough food • Excessive exercise • Vomiting or diarrhea	• *Conscious patient with gag reflex*—oral administration of some form of simple sugar, such as glucose tablets, orange juice, non-diet soda, and hard candy • *Unconscious patient*—subcutaneous, IV, or IM administration of glucagon followed by a snack or meal of complex carbohydrates and protein after blood glucose rises
Hyperglycemia (glucose > 120 mg/dl)	Gradual	• Fruity breath odor • Deep, rapid respirations • Polydipsia, polyphagia, polyuria, glucosuria • Weight loss • Dry, flushed skin • Lethargy, confusion, eventual coma	• Not enough insulin or missed insulin doses • Too much food • Lack of activity • Stress, illness, infection	• Insulin administration after checking blood glucose level • Administration of an oral hypoglycemic agent per physician recommendation • Diet control, weight loss, and exercise combined with insulin or oral hypoglycemic agents

the baby's body in the form of fat. As a result, the baby may suffer shoulder dystocia (shoulder injury) and severe hypoglycemia at birth. This baby also has a higher risk for respiratory problems, jaundice, and stillbirth. In addition, such babies are at risk for future obesity and the development of type II diabetes.

Thyroid Disorders
Hypothyroidism
ICD-9-CM code: 243 (congenital hypothyroidism), 244.9 (myxedema)

Hypothyroidism is the condition of having inadequate levels of thyroid hormone in the body. There are several types of hypothyroidism, which are named according to their cause. Congenital hypothyroidism, formerly called *cretinism*, is a congenital condition of thyroid hormone deficiency characterized by arrested physical and mental development. The term *cretin*, originally used to describe the disorder in the 18th century, was used widely in the 19th and 20th centuries.

However, the meaning of the term has more recently been deemed derogatory and is, therefore, not commonly used in medicine today. Myxedema is a severe form of hypothyroidism that develops in the older child or adult. The incidence of congenital hypothyroidism is rare in industrialized countries, due to early diagnosis and treatment of newborns. However, in many countries where diets are commonly iodine-deficient, the problem is much more prevalent.

Congenital hypothyroidism results from abnormal function of the fetal thyroid gland. In many cases, an underlying cause of hypothyroidism is dietary deficiency of iodine, an essential trace element required for synthesis of thyroid hormones. Other causes of hypothyroidism include surgical removal of the thyroid gland and some medications.

General hypothyroidism causes diminished basal metabolism. Signs and symptoms of myxedema, a term used for the collective symptoms of severe hypothyroidism, include fatigue; dry, brittle hair; cold intolerance; weight gain; constipation; mental apathy; physical sluggishness; and muscle

Patient Education

Foot and Skin Care

Type II diabetes puts a patient at increased risk for limb amputation from nonhealing wounds and ulcers. Thus, the medical assistant should provide to the patient with diabetes comprehensive patient education on foot and skin care, including:

• Inspect your skin daily, paying special attention to your feet. Use a mirror to inspect the soles of your feet.

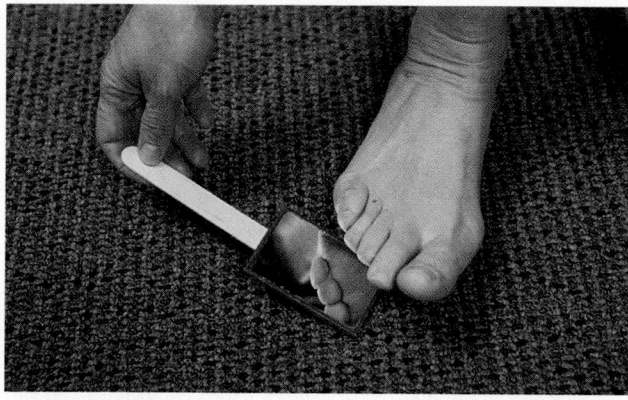

Inspection using a hand mirror

• Wash your feet daily with a mild soap and warm (not hot) water; dry thoroughly.

• Apply lotion to keep skin soft and supple.

• Trim toenails carefully, clipping straight across to avoid ingrown nails. If doing so is too difficult, have the physician trim your toenails.

• Always wear well-fitting shoes, even in the house. Break in new shoes gradually to avoid blisters.

• Never go barefoot.

• Inspect your shoes before putting them on to make sure there is nothing inside of them.

• Wear house slippers and keep a night light on to prevent foot injury when getting up during the night.

• Report redness, sores, or breaks in the skin to your physician as soon as possible.

---

aches. The character of the skin changes due to infiltration by mucopolysaccharides, giving it a waxy or coarsened appearance with nonpitting edema. Left untreated, hypothermia, coma, and death may result. Another common symptom of hypothyroidism is enlargement of the thyroid gland, sometimes called **goiter**. Congenital hypothyroidism causes poor growth and results in a very short adult. In addition, bone growth and maturation are impeded, sexual development is severely delayed, and infertility is common. (See Figure 29-3.)

Thyroid function tests detect hypothyroidism long before symptoms become apparent. A high plasma TSH and a low free T_4 index confirm the diagnosis. Treatment of most forms of hypothyroidism consists of lifelong administration of synthetic thyroid hormones. The addition of iodine to packaged table salt in many countries has alleviated the incidence of diet-related hypothyroidism, thereby reducing the incidence of goiter.

The prognosis for those with hypothyroidism is generally good, depending on how early the diagnosis is made and treatment started. In most cases, symptoms will improve or resolve.

Hyperthyroidism

ICD-9-CM code: 242.0

Hyperthyroidism is a condition of excessive levels of thyroid hormone in the body. The most common form of hyperthyroidism is called *Graves disease.* The thyroid gland produces thyroid hormones that regulate metabolism. When production of thyroid hormones increases, the body's metabolism increases. Hyperthyroidism is 10 times more common in women than in men and is more common after the age of 15. Incidence is about one per 1000 women. About 80% of patients may develop goiter.

There are several causes of hyperthyroidism, including nodular goiter, toxic adenomas, hyperemesis gravidarum (extreme nausea and vomiting during pregnancy), excessive thyroid replacement, excessive iodine intake, or pituitary adenoma. However, the most common cause is Graves disease, which is an autoimmune disorder.

Signs and symptoms of hyperthyroidism are related to stimulation of the sympathetic nervous system and increased circulating thyroxine, both of which stimulate metabolism. Signs and symptoms include tachycardia, palpitations, hypertension, tremor, anxiety, nervousness, insomnia, hyperreflexia, depression, weight loss in spite of increased food intake, heat intolerance, hair thinning, and **exophthalmos** (protruding eyeballs). (See Figure 29-4.) **Hypertrophy** (excessive growth) of the thyroid gland may also cause goiter. Thyrotoxicosis is an episode of sudden worsening of symptoms and may be life-threatening.

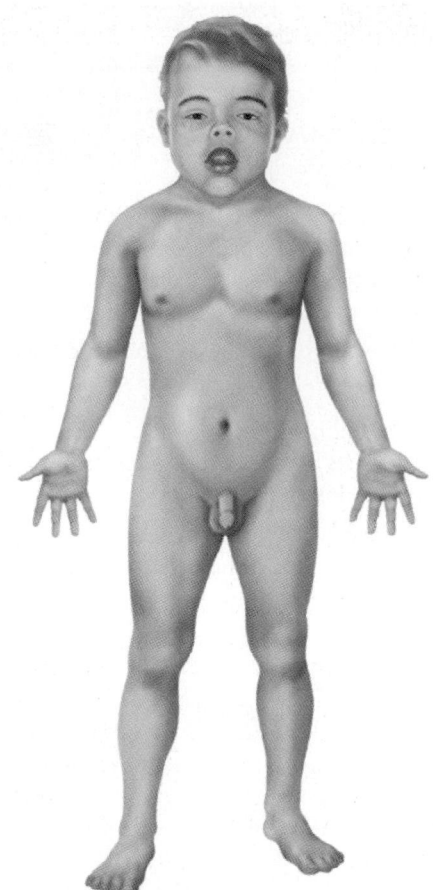

FIG 29-3 Congenital hypothyroidism.

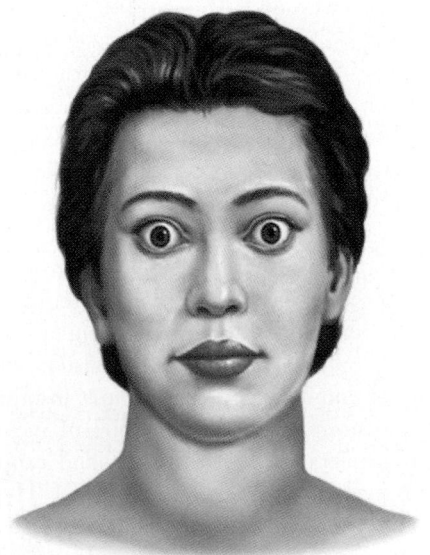

FIG 29-4 Exophthalmos (Graves disease).

Medical examination and blood tests easily detect thyroid disorders; however, early detection is vital for successful treatment. Blood tests may show a decreased TSH level and increased T_3 and T_4 levels.

Treatment of hyperthyroidism consists of medications to suppress thyroid function and surgical removal of part or all of the thyroid gland. Prevention as well as early detection and treatment are the keys to minimizing the impact of this disorder. Therefore, annual physical examinations for adults and scheduled well-baby visits for infants and children are encouraged. Prognosis for those with hyperthyroidism is generally good but is somewhat variable, depending on the underlying cause. In most cases, a balanced level of thyroid hormones can be restored.

Endocrinology Procedures

Endocrinology is a medical specialty that focuses on the study and treatment of diseases and disorders of the endocrine system. A physician who specializes in this area of medicine is an **endocrinologist.** Many patients who have endocrine disorders initially see internal medicine or family practice physicians, who then refer them to an endocrinologist. Internal medicine physicians may also be involved in follow-up care.

Assisting with Examination

To reach an accurate diagnosis, the endocrinologist must obtain a medical history, including a description of symptoms. In an examination, the medical assistant must prepare the patient by checking vital signs and obtaining a health history, which should include data regarding allergies, signs and symptoms, and medications. She should then assist the patient as needed with undressing and positioning. Patients should undress and put on the examination gown with the opening in the front. The medical assistant provides patient privacy and assists the physician as needed with the examination and performs ordered diagnostic tests. She must also assist the endocrinologist as needed with any procedures.

Patients with diabetes are commonly seen by the endocrinologist as well as physicians in nearly every other specialty area. For this reason, medical assistants help provide care for diabetic patients, regardless of where they work. Such patients commonly need ongoing education to learn about their disorder and good self-care practices. A common topic of discussion is skin and foot care because diabetes usually results in delayed wound healing and is a major reason for surgical amputation. With this in mind, medical assistants must be prepared to teach their patients how to protect and care for their skin, especially their feet. (See *Procedure 29-1: Teaching a patient to provide foot care.*)

Teaching a patient to provide foot care

Task
Teach a patient to perform daily foot care.

Conditions
- Warm water
- Mild soap
- Three or more towels
- Soft wash cloth
- Moisturizing lotion
- Hand mirror
- Emery board
- Clean, dry socks
- Shoes
- Foot rest
- Examination gloves
- Wash basins (2)
- Patient's medical record

Standards
In the time specified and within the scoring parameters determined by the instructor, the student will successfully teach the patient to perform daily foot care.

Performance Standards
1. Introduce yourself and explain the purpose of the teaching session and the importance of routine foot care, including these points:
   a. Daily skin care helps the diabetic patient maintain healthy, intact skin.
   b. Daily care enables the patient to detect skin problems early so that the physician can initiate timely intervention.
   c. Maintaining healthy skin and detecting problems early help the diabetic patient prevent limb loss caused by nonhealing wounds and infections.
2. Instruct the patient to wash his hands with lukewarm water and soap, rinse them in lukewarm water, and dry them thoroughly. Patients with peripheral neuropathy may have difficulty sensing water temperature so a cooler temperature is safest. Explain that hand washing helps prevent cross-contamination of microorganisms from the hands to the feet.
3. Instruct the patient to sit in a chair and remove his shoes and socks.
4. Wash or sanitize your hands to ensure infection control and assemble supplies, including:
   a. placing a towel or absorbent pad on the floor beneath the patient's feet (other supplies may rest on this towel)

   b. placing both basins near the patient's feet (one half full of lukewarm water with a small amount of soap added and one half full of clean rinse water)
   c. placing a footrest near the patient's feet and a towel or absorbent pad on top of it.
5. Instruct the patient to place his left foot in the basin of soapy water and let it soak for a minute or two. Explain that this allows soil particles to soften and loosen up.
6. Put on examination gloves. Use a clean, soft washcloth to wash the patient's foot, gently scrubbing all surfaces, including between the toes. Be extra gentle with any areas that are reddened, tender, or have broken skin to avoid causing further injury.
7. Guide the patient's foot from the basin of soapy water to the basin of rinse water. Gently rub all surfaces. Explain to the patient that all of the soap must be removed.
8. Place the patient's clean foot on the padded footrest and gently pat all surfaces dry, which is less likely to cause injury than rubbing. Examine the skin in all areas as you do so. Explain that dry skin is less likely to break down or harbor microorganisms and clean skin is easier to examine.
9. Hold the hand mirror below the sole of the patient's foot and ask him to examine his foot. Explain the importance of seeing every surface of his foot. Tell the patient to inspect all surfaces of the foot, including the toes, toenails, and between the toes. Explain that diabetic patients with peripheral neuropathy may have injuries they do not feel. Examination at this point also allows the foot to air-dry completely before the next step.
10. Inspect the patient's toenails for length and jagged edges. Using the emery board, file the toenails as needed to shorten and smooth the ends. (Be sure not to shorten them too much, however.) Inform the physician if the patient has extremely thick, hypertrophied toenails because a consultation with a podiatrist may be indicated. Explain that excessively long or jagged nails could result in injury from pressure or tearing. Instruct the patient to report any areas of redness, broken skin, or ulcerations to the physician as soon as possible.
11. Apply a small amount of moisturizing lotion to the patient's clean foot but not between the toes. Explain that moisturized skin is less likely to crack but that the area between the toes tends to harbor moisture and could become a breeding ground for microorganisms.

Continued

PROCEDURE 29-1—cont'd

12. Remove the examination gloves. Examine the patient's clean socks for areas of wear or hidden seams. Explain that such areas could place excessive pressure on the patient's foot.
13. Examine the patient's left shoe, including these steps:
    a. Examine the inside for any foreign objects or wear or wrinkles in the shoe lining. Explain that the inside of the shoe should be examined each time it is put on because pressure ulcers can develop quickly from pressure caused by foreign objects or wrinkles.
    b. Examine the sole of the shoe. Explain that a flat, nonskid surface provides a good base of support and is less likely to slip when walking.
    c. Explain that shoes should be worn at all times, even in the house, to prevent foot injury from stubbing the toes or stepping on objects.
    d. Explain that new shoes must be broken in slowly and carefully to prevent foot injury, blisters, or other areas of pressure or friction.

    e. Explain that slippers with nonskid soles should be kept by the bed and worn when getting up during the night and a nightlight should be kept on to prevent foot injury from stubbing the toes or stepping on objects.
14. Assist the patient as needed in putting his left sock and shoe on.
15. Instruct the patient to repeat steps 6 to 15 with his other foot, providing cueing as needed. Return demonstration provides opportunity to reinforce teaching and allows the medical assistant to verify the patient's understanding and ability to perform foot care.
16. Wash your hands and document the procedure in the patient's medical record to ensure a complete, accurate medical record.

Date	
05/11/08; 10:50 a.m.	*Pt education regarding foot care completed. Pt performed return demonstration satisfactorily. ————S. Gonzales, CMA*

Endocrine System Tests

Diagnostic tests commonly completed or ordered in the endocrinologist's office include fasting blood glucose, glucose tolerance test, glycosylated hemoglobin, urine glucose test, glucometer testing, thyroid test, thyroid scan, and radioactive iodine uptake.

Fasting Blood Glucose

The **fasting** blood glucose (FBG) test, also called a *fasting blood sugar (FBS) test*, measures glucose levels in the blood when the patient has not eaten or drunk anything for approximately 8 to 12 hours before the test. (See *Scheduling the fasting patient.*) This test can use a sample of **venous** blood, taken from a vein using a needle (venipuncture), or **peripheral** blood, taken from a finger using a lancet. Normal blood glucose levels average 70 to 110mg/dl. The medical assistant can measure blood glucose levels from a nonfasting patient as well. However, she must record how long it has been since the patient last ate. For example, if the patient ate a snack 2 hours before the test, the medical assistant should record it as "2 hours pp," which indicates that she took the sample 2 hours *postprandial,* or after eating.

Glucose Tolerance Test

The physician orders a glucose tolerance test (GTT) when she wants to evaluate how the body breaks down a concentrated amount of glucose over a period of time, such as 2, 3, or 5 hours. This test is useful for diagnosing various types of

 Front office–Back office connection

Scheduling the Fasting Patient

When scheduling a patient for laboratory tests that require a period of fasting, the administrative medical assistant should remember that some patients are vulnerable to hypoglycemia. Therefore, she should consult carefully with the patient and physician to determine the best appointment time. She should also consult with the physician about whether the patient is to take regularly scheduled medications that morning, including insulin or antidiabetic agents. In any case, she must make sure the patient understands the information regarding pretest measures as well as the reason for the test and the necessary fast. In addition, the medical assistant should remind the patient to bring a snack to eat as soon as the test is complete.

diabetes, including gestational diabetes. The patient must fast for a specified period of time before providing a blood specimen. For an oral GTT, the medical assistant must instruct the patient to drink 8 oz of a concentrated glucose solution. Glucose may also be administered IV. The medical assistant must then collect a second specimen 1/2 hour after the patient takes the glucose, and then again at 1 hour,

2 hours, 3 hours, and so on, depending on the length of the test. Typically, the medical assistant will ask the patient to collect a urine sample with each blood sample to evaluate glucose in the urine. Because patients with diabetes are unable to metabolize glucose at a normal rate, blood tests will show elevated glucose levels and urine test results may show the presence of glucose. A glucose level greater than 200 mg/dl 2 hours after a glucose challenge of 75 mg indicates a possible diagnosis of diabetes.

Glycosylated Hemoglobin

The glycosylated hemoglobin test (Hgb A1C) represents an average of blood glucose levels in the blood over the previous 4 months. This test is a good indicator of long-term control of blood glucose levels. Some glucose molecules in the blood bind to hemoglobin, which is attached to red blood cells (RBCs). The more glucose available in the blood, the more glycosylated hemoglobin is formed. The glucose remains bound to the RBCs for their normal life span, which is approximately 120 days (4 months). Therefore, this test represents blood glucose levels over 4 months. Fasting prior to this test is not necessary. The normal Hgb A1C laboratory value is 4% to 6%.

Urine Glucose Test

The urine glucose test detects glucose in a urine sample. Typically, glucose should not be present in urine. **Glucosuria** (presence of glucose in urine) indicates that the body is unable to utilize serum glucose for energy. As serum glucose levels rise to an abnormally high level, the kidneys excrete excess glucose in the urine. Therefore, glucosuria is an indirect indicator of hyperglycemia. Glucose in the urine can be detected from a random urine sample by using the dipstick method of testing.

Glucometer Testing

Blood glucose levels can be tested in the physician's office but patients can also check their own blood glucose by themselves at home, school, or work using a **glucometer.** This instrument measures the concentration of glucose in the blood, usually testing peripheral blood. Diabetic patients test their blood glucose level several times throughout the day. Although testing is slightly different for each patient, most test their glucose levels in the morning when they are fasting, before meals, and again in the evening before bedtime. (See Figure 29-5.)

Thyroid Tests

Thyroid tests evaluate hormones related to thyroid function by blood specimen analysis. Such hormones include triiodothyronine (T_3), thyroxine (T_4), thyroid stimulating hormone (TSH), and calcitonin. The patient should not need to fast but

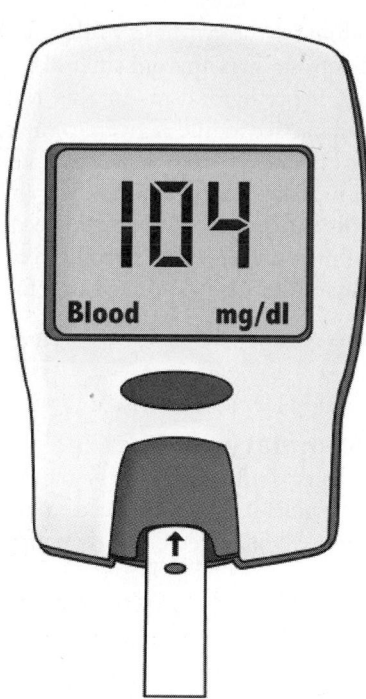

FIG 29-5 Glucometer.

should let the laboratory technician know if she is taking any thyroid medications. Normal values for a T_3 uptake test are 32% to 48.4%. Normal values for a T_4 test are 6.1 to 12.2 µg/dl. Normal values for TSH are 0.34 to 5.6 micro-international units/ml and a normal calcitonin value is less than 14 pg/ml for females and less than 19 pg/ml for males.

Thyroid Scan

A thyroid scan is a nuclear medicine study done to evaluate thyroid size, shape, position, and function. It is useful for evaluating thyroid nodules, goiter thyroiditis, or thyroid cancer. It is also helpful in differentiating masses in the neck, at the base of the tongue, and in the mediastinum. The patient must drink an oral dose of radioactive iodine or receive an IV dose of technetium. Uptake of these media by the thyroid gland and surrounding tissue reveals problems. Areas of increased uptake, called *hot spots,* are due to hyperfunctioning thyroid nodules and are not likely to be malignant. Areas of decreased uptake, or *cold spots,* are caused by hypofunctioning nodules, which are more likely to be malignant. However, determining for sure whether tissue is malignant requires tissue biopsy.

Radioactive Iodine Uptake

Radioactive iodine uptake (RAIU) is a nuclear medicine study used to evaluate thyroid function. It directly measures the ability of the thyroid gland to concentrate and retain circulating iodine for the synthesis of thyroid hormone. It is useful for diagnosing hypothyroidism and even more useful for diagnosing hyperthyroidism. In this test, a very small dose of oral radioactive iodine is given to the patient at specified intervals of time. Uptake values are measured in conjunction with measurements of circulating thyroid hormone levels to differentiate primary from secondary thyroid disease. Serial measurements are helpful in long-term management of thyroid disease and its treatment.

Chapter Summary

- Major structures of the endocrine system include the pituitary gland, pineal gland, thyroid gland, parathyroid glands, thymus gland, adrenal glands, pancreas, and ovaries and testes.
- Functions of the endocrine system include secretion of hormones that act on other glands to initiate specific processes in the body that contribute to growth and development and maintaining homeostasis.
- Major hormones of the endocrine system include growth hormone, prolactin, antidiuretic hormone, follicle-stimulating hormone, luteinizing hormone, estrogen, progesterone, testosterone, aldosterone, adrenalin, cortisol, insulin, glucagon, oxytocin, melatonin
- Common diseases of the endocrine system include diabetes mellitus (type I and type II), gestational diabetes, hypothyroidism, and hyperthyroidism.
- Common tests for endocrine system diseases and disorders are glucose testing (fasting and glucose tolerance) using blood and urine, glycosylated hemoglobin, glucometer testing, thyroid tests, thyroid scan, and radioactive iodine uptake.

Team Work Exercises

1. Divide into teams of three to five students. Each team must create an informational pamphlet for patients on one of the following topics (as assigned by the instructor). Team members must research appropriate subjects to gather the information. Consider contacting community resources as well as using online resources. Be sure to list resources on the pamphlet so that patients can obtain further information as needed. The topics include:

   a. **travel guidelines for patients with type I diabetes** (Consider out-of-country travel, need for supplies, packing and storage issues, and so on.)

   b. **exercise guidelines for patients with type I diabetes** (Include type of exercises recommended, diet guidelines, insulin administration times and sites, and so on.)

   c. **sick-day guidelines for patients with diabetes to follow when they are ill** (Include glucose testing, insulin administration, diet, fluids, when to call the physician, and so on.)

   d. **supplies for the patient with diabetes** (Include syringes, lancets, glucometers, oral agents, and so forth as well as typical pricing, where they might be obtained, and so forth.)

   e. **general dietary guidelines for patients with diabetes** (Consider recommended systems, including exchange plans, carbohydrate counting, and tracking the glycemic index. Explain the systems and describe how the individual might plan meals for a typical day. Also discuss tips for shopping and reading labels.)

2. Divide into teams of three to five students. Each team must create a skit in which the members demonstrate (by acting or role playing) the role and effect of the hormones listed below (as assigned by the instructor).

   a. insulin, glucagon, and glycogen
   b. calcium and parathyroid hormone
   c. aldosterone and antidiuretic hormone
   d. adrenocorticotropic hormone and cortisol
   e. thyroid stimulating hormone, thyroxine (T_4), and triiodothyronine (T_3)

Case Studies

1. Mrs. Popp makes an appointment for her 7-year-old daughter Rachel to see the doctor. Mrs. Popp states that Rachel is drinking much more water than usual and is also urinating more. She is wondering if the increased urination is normal due to the fact that Rachel is drinking so much more. How should the medical assistant respond?

2. Paul is a 40-year-old male who has had diabetes for the past 15 years. He currently follows a healthy diet and injects insulin as needed to control his blood glucose level. He notices that the physician orders an Hgb A1C test instead of his usual blood glucose level test and is wondering why there is a change in blood tests. What information should the medical assistant give Paul regarding his blood test?

Resources

- The Endocrine Society: *www.endo-society.org*
- Information on and support for Cushing syndrome: *www.CSRF.net*
- Information on diabetes: *www.diabetes.org*
- Information on pituitary disorders: *www.pituitary.org*
- Society for Endocrinology: *www.endocrinology.org*

Gastroenterology

Structures and Functions of the Gastrointestinal System

The gastrointestinal (GI) system consists of the alimentary canal and accessory organs of digestion. Together, these structures provide nutrients to all cells of the body.

Structures of the GI System

The structures of the GI system include the alimentary canal and the accessory organs of digestion.

Alimentary Canal

The **alimentary canal**, also known as the *digestive tract* or *gastrointestinal tract,* is the route of digestion that includes all structures from the mouth to the anus, excluding the accessory organs of digestion. At the beginning of the alimentary canal is the mouth, including the tongue, teeth, and gums. The **uvula** is a small, finger-shaped portion of soft tissue that hangs from the upper part of the mouth at the back. Continuous with the mouth is the pharynx, which is shaped like a funnel. The pharynx begins at the back of the mouth and extends to the esophagus, a long, tubelike structure that connects the mouth to the stomach, passing through the diaphragm. At the beginning of the esophagus is a small, cartilaginous flap called the **epiglottis**, which hangs between the esophagus and the trachea. At the lower end of the esophagus is a muscular opening called the *lower esophageal sphincter* (LES), also called the **cardiac sphincter** because of its location near the heart. The LES separates the esophagus from the stomach.

The abdominal cavity holds the stomach, small intestine, large intestine, rectum, and anus. This cavity is lined with a membrane called the *peritoneum.* The stomach, which is lined with **rugae**, is composed of three major areas: the fundus (upper portion), body (middle portion), and pylorus (lower portion). The pyloric sphincter, another circular muscle, lies between the lowest portion of the stomach and the small intestine.

The small intestine is a coiled tube that measures about 20 ft and consists of the duodenum (upper portion), jejunum (middle portion), and ileum (end portion). The small intestine is lined with **villi**, which are tiny, fingerlike projections surrounded by capillaries and lymph vessels. The ileocecal valve connects the ileum with the large intestine at the cecum. The large intestine includes the cecum and the colon. The cecum is a small pouch at the beginning of the large intestine. The appendix is a small, tubelike appendage that hangs from the cecum in the right lower quadrant (RLQ) of the abdomen. The cecum connects to the colon, which consists of four portions: ascending colon, transverse colon, descending colon, and sigmoid colon. The last part of the alimentary canal, the rectum, begins at the sigmoid colon and ends at the anus. (See Figure 30-1.)

Pancreas

The long, somewhat flat pancreas lies posterior and inferior to the stomach. Within the pancreas lie specialized cells called the *islets of Langerhans*. There are two types of these cells: alpha and beta cells. The pancreas also contains the pancreatic duct, which connects with the hepatic duct at the duodenum of the large intestine.

Functions of the GI System

The organs of the GI system break down food into usable nutrients through mechanical and chemical processes that break the food down into smaller pieces so the body can absorb and utilize the nutrients for all cells.

The major products of digestion are proteins, fats, vitamins, minerals, water, and glucose. Digestive enzymes called *proteases* and *lipases* break down proteins and fats. As food is digested, vitamins and minerals move into the bloodstream, which delivers water-soluble vitamins to the tissues and fat-soluble vitamins to the liver and muscle tissue for storage. Insulin is essential for enabling glucose to leave the bloodstream and enter the tissues. These products of digestion are necessary for many biochemical reactions in cells of all parts of the body.

The GI system also performs **excretion**, the process of eliminating bulk waste (feces) from the anus. These processes of digestion and excretion are carried out by the organs of the alimentary canal and the accessory organs of digestion.

Alimentary Canal

Digestion begins in the mouth as teeth mechanically break down food into smaller pieces by **mastication** (chewing). As food is chewed, or masticated, the salivary glands of the mouth secrete saliva to mix with the food. **Saliva** moistens food and contains ptyalin, a chemical that starts to break down starches. The tongue helps to form the food into a **bolus**, which is a rounded mass of masticated food that is ready for **deglutition** (swallowing). The tongue helps distinguish the taste of food. Taste buds on the surface of the tongue contain 50 to 100 taste cells, which perceive tastes of sweet, sour, salty, bitter, and umami (glutamate flavor, such as monosodium glutamate [MSG]). Each taste bud has a pore that opens to the surface of the tongue so that molecules and ions taken into the mouth can reach the taste cells. Taste cells are modified epithelial cells with microvilli that extend into the gustatory pore where the molecules and ions enter the cell. The perception of various tastes are produced by specialized nerve fibers that enter the taste cell and occupy the central portion of the cell. While it was once thought that taste buds on specific areas of the tongue sense one of the five main tastes, new research shows that the five flavors can be perceived by taste cells on all areas of the tongue. The taste cells have a life span of approximately 12 days and regenerate new cells from the base of the bud. (See Figure 30-2.)

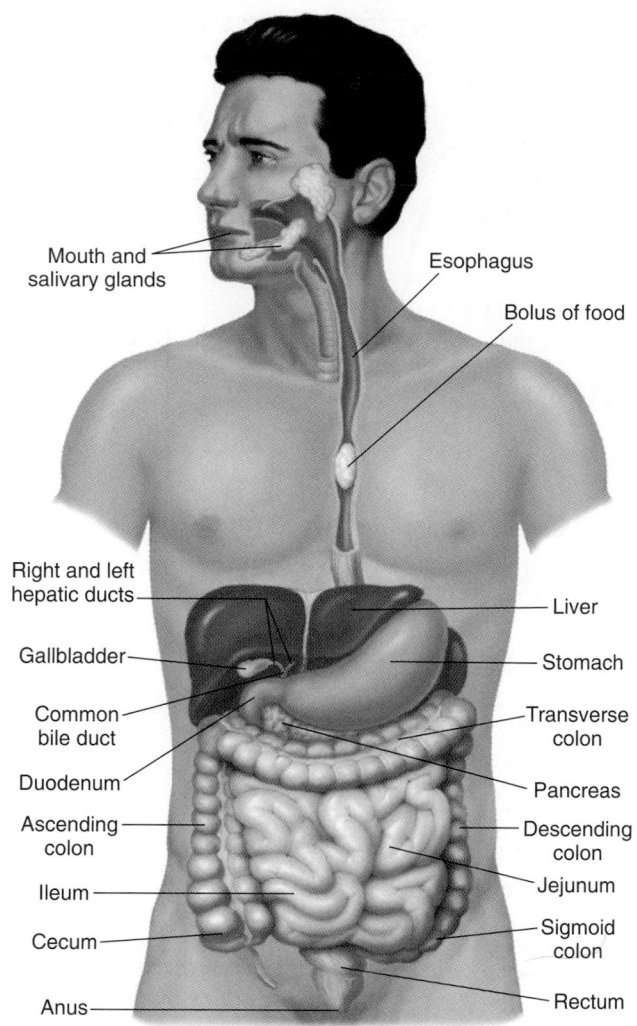

FIG 30-1 Gastrointestinal system.

Labels:
Mouth and salivary glands
Esophagus
Bolus of food
Right and left hepatic ducts
Gallbladder
Common bile duct
Duodenum
Ascending colon
Ileum
Cecum
Anus
Liver
Stomach
Transverse colon
Pancreas
Descending colon
Jejunum
Sigmoid colon
Rectum

Accessory Organs of Digestion

The accessory organs of digestion include the liver, gallbladder, and pancreas. Although these organs serve other functions for other body systems, they are referred to as *accessory organs of digestion* when discussing the GI system because they serve important functions in the digestive process.

Liver

The liver consists of two large lobes and fills the upper right and center of the abdominal cavity just below the diaphragm. It is the largest glandular organ of the body. The hepatic duct of the liver extends to the duodenum of the large intestine.

Gallbladder

The gallbladder is a 3- to 4-inch long sac on the interior surface of the liver. The gallbladder is connected to the common bile duct, which also connects to the duodenum.

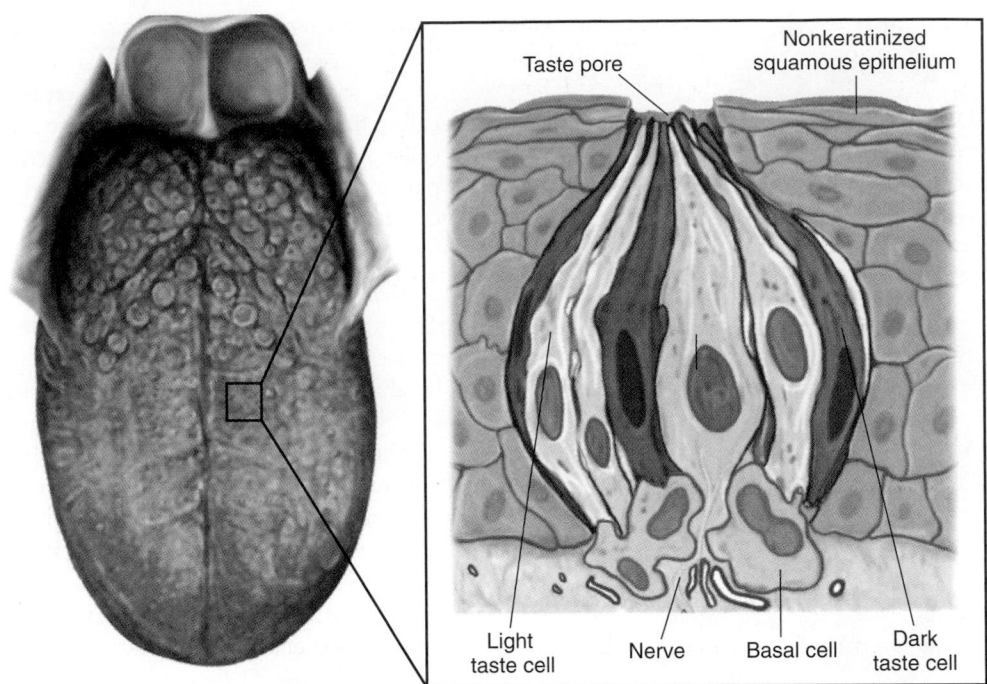

FIG 30-2 Structure of a taste bud with taste cells.

As a person swallows food, the uvula prevents the food from entering the nasal cavity. The epiglottis covers the trachea to prevent food from entering the respiratory tract. The bolus continues into the esophagus, where involuntary muscular contractions, called *peristalsis*, move the bolus downward into the stomach.

The lower esophageal sphincter lets the bolus in and prevents backflow of gastric secretions up into the esophagus. The rugae, which are folds in the internal surface of the stomach, allow the stomach to expand to accommodate large quantities of food. The fundus and body of the stomach are mostly holding areas for the food. The majority of digestion happens in the lowest portion, the pylorus. Gastric secretions within the stomach are highly acidic, with a pH around 1.7. (Some people have an elevated stomach pH due to antacid use.) These secretions continue the breakdown of food to enable the **absorption**, which is the process by which nutrients move from the digestive tract into the bloodstream. At this point in the digestive process, the food is referred to as *chyme*, a more liquid material comprised of chewed food, saliva, and digestive juices. The pyloric sphincter allows the liquid material to be released from the stomach into the small intestine a little at a time.

The villi of the small intestine increase its surface area, allowing greater absorption of water and nutrients into the blood. Most of this absorption occurs in the small intestine. (See Figure 30-3.) All other products of digestion not absorbed by the small intestine, deemed *waste*

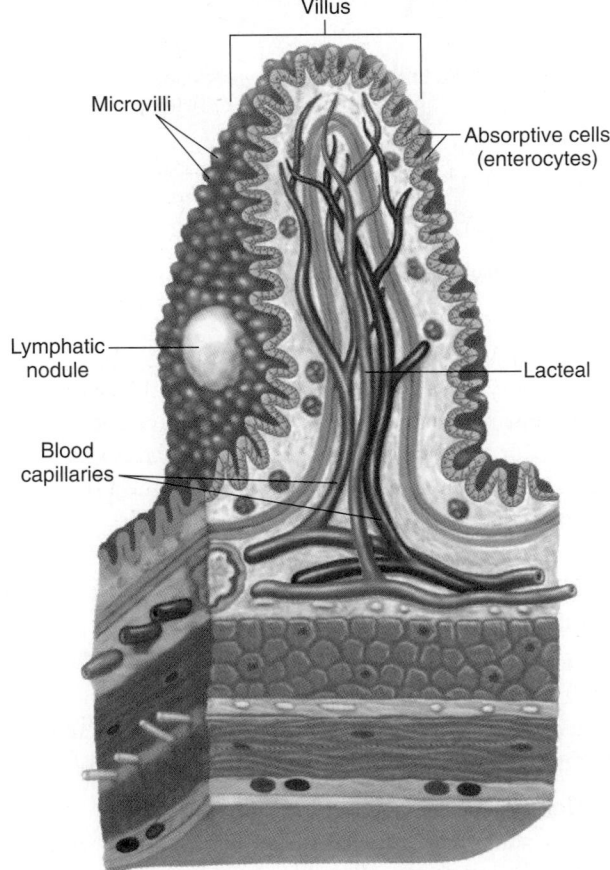

FIG 30-3 Villi of the small intestine.

products, continue into the large intestine for water absorption and elimination of bulk waste. The function of the appendix, at the junction of the small and large intestine, is unknown.

The large intestine secretes mucus to facilitate the passage of stool, the bulk waste product of digestion. No digestion occurs in the large intestine; however, it does facilitate absorption of water and some minerals. After this absorption, the large intestine facilitates the formation and elimination of stools by **defecation** (elimination of feces from the bowel).

Accessory Organs of Digestion

Although the liver, gallbladder, and pancreas are not part of the alimentary canal, these organs play vital roles in the digestion, absorption, storage, and chemical conversion of vital nutrients.

Liver

The liver is involved in digestion, absorption, storage, and excretion. Its contributions to the digestive process include:

- manufacturer of **bile**, a fat emulsifier, which it then sends to the gallbladder for storage
- production and storage of glycogen, which can be converted to glucose when needed by cells
- detoxification of drugs and alcohol, making them water soluble so they can be excreted by the kidneys
- storage of fat-soluble vitamins A, D, E, and K for use when needed by cells
- manufacture of blood lipids, such as cholesterol and other lipoproteins, that protect arterial walls from damage and transport fat-soluble substances, such as vitamins, to various tissues via the bloodstream
- destruction of old erythrocytes, recycling the iron from those blood cells, and sending it to muscles as well as back to bone marrow to make new erythrocytes and release of bilirubin, which gets excreted in feces
- use of dietary protein sources to manufacture blood-clotting proteins, such as prothrombin and fibrinogen, which aid in repair of an injured artery, vein, or capillary walls.

Gallbladder

The gallbladder acts as a storage pouch for bile. Bile, produced in the liver, is sent to the gallbladder for storage through the right and left hepatic ducts. When food that contains fat passes from the stomach to the duodenum, the gallbladder secretes the bile into the duodenum through the common bile duct to break down those fats.

Pancreas

The pancreas secretes substances into the duodenum through the pancreatic duct and directly into the bloodstream through capillaries of the islets of Langerhans.

Pancreatic enzymes and sodium bicarbonate are secreted into the duodenum to neutralize stomach acid. These pancreatic enzymes include:

- trypsin, to break down proteins
- lipase, to break down fats
- amylase, to break down carbohydrates.

The specialized cells of the islets of Langerhans secrete insulin and glucagon, two hormones that regulate blood glucose levels.

- **Insulin**, is secreted by the beta cells of the islets of Langerhans in response to increased blood glucose levels after eating. Insulin binds to glucose molecules in the bloodstream, allowing them to diffuse into the tissues.
- **Glucagon**, is secreted by the alpha cells of the islets of Langerhans in response to low blood glucose levels. Glucagon releases a storage form of glucose called glycogen from the liver. (See *Sweet mnemonic,* page 542.) Release of glycogen occurs while sleeping and fasting. (See Figure 30-4.)

Because the pancreas secretes substances into the bloodstream (insulin and glucagon) and into the alimentary canal

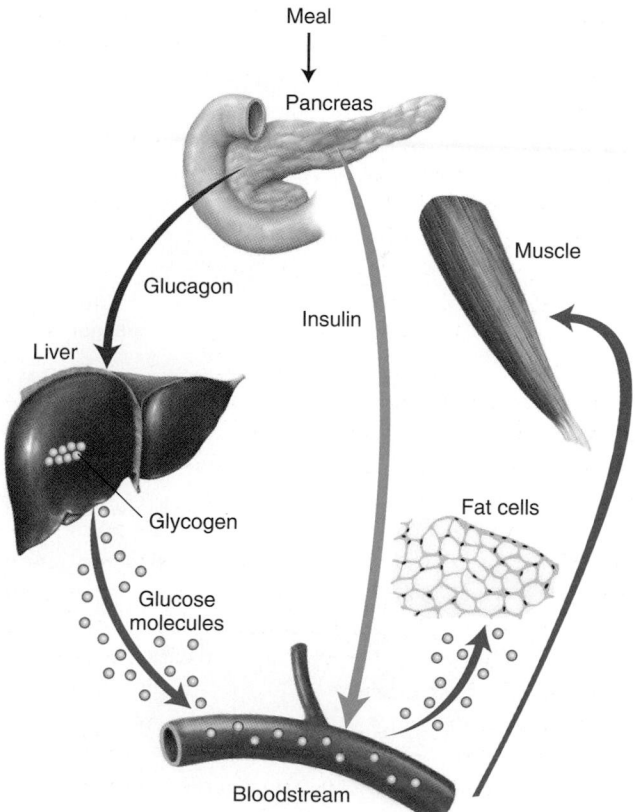

FIG 30-4 Blood glucose regulation by the accessory organs of digestion.

Sweet mnemonic

To remember which comes first, glucagon or glycogen, remember this rhyme: *Glucagon acts upon.* Glucagon acts upon glycogen to release glucose into the bloodstream.

(sodium bicarbonate and pancreatic enzymes), it is considered an exocrine (outside of the bloodstream) and endocrine (into the bloodstream) gland. For more information on the endocrine functions of the pancreas, see Chapter 29, "Endocrinology," on page 519.)

Table 30.1 | Word Elements

Element	Meaning	Example	Meaning
Combining Forms			
an/o	anus	anal (Ā-năl)	• Relating to the anus or outer rectal opening
append/o appendic/o	appendix	appendicitis (ă-pĕn-dĭ-SĪ-tĭs) appendicolysis (ă-pĕn-dĭ-KŎL-ĭ-sĭs)	• Inflammation of the appendix • Surgery to free the appendix from adhesions
bucc/o	cheek	buccal (BŬK-ăl)	• Pertaining to the cheek
cheil/o labi/o	lip	cheilitis (kī-LĪ-tĭs) labionasal (lā-bē-ō-NĀ-zăl)	• Inflammation of the lip • Pertaining to the lips and nose
cholangi/o	bile vessel	cholangioma (kō-lăn-jē-Ō-mă)	• Tumor of the bile duct
chol/e	bile, gall	choleresis (kŏl-ĕr-Ē-sĭs)	• Secretion of bile by the liver
cholecyst/o	gallbladder	cholecystitis (kō-lē-sĭs-TĪ-tĭs)	• Inflammation of the gallbladder
choledoch/o	bile duct	choledocholithiasis (kō-lēd-ō-kō-lĭ-THĪ-ă-sĭs)	• Stone in the bile duct
col/o colon/o	colon	colopexy (KŌ-lō-pĕk-sē) colonopathy (kō-lō-NŎP-ă-thē)	• Fixation of a segment of the colon to the abdominal wall • Any disease of the colon
dent/o odont/o	teeth	dentition (dĕn-TĬSH-ŭn) orthodontist (or-thō-DŎN-tĭst)	• The type, number and arrangement of teeth • Specialist concerned with positioning and alignment of teeth
duoden/o	duodenum	duodenal (dū-ō-DĒ-năl)	• Pertaining to the duodenum
enter/o	intestine	enterospasm (ĔN-tĕr-ō-spăzm)	• Intermittent painful contraction of the intestines
esophag/o	esophagus	esophagocele (ē-SŎF-ă-gō-sēl)	• Hernia of the esophagus
gastr/o	stomach	gastrectasia (găs-trĕk-TĀ-zē-ă)	• Acute or chronic dilatation of the stomach
gingiv/o	gum(s)	gingivitis (jĭn-jĭ-VĪ-tĭs)	• Inflammation of the gums
gloss/o lingu/o	tongue	glossopharyngeal (glŏs-ō-fă-RĬN-jē-ăl) lingual (LĬNG-gwăl)	• Pertaining to the tongue and pharynx (throat) • Pertaining to the tongue
hepat/o	liver	hepatitis (hĕp-ă-TĪ-tĭs)	• Inflammation of the liver
ile/o	ileum	ileostomy (ĭl-ē-ŌS-tō-mē)	• Surgery to create an opening from the ileum to the outside of the body (stoma)
jejun/o	jejunum	jejunorrhaphy (jē-joo-NOR-ă-fē)	• Surgical repair of the jejunum
or/o stomat/o	mouth	oral (OR-ăl) stomatitis (stō-mă-TĪ-tĭs)	• Pertaining to the mouth • Inflammation of the mouth
pancreat/o	pancreas	pancreatalgia (păn-krē-ă-TĂL-jē-ă)	• Pain in the pancreas

Table 30.1 | Word Elements—cont'd

Element	Meaning	Example	Meaning
pharyng/o	pharynx (throat)	**pharyngotomy** (făr-ĭn-GŎT-ō-mē)	• Incision into the pharynx
proct/o	anus, rectum	**proctologist** (prŏk-TŎL-ō-jĭst)	• Specialist in diseases and disorders of the colon, rectum, and anus
pylor/o	pylorus	**pylorodiosis** (pī-lō-rō-dĭ-Ō-sĭs)	• Dilation of the pylorus
rect/o	rectum	**rectocele** (RĔK-tō-sēl)	• Hernia of the rectum
sial/o	saliva, salivary gland	**sialolith** (sī-ĂL-ō-lĭth)	• Salivary stone
sigmoid/o	sigmoid colon	**sigmoidoscopy** (sĭg-moy-DŎS-kō-pē)	• Procedure to view the sigmoid colon
Prefixes			
dia-	through, across	**diarrhea** (dī-ă-RĒ-ă)	• Abnormally frequent discharge or flow of watery fecal matter from the bowel
peri-	around	**perihepatic** (pĕr-ĭ-hĕ-PĂT-ĭk)	• Around the liver
sub-	under, below	**sublingual** (sŭb-LĬNG-gwăl)	• Under the tongue
suffixes			
-emesis	vomit	**hematemesis** (hĕm-ăt-ĔM-ĕ-sĭs)	• Vomiting of blood
-iasis	abnormal condition	**cholelithiasis** (kō-lē-lĭ-THĬ-ă-sĭs)	• Condition of gallstones
-megaly	enlargement	**hepatomegaly** (hĕp-ă-tō-MĔG-ă-lē)	• Enlargement of the liver
-orexia	appetite	**anorexia** (ăn-ō-RĔK-sē-ă)	• Loss of appetite
-pepsia	digestion	**dyspepsia** (dĭs-PĔP-sē-ă)	• Indigestion, bad digestion
-phagia	swallowing, eating	**polyphagia** (pŏl-ē-FĀ-jē-ă)	• Eating large amounts of food, gluttony
-prandial	meal	**postprandial** (pōst-PRĂN-dē-ăl)	• Following a meal

Table 30.2 | Pathologic Terms

This table lists some of the most common pathologic terms related to the GI system with a pronunciation guide and brief definition for each.

Term	Definition	Term	Definition
appendicitis ă-pĕn-dĭ-SĪ-tĭs	Inflammation of the appendix	**dysphagia** dĭs-FĀ-jē-ă	Painful or difficult swallowing
cholelithiasis kō-lē-lĭ-THĬ-ă-sĭs	Presence of gallstones	**flatulence** FLĂT-ū-lĕns	Excessive gas in the stomach and intestines
colitis kō-LĪ-tĭs	Inflamed colon	**gastroesophageal reflux disease** găs-trō-ĕ-sŏf-ă-JĒ-ăl RĒ-flŭks dĭ-ZĔZ	Common condition where acid from the stomach flows back into the esophagus, causing discomfort and, sometimes, erosion of the lining of the esophagus
diarrhea dī-ă-RĒ-ă	Passage of loose, watery stool from the rectum		
dyspepsia dĭs-PĔP-sē-ă	Poor or painful digestion	**peritonitis** pĕr-ĭ-tō-NĪ-tĭs	Inflammation of the serous membrane that lines the abdominal cavity

Continued

Table 30.2 | Pathologic Terms—cont'd

Term	Definition	Term	Definition
polyp PŎL-ĭp	Growth projecting from a mucous membrane	pyrosis pī-RŌ-sĭs	Heartburn
pruritis proo-RĪ-tŭs	Itching, tingling		

Table 30.3 | Abbreviations

In gastroenterology, as in other areas of health care, abbreviations are commonly used. Abbreviations such as the ones listed here save time and effort in documentation and written communications.

Abbreviation	Term
ac	before meals
ALT	alanine aminotransferase (liver enzyme test)
AST	aspartate aminotransferase (liver enzyme test)
BaE, BE	barium enema
BM	bowel movement
ERCP	endoscopic retrograde cholangiopancreatography
GERD	gastroesophageal reflux disease
GI	gastrointestinal
IBD	inflammatory bowel disease
IBS	irritable bowel syndrome
IVC	intravenous cholangiogram
LFT	liver function test
NG	nasogastric
NPO, npo	nothing by mouth (Latin—*nulle per os*)
pc	after meals
PO, po	by mouth
PR	per rectum
PUD	peptic ulcer disease
SBO	small bowel obstruction

Medical Terminology Related to the GI System

Terms used the in the gastroenterology office will include the names of the organs associated with digestion, absorption, storage, and elimination of food. The medical assistant working in the gastroenterology setting will become familiar with pathologies related to the organs of the GI system. Working in these practice settings will allow the medical assistant to assist with diagnostic testing and therapeutic procedures for the GI system. To be effective in her role, a medical assistant must become well versed in the language and vocabulary that pertains to the gastrointestinal system. The following tables list common medical terminology related to the gastrointestinal system.

Common GI System Diseases and Disorders

Diseases and disorders of the GI system can cause pain and malabsorption of nutrients, adversely affect growth or maintenance of tissues, and affect overall health. The medical assistant can offer the patient resources on healthy diets, medications, and foods to avoid that promote reduction of symptoms for their specific GI ailment. There are many diseases and disorders affecting the GI system. Here are some of the most common with a summary of each, along with their corresponding ICD-9-CM code.

Disorders of the Upper GI Tract

The organs of the upper GI tract include the oral cavity, esophagus, and stomach. Disorders of these organs can cause dysphagia (difficulty swallowing) and pyrosis, commonly called *heartburn*. Patients may complain that eating is difficult and no longer enjoyable. Some of the most common diseases and disorders of the upper GI tract include gastroesophageal reflux disease, hiatal hernia, peptic ulcer disease, gastritis, and pyloric stenosis.

Gastroesophageal Reflux Disease

ICD-9-CM code: 530.81

Gastroesophageal reflux disease (GERD), commonly known as *heartburn,* is one of the most common disorders of the GI tract. It involves the backflow of acidic gastric contents into the esophagus causing pyrosis, also called *heartburn.* The tissues of the esophagus are not designed to deal with acidic gastric secretions. If prolonged exposure to these secretions occurs, the lining of the esophagus becomes irritated and causes symptoms. As many as 44% of Americans suffer from symptoms of GERD once per month and an estimated 7% to 10% have daily symptoms.

Factors that contribute to GERD include weak esophageal peristalsis, delayed gastric emptying, pyloric stenosis (narrowing of the lower portion of the stomach), hiatal hernia, obesity, smoking, alcohol, and such medications as aspirin and other nonsteroidal anti-inflammatory drugs (NSAIDs). GERD is also common in pregnant women, because the enlarging uterus exerts upward pressure on the stomach and other structures, and less-than-normal LES pressure allows the reflux of gastric contents into the esophagus.

Symptoms include heartburn, dysphagia, chronic cough, upper abdominal pain, and difficulty breathing. Symptoms worsen about 1 hour after meals, when lying down, or if intra-abdominal pressure increases, such as with coughing, belching, or physical strain. Diagnosis is based on the patient's history and clinical manifestations. Testing may include a barium swallow to detect erosion or abnormalities of the esophagus. An upper endoscopy enables visualization of the esophagus, LES, and stomach, testing of fluid pH, and biopsy of tissue for analysis.

Conservative, nonpharmacologic treatment measures include smoking cessation, weight loss, reducing or eliminating alcohol, avoiding large meals, avoiding high-fat foods or foods that reduce LES tone (such as caffeine, fat, and chocolate) 4 hours before bedtime, and elevating the head of the bed 6 in. Medication to treat GERD includes H_2-receptor antagonists, such as famotidine (Pepcid), and proton pump inhibitors, such as esomeprazole (Nexium) and omeprazole (Prilosec). If conservative measures fail, symptoms can usually be managed effectively with drug therapy. Surgical management is reserved for severe symptoms that do not respond to other measures and includes narrowing of the LES via laparoscopy. Long-term complications may include esophagitis, dysphagia, and precancerous cellular changes in the esophageal lining.

Hiatal Hernia

ICD-9-CM code: 553.3

A hernia is a protrusion of an organ or other tissue through a wall or structure that normally contains it. There are many different types and locations of hernias. A hiatal hernia is a protrusion of the stomach upward through the diaphragm, a muscle in the abdomen necessary for breathing. The incidence of hiatal hernias is greater in Western countries and increases with age, from 10% in those below the age of 40 to as high as 70% in those over 70 years of age.

A hiatal hernia occurs when the part of the diaphragm around the base of the esophagus weakens and allows a portion of the stomach to slide upward into the thoracic cavity. The cause of hiatal hernias is not always clear but contributing factors include obesity, trauma, advanced age, and anything that increases intra-abdominal pressure.

The key symptoms of hiatal hernia are the same as for GERD. Stomach fluids, which are highly acidic with a pH of 1.7, are regurgitated upward into the lower esophagus, causing pyrosis. Other symptoms may include chest pain, dysphagia, and respiratory problems if aspiration occurs. Some patients may not exhibit common symptoms but may complain of such vague symptoms as a loss of appetite or malaise. Such patients may admit some feelings of nausea or vomiting if asked but may consider such incidents unrelated.

Diagnostic studies include chest x-ray and barium study. Upper endoscopy may be done to confirm the diagnosis and check the pH of refluxed fluid. Conservative management includes weight loss; eating smaller, more frequent meals; and avoiding foods that exacerbate symptoms. Medications used to treat GERD may also be used to treat the symptoms of hiatal hernia, including H_2-receptor antagonists, such as famotidine (Pepcid). Cholinergic agents may be used to strengthen the LES. Antacids, such as aluminum hydroxide and magnesium hydroxide (Maalox, Mylanta) and calcium carbonate (Tums), are used to relieve the symptoms of heartburn associated with hiatal hernia. If conservative measures are not effective, surgical repair may be necessary.

Prognosis is generally good unless further complications arise. Complications can include a strangulated hernia, in which the protrusion of the stomach is so tight that blood supply to the tissue is restricted and tissues begin to necrotize or die. Strangulated hernias require prompt surgical intervention to avoid the development of gangrene. (See Figure 30-5.)

Peptic Ulcer Disease

ICD-9-CM code: 531.90 (gastric), 532.90 (duodenal), 530.2 (esophageal)

Ulceration occurs when an area of the protective mucous membrane lining breaks down leaving the area sensitive to the acidity of various digestive secretions. The three most common sites of ulceration are the lower esophagus, stomach, and duodenum. About 10% of Americans develop peptic ulcer disease (PUD) at some point in their lifetime and approximately 10% of emergency department patients who complain of abdominal pain are diagnosed with PUD. An estimated 50% of the world's population is infected with

A

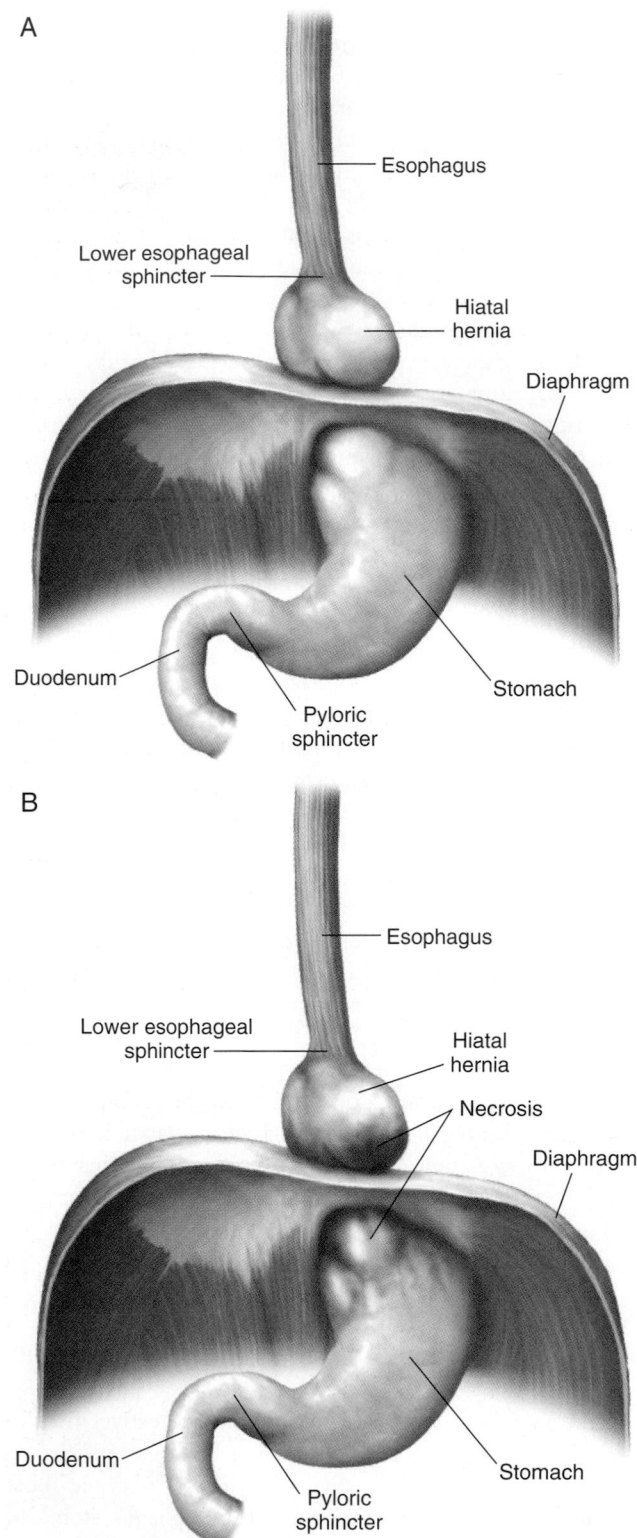

Esophagus

Lower esophageal
sphincter

Hiatal
hernia

Diaphragm

Duodenum

Stomach

Pyloric
sphincter

B

Esophagus

Lower esophageal
sphincter

Hiatal
hernia

Necrosis

Diaphragm

Duodenum

Stomach

Pyloric
sphincter

FIG 30-5 Hiatal hernia. (A) Uncomplicated hiatal hernia. (B) Strangulated hiatal hernia.

Helicobacter pylori, the bacteria responsible for most cases of peptic ulcer, although the incidence of PUD in the developed world is decreasing.

The majority of peptic ulcers result from *H. pylori* infection, which causes inflammation and breakdown of the mucosal lining of the stomach. The next most common cause of ulcer formation is the use of nonsteroidal anti-inflammatory drugs (NSAIDs), which block the production of certain prostaglandins that protect the mucosal lining of the stomach from digestive acids. Alcohol is also a contributor because it promotes acid secretion, which in excess can lead to erosion of the gastric mucosa. Smoking and eating spicy foods were once suspected to cause ulcers but have not been found to cause peptic ulcers. Although diet and stress may play a minor role in some individuals, they are not major risk factors, as was commonly believed in the past.

Symptoms of peptic ulcers include indigestion, heartburn, and epigastric pain. The most common location for a peptic ulcer is in the duodenum. Symptoms include heartburn, midepigastric pain, nausea, and vomiting, with symptoms peaking about 2 hours after eating.

Information is obtained through the health history, physical examination, and barium studies. Tests that confirm the diagnosis include a blood test or a urea breath test that reveals the presence of *H. pylori* and endoscopy, which enables direct visualization of the upper GI tract and collection of gastric contents for analysis to determine pH and the presence of blood and *H. pylori.* The physician may also perform a tissue biopsy to rule out malignancy.

The physician may prescribe antibiotics if tests confirm the presence of *H. pylori.* Other treatment measures include avoiding intake of irritating agents, such as alcohol, NSAIDs, and tobacco (which may irritate the condition even though it does not cause it) as well as such medications as H_2-receptor antagonists, antacids, and proton pump inhibitors. PUD does not generally require significant dietary changes; however, the patient should avoid any food that seems to exacerbate symptoms. Prognosis is good with early diagnosis. Potential complications include mild or severe bleeding and perforation, resulting in hemorrhage, peritonitis, and sepsis. (See Figure 30-6.)

Gastritis

ICD-9-CM code: 535.5 (use fifth digit to denote hemorrhage or no hemorrhage)
Gastritis is an acute or chronic inflammation of the lining of the stomach. In acute gastritis, the gastric mucosa is red and inflamed and can ulcerate and bleed. Chronic gastritis is found mostly in patients ages 50 and older.

The most common cause of gastritis is infection with *H. pylori,* the same bacteria that causes peptic ulcer disease. Less common causes include irritants, such as alcohol,

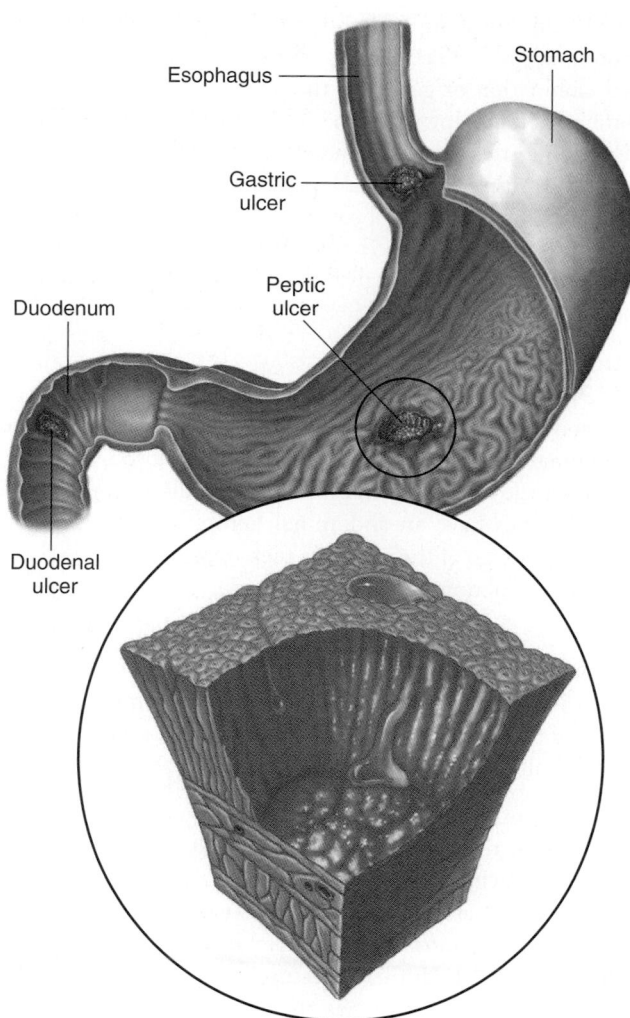

Esophagus

Stomach

Gastric
ulcer

Peptic
ulcer

Duodenum

Duodenal
ulcer

FIG 30-6 Common ulceration sites.

Emesis in the Waiting Room

Because many patients waiting to see a physician are ill—perhaps so ill that emesis (vomiting) is a possibility, the administrative medical assistant must be aware of this danger. In addition, she should have a working knowledge of blood and body secretions to protect herself and others from potentially infectious diseases.

If the administrative medical assistant is aware of a patient who may be ill, she should communicate with the clinical medical assistant to get the patient into a treatment room as quickly as possible and provide him with an emesis basin. If a room is not available, she should provide the patient with the emesis basin in the waiting room or escort him to the restroom. If a patient does vomit in the waiting area, she should clean the area immediately using proper infection control techniques.

Stomach pH testing can confirm suspected hypochlorhydria. Treatment of acute gastritis includes antibiotic therapy if *H. Pylori* is the causative agent, B_{12} injections to correct vitamin deficiency, and temporary administration of H_2-receptor antagonists to decrease acid production while the gastric mucosa heals. (See *Antacid overuse.*) Supplemental hydrochloric acid can be administered to restore digestive function of the stomach.

The prognosis for gastritis is good with proper treatment. The medical assistant should encourage patients with gastritis

Patient Education

Antacid Overuse

Many people take over-the-counter acid suppressants, also called *antacids,* to alleviate discomfort caused by overeating or eating spicy foods. However, stomach acid performs two important functions. It aids in the digestion of foods by breaking chemical bonds and inhibits the growth of bacteria.

Bacteria cannot grow in an acidic environment, so stomach acid can kill potentially harmful bacteria before they cause infection. Recent studies also indicate that prolonged stomach acid suppression contributes to osteoporosis, because stomach acid is necessary to metabolize calcium.

The medical assistant should advise patients to use over-the-counter acid suppressants sparingly to avoid poor digestion of food, decreased absorption of nutrients, and infection.

tobacco, and NSAIDs, and chronic peptic ulcers. Because it is so common in older patients, it is thought to be due in part to hypochlorhydria, a decrease in the production of stomach acid. With age or disease (such as chronic peptic ulcers), normal production of stomach acid decreases, which leaves the stomach vulnerable to irritants and infection. In addition, the decrease in acid production causes atrophy of the mucosa of the stomach, which leads to decreased production of intrinsic factor, a stomach secretion that activates vitamin B_{12}. This secondary effect of gastritis causes a vitamin B_{12} deficiency.

Patients may be asymptomatic or suffer from epigastric pain, nausea, vomiting, and hematemesis (vomiting of blood). (See *Emesis in the waiting room.*) Other symptoms include mild epigastric pain, anorexia, or intolerance to spicy and fatty foods.

Diagnosis depends on the health history and endoscopy or barium studies, which reveal the presence of inflammation.

to avoid alcohol, tobacco, and any foods that they have found to be irritating. Because the loss of gastric secretions leaves the patient at an increased risk for peptic ulcers and gastric carcinoma, the medical assistant should encourage patients to notify the physician if symptoms return.

Pyloric Stenosis

ICD-9-CM code: 537.0 (adult), 750.5 (congenital-infantile)
In pyloric stenosis, a stenosis (narrowing of the pyloric sphincter) interferes with the emptying of the stomach into the duodenum. This condition may be present at birth. It affects about 3 of every 1,000 infants, usually within the first 8 weeks of life. Boys are five times more likely than girls to suffer from pyloric stenosis. It is very rarely acquired as an adult.

In infants, a congenital hyperplasia of the mucosa and submucosa of the pylorus prevents the passage of food into the duodenum. Studies have shown that this congenital malformation could be inherited. In adults, the most common cause is scar tissue that develops around a healing gastric ulcer.

The major sign of pyloric stenosis in infants is projectile vomiting, because food cannot pass from the stomach to the duodenum. Adult symptoms include distention of the stomach and forceful projectile vomiting after eating.

Diagnosis of infants is confirmed by physical examination, which reveals a firm, nontender, mobile, hard pylorus on palpation. Palpation is most effective after the infant has vomited and when he is calm. History of forceful projectile vomiting and signs of dehydration, such as depressed fontanelles, dry mucous membranes, and decreased tearing, are also present. Adult diagnosis is confirmed by endoscopy, which shows narrowing of the pyloric sphincter. In infant and adult patients, blood tests reveal elevated electrolyte levels consistent with dehydration and acid-base imbalance.

Treatment for infants includes laparoscopic division of the muscles of the pylorus to help the passage of food. Without surgical correction, the infant will not be able to eat enough to grow and thrive. Adults can be treated with the placement of a stent to open the passage. Adult patients may be able to control symptoms with diet modification or eating small, frequent meals; however, surgical correction is commonly required.

Infants who undergo surgical correction have a good prognosis; most babies can feed 3 to 4 hours after surgery and will grow and gain weight normally. Adult prognosis is also good with diet modification and, in some cases, surgical correction.

Disorders of the Lower GI Tract

The lower GI tract is responsible for absorption of nutrients, such as minerals, and water and the synthesis of vitamin K in the large intestine. Patients with disorders of the lower GI tract commonly complain of diarrhea, constipation, or lower abdominal pain. Gas causing flatulence, the accumulation and elimination of gas from the lower intestine, is another common complaint. The medical assistant can assist the physician in the diagnosis and treatment of disorders of the lower GI tract and provide patients strategies to reduce symptoms of chronic disorders. Common diseases and disorders of the lower GI tract include abdominal hernia, appendicitis, diverticular disease, hemorrhoids, and inflammatory bowel disease.

Abdominal Hernia

ICD-9-CM code: 553.9
An abdominal hernia involves protrusion through the abdominal wall of one of the structures enclosed within it, including the intestine. An estimated 5 million people in the United States have an abdominal hernia. However, only a small percentage of these people seek treatment. Three common sites of abdominal hernias include:

- umbilicus, which accounts for 10% to 20% of all hernias
- inguinal ligament, which accounts for 75% of all hernias and is 25 times more likely in men than women
- site of previous surgery, which accounts for approximately 5% of all hernias.

An abdominal hernia can develop anywhere there is a weakness in the omentum, the musculature that lines the abdominal cavity. When this weakness results in an opening in the abdominal wall, the intestines can protrude through the opening. Contributing factors include anything that increases intra-abdominal pressure, such as heavy lifting. Umbilical hernias occur when the opening to the abdominal wall for the umbilical cord does not completely close at birth. Inguinal hernias occur when the inguinal canal, which usually closes shortly after birth, stays open, allowing abdominal structures to migrate into the canal. Rarely, women have an opening in the same region that can become herniated. Unlike the umbilical hernia, the inguinal hernia can occur in adulthood, especially at middle age and older, as a result of thinning of the tissue and loss of muscle tone in the inguinal region. Hernias at sites of previous surgeries occur because the surgical cutting of the muscle wall causes a weakness. (See Figure 30-7.)

Symptoms of abdominal hernia vary, depending on the site and severity of the hernia. Patients may notice a bulge that can be reduced by pushing on it. A person with an inguinal hernia may notice sharp pain when straining or standing. Severe pain may indicate a strangulated hernia, in which the blood supply to the herniated tissue has been cut off.

Diagnosis is usually based on physical examination findings and a description of symptoms. Radiographic studies of abdominal structures may confirm the diagnosis. Treatment depends on the type and location of the hernia as well as

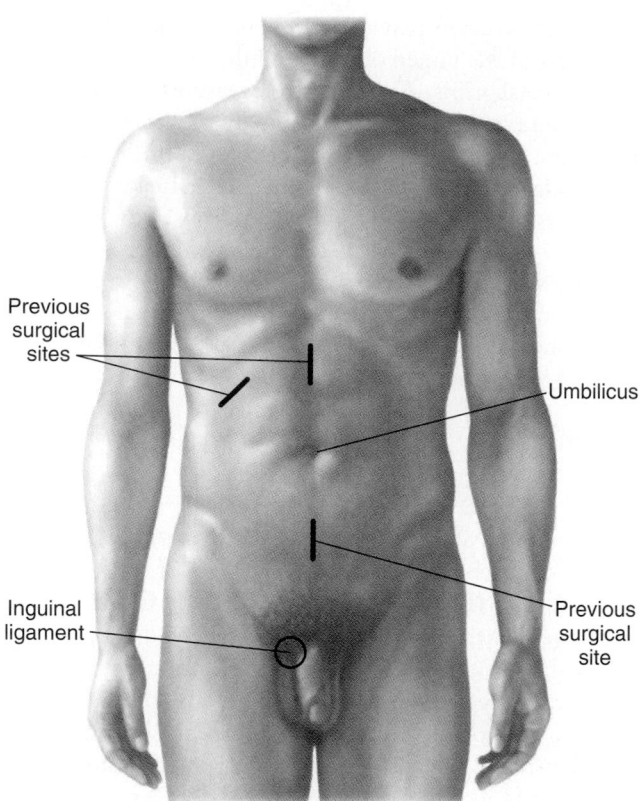

Previous
surgical
sites

Umbilicus

Inguinal
ligament

Previous
surgical
site

FIG 30-7 Common abdominal hernia sites.

may exhibit rebound tenderness to palpation at McBurney's point, a point 1 to 2 in. above and central to the right ilium and RLQ rebound tenderness. Other signs and symptoms may include fever, diarrhea, and constipation. In over half of all cases, the symptoms are less specific and pain and tenderness are more generalized.

Diagnosis is based primarily on symptoms and physical examination findings. A complete blood count (CBC) may reveal an elevated level of white blood cells (WBCs). However, radiologic tests are not helpful and exploratory surgery is usually necessary to confirm the diagnosis. The only treatment for appendicitis is surgical removal of the appendix and administration of antibiotics to prevent or resolve infection.

Prognosis is good with surgery and full recovery is expected in most cases. If the appendix ruptures before surgery, peritonitis develops, causing peritoneal abscess, infection of the reproductive organs, septicemia, and shock. In these cases, prognosis is less certain and depends on the immediate intervention.

Diverticular Disease

Diverticulosis—ICD-9-CM code: 562.10 and 562.12
Diverticulitis—ICD-9-CM code: 562.11 and 562.13
Diverticular disease includes diverticulosis and diverticulitis. Diverticulosis is a disorder in which tiny, pouchlike herniations, called *diverticula,* develop in the wall of the distal portion of the large intestine. Diverticulitis is the development of inflammation and infection of these diverticula. It is estimated that approximately half of the population has developed some degree of diverticulosis by age 60, although most people are not aware of it until they experience symptoms.

Diverticula form in the intestinal wall when increased pressure causes small herniations around small vessels and other structures that transect the wall. Contributing factors include low-fiber diet and chronic or recurrent constipation. Diverticulitis develops when the diverticula become clogged with feces, resulting in inflammation and infection.

Patients with diverticulosis are usually asymptomatic. Symptoms of diverticulitis include fever, nausea, blood-streaked stools, and left lower quadrant (LLQ) abdominal pain. Diagnosis is generally based on a description of symptoms when the patient has developed diverticulitis. Tests that confirm the diagnosis include air contrast barium enema, radiographic studies, colonoscopy, and sigmoidoscopy, which reveal diverticula and small herniations of the intestinal wall. A complete blood count (CBC) will show an elevated WBC count.

Diverticulosis is treated with dietary measures, including adequate fluid and fiber to prevent constipation and avoidance of foods containing small seeds and nuts that might lodge in the diverticula. Diverticulitis is treated with antibiotics, analgesics, and a liquid diet that allows the bowel to

patient factors, such as age and general health status. Patients may wear a truss, which is a device that reduces and holds the herniated tissue in place. However, if the patient is considered a good surgical candidate, treatment generally involves surgical repair.

If untreated, a hernia may worsen over time. Therefore, evaluation health care provider is recommended. Prognosis for a surgically repaired hernia is generally very good. A strangulated hernia is a medical emergency that requires prompt surgical intervention to prevent tissue necrosis, gangrene, and septicemia.

Appendicitis

ICD-9-CM code: 540
When the appendix becomes inflamed, the result is the condition known as *appendicitis.* Appendicitis is most common in patients between ages 10 and 40 and is the second most common cause of acute abdominal pain and surgery in the United States.

Occasionally, intestinal matter clogs the appendix, resulting in the inflammation and infection. Less than half of the patients with appendicitis develop the classic symptoms of nausea, vomiting, and severe periumbilical pain, which eventually localizes to the right lower quadrant (RLQ). Patients

rest. In cases of diverticular rupture (bowel perforation), the physician may perform surgery to resect the ruptured portion of the bowel. Additional measures include rest and stress reduction.

Prognosis for diverticulosis is good unless diverticulitis develops. Mild cases of diverticulitis usually resolve without complications. Complications may include perforation, infection, obstruction, and hemorrhage. (See *Foods that cause diverticular disease*.)

Hemorrhoids
ICD-9-CM code: 455

Hemorrhoids are varicose veins of the anal area and may be inside the rectum or on the exterior of the anal opening. They are rarely serious, but hemorrhoids are common and can be uncomfortable. It is estimated that half of adults over the age of 50 suffer from hemorrhoids.

Hemorrhoids result from constipation, which results in excessive straining during defecation, or other factors, such as pregnancy and obesity, that increase pressure on veins located in the anorectal area. Disorders that predispose people to the development of hemorrhoids include ulcerative colitis and Crohn disease.

Signs and symptoms of hemorrhoids include small bulging areas in the anal region that may be painless. However, they can easily worsen with constipation and straining to defecate. Other symptoms include pain or tenderness as well as itching. Bleeding may occasionally be present after passing stool and is usually minor.

Diagnosis is based on the health history, physical examination, and symptoms. In addition, proctoscopy, an examination of the rectum with a scope, evaluates the anal canal and rectum for internal hemorrhoids. Radiography may include a barium enema or virtual colonoscopy, which uses x-rays and computers to produce two- and three-dimensional images of the colon that reveal vein distention and possible narrowing of the lumen of the colon due to engorgement of hemorrhoidal veins. Conservative measures are aimed at treating and preventing constipation by increasing intake of dietary fluids and fiber and using of stool softeners. (See *Preventing constipation*.) Symptoms can be treated by soaking in a warm bath and applying topical anesthetics and anti-inflammatory creams. When these treatments are ineffective, a variety of measures may be used to destroy hemorrhoids, including sclerotherapy, cryotherapy, and ligation. When these measures are ineffective or when bleeding is severe, a hemorrhoidectomy is the best treatment measure.

Inflammatory Bowel Disease
Crohn disease—ICD-9-CM code: 555.9
Ulcerative colitis—ICD-9-CM code: 556.9
Irritable bowel syndrome—ICD-9-CM code: 564.1

Several disorders fall under the category of inflammatory bowel disease (IBD). These disorders include Crohn disease, ulcerative colitis, and irritable bowel syndrome (IBS). Although these disorders have some similarities, they also have some distinctive differences. In each case, diagnosis is based on presenting symptoms, barium enema, abdominal x-rays, lower endoscopy, and, possibly, tissue biopsy. Laboratory tests include CBC and stool studies. All three disorders are considered chronic in nature with no specific cure, yet all can be managed with a resulting normal or near-normal life expectancy. Even so, all three are considered risk factors for bowel cancer.

Crohn Disease

Crohn disease is inflammation and edema deep into the lining of any part of the GI tract. It affects 7 in 100,000

Patient Education

Foods That Cause Diverticular Disease

For a patient with diverticula, preventing inflammation and infection (diverticulitis) is essential. The medical assistant should teach such a patient to avoid foods that can get "stuck" in the diverticula, including:

• nuts, such as peanuts, walnuts, almonds, and cashews

• seeds, such as pumpkin and sunflower seeds

• tomatoes

• cucumbers

• strawberries

• kiwi fruit.

Patient Education

Preventing Constipation

Conservative treatment for hemorrhoids includes treating constipation. The medical assistant should teach the patient with hemorrhoids about these measures to prevent or treat constipation:

• Drink plenty of nonalcoholic, noncaffeinated fluids

• Eat a high-fiber diet (including fresh fruits, vegetables, whole grains, and bran).

• Drink prune juice.

• Use bulk-forming, nonchemical laxatives, such as Metamucil.

• Stool softeners and chemical laxatives, although available over the counter, can be habit-forming with regular use. It is important to consult with a physician when using these products.

patients in the United States. It is more prevalent in Caucasians and Jewish people and slightly more common in men than women. Most newly diagnosed patients are between the ages of 15 and 30 or 60 and 80.

The specific cause of Crohn disease is unknown. However, factors that contribute to the disease include diet, genetics, infectious agents, allergies, and psychological components. There is some evidence that it may also be an autoimmune disorder. Symptoms include chronic diarrhea, fever, weight loss, fatigue, anorexia, abdominal pain, and cramping that may localize to the right lower quadrant (RLQ).

Treatment aims at symptom management and includes administration of IV fluid and parenteral nutrition, anticholinergics and opioids to control pain and reduce bowel motility, antimicrobials for infection, corticosteroids to reduce inflammation, and surgery for perforations or to remove involved portions of the colon. Patients may also be referred to a support group or therapist. Potential complications of Crohn disease include bowel obstruction, malnutrition, adhesions, abscesses, fistulas, and fluid and electrolyte imbalance.

Ulcerative Colitis

Ulcerative colitis is a chronic inflammation of the innermost lining of the rectum and colon. This disease follows a pattern of episodes of acute symptoms alternating with periods of remission. It affects more than 500,000 Americans, usually young adults, and affects men and women equally. Incidence of the disease in people of Caucasian, Jewish, and European descent is five times higher than in other groups. This type of IBD is commonly confused with Crohn disease.

The specific cause of ulcerative colitis is unknown. Theories include heredity, antibiotic use, and autoimmune factors or environmental factors (such as urban or industrialized areas and northern climates). Symptoms include weight loss, fever, malaise, and up to 10 to 20 episodes of bloody, mucoid diarrhea per day with pain, cramping, and urgency to defecate.

Treatment for ulcerative colitis includes a nutritious, low-fiber diet and avoidance of trigger foods, which vary from patient to patient. Anticholinergics and antidiarrheals reduce bowel motility. Other medications may include bulk Metamucil, NSAIDs, sulfasalazine, mesalamine, corticosteroids, fish oil, and analgesics. Treatment may also include surgery in cases of severe hemorrhage or perforation. About 25% to 40% of people with ulcerative colitis eventually require surgery. Complications of ulcerative colitis include infection and fulminant colitis, a severe form that causes severe pain, profuse diarrhea, hemorrhage, fluid and electrolyte imbalances, and shock.

Irritable Bowel Syndrome

Irritable bowel syndrome (IBS) is a disorder of the intestine characterized by alternating episodes of constipation and diarrhea along with other GI symptoms. IBS is the most common GI disorder in the United States, accounting for more than 10% of all medical office visits. About 1 in 5 American adults suffer from IBS, and young women are most commonly affected.

The specific cause of IBS is unknown. Current theories include changes in motor or sensory nerves in the bowel, central nervous system changes, genetic factors, and hormonal influences. Symptoms include alternating diarrhea and constipation, abdominal pain, bloating, gas, distention, cramping, and heartburn. These symptoms may be aggravated by emotional stress and trigger foods, such as chocolate, milk, and alcohol.

Treatment of IBS includes avoidance of identified trigger foods, which may reduce the frequency of episodes. Antispasmodics may help reduce hypermotility. Antidiarrheal medications or laxatives may help control symptoms of diarrhea and constipation. Bulk fiber, such as Metamucil, helps minimize diarrhea and constipation. Most patients can control symptoms of IBS through medication and diet modification (avoiding trigger foods).

Disorders of the Accessory Organs of Digestion

The liver, gallbladder, and pancreas can also become diseased, cause pain, and disrupt digestion. The medical assistant can assist the physician in the diagnosis and treatment of disorders to the accessory organs of digestion by taking patient histories, scheduling laboratory and radiographic studies, and providing patient education. Common disorders of the accessory organs include viral hepatitis, cholelithiasis and cholecystitis, and acute pancreatitis.

Viral Hepatitis

ICD-9-CM code: 070.1 (hepatitis A), 070.30 (hepatitis B), 070.51 (hepatitis C, acute), 070.54 (hepatitis C, chronic), 070.52 (hepatitis D), 070.53 (hepatitis E)
Viral hepatitis is a disorder characterized by inflammatory cells in the liver. There are several types of viral hepatitis, including hepatitis A, B, C, D, and E. Diagnostic tests to determine the viral cause identify the presence of the antigen for each type of hepatitis.

Hepatitis A

Hepatitis A is caused by the hepatitis A virus (HAV), which is spread by the fecal-oral route. Risk factors for infection with HAV include living with an infected person, traveling to countries where hepatitis A is prevalent, and sharing body fluids with an infected person through sex or drug use. One-third of all Americans have evidence of past infection with HAV.

Symptoms of hepatitis A include jaundice, fatigue, abdominal pain, nausea, diarrhea, anorexia, and fever. Blood tests can confirm the presence of antibodies to hepatitis A.

Administration of immune globulin may prevent infection before exposure or treat a recent exposure (less than 2 weeks before administration). Administration of the hepatitis A vaccine conveys long-term protection against infection.

Prognosis for hepatitis A is good with treatment. The time between infection and the start of illness is approximately 28 days. Most people fully recover within 2 months. Approximately 15% of people experience relapsing symptoms for 6 months to 1 year after initial diagnosis.

Hepatitis B

Hepatitis B is caused by infection with the hepatitis B virus (HBV), which is spread through blood or body fluids. Risk factors for infection include travel to areas where HBV is common as well as IV drug use and multiple sex partners. An estimated 1.25 million Americans have chronic hepatitis B, and 20% to 30% acquired the infection during childhood. In the United States, people ages 20 to 49 are at the highest risk for the disease. Each year, approximately 5,000 Americans die from HBV infection. Worldwide, HBV is a major cause of chronic liver disease and liver cancer.

Symptoms of hepatitis B include joint pain, clay-colored feces, dark urine, abdominal pain or tenderness, nausea, anorexia, fatigue, and yellowish skin and eyes. Patients with hepatitis B will test positive for the hepatitis B antigen (HBsAg) 1 to 2 months after exposure. The hepatitis B vaccine prevents infection with HBV. Antiviral drugs treat chronic HBV infection. Although most people recover from hepatitis B, complications may include liver cancer and liver failure.

Hepatitis C

Hepatitis C occurs in acute and chronic forms. It is caused by infection with the hepatitis C virus (HCV), which is spread via the blood. Risk factors for contracting HCV include IV drug use, blood transfusion or solid organ transplant before July 1992, transfusion of clotting factors before 1987, long-term dialysis, and liver disease. Approximately 3.9 million (1.8%) Americans are currently infected. In 2003, the CDC reported 30,000 new cases of hepatitis C in the United States. About 80% of people infected with HCV are asymptomatic.

Symptoms of hepatitis C include jaundice, fatigue, abdominal pain, anorexia, nausea, fatigue, and dark urine. Tests used to confirm hepatitis C include the enzyme immunoassay (EIA) or the enhanced chemiluminescence immunoassay (CIA) test. The recombinant immunoblot assay (RIBA) test confirms positive results. There is no vaccine available for the prevention of HCV infection. Treatment for hepatitis C includes administration of interferon and ribavirin, which eliminates the virus in 50% to 80% of people. Drinking alcohol can exacerbate the disease. The mortality rate for hepatitis C is fairly low (1% to 5%). However, as many as 85% of patients with hepatitis C will develop chronic infection or chronic liver disease. Hepatitis C is the leading reason for liver transplants.

Hepatitis D

Hepatitis D is caused by infection with the hepatitis D virus (HDV). However, this form of hepatitis is only present with a coexisting HBV infection. Because testing for HDV is not routine, there is no reliable data available on its prevalence in the population. Risk factors for contracting HDV include IV drug use, hemodialysis, sexual contact with an infected person, and working in a health care or public safety setting.

Symptoms of hepatitis D include jaundice, fatigue, abdominal pain, anorexia, nausea, vomiting, joint pain, and dark urine. Blood tests reveal the presence of small and large delta antigens (HDAg-S and HDAg-L), which indicate the presence of HDV. The vaccine for hepatitis B also prevents infection with HDV. In addition, a booster of HBV immune globulin prevents infection or treats exposure at the time of diagnosis. There is no treatment for acute infection with HDV other than supportive care. Treatment for chronic hepatitis D includes administration of interferon-alfa, liver transplant, or both. Patients with hepatitis D may develop cirrhosis, and up to 20% will develop liver failure.

Hepatitis E

Hepatitis E is caused by infection with the hepatitis E virus (HEV). HEV transmission occurs via the same route as HAV, the fecal-oral route (usually through contaminated food or water). Risk factors for contracting HEV include travel to developing countries and fecal contamination of water or food. Person-to-person transmission is uncommon. Outbreaks of hepatitis E occur after heavy rainfall that disrupts and contaminates water supplies. It is prevalent in developing countries, especially those with hot climates. Hepatitis E is rare in the United States. It is most common in people from ages 15 to 40.

Symptoms of hepatitis E include jaundice, fatigue, abdominal pain, anorexia, nausea and vomiting, and dark urine. Patients with hepatitis E test positive for the hepatitis E antigen (HEV Ag). There is no treatment other than supportive care for hepatitis E.

Hepatitis E mortality rates are low. It is usually self-limiting and patients recover fully within a few weeks.

Cholelithiasis and Cholecystitis

Cholelithiasis—ICD-9-CM code: 574.20
Cholecystitis—ICD-9-CM code: 575.12

Cholelithiasis is a condition in which gallstones have developed and are present in the gallbladder, liver, biliary ducts, or all three locations. When inflammation of the gallbladder occurs along with cholelithiasis, the condition is known as *cholecystitis*. Cholelithiasis affects 20 million people in the United States, with up to 3% becoming symptomatic with cholecystitis. It occurs in both genders but most commonly affects women of childbearing age. Incidence increases with age. The ethnic groups most commonly affected include those of fair-skinned northern European descent, Native

Americans, and Hispanics. Less than 50% of people with cholelithiasis become symptomatic with acute cholecystitis.

The cause of cholelithiasis is not fully understood. Risk factors include a high-calorie, high-fat diet, obesity, oral contraceptive use, pancreatitis, and alcoholic cirrhosis. Gallstones most commonly develop from insoluble cholesterol but also from bile salts. The most common cause of cholecystitis is biliary duct obstruction by gallstones or crystallized bile sludge. The resulting increased pressure creates inflammation within the gallbladder. Other causes include infection, injury to the gallbladder, or underlying diseases such as diabetes.

People with cholelithiasis are commonly asymptomatic and may not realize that they have gallstones. If stones or sludge obstructs bile ducts, biliary colic ensues with symptoms of epigastric pain, commonly radiating into the right upper quadrant (RUQ), right shoulder, and back. Other symptoms include belching, bloating, fatty food intolerance, nausea, vomiting, muscle guarding, fever, tachycardia, jaundice, light-colored stools, dark urine, and pruritus, a tingling sensation that causes itching.

Diagnostic tests are unnecessary for cholelithiasis unless patients become symptomatic. Gallstones are commonly noted incidentally during a computed tomography (CT) scan or other tests done for other reasons. Diagnosis of cholecystitis is based on symptoms, an ultrasound that reveals wall thickening of more than 2 to 4 mm, distention, or fluid from perforation or exudates. Other tests may include oral cholecystogram, plain abdominal x-ray, or IV cholangiogram. Laboratory tests may reveal increased WBCs and, if obstruction is present, increased serum bilirubin.

If patients are asymptomatic, no treatment is indicated. However, diet should be modified to decrease fat intake. Nonsurgical treatment options that attempt to dissolve or disintegrate stones have shown limited success and are seldom used. Elective surgery may be advised for people at high risk for complications, including those with cirrhosis and portal hypertension. If a patient becomes acutely ill with cholecystitis, he may be hospitalized, placed on nothing-by-mouth status, and undergo nasogastric (NG) tube insertion. Other treatment may include antibiotics, antiemetics, analgesics, IV fluids, and electrolyte monitoring. The most definitive treatment for cholecystitis is cholecystectomy, which is the surgical removal of the gallbladder.

For patients who develop cholecystitis, prognosis is good with appropriate treatment. Complications of cholecystitis include biliary pancreatitis, perforation, and sepsis. Chronic cholecystitis may be a precursor to cancer of the gallbladder. The mortality rate for emergent cholecystectomy is 3% to 5%.

Acute Pancreatitis
ICD-9-CM code: 577.0
Acute pancreatitis is an inflammation of the pancreas. It is most common in men over age 55, possibly due to a higher rate of alcohol abuse in men than women. Black Americans are more likely than whites to develop pancreatitis. Congenital cystic fibrosis increases the risk of developing acute pancreatitis.

Acute pancreatitis is caused by pancreatic enzymes that normally remain inactive while in the pancreas and leave the pancreas through the pancreatic duct to the duodenum to digest food. In pancreatitis, the enzymes become activated while still in the pancreas and begin to digest pancreatic tissue. Chronic abuse of alcohol or an obstruction of the pancreatic duct by gallstones are the most common causes of pancreatitis. Less common causes include exposure to drugs such as diuretics and pentamidine (an antiprotozoal medication). Symptoms of acute pancreatitis include sudden onset of epigastric pain, nausea, and vomiting.

Serum analysis shows elevated pancreatic enzymes. Treatment consists of no food or drink and administration of IV fluids and electrolytes. Pain relievers and antiemetics are also administered intravenously. Feeding the patient too soon will result in a relapse of inflammation.

The degree of pancreatic inflammation can vary from mild to severe. In most patients it will resolve within a few days or weeks. However, in 5% of patients it may be so severe that multiple organ system failure, shock, and death occur. Assessment of the severity of pancreatitis is based on the evaluation of several factors. (See *APACHE II*.) These factors, along with liver function and abnormalities seen on a computed tomography (CT) scan, are used to determine prognosis.

Disorders of Nutrition
Nutritional disorders can arise from a food intolerance and an inability to absorb nutrients, as in celiac disease, or emotional disorders that compromise healthy eating habits, as

---

APACHE II

The acute physiology and chronic health evaluation II (APACHE II) system evaluates several factors to arrive at a numerical score. This score is compared to a severity scale that indicates the degree of pancreatitis. The factors evaluated include:

- body temperature
- heart rate
- mean arterial pressure
- respiratory rate
- serum creatinine and sodium levels
- arterial pH
- white blood cell count
- Glasgow coma scale
- age.

in anorexia nervosa and bulimia. Strict dietary guidelines for patients with celiac disease can help them eat foods that are tolerated and ensure adequate nutrition. Nutritional disorders that are related to body dysmorphia, in which poor eating habits result from the patient thinking she is too fat, must be treated with physical and psychological therapies to restore the body. The medical assistant can assist the physician in treating a patient with a nutritional disorder by providing the patient with nutritional information and emotional support.

Celiac Disease
ICD-9-CM code: 579.0

Celiac disease, also called *sprue* or *gluten enteropathy,* involves an intolerance to the gluten found in wheat, wheat products, oats, and barley. The intolerance to these foods causes damage to the mucosal lining of the small intestine, which hinders nutrient absorption. Celiac disease is twice as common in women as in men and affects 1 in every 133 people in the United States. Although the exact cause of celiac disease is unknown, it may be the result of an immune response.

Symptoms include abdominal distention, gas, anorexia, cramping, and steatorrhea, which is diarrhea of greasy, pale, foul-smelling stools. Other symptoms may include aphthous ulcers (small ulcers of the mouth), fatigue, and bone or joint pain. Eventually, symptoms of malnutrition related to malabsorption appear.

Blood tests reveal elevated WBC count, platelet count, and IgA level as well as increased prothrombin time and albumin level. Radiographic studies of the upper gastrointestinal system and small intestine may reveal inflammation of the mucosal lining. Definitive diagnosis is determined though tissue biopsy and improvement of symptoms while eating a gluten-free diet.

A strict gluten-free diet is the major treatment for celiac disease. However, if symptoms persist despite a change in diet, the physician may prescribe corticosteroid medication to suppress inflammation of the small intestines. Patients generally recover by strictly adhering to dietary guidelines. Complications may include osteoporosis, infertility, depression, and, later, development of abdominal cancer.

Anorexia Nervosa
ICD-9-CM code: 307.1

Anorexia nervosa is a physical and psychiatric disorder. It involves a combination of an intense fear of weight gain and severe, self-imposed restriction of food intake. Anorexia nervosa affects 0.5% to 1% of Americans, most commonly highly intelligent young women who are high achievers.

The exact cause of anorexia nervosa is not well understood. There is a psychological component and there may be a genetic one as well. Characteristics of anorexia nervosa include self-imposed starvation, dysmorphia (a distorted body image), obsession with food, and a compulsion to be thin. Malnutrition and weight loss may be mild or severe. Menstrual periods cease as body fat drops below normal.

Diagnosis is based on health history, weight loss to lower than 15% of ideal body weight, and such behaviors as eating pattern, refusal to maintain normal weight, and an intense fear of gaining weight. An electrocardiogram (ECG) may reveal arrhythmias due to electrolyte imbalance.

A team approach is vital to effective management of anorexia nervosa. Members of the team may include physicians, nurses, psychiatric-mental health professionals, and nutritionists. A primary goal is to restore normal body weight and healthy eating behaviors as well as a normalized body image. Underlying psychological issues must be addressed to prevent recurrence or worsening of symptoms. In severe cases, patients may be hospitalized for fluid, electrolyte, and nutritional replacement.

Prognosis is variable and depends on the adequacy and timeliness of interventions as well as the individual's acceptance of psychological therapy. Complications include heart failure, osteoporosis, and loss of muscle mass and strength. The mortality rate of 5% to 20% is higher than for any other psychiatric illness.

Bulimia
ICD-9-CM code: 307.51

Bulimia is a physical and psychiatric disorder. It involves a combination of obsessive eating of large quantities of food and purging behaviors. Bulimia most commonly affects women (80% of all cases) with 1% to 2% of all young women in America suffering from it.

The underlying causes of bulimia are similar to those for anorexia nervosa, including such psychological issues as a feeling of lack of control. There may also be issues of depression, conflict, anger, denial, and perfectionism. Binge and purge episodes are commonly triggered by emotional distress.

The key characteristic of bulimia is an identified pattern of binge eating (eating large quantities of food at one time) followed by purging through self-induced vomiting, excessive laxative and diuretic use, and extreme exercise. Esophagitis and gingivitis may develop and teeth may begin to erode due to frequent exposure to stomach acids. Eyes may display small broken vessels from the stress of self-induced vomiting. Weight may be normal but commonly fluctuates.

Diagnostic criteria include a pattern of binging and purging more than twice per week for at least 3 months. Patients may lose muscle mass and suffer effects of low electrolyte levels, such as cardiac arrhythmias.

In addition to psychological therapy, treatment for bulimia includes administration of antidepressants. Nutritional counseling and referral to a support group may also be helpful. Prognosis is variable and depends on the adequacy and timeliness of treatment interventions as well as the individual's acceptance of psychological therapy. Complications include heart failure and life-threatening hemorrhage caused by the rupture of esophageal vessels, the esophageal wall, or even the stomach.

Disorders That Commonly Cause Diarrhea

The causes of food poisoning and infection with *Escherichia coli*, *Campylobacter*, or *Salmonella* vary, yet all have the common key sign of diarrhea. Because health care providers begin the diagnostic process by considering a possible list of diagnoses, the physician will consider these disorders when a patient complains of diarrhea. Although the physician may use a variety of methods to confirm a diagnosis, in most cases, she will order analysis and culture of a stool specimen. All of these disorders put patients at risk for dehydration, which may become profound in some cases. Thus, measures to prevent or treat dehydration are a high priority. The medical assistant may need to instruct the patient on the proper technique for collecting a stool sample. She will also receive that sample from the patient and must adhere to OSHA guidelines regarding safety for storage and transport of body fluids.

Food Poisoning
ICD-9-CM code: 005.9

Food poisoning is a common term for a number of illnesses. Another common term for this type of illness is *dysentery*. People of any age may be affected. Food poisoning is caused by the ingestion of food that has spoiled or is contaminated by bacteria, toxins, insecticides, lead, mercury, and other substances. Common bacterial causes include *Campylobacter*, *Salmonella*, and *E. coli*. Other causes include viral and parasitic infections. The major sign of food poisoning is diarrhea, which starts 2 to 6 hours after eating the offending food. Other signs and symptoms include abdominal cramping, vomiting, fever, weakness, and headache. The term *food poisoning* and its associated ICD-9-CM code is used to diagnose a condition when the signs and symptoms point to a food-borne illness but laboratory results identifying the offending organism are not yet available. Diagnostic tests include testing emesis and blood for the suspected pathogen. Treatment depends on the infecting organism but generally includes rest and fluids. Prognosis is generally good with a full recovery being the most common outcome.

E. *Coli* Infection
ICD-9-CM code: 041.4

There are numerous strains of *E. coli*, many of which are harmless. Other strains are a common cause of intestinal and urinary tract infections. In 1982, the CDC identified a dangerous strain of *E. coli* named *O157:H7*, which refers to chemical compounds found on the bacterium's surface. It produces toxins that can cause severe damage to the intestinal lining and bloody diarrhea. There are approximately 71,000 cases of *E. coli* infection per year in the United States.

The most common source of *E. coli* O157:H7 is cattle; however, other mammals, domestic and wild, may also harbor it. People are usually infected by ingesting undercooked or raw hamburger as well as salami, alfalfa sprouts, lettuce, unpasteurized milk, apple juice, apple cider, and contaminated well water. Those swimming in contaminated water may also become infected.

Those with mild infection may be asymptomatic. Symptoms of severe infection typically begin 2 to 5 days after exposure and include bloody diarrhea and abdominal cramps, nausea, and fatigue. Other symptoms may include low-grade fever and vomiting.

Diagnosis is determined by symptoms and a stool culture. Conservative treatment for *E. coli* infection, including rest and oral fluids, is usually sufficient. In severe cases, hospitalization is needed for IV rehydration and treatment of complications.

Symptoms usually resolve within 8 days. Patients whose primary symptom is diarrhea usually recover completely. Those with more serious infections may suffer kidney impairment or failure and associated complications.

Campylobacter Infection
ICD-9-CM code: 005.8

Infection with the bacteria of the genus *Campylobacter* results in intestinal illness. According to the Centers for Disease Control and Prevention (CDC), nearly 2½ million people are affected each year by bacterial diarrheal illness caused by *Campylobacter*. Persons most commonly affected are children under the age of 5 and young adults.

There are several strains of the *Campylobacter* bacteria; however, *C. jejuni* is responsible for most cases of intestinal illness. It is spread by ingestion of contaminated food, most commonly undercooked poultry or drippings from raw poultry and contaminated water or raw milk. It may also be transmitted via infected animals and human feces.

Those infected with *Campylobacter* may be asymptomatic but usually develop diarrhea (possibly bloody), abdominal cramps and pain, fatigue, and fever. Symptoms usually appear within 2 to 5 days of exposure. Other symptoms may include nausea and vomiting.

Diagnosis is generally based on symptoms and culture of a stool specimen. Conservative treatment is usually sufficient and includes rest and fluids.

Most people recover fully after a week or so. However, those with a weakened immune system may develop septicemia. There are approximately 100 deaths each year from *Campylobacter* infection.

Salmonella Infection
ICD-9-CM code: 003.0

Salmonellosis is an intestinal infection caused by the *Salmonella* organism. Numerous types of this bacteria cause infections in animals and people. However, the species *S. typhimurium* and *S. enteritidis* are most common in the United States. An antibiotic-resistant strain known as *S. typhimurium* definitive type (DT) 104 is the next most common strain in the United States. Infections with *Salmonella* account for 1 billion dollars in direct and indirect health care costs. Outbreaks usually occur in small, contained segments of the general population or there may be large outbreaks in hospitals, restaurants, or facilities for children or the elderly. In North America and Europe, most outbreaks are reported, with approximately 40,000 cases being reported to the CDC annually.

Infection is spread via contaminated reptiles and mammals, undercooked poultry and beef, eggs, and the contaminated feces of those who are infected. Other sources may include unwashed fruits and alfalfa sprouts grown in contaminated soil.

Those infected with *Salmonella* develop symptoms within 12 to 72 hours and report fever, headache, diarrhea, and abdominal cramps. Other symptoms may include nausea, vomiting, and anorexia. Those most severely affected typically include the very young, the very old, and those with chronic illness or a weakened immune system.

Diagnosis is based on symptoms and a stool culture. Treatment includes rest and fluid replacement. (See *Treating dehydration*.) Antimicrobials are usually not needed. Severe cases may require hospitalization.

Patient Education

Treating Dehydration
To help a patient prevent or treat dehydration, the medical assistant should encourage liberal intake of recommended fluids and avoidance of fluids that exacerbate dehydration.

Recommended Fluids
- water
- fruit juice (diluted to reduce stomach irritation)
- electrolyte sports drinks (diluted to reduce stomach irritation)
- Jell-O
- popsicles
- broth.

Fluids to Avoid
- caffeinated beverages
- alcoholic beverages.

The illness usually lasts 4 to 7 days and most people recover fully without treatment. However, in some cases, severe diarrhea may result in dehydration and the need for hospitalization. A possible complication is septicemia. It is estimated that nearly $1^{1}/_{2}$ million people are infected annually, with 1,000 related deaths.

Cancers of the GI System

Cancer may develop anywhere in the GI system, although most malignancies occur in the mouth, esophagus, stomach, and colon as well as the pancreas and liver. Incidence varies with the type of cancer. Causes are variable, although tobacco use is a major contributor for nearly all types. Some forms of cancer commonly invade nearby structures by the time of diagnosis. Prognosis is generally poor in these cases. Diagnostics may include a variety of radiologic and laboratory tests. However, in most cases, tissue biopsy is needed to confirm diagnosis. Treatment nearly always involves surgical excision or resection if the cancer is still localized. However, once metastasis has occurred, surgery may only provide palliative value. Many patients also elect to undergo chemotherapy or radiation therapy for curative or palliative reasons. If patients with liver cancer qualify, they may undergo a transplant, cryoablation, or ethanol injection. With advanced malignancy of all kinds, palliative care is focused on pain relief, comfort, and maximizing function and quality of life.

Oral Cancer
ICD-9-CM code: 145.9 (mouth, unspecified)

Oral cancer includes cancerous tissue changes of any oral structure, including the lips, tongue, gums, inner cheek, or mouth floor. Oral cancer makes up 8% of all forms of malignancy, with more than 30,000 new cases diagnosed each year. It is twice as common in men as in women, and most prevalent in those over age 40. However, an elevated incidence is also seen among young men who use chewing tobacco.

Risk factors include use of chewing tobacco (80% of cases), alcohol use, poor oral hygiene, jagged teeth, and poorly fitting dentures. The most common symptom of oral cancer is the development of white, patchy lesions or mouth ulcers called *leukoplakia*. These lesions fail to heal. Such lesions are usually nontender until late in the disease process. Other symptoms include dysphagia, bleeding, referred pain to the ear or jaw, and weight loss.

Diagnosis is based on physical examination findings and tissue biopsy. Staging is done via contrast-enhanced CT scan, which may also identify bone and cartilage invasion. Treatment depends on whether the cancer is localized or has spread. Surgery to remove cancerous tissue is common and may include lymph node dissection. Radiation therapy and chemotherapy are commonly used to destroy the remaining cancer cells after surgical resection. In some cases, hyperthermia (heat therapy) is used as well.

Oral cancers tend to spread quickly and invade bone and liver and lung tissues. As a result, the 5-year survival rate for oral cancer is only 50%. More than 8,000 people in the United States die from oral cancer each year.

Esophageal Cancer
ICD-9-CM code: 150.9

Esophageal cancer develops in tissue cells in the lower esophageal lining. Such cancer is nearly always squamous cell carcinoma (SCC) but may be adenocarcinoma as well. SCC rates are highest in populations of Iran, Asia, and Africa. Adenocarcinoma rates are highest in Caucasians. Those most commonly affected are males over age 55.

Risk factors for SCC and adenocarcinoma include alcohol and tobacco use, obesity, swallowing caustic substances, poor nutrition, and GERD. Underlying disorders, such as stricture (narrowing of the esophagus) and achalasia (persistent contraction of the esophagus), are also contributing factors. Early symptoms include dysphagia, weight loss, substernal pain, the sensation of pressure or burning, and hoarseness of the voice.

Diagnosis is based on symptoms as well as x-rays, which reveal a mass, and barium swallow and tissue biopsy via upper endoscopy, which differentiate cancerous and benign lesions. Esophageal cancer is usually treated with surgery, chemotherapy, or radiation, depending on the stage of the cancer and the patient's general heath. Surgery involves an esophagectomy (removal of the esophagus) or esophagogastrectomy (removal of the lower esophagus and upper stomach).

Prognosis depends on how early the cancer is detected. There is a 30% rate of metastasis to the liver, bone, or lungs. If metastasis occurs, the prognosis becomes less favorable.

Gastric Cancer
ICD-9-CM code: 151.9

Gastric cancer occurs in tissue cells of the stomach wall. Populations with the highest rates of gastric cancer include Japanese and African American men over the age of 50.

Risk factors for the development of gastric cancer include Barrett's syndrome (replacement of the squamous epithelium of the esophagus with columnar epithelium from chronic exposure to stomach acid), infection with *H. pylori* early in life, genetics, and diet. High-risk diets include those high in complex carbohydrates but low in fresh fruits, vegetables, and fiber.

People with gastric cancer are commonly asymptomatic. As the cancer advances, symptoms include weight loss, abdominal pain, nausea, vomiting, fatigue, dysphagia, feelings of fullness, anorexia, or abdominal mass. Melena (black, tarry stools caused by the digestion of blood in the gastrointestinal tract) can also be an indication of gastric cancer.

Diagnosis is based on symptoms, health history, and contrast barium study and gastroscopy, which provide a visualization of the tumor. A CT scan may be done to detect metastasis and stage tumors. Treatment of gastric cancer depends on staging. Surgery includes a partial or total gastrectomy, radiation, or chemotherapy.

In half of all patients with gastric cancer, metastasis has occurred by the time of diagnosis. Recurrence after remission is common, with an overall 5-year survival rate of only 20%.

Colorectal Cancer
ICD-9-CM code: 154

Colorectal cancer is one of the most common types of cancer. It affects the large intestine and rectal area. Colorectal cancer is the second leading cause of cancer-related deaths in the United States, with nearly 150,000 new cases diagnosed each year. More than 90% of cases occur in persons over age 50.

Risk factors include a history of inflammatory bowel disease (IBD) and family history of colorectal cancer. Lifestyle factors may include sedentary lifestyle; a low-fiber, high-fat diet; obesity; and alcohol and tobacco use. Patients are commonly asymptomatic in the early stage. Potential symptoms include a change in bowel elimination pattern, blood in the stools, abdominal pain, pallor, anemia, and intestinal obstruction.

Diagnostic tests include fecal occult blood test to detect blood in stools and a barium enema and lower endoscopy with tissue biopsy to visualize a mass and obtain tissue for analysis. Treatment for colorectal cancer depends on the location and stage and includes surgery, chemotherapy, or radiation therapy. Newer forms of treatment also include medications that help to shrink cancerous tumors or inhibit blood flow to tumors.

Among those who experience early detection, the survival rate is 90%. However, in 61% of cases, metastasis has occurred by the time of diagnosis. More than 50,000 people die each year from colorectal cancer.

Liver Cancer
ICD-9-CM code: 155.0

Cancer of the liver is usually secondary to metastasis from other sites. Primary liver cancer is uncommon. Liver cancer is the number-one cause of cancer death in Africa and Asia and the fifth most common cancer worldwide. It is becoming more common in the United States due to the prevalence of hepatitis B and C.

Contributing factors include previous infection with hepatitis B or C. Particularly in patients with a history of chronic hepatitis B or C, the immune system attacks hepatocytes (liver cells) in an attempt to combat the virus. The repeated attack on liver cells can cause mutations in the cells and the formation of cancer. Hepatitis B and C infections contribute to 20% of all cases of liver cancer. Cirrhosis, resulting from alcohol abuse and exposure to toxins, contributes to 80% of liver cancer cases.

Symptoms of liver cancer are similar to those of chronic liver disease and include abdominal pain, hepatomegaly, weight loss, poor appetite, ascites, splenomegaly, and jaundice.

Liver function tests reveal elevated alpha-fetoprotein (AFP) over 500 g/L. Other diagnostic tests include CT or MRI scans, which reveal the presence of tumors. Biopsy for histological analysis may be done but is considered risky. Treatment of liver cancer commonly includes surgery to remove the tumor. Occasionally, the physician may consider liver transplantation. About 100 transplants occur annually for this reason. Other mainstays of treatment include chemotherapy and radiation therapy.

Liver cancer commonly metastasizes to the bones, lungs, brain, peritoneum, and adrenal glands. If metastasis is present, prognosis is poor.

Pancreatic Cancer

ICD-9-CM code: 157.9 (part unspecified)

Pancreatic cancer is a malignant tumor of the pancreas, 95% of which are adenocarcinomas, a tumor of the endocrine glands of the pancreas. The remaining 5% are tumors of the exocrine glands of the pancreas and are called *serous cystadenomas.* Pancreatic cancer, specifically adenocarcinoma, is the fourth most common cause of cancer-related death in the United States, with 32,000 deaths per year. It is most common in men ages 40 to 60.

Risk factors include family history of pancreatic cancer, high fat and meat diet, cigarette smoking, and a history of chronic pancreatitis or diabetes. Pancreatic cancer is commonly asymptomatic in the early stages and commonly goes undetected until it is advanced. Occasionally, pancreatic masses are detected when the patient is undergoing radiologic procedures for other purposes. Symptoms include abdominal pain, nausea, vomiting, weight loss, anorexia, jaundice, steatorrhea, hepatomegaly, weakness, fatigue, and diarrhea.

Diagnosis is based on health history and physical examination findings as well as abdominal ultrasound, CT scan, endoscopic retrograde pancreatography (ERCP), and a MRI scan, which enable visual confirmation of tumors. Blood testing includes liver function tests that may reveal elevated bilirubin and alkaline phosphatase, indicating bile duct obstruction (common in pancreatic cancer). A biopsy is required for definitive diagnosis. Surgery is generally useful only when pancreatic cancer is detected early or when the surgery is done for palliative purposes. Radiation and chemotherapy are commonly used.

Although serous cystadenomas respond favorably to chemotherapy, the prognosis for pancreatic cancer from adenocarcinomas is very poor. Patients who elect to undergo high-risk surgery known as the *Whipple procedure* have a 5-year survival rate of only 10% to 25%. For those who do not have this surgery, the survival rate is just over 3%.

Gastroenterology Procedures

Gastroenterology is the study of the GI system, including all structures from the mouth to the anus. A physician who specializes in the diagnosis and treatment of diseases and disorders of the GI tract and accessory organs is called a ***gastroenterologist.*** The role of the medical assistant in the gastroenterologist's office is to obtain vital signs and a health history and to assist with procedures. The medical assistant must have knowledge and understanding of the structure and function of the GI system. A thorough and complete history of the patient's symptoms is necessary for the physician to make a diagnosis, including eating habits, bowel habits, and family history. The medical assistant may be expected to administer an **enema,** a procedure in which fluid is introduced into the rectum to stimulate bowel activity and cause emptying of the lower intestines. She will also be expected to provide patient instruction for further testing and health maintenance. The gastroenterologist's office may have a standard form prepared for the medical assistant to fill in during the patient interview. (See *Common GI interview questions.*)

Assisting with Examination

The medical assistant working in the gastroenterologist's office will assist with various procedures. Because such procedures are commonly invasive and require that the patient disrobe, the medical assistant should attempt to ease the patient's anxiety by conveying a professional demeanor and attending to the patient's modesty and comfort. Such procedures include stool specimen collection with a fecal occult blood test, flexible sigmoidoscopy, and cleansing enema.

Common GI interview questions

The patient interview will vary depending on the medical specialty and the individual patient. Here are some common interview questions used during a gastrointestinal (GI) examination conducted at a gastroenterologist's office:

- Describe your typical daily meals.
- How often do you have a bowel movement?
- Do you ever experience diarrhea or constipation?
- Do you ever experience difficulty chewing or swallowing food?
- Do you ever experience heartburn?
- Do have pain before, during, or after eating?
- Does anyone in your family have stomach problems?
- Describe any stress you may have in your life.

Stool Specimen Collection

A stool specimen is commonly difficult for a patient to collect, so thorough patient instruction is essential. To enable accurate detection of bacteria, viruses, ova, or parasites in stool, the collection must not be contaminated. Specifically, urine will destroy microorganisms within the sample, so the patient must avoid allowing urine to enter the stool sample. The patient must use the sterile container and proper technique to avoid contamination. Proper patient education is vital to obtaining a useful sample. The medical assistant should instruct the patient to bring the stool sample to the office. She should then forward the sample to the laboratory for analysis. She must properly label the sample and refrigerate it if there is a delay in transport to the laboratory. (See *Procedure 30-1: Instructing the patient on collecting a stool specimen.*)

Fecal Occult Blood Test

A fecal occult blood test, sometimes referred to as a *stool card,* screens for hidden blood in a patient's stool. Because blood should not be present in any part of the colon, rectum, or anus, its presence may indicate disease. Two days before collecting the specimens, the patient must refrain from eating red meat or any food that contains red dyes and avoid intake of aspirin and aspirin products, vitamin C, and iron supplements. Intake of these things may lead to false-positive test results. The patient should also increase fiber in his diet to promote a bowel movement. Patient instruction is essential for proper collection of the specimens. Although instructions are listed on the test cards, the medical assistant should instruct the patient on the collection procedure to promote understanding. She should also be sure to tell the patient that the stool specimens should not be collected during menstruation or if bleeding hemorrhoids are present. The patient collects a stool sample and smears a small amount on the test card three different times, after which he must bring the test cards to the office for evaluation or mail them. (See Figure 30-8.) If mailed, U.S. Postal regulations permit the cards to be mailed in the mailing pouch provided, not a standard envelope. If the patient brings the cards in, the medical assistant should confirm with the patient that he followed the dietary, vitamin, and medication restrictions during the collection of the samples before she performs the test. (See *Procedure 30-2: Performing an occult blood test,* page 560.)

PROCEDURE 30-1

Instructing a patient on collecting a stool specimen

Task
Instruct a patient on how to collect a stool specimen.

Conditions
- Specimen container with lid
- Laboratory request form
- Patient's medical record
- Pen
- Plastic wrap

Standards
In the time specified and within the scoring parameters determined by the instructor, the student will successfully instruct a patient on collecting an adequate stool specimen for laboratory analysis.

Performance Standards
1. Assemble the items next to the patient to show the patient the sample container.
2. Identify the patient and explain the physician's orders for a stool sample.
3. Instruct the patient to defecate onto the plastic wrap to avoid toilet water from mixing with the sample.
4. Instruct the patient to obtain 3 to 4 tablespoons of stool (to ensure a quantity sufficient for laboratory testing) from the plastic wrap and place it in the specimen container.

5. Explain to the patient that he should be sure to avoid getting any toilet paper or urine in the container because these items could interfere with test results.
6. Tell the patient to write his name and the date and time on the container to ensure proper identification and seal the container.
7. Tell the patient to bring the sample in the closed container to the office for laboratory testing.
8. To prevent the growth of bacteria that could interfere with test results, instruct the patient to keep the sample refrigerated if he cannot transport it to the office within 2 hours.
9. Ask the patient if he understands the instructions and answer any questions he may have to ensure patient understanding and promote accurate collection procedures.
10. Document in the patient's medical record all patient education performed as well as the patient's understanding of the procedure to ensure a complete, accurate medical record.

Date	
05/26/08: 9:45 a.m.	Verbal and written instructions for stool collection given to patient. pt. understands, states he will bring sample to the office tomorrow morning. ———————————— C. Chapin, CMA

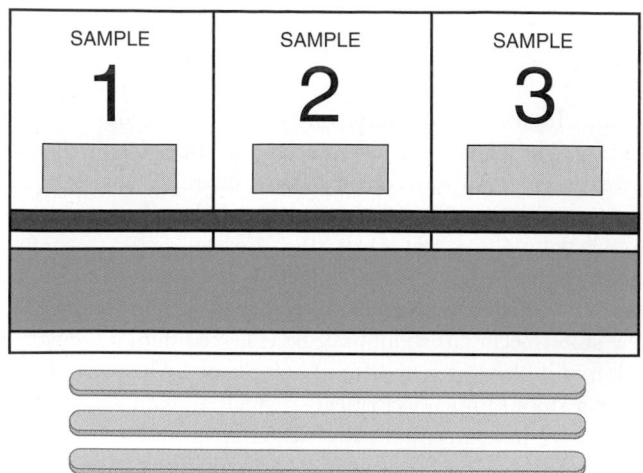

FIG 30-8 Fecal occult blood test cards.

Flexible Sigmoidoscopy

A flexible sigmoidoscopy is a procedure that uses a specialized flexible scope, called a *sigmoidoscope,* to view the sigmoid colon and obtain biopsies of tissues that may be diseased. The examination helps diagnose cancer of the colon, polyps, tumors, ulcerations, and bleeding. Polyps are areas of swelling of the mucous membrane of the colon and can cause bleeding. Although they may be benign, they can become malignant later. Therefore, removal is best to prevent malignancy.

Because the chances of a good prognosis increase with early detection, yearly flexible sigmoidoscopy is recommended for all adults after age 50.

When scheduling a patient for a flexible sigmoidoscopy, the medical assistant must give the patient instructions on how to prepare for the examination. Those instructions should include having a light, low-residue dinner the day before the procedure or a clear liquid diet the entire day before the procedure, as directed by the physician. The physician may also indicate that the patient should have an enema the night before or the morning of the procedure. (See *Cleansing enema at home.*)

The medical assistant may assist the physician with a flexible sigmoidoscopy. During the procedure, she should be sure to promote the patient's privacy and comfort. (See *Procedure 30-3: Assisting with flexible sigmoidoscopy.*)

Cleansing Enema

Although it is not a common procedure, sometimes the medical assistant will have to perform a cleansing enema to adequately prepare a patient for sigmoidoscopy. Patient home preparation for the sigmoidoscopy should clean out the colon. However, if the physician begins the rectal examination and finds that the colon is not sufficiently cleansed, a cleansing enema can be performed in the office prior to the sigmoidoscopy. (See *Procedure 30-4: Performing a cleansing enema,* page 562.)

■ PROCEDURE 30-2

Performing an occult blood test

Task
Perform an occult blood test on a stool specimen.

Conditions
- Nonsterile disposable gloves
- Hemoccult slides with stool samples (stool cards) provided by the patient
- Developer
- Timer or clock
- Biohazard bag
- Patient's medical record
- Pen

Standards
In the time specified and within the scoring parameters determined by the instructor, the student will successfully test a stool specimen for occult blood.

Performance Standards
1. Wash your hands and apply gloves to ensure infection control.
2. Open the test side of the hemoccult paper slide.

3. Place two drops of developer onto the sections of the reagent paper. To avoid contaminating the slide, be sure to avoid touching the paper with the dropper.
4. Immediately begin timing for 1 minute. At 30 seconds, watch the slide for color changes around the edges of the stool sample.
5. Place an additional drop of developer between the positive and negative control areas to ensure that the controls are in good condition.
6. At 60 seconds, compare the test areas with the control area.
7. Record the results in the patient's medical record.
8. Dispose of the cards and sample container in the biohazard bag to ensure infection control.

Date	
10/16/08; 9:30 a.m.	*Hemoccult slides 1. pos. 2. pos. 3. neg. ------- W. Jones, CMA*

Patient Education

Cleansing Enema at Home

In order to evacuate the bowel of feces, the physician will commonly order a cleansing enema for the patient. Most patients have never given themselves an enema and may be uncomfortable and unsure about the procedure. Thus, the medical assistant can teach the patient how to carry out this procedure at home.

First, the medical assistant should advise the patient to buy a Fleet enema kit at the local pharmacy or give the patient the enema kit in the office. She should instruct the patient to follow the directions on the kit and emphasize these points:

- Take your time and have privacy for the procedure.
- Use an old towel to lie on to avoid ruining bedding.
- Warm the enema solution under running water, not in the microwave, to avoid overheating the solution.
- Apply a small amount of lubricant to the tip of the nozzle before insertion to make insertion easier.
- Lie on your left side, relax, and retain the solution for 5 to 10 minutes, as directed on the package.
- Then go to the toilet to evacuate the bowels.

GI System Tests

Physicians commonly order laboratory tests to diagnose the cause of a patient's intestinal complaint. If laboratory tests are inconclusive, more invasive testing may be required, including barium studies of the upper and lower GI tract and ultrasounds of the gallbladder and internal visceral organs.

Helicobacter Pylori

The presence of *Helicobacter pylori* in the stomach is the most common cause of ulcers. The physician who suspects *H. pylori* as the cause of gastric distress can order a blood test that will detect the presence of antibodies to *H. pylori*. If the blood test is inconclusive and the physician still suspects *H. pylori*, she can order a gastric biopsy to culture and grow the bacteria. The physician will order the less invasive blood test first to avoid unnecessary patient discomfort.

Liver Function Test

A liver function test (LFT) is a blood test that determines the liver's ability to perform its many complex functions. Enzyme levels found in serum, including aspartate aminotransferase (AST) and alanine aminotransferase (ALT), indicate damage to liver cells, biliary tract obstruction, and dysfunction. When liver cells die due to liver disease, these enzymes are released into the bloodstream. Elevated AST and ALT levels can

---

PROCEDURE 30-3

Assisting with flexible sigmoidoscopy

Task
Assist the physician and the patient during sigmoidoscopy.

Conditions
- Nonsterile disposable gloves
- Flexible sigmoidoscope
- Water-soluble lubricant
- Sterile specimen container with preservative
- 4" × 4" gauze squares
- Tissue wipes
- Drape
- Biopsy forceps
- Biohazard container
- Patient's medical record
- Pen

Standards
In the time specified and within the scoring parameters determined by the instructor, the student will successfully assist the physician in a flexible sigmoidoscopy examination.

Performance Standards
1. Wash or sanitize your hands to promote infection control.

2. Assemble supplies, making sure supplies are situated for easy access by the physician. Check the light source on the sigmoidoscope to ensure that it is working.

3. Greet and identify the patient and explain the examination procedure to ensure that the procedure is performed on the correct patient and that the patient will cooperate.

4. Ask the patient if he needs to empty his bladder prior to the examination. An empty bladder reduces pressure, making the examination more tolerable.

5. Give the patient a gown and drape and ask him to remove all clothing from the waist down. Instruct him to put the gown on with the opening in the back and sit on the examination table with the drape over his lap.

6. Knock before re-entering the room to ensure patient privacy while disrobing.

7. When the physician is ready to proceed, position the patient in the Sims (left lateral) position to provide access to the rectum.

8. Drape the patient so that the corner of the drape can be lifted to expose the anus to provide warmth and privacy.

Continued

PROCEDURE 30-3—cont'd

9. Ask the patient if he is comfortable. Ask him to breathe slowly and deeply to help him relax and encourage him to relax the muscles of the anus and rectum.
10. Lubricate the physician's gloved hand for ease of examination just before the digital rectal examination.
11. To ease insertion of the sigmoidoscope, lubricate the end of it before handing it to the physician.
12. Assist the physician with suction as required.
13. Ask the patient if he is comfortable to comfort and reassure him.
14. Assist the physician with collection of a biopsy as needed. Hand the biopsy forceps to the physician and hold the specimen container to receive specimens. Do not touch the inside of the container to avoid contaminating it.
15. Place the cover on the specimen container and place the container on the counter for transport to the laboratory.
16. When the examination is complete, apply clean gloves and clean the patient's anal area with tissues to remove excess lubricant.
17. Remove your gloves and wash your hands to ensure infection control.

18. Assist the patient to a sitting position and allow him to rest to prevent postural hypotension and fainting. Ask him if he feels faint or dizzy. If he does, allow him to sit and observe him until he feels better to ensure patient safety.
19. Assist the patient off the examination table and allow him to dress and use the restroom so that the patient can expel air that was used to inflate the colon during the procedure.
20. Prepare the laboratory requisition form and accompanying specimens to ensure their proper labeling.
21. Clean the examination room to ensure cleanliness for the next patient.
22. Document the procedure in the patient's medical record.

Date	
09/26/08: 9:45 a.m.	Sigmoidoscopy with 1 bx of lesion on anterior wall at 7 inches, sent to lab. Pad placed over anal area for light bleeding. Patient instructed to call the office if bleeding continues. Follow-up when lab results receieved. ----------- -- S. Gonzales, CMA

PROCEDURE 30-4

Performing a cleansing enema

Task
Perform a cleansing enema.

Conditions
- Disposable nonsterile gloves
- Prepackaged disposable enema
- Water-soluble lubricant
- Mayo tray
- Towel
- Drape
- Tissues
- Patient's medical record
- Pen

Standard
In the time specified and within the scoring parameters determined by the instructor, the student will successfully administer a cleansing enema.

Performance Standards
1. Wash your hands to promote infection control and assemble supplies.

2. Explain the procedure to the patient to promote patient cooperation and understanding. (*Note:* Use an anatomical model or chart to explain the procedure to the patient if necessary.)
3. Ask the patient to disrobe from the waist down and put on a gown with the opening towards the back. Provide a drape and ask him to sit on the examination table with the drape across his lap.
4. Assist the patient into the Sims position (lying on his left side and bringing his right knee up towards the waist) to provide access to the rectum.
5. Remove the cover of the enema container and inspect the container to ensure that it is clean and there are no defects in the plastic that could cause discomfort.
6. Warm the enema solution to body temperature in warm water at the sink to make it easier for the patient to retain the solution.
7. Apply a small amount of lubricant to the tip of the container to ease entrance into the rectum.
8. Adjust the drape sheet to expose the buttocks.

PROCEDURE 30-4—cont'd

9. With one hand, separate the buttocks to expose the anus. Hold the enema bottle with the other hand and insert it into the anus. Point the tip of the bottle toward the patient's abdomen to follow the direction of the rectum.

10. Advise the patient to breathe deeply and slowly and to relax his abdomen to enable instillation of the solution.

11. Squeeze the bottle slowly to promote relaxation and enable the patient to retain the solution and express all of the solution into the patient's body.

12. Tell the patient that you will withdraw the enema tip and then do so slowly so that the patient is able to retain the fluid.

13. Provide the patient with a tissue to hold against the anus to prevent leaking and ask him to retain the liquid as long as possible to promote cleansing of the bowel.

14. Discard the enema container and tissues in a biohazardous waste container because these items are contaminated with body fluids.

15. Allow the patient to lie quietly for 5 to 10 minutes and then direct him to the restroom. Ask him to allow you to check the results before flushing them to ensure adequate cleansing. If the results seem inadequate, consult with the physician and repeat the procedure if necessary.

16. While the patient is in the restroom, clean the examination room in preparation for the examination or sigmoidoscopy.

17. Wash your hands to ensure infection control.

18. Document the procedure in the patient's medical record.

Date	
10/07/08; 11:45 a.m.	*Administered cleansing enema (fleet). Pt. tolerated procedure. good results. Pt. ready for sigmoidoscopy.* --- *S. Gonzales, CMA*

indicate liver dysfunction. Levels of ammonia and bilirubin found in blood are also commonly elevated in patients with liver dysfunction. The liver is also responsible for the synthesis of many blood-clotting factors; quantitative analysis of these substances can be used to assess liver damage. In addition to the blood test, the physician will observe the patient for liver dysfunction by the appearance of jaundice, a yellow discoloration of the skin due to an inability of the liver to eliminate bilirubin from the bloodstream. Further testing may include a liver biopsy if the LFT indicates dysfunction. (See *Statin drugs and the liver,* page 564.)

Upper GI X-ray

Because none of the structures of the GI tract are visible on x-ray, an upper GI x-ray involves the use of a contrast medium to help visualize organs. The medical assistant commonly schedules the procedures and sometimes assists during the procedure.

The upper GI x-ray, also known as *UGI,* views the throat, esophagus, and stomach. The examination takes 15 to 20 minutes. During the procedure, the patient must drink barium, a radiopaque substance, to increase visualization of these structures. Many physicians now use a substance similar to Alka-Seltzer combined with a small amount of water prior to the barium to introduce air into the stomach. Doing so aids the visualization of the stomach and is referred to as a *double contrast.* As the patient drinks the barium, the radiologist or technician takes the x-rays. The radiologist observes a moving picture of the flow of the liquid and takes radiologic films for a permanent record. The radiologist will dictate findings observed during the procedure. This test aids diagnosis of gastroesophageal reflux disease (GERD), hiatal hernias, dilated esophageal veins called *varices,* strictures, and tumors. This procedure as well as other GI radiologic procedures is performed in radiologic offices and outpatient departments of hospitals.

The medical assistant should prepare the patient for the procedure by telling him to eat nothing after midnight the night before the test (npo) and to take no medications for GERD. She should be sure to explain that medications for GERD will not allow the physician to see how liquid flows down the esophagus and whether it goes into the stomach or is "refluxed" back to the esophagus. The medical assistant can provide cathartics, if ordered, for the patient after the examination to help the patient excrete the barium.

Lower GI X-ray

A lower GI x-ray involves visualization of the large intestine by rectal instillation of barium sulfate. The technician instills barium into the rectum and then insufflates air into the colon to help the physician visualize the colonic mucosa. During the examination, the patient will feel a strong urge to defecate. The medical assistant can advise the patient to breathe through his mouth slowly and deeply. When the examination is over, the patient can use the toilet. The examination takes approximately 45 minutes and helps

Patient Education

Statin Drugs and the Liver

One of the many functions of the liver is to manufacture cholesterol and send it to the bloodstream. HMG-CoA reductase inhibitors, commonly called *statins,* are used to lower cholesterol in patients who are at risk for cardiovascular disease. However, because statins inhibit production of enzymes that help make cholesterol, these drugs may cause irreversible damage to the liver. Patients taking these drugs, such as atorvastatin (Lipitor), must undergo liver function tests to help prevent damage to the liver.

The medical assistant must be sure to provide proper patient education about dietary changes and increased exercise before the administration of lipid-lowering drugs to help avoid serious liver damage. The medical assistant can help her patient lower cholesterol without medications by encouraging him to:

- Increase dietary fiber, such as oats, barley, legumes, and fruit. These fibrous foods can bind to cholesterol and bile in the intestinal tract and decrease their absorption.

- Increase physical activity, which has been proven to lower levels of low-density lipoprotein (LDL)—the "bad" cholesterol—and raise levels of high-density lipoprotein (HDL)—the "good" cholesterol.

- Substitute soy for animal sources of protein, which has been proven to significantly lower serum cholesterol.

- Consume alcohol in moderation. Drinking excessive amounts of alcohol is associated with liver stress and will elevate cholesterol.

- If overweight, lose weight to decrease blood cholesterol.

diagnose polyps, diverticula, colorectal cancer, inflammatory bowel disease, and obstructions. This procedure is performed primarily in a hospital setting.

To prepare the patient for a lower GI x-ray, the medical assistant should tell him not to eat dairy products and to follow a liquid diet for 24 hours before the examination. The patient must also take a bowel preparation the night before the test. The medical assistant can advise the patient to drink the bowel preparation and remain home for the evening to enable evacuation of the bowels. The medical assistant should also tell the patient to administer a home enema on the morning of the test and verify that the contents are clear. She should advise the patient to drink plenty of fluids for 48 hours after the procedure to promote full evacuation of residual barium.

Gallbladder Ultrasound

Gallbladder ultrasound, also called *gallbladder sonography,* involves the use of sound waves with a frequency of 20,000 cycles per second. The ultrasound machine sends these sound waves into the abdomen in the area of the gallbladder to produce an image of internal body structures. Because gallstones are much denser than the gallbladder and adjacent organs, they are easy to see in the image produced. A gallbladder ultrasound can be conducted in a hospital or medical office setting.

This procedure replaces the older gallbladder x-ray that required fasting for 12 hours and ingestion of several contrast media tablets the evening before the test. Although the gallbladder ultrasound requires the patient to fast for 12 hours before the test, it requires no contrast media. The medical assistant should tell the patient to fast for 12 hours before a morning appointment or have a fat-free liquid breakfast and no lunch for an afternoon appointment.

Chapter Summary

- Structures of the GI system include the oral cavity, esophagus, stomach, and small and large intestines.
- The accessory organs of digestion include the liver, gallbladder, and pancreas.
- The functions of the GI system include the digestion, absorption, and elimination of food ingested.
- Medical assistants must be well versed in the language and vocabulary that pertain to the GI system. In addition to knowing common combining forms, they should be familiar with common abbreviations and pathological terms.
- Some of the most common disorders of the GI system include GERD, gastritis, peptic ulcer disease, IBS, hepatitis, cholecystitis (gallstones), and various cancers of the GI tract.
- Medical assistants prepare patients by assisting them as needed with undressing and positioning. They also assist the physician with examinations and procedures.
- Treatments for GI disorders vary and include medication, dietary changes, and surgery as well as psychotherapy for eating disorders.
- Diagnostic procedures include stool analysis, sigmoidoscopy, and such radiographic procedures as upper and lower GI x-ray and gallbladder ultrasound.
- Patient education is vital in diagnosing, treating, and managing disorders of the GI system.

Team Work Exercises

1. Divide into teams of three to five students. Each team must create poster illustrations or three-dimensional models of the GI system, including appropriate labels. The class or instructor can evaluate these posters to pick a winner based on accuracy, use of humor, creativity, or other criteria.

2. Divide into teams of three to five students. Each team must create a patient education pamphlet about one of the cancers of the GI system described in this chapter. Pamphlets should include:
   a. incidence of cancer
   b. early detection testing
   c. risk factors, such as behaviors, nutrition, genetics, and so forth
   d. treatments available, including medical and alternative and complementary treatments
   e. prognosis.

   Teams must provide copies of their pamphlet to the rest of the class as well as friends and family members (who are not medically trained). Each team member must ask the friend or family member questions about the information presented and note areas of confusion or lack of understanding. The teams should discuss their findings with each other and the class.

Case Studies

1. David Frenczik comes to the medical office complaining of pain in the epigastric region of his abdomen during the middle of the night. He states that he wakes with heartburn and discomfort almost every night. What is the most likely source of his discomfort? What test will the physician likely order?

2. Gretchen Holmes is a medical assistant working in the scheduling department of a gastroenterologist's office. A patient calls and states that she works in a restaurant where there has been an outbreak of hepatitis A. The patient wants to make an appointment within the next month. What should Gretchen tell this patient?

Resources

- Dahlman, D., and Bland, J.: *Why Doesn't My Doctor Know This? Conquering Irritable Bowel Syndrome, Inflammatory Bowel Disease, Crohn Disease, and Colitis.* Garden City, NY: Morgan James, 2008.
- "Digestive Wellness" (compact disc). American Media International, 2609 Tucker St. Extension, Burlington, NC 27215.
- Johnson, L.R.: *Gastrointestinal Physiology,* 7th ed. St. Louis: Mosby, 2006.
- Patient information on GI health: *www.mayoclinic.com/health/digestive-system/DG99999*
- Patient information on GI cancer: *www.caring4cancer.com*
- Patient information videos on GI health: *www.everydayhealth.com/Publicsite/Healthology/VideoTopic.aspx?category=gi*
- Sullivan, R. J., et al.: *Digestion and Nutrition.* New York: Chelsea House, 2006.

Urology and the Male Reproductive System

Learning Objectives

Upon completion of this chapter, the student will be able to:

- define and spell terms related to urology and reproduction
- identify key structures of the urinary and male reproductive systems
- describe the functions of the urinary and male reproductive systems
- describe the role of the medical assistant in urology
- identify common urological and male reproductive diseases and disorders
- list the main structures in the urinary and male reproductive systems
- identify patient education regarding diseases and disorders of the urinary and male reproductive systems
- list commonly used word elements related to the urinary and male reproductive systems
- give at least 10 examples of how new terms related to the urinary and male reproductive systems may be created by combining prefixes, suffixes, and combining forms
- describe the medical assistant's role in assisting with urological procedures
- list common tests done for urinary system diseases and disorders.

CAAHEP Competencies

Clinical Competencies
Patient Care
Prepare patients for and assist with routine and specialty examinations
Prepare patients for and assist with procedures, treatments, and minor office surgeries

General Competencies
Patient Instruction
Provide instruction for health maintenance and disease prevention

ABHES Competencies

Clinical Duties
Interview and record patient history
Prepare patients for procedures
Prepare patient for and assist physician with routine and specialty examinations and treatments and minor office surgeries
Collect and process specimens

Procedures
Teaching a patient to perform TSE
Performing urinary catheterization

Chapter Outline

Structures and Functions of the Urinary and Male Reproductive Systems
Structures of the Urinary System
Kidneys
Nephrons
Ureters, urinary bladder, and urethra
Functions of the Urinary System
Kidneys
Nephrons
Ureters, urinary bladder, and urethra
Structures of the Male Reproductive System
Functions of the Male Reproductive System
Medical Terminology Related to the Urinary and Male Reproductive Systems
Common Urological and Male Reproductive Diseases and Disorders
Urinary System Diseases and Disorders
Bacterial cystitis and urethritis

Pyelonephritis
Glomerulonephritis
Bladder cancer
Renal cancer
Wilms tumor
Hydronephrosis
Polycystic kidney disease
Renal calculi
Acute renal failure
Chronic renal failure
Male Reproductive System Diseases and Disorders
Benign prostatic hypertrophy
Prostate cancer
Testicular cancer
Epididymitis
Balanoposthitis
Prostatitis
Sexually transmitted diseases
Erectile dysfunction
Urology and Male Reproductive Procedures
Assisting with Examination
Catheterization
Renal Computed Tomography Scan
Intravenous Pyelography
Cystoscopy
Voiding Cystourethrography
Creatinine
Blood Urea Nitrogen
Renal Angiography
Vasectomy
Chapter Summary
Team Work Exercises
Case Studies
Resources

Key Terms

anuria
Absence of urine production

cystoscopy
Visual examination of the bladder

dysuria
Painful or difficult urination

filtrate
Mixture of water, electrolytes, urea, and other small molecules first filtered in the glomerulus

frequency
Need for frequent urination

hemodialysis
Artificial means of removing urea, wastes, toxins, and excess fluid from the blood

lithotripsy
Treatment that uses shock or sound waves to crush stones in the kidneys or urinary tract

micturition reflex
Bladder reflex that creates the urge to urinate

oliguria
Deficiency of urine production

peritoneal dialysis
Dialysis in which the lining of the peritoneal cavity is used as the dialyzing membrane

renal colic
Pain that radiates from the flank into the abdomen or groin area

stent
Device that holds tissue in place and maintains an opening

urgency
Sudden, nearly uncontrollable need to urinate

urinalysis
Laboratory analysis of urine

urine culture
Growth and study of microorganisms isolated from a urine specimen

urinary catheterization
Procedure that involves insertion of a sterile drainage tube into the bladder to drain or withdraw urine

vasectomy
Procedure that involves removal of a segment of the vas deferens to achieve male sterilization

Structures and Functions of the Urinary and Male Reproductive Systems

The urinary system consists of the kidneys, ureters, bladder, and urethra. It facilitates filtration of the blood, excretion of wastes, and regulation of fluid, electrolytes, acids, and bases. Structures of the male reproductive system include the penis, urethra, testes, and scrotum as well as a series of ducts and glands. These structures play an important role in reproduction.

Structures of the Urinary System
The structures of the urinary system include two kidneys, two ureters, the bladder, and the urethra. (See Figure 31-1.)

Kidneys
The key organs of the urinary system are the kidneys, which are located in the back of the abdominal cavity in the retroperitoneal space to either side of the vertebral column. The right kidney is slightly lower than the left. Each kidney is surrounded by a renal capsule made up of connective tissue and a thick layer of fat. The renal artery, vein, nerves, and ureter exit the kidneys on the medial side at the hilum. Both kidneys are highly vascular organs made up of an outer cortex and an inner medulla. Within the medulla are several oval-shaped renal pyramids, which point inward. Cupping the tip of each renal pyramid is a calyx. The area where all of the calyces join is called the *renal pelvis*. The renal pelvis narrows and joins the ureter.

Nephrons
Located primarily within the outer cortex are the nephrons. There are more than one million nephrons in each kidney. Each one is a microscopic, yet complex structure composed of an arteriole, venule, glomerulus (capillary cluster within the Bowman capsule), proximal tubule, loop of Henle, distal tubule, and capillary bed. (See Figure 31-2.)

Ureters, Urinary Bladder, and Urethra
The ureters are long, narrow tubes that connect the renal pelvis of the kidneys to the urinary bladder. The bladder is a flexible, muscular container for urine. The lining of the ureters and the bladder is uniquely designed to be flexible in accommodating varying amounts of fluid. At the base of the bladder is the exit into the urethra, a tube that varies in length, depending on the patient's sex. The male urethra is approximately 20 cm long and the female urethra is approximately 4 cm long.

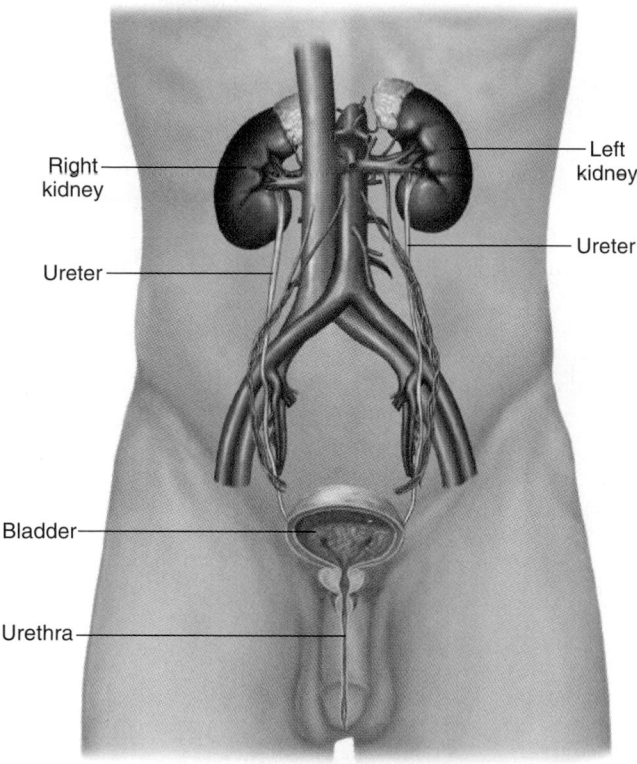

FIG 31-1 The urinary system.

Functions of the Urinary System

Each structure of the urinary system is uniquely designed and suited to its purpose. The urinary system's main functions are to filter and excrete the waste products of digestion and metabolism from the body, help to regulate blood pressure, and maintain an optimal level of fluid and electrolytes within the body.

Kidneys

The thick layer of fat in the renal capsule, which surrounds each kidney, acts as a shock absorber to cushion and protect the kidneys so that they may perform a key function of the urinary system. The highly vascular nature of the kidneys lends itself to this function, which is the filtration of blood for the elimination of wastes, excess fluids, and the regulation of electrolytes. In fact, over 20% of the blood pumped by the heart each minute passes through the kidneys. When urine is formed, it drains into the calyces, which funnel the urine inward through the renal pelvis narrows and into the ureter, which, in turn, drains urine from the kidney to the urinary bladder. In addition to filtering fluid and wastes from the body, the kidneys play active roles in maintaining blood pressure and blood pH (acidity or alkalinity). They help regulate blood pressure by retaining or excreting more fluid and electrolytes (especially sodium). They help maintain an optimal acid-base balance by retaining or excreting buffers and acids as needed.

Nephrons

The nephron has long been called the functional unit of the kidney because it is where most of the action takes place. To begin the filtration process, blood passes from a tiny arteriole into the glomerulus. The walls of the glomerulus and Bowman capsule are designed to permit optimal filtration of water, electrolytes, urea, and other small molecules. A large amount of this fluid (approximately 180 L) called *filtrate,* is created each day. However, as it moves on through the proximal tubule, loop of Henle, and distal tubule, a majority (99%) of the water and useful solutes are reabsorbed and additional wastes are excreted. After the kidneys make final adjustments in the composition of the fluid, it is called *urine*. The kidneys produce and excrete an average of 1 to 2 L of urine each day.

Ureters, Urinary Bladder, and Urethra

Urine drains from the kidneys to the bladder via the two long, narrow ureters. In the bladder, urine accumulates until the volume reaches a level that stimulates stretch receptors. These receptors initiate the **micturition reflex,** which is the urge to urinate. A person may temporarily ignore this urge. However, eventually, the increased level stimulates the

Nephron

Kidney

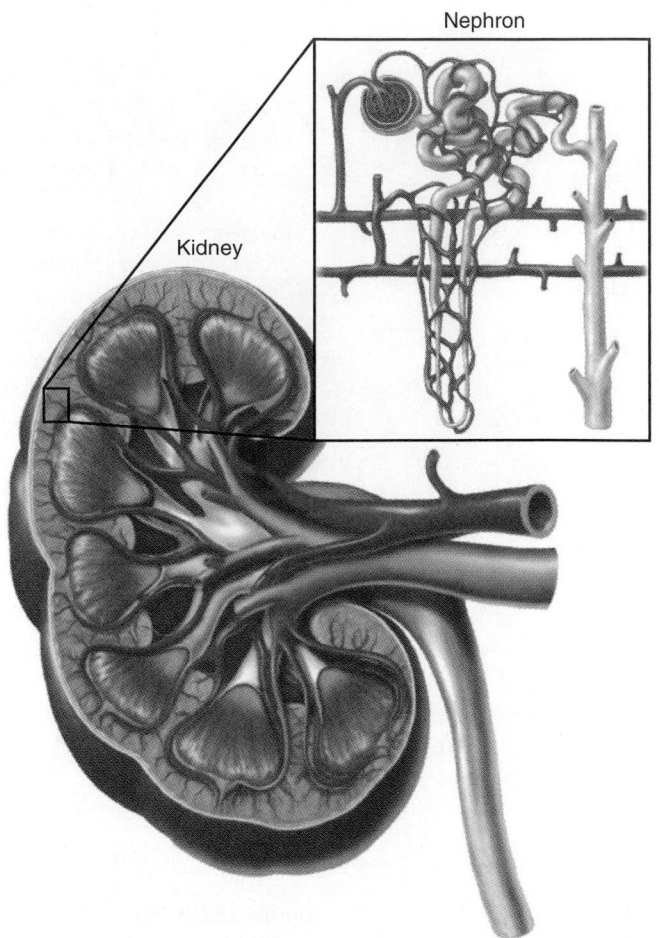

FIG 31-2 The kidney and nephron.

stretch receptors again and the urge to urinate will be even stronger. The urethra functions as a passageway for final urine elimination and emptying of the bladder. It serves a dual role in the male as a passageway for urine and for sperm mixed with seminal fluid when ejaculation occurs.

Structures of the Male Reproductive System

The male reproductive system shares some structures with other body systems, including the penis and urethra, shared by the urinary system, and the testes, shared by the endocrine system. Other structures within the male reproductive system include the prostate gland, the scrotum, and a series of ducts and glands. (See Figure 31-3.)

The scrotum is composed of two internal compartments surrounded by loose connective tissue and a smooth muscle layer. A second muscle group, called the *cremasters,* extends from the abdomen into the scrotum. Within the compartment of the scrotum are the testes. The testes are oval-shaped organs composed of an outer capsule made up

of thick, white connective tissue. The inner part is divided into 200 to 300 lobules, which contain the seminiferous tubules.

From the testes to the urethra, a series of ducts connect to each other, beginning with the seminiferous tubules, then the rete testis, efferent ductules, epididymis, vas deferens, and, finally, the ejaculatory duct, which joins with the urethra.

The urethra begins at the exit of the bladder and passes through the penis, ending at its tip. The penis is composed of three sections of erectile tissue and a distal, rounded end, which is the glans penis. A fold of skin commonly called the *foreskin* covers the glans penis. In many cultures, a procedure called circumcision is commonly practiced. In this procedure part or all of the foreskin is removed.

Functions of the Male Reproductive System

A primary function of the male reproductive system is reproduction. Sperm cells vital to this process are created and stored within the testes. They are sensitive to heat and

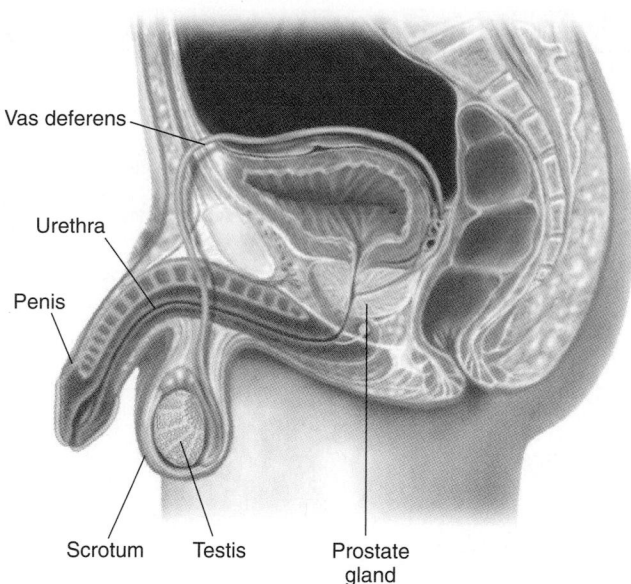

Vas deferens

Urethra

Penis

Scrotum   Testis   Prostate gland

FIG 31-3 The male reproductive system.

must live within an environment that is slightly less than normal body temperature. Therefore, prior to birth, the testes in the male fetus normally descend from the lower abdomen into the scrotum. The structures of the scrotum are designed to maintain an optimal temperature for spermatogenesis. In a cold environment, the smooth muscle of the scrotum and the cremaster muscles contract, bringing the scrotum and testes closer to the body to keep them warmer. In a warm environment, the same muscles relax and allow the scrotum and testes to descend away from the body to keep them cooler.

Spermatogenesis takes place within the seminiferous tubules of the testes. When the spermatocytes have reached a sufficient stage of maturity, they exit the testes through a series of ducts and leave the body during ejaculation.

The urethra serves a dual purpose as the exit passageway for urine and semen. However, both do not exit at the same time. During sexual activity, the internal urinary sphincter contracts to keep semen from entering the bladder and to keep urine from exiting the bladder.

During arousal, the erectile tissue of the penis becomes engorged with blood and the penis becomes firm and erect to facilitate sexual intercourse and ejaculation. The state of erection ends with ejaculation or when sexual arousal diminishes.

Secretions from a variety of sources contribute to the seminal fluid. Mucus secretions from the bulbourethral glands and the inner urethral wall lubricate the urethra and neutralize its normally acidic environment. Seminal vesicles secrete fructose and other nutrients for sperm cells as well as prostaglandin, which stimulates smooth muscle contractions in the female reproductive tract, which is thought to help move sperm through that environment. The prostate gland secretes prostatic fluid that flows through a number of ducts to the urethra and contributes an alkaline pH to help further neutralize the environment. A neutral environment is important to sperm motility because sperm need an environment that has a pH between 6.0 and 6.5 for optimal activity. Vaginal pH, by comparison, is normally between 3.5 and 4.0.

Medical Terminology Related to the Urinary and Male Reproductive Systems

Urinary and reproductive disorders are common problems that lead people to seek medical care. Whether they work in family practice offices, urgent care centers, urology clinics, or other areas, medical assistants play an important role in the provision of health care to these patients. To be effective in their role, medical assistants must become well versed in the language and vocabulary that pertain to the urinary and male reproductive systems. The following tables list common medical terminology related to these systems.

Table 31.1	**Word Elements**		
This table contains combining forms, prefixes, and suffixes related to the urinary and male reproductive systems, along with examples of terms that use the word element, a pronunciation guide, and a definition for each.			
Element	**Meaning**	**Example**	**Meaning**
Combining Forms			
bacterl/o	bacteria	**bacteriuria** (băk-tē-rē-Ū-rē-ă)	Bacteria in the urine
balan/o	glans penis	**balanitis** (băl-ă-NĪ-tĭs)	Inflammation of the glans penis

Continued

Table 31.1 | Word Elements—cont'd

Element	Meaning	Example	Meaning
Combining Forms			
cyst/o	urinary bladder	**cystoscopy** (sĭs-TŎS-kō-pē)	Visual examination of the bladder
glomerul/o	glomerulus	**glomerulopathy** (glō-mĕr-ū-LŎP-ă-thē)	Disease of the glomerulus
hemat/o	blood	**hematuria** (hē-mă-TŪ-rē-ă)	Blood in the urine
hem/o		**hemolysis** (hē-MŎL-ĭ-sĭs)	Destruction of blood
lith/o	stone	**nephrolithiasis** (nĕf-rō-lĭth-Ī-ă-sĭs)	Abnormal condition of kidney stones
nephr/o	kidney	**nephrologist** (nĕ-FRŎL-ō-jĭst)	Specialist in the study of the kidneys
ren/o		**renal** (RĒ-năl)	Pertaining to the kidneys
noct/o	night	**nocturia** (nŏk-TŪ-rē-ă)	Urination at night
olig/o	deficient	**oliguria** (ōl-ĭg-Ū-rē-ă)	Deficiency of urine (production)
orch/o	testes	**orchopathy** (ŏr-KŎ-pă-thē)	Disease of the testes
orchi/o		**orchiectomy** (ŏr-kē-ĔK-tō-mē)	Surgical removal of the testes
orchid/o		**orchidopexy** (ŏr-kĭ-dō-PĔK-sē)	Surgical fixation of the testes
test/o		**testomegaly** (tĕs-tō-MĔG-ă-lē)	Enlargement of the testes
peritone/o	peritoneum	**peritoneal** (pĕr-ĭ-tō-NĒ-ăl)	Pertaining to the peritoneum
prostat/o	prostate	**prostatoplasty** (prŏs-tă-tō-PLĂS-tē)	Surgical repair of the prostate
pyel/o	renal pelvis	**pyelonephritis** (pī-ĕ-lō-nĕ-FRĪ-tĭs)	Inflammation of the renal pelvis
py/o	pus	**pyuria** (pī-Ū-rē-ă)	Pus in the urine
spermat/o	sperm	**spermatogenesis** (spĕr-măt-ō-JĔN-ĕ-sĭs)	Producing sperm
sperm/o		**aspermia** (ă-SPĔR-mē-ă)	Condition of no sperm
urethr/o	urethra	**urethropexy** (ū-RĒ-thrō-pĕks-ē)	Surgical fixation of the urethra
ur/o	urine	**urology** (ū-RŎL-ō-jē)	Study of disorders of the urinary tract
urin/o		**urinometer** (ū-rĭ-NŎM-ĕ-tĕr)	Instrument for measuring urine
vas/o	vessel	**vasotomy** (văs-ŎT-ō-mē)	Incision into a vessel
Prefixes			
an-	without, absence of	**anuria** (ăn-Ū-rē-ă)	Absence of urine (production)
anti-	against	**antibacterial** (ăn-tĭ-băk-TĒ-rē-ăl)	Pertaining to against bacteria
dys-	painful, difficult	**dysuria** (dĭs-Ū-rē-ă)	Painful or difficult urination
poly-	many, much	**polyuria** (pŏl-ē-Ū-rē-ă)	Much urination
oligo-	deficiency	**oligospermia** (ōl-ĭ-gō-SPĔR-mē-ă)	Condition of deficienct sperm
pre-	before	**prerenal** (prē-RĒ-năl)	Pertaining to before the kidneys
trans-	through, across	**transurethral** (trăns-ū-RĒ-thrăl)	Pertaining to through or across the urethra
Suffixes			
-ary	pertaining to	**urinary** (Ū-rĭ-năr-ē)	Pertaining to urine (or the urinary tract)
-cele	herniation	**cystocele** (SĬS-tō-sēl)	Herniation of the bladder
-cidal	killing, destroying	**bacteriocidal** (băk-tĕr-ē-ō-SĪ-dăl)	Killing bacteria

Table 31.1 | Word Elements—cont'd

Element	Meaning	Example	Meaning
Suffixes			
-cyte	cell	**spermatocyte** (spĕr-MĂT-ō-sīt)	Sperm cell
-dynia	pain	**urodynia** (ū-rō-DĬN-ē-ă)	Painful urination
-ectomy	surgical removal	**prostatectomy** (prŏs-tă-TĔK-tō-mē)	Surgical removal of the prostate
-gram	record	**pyelogram** (PĬ-ĕ-lō-grăm)	Radiological record of the kidneys
-megaly	enlargement	**prostatomegaly** (prŏs-tă-tō-MĔG-ă-lē)	Enlarged prostate
-pathy	disease	**nephropathy** (nĕ-FRŎP-ă-thē)	Disease of the kidneys
-pexy	surgical fixation	**cystopexy** (SĬS-tō-pēk-sē)	Surgical fixation of the bladder
-spasm	spasm	**urethrospasm** (ū-RĒ-thrō-spăzm)	Contraction of the urethra
-tic	pertaining to	**nephrotic** (nĕ-FRŎT-ĭk)	Pertaining to the kidneys
-tripsy	crushing	**lithotripsy** (LĬTH-ō-trĭp-sē)	Crushing of a stone
-uria	urine	**oliguria** (ŏl-ĭg-Ū-rē-ă)	Deficiency of urine

Table 31.2 | Pathologic Terms

This table lists some of the most common pathologic terms related to the urinary and male reproductive systems with a brief definition for each.

Term	Definition
acute renal failure ă-KŪT RĒ-năl FĂL-yĕr	Sharp rise in the serum creatinine level of 25% or more that may last days or weeks or develop into chronic renal failure
bacterial cystitis băk-TĒ-rē-ăl sĭs-TĪ-tĭs	Inflammation of the bladder due to bacterial infection; also called *bladder infection*
balanoposthitis băl-ă-nō-pŏs-THĬ-tĭs	Inflammation of the glans penis beneath the foreskin
benign prostatic hypertrophy bē-NĬN prŏs-TĂT-ĭk hī-PĔR-trŏ-fē	Enlargement of the prostate gland caused by noncancerous cellular proliferation; also called *benign prostatic hyperplasia*
chronic renal failure KRŎN-ĭk RĒ-năl FĂL-yĕr	Progressive loss of the kidney's effectiveness in excreting waste products and regulating fluid and electrolytes; also called *chronic kidney disease*
Chlamydia trachomatis klă-MĬD-ē-ă tră-KO-mă-tĭs	Organism that causes many diseases, including genital infections in men and women
cryptorchidism krĭpt-OR-kĭd-ĭzm	Condition in which the testicles fail to descend into the scrotum
diuresis dī-ū-RĒ-sĭs	Abnormal secretion of large amounts of urine
end-stage renal disease ĔND STĀG RĒ-năl dĭ-ZĒZ	Termination of the kidneys' ability to regulate fluid and electrolytes and excrete wastes, ending in death unless transplantation occurs

Continued

Table 31.2 | **Pathologic Terms—cont'd**

Term	Definition
enuresis ĕn-ū-RĒ-sĭs	Involuntary urination during sleep; also called *bed wetting*
epididymitis ĕp-ĭ-dĭd-ĭ-MĪ-tĭs	Inflammation of the epididymis
erectile dysfunction ĕ-RĔK-tĭl dĭs-FŬNK-shŭn	Inability of a man to attain an erection adequate enough to achieve a satisfactory sexual experience; also called *impotence*
fecal incontinence FĒ-kăl ĭn-KŎNT-ĭn-ĕns	Loss of control over bowel function
glomerulonephritis glō-mĕr-ū-lō-nĕ-FRĪ-tĭs	Form of nephritis in which the glomeruli are primarily affected
glucosuria gloo-kō-SŪ-rē-ă	Glucose in the urine; also called *glycosuria*
gonorrhea gŏn-ō-RĒ-ă	Sexually transmitted infection caused by *Neisseria gonorrhoeae*
herpes simplex virus type 2 HĔR-pēz SĬM-plĕx VĪ-rŭs	Virus that causes repeated eruptions of painful vesicles on the genitals and other mucosal surfaces and on the skin
human papilloma virus HŪ-măn păp-ĭ-LŌ-mă VĪ-rŭs	Genital wart virus that is specific to humans and is a common viral sexually transmitted disease
hydronephrosis hī-drō-nĕf-RŌ-sĭs	Stretching of the renal pelvis as a result of obstruction to urinary outflow
interstitial cystitis ĭn-tĕr-STĬSH-ăl sĭs-TĪ-tĭs	Chronic condition of inflammation of the bladder lining
interstitial nephritis ĭn-tĕr-STĬSH-ăl nĕf-RĪ-tĭs	Pathologic changes in renal tissue that destroy nephrons and impair kidney function
nephritic syndrome nĕ-FRĬT-ĭk SĬN-drōm	Condition marked by increased glomerular permeability to proteins, resulting in massive proteinuria, edema, hypoalbuminemia, hyperlipidemia, and hypercoagulability
nephrolithiasis nĕf-rō-lĭth-Ī-ă-sĭs	Presence of kidney stones
nephropathy nĕ-FRŎP-ă-thē	Disease of the kidneys
nocturia nŏk-TŪ-rē-ă	Excessive need to urinate at night after going to bed
oliguria ŏl-ĭg-Ū-rē-ă	Deficiency of urine production with an output less than 400 ml/day
orchitis or-KĪ-tĭs	Inflammation of the testicle, usually caused by bacterial or viral infection; also called *orchiditis*
overflow incontinence Ō-vĕr-flō ĭn-KŎNT-ĭn-ĕns	Ineffective emptying of the bladder caused by nerve damage or other disorders, leading to urine leakage
phimosis fī-MŌ-sĭs	Stenosis of the foreskin opening so that it cannot be retracted back over the glans penis

Table 31.2 | Pathologic Terms—cont'd

Term	Definition
polycystic kidney disease pŏl-ē-SĬS-tĭk KĬD-nē dĭ-ZĒZ	Any of several hereditary disorders in which cysts form in the kidneys and other organs, eventually destroying kidney tissue and function
prostatitis prŏs-tă-TĪ-tĭs	Inflammation of the prostate gland
pyelonephritis pī-ĕ-lō-nĕ-FRĬ-tĭs	Inflammation of the kidney and renal pelvis, usually due to bacterial infection that has ascended from the urinary bladder
sexually transmitted disease SĔKS-ū-ăl-ē TRĂNS-mĭt-ĕd dĭ-ZĒZ	Any disease that may be acquired as a result of sexual intercourse or other intimate contact with an infected individual; also called *venereal disease*
spermatocele spĕr-MĂT-ō-sēl	Type of cyst that develops when the tubes that transport sperm become blocked
stress incontinence STRĔS ĭn-KŎNT-ĭn-ĕns	Involuntary urine leakage with physical stress, such as a cough or sneeze
syphilis SĬF-ĭ-lĭs	Multistage infection typically transmitted through sexual contact caused by the spirochete *Treponema pallidum*
total urinary incontinence TŌ-tăl Ū-rĭ-nār-ē ĭn-KŎNT-ĭn-ĕns	Continuous and unpredictable loss of urine
uremia ū-RĒ-mē-ă	Accumulation in the blood of metabolic by-products such as urea; also called *azotemia*
urethritis ū-rĕ-THRĬ-tĭs	Inflammation of the urethra
urinary retention Ū-rĭ-nār-ē rĭ-TĔN-shŭn	Retention of urine in the bladder due to an inability to urinate
varicocele VĂR-ĭ-kō-sēl	Presence of enlarged varicose veins within the scrotum
Wilms tumor VĬLMS TŪ-mor	Rapidly developing cancerous tumor of the kidney that usually occurs in children; also called *nephroblastoma*

Table 31.3 | Abbreviations

In urology, as in other areas of health care, abbreviations are commonly used. Abbreviations such as the ones listed here save time and effort in documentation and written communications.

Abbreviation	Term	Abbreviation	Term
ARF	acute renal failure	CRF	chronic renal failure; also called *chronic kidney disease*
BPH	benign prostatic hypertrophy; also called *benign prostatic hyperplasia*	DRE	digital rectal examination
BUN	blood urea nitrogen	ED	erectile dysfunction
CKD	chronic kidney disease; also called *chronic renal failure*	ESRD	end-stage renal disease
		GFR	glomerular filtration rate

Continued

Table 31.3 | Abbreviations—cont'd

Abbreviation	Term	Abbreviation	Term
HPV	human papillomavirus	PSA	prostatic-specific antigen
HSV	herpes simplex virus	RP	retrograde pyelogram
IVP	intravenous pyelogram	STD	sexually transmitted disease
KUB	kidney, ureter, bladder	TSE	testicular self-examination
pH	parts hydrogen (acidity or alkalinity of a substance)	TURP	transurethral resection of the prostate
		UA	urinalysis
PKD	polycystic kidney disease	UTI	urinary tract infection

Common Urological and Male Reproductive Diseases and Disorders

There are innumerable diseases and disorders of the urinary and male reproductive systems. Some of the most common urological disorders include inflammatory disorders, such as bacterial cystitis; disorders of obstruction, such as hydronephrosis; nephrotic syndrome; polycystic kidney disease; chronic renal failure; and various cancers of the urinary system. Common male reproductive disorders include benign prostatic hypertrophy, prostate or testicular cancers, sexually transmitted diseases, and erectile dysfunction.

Urinary System Diseases and Disorders
Bacterial Cystitis and Urethritis
Cystitis—ICD-9-CM code: 595.9 (unspecified)
Urethritis—ICD-9-CM code: 597.80 (unspecified)
Bacterial cystitis is an inflammation of the bladder. Urethritis is an inflammation of the urethra. These conditions commonly coexist and together constitute a urinary tract infection (UTI), sometimes referred to as a *bladder infection*. UTIs are more common in women than men because women have a short urethra (about 1½ (long), which allows microorganisms to ascend the urethra into the bladder more easily. Because of the male's longer urethra, men have fewer UTIs than women. However, they have a higher incidence of urethritis, which is the most common type of sexually transmitted disease (STD) in men.

Cystitis and other forms of UTIs are most commonly caused by bacterial invasion. The most common organisms involved are *Escherichia coli*, *Enterobacter*, *Klebsiella*, *Proteus*, and *Pseudomonas*. Other causes include such STDs as *Chlamydia trachomatis*, *Neisseria gonorrhoeae*, and herpes simplex as well as other viruses, parasites, and fungi. Contributors to the development of cystitis and urethritis include poor hygiene and sexual activity, both of which increase the likelihood of microorganisms ascending into the urinary tract.

Common symptoms of bladder inflammation include **urgency** (need to urinate urgently), **frequency** (need to urinate frequently), and **dysuria** (pain, burning, or other discomfort during urination). Other symptoms may include fever, malaise, bladder spasms, pelvic or low back pain, and cloudy, pink, or foul-smelling urine. When urethritis is caused by an STD, urethral discharge may also be present.

Diagnosis of UTI is usually based on the results of a **urinalysis** (laboratory analysis of the urine), which reveals bacteria and increased numbers of white and red blood cells. A **urine culture,** in which a laboratory examines the growth of microorganisms in a urine specimen under a microscope, may identify the causative organism. A culture of urethral discharge may also identify whether an STD is involved.

Treatment of UTI depends on the underlying cause. In the case of bacterial infection, the physician will prescribe antibiotics. Other treatment includes phenazopyridine (Pyridium), which is a urinary tract analgesic; general analgesics, such as nonsteroidal anti-inflammatory drugs (NSAIDs); and fluids to help flush the urinary tract. To help treat UTIs and to help prevent reoccurrence, the medical assistant should encourage the patient to empty her bladder soon after sexual intercourse, drink plenty of fluids (6 to 8 glasses of water each day), and drink fluids that acidify the urine and inhibit bacterial growth, such as cranberry juice. Other measures include wiping from front to back after defecation, avoiding tight-fitting clothing (which harbors moisture), and conducting routine daily hygiene. (See *Treating and preventing UTI*.)

Prognosis for UTI is good with timely diagnosis and treatment. (See *Quick urinalysis*.) Complications develop

Patient Education

Treating and Preventing UTI

The medical assistant teaching a patient with a urinary tract infection (UTI) about treatment and prevention should be sure to include these points.

Treatment

- If you think you may have a UTI, see your health care provider, who will take a brief health history, collect a urine specimen, and, possibly, conduct a physical examination.

- Drink lots of healthy fluids, such as water and juice, to help remain well hydrated and flush the urinary tract.

- Be sure to drink cranberry juice, which helps make your urine more acidic and, therefore, less hospitable to bacteria.

- Take medications as prescribed by your physician.

- Take prescribed anti-infective medication until it is gone. Do not stop taking it as soon as you feel better.

Prevention

- Continue drinking lots of fluids daily unless told otherwise by your physician.

- Urinate soon after sexual intercourse.

- Wipe from front to back after bowel movements.

- Avoid wearing tight-fitting undergarments that harbor moisture.

- Follow additional advice of your physician.

Front office–Back office connection

Quick Urinalysis

In many medical offices, if a patient complains of symptoms that could be caused by a UTI (pelvic or back pain, dysuria, urinary frequency, and so forth), the administrative medical assistant will instruct the patient to collect a urine specimen as soon as she checks in. Doing so enables the clinical medical assistant to conduct a quick urinalysis while the patient awaits examination. Because the results are available for the physician to review at the time of examination, he can make a more timely diagnosis and initiate early treatment. When the administrative and clinical medical assistants can provide specimen collection instructions and equipment to the patient, the physician is able to meet the highest standard of care.

when bacterial organisms enter other parts of the urinary tract, causing nephritis, pyelonephritis, prostatitis, and other types of infections.

Pyelonephritis

ICD-9-CM code: 590.80

Pyelonephritis is the inflammation of the renal pelvis and connective tissues. It can affect one or both kidneys. Pyelonephritis is more common in women than men because their shorter urethra makes it easier for bacteria to be introduced into the bladder.

Pyelonephritis is most commonly caused by bacterial infection from pathogens that ascend the urinary tract. The most common offender is *E. coli*. Other causes include tumors, kidney stones, and severe prostate enlargement or other obstructions that impede urine flow and create inflammation, causing an environment conducive to bacterial growth.

Signs and symptoms of pyelonephritis include sudden onset of fever, chills, nausea, and flank pain. These signs and symptoms are commonly preceded by signs of bladder infection.

Diagnosis is based on the patient's signs and symptoms and the result of urinalysis and urine culture, which reveal the presence of bacteria, casts, WBCs, and RBCs. Radiologic studies reveal enlarged, swollen kidneys.

Treatment includes IV, IM, or oral antibiotics as well as analgesics and fluids. Prognosis is usually good with early intervention, although chronic infection may lead to kidney damage.

Glomerulonephritis

ICD-9-CM code: 580 (acute), 582 (chronic)

Acute glomerulonephritis is the inflammation of the glomeruli within the kidneys. Chronic glomerulonephritis is a noninfectious disease that progresses slowly and leads to permanent kidney damage and kidney failure.

The cause of glomerulonephritis is unclear. However, it most commonly follows 1 to 2 weeks after an upper respiratory infection caused by some strains of streptococci.

Signs and symptoms of glomerulonephritis include hematuria (bloody urine), which may not be apparent to the naked eye or it may be significant enough to turn the urine a dark rust-brown or red color. Urine may also appear foamy. Other manifestations include flank pain, general malaise, anorexia, and low-grade fever. Individuals with chronic glomerulonephritis are commonly asymptomatic. Eventually, they begin to experience hypertension, hematuria, proteinuria, oliguria, azotemia (buildup of urea in the blood), malaise, nausea, vomiting, dyspnea, pruritus, and edema as renal failure progresses.

Diagnostic tests for acute and chronic glomerulonephritis are the same. Urinalysis may indicate blood, WBCs, casts, protein, or other abnormalities. Blood tests indicate elevated blood urea nitrogen (BUN), increased erythrocyte sedimentation rate (ESR), and decreased serum protein. Radiological studies may reveal kidney enlargement.

Treatment of acute glomerulonephritis may include antibiotics if streptococcal infection is still present. With both disorders, treatment measures aim to control hypertension and prevent or delay renal failure. The physician may also recommend dietary restriction of protein, sodium, and fluids.

Patients with chronic glomerulonephritis may ultimately require dialysis or kidney transplantation.

Bladder Cancer
ICD-9-CM code: 239.4

Bladder cancer is the most common form of urinary tract cancer. Most tumors develop in the bladder lining, while more invasive tumors develop in the muscle. Transitional cell carcinoma is most common in industrialized countries and squamous cell carcinomas caused by parasitic infestations are most common in developing countries. Bladder cancer is the sixth most common type of cancer and is most common in industrialized countries such as the United States, Canada, and France. Over 50,000 Americans are diagnosed with it each year and more than 12,000 die. The incidence increases with age, especially over age 55. It is three times more common in men and is more common in the Caucasian population.

The cause of bladder cancer is unknown. However, there are many contributors and risk factors, including exposure to tobacco smoke, radiation, arsenic, and other carcinogens; advanced age; chronic bladder inflammation; high-fat diet; genetics; male gender; and a history of *Schistosoma haematobium* parasitic infection. Persons at increased risk due to workplace exposures include truck drivers, machinists, printers, painters, hair dressers, and those working in the rubber, metal, leather, textile, and chemical industries.

The most common symptom of bladder cancer is hematuria (blood in the urine). Bladder cancer is generally painless and may not be obvious in early stages. Other symptoms may include urinary frequency and dysuria. Diagnosis is based on urinalysis and diagnostic imaging. Urinalysis rules out infection and identifies the presence of blood and abnormal cells. Intravenous pyelogram (IVP) enables better examination of all structures within the urinary tract. **Cystoscopy** allows visual examination of the inner bladder wall and the opportunity to take a tissue sample for biopsy, which is used to confirm the diagnosis. The physician will stage the cancer according to the tumor, node, metastasis (TNM) system. Other diagnostic tests used to determine the extent or stage of the cancer may include computed tomography (CT) scan, magnetic resonance imaging (MRI), bone scan, and ultrasound. Newer tests identify tumor markers, which are substances released by tumors. These tests are still under investigation.

Treatment varies for each patient, depending on cancer type, stage, and other health factors. Interventions include surgery, radiation, chemotherapy, immunotherapy, or a combination. Surgery may be as simple as transurethral excision of a small lesion or as complex as the surgical removal of the entire bladder, nearby lymph nodes, some of the reproductive organs or structures, and surrounding tissue.

Prognosis for bladder cancer is guarded. The 5-year survival rate for superficial bladder cancer is 85%. However, those with more invasive forms have a poorer prognosis and those with identified metastasis have a 5-year survival rate of just 5%. Because there is a high rate of recurrence, follow-up examinations, including cytology (study of tissue cells) and cystoscopy, are recommended every 3 months for 2 years and then every 6 months for another 2 years. Complications of bladder cancer and its treatment include anemia, urinary incontinence, and metastasis to other organs.

Renal Cancer
ICD-9-CM code: 189.0

Renal cancer is cancer of the kidneys. It includes renal cell carcinoma and renal pelvis carcinoma. It also includes Wilms tumor, which is a common type of kidney cancer that develops in young children. An estimated 32,000 Americans are diagnosed with renal cancer each year and an estimated 12,000 people die from renal cancer each year. It most commonly affects elderly individuals between ages 50 and 70 and affects men more than women.

The specific cause of renal cancer is not clear. However, there are a number of known risk factors, including being age 60 or over, male, or African American; using tobacco (especially pipes and cigars); being obese; having hypertension; or undergoing exposure to such toxins as solvents, asbestos, and radiation. Individuals with a history of bladder cancer and those who undergo long-term dialysis are also at increased risk.

Patients with renal cancer are commonly asymptomatic in the early stages. In later stages, the patient may experience hematuria, back pain, weight loss, fatigue, and intermittent fever.

The diagnostic process begins with routine blood and urine tests, which help the physician determine current kidney function and provide baseline data to help measure the patients' response to therapy. A complete health history and physical examination reveal signs and symptoms associated with renal cancer. Such radiologic studies as IVP, ultrasound, CT, and MRI can create detailed images of the kidneys and bladder and may detect unusual masses. Tissue biopsy, sometimes required for definitive diagnosis, reveals cancer cells.

Treatment of renal cancer includes partial or total nephrectomy via laparoscopy or more traditional surgery. When surgery is not possible, another treatment option is arterial embolization, in which the surgeon injects material to clog the main vessel leading to the kidney. This clog robs the tumor of nutrients and oxygen and relieves pain and bleeding. Radiation therapy may target and kill cancer cells and relieve the pain of metastatic cancer. Other forms of treatment include immunotherapy and chemotherapy.

Prognosis for those with renal cancer is variable and depends on the stage at the time of diagnosis. In general, the 5-year survival rate is 55%. However, those with stage 1 cancer have a 5-year survival rate of 94%. Those with stage 2 cancer have a 5-year survival rate of 65% to 75%. Those with stage 3 have a 5-year survival rate between 40% and 70%. The prognosis for those with stage 4 cancer is poor, with a 5-year survival rate of only 10%.

Wilms Tumor
ICD-9-CM code: 189.0

Wilms tumor, also known as *nephroblastoma,* is a rapidly growing type of kidney cancer that most commonly affects children between the ages of 1 and 5. Usually only one kidney is cancerous.

Wilms tumor develops from immature kidney cells that multiply and grow in an abnormal manner. There is a genetic component in some cases and the condition is commonly associated with other genetic anomalies (abnormalities).

Patients with Wilms tumor may be asymptomatic in the early stages. An abdominal mass is a common finding that may be detected by the parent when bathing or dressing the child or by the physician upon physical examination. Signs and symptoms include hematuria, weight loss, constipation, nausea, vomiting and abdominal pain, fever, anorexia, and malaise.

Diagnosis is based on physical examination, family medical history, tests of urine and blood, and diagnostic imaging. MRI, CT scan, and ultrasound are used to locate and create visual images of the tumor or other structural abnormalities. Treatment of Wilms tumor includes surgery, chemotherapy, bone marrow transplant, and radiation therapy. As with most types of cancer, the physician will order analysis of tissue cells for staging in order to determine the most appropriate course of treatment. Surgery usually includes partial or complete nephrectomy (surgical removal of the kidney) and may include removal of local lymph nodes and other

surrounding tissue. Prognosis for Wilms tumor has improved substantially in recent decades and survival is currently around 90%. Outcome is best when only one kidney is involved.

Hydronephrosis
ICD-9-CM code: 591

Hydronephrosis is not a disease but a condition. Bilateral hydronephrosis affects both kidneys. It occurs in infants, children, men, and women.

Hydronephrosis is caused by obstructed urinary outflow in which tissues of the renal pelvis are stretched due to pressure from urine accumulation. Thus, it may be caused by anything that obstructs urine outflow. It occurs in infants and children due to congenital defects. It occurs in adults due to a variety of obstructive causes, including complications of pregnancy in women and prostate enlargement in men. Obstruction may be complete or partial, unilateral (one-sided) or bilateral. Common causes of obstruction in unilateral hydronephrosis include kidney stones, blood clots, tumors, ureteral strictures or other malformations, and parasitic infestations. Causes of bilateral hydronephrosis include benign prostatic hypertrophy (BPH), neurogenic bladder, pregnancy, bladder cancer, urinary tract inflammation, and congenital malformations.

Patients with hydronephrosis are commonly asymptomatic unless kidney stones are the cause. In the case of kidney stones, patients complain of severe loin or flank pain that sometimes radiates into the lower abdomen or groin. If kidney failure develops, symptoms associated with kidney failure are present.

Radiologic tests, which may include ultrasound, IVP, and, occasionally, MRI, reveal dilation of the renal pelvis and obstruction. Blood tests may reveal creatinine and electrolyte imbalances. Urine pH may become more alkaline. In cases of complete obstruction, the kidney may be palpable on physical examination due to enlargement.

Treatment of hydronephrosis is aimed at the underlying cause, with an emphasis on restoring urine flow. The physician may order renal function studies to monitor kidney function. In the case of kidney stones, the physician may perform **lithotripsy,** a procedure in which shock waves or sound waves crush stones in the kidneys or urinary tract. The physician may also prescribe surgery to remove lodged stones or tumors or to place a **stent** (device used to hold tissue in place and maintain an opening) for urine drainage. Treatment for obstruction in the bladder outlet includes insertion of a urinary or suprapubic catheter or prostate surgery. Treatment of obstruction caused by an enlarged prostate gland usually involves prostate surgery.

If removal of the obstruction occurs in a timely manner, hydronephrosis resolves spontaneously. If restoration of urinary flow does not occur, kidney tissues dilate and atrophy and chronic renal failure may occur.

Polycystic Kidney Disease

Congenital PKD—ICD-9-CM code: 753.13
Autosomal dominant PKD—ICD-9-CM code: 753.13
Autosomal recessive PKD—ICD-9-CM code: 753.14

Polycystic kidney disease (PKD) is a group of hereditary, progressive disorders in which cysts (small sacs of fluid) form in the kidneys, eventually destroying them. Other organs may be affected, including the liver, heart, pancreas, and brain. One form of PKD usually appears early in childhood and is more severe than another form, which develops later in life. Polycystic kidney disease is the most common life-threatening hereditary disease in the United States, affecting approximately 600,000 persons. Approximately 12.5 million are affected worldwide. Incidence is higher in men, African Americans, and persons with sickle-cell disease.

PKD disorders are inherited. Autosomal recessive polycystic kidney disease (ARPKD) is more rare and deadly than autosomal dominant polycystic kidney disease (ADPKD). Children of parents with PKD have a 50% chance of getting the disease. Onset of ADPKD is usually in middle age.

Signs and symptoms of ARPKD are commonly present at birth or become apparent in early infancy. The most common signs of PKD include hypertension, hematuria, frequent kidney infections, and back or side pain. Diagnosis usually occurs after the individual begins to experience symptoms. Ultrasound and CT scan create images of the kidneys and detect the presence of cysts. Genetic testing helps definitively diagnose PKD.

There is no cure for PKD. Treatment includes measures to improve comfort and may include kidney dialysis and kidney transplant.

Many adults with PKD may be able to lead a normal or near-normal life. However, complications can occur, including hypertension, cerebral aneurysm, and renal failure. About half of those with ADPKD will develop end-stage renal disease (ESRD) by the age of 60.

Renal Calculi

ICD-9-CM code: 592

Renal calculi, also called *kidney stones*, are composed of mineral salts and cause problems when they obstruct portions of the kidneys or, more likely, a ureter. An estimated 2% to 5% of Americans develop kidney stones at some time in their lives. Caucasian males between the ages of 40 and 70 are most commonly affected. Persons with gout, hypercalcemia, hyperparathyroidism, or inflammatory bowel disease are at increased risk.

The cause of renal calculi is not fully understood in every case. One cause is hypercalciuria, an inherited condition in which excessive calcium is excreted into the urine. Another

is gout, which causes abnormal metabolism of uric acid. Other contributors include hyperparathyroidism and Crohn disease. Hyperparathyroidism affects serum calcium levels, increasing the likelihood of calcium stones. Crohn disease causes malabsorption of bile salts and fat, increasing likelihood of calcium oxalate kidney stones. Dietary contributors include excessive intake of calcium, vitamin D, oxalates, and alkali.

Patients with renal calculi are commonly asymptomatic when stones remain in the kidneys. However, when a stone moves into and obstructs a ureter, the patient experiences sudden onset of intermittent, severe pain caused by spasm of the involved ureter. The pain, which commonly radiates downward from the flank into the abdomen or groin area, is known as **renal colic.** Other symptoms include chills, fever, hematuria, and urinary frequency.

Preliminary diagnosis is based on the patient's signs and symptoms and the presence of blood in the urine. The presence of renal stones is confirmed by such radiologic tests as CT scan, ultrasound, IVP, MRI, and abdominal x-rays.

Conservative treatment of renal calculi includes opiate analgesics for pain, fluids, and smooth muscle relaxants, with the goal of enabling the patient to pass the stone in his urine. However, if the stone is too large or if the ureter is completely blocked, the physician may order surgery to remove the stone. Lithotripsy, another treatment option, involves the use of ultrasound to disintegrate the stone. (See Figure 31-4.)

Most patients are able to pass kidney stones without permanent damage. However, complete obstruction may result in hydronephrosis and potential failure of the involved kidney. Risk of recurrence is estimated at 50%.

Acute Renal Failure

ICD-9-CM code: 584

Acute renal failure (ARF) is an acute rise in the serum creatinine level of 25% or more and decreased GFR. It may last days or weeks or may develop into chronic renal disease. Approximately 3 million persons develop community-acquired ARF, meaning that it developed prior to hospitalization. A larger number of hospitalized patients develop hospital-acquired ARF. Highest rates are among those admitted to critical care and are related to advanced age, severity of illness, volume depletion, and exposure to nephrotoxic substances such as medications. Men and women are affected equally.

ARF occurs when the kidneys rapidly lose function due to some type of damage. As a result, the body retains waste products such as urea and creatinine that are normally excreted. There are many causes of ARF, which are categorized as *prerenal, renal,* and *postrenal,* depending on the physical location of the problem. Prerenal failure involves inadequate blood flow to the kidneys. Causes include hypotension caused by

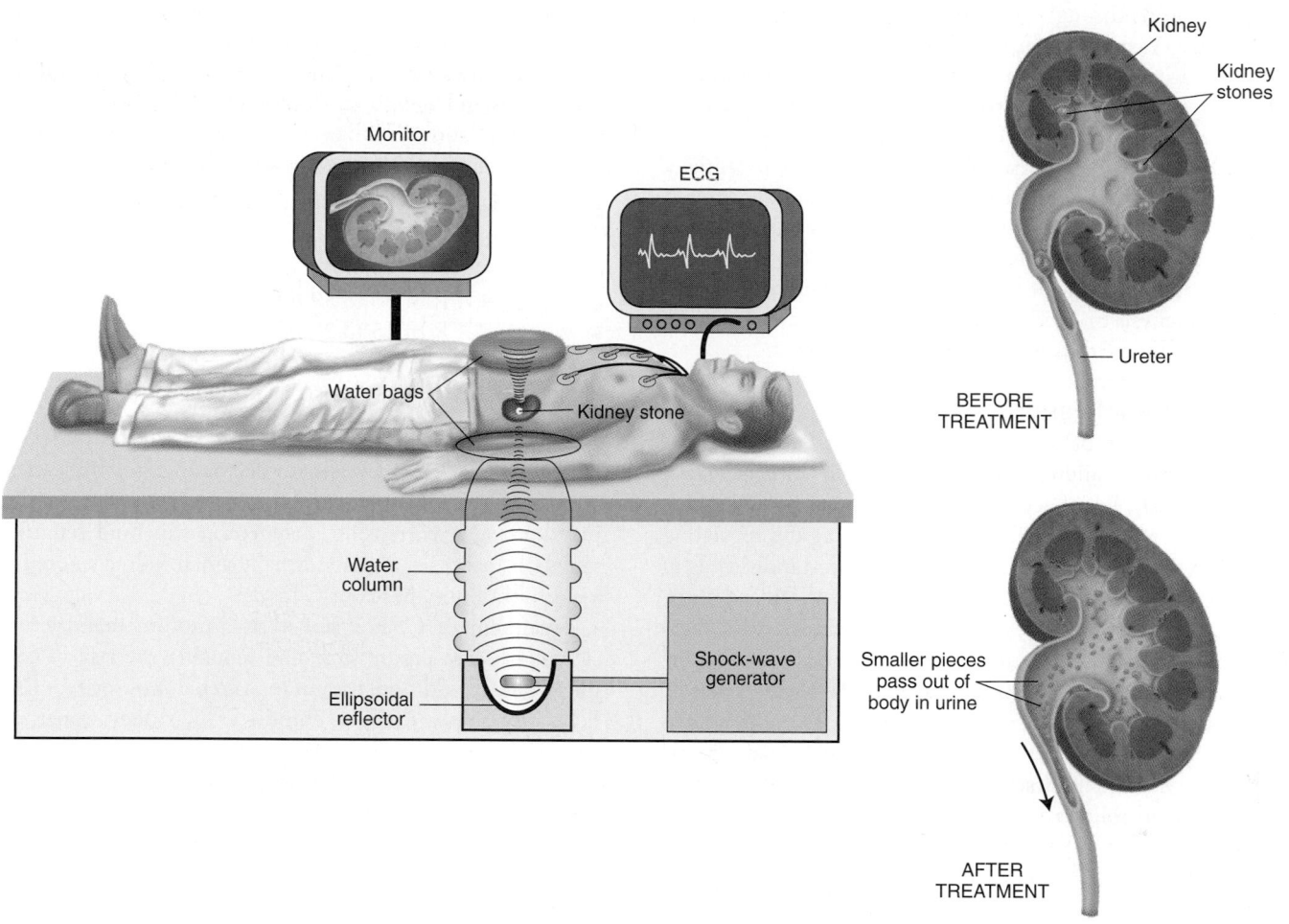

FIG 31-4 Lithotripsy.

hemorrhage, severe burns, shock or severe dehydration, liver failure, and renal vein thrombosis secondary to nephrotic syndrome. In renal failure, injury to the kidney, glomeruli, or tubules occurs. Causes of renal failure include pyelonephritis, some medications or toxins, and diseases that may damage the kidneys, such as sickle-cell disease, systemic lupus erythematosus, and multiple myeloma. In postrenal failure, an obstruction to urine outflow occurs. Causes include prostatic enlargement, kidney stones, and prostate cancer.

Common symptoms of ARF include **oliguria** (deficient urine production) or **anuria** (absence of urine production), generalized edema, altered mental status, tremors, anorexia, metallic taste in the mouth, easy bruising or bleeding, flank pain, fatigue, hypertension, and seizures. Diagnosis is based on elevated creatinine or blood urea nitrogen (BUN) values in an ill, oliguric patient. Abdominal or kidney ultrasound is the most common radiological test but others may include x-ray, CT scan, or MRI, which rule out obstruction.

Treatment of ARF is aimed at identification and treatment of the underlying cause. In many cases, the condition resolves spontaneously after the underlying cause is alleviated, such as removal, destruction, or passage of a kidney stone. Treatment also includes careful monitoring of fluid intake and output and electrolytes and administration of diuretic medications. The physician may also order diet modifications to increase carbohydrates and limit protein, sodium, and potassium intake, while ensuring adequate calories and nutrients. In some cases, temporary dialysis is also necessary.

There are two forms of dialysis: hemodialysis and peritoneal dialysis. **Hemodialysis** involves sending a patient's blood through tubes within a dialysis machine comprised of selectively permeable membranes. Just outside of the tubes is dialysis fluid which is somewhat similar in composition to human blood without the blood cells or waste products. Wastes along with excess fluid and electrolytes move from the blood across the membrane into the dialysis fluid and the machine returns the "clean" blood to the patient's body. **Peritoneal dialysis** is similar to hemodialysis except that the lining of the patient's peritoneal cavity (abdomen) is used as the dialyzing membrane. In this process, a nurse infuses dialysis fluid through a tube inserted in the patient's abdomen. Wastes then diffuse from the patient's blood vessels beneath the peritoneum, across the membrane, and into the dialysis fluid. After a specified period of time, usually 1 to 2 hours, the nurse removes the fluid.

Renal failure requires careful treatment and is potentially life-threatening. The mortality rate for hospital-acquired ARF is as high as 70% but is much lower for other groups. Infants and children with ARF have a 25% mortality rate. Some individuals may develop chronic renal failure, requiring ongoing dialysis or a kidney transplant. However, most individuals recover within several weeks or months.

Chronic Renal Failure
ICD-9-CM code: 585
Chronic renal failure (CRF), also called *chronic kidney disease* (CKD), is defined as the progressive loss of the kidney's effectiveness in excreting waste products and regulating fluid and electrolytes. An estimated 20 million individuals in the United States suffer from some degree of CRF and numbers are on the rise. The number of individuals with renal failure severe enough to require chronic dialysis or transplantation in 1999 was 340,000. However, it is estimated that by the year 2010, the number will be over 650,000. The United States has the highest rates of end-stage renal disease (ESRD), with the highest rates in the African American population. Japan follows in second place. At increased risk are elderly patients and patients with diabetes or hypertension.

Chronic renal failure develops slowly over a period of years and may result from any number of diseases that cause kidney damage. The most common causes are diabetes and hypertension, which cause at least two-thirds of all cases. Other causes include polycystic kidney disease, glomerulonephritis, analgesic nephropathy (damage caused by long-term use of analgesics, such as NSAIDs and acetaminophen), and various types of urine outflow obstruction. Risk factors include a family history of diabetes or renal failure. Also at increased risk are elderly persons and African American, Hispanic, Native American, and Pacific Islander populations.

Progression of CRF is commonly so gradual that symptoms are not evident until 90% of kidney function is lost. Symptoms are related to the development of uremia, which is the presence of increased nitrogenous waste products, especially urea, in the blood. Initial symptoms include nausea, vomiting, weight loss, fatigue, malaise, generalized pruritus, headache, and frequent hiccups. Later symptoms include oliguria, nocturia, easy bleeding or bruising, lethargy, diminished sensation in the extremities, muscle twitching, and seizures. Other symptoms might include polydipsia, pallor, hypertension, agitation, and changes in skin tone (darker or lighter).

According to the National Kidney Foundation, diagnosis is determined by checking blood pressure, urine albumin, and serum creatinine, all three of which will be elevated.

Glomerular filtration rate (GFR) is considered the most reliable indicator of renal function and is used to track the disease. Normal GFR varies by age and ranges from 116 ml/minute for patients around age 20 to 75 ml/minute for those age 70 or older. The National Kidney Foundation has categorized the severity of chronic kidney disease into five stages:

- *stage 1*—kidney damage with normal or increased GFR of greater than 90 ml/minute
- stage 2—GFR of 60 to 89 ml/minute
- *stage 3*—GFR of 30 to 59 ml/minute
- *stage 4*—GFR of 15 to 29 ml/minute
- *stage 5*—kidney failure with GFR less than 15 ml/minute or the patient is on dialysis.

Other findings may include progressively increasing creatinine and BUN levels with decreasing creatinine clearance as well as proteinuria and hyperkalemia. Other findings may include hypertension, polyneuropathy, fluid retention, metabolic acidosis, and abnormally small kidneys noted via x-ray, ultrasound, MRI, or CT scan.

Treatment of CRF is aimed at symptom management, slowing disease progression, and reducing the risk of complications. In addition, careful management of related disorders, such as heart failure, chronic UTI, kidney stones, and anemia, is essential. The physician will also prescribe dietary changes, usually including restriction of fluid, protein, and electrolytes. For individuals with end-stage renal disease, the physician will prescribe long-term dialysis and may consider kidney transplantation.

The mortality rate is highest among those with CRF severe enough to require chronic dialysis. The 5-year survival rate for this population is approximately 35%. It is even lower, at 25%, for those with underlying diabetes. Death is usually related to cardiovascular disease.

Male Reproductive System Diseases and Disorders
Benign Prostatic Hypertrophy
ICD-9-CM code: 600.2
Benign prostatic hypertrophy (BPH), also called *benign prostatic hyperplasia,* is a noncancerous growth and enlargement of the prostate gland in men. It is rare in younger men but becomes increasingly common as men age because the prostate gland increases in size with age. Incidence of symptomatic BPH is greatest in men over age 40 and is estimated at 50% for men over age 50. This rises proportionally to 80% for men over age 80. However, only a quarter of these men, approximately 300,000 per year, will seek treatment.

The cause of BPH is not fully understood; however, BPH develops in men who have elevated estrogen levels compared with relatively low testosterone levels. A substance known as dihydrotestosterone (DHT) may be a factor. DHT is synthesized from testosterone but is much more potent and plays an important role in prostate growth. As the prostate gland enlarges, it compresses the lumen, or passage, of the urethra, making it increasingly difficult for the patient to pass urine. Incomplete emptying of the bladder increases the risk of infection and other inflammatory changes to urinary tract structures.

Common symptoms of BPH are related to urethral obstruction and difficulty emptying the bladder. As a result, individuals usually complain of urgency, frequency, hesitancy, and nocturia. Patients may also notice a decrease in the force and consistency of the urinary stream. Urinary retention causes some individuals to become prone to urinary tract infections, kidney problems, and incontinence.

Diagnosis of BPH is based on the patient's description of signs and symptoms and confirmed by digital rectal examination (DRE), which reveals an enlarged prostate that is rubbery in texture. (A swollen, tender prostate indicates prostatitis, and a hard or nodular prostate may indicate cancer.) A prostate-specific antigen (PSA) blood test reveals an elevated level of prostate-specific antigen in 30% to 50% of individuals with BPH. Other diagnostic tests include rectal ultrasound, urine flow study, IVP, and cystoscopy, which help identify the degree of prostate enlargement and impedance of urine flow and differentiate benign prostatic enlargement from prostate cancer.

In some cases, initial treatment for BPH involves stabilization of kidney function by discontinuing anticholinergic drugs, treating infection, and emptying the bladder via catheterization. Further treatment for BPH aims to shrink or remove all or part of the prostate gland. In some men, the drug finasteride (Proscar) helps shrink the prostate gland. Other medications, such as terazosin (Hytrin), doxazosin (Cardura), and tamsulosin (Flomax), may act to improve urine flow and more complete emptying of the bladder in some patients. Transurethral microwave procedures employ the use of microwaves to destroy prostate tissue. Such procedures can usually be done in the medical office without general anesthesia. In a procedure called *transurethral needle ablation* (TUNA), low-level radiofrequency energy burns away part of the prostate. More invasive forms of surgery remove prostate tissue, including transurethral resection of the prostate (TURP), in which a surgeon inserts tiny surgical instruments via the urinary tract and uses them to remove prostate tissue. There are no external incisions or scars with this form of surgery. A urinary catheter must be in place postoperatively for 1 to 5 days to enable bladder irrigation and monitor urine output. Other options for surgery include laparoscopic prostatectomy, open prostatectomy, and radical prostatectomy. They are all more invasive and are generally reserved for patients with prostate cancer. They also require hospitalization and a longer recovery time.

Prognosis for BPH is generally good with adequate diagnosis and treatment. Around 5% to 10% of patients may experience some postoperative problems with sexual function and incontinence. In cases of extreme, prolonged obstruction, the ureters may dilate and hydronephrosis may develop. (See *After prostate surgery*, page 584.)

Prostate Cancer

ICD-9-CM code: 185

Prostate cancer is a malignant tumor of the prostate gland that occurs when prostate cells grow abnormally and uncontrollably. It is one of the most common forms of cancer in America. It affects 1 in 6 men, with nearly one-quarter of a million men diagnosed each year and nearly 30,000 deaths. It is rare in young men but much more common in older age groups, with over 65% of prostate cancer diagnosed in those over age 65.

The specific cause of prostate cancer is not clear. However, hormones such as testosterone are thought to play a role. Risk factors include advanced age, family history, genetics, and dietary factors. In addition, African American men are more likely to have prostate cancer; however, Caucasian men are twice as likely to die from the disease.

Patients are commonly asymptomatic in the early stages of prostate cancer. As symptoms develop, the patient may notice urinary frequency, urgency, and hesitancy; nocturia; dysuria; erectile dysfunction; painful ejaculation; hematuria; and blood in the semen. As the cancer spreads to bones and surrounding structures, the patient may complain of pain or stiffness in the lower back, hips, or upper thighs.

There is some controversy regarding the necessity of screening for prostate cancer. However, the American Cancer Society recommends that men over age 45 or 50 (depending on risk factors) undergo annual screening. Two common screening methods include digital rectal examination (DRE) and the prostate-specific antigen (PSA) test. To perform DRE, a health care provider palpates the prostate gland with a gloved, lubricated finger inserted rectally and notes irregularities in prostate gland shape, size, or texture. The PSA test detects the presence of a specific protein in the blood that is commonly elevated in the presence of prostate cancer, BPH, or prostatitis. If results of either test are abnormal, the physician will order a prostate tissue biopsy, which confirms the diagnosis if cancer cells are detected.

Treatment of prostate cancer depends on the age of the patient, aggressiveness of the cancer, and personal preference. After consultation with specialists, including a urologist, radiation oncologist, and medical oncologist, the health care team will design a treatment plan. Such a plan may include surgery, radiation, and chemotherapy. Orchiectomy (surgical removal of one or both testes) and drug therapy may reduce testosterone levels, which reduces the risk of metastasis and the aggressiveness of the cancer.

Patient Education

After Prostate Surgery

The medical assistant caring for a patient recovering from prostate surgery should emphasize to the patient that he should follow the physician's recommendations, which are tailored specifically to the patient. She should be sure to review these general guidelines:

- Be sure to rest frequently and avoid strenuous activity for the first few weeks even if you are having no pain.
- Drink lots of water to flush the bladder.
- Avoid driving or operating machinery for the time period specified by your physician.
- Avoid straining with bowel movements.
- Use these measures to avoid constipation:
  - Drink plenty of nonalcoholic, noncaffeinated fluids, including prune juice.
  - Eat a high-fiber diet, including fresh fruits, vegetables, whole grains, and bran.
  - Use bulk-forming, nonchemical laxatives, such as Metamucil.

- Be sure to consult with a physician before using stool softeners and chemical laxatives because, although they are available over the counter, they can be habit forming with regular use.
- Avoid heavy lifting.
- You may experience urinary frequency, urgency, or discomfort with urination initially. These symptoms should lessen over the next 8 to 10 weeks.
- You may experience some difficulty controlling urination initially; however, such difficulty should lessen over time,
- If you notice a mild increase in blood in your urine, you should rest and drink fluids. This increase is probably due to a loosening in the scab at the surgical site. If rest and fluids do not help or if you are concerned, call your physician.
- Although many men worry about sexual function after prostate surgery, in most cases sexual function returns fully with time.

Prognosis for prostate cancer is variable, depending on the cancer stage, Gleason score (microscopic appearance of cells), and PSA level. Overall, the 5-year survival rate for all types of prostate cancer is just over 70% and the 10-year survival rate is around 55%. For those whose cancer has already spread at the time of diagnosis, the 5-year survival rate is only 30%.

Testicular Cancer

ICD-9-CM code: 186.9

Testicular cancer is a malignancy of the testicle that occurs when cells grow abnormally and uncontrollably. It usually affects only one testicle and is the most common form of cancer in young males between the ages of 18 and 32, and the incidence is increasing. Approximately 7600 Americans are diagnosed and 400 die each year. Incidence is higher in Caucasians than other groups.

The specific cause of testicular cancer is unclear. Risk factors include a history of cryptorchidism (undescended testicle), infection with HIV or AIDs, age between 15 and 34, Caucasian race, and a family history of testicular cancer.

Patients with testicular cancer may be asymptomatic in the early stages. Signs and symptoms include a lump or enlargement in the testicle, which may or may not be painful; a dull ache within the groin or abdomen; a feeling of heaviness within the scrotum; scrotal edema; testicular or scrotal pain or discomfort; breast enlargement; fatigue; and malaise.

Diagnosis is generally made after the patient has noticed a lump or other abnormality and then seeks medical care. A physician may also note a lump during a regular health examination. Testicular ultrasound is highly effective in identifying testicular cancer. It helps the physician examine shape, size, and density of the testicles as well as any other masses. A solid mass is a sign of a malignant tumor, because most other testicular conditions involve the presence of fluid. If findings are suspicious, tissue biopsy confirms the diagnosis. Blood tests to detect alpha-fetoprotein (AFP) and human chorionic gonadotropin (HCG), two proteins called *tumor markers*, in blood may indicate the presence of a testicular tumor. A CT scan may be done to help stage the cancer and identify whether it has spread to other organs.

Treatment for testicular cancer depends on the type of cancer identified and whether it has spread. Surgical intervention usually includes orchiectomy and removal of local lymph nodes. Treatment also includes radiation therapy, chemotherapy, and, sometimes, bone marrow transplantation.

Prognosis for testicular cancer is good when it is diagnosed early, but declines as the cancer becomes more advanced. (See *Concerns about testicular cancer.*) Overall, there is a 95% rate of successful treatment. Because cancer is usually limited to one testicle, men are usually able to retain normal sexual function and fertility. (See *Procedure 31-1: Teaching a patient to perform TSE.*)

Patient Education

Concerns About Testicular Cancer

The medical assistant should encourage male patients to perform monthly testicular self-examination (TSE). Performing the TSE enables the patient to become familiar with how these tissues normally feel. By doing monthly examinations, the patient will notice changes early.

The medical assistant should instruct the patient to report to the physician any changes that persist for more than 2 weeks so that he can evaluate the changes. In addition, the medical assistant should inform the male patient that other disorders besides cancer may explain testicular changes, including:

- benign masses, such as hernias, inflammation, fluid, and cysts
- inflammation of structures, such as the epididymis
- varicocele, which is the presence of enlarged veins (varicose veins) within the scrotum
- orchitis, which is inflammation of the testicle caused by bacterial or viral infection
- spermatocele, a type of cyst that develops when the tubes that transport sperm become blocked.

PROCEDURE 31-1

Teaching a patient to perform TSE

Task

Teach a male patient to perform a testicular self-examination (TSE).

Conditions

- TSE pamphlet
- Examination model
- TSE shower card

Standards

In the time specified and within the scoring parameters determined by the instructor, the student will successfully teach a male patient to perform a testicular self-examination.

Performance Standards

1. Greet and identify your patient to prevent errors. Introduce yourself and explain the procedure to ease patient anxiety.
2. Wash or sanitize your hands to ensure infection control and assemble supplies.
3. To motivate the patient, explain the rationale for regular performance of TSE, including:
   a. Testicular cancer commonly goes undetected in the early stages because many patients experience no discomfort.
   b. Regular monthly exam allows him to note any changes in a timely manner.
   c. Examinations should begin during puberty.
   d. Examination is easiest during a warm bath or shower.
4. Using the examination model, demonstrate examination of the testes:
   a. Hold the scrotum in the palms of the hand and feel one testicle.

   b. Apply gentle pressure while rolling it between the fingers.
   c. Note any hard, painless lumps.
5. Using the examination model, demonstrate examination of the epididymis:
   a. Locate the circular-shaped cord behind the testis.
   b. Feel for any hard lumps.
6. Using the examination model, demonstrate examination of the vas deferens:
   a. Locate the firm, movable, smooth tube that runs upward from the epididymis.
   b. Feel for any hard lumps.
7. Repeat the demonstration of examination on the other side to reinforce learning.
8. Have the patient demonstrate TSE using the model to reinforce learning and enable correction or clarification as needed.
9. Give the patient a TSE pamphlet, which provides the patient with a source of information he can refer to as needed. and shower card. Instruct him to hang the card in his shower to remind him to perform monthly TSE, establish a regular routine of TSE performance, and keep instructions at hand.
10. Record TSE education in the patient's medical record to ensures a complete, accurate medical record.

Date	
03/17/08. 10:30 a.m.	*TSE teaching done. Patient given pamphlet and shower card.* ————————————————————*S. Gonzales. CMA*

Epididymitis

ICD-9-CM code: 604.90

Epididymitis is the inflammation or infection of the epididymis, a duct on the surface of the testicle. It affects over half a million men between ages 19 and 35 each year.

Epididymitis is commonly caused by a sexually transmitted disease. Causative organisms typically include *Neisseria gonorrhoeae* and *Chlamydia trachomatis*. Other organisms include *Staphylococcus* and *E. coli*. Epididymitis can also result as a complication of a urinary tract infection, prostatitis, and injury associated with surgery or the chronic presence of a urinary catheter.

Signs and symptoms of epididymitis include abdominal or flank pain or more localized pain in the testicle or scrotum. Other manifestations may include edema, dysuria, urinary frequency and urgency, urinary retention, fever, chills, discharge, and symptoms of urethritis.

Diagnosis is based on physical examination findings and the results of urinalysis and urine culture, which reveal the presence of bacteria and WBCs. Blood tests may also indicate an elevated WBC count. In some cases, regular or color-coded Doppler ultrasound reveals a thickened, enlarged epididymis and increased Doppler wave pulsation.

While a potential complication of epididymitis is sterility, prognosis is usually good with timely diagnosis and treatment.

Balanoposthitis

ICD-9-CM code: 607.1

Balanoposthitis, also called *balanitis*, is the inflammation of the glans penis and foreskin covering the glans penis. General incidence is unclear. However, one study found that 11% of male genitourinary clinic attendees had this disorder.

Balanoposthitis is most commonly caused by fungal infection but bacterial pathogens may also be involved. Organisms include the *Candida* species as well as *Bacteroides, Gardnerella,* and beta-hemolytic streptococci. They proliferate in the presence of smegma (a thick, cheesy, odoriferous secretion). The result is localized inflammation and edema. It develops most commonly in uncircumcised men with poor hygiene.

Signs and symptoms of balanoposthitis include tenderness, itching, redness, edema, and ulceration of the glans penis and foreskin; and meatal stenosis and phimosis (stenosis of the foreskin opening so that it cannot be pushed back over the glans penis).

Diagnosis is usually based on physical examination findings. Laboratory studies may include culture of urethral discharge and microscopic evaluation to identify the pathogen involved.

Treatment depends on the cause and usually includes daily retraction and cleaning of the foreskin and application of antibiotic or antifungal cream. The physician may also prescribe oral antibiotics. The physician may also recommend circumcision for those patients with phimosis to prevent recurrence.

Prostatitis

ICD-9-CM code: 601.0 (acute), 601.1 (chronic)

Prostatitis is the acute or chronic inflammation of the prostate gland, a small organ located below the bladder and similar in shape and size to a walnut. It is most common in men over the age of 50.

Prostatitis is categorized according to whether it is acute; chronic; includes conditions known previously as prostatodynia, chronic pelvic pain syndrome, and nonbacterial prostatitis or whether the individual is symptomatic or not. Prostatitis usually develops secondary to bacterial growth after the development of a UTI. Causative organisms include *N. gonorrhoeae, E. coli, Staphylococcus, Pseudomonas,* or *Streptococcus.*

Signs and symptoms include fever, chills, urethral discharge, dysuria, malaise, myalgias (muscle aches), and perineal discomfort. Upon examination, the prostate gland is tender and enlarged. Culture of prostatic secretions help identify the causative organism so that appropriate antibiotics can be selected. Treatment includes an extended course of antibiotics, opiate analgesics, and antispasmodics to relieve discomfort. Prognosis is very good for acute prostatitis. The prognosis for chronic prostatitis is less certain because complications may occur, including urethritis, epididymitis, and cystitis.

Sexually Transmitted Diseases

Chlamydia—ICD-9-CM code: 079.98
Gonorrhea—ICD-9-CM code: 098.0
Genital herpes, HSV-2—ICD-9-CM code: 054.10
HPV—ICD-9-CM code: 078.1
Genital syphilis—ICD-9-CM code: 091.0 (primary)
Secondary syphilis—ICD-9-CM code: 091.1 (unspecified)
Latent syphilis—ICD-9-CM code: 097.1 (unspecified)

Sexually transmitted diseases (STDs) are a group of diseases transmitted through sexual intercourse or other intimate contact with infected individuals. Viruses that most commonly cause STDs include human papillomavirus (HPV), herpes simplex virus (HSV), and hepatitis A, B, and C. The HPV virus is actually a group of more than 100 tumor viruses that can cause tissue growths on the surface of skin and mucous membranes and in some cases are responsible for cervical cancer in women.

Other organisms that often cause STDs include *Chlamydia trachomatis* and *Neisseria gonorrhoeae.* In nearly all cases, infection is spread through direct contact with lesions or other body fluids. Some types of STDs, such as syphilis, are becoming less common, but others have become epidemic. HPV has become the most common STD in the United States today, with more than 50% of all sexually active men and women becoming infected at some time. An estimated 20 million Americans between the ages of 15 and 49 are currently infected and over 6 million become newly infected each year. Young inner-city teens are most at risk for contracting gonorrhea, and nearly 400,000 cases are reported annually in the United States. An estimated 90 million people worldwide are infected with the genital herpes virus.

Symptoms of STDs vary with the organism involved. In some cases, patients are asymptomatic. In general, symptoms of bacterial STDs include urethral or vaginal discharge, dysuria, and pelvic pain. Symptoms of herpes simplex include local pain, itching, burning, dysuria, and a rash of small vesicles or pustules. Individuals with HPV infection are commonly asymptomatic unless they notice tissue growths, sometimes called warts, in the anogenital area. In many cases, HPV is only detected through an abnormal result from a routine Pap test.

Diagnosis of an STD is usually based on culture of vaginal or urethral discharge, examination of lesions, and the patient's description of symptoms. Antibiotics are used to treat bacterial STDs. Treatment of viral STDs is more challenging. In some cases, antiviral medication helps minimize viral shedding and lessens symptoms; however, a complete cure is usually not possible. Patients should refrain from sexual contact with others until treatment is complete. Sexual contacts should be identified for culture and treatment if necessary.

Prognosis for bacterial STDs is good with timely diagnosis and treatment. Prognosis for viral STDs is generally good with adequate self-care measures; however, because a cure is usually not possible, complications may occur. Some STDs can be passed to infants at birth, resulting in blindness or respiratory problems. HPV is the most common cause of cervical cancer in women.

Erectile Dysfunction
ICD-9-CM code: 607.84 (organic origin), 302.72 (inhibited sexual excitement)
The term *erectile dysfunction* (ED), also called *impotence,* is a general term that describes a number of disorders, all of which impact the ability of a man to attain an erection adequate enough to achieve a satisfactory sexual experience. Episodic ED occurs at some time to most men and is not considered problematic from a medical standpoint. As men age, some changes in erectile function are common, including loss of rigidity, need for more stimulation, less intense orgasm, and need for increased recovery time between erections. However, when problems with ED become chronic or reoccur frequently, they can be a sign of a physical or emotional problem. Men who experience ED that lasts longer than 2 months are encouraged to see their health care provider. ED is most common in men over the age of 65 but can occur at any age. Incidence is higher in men who smoke

or abuse alcohol or other drugs and those with diabetes and cardiovascular disease.

Causes of ED fall into two categories: physical and psychological. Common physical causes include disorders that affect nerve function, such as diabetes, spinal cord injury, and multiple sclerosis. Other disorders that may cause ED are cardiovascular disease or hormonal problems. ED may also be caused by adverse effects of medication, surgical complications, and drug and alcohol abuse. Psychological causes include fatigue, depression, stress, anxiety, and negative feelings toward or lack of interest in the sexual partner.

The main symptom of ED is difficulty developing or maintaining a full erection throughout intercourse. In order to diagnose ED, the physician must gather a health history, including a description of symptom onset and pattern and information about other medical conditions, medications, and recent physical and emotional events. Blood tests check hormone levels, such as testosterone, and help rule out underlying disorders, such as diabetes. The physician may adjust current medications to determine whether they are a factor. Ultrasonography can evaluate circulation. Neurological evaluation checks for nerve damage. Other tests include cavernosography to visualize the corpus cavernosum and cavernosometry to measure vascular pressure in the penis.

Treatment of ED depends on the underlying cause. Psychological causes are treated with counseling and, in some cases, medication. When ED is caused by medications, a change in dose or switch to another medication may resolve the problem. Treatment of physical causes is tailored to the individual disorder. There are numerous medications on the market for the treatment of ED, including sildenafil (Viagra), tadalafil (Cialis), and vardenafil (Levitra). These drugs relax smooth muscle in the penis, enabling greater blood flow, which results in increased quality of an erection when physical and psychological stimulation occur. Other treatments include testosterone replacement therapy, surgery, penile implants, and needle-injection therapy.

Prognosis for ED is variable. In many cases, it may resolve completely with appropriate treatment. In other cases, it may not fully resolve but can be lessened. (See *Teaching about ED,* page 588.)

Urology and Male Reproductive Procedures

Urology is a medical specialty that focuses on the study and treatment of diseases and disorders of the urinary and male reproductive systems. A physician who specializes in this area of medicine is a urologist. Many patients who have urological disorders initially see family practice physicians who then refer them to a urologist.

Teaching About ED

Erectile dysfunction (ED) is a personal subject and many men feel embarrassed about discussing it. However, the medical assistant should encourage male patients to discuss their concerns with the physician. When teaching about ED and treatment, the medical assistant should be sure to include these points:

- Many forms of treatment for ED are available. Discuss your concerns with the physician to identify a treatment plan that is right for you.

- Many unapproved treatments are promoted on television and the Internet. However, many of them do not work and some can actually harm you. Therefore, please talk with your physician prior to trying any of them.

- Even approved treatment methods are not right for everyone. Therefore, you should never use someone else's prescription medication. For example, if you have had a stroke, heart attack, or heart rhythm problem within the past 6 months, some medications could harm you.

- Never take sildenafil (Viagra), tadalafil (Cialis), or vardenafil (Levitra) with nitrate medications such as nitroglycerine because you could experience heart and blood pressure problems.

- It may take time to experience the full benefit of some medications, so do not be disappointed if you do not experience optimal results with the first dose.

- Because the key to a mutually satisfying sexual relationship with your partner is communication, discuss your concerns with your partner and seek counseling if needed.

The medical assistant will help the urologist with examinations as well as procedures, diagnostic tests, and patient education. Urinalysis, urine culture, and 24-hour urine specimens are essential components in diagnosing urological diseases and disorders. Methods for collecting urine specimens include the clean-catch, midstream method or catheterization, depending on the necessity for a sterile specimen, the patient's ability to comply with the physical demands of collecting a clean-catch specimen, and the physician's preference. (For more information on urine collection and analysis, see Chapter 44, "Urinalysis," on page 923.)

Assisting with Examination

The medical assistant prepares patients for examination by checking vital signs and obtaining a health history, which should include data regarding allergies, symptoms, and medications. In most urology offices, the medical assistant will routinely ask the patient to collect a urine specimen each time the patient checks in. Therefore, the medical assistant should become well versed in instructing patients how to obtain a clean-catch, midstream specimen. She should then assist the patient as needed with undressing and positioning. For physical examination of the urinary tract, female patients should be placed on the examination table in the dorsal recumbent position. If the physician is male, then a female assistant should remain in the room. Male patients are seated on the examination table. In both cases, unless a urine specimen is to be obtained by catheterization, the medical assistant should encourage patients to empty their bladders before the examination.

The medical assistant provides patient privacy and assists the physician as needed with the examination and performs ordered diagnostic tests. When examining a male patient, the physician uses inspection and palpation to examine the foreskin (if the patient is not circumcised), glans, penis, and scrotum for abnormal tenderness or masses. The physician may ask the medical assistant to dim the lights if he uses a transilluminator. The physician will typically perform a hernia check as well as a rectal examination, which allows the physician to palpate the prostate gland, noting the presence of enlargement, asymmetry, nodules, or other abnormalities.

Catheterization

Urinary catheterization is a procedure in which a sterile drainage tube is introduced into the bladder through the urethra to drain or withdraw urine. There are distinct advantages and disadvantages to obtaining a urine specimen by urinary catheterization. Disadvantages include invasiveness and the risk of introducing microorganisms into the urinary tract of the patient, in addition to the potential embarrassment experienced by the patient. However, advantages include the ability to obtain a more reliable specimen, particularly when the patient has some form of disability that might interfere with her ability to collect a clean-catch specimen properly. In any case, the medical assistant who performs the catheterization should use measures to protect the privacy and dignity of the patient and follow aseptic technique to protect the quality of the specimen obtained and protect the patient from infection.

Medical assistants should perform catheterizations only under a physician's order and only if she has been specifically trained in this procedure. Catheters are available in a variety of brands, types, and sizes. Medical offices and hospitals commonly stock size 14 to 20 for adults and size 8 to 10 for children. In the rare event that an adult suffers from urethral stenosis, the medical assistant may need to use a child's size. Although the physician will occasionally specify the type of catheter to use, the medical assistant will more commonly use her discretion to determine the appropriate catheter. Therefore, the medical assistant must choose carefully and take into consideration the patient's age, size, and gender and the rationale for the catheterization. If the purpose is simply to empty the patient's bladder, as when a patient is suffering from urinary retention, she should choose a straight catheter, sometimes called an *in-and-out catheter*. Some medical offices stock sterile catheterization kits that contain needed supplies. In such kits, the plastic supply container doubles as a urine collection tray. These kits usually contain a medium-size pair of sterile gloves; povidone-iodine swabs; water-soluble lubricant; a specimen container, lid, and label; and two drapes, one of which is fenestrated (has a small window in it). The kit may or may not include the catheter itself.

If the patient is female and the sole purpose of the catheterization is to obtain a urine specimen, then the medical assistant may use a minicatheter, also called a *fem-cath*. If the catheter must remain in place for a period of time, the medical assistant should choose an indwelling catheter. These catheters have a port for injecting a small amount of sterile water to inflate a small balloon near the tip of the catheter. The balloon helps secure the catheter in the patient's bladder, although the external catheter tubing should always be secured to the patient's leg with a catheter strap for the patient's safety and comfort.

Some patients may have difficulty lying supine for catheterization, especially if they are elderly or have such medical conditions as severe arthritis or heart failure. In such cases, a male patient can be positioned in a semi-Fowler position if necessary. However, such a position will not work with female patients, because it makes it impossible for the medical assistant to locate and visualize the patient's urethra. For the female patient unable to lie supine, the medical assistant can assist the patient into the side-lying position. If the medical assistant stands behind the patient, she will have good view and access to the patient's urethra. However, this technique does require a second assistant to help support the patient's upper leg.

Whenever the patient is a male with an enlarged prostate, a coudé catheter is a good option. It is slightly more rigid, has a slight curve near the tip, which is more rounded in shape. (See Figure 31-5.) It was designed specifically for such patients and more easily slips by the enlarged prostate to enable successful catheter insertion. (See *Procedure 31-2: Performing urinary catheterization*, page 590.)

Many urology tests aid in the diagnosis of urinary and reproductive disorders. Some of the most common tests include renal computed tomography, intravenous pyelography, cystoscopy, cystourethrography, creatinine, blood urea nitrogen, and renal angiography.

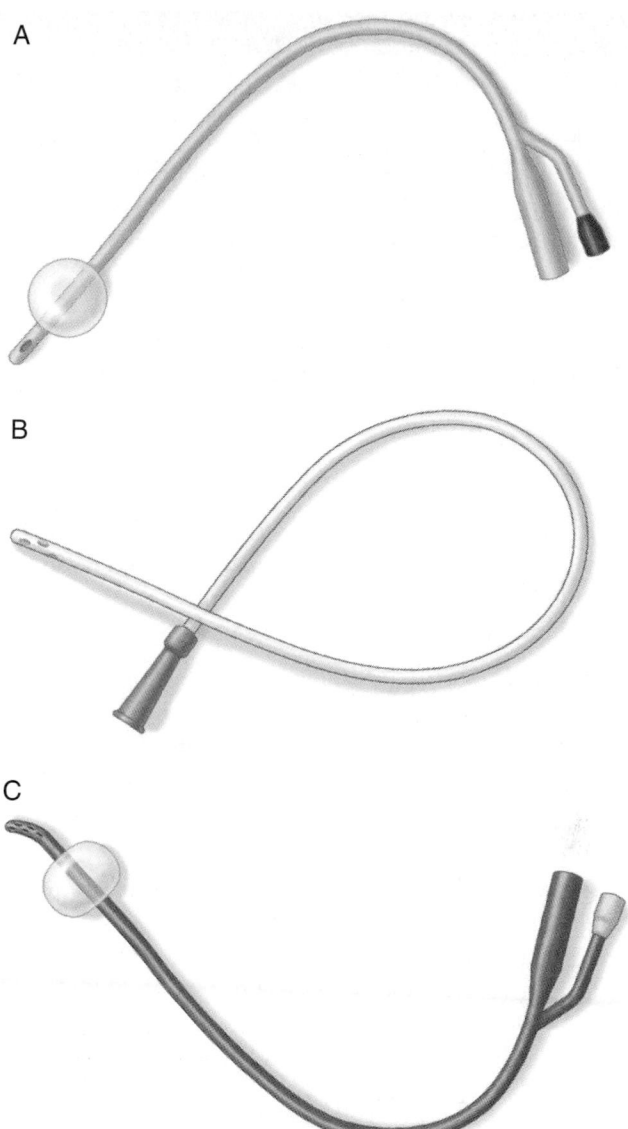

FIG 31-5 Catheters. (A) Indwelling. (B) Straight. (C) Coudé catheter.

Renal Computed Tomography Scan

A renal computed tomography (CT) scan is a painless radiological procedure in which multiple x-ray beams and detectors rotate around the patient to produce three-dimensional cross-sectional views of the kidneys. This procedure provides more detail than standard x-rays and is useful in identifying lesions, abscesses, fluid accumulation, kidney stones, obstructions, and tumors. It can also aid in needle placement for a kidney biopsy.

The scan may or may not include administration of a contrast dye, a radioactive substance administered intravenously or orally that causes the tissue being studied to show up more clearly. Patients who are or may be pregnant; those allergic to contrast dye, iodine, or shellfish; or those sensitive

PROCEDURE 31-2

Performing Urinary Catheterization

Task
Perform urinary catheterization on a patient.

Conditions
- Light source
- Laboratory slip
- Ink pen
- Nonsterile waterproof underpad
- Sterile urethral catheterization kit containing:
  - Straight catheter
  - Drapes
  - Tray
  - Gloves
  - Lubricant
  - Povidone-iodine swabs or cotton balls and povidone-iodine solution
  - Specimen container and label

Standards
In the time specified and within the scoring parameters determined by the instructor, the student will successfully perform catheterization on a patient to empty the bladder or collect a urine specimen.

Performance Standards
1. Wash or sanitize your hands to ensure infection control and assemble supplies.
2. Greet and identify your patient to prevent errors. Introduce yourself and explain the procedure to ease patient anxiety.
3. Ask the patient about allergy to iodine. If the patient is allergic, omit the povidone-iodine from this procedure to prevent an allergic reaction.
4. Instruct the patient to remove clothing below the waist, including undergarments, to facilitate efficient performance of the procedure. The patient may keep socks on if desired to help stay warm. Assist the patient as needed.
5. Assist the patient into the dorsal recumbent position and drape the patient for warmth and privacy, leaving the genital area exposed to help facilitate visualization of the urethra in female patients. (*Note:* Other than a pillow for the head, the patient should lie completely flat.)
6. For the female patient who is unable to lie completely flat or abduct her hips, consider an alternative side-lying position, which requires a second assistant to support the patient's upper leg. This position is more comfortable for these patients and increases the medical assistant's success in locating the female urethra and successfully completing the procedure.

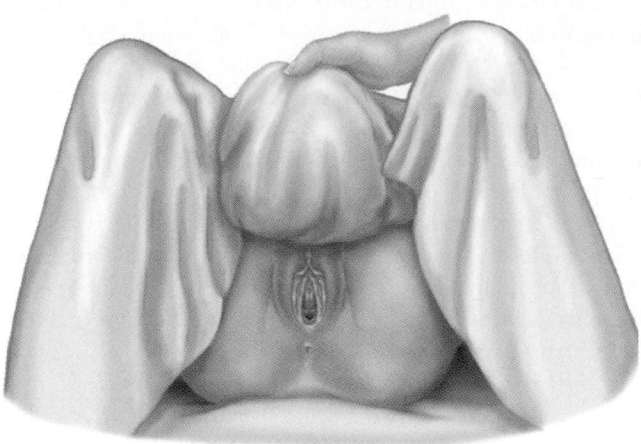

Place the patient in a flat, dorsal recumbent position and apply drapes for warmth and privacy.

7. Adjust the light source on the genital area. If an adjustable lamp is not available, have an assistant hold a flashlight. Good lighting is critical in identifying the urethra.
8. Place the nonsterile waterproof underpad under the patient's buttocks to absorb excess moisture.
9. To reduce the risk of infection to the patient and ensure a good-quality urine specimen, provide perineal hygiene as needed, including:
   a. Apply nonsterile gloves.
   b. Wash the perineal area with warm water and soap.
   c. Dry the perineal area with a towel.
   d. Remove and dispose of gloves.
   e. Wash your hands.
10. Open the catheter kit on a clean, dry, uncluttered surface using sterile technique to ensure infection control. Using a Mayo stand or other small wheeled table is optimal because it provides an efficient, movable work surface.
11. Keep the plastic bag that contained the kit nearby to use as a waste receptacle to enable efficient disposal of waste during the procedure.
12. Remove the sterile gloves from the kit and put them on to arrange sterile supplies within the kit without contaminating them.
13. If the physician's order does not include a specimen, remove the specimen container, lid, and label and set them aside to avoid cluttering the work space with unnecessary items.
14. If the order does request a specimen, place the label aside and put the specimen container and lid on a sterile surface within easy reach.

15. Open the sterile lubricant package. Grasp the catheter and apply the lubricant to the distal 1" to 2" of the catheter to ease catheter insertion and minimize patient discomfort. Place the catheter back inside the urine collection tray. Dispose of the lubricant wrapper.

16. Open the povidone-iodine swab packet and pull the swabs most of the way from their package. If the kit contains cotton balls, rather than swabs, place them in the sterile container and pour the povidone-iodine solution over them. Preparing all items ahead of time increases efficiency and decreases anxiety, stress, and the risk of contamination during the procedure.

17. Grasp the sterile drape so that two of the corners are wrapped around your hands to avoid contaminating your sterile gloves. Place the drape with the water-proof side down just under the patient's buttocks to provide a sterile area near the genital areas to place supplies and help ensure infection control. Ask the patient to lift her buttocks slightly if possible to facilitate this process.

18. Grasp the fenestrated drape and allow it to unfold without touching a nonsterile surface. Place it over the patient's genital area so that the genitals are visible through the window. (*Note:* Some providers prefer not to use a drape for female patients because the fenestrated drape may shift during the procedure and become a hindrance.)

19. Move the sterile tray by holding the inside with fingers extended outward against the sides and place it on the sterile drape near the client's buttocks to place needed items close at hand.

20. If the order requests a specimen, place the specimen container upright next to the urine collection tray on the sterile drape.

Female patients

21. With your nondominant hand, separate the *inner* labia as widely as possible so that the urethral meatus is visible. This hand is now considered contaminated and must remain in place until the catheter is fully inserted.

22. With your dominant hand, grasp the povidone-iodine swabs (or soaked cotton balls) and wipe from top to bottom on one side of the inner labia.

23. Grasp another swab (or cotton ball) and wipe from top-to-bottom on the other side of the inner labia.

24. Grasp another swab (or cotton ball) and wipe from top-to-bottom over the urinary meatus. Cleaning the area in this way reduces the presence of microorganisms and the risk of infection to the patient and increases the quality of the urine specimen.

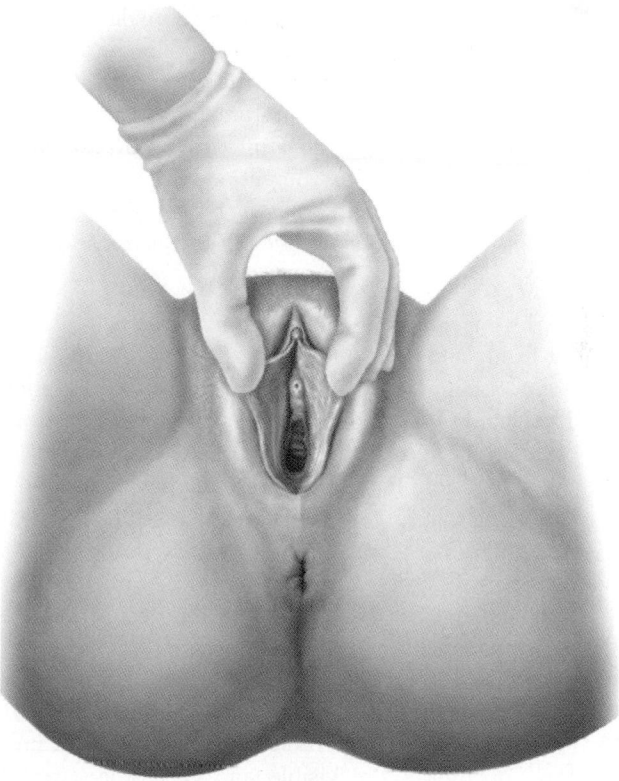

Wrap the corners of the sterile drape around your sterile gloved hands as you position the drape.

Separate the inner labia as widely as possible in order to view the urethral meatus.

Continued

PROCEDURE 31-2—cont'd

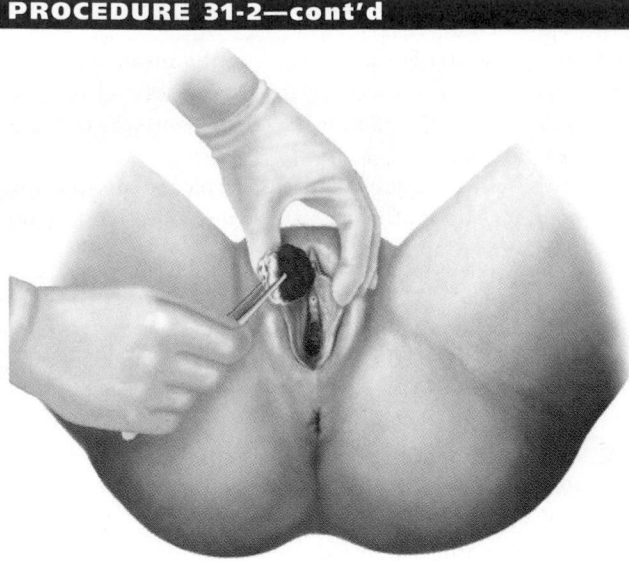

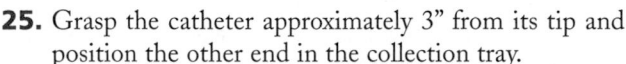
Separate the inner labia as you cleanse with povidone-iodine swabs.

25. Grasp the catheter approximately 3" from its tip and position the other end in the collection tray.
26. Ask the client to cough or bear down to make the urethral opening more visible and relax the external sphincter, making catheter insertion easier.
27. Hold the catheter at a slight upward angle (pointing toward the patient's umbilicus) to help the catheter slide into the urethra, rather than the vagina. Insert the lubricated tip into the urethra approximately 2" or until urine begins to flow into the collection tray. Release the labia with your nondominant hand and grasp the catheter, being sure *not* to let go of it because the catheter will quickly slide out if it is not secure.

Male patients
28. With your nondominant hand, grasp the penis gently yet firmly and use gentle traction in an upward direction to straighten the urethra, making insertion easier. This hand is now contaminated and must remain in place until the catheter is fully inserted.
29. With your dominant hand, grasp the povidone-iodine swabs (or soaked cotton balls) and wipe in a circular pattern from the meatus outward. Repeat this step two more times to reduce the presence of microorganisms and the risk of infection to the patient and increase the quality of the urine specimen.
30. Grasp the catheter approximately 3" from its tip and position the other end in the collection tray.
31. Ask the client to cough or bear down to make the urethral opening more visible and relax the external sphincter, making catheter insertion easier.

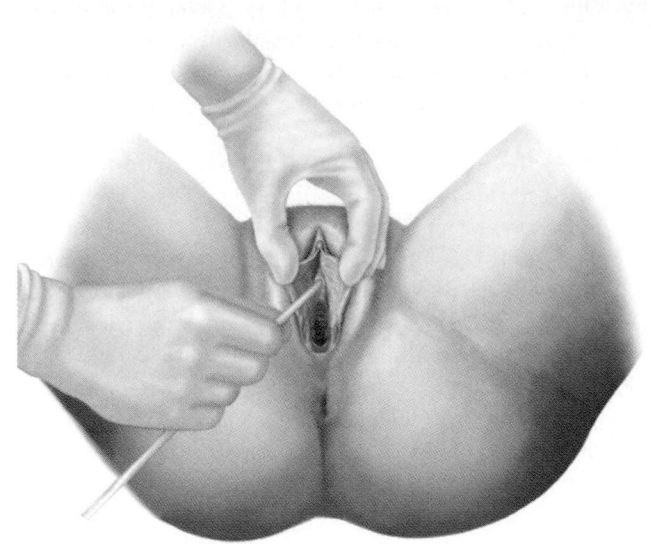
Insert the catheter at a slight upward angle.

32. Insert the lubricated tip of the catheter into the urethra until urine begins to flow into the collection tray. (*Note:* For some men, you may need to insert nearly all of the catheter.)

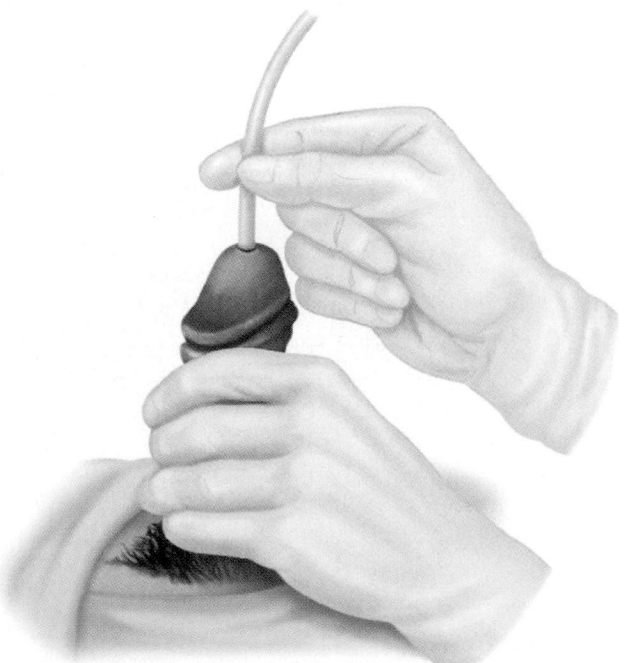
Continue inserting the catheter until urine begins to flow.

PROCEDURE 31-2—cont'd

33. Release the penis with your nondominant hand and grasp the catheter to hold it securely for the remainder of the procedure because the catheter will quickly slide out if it is not secure.

All patients

34. If the order requires a specimen, follow these steps:

　a. Use your dominant hand to temporarily crimp the catheter.

　b. Move it over the specimen container.

　c. Uncrimp the catheter and allow urine to flow into the specimen container.

　d. Crimp the catheter once more and move it back over the collection tray.

　e. Resume draining urine into the collection tray until the patient's bladder is empty.

35. When urine flow has stopped, gently remove the catheter from the urethra and dispose of it.

36. Dispose of supplies, remove your gloves, and wash your hands to ensure infection control.

37. Secure the lid to the specimen container. Note the total amount of urine collected in both containers and then discard the excess urine in an approved manner. If the

patient has been experiencing urinary retention, the physician will want to know the total volume retained.

38. Assist the patient off of the examination table and with dressing if necessary.

39. Write the patient identification data on the specimen label and affix it to the side of the specimen container, not the lid, because the laboratory processes many specimens at one time and the lid may become separated from container.

40. Complete the laboratory slip, package it with the specimen in the approved manner, and send it to the laboratory according to facility policy. Correct identification is critical to ensuring accurate results are recorded for each patient.

41. Document the procedure in the patient's medical record to ensure a complete, accurate medical record.

Date	
11/20/08: 8:30 a.m.	*Straight cath done using aseptic technique, 550 ml clear, yellow urine obtained, specimen sent to lab. --------------------* *---W. Jones, CMA*

to medications should discuss these issues with their physician before undergoing a renal CT scan. If the scan does involve a contrast dye, the medical assistant should instruct the patient to refrain from eating or drinking for a period of several hours before the test. The general steps of a renal CT scan include:

- The patient must remove clothing, jewelry, and other objects that may interfere with the procedure and put on a gown.
- If the test involves a contrast dye, a nurse will insert an intravenous (IV) line in the patient's hand or arm. For oral contrast, the patient must drink a liquid that includes the contrast. The nurse should tell the patient that he may briefly feel a warm, flushing sensation, salty or metallic taste in his mouth, headache, nausea, or vomiting.
- The patient must lie on a table that slides into the large, circular opening of the scanner.
- The technologist will be nearby in a separate room where the controls are located but will be able to view the patient through a window. The technologist will also be able to communicate with and hear the patient through a speaker system.
- As the scanner begins to rotate, the patient will hear clicking sounds. The technologist should reassure the patient that these sounds are normal.

- The scanner transmits the x-ray information to the computer, which converts the information into an image that the radiologist will interpret.
- The technologist will instruct the patient to lie very still during the procedure and to briefly hold his breath at various times.
- When the procedure is completed, the IV line is removed and the patient is asked to wait briefly while the radiologist verifies the clarity of the scan.

Intravenous Pyelography

Intravenous pyelography (IVP), also known as an *intravenous pyelogram* or *intravenous urogram* (IVU), is a radiological procedure used to identify abnormalities of the structures of the urinary system, including the kidneys, ureters, and bladder. It is the most common procedure to identify urinary tract dysfunction or kidney disease. It is typically done to investigate the cause of hematuria and to identify tumors or lesions. This procedure begins with injection of a radiopaque contrast dye, and then a series of x-rays taken over a 30-minute period record the progress of the dye as it filters through the kidneys. The radiologist will examine the x-rays for the shape, size, position, and equal filtration and flow of the kidneys. She will also examine the ureters for symmetry and smooth appearance and the bladder for a smooth appearance and complete emptying. Regular IVPs are less common than in the past. Instead, CT scans are replacing them or combined with IVPs because this procedure obtains better images with greater detail.

Cystoscopy

Cystoscopy is a procedure in which a cystoscope is introduced into the urethra and bladder to facilitate visual examination of the bladder wall, obtain tissue for biopsy, examine the ureters, locate and remove kidney or bladder calculi (stones), place stents, and distend (stretch) the bladder or dilate the ureters or urethra. This procedure may take place in the physician's office with or without topical anesthesia if simple visualization is planned. If the physician orders bladder distention (stretching) or biopsy, the procedure must take place in an operating room under general anesthesia.

A cystoscope is generally the diameter of a pencil with a lighted tip. It may also have a second lumen (tube) for inserting instruments to obtain tissue specimens or treat urinary problems. Typical reasons for cystoscopy include the diagnosis and treatment of such conditions as interstitial cystitis (chronic inflammatory condition), frequent UTIs, unexplained hematuria, overactive bladder or urinary incontinence, unusual findings in a urinalysis, urinary blockages, stones, polyps, tumors, or cancer. There is usually no special preparation for a cystoscopy unless general anesthesia is planned, in which case the medical assistant should instruct the patient to avoid eating or drinking anything for a specified period of time beforehand.

For the procedure, the medical assistant should instruct the patient to undress and put on an examination gown. The medical assistant should then help the patient assume the dorsal recumbent or lithotomy position and provide draping for warmth and privacy. She may also clean the genital area to reduce microorganisms and apply a topical anesthetic if ordered. When the physician inserts the cystoscope, the patient may feel a brief pinching sensation in the urethra. The physician may instill a sterile liquid, such as water or saline, into the bladder to fill it so that he can better visualize the bladder wall. This liquid may cause mild discomfort for the patient and the urge to urinate. The medical assistant should reassure the patient that the sensation will pass soon and that the physician will drain the liquid shortly. The entire procedure usually takes 20 minutes or less.

The medical assistant should explain to the patient that, after the procedure, he may notice burning with urination or presence of blood in his urine. Less commonly, he may notice mild abdominal pains caused by bladder spasms. These spasms rarely last for more than 24 hours; however, the patient should report them to the physician if they continue for more than a couple of days. The medical assistant should also encourage the patient to drink 1 L (approximately 1 qt) of water over the next 2 hours to reduce the risk of infection. He may also use mild heat in the form of a warm bath or the application of a warm washcloth to ease temporary discomfort.

Voiding Cystourethrography

Voiding cystourethrography examines the bladder and urethra as the bladder fills and empties. It helps identify structural abnormalities, urine flow abnormalities such as ureteral reflux, the cause of repeated UTIs, prostate enlargement, and causes of urinary incontinence. As with other procedures, the patient should notify her physician if she is or might be pregnant, is breastfeeding, or might be allergic to contrast dye. The medical assistant should also ask the patient about her use of bismuth-containing medications, such as Pepto-Bismol, or a history of using barium contrast dye within the past 4 days, because they may interfere with test results.

Prior to the procedure the medical assistant should instruct the patient to remove her clothes, put on a gown, and empty her bladder. The medical assistant should then help the patient assume the dorsal recumbent position and provide draping for warmth and privacy. She may also clean the genital area to reduce microorganisms. The physician will then insert a urinary catheter and slowly instill a radiopaque dye into the bladder until it is full. The physician will then take x-rays with the patient standing, sitting, and lying down. The physician will then remove the catheter. The medical assistant should instruct the patient to urinate while the x-rays are taken. The test usually takes 45 minutes or less and is generally not painful, although the patient may find the procedure uncomfortable at times due to positioning requirements and the feeling of a full bladder.

The medical assistant should explain to the patient that, after the procedure, she may notice burning with urination or presence of blood in her urine. Less commonly, she may notice mild lower abdominal pain. This pain rarely lasts for more than 24 hours; however, the patient should report it to the physician if it continues for more than a couple of days. The patient should also report problems with urine leakage, foul-smelling urine, flank pain, fever or chills, and nausea or vomiting. The medical assistant should encourage the patient to drink fluids to reduce risk of infection.

Creatinine

Creatinine is the decomposition product of metabolism of a substance called *phosphocreatine,* a source of energy for muscle contraction. Small amounts of it are normally found in urine and blood. Increased quantities are found in advanced stages of renal disease. The normal creatinine level is 0.5 to 1.4 mg/dl.

Blood Urea Nitrogen

Blood urea nitrogen (BUN) is a test that measures the amount of nitrogen in the blood that comes from the waste product urea and reflects the balance between its production and excretion. It is normally removed from blood and excreted by the kidneys in urine. Normal BUN levels are generally between 6 and 19 mg/dl. When evaluating kidney function, physicians commonly order the BUN test along with creatinine.

Renal Angiography

Renal angiography, also called *renal arteriography,* is a procedure in which a contrast dye injected through a catheter into the renal vessels makes them visible on a radiological machine called a *fluoroscope.* This procedure detects vascular abnormalities, evaluates renal disease, and examines the kidneys before or after transplantation.

Prior to the procedure, the medical assistant may instruct the patient to avoid eating or drinking for 12 hours. Immediately before the procedure, she should instruct the patient to undress and put on an examination gown. During the procedure, the medical assistant should instruct the patient to lie very still. After the radiologist injects a local anesthetic near the site to be used (an artery in the arm or leg), he will thread a catheter through the aorta and into the renal artery. He then injects a contrast dye through the catheter and takes a series of x-rays as the dye circulates through the kidneys. The physician will then remove the catheter and apply pressure to stop any bleeding. During this time, the medical assistant should measure the patient's vital signs and instruct her to rest. She should also instruct the patient to rest after discharge, avoid physical exertion for 24 hours, and report any excessive signs of bleeding or swelling.

Vasectomy

The most common male reproductive procedure performed in the medical office is the **vasectomy,** which is a surgical procedure performed to sterilize a man. The physician performs it in the office using a local anesthetic. In this procedure, the surgeon makes a small incision in the scrotum and lifts and removes a small section of the vas deferens. The surgeon then sutures or clips the ends of the vas deferens and closes the area with sutures. (See Figure 31-6.)

After the procedure, the medical assistant should instruct the patient to rest for a couple of days and use cold application and analgesics such as ibuprofen for discomfort. She

should also tell the patient that some sperm may remain in the ducts and that it can take up to 1 month for all sperm to be gone. The patient should provide two specimens for a sperm count 4 to 6 weeks apart. Until these tests verify sterility, the patient should use some means of contraception. (See *Confirming sterility.*)

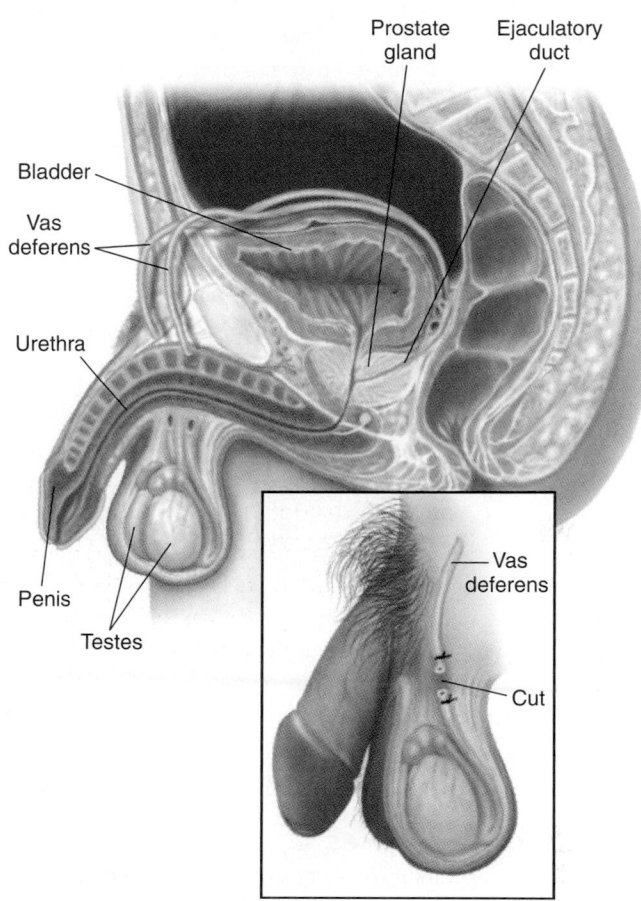

FIG 31-6 Vasectomy.

Patient Education

Confirming Sterility

The medical assistant may need to explain to a patient that he must bring in two separate semen specimens 4 to 6 weeks apart after undergoing a vasectomy for testing. The physician cannot confirm sterility until the patient provides these specimens. The medical assistant should be sure to explain to the patient that he does not have to completely fill the specimen cup.

Chapter Summary

- The urinary system is responsible for filtering excessive fluid and wastes from the blood and maintaining a healthy acid-base balance. Key structures of the urinary system include the kidneys, ureters, bladder, and urethra.
- The male reproductive system is responsible for procreation and regulation of several of the hormones in the body and shares many of the same structures with the urinary system.
- Medical assistants must be well versed in the language and vocabulary that pertain to the urinary and male reproductive systems. In addition to knowing common word elements, they should be familiar with common pathological terms and abbreviations.
- Some of the most common disorders of the urinary system include bacterial cystitis and urethritis, bladder cancer, renal cancer, Wilms tumor, nephrotic syndrome, hydronephrosis, polycystic kidney disease, renal calculi, acute renal failure, and chronic renal failure.
- Some of the most common disorders of the male reproductive system include BPH, prostate cancer, testicular cancer, STDs, and ED.
- Urology is a medical specialty that focuses on the study and treatment of diseases and disorders of the urinary system. Medical assistants assist physicians in urology with patient examinations, diagnostic testing, and procedures.
- A common procedure done in the urology office is urinary catheterization. The physician may order catheterization to empty the bladder or collect a urine specimen.
- Vasectomy is a surgical procedure to achieve male sterilization. Follow-up testing is essential to confirming sterility.

Team Work Exercises

1. Medical assistants must sometimes discuss personal subjects with patients. Doing so can be uncomfortable for the patient and medical assistant. However, the medical assistant can reduce discomfort for both parties by speaking in a sensitive, kind, clear manner and projecting a professional demeanor. The medical assistant will be more successful in achieving this goal if she practices discussing these topics with classmates first. Divide into groups of three to five students each. Each team must complete one of these assignments (as assigned by the instructor):
   a. Collection of a urine specimen is a common task for administrative and clinical medical assistants. Write up a set of instructions that would be clear and understandable to the average patient. Read the instructions to the rest of the class and solicit their suggestions for improvement or changes.
   b. Write up postprocedure instructions that would be clear and understandable to a patient who has just undergone a vasectomy. Instructions should address self-care and follow-up testing. Read the instructions to the rest of the class and solicit their suggestions for improvement or changes.
   c. Write up a set of instructions and discussion points on self-care and prevention activities for UTI. Make sure the instructions would be clear and understandable to the average patient. Read the instructions to the class. Solicit their suggestions for improvement or changes.
   d. Write up a set of instructions and discussion points on self-care and prevention activities for STDs. Make sure the instructions would be clear and understandable to the average patient. Read the instructions to the class. Solicit their suggestions for improvement or changes.
2. Divide into groups of three or four students and select one of the following tests:
   a. renal computed tomography
   b. kidney ureter-bladder films (KUB x-ray)
   c. intravenous pyelography (IVP)
   d. cystoscopy
   e. cystourethrography (voiding)
   f. creatinine clearance
   g. blood urea nitrogen (BUN)
   h. angiography (renal).
   Gather as much information about the test as you can from this text, other medical books, the Internet, and your local medical clinic. Create a teaching poster and present your information to the class. Be sure to address the most common reasons the test is ordered, any preparation the patient must complete before the procedure, a description of the actual procedure, description of the typical findings (normal and abnormal), and any postprocedure information or activities the patient must know about. Be sure to create a poster that is colorful and visual (with illustrations, photos, and so forth) and that presents information in an organized manner.

Case Studies

1. Rick Bell is a 52-year-old man who is a regular patient at the clinic. He calls in the morning stating that he has been awake since 4 a.m. with intermittent, severe pain in his right flank that sometimes radiates down into his groin. The physician suspects that Mr. Bell may have a kidney stone. What testing will the physician probably order to rule out or confirm this diagnosis? When the physician confirms a diagnosis of nephrolithiasis, what treatment options will be considered? If the physician asks Mr. Bell to try to pass the stone naturally, what instructions should he receive? If the stone totally obstructs the ureter, what complicating condition could result?

2. Howard Jameson comes to the medical office to discuss concerns about ED with his physician. List some potential causes and contributors to this condition. What data will the physician gather to formulate a diagnosis? Mr. Jameson is interested in trying one of the currently available prescription medications to help with this problem. List these medications. Describe how these medications work. Describe what patient education Mr. Jameson should receive if he decides to use one of these medications.

Resources

- Information on prostate cancer: *www.prostatecancerfoundation.org* and *www.nci.nih.gov/cancertopics/types/prostate*
- Information on testicular cancer: *www.nci.nih.gov/cancertopics/types/testicular*
- National Kidney Foundation: *www.kidney.org*
- Senior health: *http://seniorhealth.about.com/od/sexandsexuality/Sex_and_Sexuality_for_Seniors.htm*
- Urology patient education information: *www.urologyhealth.org*

Obstetrics and Gynecology

Learning Objectives

Upon completion of this chapter, the student will be able to:

- define key terms related to obstetrics and gynecology (OB-GYN)
- describe the function of the female reproductive system
- identify the structures of the female reproductive system
- identify the role of the medical assistant in OB-GYN
- identify instruments used during a gynecological examination
- assist with examinations and procedures
- explain diagnostic procedures related to OB-GYN
- describe prenatal and postpartum care
- calculate estimated due date (EDD)
- define the stages of labor
- list common complications of pregnancy
- describe menopause
- identify common diseases and disorders related to OB-GYN
- identify common laboratory tests related to OB-GYN
- provide patient education
- perform patient teaching for breast self-examination.

CAAHEP Competencies

Clinical Competencies
Diagnostic Testing
  CLIA-waived tests
Patient Care
  Prepare and maintain examination and treatment areas
  Prepare patients for and assist with routine and specialty examinations

General Competencies
Legal Concepts
  Establish and maintain the medical record
  Document accurately
Patient Instruction
  Instruct individuals according to their needs
  Provide instruction for health maintenance and disease prevention
  Identify community resources

ABHES Competencies

Communication
  Be impartial and show empathy when dealing with patients
  Adapt what is said to the recipient's level of comprehension
  Serve as a liaison between the physician and others
Clinical Duties
  Interview and record patient history
  Prepare patients for procedures
  Apply principles of aseptic techniques and infection control
  Take vital signs
  Prepare and maintain examination and treatment areas
  Prepare patient for and assist physician with routine and specialty examinations and treatments and minor office surgeries
  Collect and process specimens
  Perform selected CLIA-waived tests (i.e., "kit" tests such as pregnancy, quick strep, dip sticks) that assist with diagnosis and treatment
  Dispose of biohazardous materials
  Practice standard precautions
Legal Concepts
  Determine needs for documentation and reporting
  Document accurately
Instruction
  Instruct patients with special needs
  Teach patients methods of health promotion and disease prevention

Procedures

  Providing instruction on breast self-examination
  Preparing a patient for and assisting with a gynecological examination

Chapter Outline

Structures and Functions of the Female Reproductive System
  Structures of the Female Reproductive System
    Internal structures
    External structures
    Breasts
  Functions of the Female Reproductive System
    Internal structures
    External structures
    Breasts
Female Reproductive Cycle
  Menstruation
    Follicular phase
    Luteal phase
    Menstrual phase
  Pregnancy
  Birth Process
  Menopause
Medical Terminology Related to the Female Reproductive System
Common Obstetric and Gynecological Diseases and Disorders
  Vaginal Infections
    Candidiasis
    Chlamydia
    Genital herpes
    Genital warts
    Gonorrhea

Key Terms

abortion
Spontaneous or induced termination of pregnancy before the fetus reaches a viable age

adenomyosis
Benign invasive growth of endometrial tissue into the myometrium

Bartholin glands
Two small glands located at the opening of the vagina

blastocyte
Group of cells in early gestation that will form an embryo

coitus
Sexual intercourse

colposcope
Instrument used to examine the tissues of the vagina and cervix

colposcopy
Examination of vaginal and cervical tissues by means of a colposcope

conception
Time at which an ovum is fertilized

dilation
Increase in size

effacement
Thinning of the cervix during labor

endometrium
Mucous membrane that lines the uterus

episiotomy
Incision made into the perineum to facilitate delivery of a baby

estrogen
Hormone that stimulates female characteristics

fetus
Term used to describe a developing human in utero from 9 weeks' gestation (after the embryonic stage) until birth

fundus
Area of the uterus above the openings to the fallopian tubes

gestation
Time from conception to birth

gravidity
Total number of pregnancies

hormone
Chemical substance released from a gland or organ

lactation
Process by which a mother produces milk for her newborn infant

mammary glands
Milk-producing glands in a female

menarche
Age of first menstruation or the onset of menstruation

menopause
Permanent cessation of menstruation, usually occurring between ages 38 and 58

menstruation
Female cycle of producing and expelling the unfertilized ovum

neonate
Newborn from birth to 1 month of age

ovaries
Glands that produce ova, the cells from the female necessary for procreation

Papanicolaou test
Test used to detect cancer of cervical cells

perineum
Area between the vaginal opening and anus

placenta
Uterine structure that is connected to the fetus by the umbilical cord and from which the fetus obtains nourishment and oxygen

postpartum
Time from birth up to 6 weeks

prenatal
Time of gestation before birth

progesterone
Hormone that prepares the uterus for pregnancy

prolactin
Hormone that stimulates breast development and production of milk

zygote
Fertilized ovum

Structures and Functions of the Female Reproductive System

The female reproductive system includes ovaries, fallopian tubes, a uterus, a vagina, a vulva, a clitoris, labia, and a perineum. The female reproductive system houses the organs necessary for the reproduction of another human. It also manufactures **hormones**, which are chemicals secreted into the bloodstream that cause reactions. The female reproductive system produces the hormones that are necessary for the development and functioning of reproductive organs.

Structures of the Female Reproductive System

The female reproductive system is made up of internal structures and external structures.

Internal Structures

Internal organs and structures of the female reproductive system include the ovaries, fallopian tubes, fimbriae, uterus, cervix, vagina, endometrium, and myometrium. (See Figure 32-1.)

The **ovaries** are flat, oval-shaped structures located on each side of the uterus in the lower abdominal cavity, attached to the broad ligament. The ovaries contain the graafian follicles, in which are the immature ova, or eggs. The two fallopian tubes extend approximately 4" from the sides of the superior lateral surface of the uterus toward the ovaries. Although the fallopian tubes do not connect to the ovaries directly, they are attached to the broad ligament for stability. Each fallopian tube ends with wavelike structures called *fimbriae.*

The uterus is a thick-walled, muscular organ located posterior to the urinary bladder and anterior to the rectum. The uterus consists of the **fundus**, the rounded upper portion; the corpus, the body of the uterus; and the cervix, the narrowed section that opens into the vagina. The cavity of the uterus is triangular in shape and the innermost lining is called the *endometrium.* The myometrium, or muscular tissue of the uterus, consists of muscle fibers that run in many directions, including circular, longitudinal, and diagonal.

External Structures

The external structures of the female reproductive system, also called the *vulva*, include the clitoris, urethral meatus, labia, mons pubis, and **Bartholin glands**. (See Figure 32-2.) This area in men and women is also called the *perineum*.

The clitoris, made up of elongated erectile tissue, is located beneath the anterior aspect of the labia. The urethral meatus, located posterior to the clitoris and anterior to the vaginal opening, is the opening to the urinary bladder. The labia, which cover the clitoris, urethral meatus, and vaginal opening, consists of two layers. The labia minora is a thin layer of tissue that extends from the anterior clitoris to the posterior aspect of the vaginal opening. The labia majora lies

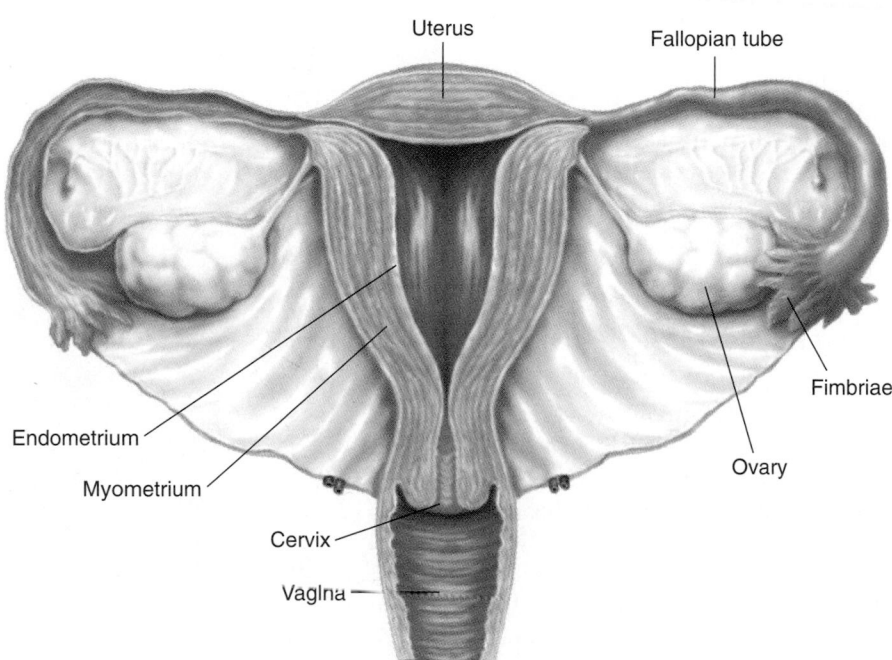

FIG 32-1 Internal structures of the female reproductive system.

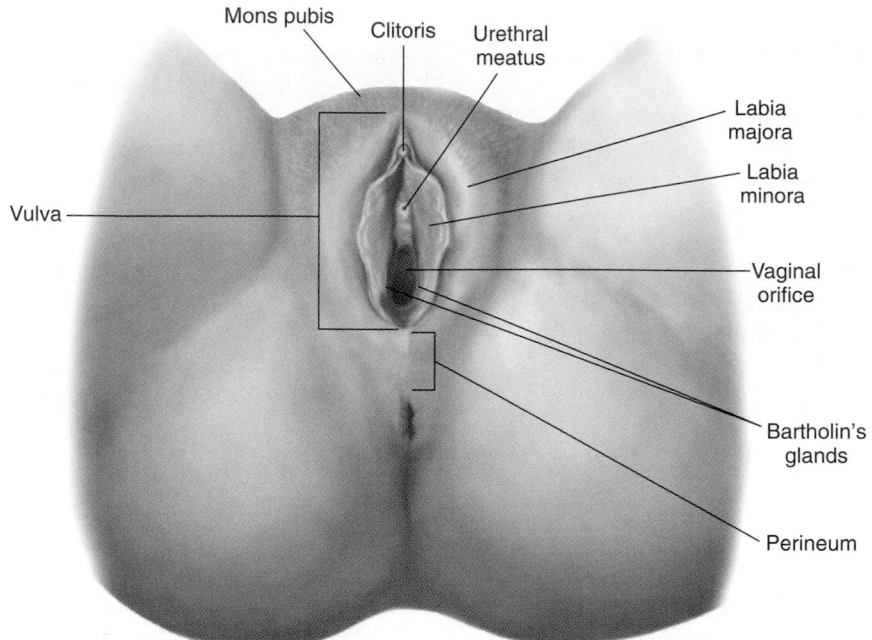

FIG 32-2 External structures of the female reproductive system.

on either side of the labia minora and forms the lateral borders of the vulva. In the adult female, the labia majora and mons pubis, the pad of fatty tissue that covers the pubic symphysis (or *pubic bone*), is covered in coarse hair.

Breasts

During puberty, increased secretion of estrogen causes breasts to develop. (See Figure 32-3.) The center of each breast has a region of pigmented tissue called the *areola*. At the center of the areola is the nipple. Inside each breast are 15 to 20 lobes of glandular tissue, including **mammary glands**, which are the milk-producing glands in a female. This glandular tissue is surrounded by connective and adipose tissue.

Functions of the Female Reproductive System

The primary function of the female reproductive system is to bear offspring, that is, produce another human being. The internal and external organs and structures of the female reproductive system all function toward achieving this ultimate goal.

Internal Structures

Ovaries are the primary sex organs in females. Ovaries produce ova, one-half of the necessary components of a new life. They also produce two female hormones:

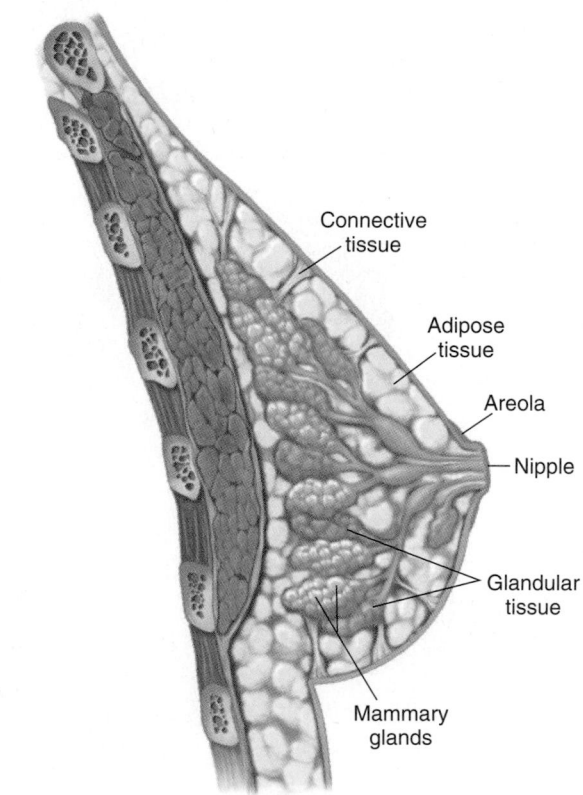

FIG 32-3 Cross-section of the female breast.

- **Estrogen** acts to develop the female reproductive organs during puberty, produces secondary sexual characteristics such as breasts and pubic hair, and prepares the uterus for a fertilized egg.
- **Progesterone** is responsible for the changes in the **endometrium**, the lining of the uterus, which allows for implantation of the **blastocyte** (the developing embryo).

The fallopian tubes are the pathways through which the ovum travels from an ovary to the uterus. The wavelike fimbriae on the ends of the fallopian tubes help direct the ovum from the ovary into the tube. As the ovum travels down the tube, the ovary secretes estrogen and progesterone to change the endometrial tissue of the uterus to be more receptive to implantation of the ovum.

The cervix and uterus house and protect the developing fetus. The muscular tissue of the uterus is able to expand during pregnancy to accommodate the growing fetus. The cervix will dilate during the birth process to allow delivery of the fetus. The multidirectional muscles of the myometrium also enable forceful contraction of the uterus during the birth process.

External Structures

The labia protect other external and internal structures. The clitoris responds to stimulation, causing orgasm. The vagina acts as the passageway for the penis during sexual intercourse and as the birth canal during the birth process.

Breasts

The connective tissue of the breasts provides support and the adipose tissue provides insulation. The amount and distribution of the adipose tissue determine the size and shape of the breasts. However, the role of the breasts in reproduction is nourishing the **neonate**, or newborn baby, with the mother's breast milk, a process called *lactation*.

The mammary glands of the breasts are the organ of milk production in response to the later part of pregnancy and after giving birth. During pregnancy, the breasts respond to four hormones:

- Estrogen increases the size of the breasts.
- Progesterone stimulates the development of the duct system (for lactation).

Breastfeeding for a healthy baby and mother

The American Association of Pediatricians (AAP) recommends breastfeeding exclusively for the first 6 months of an infant's life. At 6 months of age, the mother can introduce solid food; however, the AAP recommends that breastfeeding continue to age 12 months. The health benefits associated with breastfeeding for this length of time or longer are significant for the baby and the mother.

Benefits for Baby

New research shows that babies who are exclusively breast-fed for 6 months are less likely to develop infections, respiratory illnesses, diabetes, sudden infant death syndrome (SIDS), asthma, allergies, some cancers, and, possibly, childhood obesity. Benefits of breastfeeding for babies include:

- physical closeness to the mother's body that helps create an emotional bond between the infant and mother
- more easily digested by the baby than formula
- no preparation required and always available
- all the nutrients, calories, and fluids that a baby needs to be healthy
- growth factors that ensure the development of the baby's organs
- many substances (that formula does not have) to protect the baby from various disorders, including:
  - ear infection
  - diarrhea
- pneumonia, wheezing, and bronchiolitis
- bacterial and viral infections such as meningitis.

Benefits for Mother

For some mothers and babies, breastfeeding goes smoothly from the start. For others, it takes a little time and several attempts to get the process going effectively. Like anything new, breastfeeding takes some practice. These difficulties and adjustments are perfectly normal. The medical assistant should reassure a new mother who is struggling with breastfeeding and encourage her to talk to her doctors and nurses as well as her pediatrician. Other helpful resources include a lactation specialist and a breastfeeding support group. Benefits of breastfeeding for the mother include:

- releases hormones in the body that promote mothering behaviors
- returns the uterus to the size it was before pregnancy more quickly
- may help with weight loss because milk production uses calories
- delays return of the menstrual period, helping to keep iron in the body
- reduces the risk of ovarian and breast cancers
- keeps bones strong, which helps protect against bone fractures in older age.

- **Prolactin** stimulates the production of milk.
- Oxytocin promotes the ejection of milk from the glands. (See *Breastfeeding for a healthy baby and mother*.)

Female Reproductive Cycle

The female reproductive system follows a cycle that parallels the life span. The cycle includes menarche, menstruation, pregnancy and childbirth (for some women), and menopause. The timing of these stages varies from woman to woman; however, the cycle will follow this order for every woman.

Menstruation

Menarche, the onset of menstruation (or *menstruation*), varies in adolescent females from age 9 up to age 17. The average age of menarche is age 13. **Menstruation**, also called the *menstrual cycle*, is a normal body process that occurs approximately every 28 days. The body gets rid of the thickened endometrial tissue that develops each month in preparation for pregnancy. The 28-day cycle occurs in three phases:

- follicular
- luteal
- menstrual.

Follicular Phase

In the follicular phase, the hypothalamus of the brain secretes gonadotropin-releasing hormone (GnRH), which stimulates the anterior pituitary gland to secrete follicle-stimulating hormone (FSH) and luteinizing hormone (LH). These hormones act on the graafian follicles of the ovaries, to secrete estrogen, which stimulates the growth and thickening of the endometrium of the uterus. In between 9 to 14 days, the graafian follicle ripens and bulges out of the ovarian wall in a process called ovulation. The wall becomes thinner until the ovum ruptures the wall and is released into the abdominal cavity. The spot of rupture on the ovary, now called the *corpus luteum*, begins to secrete progesterone, which acts on the endometrium to prepare it for pregnancy. The emergence of the ovum ends the follicular phase.

Luteal Phase

In the luteal phase, the ovum is propelled toward the fallopian tubes by the wavelike action of the fimbriae. During this phase, progesterone produced by the corpus luteum continues to cause extensive growth of the functional layer of the endometrium. If fertilization of the ovum, also called *conception*, occurs, the corpus luteum will secrete human chorionic gonadotropin (HCG). If no conception occurs, the corpus luteum does not secrete HCG and, instead, atrophies into a mass of fibrous tissue called the *corpus albicans*. In the absence of HCG and decreasing progesterone levels, the endometrium begins to deteriorate and menstruation begins.

Menstrual Phase

The third and final phase is the menstrual phase. In this phase, the uterus discharges necrotic endometrial tissue, mucus, and blood engorgement of the endometrium. The menstrual phase lasts between 5 to 7 days, after which the follicular phase begins again. (See Figure 32-4.)

Pregnancy

Fertilization is the process of one sperm penetrating an egg and forming a **zygote**. The resulting zygote has 23 chromosomes from the ovum and 23 chromosomes from the sperm and is a unique new being. The cell begins to grow and multiply immediately as it travels down the fallopian tube. The zygote reaches the uterus in 4 to 6 days and implants in the uterine endometrium. Implantation of the zygote causes a change in the menstrual cycle. The ovaries release high levels of estrogen and progesterone, causing the endometrium to be receptive to implantation. The corpus luteum secretes inhibin, which inhibits secretion of FSH in the anterior pituitary gland, and relaxin, which prevents contractions of the myometrium, increasing the likelihood of implantation of the zygote. The resulting low level of FSH along with low levels of LH prevents stimulation of a new follicle and disrupts the 28-day menstrual cycle. Secretions from the fallopian tubes and uterine glands provide nutrients for the developing zygote. After implantation, the **placenta**, the organ of nutrition for the growing zygote, forms within the wall of the uterus.

As the zygote develops into an embryo and then a fetus, the placenta also grows to provide nourishment and supply oxygen. The placenta begins forming early after conception and is completely formed by 12 weeks' gestation. The mature placenta is approximately 7" in diameter and is in the shape of a flat disc. It adheres to the wall of the uterus and connects to the developing fetus through the umbilical cord. The umbilical cord contains two arteries and one vein; the arteries supply oxygen and nutrients to the fetus while the vein removes carbon dioxide and wastes. The placenta secretes human chorionic gonadotropin (hCG), a hormone that stimulates the corpus luteum of the maternal ovary so that it will continue to secrete estrogen and progesterone. As the placenta increases in size, it will secrete estrogen and progesterone itself and hCG levels in the bloodstream will drop. Estrogen will prevent the secretion of FSH and LH (from the anterior pituitary gland), which prevents the normal menstrual cycle. Progesterone will prevent contractions of the uterus that would result in a miscarriage.

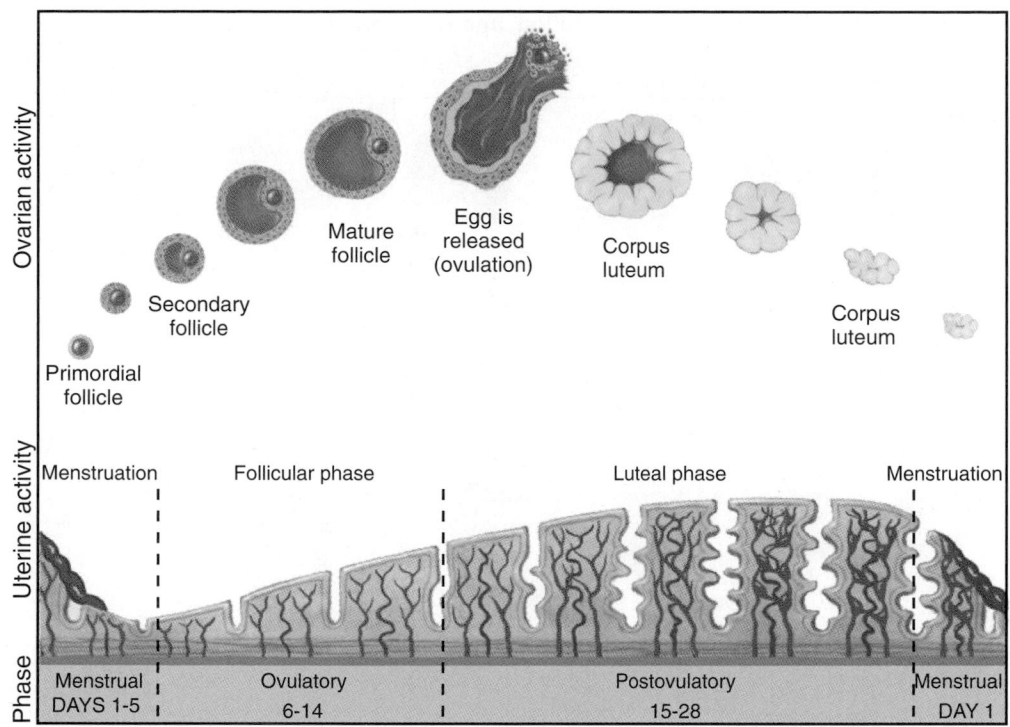

FIG 32-4 Phases of the menstrual cycle.

Pregnancy, also called **gestation**, is broken into three equal time periods, called *trimesters*. The first trimester of pregnancy, called the *embryonic and early fetal period*, begins 2 weeks after fertilization when the zygote is well established in the uterus and lasts to 9 weeks' gestation. During this period, the zygote becomes an *embryo* and develops all its tissues and organs. The pregnant patient should establish obstetrical care early in the **prenatal** period, the period during pregnancy and before birth. Ideally, the patient should establish regular prenatal care with an obstetrician early in the first trimester.

At 9 weeks' gestation, the embryo is called a **fetus**. By 12 weeks, the ultrasound technician or obstetrician can determine the sex of the embryo using ultrasonography. The medical assistant can advise the pregnant patient that her body as well as that of the developing fetus is changing. Because of these changes, she will most likely experience symptoms during the first trimester, such as fatigue, nausea, vomiting, breast tenderness, urinary frequency, constipation, and insomnia. The medical assistant and physician can encourage the patient to get proper rest, drink plenty of fluids, exercise regularly, and eat small, frequent meals to minimize symptoms.

During the second trimester, at 15 to 28 weeks' gestation, the uterus has expanded to above the umbilicus and the expectant mother can feel the first fetal movements.

By 20 weeks, the fetus can open its eyes; by 24 weeks the fetus can hear sounds made outside the uterus. As the second trimester progresses, fetal movements become vigorous, and the mother can note when the fetus is sleeping or awake. At this time, fetal growth is rapid; by the end of the second trimester, the fetus has developed eyelashes and eyebrows and subcutaneous fat deposits. Even so, the fetus at this stage is not yet ready for birth because it still weighs less than 2 lb. If it were born at 23 weeks, it would have a 1 in 10,000 chance of surviving.

During the third trimester, the fetus adds more subcutaneous fat, the testes descend in males, and the lungs grow toward full development. Maternal weight gain can be in excess of 1 lb per week. The patient may experience lower back pain and fatigue, due to the increase in fetal size and quantity of amniotic fluid. The medical assistant can encourage her patient to rest and elevate her feet if she experiences swelling, or edema. The physician must monitor weight gain and blood pressure to detect the possible onset of preeclampsia, a complication in late-term pregnancy. By the end of the seventh month, or 28 weeks' gestation, the fetus has typically moved into the head-down position in anticipation of birth. At full term, 38 to 40 weeks' gestation, the average weight of the fetus is 7½ lb. (See Figure 32-5.)

Period of dividing zygote, implantation, and bilaminar embryo (in weeks)

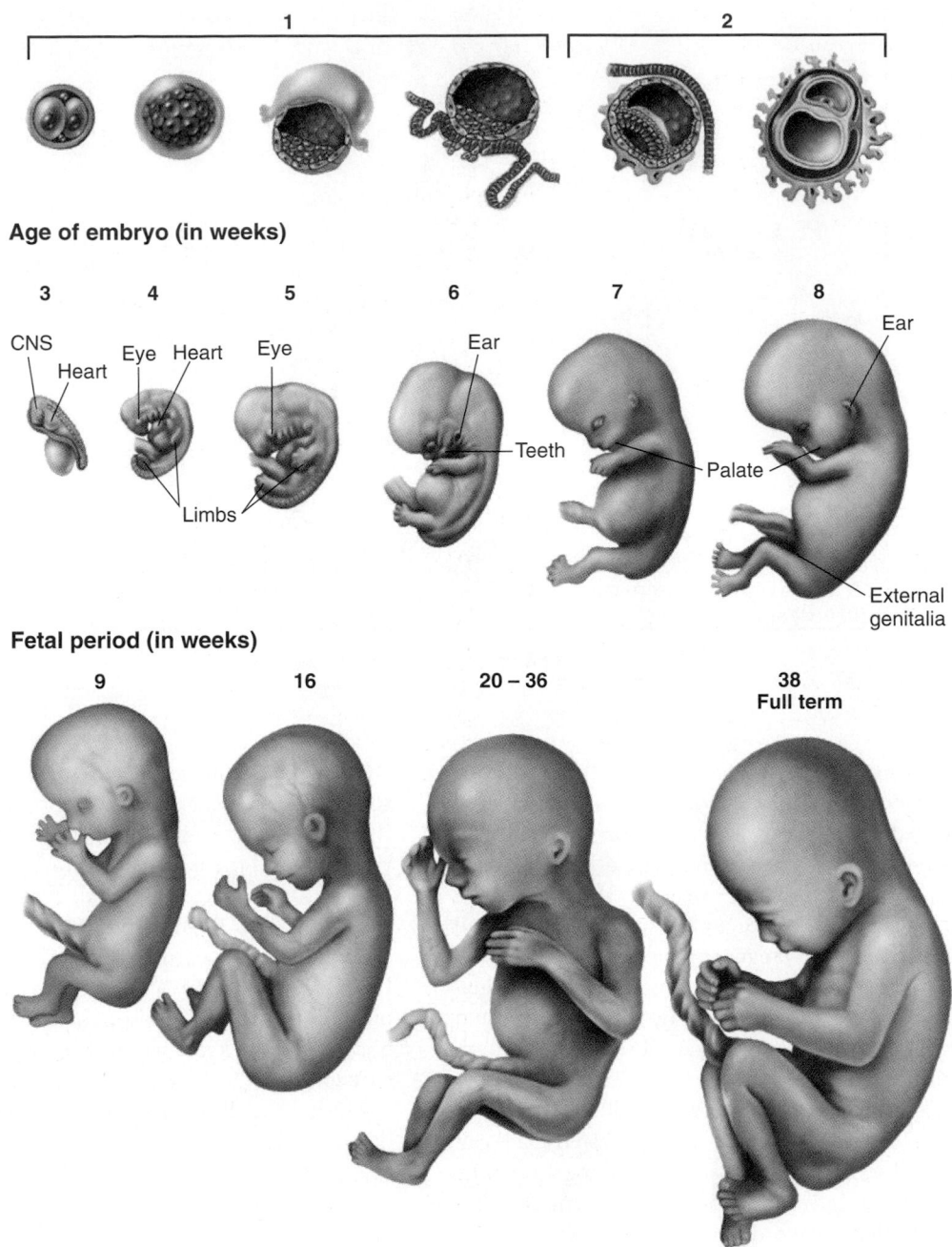

Age of embryo (in weeks)

Fetal period (in weeks)

FIG 32-5 Stages of embryonic and fetal development.

Birth Process

Toward the end of gestation, the placental secretion of progesterone decreases, while the levels of estrogen remain high. The myometrium will start to gently contract at irregular intervals. These early contractions that do not directly precede labor are called *Braxton Hicks contractions*. The beginning of labor and delivery is usually signaled by the expulsion of the mucus plug that developed in the cervix to protect the fetus from organisms in the vagina. After the expulsion of the mucus plug, the amniotic fluid from the uterus may start to leak slowly or may rush out of the body more quickly. The uterus will begin more rhythmic contractions due to a drop in the secretion of progesterone from the placenta.

The first stage of active labor starts with dilation and effacement of the cervix. The contractions of the uterus force the amniotic sac into the cervix, causing **dilation**, or expansion, of the diameter of the cervical opening. The degree of cervical dilation is measured in centimeters from 1 to 10 cm. At 10 cm, the cervix is large enough to accommodate delivery. Cervical **effacement** is the thinning of the cervix as the opening of the cervix (called the *internal os*) is pulled up into the lower portion of the uterus. This effacement further accommodates delivery. Uterine contractions increase in intensity in this stage and come at more frequent intervals. This first stage of labor can last from 1 to 24 hours. Depending on the amount of time and the intensity of contractions, the patient may become exhausted. During this time, a nurse can provide analgesics or local anesthetics to the patient to help ease her discomfort.

The second stage of labor involves delivery of the infant. In this stage, the posterior pituitary gland secretes oxytocin, a powerful hormone that causes even more forceful contraction of the uterus. During these contractions, the woman will feel the need to "push," or bear down on these contractions. Eventually, as the woman bears down, the top of the baby's head will appear at the cervical opening, called *crowning*. After the mother delivers the baby's head, she will deliver the shoulders. Just before delivery of the shoulders, the baby's head appears to rotate to the side. After the mother delivers the shoulders, the body of the baby passes easily through the opening, completing the second stage of labor.

In the third stage of labor, the placenta detaches from the uterine wall, and the uterus expels it from the body, usually with a few more contractions. The uterus will continue to contract after delivery of the placenta to constrict open blood vessels and control bleeding. If the physician performed an **episiotomy**, an incision into the perineum to ease delivery, or tearing of the perineum occurred during the birth process, the patient may require sutures to the perineum.

Menopause

The menstrual cycle continues throughout a woman's life until a period called *menopause*, the normal cessation of menstruation. Menopause will occur naturally in most women approximately 40 years after menarche. The menstruation may stop suddenly or the flow and frequency of menstruation may decrease gradually. Removal of the uterus or ovaries causes surgical menopause, which occurs immediately after the surgery.

Symptoms of menopause vary widely in severity, begin soon after the ovaries stop functioning, and may last from a few months to several years. Signs and symptoms of menopause can include:

- hot flashes, chills, night sweats
- excitability
- fatigue, apathy, mental depression, crying episodes
- insomnia
- vertigo
- headaches
- numbness, tingling, myalgia
- urinary and gastrointestinal disturbances.

Treatment of menopausal symptoms may include hormone replacement therapy (HRT). However, because of the risks associated with this drug therapy, the patient and physician must determine whether or not it is a viable option. The physician and medical assistant should encourage a menopausal patient to maintain a diet high in calcium, vitamins, and minerals. Such a diet will help her naturally reduce menopausal symptoms.

Medical Terminology Related to the Female Reproductive System

The female reproductive system is complex and changes throughout a woman's life. The patient will seek care during her years of menstruation, pregnancy, menopause, and postmenopause. To be effective in their role, medical assistants must become well versed in the language and vocabulary that pertains to the female reproductive system. The following tables on pp. 608–610. list common medical terminology related to the female reproductive system.

Table 32.1 | Word Elements

This table contains combining forms, prefixes, and suffixes related to the female reproductive system, along with examples of terms that use the word element, a pronunciation guide, and a definition for each.

Word Element	Meaning	Example	Meaning
Combining Forms			
amni/o	amniotic sac	**amniocentesis** (ăm-nē-ō-sĕn-TĔ-sĭs)	transabdominal puncture of the amniotic sac
cervic/o	neck; cervix	**cervicitis** (sĕr-vĭ-SĬ-tĭs)	inflammation of the cervix
colp/o	vagina	**colpoptosis** (kŏl-pŏp-TŎ-sĭs)	prolapse of the vagina
galact/o	milk	**galactopoiesis** (gă-lăk-tō-poy-Ē-sĭs)	milk production
gynec/o	woman, female	**gynecology** (gī-nĕ-KŎL-ō-jē)	study of diseases of the female reproductive system and the breasts
hyster/o	uterus (womb)	**hysterectomy** (hĭs-tĕr-ĔK-tō-mē)	surgical removal of the uterus
lact/o	milk	**lactation** (lăk-TĀ-shŭn)	production and release of milk by mammary glands
mamm/o	breast	**mammography** (măm-ŎG-ră-fē)	radiographic imaging of the breast
mast/o	breast	**mastectomy** (măs-TĔK-tŏ-mē)	surgical removal of the breast
men/o	menses, menstruation	**menopause** (MĔN-ō-pawz)	permanent cessation of menstrual activity
metr/o	uterus (womb); measure	**endometrium** (ĕn-dō-MĔ-trē-ŭm)	mucous membrane that lines the uterus
nat/o	birth	**prenatal** (prē-NĀ-tăl)	occurring before birth
oophor/o	ovary	**oophorectomy** (ō-ŏf-ō-RĔK-tō-mē)	excision of an ovary
ovari/o	ovary	**ovariotubal** (ō-vā-rē-ō-TŪ-băl)	concerning the ovary and oviducts
perine/o	perineum	**perineoplasty** (pĕr-ĭ-NĔ-ō-plăs-tē)	reparative surgery on the perineum
salping/o	tube (fallopian or eustachian)	**salpingocele** (săl-PĬNG-gō-sēl)	hernia of the fallopian tube
vagin/o	vagina	**vaginapexy** (văj-ĭn-ă-PĔK-sē)	repair of a relaxed or prolapsed vagina
Prefixes			
ante-	before, in front of	**antepartum** (ăn-tē-PĂR-tŭm)	period of pregnancy between conception and onset of labor
dys-	bad; painful; difficult	**dysmenorrhea** (dĭs-mĕn-ō-RĒ-ă)	pain associated with menstruation
endo-	in, within	**endometrium** (ĕn-dō-MĔ-trē-ŭm)	mucous membrane that lines the uterus
multi-	many, much	**multipara** (mŭl-TĬP-ă-ră)	woman who has delivered more than one viable infant
post-	after	**postmenopausal** (pōst-mĕn-ō-PAW-zăl)	time period after permanent cessation of the menstruation
pre-	before	**precoital** (prē-KŌ-ĭ-tăl)	prior to sexual intercourse
primi-	first	**primigravida** (prī-mĭ-GRĂV-ĭ-dă)	woman during her first pregnancy

Table 32.1 | Word Elements—cont'd

Word Element	Meaning	Example	Meaning
Suffixes			
-arche	beginning	**menarche** (mĕn-ĂR-kē)	first menstrual period; onset of menstruation
-cele	hernia	**uterocele** (ū-TĔR-ō-sēl)	hernia of the uterus
-gravida	pregnancy	**nulligravida** (nŭl-ĭ-GRĂV-ĭdă)	woman who has never conceived a child
-para	to bear (offspring)	**unipara** (ū-NĬP-ă-ră)	woman who has had one pregnancy to 20 weeks' duration or longer
-rrhea	to flow, to discharge	**amenorrhea** (ă-mĕn-ō-RĒ-ă)	abnormal absence of menstruation
-salpinx	tube (fallopian or eustachian)	**pyosalpinx** (pī-ō-SĂL-pĭnks)	pus in the fallopian tube
-tocia	childbirth, labor	**dystocia** (dĭs-TŌ-sē-ā)	difficult or painful childbirth

Table 32.2 | Pathologic Terms

This table lists some of the most common pathologic terms related to the female reproductive system with a brief definition of each.

Term	Definition
adenomyosis ăd-ĕ-nō-mī-O-sĭs	benign invasive growth of endometrial tissue into the myometrium
amenorrhea ă-mĕn-ō-RĒ-ă	absence of menstruation or monthly period
dysmenorrhea dĭs-mĕn-ō-RĒ-ă	painful menstruation
eclampsia ĕ-KLĂMP-sē-ă	disorder of pregnancy marked by hypertension, convulsions, and coma
endometriosis ĕn-dō-mē-trē-O-sĭs	growth of endometrial tissue outside of the uterus, commonly on adjacent organs
fibroids FĪ-broyds	benign uterine tumors
gestational diabetes jĕs-TĀ-shŭn-ăl dī-ă-BĒ-tēz	diabetes mellitus that occurs during pregnancy
menorrhagia mĕn-ō-RĀ-jē-ă	menstrual bleeding that is excessive in amount of blood and number of days of menstruation
placenta previa plă-SĔN-tă PRĒ-vē-ă	condition in which the placenta is located over the cervical opening to the vagina
preeclampsia prē-ĕ-KLĂMP-sē-ă	condition during pregnancy characterized by increasing blood pressure, proteinuria, and edema
uterine prolapse Ū-tĕr-ĭn PRO-lăps	protrusion of the uterus through the vagina
sexually transmitted disease SĔK-shū-ă-lē TRĂNS-mĭt-ĕd dĭs-ĒZ	infection that spreads by sexual contact

Table 32.3 | Abbreviations

In obstetrics and gynecology, as in other areas of health care, abbreviations are commonly used. Abbreviations such as the ones listed below save time and effort in documentation and written communications.

Abbreviation	Term
C-section	cesarean section
D&C	dilatation and curettage
FSH	follicle-stimulating hormone
GYN	gynecology
IUD	intrauterine device
IVF	in vitro fertilization
LH	leutinizing hormone
LMP	last menstrual period
OB-GYN	obstetrics and gynecology
OC	oral contraceptive
Pap test	Papanicolaou test
PID	pelvic inflammatory disease
STD	sexually transmitted disease
STI	sexually transmitted infection
TAH	total abdominal hysterectomy
TAH-BSO	total abdominal hysterectomy with bilateral salpingo-oophorectomy

Common Obstetric and Gynecological Diseases and Disorders

There are innumerable diseases and disorders of the female reproductive system. Some of the most common include vaginal infections, menstrual disorders, uterine disorders, complications of pregnancy, infertility, fibrocystic breast disease, and cancer.

Vaginal Infections

Infections of the vagina, or *vaginitis,* may be acquired through sexual contact or as an adverse effect of medications, such as antibiotics or steroids. The medical assistant should keep in mind that the patient with a vaginal infection may be embarrassed by the odor that can accompany infection or may be irritable due to inability to sleep from symptoms of itching, burning, and pain. Although a symptomatic patient may be irritable, she will appreciate the care and concern of the professional medical assistant who helps the physician resolve the patient's discomfort as quickly as possible. If left untreated, many vaginal infections can migrate up the reproductive tract and cause further infection and possible infertility. Common vaginal infections include candidiasis, chlamydia, genital herpes, genital warts, gonorrhea, syphilis, AIDS, trichomoniasis, and Bartholin gland cyst.

Candidiasis
ICD-9-CM code: 553.3
Candidiasis, also known as a *yeast infection,* is infection of the vagina by the *Candida albicans* pathogen. Nearly 75% of all adult women have experienced symptoms of a yeast infection. In addition, studies show that up to 19% of women may have experienced yeast infection without symptoms. (See Figure 32-6.)

While infection with *C. albicans* can occur in other areas, such as the mouth (thrush), vaginal candidiasis usually occurs when the normal flora of the vaginal area has been disrupted. Causes of such disruption include antibiotic therapy, oral contraceptives, diabetes, clothing or undergarments that are too tight, and steroid therapy. Vaginal candidiasis during pregnancy is common, possibly as a result of increased estrogen levels. The most common cause of candidiasis is use of antibiotics. Although the intended effect of antibiotic therapy is to kill harmful bacteria, it also kills helpful bacteria (normal flora) as well. The resulting disruption of normal flora allows *C. albicans* to overgrow, possibly leading to infection.

Signs and symptoms of vaginal candidiasis include pruritus and an odorless, white vaginal discharge that may be described as cottage cheese-like. Other patients may complain of burning with urination (dysuria). The physician

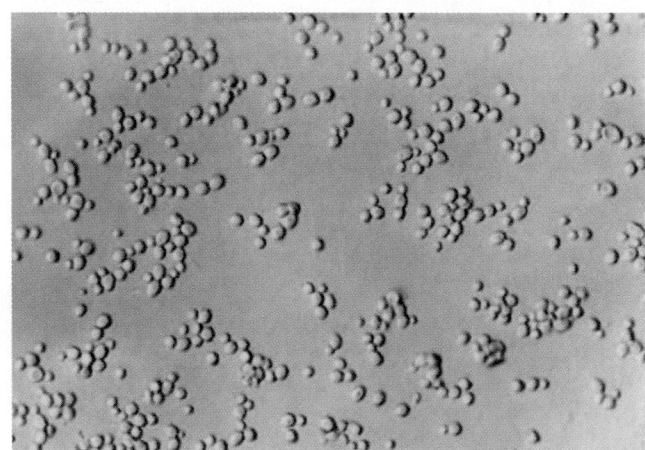

FIG 32-6 *Candida albicans.*

determines a diagnosis using a procedure called a *wet preparation* or *wet prep*. Using a speculum to open the vagina, the physician obtains a specimen from the vagina with a wooden applicator. She then places the specimen on a clean glass slide, adds 10% potassium hydroxide (KOH), and applies a glass cover slip. Positive results reveal groups of *C. albicans* cells, which have a characteristic appearance when viewed with a microscope.

Treatment for vaginal candidiasis includes the use of vaginal antifungal drugs in oral form, such as fluconazole (Diflucan) or a vaginal cream or suppository, such as clotrimazole (Gyne-Lotrimin) or miconazole (Monistat). Topical creams can also be applied to the outer area if irritation is present. Typically, treatment is restricted to the female patient. However, if the infection recurs, treatment of a sexual partner may be necessary. To prevent reoccurrence of candidiasis while taking antibiotics, patients should eat active yogurt cultures and drink acidophilus milk to replenish "good" bacteria in the vagina.

With treatment, 90% of *C. albicans* infections resolve. However, patients who are immunocompromised, such as those with cancer or HIV or those with diabetes may require a longer antifungal treatment regimen.

Chlamydia
ICD-9-CM code: 553.3
Although chlamydia is a type of bacterial vaginal infection, it is also considered a sexually transmitted disease (STD) or sexually transmitted infection (STI). It is one of the most commonly transmitted STDs in North America, affecting 3 to 9 million people per year. It is thought to be present in 10% of all college students and in half of all patients with pelvic inflammatory disease. The Centers for Disease Control and Prevention (CDC) recommends yearly chlamydia screenings for sexually active women under age 26. Up to 75% of females are asymptomatic, giving chlamydia its name as the "silent" STD.

Chlamydia is caused by the pathogen *Chlamydia trachomatis*, which is spread through sexual contact. Symptomatic patients may complain of purulent vaginal or urethral discharge, pain in the genital area, itching, and dysuria.

Diagnosis can be obtained from cultures, such as the wet preparation. Treatment may include antibiotic therapy for a minimum of 1 week with erythromycin, azithromycin (Zithromax), doxycycline (Vibramycin), or tetracycline (Sumycin). If acquired during pregnancy, chlamydia will also spread from the mother to the fetus during delivery and can cause conjunctivitis, pneumonia, or even blindness. (*Note:* Tetracycline is contraindicated in the pregnant patient. A pregnant patient should be prescribed "mycins" only.) The medical assistant should instruct the patient diagnosed with chlamydia to abstain from sexual intercourse to avoid infecting her partner and to prevent reinfection.

If left untreated, chlamydia can migrate up the reproductive tract, causing inflammation and scarring of the fallopian tubes, resulting in permanent infertility. In addition, women with an active chlamydia infection are more susceptible than noninfected women to infection with the human immunodeficiency virus (HIV) if they are exposed to the virus.

Genital Herpes
ICD-9-CM code: 553.3
Genital herpes is a sexually transmitted infection with the herpes simplex virus 2. It affects 85 to 90 million people worldwide. It is spread by sexual contact with an infected person. Symptoms of genital herpes include local pain and itching, burning, dysuria, and tingling or shooting pains 1 to 2 days before eruption of the rash. The rash is characterized by reddened patches with small vesicles in the genitorectal region. Some patients complain of fever and malaise during an outbreak. The rash lasts for approximately 10 days and is most contagious when the vesicles rupture during this time. However, asymptomatic shedding of the virus can cause transmission in the absence of an outbreak.

Tests used to confirm HSV diagnosis use a sample of cells or fluid, most commonly from lesions in the genital area or, less commonly, from spinal fluid, blood, urine, or tears. There are two tests that confirm HSV infection:

- Herpes viral culture tests cells or fluid from a fresh lesion. The physician collects the sample with a cotton swab and places it in a culture cup. It is the most specific method of determining infection and is, therefore, the most common test performed.
- Herpesvirus antigen detection tests cells from a fresh lesion. The physician scrapes some cells from a fresh lesion and smears them on a microscope slide. Herpesvirus antigens are visible through the microscope on the surface of cells infected with the herpesvirus. The physician may order this test along with a viral culture.

There is no cure for genital herpes; treatment with oral acyclovir (Zovirax), famciclovir (Famvir), or valacyclovir (Valtrex) can be used for the initial outbreak and subsequent infections. Although these antivirals shorten the duration of the lesions, patients must be aware that the outbreak can return. The medical assistant should advise patients to abstain from sexual contact during an outbreak to prevent transmission to their partners. Genital herpes can also be transmitted from mother to fetus during delivery and can cause respiratory illnesses, retinal infection, encephalitis, or death of the neonate. Pregnant women with genital herpes can schedule a Cesarean delivery or take acyclovir to suppress the infection until after birth. Women with genital herpes have an increased risk of cervical cancer and should get yearly Papanicolaou (Pap) tests.

Genital Warts

ICD-9-CM code: 553.3

A wart is a hypertrophy, or overgrowth, of the papillae and epidermis. Warts are small, soft, pink, raised, painless growths. Around 1 million people in the United States suffer from genital warts each year.

Unlike warts that can appear on the hands or the feet, genital warts are sexually transmitted. Genital warts are caused by the human papillomavirus. The warts may be a single growth that becomes cauliflower-like; they can spread to the perianal area. Most patients are asymptomatic, but some will report itching and burning.

The physician diagnoses genital warts primarily by visual inspection. The diagnosis is confirmed if warts turn whitish in color when swabbed with acetic acid (vinegar). There is no complete cure for genital warts. Although topical podophyllin or laser surgery can be used to destroy genital warts, they may return after treatment. Treatment should be administered weekly until all warts are removed. After successful treatment, the patient should schedule a follow-up examination in 3 months. The medical assistant should instruct the patient to abstain from intercourse or use a condom to prevent infecting her partner. The lesions may disappear without treatment; however, active infection may still be present and transmission to a partner is possible. The patient should undergo testing for human immunodeficiency virus (HIV) and other STDs and a Pap test every 6 months because genital warts increase her risk of cervical cancer.

Gonorrhea

ICD-9-CM code: 553.3

Gonorrhea is a sexually transmitted disease caused by the pathogen *Neisseria gonorrhoeae*. Sexually active teens are at the highest risk for contracting gonorrhea. Co-infection with chlamydia is common and is estimated to occur in 30% of patients with gonorrhea. The CDC estimates that more than 700,000 persons in the United States acquire new gonorrhea infections each year. Only about half of these infections are reported to the CDC. In 2006, the rate of reported gonorrhea infections was 120.9 per 100,000 persons.

Because the *N. gonorrhoeae* bacteria die with exposure to air, gonorrhea is spread only through direct sexual contact. Women with gonorrhea are commonly asymptomatic but may experience a greenish-yellow discharge from the cervix. If the fallopian tubes are affected, the patient may experience lower abdominal pain. Symptoms can also include swollen glands and a milky discharge from the anus.

Three main tests are used to diagnose gonorrhea. The physician can use a swab to obtain a sample from the most likely site of infection (such as the cervix, penis, urethra, rectum, or throat). Laboratory analysis of the specimen will reveal the presence of *N. gonorrhoeae*. If the most likely site is the cervix or urethra, a urinalysis will also reveal presence of the bacterium. A Gram stain performed on a sample from the cervix or urethra, which can be done in the physician's office, will also reveal *N. gonorrhoeae*.

Because of the increasing resistance of *N. gonorrhoeae* to fluoroquinolones, the CDC currently recommends only cephalosporins to treat the disease. Such treatment may be administered through a single injection or single-dose pill. The medical assistant should emphasize to the patient the importance of completing the full course of antibiotics to prevent reinfection. She should also direct the patient to avoid contact with any discharge, because her eyes can become infected as well, and to refrain from sexual contact while being treated. After treatment, vaginal cultures ensure that the infection is gone. All people who have had sexual contact with the patient should be tested. The medical office must report all cases of gonorrhea to the local public health department.

Pregnant patients with a known case of gonorrhea cannot deliver vaginally, because the bacteria can cause blindness in the neonate. Because many women are asymptomatic, routine treatment includes administration of silver nitrate solution to every neonate's eyes immediately after birth to kill the bacteria if present. If left untreated, gonorrhea can cause pelvic inflammatory disease (PID) and permanent sterility.

Syphilis

ICD-9-CM code: 553.3

Syphilis is a multistage infection caused by the spirochete *Treponema pallidum*. Syphilis is a sexually transmitted disease that is most commonly seen in teens, young adults, abusers of illicit drugs, and patients with HIV infection. Syphilis is most prevalent in sexually active adults between ages 20 and 29. In the United States, health officials reported over 36,000 cases of syphilis in 2006, including 9,756 cases of primary and secondary syphilis.

Syphilis is transmitted from person to person by direct contact with skin and mucous membranes. The spirochetes can penetrate the skin and enter regional lymph nodes, spreading throughout the entire body. After an incubation period of 10 days to 2 months, painless ulcers, or *chancres*, appear in the primary stage of syphilis. The chancres are highly infectious and mostly appear on the genitals.

In the secondary stage, a widespread body rash appears with symptoms of fever, headaches, malaise, and inflammation of the lymph nodes. Moist, broad papules filled with infectious fluid appear along the perineum. Shallow ulcerations in the mouth can also appear. If left untreated, secondary syphilis can progress to the third stage.

Tertiary syphilis includes tissue damage to the aorta, central nervous system, bones, and skin. Permanent damage can include aortic aneurysm, meningitis, sensory and gait deficits, and damage to the optic nerve, causing blindness.

Diagnosis is made through a polymerase chain reaction test, available mostly at research hospitals, which detects antibodies to *T. pallidum* in blood, body fluid, or tissue. Treatment consists of long-acting preparations of penicillin. The duration of treatment depends on the stage of syphilis and any co-infections, such as HIV. Doxycycline or tetracycline are substitutes if the patient is allergic to penicillin. The medical assistant should advise the patient to avoid sexual contact during treatment and refer the patient to the local public health agency to contact and locate all sexual partners.

If diagnosed and treated during the primary or secondary stage, the patient will suffer no permanent damage. Late-stage syphilis can lead to long-term health problems, such as heart and blood vessel damage (including aneurysm and aortitis) and damage to skin and bones.

AIDS

ICD-9-CM code: 042 (excludes asymptomatic HIV infection status V08)

Acquired immune deficiency syndrome (AIDS) is the most advanced stage of infection with human immunodeficiency virus (HIV). The late stage of the condition leaves the body unable to fight opportunistic infections and tumors. In the United States, 40,000 new cases of AIDS are reported each year; worldwide, more than 25 million people have died from AIDS, making it the most deadly epidemic in history.

Human immunodeficiency virus (HIV), a retrovirus containing ribonucleic acid (RNA), causes AIDS. HIV is spread from person to person via direct contact with blood, semen, vaginal secretions, or breast milk. People at increased risk for HIV and AIDS are those with multiple sexual partners and those who abuse intravenous drugs.

Symptoms of HIV include opportunistic infections, those that a healthy immune system could defend against. Signs and symptoms of these infections include fatigue, fever, chills, night sweats, oral ulcerations, dyspnea, dysphagia, anorexia, pneumonia, diarrhea, weight loss, confusion, and dementia.

HIV is diagnosed by a blood test that confirms the presence of anti-HIV antibodies (IgG and IgM) and the HIV p24 antigen. AIDS is diagnosed as a later stage of HIV when the CD4+ helper T-cells are at a count of 200 or less (normal value is 1600). There is no cure for HIV. Treatment includes antiviral medications, such as AZT-zidovudine.

Without treatment, the average time of survival after infection with HIV is 9 to 11 years. With treatment, the average life expectancy for newly diagnosed HIV infection is 20 years. The prognosis for AIDS varies from patient to patient. Some die in a very short time; others live for several years with a T-cell count of less than 200. The medical assistant should encourage patients who engage in behaviors at high risk for contracting HIV to get tested for HIV prior to pregnancy. If an HIV-positive patient does become pregnant, antiretroviral therapy should begin as soon as possible to reduce risk of transmission to the developing fetus. Breastfeeding is contraindicated for HIV mothers because it is known to transmit the virus to the neonate.

Trichomoniasis

ICD-9-CM code: 553.3

Trichomoniasis is an infection of the vagina with the protozoa *Trichomonas vaginalis*. Symptoms of trichomoniasis include frothy white or yellow vaginal discharge with a characteristic foul odor. Occasionally, trichomoniasis is asymptomatic. Diagnosis is obtained by a wet preparation, which confirms the presence of *T. vaginalis*.

Treatment with oral metronidazole (Flagyl) will kill the protozoa. If left untreated, trichomoniasis can cause an inflamed cervix and urethra. The medical assistant should instruct the patient to refrain from drinking alcohol during treatment with metronidazole, because confusion and psychosis can occur. Flagyl is contraindicated during the first trimester of pregnancy, due to potential damage to the developing fetus. First-trimester pregnant and breast-feeding patients can be treated with clotrimazole vaginal suppositories for temporary relief. The medical assistant can encourage her patient to contact her sexual partners to inform them of the diagnosis and initiate treatment.

With treatment, a full recovery from infection is common. Previous infections can increase the risk of HIV transmission and delivering a baby with low birth weight. In addition, the patient with trichomoniasis is at greater risk for cervical cancer because of the damage to cervical cells.

Bartholin Gland Cyst

ICD-9-CM code: 616.3

The Bartholin glands are two small mucous glands located in each lateral wall of the vestibule of the vagina. These glands secrete a lubricating fluid for intercourse. Approximately 2% of women develop a Bartholin gland cyst, and 85% of those cases occur during a woman's reproductive years.

Occasionally, the ducts of one or both of the Bartholin glands become blocked, although the cause of blockage is unknown. If blockage occurs, the lubricating fluid cannot leave the gland, causing it to become inflamed and tender, forming a cyst.

Signs and symptoms of Bartholin gland cyst include a tender or painful lump near the vaginal opening, discomfort while walking or sitting, pain during intercourse, and fever. Visual inspection reveals an inflamed gland, which confirms the diagnosis.

The medical assistant can instruct the patient to try applying warm compresses to the area in an effort to open the duct and express the fluid. If this treatment is unsuccessful, the physician may lance the gland with a scalpel and insert a small rubber tube to facilitate drainage. The patient must leave the drain in for a prescribed period of time, which varies based on the severity of the occlusion to the duct. The patient must then return to the office so that the physician can remove the drain.

The cyst should not return, because the duct remains open after removal of the drain. The medical assistant should instruct the patient to abstain from intercourse until the drain is removed.

Menstrual Disorders

Many women experience symptoms related to menstruation. Intensity of symptoms can vary greatly. If possible, treatments are directed at decreasing symptoms without disrupting fertility. Common menstrual disorders include dysmenorrhea, amenorrhea, ovarian cysts, premenstrual syndrome, and toxic shock syndrome.

Dysmenorrhea
ICD-9-CM code:625.3

Dysmenorrhea is pain in the lower abdominal and pelvic area associated with menstrual flow. It is most common in women in their 20s and early 30s.

Causes of dysmenorrhea include hormonal imbalances, endometriosis, uterine fibroids, PID, and uterine malposition. Signs and symptoms include headache, nausea, vomiting, fatigue, and diarrhea. The patient may also complain of lower back pain and body aches. Symptoms typically begin 12 to 24 hours before menstruation begins and continue for 3 to 5 days.

Diagnosis of dysmenorrhea depends on the health history. The patient suffering from dysmenorrhea will report an inability to go to work or school on some days during menstruation each month due to headache, backache, fatigue, and nausea. She may report that the quantity of blood is unmanageable even with a combination of extra-absorbent tampons and overnight sanitary pads.

Treatment may include analgesics, warm or cold compresses, medications to reduce uterine contractions, or oral contraceptives, which suppress ovulation and, therefore, decrease symptoms. The medical assistant can advise her patient to get plenty of rest and avoid caffeine and alcohol. A healthy diet and moderate physical exercise have also been shown to lessen symptoms of dysmenorrhea.

Some women experience a sharp decrease in symptoms of dysmenorrhea after pregnancy. Others experience a more gradual decrease with increasing age.

Amenorrhea
ICD-9-CM code: 626.0

Amenorrhea is the absence of menstruation in a woman between the ages of 16 and 40. Amenorrhea affects 2% to 5% of all women of childbearing age in the United States.

Causes of amenorrhea include hypothalamic, pituitary, and endocrine dysfunction; congenital or acquired abnormalities of the reproductive tract; or an eating disorder that causes extreme weight loss. Symptoms include absent menstruation for 3 or more consecutive months (in the absence of pregnancy or breastfeeding).

Treatment is directed at the cause of the lack of menstruation. HRT can regulate hormonal disruptions. In the case of anorexia or bulimia, the medical assistant should provide the patient with referrals for psychotherapy. Amenorrhea is reversible with treatment.

Ovarian Cysts
ICD-9-CM code: 620.2

Ovarian cysts are sacs of fluid or semisolid masses that grow within the ovary. They can form any time between puberty and menopause, including during pregnancy. In the United States, nearly all premenopausal women have ovarian cysts and around 14% of postmenopausal women have them. A related disorder, polycystic ovary syndrome (PCOS), is an endocrine disorder that causes irregular ovulation, lack of menstruation, and secretion of excessive amounts of androgenic (male) hormones. The suppression of ovulation makes this syndrome a major cause of infertility. PCOS affects approximately 10% of all women in the United States.

The definitive cause of ovarian cysts is unknown. Hypothyroidism and early age of menarche may contribute to the development of ovarian cysts. The cause of polycystic ovary syndrome is also unclear. However it is linked to a decrease in FSH as well as abnormally high levels of testosterone, estrogen, and luteinizing hormone.

Most ovarian cysts are asymptomatic and benign. Larger cysts or cysts that occur in groups on the ovary can produce symptoms of lower back pain, nausea, vomiting, and abnormal uterine bleeding. Women with polycystic ovary syndrome are commonly diagnosed while being evaluated for infertility or absence of menstruation. Symptoms of this syndrome include acne, hyperinsulinemia, obesity, type 2 diabetes, male pattern baldness, and hirsutism (excessive body hair). The emotional effects of increased body hair and skin eruptions may adversely affect body image in young women. Because the follicles of the ovaries are not stimulated each month, absent menstruation is a common sign. Ultrasound confirms the diagnosis by revealing cysts.

Treatment with oral contraceptives, which suppress ovulation and thus cause changes to the ovary, can slow the growth of ovarian cysts, reducing symptoms. If oral contraceptives do not control symptoms, the physician may perform a laparoscopic procedure to drain or remove the cysts. Emergency surgical removal is indicated if a large cyst ruptures or the ovary twists and blood supply to the ovary is compromised. Symptoms of this emergency condition include acute abdominal pain and massive intraperitoneal hemorrhage. Treatment of polycystic ovary syndrome is directed at normalizing hormone ratios and reestablishing normal menstrual cycles. Treatment for diabetes and obesity should accompany hormone therapy. With hormone therapy, masculinization will also decrease. With proper treatment to balance hormones, pregnancy is possible for patients with PCOS.

The prognosis for ovarian cysts varies with age. Around 66% of women under age 20 who undergo treatment for ovarian cysts experience a reduction in cyst size and symptoms. About 75% of patients ages 21 to 49 experience a reduction in symptoms and size without treatment; 7% of women in this age group are diagnosed with ovarian cancer. The rate of cancer increases with age, so surgical removal of the cysts is recommended for postmenopausal women. In women age 80 and older, 60% of ovarian cysts show signs of cancer. Even so, surgery may not be warranted due to the patient's age.

Premenstrual Syndrome
ICD-9-CM code: 625.4
Premenstrual syndrome includes a range of symptoms that generally occur 7 to 14 days before menstruation begins. The severity of symptoms varies greatly and can include behavioral, neurological, respiratory, gastrointestinal, and musculoskeletal complaints. About 30% to 50% of women ages 22 to 40 suffer premenstrual syndrome.

The cause of premenstrual syndrome is unknown. Increased levels of antidiuretic hormone are known to cause the signs and symptoms of fluid retention, bloating, headaches, and central nervous system symptoms. However, the cause of increased ADH is unknown. Behavioral complaints include depression, irritability, lethargy, and nervousness. Neurological complaints include headache, dizziness, fainting, and numbness in the extremities. Respiratory complaints include exacerbation of asthma, allergic rhinitis, and cold symptoms. Gastrointestinal complaints include diarrhea, constipation, abdominal cramping and bloating, temporary weight gain, and increased appetite. The patient may also experience an increase in acne and breast pain, tenderness, or enlargement.

Diagnosis is based on the patient's symptoms. A report of relief from symptoms on days 4 through 13 of the menstrual cycle confirms the diagnosis. Treatment is directed at reducing symptoms. The only definitive cure for PMS is hysterectomy, including removal of the ovaries. Thus, most patients manage symptoms with over-the-counter (OTC) medications, diet, and exercise. Medications can include diuretics, analgesics, stimulants such as caffeine, and antihistamines. OTC combination products such as Midol or Pamprin contain various combinations of medications to relieve symptoms. The medical assistant can advise her patient to discuss medication options with the physician and to record which OTC medications best reduce her symptoms.

Women with PMS generally experience no long-term complications from the disorder, other than the continuing cycle of symptoms near the onset of menstruation. PMS alone is not linked to a decrease in fertility.

Toxic Shock Syndrome
ICD-9-CM code: 040.89
Toxic shock syndrome (TSS) is a rare disorder caused by an exotoxin, a dangerous substance produced by bacteria. The causative agents are *Staphylococcus aureus* and *Streptococcus pyogenes*. The CDC estimates that between 1 and 17 menstruating females out of 100,000 will get TSS.

Although other sources of infection can result in TSS, it is most prevalent in young women who use tampons during menstruation. The toxin produced by *S. aureus* and *S. pyogenes* requires a neutral pH and protein-rich environment, which is provided by menstrual blood. The insertion of a tampon allows air to enter the vagina, making the normally anaerobic vagina aerobic. This air provides oxygen for further growth of the toxin. TSS may rarely develop through infection from cuts, surgical incisions, or burns on the skin. However, most people exposed to the toxin-producing strains of *S. aureus* and *S. pyogenes* do not develop TSS because of antibodies to these toxins in the normal flora of the skin.

Symptoms include fever of 102°F or greater and diffuse, erythematous rash followed by peeling of the skin 1 to 2 weeks after onset of the rash. The patient may experience hypotension and syncope; gastrointestinal disturbances, such as diarrhea and vomiting; and muscle aches and pains.

Treatment with nafcillin or oxacillin will not affect the initial syndrome but may prevent its recurrence. The medical assistant can advise her patients who use tampons to change them often and discontinue their use if fever develops during use. Symptoms may progress to renal and hepatic failure. About 5% to 15% of TSS cases are fatal. Patients who have been successfully treated for TSS should never use tampons again because they are at an increased risk for recurrence.

Uterine Disorders
The healthy uterus has the ability to cleanse itself with menstrual flow and secretion of normal mucus. Infections of the uterus can be caused by sexually transmitted diseases, poor hygiene, or untreated vaginal infection. Uterine disorders may also be caused by growth of abnormal tissues and uterine malposition. Common uterine disorders include endometriosis, PID, uterine fibroids, and uterine prolapse.

Endometriosis
ICD-9-CM code: 617.9 (site unspecified)
Endometriosis is the growth of endometrial tissue outside of the uterus. Normally, the endometrium grows thicker in response to hormonal changes during the menstrual cycle. The uterus sheds the active endometrial layer during menstruation. In some women, endometrial tissue can grow outside of the uterus, affecting the ovaries, ligaments, and peritoneal tissues. (See Figure 32-7.) Endometriosis occurs in 7% to 10% of menstruating women worldwide. It can persist, though rarely, in postmenopausal women.

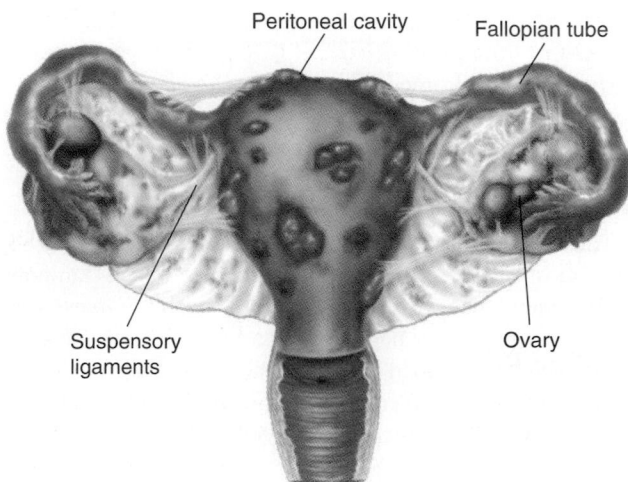

Peritoneal cavity   Fallopian tube

Suspensory
ligaments   Ovary

FIG 32-7 Sites of endometriosis.

Although the cause of endometriosis is unknown, it is thought that either endometrial cells migrate during fetal development or the cells that are shed during menstruation are possibly expelled out of the fallopian tubes during menstruation. Recent trauma or uterine surgery are other possible causes.

Endometrial tissue that grows outside of the uterus is not shed and can cause pain in the abdomen, pelvis, and vagina. Pain ensues 5 to 6 days before menstruation and lasts until 3 to 4 days after the menstrual period. The degree of pain and discomfort varies, depending on the quantity of tissue growth and its location. Diagnosis is based on visual examination via laparoscopy or biopsy, which reveal endometrial tissue outside of the uterus.

Treatment options vary based on the patient's age and her desire to preserve her fertility. Surgical removal of endometrial cysts can clear ovaries and fallopian tubes, restoring fertility. Oral contraceptives can suppress ovulation and, therefore, reduce symptoms. If fertility is not necessary, the physician may prescribe danazol (Danocrine) to inhibit the pituitary release of gonadotropins. Alternatively, the physician may prescribe leuprolide (Lupron) or nafarelin (Synarel) to suppress gonadotropin-releasing hormone (GnRH) production. These medications cause decline of FSH and LH, which decreases ovarian function and can induce an early menopause. If the patient decides that she no longer wants to bear children, severe cases of endometriosis are treated with complete hysterectomy, including the removal of the uterus, fallopian tubes, and ovaries.

The main complication of endometriosis is impaired fertility. Around 30% to 50% of women who experience infertility are diagnosed with endometriosis. For patients who are able to decrease the amount of endometrial tissue growth outside the uterus, pregnancy is possible (if desired).

Severe endometriosis can cause bowel and urethral obstructions, which adversely affect the urinary and GI systems.

Pelvic Inflammatory Disease
ICD-9-CM code: 553.3

Pelvic inflammatory disease (PID) describes any acute or chronic infection of the female reproductive system, including the vagina, cervix, uterus, fallopian tubes, and ovaries. More than 1 million women in the United States are affected by PID each year. It is most common in teenagers.

PID can be caused by an untreated vaginal infection in which the infection ascends into the internal reproductive organs. The longer the infection goes untreated, the further it ascends, affecting more of the reproductive tract. The fallopian tubes may become blocked with pus or scar tissue, causing infertility. Common pathogens that cause PID include *Neisseria gonorrhoeae* and *Chlamydia trachomatis.*

The patient may be asymptomatic or experience such signs and symptoms as purulent vaginal discharge, odor, fever, malaise, lower abdominal pain, dysuria, nausea, vomiting, and heavy bleeding.

Culturing the discharge and identifying the causative organism confirm the diagnosis. Treatment includes antibiotic or antifungal medications as indicated by the causative organism. The medical assistant should encourage her patient to discuss STDs with her sexual partners, because they will most likely also be infected.

Because PID may be asymptomatic, infection may progress untreated. Prolonged infection causes sterility through scarring of the fallopian tubes, ovaries, and uterus. The infection also increases the chances of a tubal pregnancy.

Uterine Fibroids
ICD-9-CM code: 218.9 (unspecified)

Uterine fibroids are benign, smooth tumors made of muscle and fat, called *leiomyomas.* They grow in size during the reproductive years and may regress after menopause. Noncancerous tumors of the uterus are the most common tumor found in women. In the United States, about 20% to 40% of women age 35 and older have uterine fibroids. African American women are at greater risk. Fibroids are the most common cause of hysterectomy in premenopausal women. (See Figure 32-8.)

The cause of uterine fibroids is unknown. They are typically asymptomatic until age 30 but cause symptoms later as they grow in size and number. Uterine fibroids most commonly occur in clusters and symptoms are related to their specific location. Those that encroach on the bladder region will produce urinary frequency and dysuria; those that encroach on the rectum can cause spasm of the anal sphincter. The patient may feel an abdominal fullness due to enlargement of the uterus. The most common site of uterine fibroids is within the endometrium. Such fibroids can cause

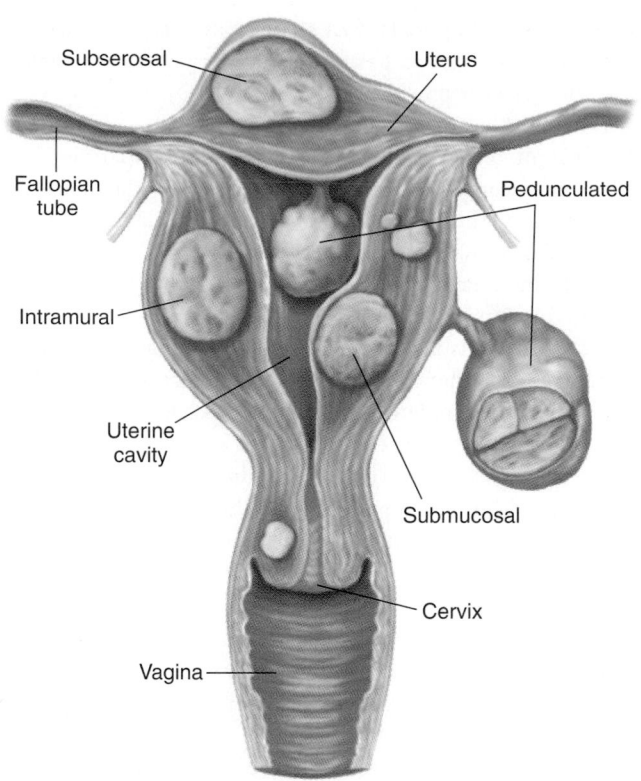

FIG 32-8 Types of uterine fibroids.

menorrhagia (excessive menstrual flow) and dysmenorrhea. If the fibroid is attached to the uterus by a stalk, pain is caused by uterine contractions in an attempt to expel the fibroid.

Diagnosis is based on the patient's report of symptoms and visualization by ultrasound confirms the diagnosis. Ultrasound is the most common diagnostic tool because it is minimally invasive and available in most medical offices. Less commonly, a MRI or hysteroscopy is used to confirm the presence of fibroids. Ultrasound may also serve as an assessment tool to determine if fibroids are growing in size and number.

Asymptomatic fibroids should be left untreated and observed for changes throughout the patient's life. Treatment of fibroids that cause symptoms includes oral administration of luteinizing hormone-releasing hormone (LHRH), which causes the fibroids to shrink. If the patient no longer wants to preserve fertility, uterine ablation can debulk endometrial fibroids. The ablation procedure is a one-day surgery under general anesthesia. In the procedure, the surgeon fills the uterine cavity with heated fluid that destroys the active layer of the endometrium. If uterine fibroids are connected by a stalk, the surgeon removes them before the ablation. As a result of the ablation, the fibroid's blood supply is diminished and the tumor will shrink.

Treatment of uterine fibroids is commonly successful. Depending on their location, fibroids may impact fertility.

Most women who experience uterine fibroids and infertility also suffer from other disorders, such as decreased production of ova.

Uterine Prolapse
ICD-9-CM code: 618.1

Uterine prolapse is the displacement of the uterus downward into the cervix. In the United States, approximately 14% of women who have given birth at least once have some degree of uterine prolapse. African American women have the lowest risk; Hispanic women have the highest risk. Parity and obesity increase the risk of uterine prolapse.

Causes of uterine prolapse include age, weakening of the musculature, pelvic tumors that press the uterus downward, traumatic vaginal delivery, or chronic constipation and straining. The patient may experience an inability to empty her bladder or be asymptomatic.

Diagnosis is based on physical examination. During the examination, the physician asks the patient to bear down. This pressure causes the cervix to protrude out through the vaginal opening. There are three stages of uterine prolapse:

- mild—protrusion of the cervix into the lower portion of the vagina
- moderate—protrusion past the vaginal opening
- severe—protrusion of the entire uterus past the opening of the vagina. (See Figure 32-9.)

Surgical correction, called *uteropexy,* can lift the uterus into its normal position. After surgical correction, most patients experience no further problems, but some women

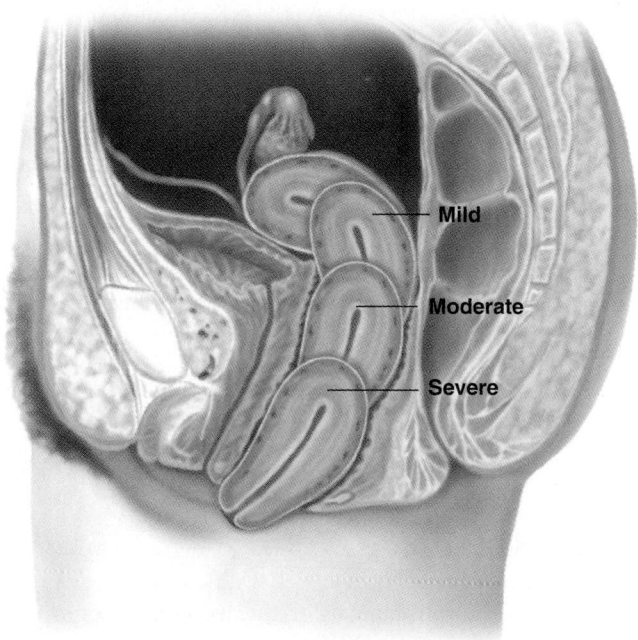

FIG 32-9 Three stages of uterine prolapse.

suffer from recurrent prolapse and require additional surgical correction.

Complications of Pregnancy

Many women enjoy a healthy pregnancy and deliver a child without complication. Unfortunately, some pregnancies are difficult for the mother or fetus or both. Some pregnancies are unsuccessful and the patient does not deliver a live infant. In the event of complications, the medical assistant and physician can work together to treat the patient in a compassionate manner and educate her as needed. Common complications of pregnancy include ectopic pregnancy, abortion, gestational diabetes, placenta previa, abruptio placentae, and eclampsia.

Ectopic Pregnancy
ICD-9-CM code: 633.9

Ectopic pregnancy involves implantation of a fertilized ovum in places other than the uterine wall. Most ectopic pregnancies occur in the wall of the fallopian tube; however, it may occur in other places, including the cervix, abdomen, and ovaries. Ectopic pregnancy occurs in approximately 1% of all pregnancies. About 98% of these cases involve implantation in the fallopian tube.

Normally, fertilization occurs in the outer one-third of the fallopian tube. The corpus luteum releases secretions from the glands within the tubes, and the fertilized cell, now called a zygote, normally moves from the fallopian tube into the uterus for implantation. If the zygote does not move into the uterus and begins to implant into the wall of the fallopian tube, it will not be able to grow and develop in the narrow space of the tube. As the cells begin to divide and the zygote grows in size, the patient may experience sharp pain, fever, and bleeding.

Diagnosis is based on a positive urine pregnancy test (indicating the presence of hCG in urine) and a blood test also indicating the presence of hCG. Abdominal ultrasound shows an empty uterus and may show a gestational sac with a fetal heart within the fallopian tube.

Approximately 50% of ectopic pregnancies result in miscarriage and require no surgical intervention. The other 50% require surgical removal of the embryo to prevent rupture of the tube and infection.

The patient may be able to conceive again if there is no damage to the other fallopian tube. The medical assistant can comfort the patient; the physician can also console the patient and explain when she can try to conceive again.

Abortion
ICD-9-CM code: 632

Abortion is the spontaneous or therapeutic loss of a pregnancy that is less than 20 weeks' gestation. Spontaneous abortion, also called *miscarriage,* occurs in 30% of all first pregnancies and up to 15% of all pregnancies. Some miscarriages occur so early in gestation that the patient is unaware that she was ever pregnant.

The most common cause of spontaneous abortion is an error in fetal development that is incompatible with life. Other causes include abnormalities of the placenta, endocrine disturbances, acute infectious disease, severe shock, or trauma. Signs and symptoms of a spontaneous abortion include abdominal cramps, vaginal bleeding, and passage of clots of tissue.

If the patient is aware of the pregnancy, diagnosis is confirmed by examination of expelled fetal tissue. Ultrasound may confirm complete expulsion of tissue. The medical assistant must monitor the vital signs of a patient who suffers a spontaneous abortion to ensure that the blood loss does not indicate tearing damage to the uterus. The medical assistant can submit any tissue that the patient passes and collects for examination in the laboratory. The physician must also examine the patient for shock and sepsis. If the abortion is incomplete and fetal tissue is still present in the uterus, the patient must undergo dilatation and curettage (D&C) to eliminate any remaining tissue that could cause infection.

A patient may decide to end her pregnancy for emotional or physical reasons. Women who are victims of rape or incest, have an unplanned pregnancy, or have a medical condition that will compromise the pregnancy (such as cardiac or kidney disease) may elect a therapeutic abortion. In addition, if genetic defects are detected in the fetus, the patient may decide to end the pregnancy. The patient who elects to have an abortion may have some of the same emotional reactions as a patient who suffers a spontaneous abortion. The medical assistant must comfort and support her patient's emotional needs in both forms of unsuccessful pregnancies. (See *Emotional support after abortion.*)

Prognosis for surgical and spontaneous abortion in the first trimester of gestation is usually good. The patient should recover and, if no underlying fertility issues are present, should be able to become pregnant in the future. Second- or third-trimester abortions can have complications resulting from hemorrhage and damage to internal organs, which may lead to an inability to become pregnant. Unsafe abortions, performed illegally, commonly by unqualified individuals, are a public health concern worldwide due to the high incidence of incomplete abortion, sepsis, hemorrhage, and damage to internal organs. The World Health Organization estimates that 19 million unsafe abortions are performed annually and 68,000 deaths occur as a result each year.

Gestational Diabetes
ICD-9-CM code: 648.8

Gestational diabetes is the development of type 2 diabetes mellitus in a woman during pregnancy when she did

Emotional support after abortion

The medical assistant caring for a patient who has experienced a spontaneous or elective abortion must try to ease the patient's anxiety and help her cope with the loss of the pregnancy. Whether she has miscarried or has elected to end the pregnancy for physical, economic, or other personal reasons, the patient must process the experience emotionally. The emotional response of the individual patient may vary from grief and anger to guilt, depression, sadness, or even relief. The medical assistant can refer the patient to the many support groups that are available online and through local organizations. Some other resources include:

- *http://www.fertilityplus.org/faq/miscarriage/resources.html*
- *http://www.bellaonline.com/subjects/6461.asp*
- Cohen, J.: *Coming to Term: Uncovering the Truth about Miscarriage.* New Brunswick, NJ: Rutgers University Press, 2007.
- McLaughlin, S.: *Surviving Miscarriage: You Are Not Alone.* Bloomington, IN: iUniverse, Inc., 2005.

not have diabetes before becoming pregnant. In the United States, gestational diabetes occurs in about 4% to 8% of pregnancies and usually resolves after the woman gives birth.

Pregnancy brings on many changes in a patient's body, including how the body uses glucose. The cells of the body may also become resistant to insulin, causing them to be starved of needed glucose. Some patients who have normal blood glucose metabolism when not pregnant develop diabetes during pregnancy. Patients at risk for gestational diabetes include women over age 25, women who are overweight at the onset of pregnancy, and women who have a family history of diabetes. Women who have miscarried or given birth to very large babies are at increased risk. Because there is a high incidence of diabetes among Native Americans, African Americans, Pacific Islanders, and Mexican Americans, patients from these ethnic groups are also at an increased risk for developing gestational diabetes. Signs and symptoms of gestational diabetes are the same as diabetes in the nonpregnant patient, including extreme thirst, fatigue, dehydration, and sudden weight loss or gain.

Although not all pregnant women are considered at risk for gestational diabetes, all obstetric patients should undergo screening to prevent damage to the fetus and the mother. Such screening involves an oral glucose tolerance test for all patients at 24 to 28 weeks' gestation. The test shows the patient's ability to metabolize a specific load of glucose over time. After fasting for at least 12 hours, the patient must first undergo blood testing to determine the fasting blood glucose value. She must then drink a specific dose of a glucose solution, and, an hour later, provide another blood sample for testing to evaluate how much glucose has left the bloodstream and entered the cells. If the blood glucose level is elevated at 1 hour after ingestion of the solution, it indicates poor glucose metabolism and requires a more comprehensive 3-hour test. In the 3-hour test, the patient must continue fasting, drink more of the glucose solution, and provide blood samples at 1-, 2-, and 3-hour intervals. Blood glucose levels should peak within the first hour after drinking the glucose and then begin to drop. Normal blood glucose values are 60 to 100 mg/dl when fasting, less than 200 mg/dl at 1 hour, and less than 140 mg/dl at 2 hours. Because the patient must remain at the hospital or laboratory for an extended period of time, the medical assistant should suggest that she bring reading materials.

Treatment of gestational diabetes includes a calorie-restricted diet, regular exercise, blood glucose monitoring, and, possibly, insulin injections (depending on severity) to maintain normal blood glucose levels. Oral hypoglycemic medications are contraindicated during pregnancy and should not be administered.

Although gestational diabetes usually subsides after the patient gives birth, the patient has a 50% chance of developing type 2 diabetes later in life. If left untreated, gestational diabetes can cause fetal developmental problems resulting from macrosomia (excessively large fetus). In addition, the mother is at increased risk for hypertension, eclampsia, and the need for cesarean delivery.

Placenta Previa
ICD-9-CM code: 641.00

Placenta previa is the implantation of the placenta, the organ of nutrition for the developing fetus, in the lower uterine segment. The placenta normally adheres to the central or upper portion of the uterine wall. Upon labor, the fetus leaves the uterus before delivery of the placenta. However, if the placenta implants in the lower uterine segment, it can obstruct delivery of the fetus. Placenta previa occurs in approximately 1 out of every 200 pregnancies. There are three degrees of placenta previa:

- centralis, where the placenta completely covers the cervix
- marginalis, where the placenta partially obstructs the cervix
- lateralis, where the cervix is not obstructed by the placenta but the placenta is placed low enough to possibly obstruct a vaginal delivery of the fetus. (See Figure 32-10.)

The cause of placenta previa is unknown but advanced maternal age (age 35 and older), increased parity (number of pregnancies), and previous uterine surgery, including cesarean section (regardless of incision type), increase the risk.

Signs and symptoms of placenta previa include slight hemorrhage with recurrent severity in the seventh or eighth month of pregnancy. Gradually, the patient will experience

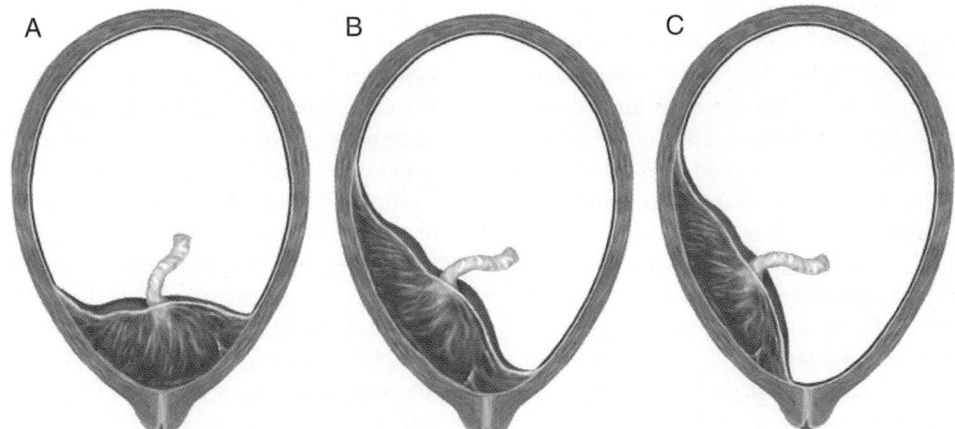

FIG 32-10 Placenta previa. (A) Centralis. (B) Marginalis. (C) Lateralis.

anemia, pallor, rapid weak pulse, air hunger, and low blood pressure. Diagnosis is obtained using ultrasound.

Treatment prior to delivery should include hospital bedrest and treatment of anemia. Vaginal examination is deferred, if possible, until 36 weeks' gestation to prevent infection. Vaginal delivery may be attempted in cases of placenta previa marginalis and lateralis, but not for the centralis form. If vaginal delivery is attempted, the obstetrician will order a "double set-up," where all equipment and personnel are available for emergency cesarean delivery. Immediate postpartum care includes monitoring the mother closely for continued bleeding and administering prophylactic antibiotics because of the high risk of infection.

The risk of complications increases with the severity of placenta previa and can include medical problems for the neonate secondary to blood loss, small birth weight due to restriction of space to grow in utero, and increased incidence of congenital anomalies. Risks to the mother include

life-threatening hemorrhage, cesarean delivery, increased risk of postpartum hemorrhage, and increased risk of placenta accreta (in which the placenta attaches directly to uterine muscle, requiring surgical removal).

Abruptio Placentae
ICD-9-CM code: 641.20

Abruptio placentae is the sudden, premature detachment of the placenta from the uterine wall. It is estimated that 1 in 120 births are complicated by placental abruption. There are three levels of abruption:

- Grade 1 is detachment of less than 20% of the surface of the placenta.
- Grade 2 is detachment of 20% to 50% of the placental surface.
- Grade 3 is detachment of more than 50% of the placenta. (See Figure 32-11.)

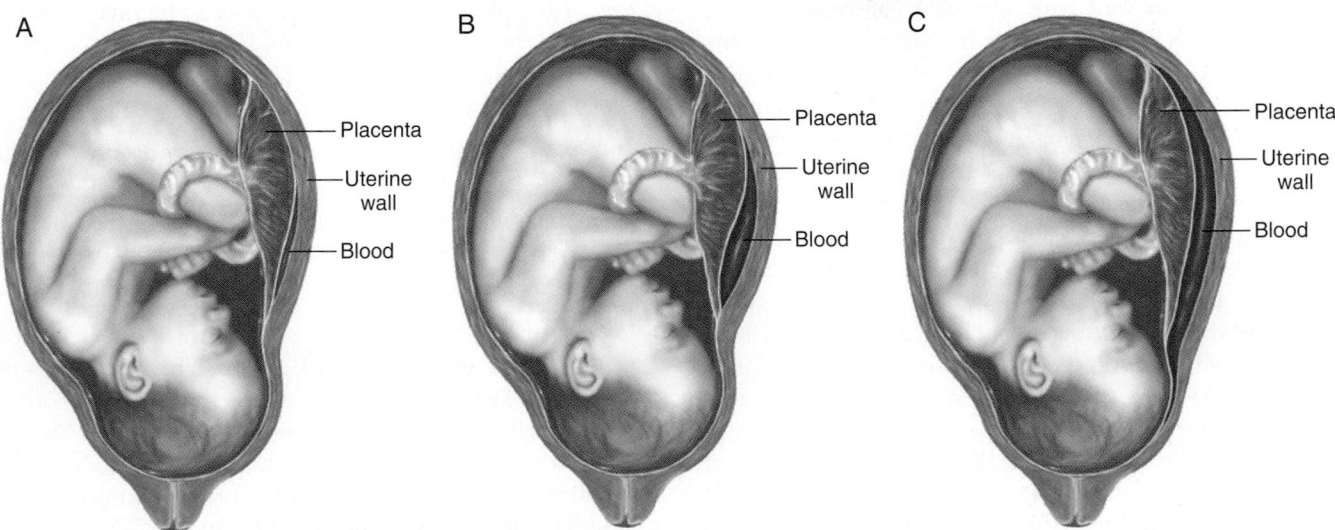

FIG 32-11 Abruptio placentae. (A) Grade 1. (B) Grade 2. (C) Grade 3.

The cause of abruptio placentae is unknown; however, cocaine abuse and toxemia increase the risk. Symptoms of mild abruption (grade 1) include vaginal bleeding, uterine tenderness, and mild tetany (muscular spasm). Grade 2 symptoms include those of grade 1 as well as fetal distress, because the fetus is not getting enough oxygen and nutrition. In grade 3, uterine tetany is severe, the mother is in shock, and the fetus dies due to lack of oxygen.

Diagnosis is usually made when the patient reports painless bleeding during the third trimester. Ultrasound provides a visual confirmation of the diagnosis.

Treatment of abruptio placentae varies with the severity of detachment. Women with a grade 1 detachment may be restricted to bedrest and undergo monitoring to prolong the pregnancy to a safe gestational age for the fetus. Administration of betamethasone, a drug that expedites development of fetal lungs, may be necessary if the fetus must be delivered early. Grade 2 detachment at or near term is treated by delivery of the fetus, either by vaginal induction or cesarean section. Because grade 3 detachment results in the death of the fetus, treatment aims to care for the mother.

Depending on the degree of separation, abruptio placentae causes fetal death in 20% to 40% of cases. It can also cause maternal death, due to shock and hemorrhage. In cases of hemorrhage, an emergency hysterectomy may be necessary to save the mother's life. About 40% to 50% of infants who survive abruptio placentae experience complications, which range from mild to severe. Women who have had the condition are more likely to have reoccurrence in subsequent pregnancies.

Eclampsia
ICD-9-CM code: 642.60

A condition called *pre-eclampsia* is characterized by severe hypertension in pregnancy. If left untreated, pre-eclampsia can progress to eclampsia, which includes convulsions and coma. About 3% to 5% of all pregnant women suffer from pre-eclampsia. Of those women, 1 in 20 progress to eclampsia.

The causes of pre-eclampsia and eclampsia are unknown. However, the risk is greater in teen pregnancy, first-time pregnancy, women age 35 and older, African American women, and women with multiple fetuses or a history of diabetes, hypertension, or renal disease.

Signs and symptoms of pre-eclampsia include hypertension, proteinuria, and edema. Progression to eclampsia is indicated by severe muscle aches, severe agitation, one or more grand mal seizures, coma, and convulsions. Without treatment, seizures may recur within minutes. Severe right upper quadrant pain, indicative of hepatic edema, and generalized abdominal pain may also be present.

Blood tests used to diagnose pre-eclampsia include creatinine to assess kidney function. Monitoring of blood pressure and breathing is important as well. Difficulty breathing can be a sign of pre-eclampsia or eclampsia.

Treatment is directed at managing seizures, monitoring blood pressure, and continuing the pregnancy for as long as possible. The patient must be hospitalized and an indwelling catheter inserted. Hourly monitoring of urinary output is necessary to diagnose renal failure. The hospitalized patient is given IV magnesium sulfate in an attempt to stop seizures. Induction of labor and cesarean section are necessary if blood pressure becomes dangerously high.

Eclampsia is the most serious complication of pregnancy and can lead to maternal and fetal death. Organ damage can involve the kidneys, liver, brain, and placenta. Damage to the placenta includes infarcts, thromboses, and hemorrhages. The developing fetus may suffer severe developmental delays due to inadequate supplies of blood, oxygen, and nutrition from the damaged placenta.

The medical assistant should monitor the patient's blood pressure and encourage her to keep regular obstetric appointments in an attempt to diagnose pre-eclampsia and avoid life-threatening eclampsia.

Cancers of the Female Reproductive System

Some of the most common forms of cancer are cancers of the female reproductive system, including breast cancer, cervical cancer, uterine cancer, and ovarian cancer.

Breast Cancer
ICD-9-CM code:174.9 (primary)

Breast cancer is the growth of abnormal cells in the tissue of the breast. It usually forms in the lactiferous ducts, the tubes that carry milk to the nipple, and the lobules, the glands that produce the milk. Breast cancer is the second leading cause of cancer death in women in the United States. According to the American Cancer Society, 1 in 8 women develop breast cancer and 1 in 28 risk death from the disease. Breast cancer occurs most commonly in women age 35 and older. It is the leading cause of death in American women ages 40 to 55.

The exact cause of breast cancer is unknown. Scientists have discovered a link between breast cancer and the two genes, BRCA-1 and BRCA-2. Discovery of these genes shows that breast cancer has some genetic predisposition; however, that does not indicate the only cause of breast cancer is genetic. Risk factors for breast cancer include:

- family history of breast cancer or presence of BRCA-1 or BRCA-2
- early onset of menstruation (age 12 or earlier) or late menopause (age 55 or later)
- never having children or having a first child after age 35
- high-fat diet, obesity, and alcohol intake
- history of endometrial or ovarian cancer
- use of estrogen replacement therapy or oral contraceptives
- history of fibrocystic breast disease.

Signs and symptoms of breast cancer include a dominant breast mass, bloody or brown discharge from the nipple, and breast nodules or irregularities. The breast mass is usually painless and freely moveable in the early stage but later becomes fixed.

If done regularly, breast self-examination (BSE) is the most reliable method for early detection of breast cancer. If the patient palpates a painless lump in her breast during BSE, the physician will conduct a breast examination and further testing to confirm the diagnosis. A mammogram can confirm the presence of a breast mass. It can also detect tumors that are too small to palpate. About 70% of masses found by mammography are benign. If a mass is found, a fine needle aspiration can be used to determine if the mass is solid or a fluid-filled cyst. A biopsy of the tissue evaluates the cells for malignancy. Upon confirmation of a breast cancer diagnosis, the physician will assess the stage, or progression, of the disease. Staging involves assessment of the size of the tumor and metastasis to the chest wall, skin, axilla, or distant sites. (See *Cancer staging*.)

Treatment for breast cancer is based on the stage of the disease, the patient's age, and whether she is currently menstruating or in menopause. Treatments include various combinations of surgery, radiation, chemotherapy, and hormone therapy:

- *Lumpectomy* involves removal of the tumor, surrounding tissue, and, possibly, adjacent lymph nodes (for testing) through a small incision. Lumpectomy is a treatment for small, well-defined lesions and is effective in early stage breast cancer.
- *Partial mastectomy* involves removal of the tumor, a wedge of surrounding normal tissue, skin and fascia, and, possibly, axillary lymph nodes. This procedure is used for early stage breast cancer with small, well-defined lesions. Radiation or chemotherapy is common after surgery to destroy undetected diseased tissue in the breast.
- *Total mastectomy* involves surgical removal of the entire breast and is done if the cancer is confined to the breast tissue and no lymph node involvement is noted. If the patient does not have advanced disease, surgery can be performed for cosmetic reconstruction.
- *Modified radical mastectomy* involves removal of the entire breast, axillary lymph nodes, and chest fascia. This procedure is used for advanced stages of breast cancer that may include metastasis to lymph nodes or adjacent tissues. If cancer has spread to the lymph tissue, radiation and chemotherapy are used to destroy more cancer cells. This procedure replaces the older radical mastectomy procedure, where chest muscles were also removed. This newer procedure allows the patient more function and upper body strength after surgery.
- *Radiation therapy* involves the administration of radioactivity externally via external beam radiation or internally via brachytherapy, which places radioactive substances near or within cancerous cells. Radiation therapy destroys malignant cells. The radiation directed at the tumor and a margin of healthy tissue around it ensures that all of the malignant cells are affected. Radiation therapy can also be used before or after surgery to destroy small, early stage tumors. Before surgery, it weakens cancerous tissue, making it easier to remove. After surgery, it treats the local area to kill any remaining cancer cells and prevent recurrence.
- *Chemotherapy* involves the use of drugs (cytotoxins) to kill cancer cells. It can be used alone or in combination with surgery or radiation therapy. Chemotherapy is administered in a hospital, a physician's office, or the patient's home. The drugs can be administered orally, IM, subcutaneously, or IV. Cyclophosphamide, methotrexate, and fluorouracil are commonly administered in combination.
- *Hormone therapy* involves administration of antihormonal drugs, including tamoxifen, aminoglutethimide, and fluoxymesterone. Breast cancer cells are thought to grow in response to such hormones as estrogen and progesterone, so these drugs suppress production of those hormones. Hormone therapy is generally offered only to women who are postmenopausal.

Prognosis is based primarily on the tumor's stage. Patients with large tumors that have metastasized to lymph nodes, the chest wall, or distal organs have a poor prognosis. Patients with smaller tumors with no metastasis have better outcomes. Complications include metastasis to secondary tumors and adverse effects of chemotherapy, including nausea, vomiting, immunosuppression, fatigue, and hair loss. Because early diagnosis and treatment of cancer provides the best outcome, the medical assistant should emphasize

---

Cancer staging

Cancer staging is used in cancers of the female reproductive system as well as cancers of other organ systems. Staging indicates the extent of the spread of cancerous tumors and provides standardized descriptions of tumors, treatment recommendations, and outcomes. It is used to create criteria for including patients in clinical trials and determine a treatment regimen as well as a prognosis.

The universally used tumor, node, metastasis (TNM) staging system is based on three factors:

- tumor (T)—size or extent of local spread of a primary tumor
- node (N)—presence or absence and extent of regional or distal lymph node metastasis
- metastasis (M)—presence or absence of distant metastasis (cancer in other organs).

the importance of routine cancer screenings to all her patients.

Cervical Cancer

ICD-9-CM code: 180.9 (primary)
Cervical cancer is an abnormal growth and development of the cells of the cervix. Cervical cancer is the third most common cancer of the female reproductive tract, causing 5% of all cancer deaths in women. About 80% of all cervical cancers are squamous cell carcinomas (changes in the surface cells of the cervix) and the remaining 20% are adenocarcinomas (changes in the cells of the mucus-producing glands of the cervix). Very few cases of cervical cancer involve both types of carcinoma. Most women who get cervical cancer are in their 50s; however, younger women can also get cervical cancer.

The cause of cervical cancer is unknown. Factors contributing to cervical cancer include smoking tobacco, early age intercourse, multiple sexual partners, herpes simplex 2 virus, and a history of more than one pregnancy. Because some strains of human papilloma virus (HPV) are carcinogenic to the cervix, many patients with HPV infection contract cervical cancer. (See *Cervical cancer and HPV.*)

Early cervical cancer is asymptomatic. Pap test screening enables a diagnosis before symptoms appear so that treatment can begin early. The Pap test detects abnormal cellular changes with a 95% accuracy rate. Later stage cervical cancer signs and symptoms include abnormal vaginal bleeding, persistent discharge, and pain and bleeding after intercourse.

Treatment for cervical cancer varies from cryosurgery to laser treatments to eliminate intraepithelial cancer cells.

Cervical cancer and HPV

In 2006, researchers identified a history of human papilloma virus (HPV) as the most significant risk factor for cervical cancer. In response to these findings, the federal government issued a policy recommending immunization against HPV for all sexually active females. The immunization, a three-shot series, can be given to girls as young as age 8 to establish immunity prior to sexual activity.

Because the federal government recommends administration of the vaccine to girls at a very young age, the policy is considered somewhat controversial. Some parents may feel the vaccine encourages or sanctions sexual activity at an early age. In addition, although the statistical correlation between HPV and cervical cancer is significant, there is no definitive proof to date that HPV causes cervical cancer.

The HPV vaccine (Gardasil) is currently available in most gynecologists' offices.

Conization (removal of a cone-shaped section of cervical mucous membrane cells), surgical resection, radiation, and chemotherapy treat cancer that has grown deeper into the cervix. Hysterectomy is a treatment option for women with preinvasive cervical cancer who do not wish to preserve fertility. The survival rate for patients with preinvasive cancer is almost 100%. For patients with invasive cervical cancer, the survival rate is approximately 91%. About 35% of patients with invasive cervical cancer experience recurrence.

Uterine Cancer

ICD-9-CM code: 179 (primary)
Uterine cancer is called an *adenocarcinoma* because it begins in the endometrial cells of the uterus, usually in the glandular tissue. It is the most common malignancy of the female reproductive system. Uterine cancer typically affects postmenopausal women between ages 50 and 60. The incidence is more common in white women but the death rate is higher in black women.

Signs and symptoms include bleeding in the postmenopausal patient; yellow, watery discharge with a foul odor; and cramping or pressure in the abdomen or pelvis. Results of a uterine biopsy, when viewed under a microscope, will show cellular changes consistent with cancer. If the biopsy is inconclusive, the physician will perform a D&C to obtain an adequate sample to determine malignancy.

Treatment for uterine cancer is most commonly a total hysterectomy to prevent recurrence of cancer to any of the reproductive organs. The physician may prescribe radiation therapy before surgery if the tumor is poorly defined. The physician may also prescribe chemotherapy after surgery to prevent growth of cancer in adjacent organs. Administration of progesterone before surgery reduces uterine bleeding during the procedure.

The 1-year survival rate for uterine cancer is 92% and the 5-year survival rate varies from 65% to 70%, based on the time of diagnosis.

Ovarian Cancer

ICD-9-CM code: 183.0 (primary)
Ovarian tumors arise from three different types of ovarian cells:

- *Epithelial tumors*, which are changes to the surface cells of the ovary, are the most common type of ovarian cancer.
- *Germ cell tumors* are abnormal changes to the cells that produce the ova.
- *Stromal tumors* are abnormal changes to cells of the connective tissue that holds the ovary together and produces estrogen and progesterone.

Ovarian cancer accounts for 4% of all cancers among women. About 85% to 90% of ovarian cancers arise from the surface epithelium of the ovary. The other 10% to 15% arise as germ cell tumors from the ova within the ovary. Germ cell tumors usually occur in younger women, even prepubescent girls. Epithelial tumors most commonly affect women ages 40 to 65. Many patients who develop ovarian cancer have the BRCA-1 or BRCA-2 gene, suggesting that they have a hereditary predisposition to ovarian cancer.

Early stage symptoms include mild abdominal pain, abdominal bloating, diarrhea or constipation, indigestion, gas, upset stomach, fatigue, and abnormal menstrual or vaginal bleeding. Because these symptoms are vague, many patients do not get diagnosed in the early stages. Most cases are diagnosed when the disease has already progressed and symptoms include a buildup of fluid in the abdominal cavity (ascites); shortness of breath; dry, persistent cough; nausea; vomiting; abdominal tumors; and weight loss.

Treatment depends on the stage and grade of the tumor and includes surgical removal of the entire reproductive system and affected adjacent tissues, such as the regional lymph nodes and omentum. The physician may prescribe radiation and chemotherapy to kill cancer cells that have spread to adjacent organs and cannot be surgically removed. (See *Taking care during radiation and chemotherapy*.)

Because most ovarian cancers progress to a late stage before diagnosis, only 25% of patients survive for 5 years.

Other Disorders of the Female Reproductive System

Other disorders of the female reproductive system include infertility and fibrocystic breast disease. The medical assistant can assist the physician in diagnosis, treatment, and patient education related to these disorders.

Infertility
ICD-9-CM code: 628.9 (unspecified origin)
Infertility is an inability to achieve pregnancy after trying to conceive for a period of 1 year or more. The condition affects 20% of all couples and may be caused by a problem in the male or the female. Infertility can be:

- primary, which is the inability of a woman to conceive her first child
- secondary, which is infertility in a woman who previously conceived.

Female causes of infertility vary from hormonal imbalances that suppress ovulation to structural problems, such as blocked fallopian tubes or uterine malposition. Eating disorders or nutritional disorders may also decrease the chance of successful conception.

Diagnosis of the cause of infertility is based on a comprehensive health history of both partners with assessment of their usual timing for intercourse. Female assessment includes evaluation of ovulation by charting basal body temperature. Laparoscopic examination of the ovaries, fallopian tubes, and uterus may reveal structural abnormalities. Blood tests include an evaluation of hormone levels, which may indicate under- or overproduction of one or more of the female hormones. Hormonal balance is necessary for normal ovulation, implantation of the ova, and successful pregnancy.

Treatments for infertility vary. Nonsurgical treatments are directed at correcting hormonal imbalances that suppress

---

Patient Education

Taking Care During Radiation and Chemotherapy

Radiation and chemotherapy are used to kill cancer cells. Unfortunately, these treatments also kill healthy cells of the body. Both regimens can cause such symptoms as nausea, vomiting, diarrhea, hair loss, fatigue, stomatitis (inflammation of the tissues of the mouth), tissue necrosis, and weakening of the immune system.

The medical assistant should advise her patient undergoing radiation and chemotherapy to:

- eat cool, soft, bland foods to reduce nausea and prevent vomiting
- eat iron-rich foods or take a multivitamin and mineral combination to replace red blood cells (RBCs) lost during treatment and maintain tissue oxygenation
- use acupuncture to treat nausea and stimulate appetite

- use a soft toothbrush to avoid gum irritation and infection and apply a topical, over-the-counter antibiotic to the gums
- use an electric razor to avoid cutting the skin and increasing the risk of infection
- rest often—radiation and chemotherapy cause fatigue—and ask friends or family to help with daily chores and driving to the hospital or clinic for treatments
- report symptoms of infection, such as fever, cough, sore throat, and dysuria, so that the physician can initiate treatment of infection or stop radiation or chemotherapy to allow the patient's body to fight the infection
- report sudden headaches, which can indicate intracranial bleeding; a situation needing immediate attention.

ovulation or make it impossible for the embryo to implant in the uterus. Surgical treatments include in vitro fertilization, where ova are harvested and fertilized outside of the mother's body and then implanted in the uterus.

An obstetrical medical practice waiting room is commonly filled with pregnant patients; this environment can be stressful to the woman trying to conceive, as can the fact that treatments for infertility are expensive and often not covered by medical insurance. Patients who are experiencing infertility may be depressed and extremely emotional. The medical assistant can listen to and comfort her patient who is trying to conceive.

The success rates for infertility treatment depend on the cause, the age of the couple, and any underlying health problems that may impact fertility. The CDC reports that assisted reproductive therapy is successful in 38% of women under age 35, 30% of women ages 35 to 37, 20% of women ages 38 to 40, and only 11% in women age 41 and older.

Fibrocystic Breast Disease
ICD-9-CM code: 610.1

Fibrocystic breast disease is the presence of multiple lumps in the breast, consisting of fibrous tumors or fluid-filled cysts. About 33% of women ages 30 to 50 and 50% of all women at some point in their lifetime will develop fibrocystic breast disease.

Causes of fibrocystic breast disease are unknown and may be related to normal aging. Symptoms include palpable, firm, well-defined, painless nodules in the breast. The cysts may be more tender than the fibroids and tenderness may increase in relation to the menstrual cycle. Over time, the fluid-filled cysts enlarge and become fibrous, increasing in density and firmness.

Diagnosis is confirmed by a manual breast examination and mammography. Treatments for fibroids include needle aspiration of fluid-filled cysts. After aspiration, the cysts rarely refill with fluid. The medical assistant should advise patients to reduce intake of caffeine and dietary fat, which are known to exacerbate fibrocystic breast disease. If dietary changes decrease the symptoms and the patient can maintain these changes, recurrence of cysts may be avoided. Although the presence of fibroids does not increase the risk of breast cancer, their presence may interfere with the diagnosis of breast cancer by mammogram.

Obstetric and Gynecological Procedures

Obstetrics and gynecology (OB-GYN), two separate specialties that are commonly combined, is also called *women's health*. Obstetrics is the specialized branch of medicine involving the treatment and care of a pregnant female. The physician who specializes in obstetrics is called an *obstetrician*. Gynecology is the specialized branch of medicine involving the female reproductive system. The physician who specializes in diagnosing and treating diseases and disorders of the female reproductive system is called a *gynecologist*.

Medical assistants working in OB-GYN, or women's health, obtain vital signs and histories on all patients; assist with Pap tests, pelvic examinations, and breast examinations; and perform routine laboratory tests, such as urinalysis and pregnancy tests. (See *Common OB-GYN interview questions*.) In this area, patient education is an important part of the medical assistant's job. The medical assistant should instruct patients to perform a breast self-examination every month.

Prenatal Care

Obstetric care ideally begins early in pregnancy, continues through the pregnancy, and ends in the **postpartum** period, the period extending several weeks after delivery. Ideally, care ends with a checkup at 2 weeks postpartum, which enables the obstetrician to monitor the patient's progress throughout the pregnancy and provides many opportunities for the patient to ask questions and obtain information. The medical assistant can play a major role in educating these patients.

Initial Visit

During the initial prenatal visit, the medical assistant or obstetrician will obtain a complete health history, including medical, surgical, family, and obstetric history. The obstetric history includes:

- **gravidity**, which is how many times the patient has been pregnant
- number of live births (indicated by the term *para*)
- number of spontaneous and elective abortions (indicated by the term *ab*).

So, if a woman experienced 3 pregnancies, 2 births, and 1 miscarriage, she would be designated as a *gravida 3, para 2, ab 1*.

Common OB-GYN interview questions

The medical assistant working in an obstetric-gynecological (OB-GYN) office should be sure to include these questions when taking a health history:

- When was the first day of your last menstrual period (LMP)?
- Are you sexually active?
- Do you use birth control?
- When was your last Pap test?
- Do you do monthly breast self-examinations?

In addition to establishing the patient's history, the obstetrician can determine the expected date of delivery (EDD) using Nägele's rule. (See *Nägele's rule*.) Many offices have an EDD wheel, which automatically computes the EDD using Nägele's rule. (See Figure 32-12.)

Also during the initial visit, the obstetrician will perform a complete breast, abdominal, pelvic, and rectal examination. The medical assistant must check vital signs, including weight, and perform baseline laboratory tests. Tests include:

- complete blood count (CBC)
- urinalysis
- rubella
- RPR
- Blood typing and Rh
- Pap test
- screening tests for chlamydia, gonorrhea, group B beta *Streptococcus*, hepatitis B and, possibly, HIV.

At the first prenatal visit, the medical assistant should educate her patient verbally and through written materials on pregnancy, food choices, and how her body will change over the course of the pregnancy. (See *Supplements during pregnancy*.) The medical assistant can also set future appointments and help establish a trusting relationship between the patient and the staff. The patient who feels comfortable with the physician and staff will be more

Nägele's rule

Nägele's rule is a formula that uses the first day of the last menstrual period (LMP) to determine the estimated date of delivery (EDD) of an infant. Here is the formula:

LMP + 7 days − 3 months + 1 year

So, for a woman whose LMP was July 12, 2008, the EDD would be:

July 12 + 7 days = July 19
July 19 − 3 months = April 19
April 19 + 1 year = April 19, 2009
EDD = April 19, 2009

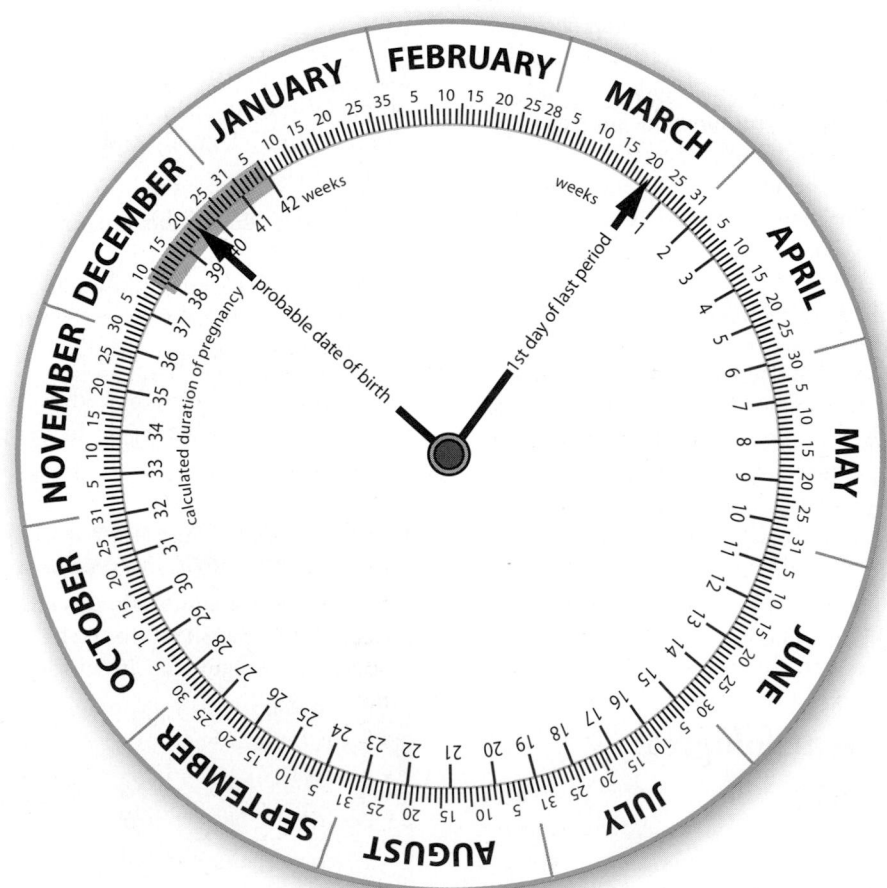

FIG 32-12 EDD wheel used to compute estimated date of delivery.

Supplements during pregnancy

Most obstetricians advise their pregnant patients to take prenatal vitamin supplements during pregnancy and lactation to ensure that the developing fetus or growing infant receives the nutrients necessary for proper growth and development. Prenatal vitamins contain higher doses of folate, iron, and calcium than regular vitamin-mineral supplements, which aids in:

- fetal red blood cell development (iron)
- fetal bone and tooth development (vitamin D and calcium)
- deoxyribonucleic acid (DNA) and ribonucleic acid (RNA) synthesis (folate, vitamin B_{12}, iron, and zinc).

These supplements are especially beneficial if a woman experiences nausea, food aversions, or vomiting or has poor eating habits in general. The patient who is carrying multiple fetuses, smokes cigarettes, or uses illicit drugs is especially in need of vitamin and mineral supplementation.

initiate early treatment of potentially harmful conditions, confirm the due date, and identify the sex of the fetus.

After the medical assistant has conducted the interview and examination, she must prepare the patient for the physician's examination. The medical assistant must ask the patient to change into an examination gown with the opening directed to the front. When the patient has finished changing, the medical assistant must knock on the door and then help the patient onto the examination table, if she needs assistance. The medical assistant should support the patient and be ready to assist the physician as she conducts the examination, which includes:

- measurement of the fundal height, or how much the top of the uterus has grown upward, to determine normal growth, excessive fundal height (which can indicate multiple fetuses or excess amniotic fluid), or limited fundal height (which can indicate poor fetal development or fetal death)
- measurement and recording of fetal heart rate using a fetoscope or Doppler fetal pulse monitor to ensure fetal circulation and detect multiple fetuses

likely to keep prenatal appointments, ask questions, and share health information.

Routine Prenatal Visits

At each visit, the medical assistant must follow a set format to ensure consistent evaluation of the mother's health and development of the fetus. This format includes:

- Interviewing the patient and recording any complaints, such as food intolerances, nausea, vomiting, and fatigue. Early treatment of problems can reduce symptoms and avoid more serious complications later in the pregnancy.
- Requesting a urine sample and testing for glucose and protein. Glucose in the urine is an indication of diabetes or poor blood glucose control (hypoglycemia or hyperglycemia). Protein in the urine is an indication of kidney disorders, such as urinary tract infection, glomerulonephritis, and nephritis, or other pregnancy-related disorders, such as preeclampsia, eclampsia, and toxemia.
- Measuring the patient's weight and recording the findings. Weight gain reflects the mother's nutrition and the related health of the fetus. Excessive weight gain could be due to overnutrition, poor eating habits, or fluid retention. Inadequate weight gain can compromise the growth and development of the fetus. (See *Weight gain during pregnancy*.)
- Measuring and recording the patient's vital signs. Changes in blood pressure may indicate hypertension and other complications.
- Checking the patient's medical record to ensure that all laboratory test results are included. Laboratory findings help

Weight gain during pregnancy

Most physicians recommend that a pregnant woman should gain no more than 35 lb during her entire pregnancy. Excess weight gain during pregnancy can cause hypertension, increased stress on the heart, and gestational diabetes. Excess weight gain also puts the mother at risk for diabetes, heart disease, orthopedic injuries, and reduced self-esteem related to excess body weight after pregnancy.

In addition to the weight contributed by the growing fetus, weight gain during pregnancy is also the result of the growing placenta, uterus, and breasts as well as amniotic fluid, increased blood volume, and increased fat in the breasts for breastfeeding and in the thighs to support the growing fetus. Following is a breakdown of the average values for each element involved in weight gain for a pregnant woman who gains 20 lb during pregnancy. Although the baby may contribute a few more pounds, the placenta, uterus, and breasts remain fairly steady, regardless of other factors. Thus, the majority of additional weight gain is typically in additional fat and fluid.

Total weight of baby	7.5 lb
Placenta	1.0 lb
Enlarged uterus	2.0 lb
Enlarged breasts	1.5 lb
Additional fat and fluid	8.0 lb
Total	**20.0 lb**

- internal examination of the patient, which is not performed at every visit but is used to assess the cervix to determine pregnancy or cervical dilation and effacement
- patient education, including asking the patient if she has questions or concerns and educating her about teratogens

(any drug or chemical that can cause damage to the developing embryo) to empower the patient to make the best decisions for her baby and her own health (See *Food and drug safety during pregnancy*.)

- orders for further testing, such as a fetal ultrasound, to determine the health and development of the fetus.

Food and drug safety during pregnancy

The medical assistant and physician need to educate the patient on the risks of teratogens, any drug or chemical that can cause damage to the developing embryo. There are several categories of teratogens that the pregnant woman should be aware of, including:

- environmental contaminants
- alcohol
- tobacco
- some medications.

Environmental Contaminants

The most common environmental contaminants that impact pregnancy are lead and mercury. Lead and mercury easily cross the placental barrier and can inflict severe damage on the developing fetal nervous system. Infants and young children whose mother was exposed to lead or mercury during pregnancy show signs of delayed mental and psychomotor development, behavior problems, and impaired hearing. Fetal exposure to lead is also linked to low birth weight. Although fatty fish contains omega-3 fatty acids, which are beneficial to the mother and developing fetus, many types of fatty fish contain high levels of mercury. The medical assistant should advise her pregnant patients to avoid eating shark, swordfish, king mackerel, and tilefish during pregnancy and lactation. She should also advise her patient to avoid exposure to lead by following these measures:

- having the water in the home tested for lead
- using only cold water for drinking, cooking, and making formula, because cold water absorbs less lead
- avoiding storing acidic foods or beverages (such as orange juice or vinegar) in ceramic dishware
- storing canned food after opening in a lead-free container.

Alcohol

Alcohol is unsafe for pregnant women to consume in any dosage. At high dosages, alcohol consumption will cause fetal alcohol syndrome (FAS), a collection of characteristics that include a small head with multiple facial abnormalities; small eyes with short slits; a wide, flat nasal bridge; a midface that lacks a groove between the lips and nose; and a small jaw. The affected child commonly exhibits persistent growth retardation, hyperactivity, and learning deficits. The neonate with FAS may experience alcohol withdrawal symptoms during the first few days of life. No quantity of alcohol consumption is safe during pregnancy; all physicians recommend abstaining from alcohol during pregnancy.

Tobacco

Smoking during pregnancy or exposure to second-hand smoke has been linked to low fetal birth weight, abruptio placentae, and premature birth.

Medications

In addition to the dangers of alcohol and cigarettes, the medical assistant should explain to her patient that many medications are contraindicated during pregnancy. Medication safety during pregnancy is grouped into five categories by the U.S. Food and Drug Administration (FDA):

- A—No harm has been demonstrated in well-designed studies of pregnant and lactating women (for example, folic acid supplements).
- B—Without known risk in human pregnancy or breastfeeding; studies in laboratory animals have been performed with positive or negative effects but no known demonstrable risk in pregnancy is yet known (for example, amoxicillin, a commonly used antibiotic, and acyclovir, an antiviral medication used for herpes).
- C—Use in human pregnancy or breastfeeding has not been adequately studied; risk of usage cannot be excluded but has not been proven (for example, albuterol, hydrocodone, omeprazole, and verapamil).
- D—Known to cause fetal harm when administered during pregnancy or harm to infants during breastfeeding (for example, tetracycline antibiotics).
- X—Contraindicated during pregnancy; evidence of risk has been accrued from clinical trials or postmarketing surveillance (for example, isotretinoin, thalidomide, and warfarin).

Lactation Consultation

During the last trimester of pregnancy, the medical assistant should ask her patient if she will bottle feed or breastfeed her baby. She should give the patient who plans to breastfeed written information, such as pamphlets, as well as video instruction if available. The medical assistant can also provide a referral to a lactation consultant with whom the patient can meet in the hospital after the birth or prior to the birth of her baby for a one-on-one consultation or a series of classes.

The medical assistant should encourage patients to try breastfeeding because it is beneficial for the mother and infant. Maternal antibodies contained in breast milk will protect the baby from many childhood illnesses. Studies have also shown that breastfed babies are less likely to suffer from high cholesterol, obesity, diabetes, allergies, and asthma. Breastfeeding also stimulates uterine contractions and helps the uterus return to pregravid (prepregnancy) size. The medical assistant should also make the patient aware of her additional nutritional requirements while breastfeeding. (See *Breastfeeding diet.*)

Assessment of the Neonate

Immediately after delivery, the obstetrician suctions the infant's nose and mouth and clamps and cuts the umbilical cord. Rapid changes in the respiratory and circulatory systems are evident as the infant becomes independent of the mother's circulation. The infant inhales and starts to breathe spontaneously. Carbon dioxide (CO_2) levels in the infant's blood rise and stimulate the respiratory center of the brain in the medulla. Full expansion of the lungs may take up to 7 days after birth. Respiration during the first few days of life is rapid—up to 40 respirations per minute. Breathing stimulates blood circulation in the neonate and the bluish color of the neonate's skin changes to a normal skin tone within a few minutes. Because the neonate's liver is not fully developed, his skin may look yellow, or *jaundiced,* due to an inability to excrete bilirubin. The obstetrician or pediatrician will assess the neonate at 1 and 5 minutes after birth. (For more information on neonatal assessment, see Chapter 33, page 641.)

Postpartum Visit

The postpartum visit is approximately 6 weeks after vaginal delivery or 2 to 3 weeks following a cesarean delivery. The medical assistant must weigh the patient and check her vital signs. The physician examines the perineum. If an episiotomy was performed, the physician checks to assess proper healing; if cesarean section was necessary, the physician assesses the sutures of the incision. The physician also performs a breast and pelvic examination and discusses birth control options with the patient. (See *Contraception,* page 630.)

Assisting with the Gynecological Examination

The gynecological examination consists of vital signs assessment, height and weight measurement, breast examination, and pelvic examination, which often includes a Pap test. The patient should undergo examination annually to avoid delaying treatment of reproductive system abnormalities.

When preparing a patient for the gynecological examination, the medical assistant must measure and record the patient's weight and height, record the date of the patient's LMP, and obtain vital signs and a health history. The patient undergoing a gynecological examination should not be menstruating. To prepare the patient for the examination, the medical assistant should advise her to void or instruct her on collecting a urine specimen if required. The patient will be more comfortable during the examination if she has an empty bladder. When taking the gynecological history, the medical assistant must be sure to ask about certain subjects, including:

- menstrual cycle
  - age at menarche (if the patient is new to the practice)
  - regularity
  - amount and duration of flow
  - history of menstrual symptoms and previous treatments

Breastfeeding diet

The average lactating mother produces 25 oz of milk per day. In order to maintain this rate of production, she must take in an extra 500 calories each day for the first 6 months of lactation. As the infant tapers his nursing and adds more solid foods to his diet, the need for extra calories decreases.

The medical assistant can help her patients make good nutritional choices by offering information on healthy foods. Dietary requirements for a nursing mother in the first 6 months of lactation include:

- additional carbohydrates, such as whole grains, fruits, and vegetables, to replace glucose used to make lactose in breast milk

- intake of protein and fatty acids, such as fish (other than those on the list to avoid), chicken, tofu, and legumes, at the same level as in the late stage of pregnancy

- intake of adequate fluids, such as water, juice, and herbal or decaffeinated tea, and fiber, such as whole grain breads and pastas, to prevent maternal dehydration and constipation

- avoidance of alcohol, caffeine, and many prescribed medications.

Contraception

The gynecological patient may request information on contraception (birth control). Methods for preventing pregnancy vary in their level of risk, convenience, and effectiveness. The medical assistant can offer her patient information on the various types of birth control so that she can make an informed decision with her physician.

The following table lists some of the most common methods of contraception, along with a description, rate of effectiveness, contraindications, and adverse effects for each.

Type	Description	Effectiveness	Contraindications	Adverse Effects
Abstinence	Refraining from sexual intercourse	100%	• None	• None
Surgical sterilization	In females, cutting the fallopian tubes and cauterizing the ends (tubal ligation); in males, surgical resection of the vas deferens (vasectomy)*	100%	• None	• None
Diaphragm, cervical cap	Barrier method that involves insertion of a rubber disk that is roughly the size of a baseball (diaphragm) or a thimble (cap) over the cervix	89% to 98%	• Latex, rubber, or spermicide allergy in either partner • Uterine prolapse • Cystocele	• Increased risk of UTI (diaphragm) • Increased risk of abnormal Pap test result (cap)
Condom	Barrier method that uses a rubber or latex sheath that fits over the penis	90% to 98%	• Latex or spermicide allergy in either partner	• Possible allergic response to spermicide or latex
Female condom	Barrier method that uses a latex pouch suspended from an inner ring that fits over the cervix	75% to 97%	• Latex or spermicide allergy in either partner	• Possible allergic response to spermicide or latex

*In some cases, vasectomy can be reversed.

Contraception—cont'd

Type	Description	Effectiveness	Contraindications	Adverse Effects
Intrauterine device (IUD)	T-shaped copper or plastic wire that a physician inserts into the uterus, which causes endometrial inflammation, thus preventing implantation of a fertilized egg	94% to 98%	• Cervicitis • Vaginitis • History of STDs, ectopic pregnancy, endometriosis, or pelvic infection	• Increased risk of PID • Spotting in 10% to 15% of users
medroxyprogesterone (Depo-Provera)	Prescription medication administered via IM injection (150 mg every 3 months) that inhibits development of a follicle and prevents ovulation	99.5%	• Not recommended if the patient wants to become pregnant within 1 year • Breast cancer • Liver disease	• Headache, weight gain, depression • Return of fertility may take 12 to 18 months
Oral contraceptives	Oral medication taken daily that suppresses ovulation and induces endometrial atrophy	99%	• Coronary artery disease • Thrombolytic disorder • Breast, liver, reproductive tract cancer • Smoking • Diabetes • Sickle cell anemia	• Nausea • Breakthrough bleeding • Breast tenderness and fluid retention • Hypertension, elevated blood lipids, and blood clots • Stroke
Contraceptive patch (Ortho-Evra)	Transdermal patch applied once per week for 3 weeks and nothing for the 4th week of the menstrual cycle that suppresses ovulation	99%	• Coronary artery disease • Thrombolytic disorder • Breast, liver, reproductive tract cancer • Smoking • Diabetes • Sickle cell anemia	• Nausea • Breakthrough bleeding • Breast tenderness and fluid retention • Hypertension, elevated blood lipids, and blood clots • Stroke

- urinary symptoms
  - frequency
  - itching and burning
- vaginal pain or discharge
- breast health (if the patient has felt any lumps and date of last mammogram)
- date of last Pap test
- sexual history, including history of STDs
- number of pregnancies and live births
- date of LMP
- social history, including smoking and alcohol use
- medications the patient is presently taking, including oral contraceptives
- any questions the patient has for the doctor (include on note in the medical record).

After the medical assistant records the gynecological history, she should provide the patient with a gown and drape and ask her to undress completely, put on the gown with the opening in the front, and use the drape to cover her legs.

Breast Examination

When the physician is ready to begin the examination, the medical assistant should assist the patient into the supine position. The physician or nurse practitioner will begin by performing the breast examination and may use this time to explain to the patient how to do her own breast self-examination (BSE). The provider commonly asks the medical assistant to teach the patient how to do a BSE with the use of a model breast or written instructions. (See *Procedure 32-1: Providing instruction on breast self-examination.*)

Pelvic Examination

The physician or nurse practitioner talks with the patient to answer questions and establish rapport. The provider should

---

PROCEDURE 32-1

Providing instruction on breast self-examination

Task
Instruct the patient on how to conduct a breast self-examination.

Conditions
- Breast model, written patient instructional brochure, or both
- Patient's medical record
- Pen

Standards
In the time specified and within the scoring parameters determined by the instructor, the student will successfully instruct the patient on how to conduct a breast self-examination.

Performance Standards
1. Greet and identify the patient.
2. Discuss the importance of performing a breast self-examination as a way to detect breast lumps.
3. Explain to the patient that she should perform a breast self-examination monthly and that the best time to conduct the examination is in the middle of her menstrual cycle because her breasts are likely to be less tender at that time. Suggest to the patient that she use a calendar to remind her to do the examination monthly.
4. Instruct the patient to stand in front of a mirror with her shoulders straight and arms on her hips. Tell her to look at each breast for changes in size, shape, or color; dimpling or puckering; redness; rash; swelling; changes in nipple shape; or discharge from the nipple. Such abnormalities may be an indication of breast pathology.
5. Tell the patient that she should next raise her arms and repeat step 4 to get a clear view of her breasts.
6. Instruct patient to inspect her nipples for discharge by squeezing them.
7. Explain to the patient that she should also inspect her breasts by lying down on a bed to allow access to all parts of the breast and palpating each breast for lumps.
   a. The patient should palpate the left breast with the first two fingers of the right hand and the right breast with the first two fingers of the left hand. Using the opposite hand enables the patient to palpate the entire breast.
   b. The patient should cover the entire breast, using the same starting point and going in a back-and-forth motion. You can suggest to the patient starting at the nipple and going in a circular motion from inside to outside or starting at the upper portion of the armpit and moving back and forth, covering the entire breast. Performing the procedure consistently ensures that the entire breast is evaluated.
   c. Instruct the patient to check for lumps in her armpits as well as the area above the breast around the collarbone. Lumps in these areas can also be an indication of breast pathology.

PROCEDURE 32-1—cont'd

8. Explain to the patient that she is looking for a small, hard, round lump and that as she performs the procedure on a regular basis, she will begin to see a pattern in her breasts and feeling a lump will become easier.

9. If available, use a breast model to demonstrate the proper technique for inspecting for lumps. A breast model will also contain simulated lumps for the patient to feel.

10. Give the patient an instructional brochure to take home. Written instructions will reinforce understanding of the procedure and aid in patient compliance.

11. Ask the patient if she has any questions and remind her to call the office immediately if she feels a lump. Early detection and treatment can prevent the spread of breast cancer.

12. Document the patient education in the patient's medical record.

Date	
08/19/08; 1:15 p.m.	*Pt. instructed on SBE and given written instructions.* ---- --J. Morgan, CMA

try to make the patient feel comfortable and not rushed. If the provider is male, the medical assistant commonly stays in the room during the pelvic examination, even if the provider does not require her assistance. For the pelvic examination, the medical assistant should assist the patient into the lithotomy position with her feet in stirrups. Because this position can be uncomfortable for the patient, the medical assistant should wait until the physician is ready to do the examination before assisting the patient into this position. She should make sure the patient's buttocks are at the edge of the table and assist her as necessary to reassure and support her.

As the examination continues, the physician may ask the medical assistant to hand her each instrument. It is the responsibility of the medical assistant to make sure all instruments have been properly cleaned or sterilized and are available to the physician. The medical assistant should also label all specimens accurately before taking them to the laboratory. During the examination, the physician will perform a bimanual pelvic examination. The physician places two fingers (pointer and ring fingers) inside the vagina and pushes down on the abdomen superior to the fundus (top of the uterus) with the other hand. (See Figure 32-13.)

The physician will then insert a vaginal speculum into the vagina to retract the walls of the vagina in order to obtain a specimen for the Papanicolaou (Pap) test. (See Figure 32-14.)

In addition to the vaginal speculum, a uterine curette, biopsy forceps, and uterine sounds are used for various gynecological procedures.

Pap Test, KOH Preparation, and Wet Preparation

The **Papanicolaou (Pap) test**, also called *Pap smear*, is used to detect cancer cells in the cervix. Named after George Nicholas Papanicolaou, the Pap test helps diagnose cervical cancer so treatment can begin early. An older version of the test involved collecting cells and smearing them on a slide and spraying a fixative. A newer version of the Pap test involves scraping the patient's cervix with a cytology brush

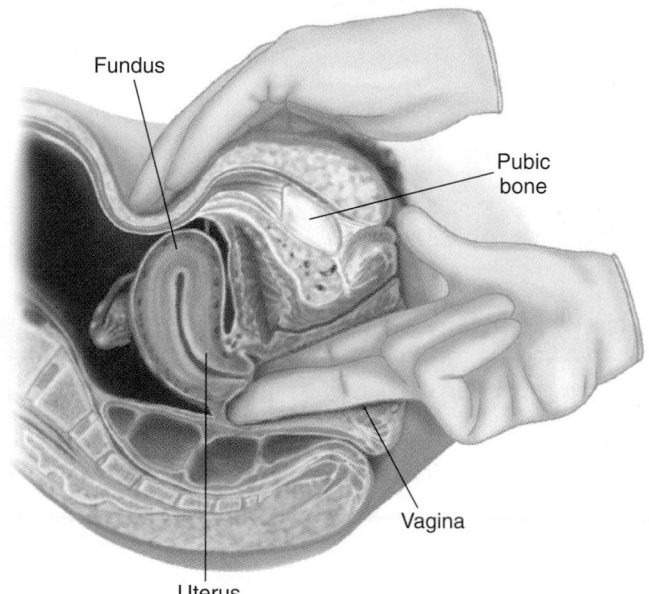

FIG 32-13 Bimanual pelvic examination.

and then immediately placing the brush in a vial of transport fluid.

The potassium hydroxide (KOH) preparation is used to diagnose fungal infection. The wet preparation is used to diagnose yeast, bacteria, and *Trichomonas* infections. Because both of these tests involve taking a sample of vaginal discharge, the physician performs them at the same time as the Pap test. (See *Procedure 32-2: Preparing a patient for and assisting with a gynecological examination*, pages 634 and 635.)

Common Gynecological Surgical Procedures

Gynecologists commonly treat pathologies of the vagina, cervix, and uterus with minor surgical procedures. Some procedures are offered in the physician's office and some require an outpatient hospital setting, where the patient is

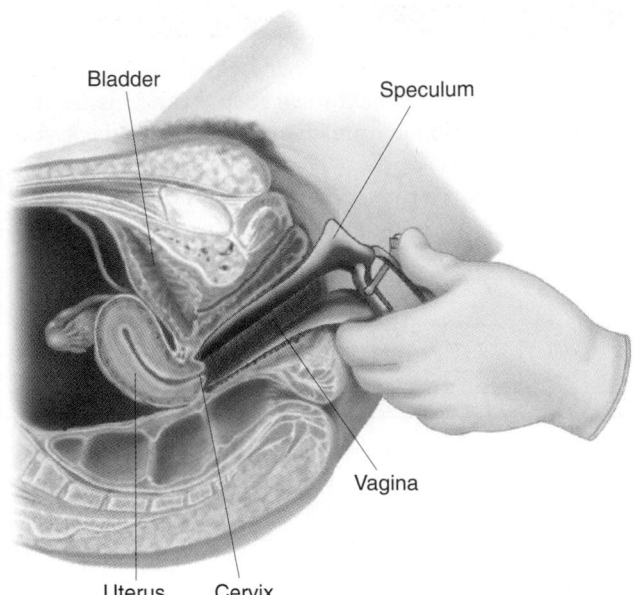

FIG 32-14 Speculum retracting the walls of the vagina to obtain a specimen for the Pap test.

discharged on the same day as the procedure. More complicated procedures, such as a hysterectomy, require overnight hospitalization and observation.

Cryosurgery

Cryosurgery is a surgical technique that uses extremely cold probes to destroy unwanted, cancerous, or infected tissues. The physician may choose to treat the cervix with cryosurgery in cases of cervical erosion, when cervical tissue grows downward into the endocervical canal, or chronic inflammation of cervical epithelial tissue due to infection. Cryosurgery uses a special machine that flows liquid nitrogen through a probe to freeze and destroy the unwanted tissue. With the patient in the lithotomy position, the physician cleans the cervix with a cotton swab soaked in sterile saline solution to remove mucus and cellular debris. Then the physician places the probe against the cervix and turns on the machine. The liquid nitrogen freezes the area in about 3 minutes. The patient may feel discomfort similar to menstrual cramping during the procedure and may take an analgesic after the procedure as directed by the physician. The medical assistant should advise the patient that

---

▪ PROCEDURE 32-2

Preparing a patient for and assisting with a gynecological examination

Task

Prepare a patient for and assist with a gynecological examination that includes a Papanicolaou (Pap) test.

Conditions

- 3 pairs of gloves
- Lubricant
- Tissues
- Patient gown and drape
- Disposable vaginal speculum
- Light source
- Pap test container
- Cytology requisition form
- Biohazard specimen transport bag
- Specimen collection swab, cytobrush, or cervical scraper
- Biohazardous waste container
- Pen
- Patient's medical record

Standards

In the time specified and within the scoring parameters determined by the instructor, the student will successfully prepare a patient for a gynecological examination, assist the physician with the examination, and prepare for and process a Pap test.

Performance Standards

1. Wash or sanitize your hands and assemble the supplies, making sure supplies are situated for easy access by the physician. Label the specimen bottle and complete the cytology requisition form, being sure to list the source of the specimen (vaginal or cervical).

2. Greet and identify the patient and explain the examination procedure to ensure accurate results.

3. Instruct the patient on how to collect a urine specimen, if required. If a urine specimen is not required, ask the patient if she needs to void, because a full bladder may cause discomfort during the examination.

4. Obtain and record proper patient history, vital signs, and height and weight.

5. Instruct the patient to remove all clothing and advise her on the proper way to put on the gown (with the opening in the front) and to wrap the drape around her waist. Leave the room to allow the patient to undress, unless the patient requires your assistance.

6. Notify the physician when the patient is ready for examination.

7. Knock before re-entering the room to ensure patient privacy.

PROCEDURE 32-2—cont'd

8. Assist the patient into the supine position for breast examination and then into the lithotomy position for the gynecological examination, redraping as necessary.
9. Check the light source for the physician and make sure the supplies are readily available.
10. Put on gloves and assist the physician in the examination as needed.
11. Lubricate or warm the speculum according to office policy and hand it to the physician. Support patient as necessary.
12. Hand the cytobrush or other specimen collection swab to the physician.
13. Open the bottle so the physician can insert the cytobrush into the bottle. Swirl the cytobrush in the solution 10 times. Withdraw the cytobrush from the bottle, being sure to tap it against the side of the bottle to dislodge the cells from the cytobrush.
14. Dispose of the cytobrush in the biohazardous waste container to ensure infection control.
15. Secure the lid on the bottle.
16. If a wet mount sample is required, follow these steps:
    a. Hand the cotton-tipped applicator to the physician.
    b. After the physician takes a sample of the vaginal discharge, take the applicator from the physician and immediately put it into a test tube containing 0.5 ml of sterile saline solution.
    c. Vigorously mix the applicator in the test tube, pressing the tip of the applicator against the sides of the test tube to ensure that an adequate quantity of the sample is transferred to the test tube.
    d. Place a drop of the solution on a microscopic slide and add a coverslip.
    e. Place the slide on the microscope for the physician to view.

17. If a KOH preparation is required, follow the steps for a wet mount and add a few drops of 10% potassium hydroxide (KOH) to the microscope slide before adding a coverslip.
18. Apply lubricant to the physician's gloved index and middle fingers. Support the patient as necessary while the physician performs the bimanual examination.
19. After the physician completes the bimanual examination, hand a new pair of gloves to the physician for the rectal examination to avoid contaminating the rectal area with vaginal secretions.
20. When the physician has completed the examination, assist the patient out of the stirrups and back onto the examination table. Provide tissues to the patient to wipe away any lubricant before she gets dressed.
21. Explain to the patient that she may get dressed and tell her where to dispose of the gown and drape.
22. Explain to the patient how the office will communicate the test results to her, based on office policy, and release the patient.
23. Process the bottle and cytology requisition form for proper transport to the laboratory.
24. Wash your hands to ensure infection control.
25. Document the examination and Pap test, as well as other tests if performed, in the patient's medical record to ensure a complete, accurate medical record.
26. Clean up the examination room according to proper disposal techniques to ensure infection control and cleanliness for the next patient.

Date	
05/30/08: 9:45 a.m.	*Annual gynecological examination with ThinPrep Pap test.* --*J. Morgan. CMA*

---

discharge after the procedure is normal and will last from 1 week to 1 month. The patient should avoid using tampons and engaging in sexual intercourse for 1 month after the procedure. The patient should report to the physician any foul odor in the discharge, which is an indication of infection, or heavy bleeding.

Laparoscopy

For patients with suspected endometriosis, ovarian cysts or tumors, or other local internal pathologies, the physician may view the internal reproductive organs with a laparoscope. The physician performs a laparoscopy in an operating room with the patient under general anesthesia. The scope is inserted into the patient's body through a small incision next to the umbilicus or the vagina. The physician must explain the procedure to the patient beforehand and answer any questions she may have. The medical assistant can schedule the laparoscopy and advise the patient not to drink or eat after midnight the night before the procedure.

Dilatation and Curettage

The physician performs a dilatation and curettage (D&C) to remove the contents of the uterus in the case of an incomplete abortion and to examine the endometrial tissue in the case of excessive menstrual bleeding. In the procedure, the physician dilates the cervix and scrapes away the endometrial tissue. A D&C is performed in an operating room with the patient under general anesthesia. The physician will explain the procedure to the patient and answer any questions. The medical assistant can schedule the D&C and advise the patient not to drink or eat after midnight the night before the procedure.

Uterine Ablation

A patient suffering from dysmenorrhea (painful, difficult menstruation) who does not wish to preserve fertility can benefit from a uterine ablation. Uterine ablation destroys the entire thickness of the endometrium (active layer of the uterus) and some superficial myometrium (muscle layer of the uterus). The glandular material within the endometrium responds to hormonal changes each month that cause the menstruation. Removal of the active layer causes menstruation to cease. Some women will continue to have a menstruation after the procedure since some glandular tissue may be present in the myometrium, a condition called **adenomyosis**. Uterine ablation is performed in an operating room with the patient under general anesthesia and in an outpatient hospital setting. The physician fills the uterine cavity with heated fluid that destroys the active layer of the endometrium. The fluid is introduced into the uterus via a balloon or free flow of fluid. In either case, the physician will drain the fluid through the tube to prevent burning the external vaginal tissues. When scheduling a uterine ablation, the medical assistant should ask the patient to have someone drive her to the hospital or surgical center. The patient should be instructed to have nothing to drink or eat after midnight the night before the procedure.

Hysterectomy

Hysterectomy is the surgical removal of the uterus. In addition, the fallopian tubes and ovaries are sometimes removed in a procedure called a *salpingo-oophorectomy*. Hysterectomy is the second most common abdominal surgery for women in the United States. Over 600,000 hysterectomies are performed every year, and one in three women has a hysterectomy by the age of 60.

The removal of the uterus can be complete or partial:

- *Complete*, or *total, hysterectomy* is the most common form of the procedure. It involves the removal of the cervix as well as the uterus.
- *Partial*, or *subtotal, hysterectomy* is the removal of the upper portions of the uterus, the fundus and the corpus, leaving the cervix in place.
- *Radical hysterectomy* is the removal of the uterus, cervix, upper part of the vagina, and the supporting connective tissue. This form of hysterectomy is performed in cases of cancer.

Hysterectomy is indicated in cases of uterine fibroids, endometriosis, adenomyosis (glands embedded in the myometrium causing bleeding), vaginal prolapse, heavy menstrual bleeding, uterine cancer, advanced cervical cancer, ovarian cancer, and uncontrollable postpartum bleeding. A patient may elect to have a hysterectomy if she has a strong family history of reproductive cancers, especially if she is tested and has BRCA1 or BRCA2, the two genes responsible for breast cancer.

The surgeon performs a hysterectomy through an abdominal incision, if the uterus is very large or there is a large amount of scar tissue, or through the vagina, if the uterus is small and easy to remove. In a laparoscopic supracervical hysterectomy (LSH) the surgeon uses a lighted laparoscope to aid removal of the uterus in small pieces through small incisions in the abdomen. This method allows the surgeon to remove a larger uterus with a smaller abdominal incision. In a laparoscopically assisted vaginal hysterectomy (LAVH), the surgeon removes the uterus through the vagina and uses the scope to examine the area for possible pathology to adjacent organs or tissues.

Complications of hysterectomy include blood clots; postsurgical infection; excessive bleeding; damage to the urinary tract, bladder, or rectum; and early onset of menopause. The gynecologist will advise the patient to abstain from sexual activity for 6 weeks after surgery. If the cervix is still intact, the gynecologist will advise the patient to have regular Pap tests to detect possible cervical cancer or dysplasia. Premenopausal women who have hysterectomy with salpingo-oophorectomy will experience a sudden onset of menopause. Women who undergo hysterectomy without removal of the ovaries may experience menopause sooner, but not immediately after surgery. For many women, a hysterectomy alleviates years of suffering from excessive uterine bleeding. Unless the patient has uncontrolled postpartum bleeding or cancer, she does not have to rush to a decision about hysterectomy. The medical assistant can provide the patient with information on the procedure, recovery, and alternatives to hysterectomy. (See *Alternatives to hysterectomy*.)

Diagnostic Testing in Pregnancy

A patient may tell the medical assistant that she did a home pregnancy test and got a positive result or she just feels that she may be pregnant. The medical assistant can then confirm the pregnancy by using a urine pregnancy test. The test results are clearest on a first morning urine sample, but accurate results can be obtained with urine obtained later in the day. Detection of human chorionic gonadotropin (HCG) indicates the presence of a placenta and, therefore, confirms pregnancy. The medical assistant can perform the urine test at the onset of the physical examination. Testing in the medical office is the same as a home urine pregnancy test; accurate results depend on following instructions.

In addition to routine examinations, the physician may order additional testing to further understand the development of the fetus and initiate early treatment if abnormalities are diagnosed. Such tests include fetal ultrasound, amniocentesis, and chorionic villus sampling.

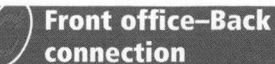
Fetal Ultrasound

During the course of a woman's pregnancy, the physician may order a fetal ultrasound for various reasons. The ultrasound can confirm multiple pregnancies and determine fetal age, position, and sex. It can also detect such fetal abnormalities as defects in the heart or other organs.

A fetal ultrasound may be vaginal or abdominal. The medical assistant should instruct the patient to drink at least 32 oz of water 1 hour before the test because a full bladder enhances visualization of the fetus. If the ultrasound is performed at 12 weeks' gestation or later, the physician can determine the sex of the fetus. The patient may choose to know the sex of the fetus or may elect to be "surprised" when the baby is born. If the patient does not want to know the sex of her baby, the medical assistant should be sure to note this wish in her medical record. (See *Coding ultrasound.*)

Amniocentesis

Amniocentesis is performed at 16 to 18 weeks' gestation. The physician inserts a hypodermic needle into the amniotic sac and extracts a sample of 10 to 20 ml of amniotic fluid. The laboratory examines the chromosomes of fetal cells present in the fluid to identify possible chromosomal abnormalities, such as Down syndrome. Because the risk of having a child with Down syndrome increases with maternal age, many physicians routinely order amniocentesis for patients over age 35.

Chorionic Villus Sampling

In chorionic villus sampling (CVS), the physician inserts a biopsy catheter through the vagina and cervix to collect a small portion of the chorionic villi, the vascular projections from the chorion that form the fetal portion of the placenta.

Microscopic and chemical examination of the sample evaluates the chromosomal, enzymatic, and DNA status of the fetus. The physician performs this procedure, if necessary, at 8 to 12 weeks' gestation. CVS is not a routine procedure because it is more invasive than amniocentesis. A woman who experienced miscarriage or gave birth to a baby with chromosomal abnormalities is considered high-risk and, therefore, may require CVS.

Common Gynecological Diagnostic Tests

The gynecologist may order diagnostic tests to detect infection or early stages of cancer. The medical assistant must assist the physician and comfort the patient during and after testing and provide patient instruction as needed. Common gynecological diagnostic tests include amplified DNA probe test, endometrial biopsy, and mammography.

Amplified DNA Probe Test

An amplified DNA probe test detects for chlamydia and gonorrhea. The test is available for men and women. The female patient must be tested prior to the gynecological examination because the lubricant used during examination interferes with test results. The Probe TEC pink kit contains preservatives, one large swab, one culturette, and instructions. In the procedure, the medical assistant hands the large swab to the physician, who uses it to clean the cervix, removing mucus, blood, and cellular debris that could interfere with test results. The medical assistant then discards the large swab. The physician then inserts the culturette into the cervical canal and rotates the swab for 15 to 30 seconds.

The physician breaks off the swab into the liquid in the transport tube and caps the tube. The medical assistant should comfort and reassure the patient during the procedure.

Colposcopy with Biopsy

If a Pap test returns an abnormal result, the physician performs a colposcopy, which is visualization of the vagina and cervix using a specialized instrument called a **colposcope**. With the patient in the lithotomy position, the physician cleans the vagina with a long cotton-tipped applicator moistened with sterile saline. Using another swab, she then cleans the cervix with acetic acid, which dissolves cervical mucus, aiding in visualization of normal and abnormal cells. The medical assistant should reassure the patient that the acetic acid will not burn. The physician then introduces the colposcope into the vagina and examines the cervix. Because lubricant blurs images of the tissues, the physician cannot use it to aid insertion of the colposcope.

If the physician sees an area of abnormal tissue, she will perform a cervical punch or cone biopsy. The cervical punch biopsy removes small pieces of tissue with a cervical punch biopsy forceps. Because the tissue samples are small and the procedure is quick, a topical anesthetic can be used. If the physician suspects a more invasive cancer, she can obtain a larger sample with a cone biopsy. The cone biopsy requires a local anesthetic injection and can be used to remove an entire lesion. (See Figure 32-15.)

The physician may cauterize the tissue to control bleeding. After obtaining the sample, the physician packs the vagina with sterile packing, applying a thick substance,

called *Monsel's solution*, with cotton swabs to the cervix to control bleeding. The yellow solution turns black upon exposure to blood. Thus, the patient can expect to see a coffee-ground discharge. The medical assistant must place the specimen in a container of formalin, label it, complete the requisition form, and send it to the pathology laboratory for analysis.

The medical assistant should tell the patient when the results will be available and confirm a phone number where the patient can be reached. She should also explain to the patient that she may experience some discomfort or cramping after the procedure. She should also advise the patient to refrain from exercising or lifting heavy objects for 24 hours and to keep the packing material in the vagina for 24 hours and report any bleeding that is greater than a normal menstrual period. The patient should also report any fever or signs of infection. (See *LEEP*.)

Endometrial Biopsy

The physician may perform an endometrial biopsy to determine the cause of postmenopausal bleeding. Because the postmenopausal patient no longer ovulates, the endometrium should not proliferate and cause bleeding. Postmenopausal bleeding may indicate polycystic ovaries. Estrogen replacement therapy (ERT) may also be a cause. High levels of estrogen stimulate endometrial hypertrophy and bleeding. If the patient with postmenopausal bleeding is taking ERT, the physician may decrease the dosage to determine if doing so will resolve the bleeding before performing an endometrial biopsy.

In an endometrial biopsy, the physician cleans the cervix with povidone-iodine solution. Before the procedure, the medical assistant should make sure the patient does not have an iodine allergy. If the patient is allergic to iodine, the physician will use a chlorhexidine (Hibiclens) solution. Then the physician pushes a long, strawlike tube that houses a sampling device into the cervical os (the opening of the

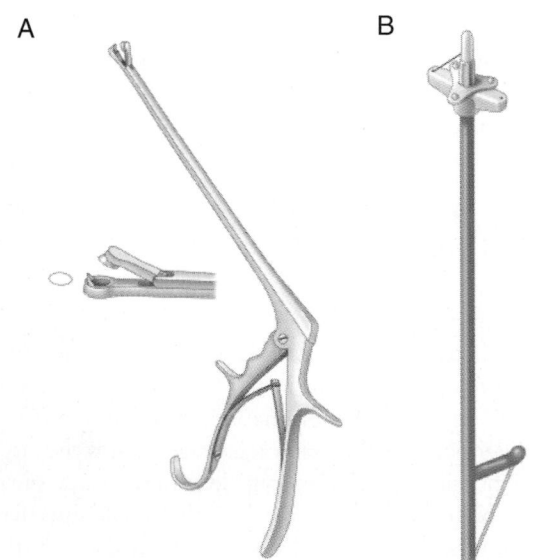

FIG 32-15 Biopsy forceps. (A) Punch biopsy forceps. (B) Cone biopsy forceps.

LEEP

Some physicians prefer to perform a loop electrosurgical excision procedure (LEEP), which is less invasive than a colposcopy. In this procedure, the physician injects a local anesthetic into the cervix and places a wire loop in the vagina. A high-frequency electrical current runs through the loop and burns off abnormal tissue from the cervix and cervical canal. The LEEP procedure is a diagnostic tool, a method of obtaining biopsy specimens, and a treatment (removal of abnormal cells). Because the electrical current cauterizes tissue, this procedure causes less bleeding than a cervical punch or cone biopsy.

cervix) and then the uterus. When the tube enters the uterus, the physician pulls back on a plunger, creating suction that pulls a sample of endometrial tissue from the uterine wall into the sampling device. The physician removes the tube and device and hands it to the medical assistant. The medical assistant puts the sampling device into a container, labels the container with the appropriate patient information, and completes a requisition form for transport to the pathology laboratory. The procedure is quick and almost painless. The medical assistant should explain to the patient that she may experience some cramping and can use an analgesic for pain as directed by the physician.

Mammography

Mammography is considered one of the most effective methods for early detection of breast cancer when used in combination with breast self-examination. It is recommended that women receive their first mammogram at age 40 and have follow-up mammograms yearly or as directed by their physician. A mammogram is taken by positioning the patient's breast on a mammography machine. Pressure is first applied from the top and bottom of the breast and then laterally from each side to flatten the breast, aiding in imaging. The patient may experience some discomfort and slight bruising. When scheduling the mammogram, the medical assistant can give written as well as verbal instructions. (See *Mammography preparation*.)

Chapter Summary

- The female reproductive system houses the organs necessary for the reproduction of another human and manufactures the hormones necessary for the development and functioning of the reproductive organs.
- Medical assistants must be well versed in the language and vocabulary that pertains to the female reproductive system. In addition to knowing common word elements, they should be familiar with common pathological terms and abbreviations.
- Obstetric patients should receive routine prenatal care and education to promote the health both of the mother and the developing fetus.
- Gynecological patients need health screenings and education regarding reproductive health, early diagnosis of cancers, and general health promotion.
- Common disorders of the female reproductive system include vaginal infections, including STDs and bacterial and fungal infections; menstrual disorders; uterine disorders; cancer; complications of pregnancy; infertility; and fibrocystic breast disease.
- Common diagnostic tests include the Pap test, breast self-examination, biopsy, and mammogram.
- Common treatment procedures include cryosurgery, ablation, hormone therapy, and surgical correction.

Team Work Exercises

1. Divide into two groups. Research the HPV vaccination and debate the advantages and disadvantages of administering the vaccine to 8-year-old girls. Include such topics as vaccine safety, vaccine efficacy, and social and moral implications. Does giving the vaccine to girls encourage promiscuity?
2. Divide into four groups. Each team must create posters and computer presentations on one of the topics given here. All teams must host a women's health fair at the school to present the information. Topics include:
   a. breast cancer prevention (early diagnosis)
   b. nutrition for women
   c. STD prevention
   d. prenatal care.

 Patient Education

Mammography Preparation

The medical assistant should provide education and instruction on mammography to a patient before the examination. She should be sure to include these instructions:

- If possible, do not schedule the examination immediately before or during the patient's menstrual cycle. Breasts are commonly tender at this time, so the examination would be more uncomfortable.

- The test requires the patient to stand for approximately 15 minutes. Accommodations can be made for a patient who cannot stand for that amount of time.

- Avoid caffeine for several days before the test to reduce the risk of swelling and soreness, which caffeine exacerbates.

- Do not use any lotions, powders, antiperspirants, or deodorants on the morning of the test, because these products may interfere with the image produced.

- The machine will compress each breast first from top to bottom and then from side to side. The patient may experience some discomfort; however, full compression allows for an accurate picture of the breast.

- Clothing from the waist up must be removed for the test. Slacks and comfortable shoes are recommended.

- The patient may take an analgesic, as directed by the physician, after the examination if she is sore or experiences pain.

Case Studies

1. Cheryl is a 42-year-old mother of three who is interested in permanent contraception. Her husband is unwilling to have a vasectomy. Cheryl is considering tubal ligation but also wants information on pharmaceutical methods of birth control. What information can the medical assistant give to Cheryl?

2. Cynthia calls the office complaining of pain and bleeding after her LEEP procedure 6 days ago. What should the medical assistant discuss with the patient regarding normal aftercare for a LEEP procedure? Does she need to be seen by the physician? Explain your answer.

Resources

- General information on the female reproductive system: *www.nlm.nih.gov/medlineplus/femalereproductivesystem.html*

- Information on breast cancer: *www.cancer.gov/cancerinfo/types/breast* and *www.nationalbreastcancer.org*
- Information on HPV and the HPV vaccine: *www.emedicine.com/MED/topic1037.htm* and *www.gardasil.com*
- Information on infertility: *www.resolve.org/site/PageServer?pagename=lrn_home*
- Information on menopause: *www.nlm.nih.gov/medlineplus/menopause.html* and *www.menopause.org/default.htm*
- Information on seafood safety during pregnancy: *http://www.epa.gov/waterscience/fish/advice*
- STD information from the CDC: *www.cdc.gov/std*

Pediatrics

Learning Objectives

Upon completion of this chapter, the student will be able to:

- define, spell, and pronounce terminology related to pediatrics
- identify the role of the medical assistant in pediatrics
- review normal growth and development
- identify reasons for a well-child examination
- describe a sick-child examination
- differentiate between adult and pediatric vital sign values
- obtain pediatric vital signs
- chart growth and development on male and female charts
- identify common screening tests for pediatric patients
- identify a state-mandated immunization schedule
- perform immunization injections
- identify vitamin supplements
- identify common childhood illnesses
- provide patient education regarding safety for pediatric patients.

CAAHEP Competencies

Clinical Competencies
Patient Care
Obtain vital signs
Prepare and maintain examination and treatment areas
Prepare patients for and assist with routine and specialty examinations
Prepare patients for and assist with procedures, treatments, and minor office surgeries
Maintain medication and immunization records

ABHES Competencies

Clinical Duties
Interview and record patient history
Prepare patients for procedures
Take vital signs
Prepare and maintain examination and treatment area
Maintain medication and immunization records
Perform capillary puncture
Obtain throat specimen for microbiological testing
Perform urinalysis

Procedures
Collecting a urine specimen from an infant

Chapter Outline
Pediatric Patients
Growth and Development
Medical Terminology Related to Pediatrics
Common Pediatric Diseases and Disorders
Communicable Pediatric Diseases and Disorders
Common cold
Conjunctivitis
Croup
Diarrhea
Impetigo
Influenza virus
Otitis media
Respiratory syncytial virus
Strep throat
Oral thrush
Chickenpox
Warts
Noncommunicable Pediatric Diseases and Disorders
Allergies
Eating disorders

Asthma
Behavioral disorders
Autism
Down syndrome
Constipation
Failure to thrive
Cerebral palsy
Eczema
Scoliosis
Obesity
Lead poisoning
Phenylketonuria
Pediatric Procedures
Assisting with Examination
Vital signs
Vision screening
Hearing screening
Well-child examination
Sick-child examination
Reporting Abuse
Physical abuse
Sexual abuse
Neglect
Immunizations
Vaccine registry
Objections to vaccination
Pediatric Laboratory Tests
Urinalysis
Hemoglobin and hematocrit
Rapid Strep test
Nutritional Counseling
Birth to 6 months
6 months to 1 year
Age 1
Ages 2 to 5
School-age children
Adolescents
Vitamin and mineral supplements
Chapter Summary
Team Work Exercises
Case Studies
Resources

Pediatric Patients

Pediatrics is a specialty branch of medicine dealing with the care and treatment of children, including the:

- **neonate**, or newborn, from birth to age 28 days
- **infant**, from age 1 month to 1 year
- **child**, from age 1 year to age 12 years (or onset of puberty)
- **adolescent**, from age 12 (or onset of puberty) to 18 years (or full growth).

A **pediatrician** is a medical doctor who specializes in diagnosing and treating diseases and disorders of these patients. The medical assistant or nurse, as instructed by the pediatrician, will administer **vaccines**, which are preparations usually provided via injection that immunize a child against contracting various childhood illnesses, some of which can be life-threatening or impact normal growth and development.

Growth and Development

Physical and intellectual growth and development begin at conception and continue through life. Growth can be evaluated by measuring physical aspects, such as height, weight, and head circumference, as well as by assessing development of language, social skills, and gross and fine motor skills. (See *Developing motor skills*.) A neonate grows at a rapid rate physically and intellectually. He changes almost daily by gaining weight and learning how to identify sounds and faces. The pediatrician assesses changes as a child grows, identifying normal and abnormal developments. Early indications of a developmental delay alert the pediatrician to address this concern.

Medical Terminology Related to Pediatrics

Terms used the in the pediatric office will include those that relate to growth and development; diseases common to neonates, infants, children, and adolescents; and procedures regularly performed as part of pediatric practice. Working in these practice settings will afford the medical assistant the opportunity to assist with diagnostic testing and therapeutic procedures performed on neonates, infants, children, and adolescents. To be effective in her role, a medical assistant must become well versed in the language and vocabulary that pertain to pediatrics. The following tables list common medical terminology related to pediatrics.

Developing motor skills

Motor skills are particular skills of movement that a child acquires as he grows and develops. These motor skills are categorized as *gross* or *fine*. *Gross motor skills* are those skills that show the development of control over large muscle groups, producing large movements, such as rolling over. *Fine motor skills* show control over smaller muscle groups, producing more exact movements, such as putting finger and thumb together to grasp an object.

The following table lists gross and fine motor skills along with the age of normal development.

Age in Months	Gross Motor Development	Fine Motor Development
2	• Can lift head briefly in prone position	• Follows object vertically when in supine position
4	• Rolls front to back • Can hold head up in prone position with arms extended	• Brings toys to mouth • Looks at objects in hand
6	• Sits leaning with arms forward • Bears full weight on legs when held in standing position	• Reaches for toys with one hand • Reaches after a dropped toy
10	• Walks using two hands on a rail or furniture • Lets self down from standing with partial control	• Performs a thumb-finger grasp of small objects • Grasps toys by handles
12	• Walks a few steps • Stands well alone • Climbs stairs on hands and knees	• Helps to turn pages in a book • Imitates scribbling
15	• Walks well • Moves on hands and knees backwards down stairs • Can get to standing position without support	• Stacks two or three 1" cubes • Scribbles with colors on paper • Attempts feeding self with spoon
24	• Jumps • Kicks ball • Throws ball overhand	• Turns door knobs • Stacks six to seven cubes

Table 33.1 | Word Elements

Element	Meaning	Example	Meaning
Combining Forms			
ped/o	child	**pediatrician** (pē-dē-ă-TRĬSH-ăn)	Specialist in the diagnosis and treatment of children
gen/o	formation, production; origin	**congenital** (kŏn-JĔN-ĭ-tăl)	Present at birth
immun/o	protection from or resistance to disease	**immunization** (ĭm-ū-nĭ-ZĀ-shŭn)	Protection from disease in the form of vaccination
juven/o	young	**juvenile** (JŪ-vĕ-nīl)	Pertaining to childhood
nat/o	birth	**prenatal** (prē-NĀ-t'l)	Before birth
Prefixes			
neo-	new	**neonate** (NĒ-ō-nāt)	Infant from birth to 28 days
Suffixes			
-iatric	medicine, medical profession, treatment	**pediatrics** (pē-dē-ĂT-rĭks)	Concerning the treatment of children
-plasia	formation, growth	**dysplasia** (dĭs-PLĀ-zē-ă)	Abnormal development
-trophy	growth, development	**atrophy** (ĂT-rō-fē)	Lack of development or growth, decrease in size of an organ or tissue

Table 33.2 | **Pathologic Terms**

This table lists some of the most common pathologic terms related to pediatrics with a pronunciation guide and brief definition for each.

Term	Definition
anorexia nervosa ăn-ō-RĔK-sē-ă nĕr-VO-să	Psychological disorder characterized by self-starvation and morbid fear of weight gain
asthma ĂZ-mă	Condition marked by recurrent attacks of dyspnea (difficulty breathing) with wheezing due to bronchial spasm
attention deficit disorder ă-TĔN-shŭn DĔF-ĭ-sĭt	Behavior marked by the inability to focus attention for short periods of time or engage in quiet activities
attention deficit hyperactive disorder ă-TĔN-shŭn DĔF-ĭ-sĭt hī-pĕr-ĂC-tĭv	Behavior marked by the inability to focus attention or engage in quiet activities and uncontrolled compulsive behavior
bronchiolitis brŏng-kē-ō-LĪ-tĭs	Inflammation of the bronchioles (small passages of the bronchial tree)
bulimia nervosa bū-LĔM-ē-ă nĕr-VO-să	Psychological disorder characterized by compulsive overeating followed by self-induced vomiting or misuse of diuretics and laxatives
cerebral palsy SĔR-ĕ-brŭl PAWL-zē	Disorder characterized by muscle weakness, loss of control, spastic muscle; due to birth defects or infection acquired soon after birth.
constipation kŏn-stĭ-PĂ-shŭn	Difficultly defecating due to hard, compacted stools
Down syndrome	Mild to moderate mental retardation and physical characteristics due to three copies (trisomy) of chromosome 21
failure to thrive	Health status assigned to infants with insufficient weight gain
febrile FĔ-brĭl	Pertaining to fever
obesity ō-BĔ-sĭ-tē	Body weight that is 20% or more over the patient's ideal weight
otitis media ō-TĪ-tĭs	Presence of infectious fluid in the middle ear
pediculosis pē-dĭk-ū-LO-sĭs	Parasitic skin disorder caused by lice
scoliosis skō-lē-O-sĭs	Lateral curvature of the spine
stridor STRĪ-dor	Shrill, harsh respiratory sound heard during inhalation or in the presence of obstruction to the larynx
tonsillitis tŏn-sĭl-Ī-tĭs	Inflammation of the tonsils, usually due to a viral infection

Table 33.3 | Abbreviations

In pediatrics, as in other areas of health care, abbreviations are commonly used. Abbreviations such as the ones listed below save time and effort in documentation and written communications.

Abbreviation	Term
ADD	attention deficit disorder
ADHD	attention deficit hyperactive disorder
AGA	appropriate for gestational age
APGAR	activity, pulse, grimace, appearance, respiration
BSA	body surface area
DDH	developmental dysplasia of the hip
DPT	diptheria, pertussis, and tetanus (combination vaccine)
Hep B	hepatitis B vaccination
HiB	*Haemophilus influenzae* type B vaccine
IPV	inactivated poliovirus vaccine
MMR	measles, mumps and rubella (combination vaccine)
PCV	pneumococcal conjugate vaccine
PDA	patent ductus arteriosis
Peds	pediatrics
ROP	retinopathy of prematurity
SIDS	sudden infant death syndrome

Common Pediatric Diseases and Disorders

There are innumerable pediatric diseases and disorders. Some of the most common are discussed below, grouped by communicable and noncommunicable diseases and disorders.

Communicable Pediatric Diseases and Disorders

Communicable diseases and disorders are those that are spread from one person to another via droplets from exhaled air, blood, body fluids, and contact with a surface that the infected person has touched. Children are more susceptible to communicable diseases and disorders because they are less likely to follow or be able to follow precautions such as proper hand washing. In addition, young children are prone to putting objects in their mouths, which greatly increases the likelihood of transmission of pathogens from the object to the child's mouth or from the child's mouth to the object. (See *Communicating about communicable diseases*.)

Some of the most common pediatric communicable diseases and disorders include the common cold, conjunctivitis, croup, diarrhea, impetigo, influenza virus, otitis media, respiratory syncytial virus, *Strep* throat, thrush, chickenpox, and warts.

Common cold

ICD-9-CM code: 460

The common cold is actually a group of symptoms that may be caused by several viruses. Young children are especially susceptible to common colds because their immature immune systems have not yet developed resistance to most of the viruses that cause them. Children, especially preschoolers, can have a cold 8 to 10 times per year, more than double the amount of the average adult, who has a cold 2 to 4 times per year.

Although the most common cause of colds is the rhinovirus, more than 200 viruses can cause a cold. Symptoms appear 1 to 3 days after exposure to a cold virus and can include:

- runny or stuffy nose
- sore throat
- coughing, sneezing, and congestion
- body aches and mild headache
- watery, itchy eyes
- low-grade fever (up to 102°F)
- mild fatigue.

Diagnosis is based on physical examination and history of signs and symptoms. Treatment for the common cold

Front office–Back office connection

Communicating About Communicable Diseases

In order to stop the spread of communicable diseases in the reception area of the pediatric medical office, the administrative and clinical medical assistants must work together. When a pediatric patient suspected of having a communicable disease visits the office, the administrative medical assistant should immediately check with the clinical medical assistant in order to remove the child from the waiting room to an examination room as soon as possible. In the reception area, where there are many patients who are well and ill, infection control is only minimally possible. In an examination room, infection control measures are in place that will more successfully inhibit the spread of disease.

involves rest and fluids. The discharge from the child's nose may become thick and yellow or green in color as the cold runs its course. The medical assistant should assure the parent or caregiver not to be alarmed by the nasal discharge. She should also advise them to contact the physician if the child's symptoms do not resolve within 1 week. In addition, she should teach caregivers and patients about infection prevention techniques. (See *Preschool prevention practices*.) Persistent viral colds can result in bacterial infection in the lungs, sinuses, or ears, which requires treatment.

Conjunctivitis
ICD-9-CM code: 372.30

Conjunctivitis, commonly called *pink eye,* is an inflammation or infection of the conjunctiva, which is the transparent membrane that lines the eyelid and part of the eyeball. A recent study estimated 4% of school children and 6% of high schoolers see a physician for conjunctivitis each year.

Causes of conjunctivitis include a bacterial or viral infection, an allergic reaction, or irritation by a foreign object in the eye. Inflammation of the small blood vessels in the conjunctiva cause the sclera, or white of the eye, to appear pink or red, giving it the name *pink eye.*

The most common signs and symptoms of conjunctivitis include:

- itchiness in one or both eyes
- redness in one or both eyes
- sensitivity to light
- blurred vision
- gritty feeling in one or both eyes

- yellow or green discharge in one or both eyes that forms a crust during the night
- tearing.

Bacterial conjunctivitis is the most common form found in children. It commonly produces a thick, yellow-green discharge and may be associated with a respiratory infection or a sore throat. The viral form shares the same signs and symptoms as the bacterial form except it does not develop a yellow or green discharge.

Treatment for bacterial conjunctivitis consists of antibiotic eye ointment for infants and young children and eye drops for older children. An ointment is commonly easier to administer to an infant or young child than eye drops. The medical assistant should provide thorough patient teaching on eye care. (See *Teaching about eye care.*) Antibiotics are not effective in treating viral conjunctivitis. However, warm compresses to soothe the eye may provide symptomatic relief until the virus resolves. With treatment, conjunctivitis usually resolves within 3 to 5 days without long-term implications for vision or eye health.

A neonate may be born with an incompletely opened tear duct, which causes the infection. A neonate's eyes are susceptible to bacteria normally present in the mother's birth canal. In rare cases, these bacteria can cause infants to develop a serious form of conjunctivitis known as *ophthalmia neonatorum,* which requires immediate treatment to preserve sight. To prevent this serious complication, most hospital policies require administration of a preventive antibiotic, such as erythromycin ointment, to the eyes of every neonate.

Croup
ICD-9-CM code: 646.4

Croup is a severe, viral respiratory illness that involves swelling and edema of respiratory passages. Because children under age 5 have small airways, they are most susceptible to croup.

Croup may be caused by several viruses, most commonly the parainfluenza virus and, less commonly, respiratory syncytial virus (RSV), the measles virus, or other viruses. Croup is rarely caused by a bacterial infection.

Croup is marked by a harsh, repetitive cough caused by swelling and edema around the larynx (vocal cords) and trachea. The sound is similar to the noise of a barking seal. Attacks of croup commonly wake a sleeping child as he gasps for breath; the experience can be frightening for the parent or caregiver and the child.

Because the cause of the croup is viral, treatment is directed at keeping the child comfortable and allowing the body to fight the infection. (See *Home care for croup*.) Because it is contagious, hand washing and cleaning surfaces touched by the infected child can prevent spreading croup to siblings or other children. Croup is also sometimes

---

 Patient Education

Preschool Prevention Practices

Because cold viruses are highly contagious, preschoolers who spend a lot of time with their peers are repeatedly exposed to the common cold. However, teaching prevention will reduce the number of colds. The medical assistant should teach the young child to wash his hands and cover his mouth and nose when he sneezes. Adults and children should not share towels, face cloths, or drinking glasses with infected people.

To teach hand washing techniques to a child, the medical assistant can show parents and children how hand washing can be fun. She can teach the child to sing while he washes his hands. Singing "Happy Birthday" or a favorite nursery rhyme while hand washing will ensure that the child spends enough time lathering and rinsing his hands to remove possible pathogens that cause disease.

Patient Education

Teaching About Eye Care

When treating bacterial conjunctivitis, the medical assistant should show the parent or caregiver how to administer ointment or drops properly. She must tell the caregiver to take care not to touch the container to the contaminated eye. She should also explain to the caregiver that the child should not attend school or day care until she has been treated for 24 hours to prevent spread of infection throughout the school. In addition, she should explain that frequent hand washing can prevent transmission from one eye to the other eye or to classmates and family members.

Sometimes a child is born with a blockage in one or both tear ducts. If left untreated, this condition can lead to infection, because the damaged duct does not allow the eye to drain and clean the area. The pediatrician or medical assistant should instruct the caregiver to clean and massage the blocked duct. To clean the duct and the eye, the caregiver should use a moistened clean cotton ball or washcloth with warm (not hot) water, wiping away drainage around the eye from the inner canthus to the outer part of the eye. If ordered by the physician, the medical assistant should also instruct the patient to massage the tear duct two to three times each day for several months, according to the physician's order. If ordered, the medical assistant can demonstrate the proper technique by massaging the duct in an upward motion from the side of the nose to the inner canthus of the eye.

Patient Education

Home Care for Croup

The medical assistant can instruct parents or caregivers on proper home care for children with croup. She should instruct the parent to provide plenty of fluids and encourage lots of rest. She should also instruct the parent to administer moist air using a humidifier or running a hot shower and sitting in the bathroom with the child to help him to breathe more easily. Because breathing is difficult, the child could become anxious. The medical assistant should instruct the parent or caregiver to remain calm while administering moist air to help the child relax and avoid panic.

While most cases of croup can be treated at home, the medical assistant should instruct parents to bring the child in if he:

- makes noisy, high-pitched breathing sounds when inhaling (stridor)

- has difficulty swallowing (dysphagia) or begins to drool

- is extremely irritable or agitated

- has difficulty breathing (dyspnea)

- develops blue or grayish skin around the nose, mouth, or fingernails (cyanosis).

treated with corticosteroids to decrease inflammation in the airway.

While croup is usually self-limiting, it occasionally results in death from complete obstruction of the airway. Also, if treatment includes corticosteroids, immune suppression from such medication can result in secondary infections.

Diarrhea

ICD-9-CM code: 787.91

Diarrhea is the elimination of large amounts of watery stool and mucus from the gastrointestinal tract. Because the causes of diarrhea vary, its incidence is common across all populations, regardless of age, sex, race, and socioeconomic status. Outbreaks of diarrhea may occur within a family or at a day care center, where widespread transmission of the offending pathogen causes the condition in many people.

The most common cause of diarrhea in children is an infection with various forms of bacteria, viruses, or parasites. Less commonly, it may be caused by food allergy or adverse reactions to medications. Because the body is focused on

ridding itself of the offending organism, the digested food, called *chyme*, moves too quickly through the digestive tract to provide sufficient time for the intestines to absorb water. The irritated, inflamed lining of the digestive tract secretes mucus to protect the surface of the intestines from the irritant. The result is watery stool with strings of mucus. Diarrhea may accompany another illness, such as the flu, or may be present with no other symptoms.

Diagnosis is based on the parent or caregiver's report that the child has had two or more loose or watery stools within a 24-hour period. If bloody stool is present, the pediatrician will order collection of a fecal sample to identify the causative agent.

Treatment of diarrhea aims to replenish fluids and remove the cause of diarrhea, including removing foods or medications if they are the cause. If stool cultures are positive for bacteria, the pediatrician will prescribe an antibiotic.

In addition to replenishing fluids, an infant or a child recovering from diarrhea must eat. Withholding food can damage or cause atonia (loss of muscle tone) in the intestines. An infant should also continue to take breast milk or formula. Although the infant's appetite may be poor if diarrhea is due to a cold or flu, the parent or caregiver should continue to offer food. The parent or caregiver of a toddler and older child should feed him a mild diet that is high in carbohydrates. The child should avoid soda, juice, and sports drinks, because they lack electrolytes and contain sugar, which can cause further diarrhea. (See *Home treatment for diarrhea*.)

The day after an infant or young child comes into the pediatric office with diarrhea, the medical assistant should check in with the parent or caregiver by telephone. The medical assistant can ask the parent if the diarrhea is subsiding and if the child is eating, drinking, and producing urine. The medical assistant should instruct the parent to bring the child back into the office if the parent sees no improvement at home. If the infant or child's diarrhea causes severe dehydration, the pediatrician may decide to admit the child to the hospital to administer IV fluids and electrolytes.

Most cases of diarrhea resolve with dietary changes. If diarrhea is left untreated, it could lead to decreased pulse rate, hypotension, diminished urine output, kidney failure, confusion, acidosis and, possibly, death.

Impetigo
ICD-9-CM code: 684

Impetigo is a common, highly contagious skin infection. Impetigo accounts for 10% of all skin problems seen in the pediatric office. It is most prevalent in warm, humid environments and is rarely seen in northern states during the winter months. It is most common in preschoolers and commonly spreads through day care centers and preschools.

Impetigo appears as small, fluid-filled vesicles around the mouth or nose. The vesicles quickly enlarge and rupture, excreting a yellow exudate. The lesions then crust over and the crusty area is inflamed and moist.

The cause of impetigo is infection with the *Streptococcus* or *Staphylococcus aureus* pathogen. It is easily spread because

---

⬛ Patient Education

Home Treatment for Diarrhea

When a child has diarrhea, the medical assistant can advise the caregiver on several measures to treat it at home, including avoiding the P foods and dairy, ensuring hydration, providing a mild diet high in carbohydrates when the child is recovering, and looking for signs of serious dehydration or other signs that require a visit to the physician.

P foods and dairy

When a child is suffering from diarrhea, the first care measure the caregiver can institute is eliminating certain foods from the child's diet that stimulate peristalsis (movement of food through the digestive tract). An easy way to remember these foods is to remember the letters *P* and *D*. Most fruits that start with the letter *P*, such as prunes, peaches, and pears (as well as *a*pricots) will exacerbate diarrhea. In addition, the caregiver should eliminate *d*airy, such as milk, cheese, and yogurt, for the same reason.

Hydration

Prolonged diarrhea will cause dehydration, electrolyte imbalance, and diaper rash in infants. The medical assistant can educate parents to look for the signs of dehydration that accompany diarrhea, including:

• lack of tears when crying

• lethargy

• few wet diapers

• dry mouth and lips

• weight loss

• irritability.

The pediatrician may recommend the use of oral rehydration products, such as Pedialyte or Infalyte. The medical assistant should instruct the caregiver to give small amounts of these products, approximately 3 tablespoons, every 15 minutes. She should also be sure to tell the caregiver never to give infants or small children over-the-counter antidiarrheal medications, such as Pepto-Bismol or Imodium, because they can decrease bowel motility and cause respiratory depression and drowsiness. These products are designed and dosages are given only for older children and adults.

BRAT for recovery

When a toddler or older child is recovering from diarrhea, the caregiver should provide foods that are high in carbohydrates, to help enhance fluid and sodium absorption, and mild, to avoid irritating the intestines. For this reason, most pediatricians recommend the *BRAT* diet, which consists of:

• *B*ananas

• *R*ice

• *A*pplesauce

• *T*oast.

When to come to the office

The medical assistant should advise the parent or caregiver to bring a young child who has diarrhea for more than 2 days to see the physician to determine the cause and appropriate treatment.

the rash is pruritic (itchy). Thus, when scratched, it spreads to other areas on the child's face and to other family members.

The pediatrician will prescribe topical antibiotic ointment to kill the offending organism. The medical assistant should instruct patients and parents to wash hands frequently and refrain from sharing drinking glasses, towels, or facecloths to prevent spreading the infection.

Most cases of impetigo completely resolve with treatment. As the lesions heal, they appear red; however, permanent scarring is rare. Rarely, cellulitis and lymphadenitis occur, prolonging treatment. Acute poststreptococcal glomerulonephritis is a rare but serious complication.

Influenza Virus

ICD-9-CM code: 487.1

Influenza is a respiratory viral infection that attacks the nose, throat, bronchi, and lungs. According to the Centers for Disease Control and Prevention (CDC), as many as 36,000 Americans die each year of complications of influenza and more than 200,000 are hospitalized. Young children, patients with weakened immune systems, patients with chronic illnesses, and the elderly are especially vulnerable.

Children who are taking medications that suppress the immune system have an increased risk of contracting influenza. Also, those with asthma or other chronic lung disease, cardiovascular disease, diabetes, chronic kidney disease, HIV infection, or sickle-cell anemia are also at increased risk.

The flu is caused by three types of viruses:

- influenza type A, which is responsible for the deadly influenza pandemics (worldwide epidemics) that strike every 10 to 40 years
- influenza type B, which can cause smaller, more localized outbreaks that generally occur every 3 to 15 years
- influenza type C, which is the least common form and causes only mild symptoms.

Each type encompasses many different strains. Types A or B cause the flu that circulates almost every winter and, occasionally, a stronger strain of these types causes a deadly pandemic or more serious local outbreak. Types A and B are constantly changing, with new strains appearing regularly, whereas type C is more stable. All three types of influenza virus are transmitted through the air in droplets when someone with the infection coughs, sneezes, or talks. These droplets spread throughout the immediate environment of the infected person, landing on objects (such as toys and doorknobs), the hands of the infected person, or the hands or face of another person. Transmission occurs when another person touches a contaminated object and then touches her eyes, nose, or mouth. A person can also breathe the droplets into the respiratory tract from the air before they land. The medical assistant should instruct parents or caregivers of pediatric patients to prevent transmission by frequently washing everyone's hands and toys as well as other objects used by the infected person. In addition, parents should try to prevent the sharing of toys between infected and uninfected children.

Initially, the flu may seem like a common cold, with a stuffy or runny nose, sore throat, headache, or fatigue. However, unlike the common cold virus, influenza symptoms appear quickly and are more severe than the common cold. Signs and symptoms of the flu in children include:

- fever can be as high as 103° to 105°F
- diarrhea and vomiting
- chills and sweats
- headache
- dry cough
- muscle aches and pains in the back, arms, and legs
- weakness, fatigue, and lethargy
- nasal congestion
- loss of appetite.

Once a patient has had the flu, he develops antibodies to the specific virus that caused it. These antibodies will prevent recurrence of symptoms if the infection occurs again. However, those antibodies do not protect against new strains of the virus. The patient can also obtain antibodies from a flu vaccine. The vaccine contains the virus in an attenuated (weakened) form so that the body will develop antibodies to it but will not suffer from flu symptoms. Thus, when the patient comes in contact with that strain of the virus, the immune system is ready to fight off the infection. Infants and young children (as well as people over age 65) are considered at high risk for complications of influenza. Thus, for these patients, physicians recommend an annual flu vaccination, which is safe for children over age 6 months, according to the CDC.

Otitis Media

ICD-9-CM code: 382 (use 4th and 5th digits for further classification)

Otitis media is an infection of the middle ear. It occurs most commonly in babies and children between ages 4 months and 5 years. Otitis media accounts for an estimated 16 million pediatric visits each year in the United States. About 17% to 20% of American children have had at least one case of otitis media by age 2.

Normally, the middle ear is filled with air; in otitis media, infection causes fluid to collect behind the tympanic membrane. Infection in children is typically caused by an immature immune system and frequent viral upper respiratory infection. In addition, collection of this fluid is more common in children because the position of the eustachian tube is more horizontal, allowing fluid to collect behind the tympanic membrane, rather than drain.

As more fluid is produced by the infection, increased pressure on the tympanic membrane causes pain. The fluid may be serous (clear) or purulent (pus-filled). While both serous and purulent otitis media cause pain, the purulent form can cause fever as well. An infant or young child with otitis media who cannot yet talk may pull at her ear or simply cry inconsolably. Fever and cough may accompany otitis media.

Diagnosis of the infection is confirmed by physical examination of the tympanic membrane using an otoscope. A healthy tympanic membrane is gray and shiny; an infected tympanic membrane appears inflamed, bulging, pink or red, and dull. (See Figure 33-1.) The child may also cry when the otoscope is inserted into the ear due to pain. If fluid is present in the canal, the pediatrician may order a culture to determine the causative pathogen.

In the past, the standard treatment for otitis media was administration of antibiotics. However, the overuse of antibiotics has led to resistant strains of bacteria, thus lessening the effectiveness of antibiotics overall. Thus, many pediatricians refrain from prescribing antibiotics in cases of mild or moderate infection and recommend treating pain with acetaminophen and a decongestant to promote drainage. (See *Home care for otitis media.*)

A child with recurrent ear infections, hearing loss, or other health conditions may require antibiotics or a tympanostomy. Tympanostomy is a surgical procedure that creates an opening in the tympanic membrane to insert a small tube, which facilitates drainage of fluid. (See Figure 33-2.) Patients with chronic otitis media may require a tympanostomy to prevent hearing loss from permanent damage to the ossicles of the ear.

Patient Education

Home Care for Otitis Media

Most parents or caregivers who take their child to see a pediatrician for otitis media expect to receive a prescription for antibiotics. To avoid overuse of antibiotics, most pediatricians now recommend treating mild otitis media with pain relievers and decongestants. Thus, the medical assistant should encourage the parent to try to manage the ear infection with home care. She should advise the parent to call the pediatrician if the child develops a fever or severe pain, which are signs of a more advanced infection that would most likely require antibiotics. Attempting to provide home care at the onset of symptoms may clear the infection, precluding the need for antibiotics. By treating fewer ear infections with antibiotics, the patient is less likely to develop resistance to antibiotics from repeated use.

The medical assistant should educate the parent on how to treat an ear infection at home, including methods of pain relief, such as:

- pain reliever, as directed by the physician
- applying warm compresses to the affected ear
- putting a hairdryer on a low setting and gently warming the affected ear
- massaging the temples, nasal sinuses, and mastoid (behind the ear), which can also relieve congestion.

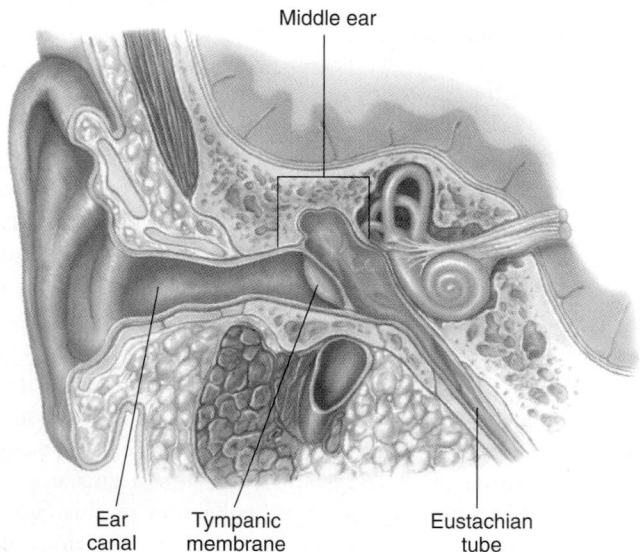

FIG 33-1 Tympanic membrane in otitis media.

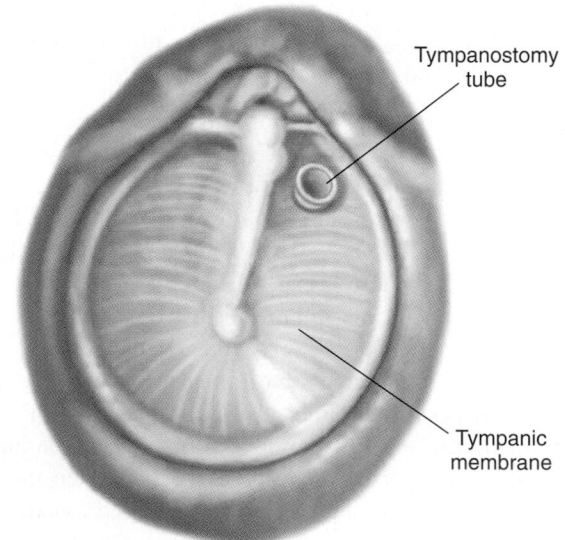

FIG 33-2 Tympanostomy.

Respiratory Syncytial Virus
ICD-9-CM code: 079.6

Respiratory syncytial virus (RSV) is a virus that causes infections of the respiratory tract and the lungs. It is so common that most children have been infected with the virus by the time they reach age 2. It is the leading cause of serious respiratory infection in infants and children. Children at higher risk for RSV include those with weakened immune systems (such as from chemotherapy or transplantation) or congenital heart or lung disease, those born prematurely or with a low birth weight, and those attending child care or who have siblings attending child care. Infants who are exposed to cigarette smoke or high levels of air pollution are also at increased risk for developing RSV.

RSV is caused by exposure to the virus and is spread by respiratory secretions of infected persons. Signs and symptoms of severe RSV in young children include:

- fever of 103°F or higher
- severe cough
- wheezing (high-pitched noise usually heard on exhalation)
- tachypnea (rapid breathing)
- marked drawing in of the chest muscles and skin between the ribs, which indicates dyspnea (difficulty breathing)
- orthopnea (breathing is eased by sitting, rather than lying down)
- cyanosis (bluish color of the skin due to lack of oxygen)
- poor appetite.

In older, healthy children and adults, the symptoms of RSV are that of the common cold, including runny nose or congestion, dry cough, sore throat, low-grade fever, mild headache, lethargy, and malaise.

In severe and mild cases, signs and symptoms typically appear about 4 to 6 days after exposure to the infection. The same precautions to prevent transmission of the common cold apply to RSV, including hand washing and not sharing towels, facecloths, and drinking glasses.

Diagnosis of RSV is determined by sputum analysis, which reveals presence of the virus, viral antigens, or viral RNA. Treatment for severe RSV includes acetaminophen for discomfort and fever and hospitalization to administer intravenous fluids and electrolytes as well as oxygen therapy and, sometimes, mechanical ventilation. Ribavirin aerosol may be used to treat some patients with severe RSV. Treatment for less severe RSV includes fluids and acetaminophen.

Most children completely recover from RSV in 8 to 15 days. Death from RSV infection is relatively rare; however, it can cause death in high-risk infants under age 6 months. RSV in infancy may increase a child's risk of developing asthma and allergies as they age. RSV in children ages 3 and under

can lead to a lower respiratory tract illness, such as pneumonia (inflammation of the lungs) and bronchiolitis (inflammation of the bronchioles). RSV is the most common cause of these disorders.

Strep Throat
ICD-9-CM code: 034.0

Strep throat is an infection that causes throat soreness, inflammation and tenderness of cervical lymph glands, and fever. It can occur at any age; however, it is rarely seen in children younger than age 3.

Strep throat is caused by infection with group A *Streptococcus* bacteria. Family members who carry the *Streptococcus* bacteria may be asymptomatic (experience no symptoms). These family members can pass the infection to children, who then experience repeated infection. Some people, called *carriers*, harbor the *Streptococcus* bacteria in their throats but never experience symptoms.

Signs and symptoms of *Strep* throat in infants and small children include sleeplessness, irritability, fever, refusal to breastfeed or drink from a bottle or cup, and, occasionally, a fine, red rash on the torso, arms, and legs.

Throat culture confirming the presence of *Streptococcus* diagnoses the condition. Treatment of *Strep* throat involves administration of antibiotics. Treatment is the same for younger and older children. The medical assistant should encourage the parent or caregiver to administer the entire prescription of antibiotics to avoid superinfection.

(See *Antibiotics and superinfection page 652*.) If the parent tells the medical assistant that she cannot afford to purchase the entire prescription, the medical assistant should investigate offering samples to the parent. Additionally, the medical assistant can investigate social services available in her state to ensure that her patient gets the proper medication. The medical assistant should also explain the dangers of sharing prescriptions. The pediatrician prescribes the medication for one patient only. Splitting a medication between two children can cause superinfection. Also, the medication may be contraindicated for the other child due to an allergy, a medical condition, or a possible drug interaction with another medication the child is taking. In addition to the prescribed antibiotics, cool fluids will soothe the throat and prevent dehydration.

Most cases of *Strep* throat resolve with treatment. However, recurrence is common, in part because it is so easily spread to other family members and friends. The recurrence of *Strep* throat is likely not a sign of an underlying problem with the child's immune system. Complications of *Strep* throat include rheumatic fever, which produces skin rash, joint inflammation, and, possibly, damage to heart valves. Kidney damage and inflammation can result from lack of treatment.

Antibiotics and superinfection

When the pediatrician prescribes antibiotics to a patient, the medical assistant should advise the parent to give the child the entire prescription to avoid superinfection. A superinfection occurs when the patient takes some of the antibiotic but stops taking it when she starts feeling better, rather than completing the entire course of medication as prescribed. In such a case, the antibiotic the patient takes only kills the weakest bacteria. The stronger bacteria survive and reinfect the patient, who experiences a rebound of symptoms, which are commonly much worse than the initial infection.

In addition, the remaining bacteria may acquire resistance to the antibiotic, forcing the physician to find a stronger antibiotic to kill the remaining bacteria. If the patient or another child whom the patient infects has had many infections and taken many different antibiotics, the physician may not be able to find an antibiotic to treat the infection effectively.

Oral Thrush

ICD-9-CM code: 112.0 (neonate 771.7)

Oral thrush is a fungal infection of the mouth. Although it can affect anyone, it occurs most commonly in babies and toddlers. The infection usually occurs within the first 6 months of life.

Oral thrush is caused by *Candida albicans*. Most healthy people have a small amount of fungus in the mouth and digestive tract, but the normal flora of the GI tract keep the fungus in balance. Oral thrush and other *Candida* infections occur when antibiotics disturb the natural balance of microorganisms in the body or the immune system is weakened by disease or immunosuppressive drugs, such as prednisone.

Oral thrush causes creamy white lesions, usually on the inner cheeks and tongue. The lesions can be painful and may bleed slightly when scraped or when brushing the child's teeth. A healthy neonate with oral thrush usually develops symptoms during the first few weeks of life. In addition to the distinctive white lesions in the mouth, the parent or caregiver may notice that the infant is irritable and fussy and may not want to eat. During breastfeeding, the neonate can pass the infection to the mother. Occasionally, oral thrush may spread to the roof of the mouth, gums, tonsils, or back of the throat.

Treatment of oral thrush consists of administration of an antimycotic, such as fluconazole (Diflucan), which caregivers can administer to infants and children as a liquid. Although the baby may be fussy, the parent or caregiver should try to continue the normal feeding schedule.

Oral thrush is a minor problem for healthy children, but for those with weakened immune systems, symptoms of oral thrush may be more severe, widespread, and difficult to control. Uncontrolled thrush may lead to diaper rash and vaginal yeast infections. Severe complications that spread to the esophagus, brain, heart, and joints are rare but may occur in immunocompromised infants, such as those with HIV.

Chickenpox

ICD-9-CM code: 052.9

Chickenpox is a highly contagious virus that causes fever and a rash. Prior to the vaccine developed in 1995, approximately 4 million Americans (mostly children) contracted chickenpox each year. Widespread administration of the vaccine reduced the number of cases and hospitalizations. The virus is highly contagious for people who are not immune—children or adults who have not previously had chickenpox or the vaccine.

Chickenpox is caused by the varicella-zoster virus, which is part of a group of viruses called *herpesviruses*. The virus spreads easily from person to person through direct contact with the rash or by droplets dispersed into the air by coughing or sneezing. (See *Chickenpox will not wait.*)

Signs of chickenpox include the classic red, itchy rash on the face, scalp, chest, and back. The rash can also spread to the entire body, including the throat, eyes, and vagina. The chickenpox rash usually appears less than 2 weeks after exposure to the virus and begins as superficial spots. These spots quickly turn into small, fluid-filled blisters that break open and crust over. New spots continue to appear for several days and may number in the hundreds. Itching may range from mild to intense. The rash may be preceded or accompanied by:

- fever
- abdominal pain or loss of appetite
- mild headache
- malaise, lethargy, and irritability

Front office–Back office connection

Chickenpox Will Not Wait

Because children with chickenpox are highly contagious, the administrative medical assistant should work quickly with the clinical medical assistant to get him into a treatment room immediately. He should not wait in the waiting room with the other children. If a parent calls the office suspecting that her children have chickenpox, the administrative and clinical medical assistants should coordinate examinations so that a treatment room is waiting for the patients when they arrive.

- mild cough and runny nose for the first 2 days of illness before the rash appears. A person who has chickenpox can transmit the virus for up to 48 hours before symptoms appear and remains contagious until all spots crust over.

Treatment for chickenpox involves acetaminophen for pain and fever and rest at home. Children with chickenpox should not go to school until all lesions have crusted over. The medical assistant should instruct the parent or caregiver to call the office if any of the more severe effects occur, including:

- marked increase in warmth, tenderness, or redness of the rash, which possibly indicates a secondary bacterial skin infection
- spread of the rash to one or both eyes
- dizziness or disorientation
- rapid heartbeat or shortness of breath
- tremors or loss of muscle coordination
- stiff neck
- worsening cough
- vomiting
- fever higher than 103°F.

Chickenpox usually lasts about 2 weeks and rarely causes complications. Although the disease is generally mild in healthy children, it can be serious for anyone. There is no way to know which infected child or adult will develop a severe case. Thus, most states have made administration of the chickenpox vaccine a requirement for attendance in public school. The medical assistant should advise her patients on their state's mandate for vaccination. For most patients, the chickenpox vaccine is a safe, effective way to prevent chickenpox. In the small number of cases when the vaccine does not stop chickenpox completely, the resulting infection is much milder than it would have been without the vaccine. Many people who experience chickenpox as a child will contract shingles, a reemergence of the varicella-zoster virus that usually occurs in older adults.

Warts
ICD-9-CM code: 078.10
Common warts are noncancerous skin growths. Children and teens are susceptible to common warts. Approximately 4% of 9- to 14-year-olds in the United States develop common warts.

Warts are caused by human papillomavirus (HPV). HPV causes a rapid growth of cells on the outer layer of skin. These growths are small, fleshy, grainy bumps that are rough to the touch and usually painless. Warts may occur singly or in multiple clusters. They commonly contain one or more tiny black dots, which are small, clotted blood vessels. They usually occur on the hands or fingers or near the fingernails. Nail biting can also cause warts to spread on to the fingertips and around the nails.

Diagnosis is based on physical examination. Treatment for warts at home can include over-the-counter wart dissolving medication that contains salicylic acid. Another effective home remedy involves wrapping the wart in duct tape. Destroying the wart helps prevent common warts from spreading to other parts of the body or to other people. If these treatments are ineffective, the physician may freeze the wart with liquid nitrogen or burn it with electrocautery to remove it. Unless the warts are large or extremely uncomfortable, surgical removal is generally avoided. Surgery can cause a permanent scar and subsequent warts can be more severe because they can grow over the scar tissue.

Because warts are caused by a virus, they may recur after treatment and can become a persistent problem. The medical assistant should instruct patients and their parents to notify the physician if warts are painful or rapidly multiplying, because these signs may indicate a suppressed immune system or skin cancer, which require immediate evaluation and treatment.

Noncommunicable Pediatric Diseases and Disorders
Noncommunicable disorders are those that are not transmitted via contact with other people. These disorders may have a genetic component or may be the result of the environment, trauma before or at birth, inappropriate nutrition, and other factors. Some of the most common noncommunicable pediatric diseases and disorders include allergies, anorexia or bulimia nervosa, asthma, attention deficit disorder, autism, Down syndrome, constipation, failure to thrive, cerebral palsy, eczema, scoliosis, obesity, lead poisoning, and phenylketonuria.

Allergies
ICD-9-CM code: 995.3 (unspecified)
An allergy is a response by the immune system to a substance that it perceives as harmful. About 11% of the U.S. population has an allergy to one or more substances. Children are more likely to have allergies before age 10. After that age, symptoms typically decrease.

The first time that the substance is introduced into the body, the body manufactures antibodies to fight the substance. After the initial contact, any time that the allergen is introduced into the body, the antibodies begin to attack. Antibody formation causes a release of histamine and prostaglandins. The combined effects of histamine and prostaglandins production can cause these reactions:

- Histamine causes mucous membranes to secrete. The patient will develop a runny nose and itchy, watery eyes.
- Prostaglandins cause constriction of smooth muscle, such as the bronchioles, which results in constriction of the airways and difficulty breathing.

- Capillary permeability increases, which pushes fluid out of the bloodstream and into the tissues, causing a drop in blood pressure.

Common allergens include dust, animal hair, pollen, stings from such insects as bees or wasps, drugs, and such foods as peanuts, tree nuts, wheat, eggs, milk, soy, and fish or shellfish. Common signs and symptoms of an allergic reaction include hives, eczema, hay fever, and asthma.

Skin testing is the most common type of test used to identify potential allergens causing a reaction. One type of skin test, called the *scratch test*, involves placing a small amount of a common allergen on the skin's surface and scratching the area so that the substance is introduced under the skin. The result is positive if the skin in that area reacts with swelling and redness. Another allergy test, called the *radioallergosorbent test* (RAST), measures specific allergy-related substances in the bloodstream. (For more information on allergy testing, see Chapter 25, page 411.)

Mild allergic responses in children can be treated with antihistamines and behavior changes to avoid the offending allergen. Childhood food allergies to eggs, milk, and soy may diminish with age. However, allergies to such foods as peanuts are commonly more severe and the child is less likely to outgrow such an allergy. (See *Food allergies at school*.)

Severe allergic reactions to substances such as bee stings or certain medications can cause anaphylactic shock, which is a medical emergency. In anaphylactic shock, the patient experiences bronchial constriction, increased mucus production, and increased capillary permeability, which can cause severe dyspnea and dangerously low blood pressure. A child with severe allergies should wear a medical alert bracelet, which explains the child's allergies to medical personnel and others who need the information to treat the patient (See Figure 33-3.) In addition, the child should carry an Epi-Pen, which is a prefilled syringe of epinephrine for use if the child is exposed to the allergen. Epinephrine causes an increase in

heart rate and blood pressure. The medical assistant should instruct parents on the use of the Epi-Pen. She should also teach the child how to use it himself if he is old enough to understand. The medical assistant should emphasize that the child should have the Epi-Pen with him at all times. She must emphasize to the patient and parents that avoiding the allergen is the primary goal. If the child comes in contact with the allergen and uses the Epi-Pen, he must undergo examination by a physician immediately. (See Figure 33-4.)

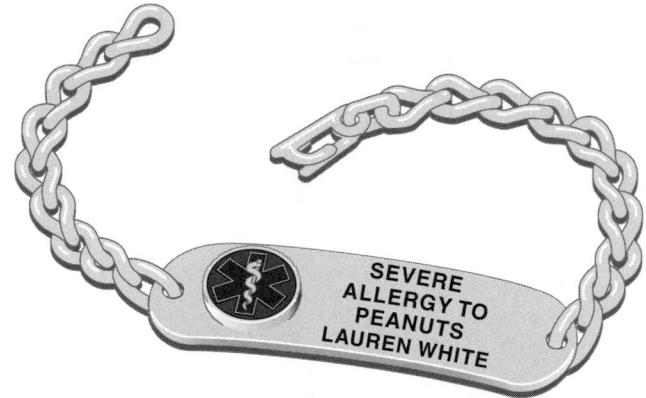

FIG 33-3 Medical alert bracelet.

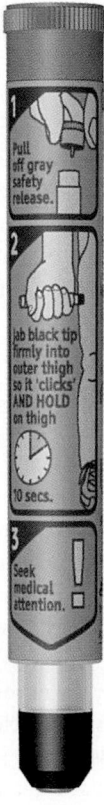

FIG 33-4 Epi-Pen.

Food allergies at school

Allergy to peanuts is severe in many children, so much so that many schools offer a "peanut-free" section of the school cafeteria and ban peanut butter or other peanut products in the classroom. Most schools also require an ingredient list for snacks prepared by a student or parent that will be shared with the entire class, such as birthday cupcakes or brownies. Some schools even discourage such foods for celebrations and encourage instead handing out pencils, stickers, or other inexpensive items instead. In addition, schools try to discourage children from trading foods at school.

Eating Disorders

Anorexia nervosa—ICD-9-CM code: 307.1
Bulimia nervosa—ICD-9-CM code: 307.51

Anorexia nervosa and bulimia nervosa are psychological disorders marked by altered eating behaviors. In anorexia nervosa, the patient suffers extreme weight loss due to self-starvation. In bulimia nervosa, self-starvation also occurs; however, this disorder is characterized by a cycle of starvation, binge eating, and purging of the food by forced vomiting or use of laxatives or other medications to forcibly expel the food from the body. An anorexic or bulimic patient may also engage in excessive exercise in an attempt to lose weight. Anorexia and bulimia are typically pediatric disorders that mainly occur in girls, with a peak onset period from ages 12 to 14.

Anorexia nervosa and bulimia nervosa may be caused by emotional disorders that create extreme anxiety about physical appearance and a distorted body image. Certain personality traits, such as perfectionism or overachieving, also predispose a person to developing an eating disorder. In addition, recent research suggests genetic, nutritional, or neurobiological links. Some research shows that eating disorders may have a genetic link because a sibling of a person who experiences anorexia or bulimia is more likely to develop an eating disorder. Researchers have also connected these disorders to a decrease in the amount of the neurotransmitter serotonin. A link has also been made between zinc deficiency, which causes decreased appetite, and deficiency of other nutrients, such as tyrosine and tryptophan, both precursors of neurotransmitters, and vitamin B_1. Deficiency in these nutrients contributes to a cycle of malnutrition.

The typical anorexic or bulimic patient is a high achiever and a perfectionist. An anorexic patient is usually extremely thin. In bulimia, the patient may be thin, overweight, or normal weight, making the condition more difficult to diagnose.

Diagnosis is based on physical examination findings and the health history. The anorexic patient will typically refuse to maintain a normal body weight and may weigh less than 85% of normal body weight for height. She may express a fear of gaining weight and describe her body as too fat, denying the seriousness of her current low body weight. She may also experience absence of three or more consecutive menstrual cycles due to her reduced body weight. Diagnosis of the bulimic patient is more difficult because she is not necessarily underweight and the patient may be ashamed and unwilling to discuss her behavior. Physical findings in bulimia include erosion of gum tissues and esophageal damage from forced vomiting. Diagnosis is based on these findings as well as a detailed health history, which may reveal fatigue, lethargy, signs of depression, low self-esteem, previous suicide attempt, or general demeanor of apathy. As with the anorexic patient, the bulimic patient may have missed menstrual cycles.

The pediatric medical assistant should be aware of the need for specialized care of her anorexic or bulimic patient. Parents and patients should be given referrals for appropriate treatment. Structured programs designed for patients with eating disorders can include:

- nutritional counseling
- behavioral therapy
- family therapy
- group therapy
- psychological and psychiatric consultation.

Prognosis for anorexia nervosa and bulimia nervosa depends on the severity of the disorder and how long it has been occurring before treatment. Approximately 6% of diagnosed anorexic and bulimic patients eventually die from complications related to organ failure and from suicide. Girls with anorexia may experience amenorrhea (absence of a menstrual period) or delay of menarche (first menstrual period). Other complications of anorexia include osteoporosis, low body temperature, lethargy, slow heart rate, dry skin, brittle nails, development of fine body hair called *lanugo*, and infertility. In bulimia, repeated forcing of food from the stomach to the esophagus can cause esophageal ulcers, bleeding, bleeding gums, gingivitis, dental caries (cavities), and an absent gag reflex. The subsequent fluid and electrolyte imbalance can result in cardiac arrhythmia.

Asthma

ICD-9-CM code: 493.0 (childhood asthma; use 5th digit)

Asthma is a disorder characterized by inflammation and spasm of the bronchi, increased mucus secretions in the bronchi, and narrowing of the airway. Asthma affects about 15% of all children in the United States, making it the most common chronic disease in children and the most common disorder seen in the pediatric office.

Specific causes of asthma vary and triggers can include cigarette smoke, cold viruses, exercise (called *exercise-induced asthma*), and environmental allergies. Regardless of the trigger, the patient will experience difficulty inhaling and exhaling, shortness of breath, wheezing, tightness in the chest, difficulty speaking, and anxiety. In some cases, intermittent episodes of severe symptoms, called *asthma attacks*, can occur. Coughing may also occur at the onset of an episode.

Diagnosis of asthma is based on patient history and clinical findings. Tests include spirometry, which measures the amount of air entering and leaving the lungs. Because many patients with chronic asthma exhibit normal results with spirometry, patients may also be asked to conduct a peak expiratory flow (PEF) test, which measures the exchange of air, twice per day for about 2 weeks. The patient should take the PEF test each morning upon waking and before taking bronchodilators. Although peak flow varies normally, a variability greater than 20% confirms a diagnosis of asthma.

A patient who suffers from eczema or other allergic conditions is at greater risk for developing asthma. Because airway function tests are not always possible on small children, diagnosis may be confirmed by a positive response to treatment.

Treatments for asthma include bronchodilators using an inhaler or nebulizer, anti-inflammatory medications, and avoidance of common triggers. Some patients periodically suffer from asthma "attacks," which are the sudden, severe inability to catch a breath and require the immediate use of an inhaler. Patients who experience more than two asthma attacks per week should be referred to a respiratory specialist. The medical assistant should demonstrate use of an inhaler or nebulizer to patients and caregivers. (For more information on how to use an inhaler or nebulizer, see Chapter 28, page 495.)

Prognosis for childhood asthma is generally good, with 54% of patients outgrowing asthma after 10 years. With proper treatment, the extent of permanent lung damage is minimal.

Behavioral Disorders

Attention deficit disorder—ICD-9-CM code: 314.00
Attention deficit hyperactivity disorder—ICD-9-CM code: 314.01

Attention deficit disorder (ADD) and attention deficit hyperactivity disorder (ADHD) are behavioral disorders. In ADD, a patient displays an inability to focus attention for short periods of time and has trouble prioritizing and completing tasks. In ADHD, the patient also has trouble focusing and finishing tasks and, in addition, has trouble sitting still for long and prefers to be moving around. Although the disorder can be familial, no genetic factor has yet been identified; boys are 10 times more likely to suffer from ADD or ADHD than girls.

Signs of ADD and ADHD include an inability to organize school supplies, books, and personal items and trouble prioritizing time. In addition, the patient with ADHD is unable to sit still and is excessively active.

Diagnosis of ADD or ADHD involves a patient interview by a pediatrician or psychologist, noting the following findings:

- ADD (must exhibit at least six behaviors to a degree that is considered abnormal)
  - often fails to give close attention to details or makes mistakes in schoolwork
  - has difficulty sustaining attention in tasks
  - seems not to listen
  - fails to follow instructions or finish work
  - is unorganized
  - has difficulties with schoolwork or homework

- loses things, such as school assignments, books, and tools
- is easily distracted
- is forgetful about daily activities

- ADHD (must exhibit at least six behaviors to a degree that is considered abnormal)
  - is fidgety and squirms
  - does not stay seated
  - runs or climbs excessively or has feelings of restlessness (in older children)
  - has difficulty playing quietly
  - is often "on the go" or acts as if "driven by a motor"
  - often talks excessively
  - blurts out answers to questions
  - has difficulty waiting in lines or taking turns
  - often interrupts or intrudes on others.

There is no known cure, but medication and counseling can help the child focus. Medications may include atomoxetine (Straterra) or the combination drug dextroamphetamine and amphetamine (Adderall). The physician may recommend restricting food additives if they are found to contribute to the child's hyperactivity. Symptoms of ADD and ADHD usually subside or completely disappear with age.

Autism

ICD-9-CM code: 299.0

Autism is a bioneurological developmental disability. Males are four times more likely to suffer from autism than females. Autism is usually not diagnosed until age 3 or later. The National Autism Association reports that 1 child in 150 is affected by autism.

The cause of autism is unknown. However, recent studies have suggested there may be a link between autism and thimerosal, a mercury compound used as a preservative in childhood vaccines.

Symptoms of autism can include:

- failure to make eye contact
- repetitive behaviors such as rocking
- delayed language development
- poor cognitive function
- extreme agitation with changes in routine
- preference for solitary play activities
- indifference or lack of attachment to people.

Diagnosis of autism is based on behaviors defined in the *Diagnostic and Statistical Manual of Mental Disorders,* 4th edition (DSM-IV). To meet the criteria, the patient must exhibit at least two symptoms of impaired social interaction, at least one symptom of impaired communication, and at least one symptom of repetitive behavior.

Early intervention by a referral to specialists will initiate therapies that can increase the child's speech development and interactions with others. The medical assistant should be aware of the signs of autism and note such observations for the pediatrician, who can make referrals for testing and treatment as appropriate.

Down Syndrome
ICD-9-CM code: 758.0

Down syndrome, or *trisomy 21,* is a common chromosomal disorder that causes delays in physical and intellectual development. It occurs in 1 out of every 800 children born each year and occurs in all populations, regardless of race, sex, or socioeconomic status.

Down syndrome is caused by an error in cell division during conception that results in the presence of an extra (or part of an extra) 21st chromosome. It is also related to advanced maternal age at the time of pregnancy. The risk of conceiving a child with Down syndrome for mothers who conceive at age 40 is more than seven times higher than mothers who conceive at age 35. Down syndrome causes distinctive physical characteristics, including:

- small head with a flat facial profile
- mouth that tends to hang open
- large tongue with a high arched palate
- slanted eyes with irises that contain Brushfield spots
- hypotonia (weak muscle tone)
- congenital heart defects (common).

Patients with Down syndrome will likely suffer from other health problems, including:

- cognitive impairment (varies in degree)
- sexual development delayed or incomplete (common)
- visual problems such as cataracts and strabismus
- hearing problems
- decreased resistance to infection
- high risk of developing leukemia.

Infants are diagnosed with Down syndrome at birth due to its distinctive physical characteristics. There is no cure for Down syndrome. Treatment aims to monitor development and address complications. Because a child with Down syndrome experiences developmental delays, an accurate record of her individual development is vital. Accompanying physical problems, such as heart defects and vision or hearing impairments, should be treated along with the regular well-baby and well-child visits. It is extremely important for patients with Down syndrome to receive vaccinations because they are more susceptible to infection. When age appropriate, the medical assistant or parent can explain the importance of hand washing and proper hygiene to the patient.

In the past, life expectancy for people with Down syndrome was severely limited. However, with early intervention and advances in treatment for complications, people with Down syndrome can live into their 40s or 50s. However, people with Down syndrome are at increased risk for developing Alzheimer disease after age 40.

Constipation
ICD-9-CM code: 564.0

Constipation is a condition in which a person has hard stools that are difficult to expel. Defecation is commonly painful and infrequent. Constipation occurs in approximately 2% of the general population but is most prevalent in children. Women and elderly persons also suffer more bouts of constipation than young men.

Children and adolescents who suffer from chronic constipation are probably not eating enough fiber or drinking enough water. Medications can also cause constipation. Signs and symptoms include hard, dry stools that are hard to pass and an infrequent urge to defecate. Because babies and young children are not able to communicate sensations of pain or difficulty passing stool, the parent or caregiver may notice the child straining and turning red when trying to defecate. The parent may also note the child holding his abdomen or complaining of a bellyache. Stools that the child is able to pass may be small lumps that look like nuts.

The medical assistant can encourage the child with constipation and his parent to make changes to the child's diet to relieve constipation. (See *Dietary changes to relieve constipation,* page 658.) If dietary changes are inadequate, the physician may prescribe a stool softener. The medical assistant must advise the parent to avoid giving too much stool softener to the child, because it could cause diarrhea and dehydration.

Most children with constipation respond favorably to dietary changes and normal bowel function returns. In some cases, constipation can lead to hemorrhoids or anal fissures (tears around the skin of the anus due to stretching of the sphincter muscle). Rectal bleeding may occur from hemorrhoids and anal fissures. The medical assistant should instruct the parent or caregiver to bring the child to the pediatrician if she notices blood in the child's diaper or underwear. In severe cases, constipation can lead to a bowel obstruction. If the bowel obstruction ruptures, surgical repair is necessary.

Failure to Thrive
ICD-9-CM code: 783.41

Failure to thrive (FTT) is a condition of insufficient weight gain according to standardized growth charts. Children experience irregular growth patterns, gaining height and weight in irregular intervals, commonly called *growth spurts.* So long as toddlers are growing and developing, there is little cause for concern. However, infants who do not gain sufficient weight will not develop normally. Although the

Patient Education

Dietary Changes to Relieve Constipation

The medical assistant should teach the pediatric patient and his parent or caregiver about foods that cause constipation and others that help alleviate it.

Foods to encourage

- apples
- oranges
- high-fiber cereals
- high-fiber, whole-grain bread
- apple juice or prune or plum juice
- water

Foods to Avoid

- bananas
- pudding
- cheese
- rice
- white bread

exact incidence of FTT is not known, approximately 10% of children under age 2 who have parents with psychological problems and low socioeconomic status exhibit FTT. The FTT category includes infants whose weight is under the third percentile.

The most common cause of failure to thrive is inadequate nutrition. Colicky babies, mothers who used alcohol or had poor nutrition during pregnancy, and new mothers who experience fatigue and postpartum depression can all contribute to FTT. Causes can also include cleft palate, which affects the infant's ability to suck, or malabsorption disease, which compromises the body's ability to absorb formula or breast milk. Social and economic factors that can promote FTT include poverty, drug and alcohol abuse, depression, abuse, and immature parents. To identify a child with feeding problems, the medical assistant can use the PEACH survey. (See *Identifying feeding problems*.)

The medical assistant can help an infant with FTT by reporting suspected abuse, neglect, or drug abuse to social services and offering resources for financial assistance. Most states have programs for food stamps or nutritional assistance.

Prognosis for the child with FTT depends on the cause. Infants who have malabsorptive disease treated with diet modification or cleft palate that is surgically corrected have good outcomes. FTT due to abuse and neglect can lead to permanent lack of growth and possible long-term developmental

delay. The length of time of the abuse or neglect impacts the long-term outcome.

Cerebral Palsy
ICD-9-CM code: 343.9

Cerebral palsy (CP) is a disorder of the brain that affects posture, balance, and movement. According to a March 2008 study by the CDC, CP occurs in 1 of every 278 children. The study also found that boys have a higher risk for CP as do African Americans and children from low- or middle-income families.

The cause of CP is an injury to or error in development of the areas of the brain that control posture, balance, and movement. The cause may be:

- congenital due to:
  - genetic disorder that is present at birth
  - infection during pregnancy (meningitis)
  - jaundice in the neonate
  - Rh incompatibility
- acquired due to:
  - brain injury (head trauma at birth or after)
  - infection in neonate (meningitis).

CP is characterized by a wide variety of symptoms, including lack of muscle control, muscle weakness, spastic muscles, delayed development, mental retardation, and hearing and vision problems. The disorder appears within the first few years of the patient's life and does not worsen over time.

The pediatrician can diagnose the patient with CP based on physical examination findings. Lack of muscle tone, or *floppy baby syndrome*, is an indication of CP. The pediatrician can refer patients to physical, speech, and occupational therapy to maximize potential function. The pediatrician still provides routine care to the patient, while the patient benefits from therapies specifically designed for his needs.

The prognosis for CP is very individualized. With supportive treatments such as medications, surgery, and assistive devices, each patient with CP can reach her individual potential. Some complications of CP include seizures, which affect 50% of children with CP, mental retardation, learning disabilities, and ADHD.

Eczema
ICD-9-CM code: 692.6

Eczema, or *atopic dermatitis*, is an inflammatory skin disease. Patients with allergies or family history of asthma, allergies to foods, and outdoor allergies are more susceptible to developing eczema. Pediatricians diagnose eczema in about 1 in 10 children in the United States, usually within the infant's first few months of life. It is somewhat more prevalent in Asian Americans and African Americans.

Identifying feeding problems

The medical assistant can help identify feeding problems in children from birth to age 5 by using the Parent Eating and Nutrition Assessment for Children with Special Health Needs (PEACH) survey. Parents who have a child who is not reaching developmental milestones and gaining adequate weight can also use the PEACH survey to identify nutritional deficiencies that might be affecting the child's overall health. The survey contains 17 "yes" or "no" questions. Each question with a yes answer is assigned a score from 1 to 4. A total score of 4 or more indicates a probable nutritional problem.

PEACH Survey

Agency: _Head Start_   **Date:** _10/15/09_
Child's name: _Ling Su Chen_   **Date of birth:** _12/22/07_
Address: _14 Roberts Ave. Blueville CT 06000_   **Phone #:** _860-555-8752_

Please circle YES or NO for each question as it applies to your child. Circle the points for each yes.

1. Does your child have a health problem (do not include colds or flu)? If yes, what is it?
   (YES) NO (1)
   cerebral palsy

2. Is your child: _____ small for age, _X_ too thin, or _____ too heavy? (If you check any of the above, please circle YES.)
   (YES) NO (3)

3. Does your child have any feeding problems? If yes, what are they?
   (YES) NO (3)
   difficulty swallowing

4. Is your child's appetite a problem If yes, describe:
   YES (NO) 1
   she gets hungry, although sporadically

5. Is your child on a special diet? If yes, what type of diet?
   YES (NO) 2

6. Does your child take medicine for a health problem (do not include vitamins, iron, or fluoride)? Include name of medicine(s).
   YES (NO) 1

7. Does your child have food allergies? If yes, to what foods?
   (YES) NO (1)
   strawberries

8. Does your child use a feeding tube or other special feeding method? If yes, explain:
   YES (NO) 4

9. Circle YES if your child does not eat any of these foods: _____ milk, _____ meats, _____ vegetables, _____ fruits. (Check all that apply.)
   YES (NO) 1

10. Circle YES if your child has problems with _____ sucking, _X_ swallowing, _____ chewing, _____ or gagging. (Check all that apply.)
    (YES) NO (3)

11. Circle YES if your child has problems with _X_ loose stools, _____ hard stools, _____ throwing up, _____ spitting up (Check all that apply.)
    (YES) NO (3)

12. Does your child eat clay, paint chips, dirt, or anything else that is not food? If yes, what?
    YES (NO) 2

13. Does your child refuse to eat, throw food, or do other things to upset you at mealtime? If yes, explain:
    YES (NO) 2

14. For infants under 12 months who are bottle fed: Does your child drink less than 3 (8-ounce) bottles of milk per day?
    YES NO 1

15. For children over 12 months (Check if applies and circle the YES).
    Is your child not using a cup?_____ Is your child not finger feeding?_____
    YES (NO) 1

16. For children over 18 months: Does your child still take most liquids from a bottle?
    YES (NO) 2

17. Circle YES if your child is not using a spoon.
    YES (NO) 2

Total points for YES answers = _14_

The cause of eczema is unknown; however, there are several possible triggers, including food, environmental irritants, and stress. The rash appears as a vesicular rash on the face, neck, elbows, or behind the knees and ears. Diagnosis of eczema is based on physical examination of the rash.

Treatment is directed at reducing the frequency and number of eruptions by avoiding triggers. Topical corticosteriods, such as hydrocortisone (Dermacort), and oral antihistamines, such as diphenhydramine (Benadryl), fexofenadine (Allegra), and cetirizine (Zyrtec), are used to control itching. If secondary staphylococcal infection occurs (due to scratching), the physician may prescribe oral antibiotics. The medical assistant can instruct the parents on how to monitor the patient's skin and record possible triggers by keeping a diary. If avoidance of triggers clears the skin, the parents or caregiver can treat the child at home. The medical assistant should instruct parents to contact the physician if the child:

- cannot sleep or is distracted from his daily routines
- complains that his skin is extremely painful
- scratches and causes bleeding or possible infection
- does not find relief from self-care, such as avoidance of triggers and use of unscented lotions.

Childhood eczema commonly clears with age. More than half of children with eczema will completely recover by their teenage years. Complications of eczema include *Staphylococcus* infection, which may be caused by the patient scratching the skin, leaving open areas in the skin where bacteria can colonize.

Scoliosis
ICD-9-CM code: 737.30
Scoliosis is an abnormal lateral (side) curvature of the spine. The condition usually appears in adolescence, during periods of rapid growth. School nurses commonly screen for scoliosis and refer patients to their physician. About 2% to 3% of Americans have a curvature greater than 10 degrees. Curvature greater than 20 degrees affects 1 in 2500 Americans. Scoliosis is more common in adolescent girls and occurs in males most commonly in infancy.

A pediatrician, chiropractor, or osteopath will usually perform the assessment using physical examination. The practitioner observes the patient from the back while she bends forward at the waist. A positive finding for scoliosis is observed when a discrepancy in hip and shoulder height is observed upon forward bending.

Treatments can include asymmetrical exercises to stretch and strengthen and application of a brace, cast, traction, or electrical muscle stimulation. Severe scoliosis may require surgical correction.

Prognosis depends on the likelihood of progression of the curvature. Patients who have not yet reached skeletal maturity are more likely to have progressive curvature. Severe, uncorrected scoliosis can compromise respiration, due to compression of the diaphragm on one side. Fertility in females may be compromised if the rib cage will not allow uterine expansion in late pregnancy.

Obesity
ICD-9-CM code: 278.00
Obesity is defined as a body mass index (BMI) over 30. (For more information on body mass index, see Chapter 37, page 777.) Childhood obesity has become more and more prevalent over the past 30 years. In the United States, about 30% of children age 5 and older are obese.

Causes of obesity in general vary and can include lifestyle factors as well as endocrine disorders. However, in childhood obesity, endocrine disorders are rarely the cause. Instead, a diet high in sugar and fat combined with a lack of exercise are the clear causes.

The medical assistant can give the parents, caregivers, and child nutritional guidelines for health and weight management and a list of community resources. She should also encourage families to help children lose weight by engaging in exercise, limiting television watching and computer time, and limiting intake of foods with little nutritional value or high sugar and fat content.

Although obesity in itself is not a disorder with a prognosis, the complications associated with it can limit life expectancy if they remain unaddressed. For example, type II diabetes, high cholesterol, and hypertension, which were once complications of obesity seen only in adults, are now seen in children.

Lead Poisoning
ICD-9-CM code: 984.9
Lead poisoning, or *plumbism,* is a chronic disorder caused by poisoning by ingestion or inhalation of lead-contaminated paint, soil, or dust. According to the CDC, approximately 2% of children between ages 1 and 5 contract lead poisoning. Children of lower socioeconomic status are at greater risk of contracting lead poisoning. Because lead competes for absorption with many vitamins and minerals, such as iron, calcium, zinc, vitamin C, and vitamin D, the malnourished child will absorb more lead due to low intake of these nutrients. In addition, the empty stomach of a hungry child will absorb more lead if it is consumed.

In the body, lead interferes with minerals, such as iron, calcium, and zinc. It replaces these minerals and disrupts their normal function. In the bloodstream, lead replaces iron in the hemoglobin of RBCs, making them unable to carry oxygen to tissues. In bone, lead interferes with the absorption of the calcium needed to make bone cells. Decreased zinc absorption causes immune suppression.

Signs and symptoms of lead poisoning include recurrent episodes of diarrhea, irritability, and fatigue. Because these symptoms are similar to those of iron deficiency anemia, the two are commonly confused. In fact, iron deficiency anemia and lead poisoning are often diagnosed together in children of low socioeconomic backgrounds.

Diagnosis is based on blood sample analysis for lead (PbB). Lead levels greater than 60 to 70 micrograms/dl of whole blood indicates poisoning. Treatment includes chelation therapy, which involves injection of a chelating agent that binds to lead, making it water soluble so the child can excrete it in urine. Because children with lead poisoning usually have an iron deficiency, iron supplementation typically accompanies chelation therapy. In addition, the identified sources of lead in the child's environment should be removed to prevent further poisoning. (See *Lead poisoning prevention*.)

Prognosis is based on the child's lead levels and how long the child ingested lead before diagnosis and treatment. Outcomes vary from severe, such as permanent reduction in IQ and permanent brain damage that can affect nerves and muscles, to mild, which can include complete recovery that could take months to years. In addition, lead poisoning further suppresses the children's immune system, leaving them little protection from infectious diseases.

Phenylketonuria

ICD-9-CM code: 270.1

Infants born with phenylketonuria (PKU) have an inability to properly use protein, specifically the amino acid called *phenylalanine*. It is estimated that 1 in every 70 persons is a carrier for PKU and that the disorder affects 1 in every 15,000 to 20,000 infants born in the United States.

Normally, when a person eats proteins, her body breaks down the proteins into separate amino acids. In a patient with PKU, one of the enzymes that changes phenylalanine into another amino acid, tyrosine, is missing. As a result, the amount of phenylalinine accumulates in the blood. This increase in phenylalanine in the blood prevents the infant's brain from growing and developing normally. In addition to increased levels of phenylalanine, other symptoms of PKU include skin rash, irritable behavior, and a musty body odor.

A PKU test, mandated by most states, is typically performed before the baby leaves the hospital but may be done after discharge or if the newborn was delivered at home. A simple blood test diagnoses the disorder.

Early diagnosis of the disorder allows parents to put the child on a special diet that is very low in phenylalanine, including phenylalanine-free formula, careful tracking of intake of fruits and vegetables and cereals, breads, and pastas, and elimination of foods that are high in protein, such as dairy products, beans, nuts, meat, eggs, and fish. In addition, as the PKU patient ages, she should avoid the artificial

---

 Patient Education

Lead Poisoning Prevention

The Centers for Disease Control and Prevention (CDC) recommends that health care providers continue their traditional role of providing anticipatory guidance on lead poisoning as part of routine well-child care, assessing the risk of exposure to lead, conducting blood lead screenings in children, and treating children who have elevated blood lead levels (BLLs). In addition, the CDC urges health care and social service providers to expand their roles to keep abreast of research data that clarify the relationship between lead exposure and neurocognitive development in children. They can also strongly advocate for children and foster lead exposure prevention by helping facilitate implementation of specific strategic plans to eliminate childhood lead poisoning in their local and state communities. Health care and social service providers are highly effective child advocates, and their active participation in the process provides the expertise and leadership needed to reach this goal. The CDC recommends health care and social service providers to:

- provide culturally appropriate education to all pregnant women and families with young children about the principal sources of lead and ways to reduce exposure
- target outreach, education, and screening programs to populations with the greatest risk of lead exposure
- become aware of, and actively support, lead poisoning elimination efforts in the community
- express concern to federal, state, and local policy and decision makers that children live in a lead-safe environment, actively support legislation and regulatory initiatives, and advocate for lead-safe, affordable housing by supporting appropriate legislation
- become aware of and comply with lead screening policies issued by Medicaid or state and local health departments
- ensure training of staff members engaged in housing renovation or rehabilitation in lead-safe work practices.

sweetener aspartame, which breaks down into two amino acids, including phenylalanine.

The length of time phenylalanine levels remain high is directly proportional to the extent of brain damage and disability. Thus, untreated PKU will cause progressive mental retardation. However, because most cases are identified with neonatal screening, the more serious complications of PKU are rarely seen.

Pediatric Procedures

The medical assistant working in a pediatric office must be able to listen well, speak clearly, and have a solid understanding of a child's normal growth and development in order to effectively interact with pediatric patients and their parents or caregivers. Because pediatric patients may be fearful of the medical office, the medical assistant should try to minimize fear and promote an atmosphere of trust and comfort. For example, when the medical assistant explains procedures to the child and speaks at the child's level of understanding, the child will be relaxed and more likely to cooperate during the interview, examination, or procedure.

When asking questions regarding the patient's health, she should address questions to the child and parent or caregiver, including both in the conversation. If the patient is very young, the medical assistant may want to ask the parent or caregiver what she thinks the problem is. When a parent or caregiver states, "Something is just not right," the medical assistant should take note and listen attentively as the parent or caregiver explains the symptoms she is noticing in the child. The parent or primary caregiver is the best judge of the daily activities of the child and is better able to notice when something "different" is happening—even if changes are subtle. When directing questions to an older child, the medical assistant should encourage the patient, not the adult, to answer the questions if possible. As the pediatric patient ages, usually around age 12, the medical assistant may find it necessary to speak with the patient alone.

The medical assistant should always be truthful with a child regarding any examination or procedure. If a procedure may be painful, she should share that information with the child and the parent or caregiver, assuring them that she will be there for support and encouragement. It may help to encourage the child to express his concerns. In addition, allowing the child to touch and hold pieces of equipment to be used, such as a stethoscope, can create an environment of safety, promoting a healthy relationship between the pediatrician's office and the patient. When explaining examinations or procedures, the medical assistant should avoid using medical terms and abbreviations that the patient and parent or caregiver may not understand.

If a medical assistant does not feel comfortable picking up and holding infants, she should practice using a doll at first and then ask relatives or friends if they would allow her to pick up and hold their infant. The medical assistant must convey confidence to the patient as well as the parent or caregiver.

In the pediatric office, the medical assistant may assist with examinations, perform immunizations and basic laboratory tests, and assist the physician with procedures.

Assisting with Examination
In assisting with the pediatric examination, the medical assistant will obtain vital signs, plot a patient's growth on a chart, and screen for vision and hearing as well as assist the pediatrician with his examination.

Vital Signs
Measurement of vital signs for a child is the same as for an adult, with slight changes in equipment to account for the smaller size of the patient. However, normal values for pediatric vital signs change as the patient grows from infancy through adolescence. Height and weight scales and blood pressure cuffs for a child function in the same manner as those for an adult but are fitted to the pediatric patient.

The medical assistant will measure pediatric vital signs routinely at each office visit. As with adults, pediatric vital signs include height, weight, temperature, respirations, and pulse and also include head circumference. (For more information on the procedure for vital signs measurement, see Chapter 21, page 319.) Blood pressure is not usually assessed until the child is approximately 3 years old. This practice may vary with pediatricians and individual patients. Special examinations may require a blood pressure reading, such as an examination for summer camp or a sports physical.

Height
Equipment for measuring height must be accurate, stable, and fixed. The medical assistant should measure the height, or length, of a child less than age 2 with the child lying down in the supine position, which enables a more accurate measurement. Standard growth charts developed for younger children account for this type of measurement. The medical assistant should ensure that the examination paper on the table is clean and then lay the child down on the paper. Using a pen, she should first make a mark on the examination paper at the crown of the child's head. Then, after ensuring that the child's leg is fully extended and that the child hasn't moved from the initial mark, quickly mark the paper at the heel of the child's foot. The medical assistant should then ask the parent or caregiver to pick up the child and then measure between the marks on the paper.

Children older than age 2 can stand erect against a standing scale or ruler mounted on the wall. The medical assistant should be sure to have the patient remove his shoes before taking the measurement. (See Figure 33-5.) Because accuracy is essential, the medical assistant should measure again if she is unsure of her initial measurement. She should record the length or height of the patient in inches and centimeters in the patient's medical record.

Weight

The medical assistant should weigh the infant without a diaper. If it is necessary to weigh the child with a diaper, the medical assistant should subtract the weight of the diaper after weighing the child. The medical assistant should ask children older than age 2 to stand on a scale. The older child can remain clothed for weight measurement, although his shoes should be off. Because weight gain in older children is more gradual and usually measured only yearly, the amount that clothing would add to the measurement is negligible. (See Figure 33-6.) Some children may refuse to stand on the scale. If a child is unwilling, the medical assistant should ask the parent or caregiver to hold the child in her arms, note the weight of both of them, weigh the parent alone, and then subtract the difference to arrive at the child's weight.

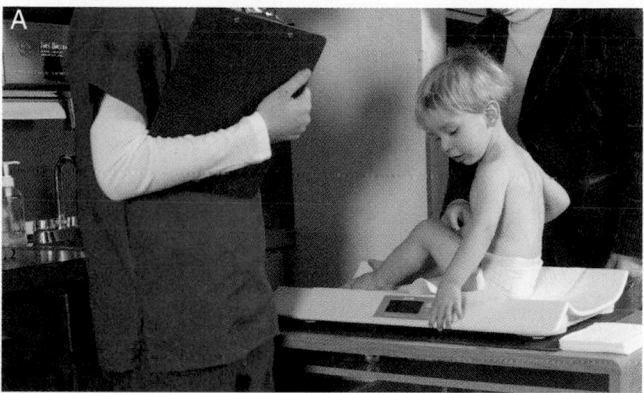

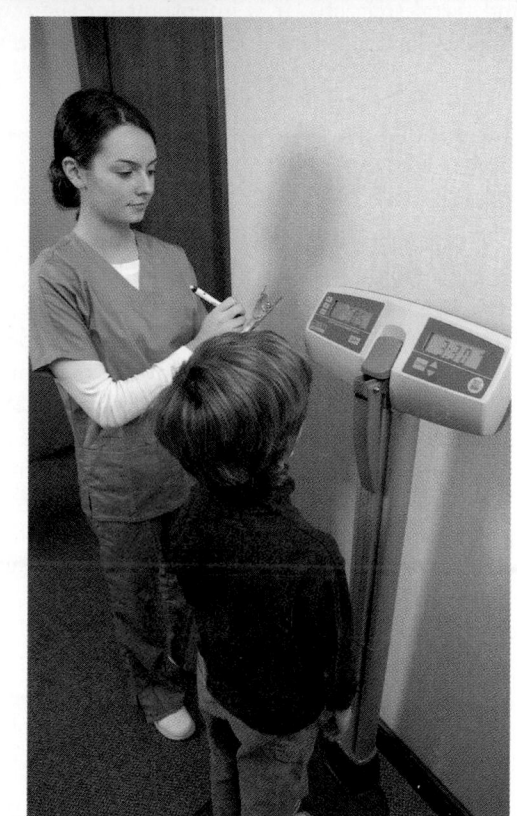

FIG 33-6 Measuring pediatric weight. (A) Measuring an infant. (B) Measuring an older child.

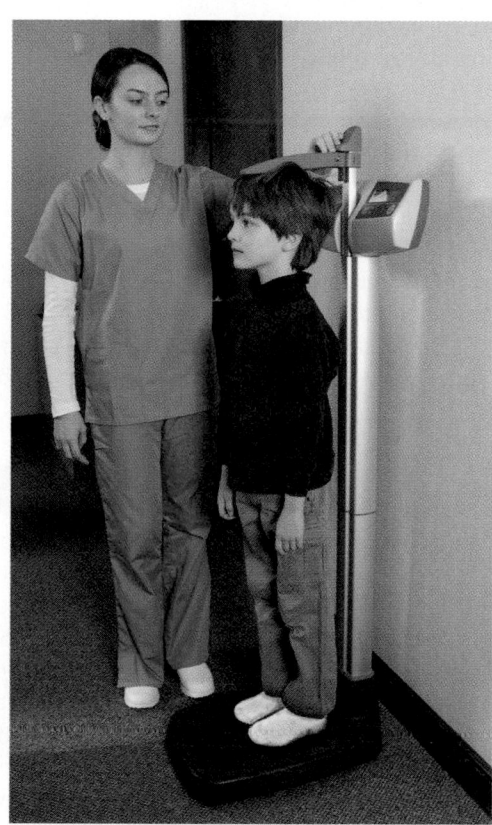

FIG 33-5 Measuring pediatric height for a child over age 2.

(See *Help with pediatric vital signs*, page 664.) As with height, accuracy is essential, so the medical assistant should weigh the child twice if necessary to be sure. She should record the child's weight in pounds and kilograms in the patient's medical record and on the growth chart. (See *Plotting growth*, page 664.) Regardless of the patient, the medical assistant should balance and check the scale for accuracy before every use. In addition, the medical office should coordinate professional calibration of all the scales annually.

Temperature

Body temperature can be measured in Celsius (C) or Fahrenheit (F). Methods of obtaining temperature will vary greatly from office to office. Digital and electronic thermometers are commonly used in pediatrics as well as other areas because they are easy to use and provide a quick reading. The American Academy of Pediatrics (AAP) has discouraged the use of mercury thermometers since 2001. The medical assistant must be sure to use the correct thermometer for the specific route by which she needs to obtain a temperature. Routes for obtaining pediatric temperature include axilla (armpit), oral (mouth), tympanic (ear), and rectal (rectum). It is important for the medical assistant to understand the equipment, so, if necessary, she should read the manufacturer's instructions for the type of thermometer she uses.

To measure axillary temperature, the medical assistant places the thermometer under the infant's or child's arm in the armpit area, or *axilla,* holding it tightly in place with the arm held against the patient's body. She should hold the thermometer in this spot for approximately 1 minute. The axillary method is best for infants older than age 3 months. If the axillary temperature is 99.0°F or higher, the medical assistant should recheck the temperature by using the rectal method for accuracy. She should then document the patient's temperature by recording the number and stating that she obtained the temperature using the axillary method.

To measure oral temperature, the medical assistant places an oral thermometer into the patient's mouth. She should place most oral thermometers under the tongue or in the cheek for 30 seconds to 1 minute and instruct the child to close his lips around the probe without biting down. The child must be old enough to understand these instructions, usually around age 4 or 5. The medical assistant should hold the thermometer in place until the reading is complete, approximately 1 minute (some types are less than 1 minute). She should record the patient's temperature in the medical record, including that she obtained the temperature using the oral route. The medical assistant should not try to obtain an oral temperature if the patient cannot hold the thermometer in his mouth, mouth sores are present, the patient has a history of seizures, or the patient cannot breathe through his nose.

The medical assistant obtains a tympanic temperature by placing a tympanic thermometer into the ear canal. The AAP does not advise using this method for children under age 2. The thermometer measures the heat from the tympanic membrane (eardrum). When using this method in a child, the medical assistant must straighten the ear canal by pulling the pinna (outer cartilage) of the ear down and back. She should then hold the tympanic thermometer in place until a reading appears on the screen or she hears a beep,

---

Front office–Back office connection

Help with Pediatric Vital Signs

The clinical medical assistant may need help from the administrative medical assistant to obtain accurate pediatric vital signs if a child is uncooperative and the parent or caregiver does not wish to help. Some offices establish a special phrase or code word to use to indicate that the back office needs additional help. For example, the clinical medical assistant might discreetly say to the administrative medical assistant, "Staff for room two," or even simply, "Assist in room two." Using these types of phrases will enable the clinical medical assistant to avoid using negative words, such as "difficult patient," within earshot of the patient in the examination room or others in the reception area.

All staff members of the pediatric office should work together to make the patient's visit as pleasant as possible and give the physician the necessary information to make accurate decisions regarding the patient's health.

Plotting growth

The medical assistant must use a standardized growth chart to record a patient's height and weight and another chart for head circumference. These charts were developed based on an average of height, weight, and head circumference for breast-fed and formula-fed infants and children in the United States. The charts are age and sex specific.

The medical assistant should always double-check the measurements before plotting them on the chart. The physician uses this information to compare the patient to other children of the same sex and age. From this comparison, the physician can determine if the child is achieving average growth.

To plot the patient's measurements, the medical assistant must use the appropriate graph for the patient's sex and age group. For example, the following chart shows the growth of a boy from birth to age 3 (36 months). The medical assistant has plotted the boy's height at age 36 months as 37½" and his weight as 31 lb, 8 oz. There is space to record head circumference on the chart; however, the medical assistant should not graph that measurement.

Plotting growth—cont'd

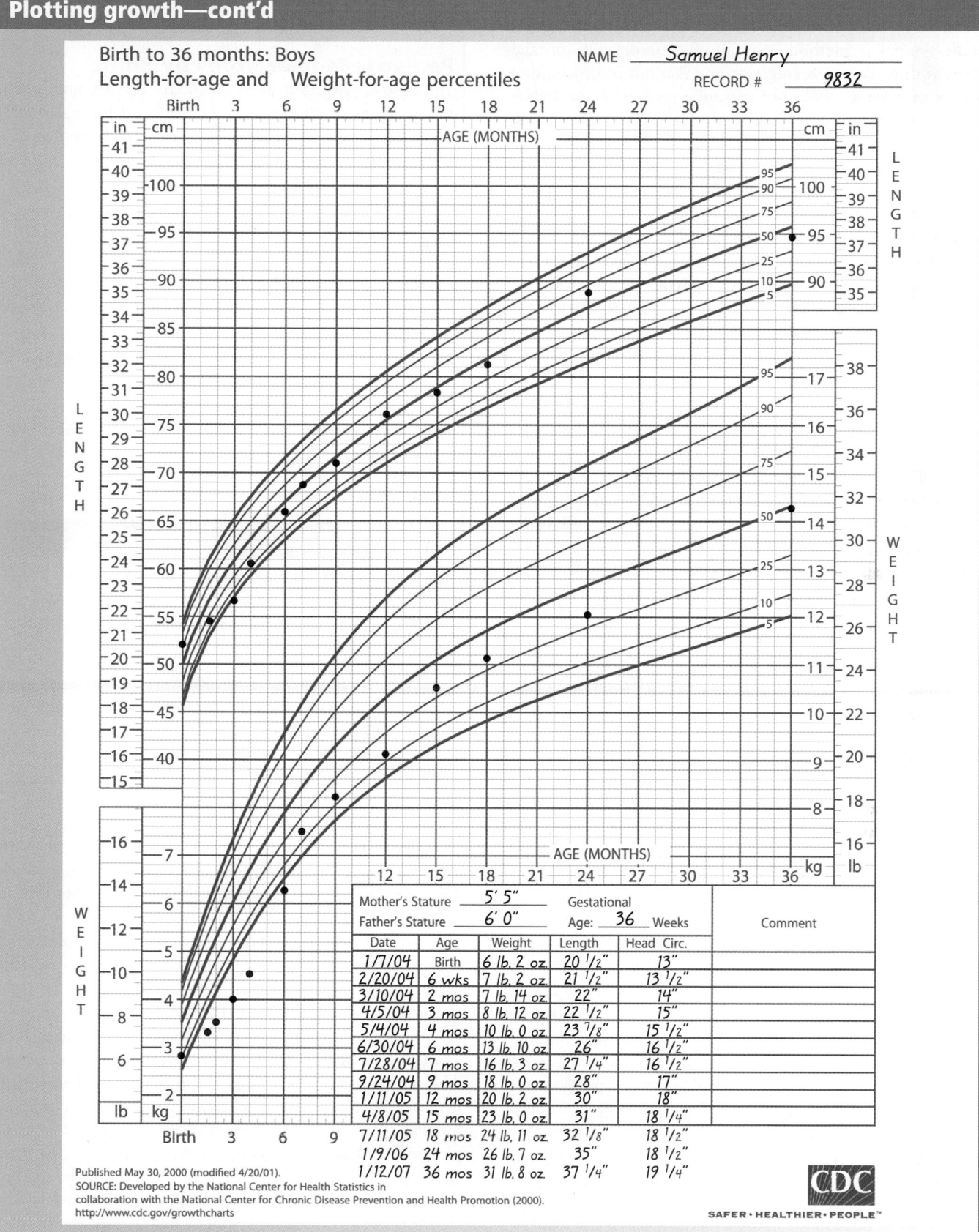

Birth to 36 months: Boys
Length-for-age and   Weight-for-age percentiles

NAME   *Samuel Henry*
RECORD #   ___9832___

Mother's Stature ___5' 5"___
Father's Stature ___6' 0"___
Gestational Age: __36__ Weeks

Comment

Date	Age	Weight	Length	Head Circ.
1/7/04	Birth	6 lb, 2 oz.	20 1/2"	13"
2/20/04	6 wks	7 lb, 2 oz.	21 1/2"	13 1/2"
3/10/04	2 mos	7 lb, 14 oz.	22"	14"
4/5/04	3 mos	8 lb, 12 oz.	22 1/2"	15"
5/4/04	4 mos	10 lb, 0 oz.	23 7/8"	15 1/2"
6/30/04	6 mos	13 lb, 10 oz.	26"	16 1/2"
7/28/04	7 mos	16 lb, 3 oz.	27 1/4"	16 1/2"
9/24/04	9 mos	18 lb, 0 oz.	28"	17"
1/11/05	12 mos	20 lb, 2 oz.	30"	18"
4/8/05	15 mos	23 lb, 0 oz.	31"	18 1/4"
7/11/05	18 mos	24 lb, 11 oz.	32 1/8"	18 1/2"
1/9/06	24 mos	26 lb, 7 oz.	35"	18 1/2"
1/12/07	36 mos	31 lb, 8 oz.	37 1/4"	19 1/4"

Published May 30, 2000 (modified 4/20/01).
SOURCE: Developed by the National Center for Health Statistics in
collaboration with the National Center for Chronic Disease Prevention and Health Promotion (2000).
http://www.cdc.gov/growthcharts

CDC
SAFER · HEALTHIER · PEOPLE™

depending on the device used, and record the patient's temperature in the medical record, including the method used. The tympanic method may be uncomfortable for the patient if he has an ear infection and it is not recommended if there is a large amount of **cerumen** (yellowish waxy substance secreted in the ear canal, also called *earwax*) present in the canal.

The medical assistant obtains a rectal temperature on infants under 3 months of age and when requested by the physician. This method requires a rectal thermometer, which she inserts into the patient's rectum. The rectal route is the most accurate temperature reading for children under age 2 years. However, because most patients do not like this method, many offices use alternatives. The medical assistant should wash her hands and apply gloves before starting this procedure. To measure rectal temperature, the medical assistant must place the patient in a prone or side-lying position and add lubricant to the thermometer to ease insertion. She should insert the thermometer slowly, without force, to approximately 1" (2.5 cm). She should continue to hold the thermometer in place for a specified amount of time, usually about 1 minute. She must never leave the child unattended while checking rectal temperature. She should then remove the thermometer and note the reading, wipe away excess lubricant, and document the patient's temperature, being sure to record the rectal route. Rectal temperature greater than 100.5°F in children less than 3 months of age requires immediate attention. The medical assistant should not use the rectal route if the patient has diarrhea, hemorrhoids, or any other disorder than may make this procedure uncomfortable. (See *Pediatric temperatures by route*.)

Respirations

When the infant is resting calmly, the medical assistant should measure respirations by watching the rise and fall of his chest and abdomen. During inspiration, the chest rises and, during expiration, it falls. One inspiration and expiration count as one respiration. Respirations are sometimes difficult to count in neonates and infants because these rates are more rapid than an adult's. Average respirations for an adult are 12 to 20 breaths (respirations) per minute, and normal respirations for an infant or young child can be 30 to 60 breaths/minute. (See *Normal pediatric respiratory rates*.) If the patient is crying or fearful, the results may be inaccurate. If necessary, the medical assistant should attempt to calm the patient or ask the parent or caregiver to try to calm the patient. She should count respirations for 1 full minute and record the number in the patient's medical record.

Pulse

Pulse, or *heart rate,* is commonly described as the "lub dub" identifying sounds made by the valves in the heart as

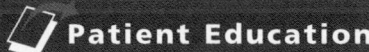

Patient Education

Pediatric Temperatures by Route

The medical assistant can explain to parents and caregivers of small children that the route of measurement will affect the normal range for a child's temperature. Here are the normal ranges for each route:

- axillary—94.5° to 99.1°F (34.7° to 37.3°C)
- oral—95.9° to 99.5°F (35.5° to 37.5°C)
- tympanic—94.5° to 99.1°F (34.7° to 34.3°C)
- rectal—97.9° to 100.4°F (36.6° to 38°C).

Fever in children is classified as temperature of 100.5°F (36.6°C) or higher. The medical assistant should instruct parents and caregivers on how to accurately obtain their child's temperature. In addition, she should warn parents about some methods that garner questionable results, including fever strips placed on the forehead and other types of disposable thermometers, which are not as accurate.

Normal pediatric respiratory rates

Because a child's normal respiratory rate varies as he grows, the medical assistant must know the normal values for infants, children, adolescents, and adults. These values include:

- neonates and infants—30 to 60 breaths/minute
- children ages 1 to 7 years—18 to 30 breaths/minute
- older children ages 8 to 18 and adults—12 to 20 breaths/minute.

the chambers relax and contract. Heart rate in neonates and infants is higher than in older children and adults. The average pulse in adults is 60 to 72 beats/minute and the average pulse in infants and young children can be 100 to 160 beats/ minute. The medical assistant must count the pulse in pediatric patients for 1 full minute. (See *Normal pediatric pulse rates*.) She must also monitor the rhythm of the pulse, noting if it is regular or irregular.

To measure the pulse of a patient under age 5, the medical assistant should measure the apical pulse with a stethoscope. The apical pulse site is located at the apex of the heart at the fifth intercostal space to the left of the sternum. The medical assistant may need to count rib spaces for accuracy and placement of the stethoscope by palpating the patient's chest. The medical assistant can measure the pulse in children over age 5 by palpating the radial or brachial artery and counting for 1 minute. She should then record the number

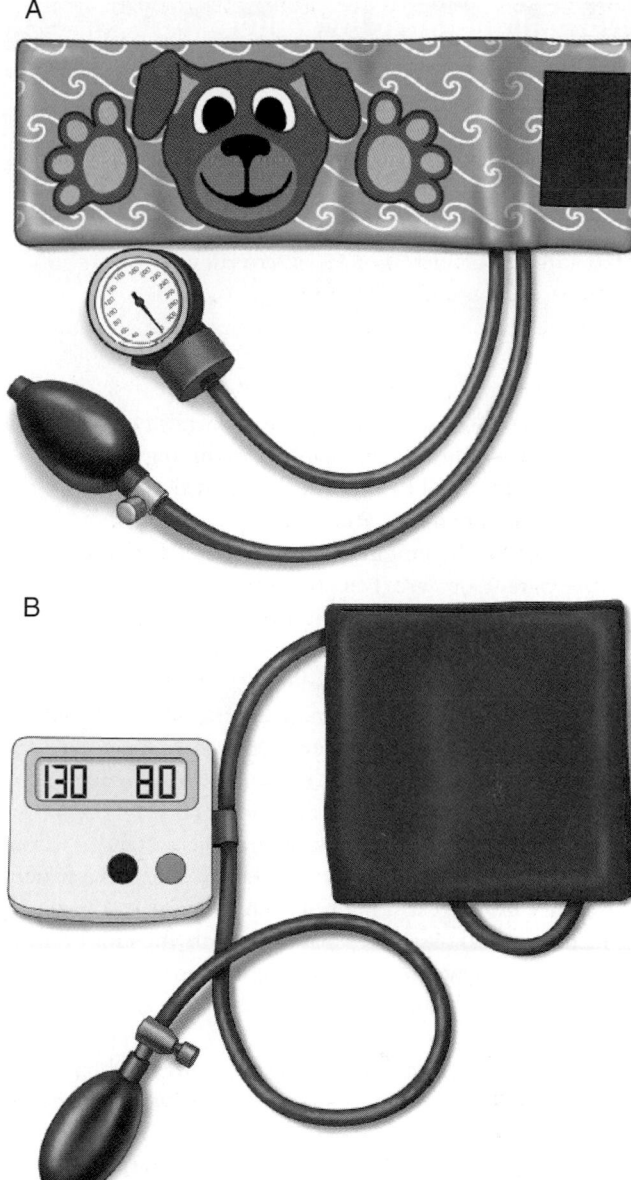

FIG 33-7 Pediatric sphygmomanometers. (A) Aneroid. (B) Digital.

in the patient's medical record along with the rhythm and method of measurement.

Blood Pressure

Blood pressure measurement is routine in pediatric patients after age 3. Blood pressure is measured in millimeters of mercury (mm Hg). The measurement is uncommon in the neonate unless the pediatrician suspects an abnormality. Blood pressure in children is lower than in adults. As a child grows in age and size, normal values increase and, eventually, approach normal adult values, which are 120 to 139/80 to 89 mm Hg. (See *Normal pediatric BP values,* page 668.)

To obtain the blood pressure of a pediatric patient, the medical assistant must make sure the blood pressure cuff is the appropriate size. Using the wrong size may cause the blood pressure reading to be falsely high or low. To measure blood pressure, the medical assistant can use a digital or an aneroid sphygmomanometer. (See Figure 33-7.) The medical office may have a wall-mounted device in each examination room or a stand that the medical assistant can move from one room to another. If the medical assistant is uncertain about how to use the equipment, she should read through the manufacturer's instruction manual.

Because a young child may be frightened of the equipment and what it will do, the medical assistant should explain to the patient that the cuff will give their arm a "hug" and then the hug will lessen while she listens with her stethoscope. She should make sure the patient's arm is resting and the patient is relaxed. If the medical assistant has difficulty obtaining a blood pressure measurement, she can use a handheld Doppler ultrasound device, which measures the blood flow in the major arteries and veins of the arms or legs. She must place the Doppler probe over the artery where she would normally place the stethoscope to magnify the sounds, making them easier to hear. After she measures the blood pressure, the medical assistant should record the number in the patient's medical record, being sure to include which of the patient's arms she used.

Head Circumference

The medical assistant should measure head circumference at every well-child examination starting at birth and continuing until age 3. Typically, the medical assistant should measure head circumference last, because most infants and children become upset when the medical assistant places the measuring device around their heads, which makes accurate measurement of temperature, pulse, respirations, and blood pressure difficult. The medical assistant should measure at least twice for accuracy, asking the caregiver or another medical assistant for help if needed to stabilize the

Normal pediatric BP values

The normal resting blood pressure (BP) rate for children varies from birth to adolescence. Normal resting pediatric BP rates include:

- birth to age 1—95/70 mm Hg
- toddler to school-age child—100/70 mm Hg
- children ages 6 to 13—110/74 mm Hg
- children ages 14 to 18—120/76 mm Hg.

child's head. She should place the measuring tape on the most prominent points of the head, including the forehead and occipital bone. The medical assistant should record the measurement in inches and centimeters. She should also make a copy of the height, weight, and head circumference for the parent or caregiver and encourage her to keep a record at home.

Vision Screening

To perform a pediatric vision screening test, the medical assistant will use the Snellen eye chart. The pediatric Snellen chart has pictures for the patient to identify or the letter E pointing in different directions. (See Figure 33-8.) The medical assistant must ask the patient to stand 20" from the chart and should conduct the test by asking the patient to identify the largest item and then progress to the smallest. The medical assistant's patience with the child during the examination will promote cooperation. If the child views the examination as fun or a game, he will be interested and involved in the testing.

Early diagnosis and treatment of vision problems will help the child with schoolwork and participation in activities. If the child requires corrective lenses for vision problems, the pediatrician will refer the patient to an optometrist. Durable corrective lenses that resist breakage and scratches are best for children so they can participate in sports and other activities without worry or risk of injury from broken lenses.

Hearing Screening

The medical assistant may perform a hearing screening in the pediatric office or at a school. Hearing testing for infants and small children who cannot follow specific instructions involves assessment using visual reinforcement audiometry (VRA). In this test, the child sits on the parent's lap in the center of the testing room with speakers having toys mounted inside to the right and left of the child. When the child responds correctly by turning toward the source of a sound, the tester can animate the toy in that speaker as a positive reinforcement for responding to the sound. As the

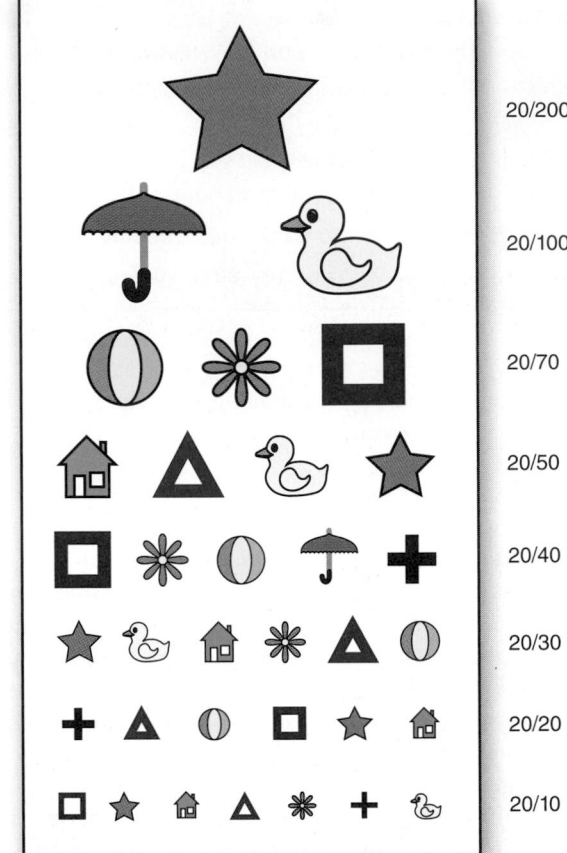

	20/200
	20/100
	20/70
	20/50
	20/40
	20/30
	20/20
	20/10

FIG 33-8 Pediatric Snellen charts.

child becomes conditioned to seeing the animated toy when he hears the sound, he will indicate hearing ability by turning to the toy whenever he hears the sound (before the animation). Older children who can follow instructions are tested using the same audiometer as adults. (For more information on audiometry testing, see Chapter 36, page 745.)

Early diagnosis of hearing problems is important for the child's performance in school and her interactions with friends and family. Some hearing deficits are related to infection and can be treated and resolved. Other hearing problems may not be reversible; however, treatment with a hearing aid may enable the child to overcome the disadvantages of hearing loss.

Well-Child Examination

Well-child examinations should occur at regular intervals to assess growth and development. The goals of a well-child examination are to:

- establish a trusting relationship between the pediatric patient, his parents or caregivers, and health care professionals

- promote health through education and immunizations
- prevent problems and diseases
- provide early detection of problems if present.

Well-child examinations are also a time to reinforce healthy behaviors and provide caregivers with education regarding nutrition, safety, sleep, development, and discipline. (See *Teaching wellness and prevention.*) During the well-child examination, the pediatrician will do a head-to-toe physical examination, including general appearance, eyes (basic examination), ears, muscle tone, reflexes, spinal alignment, and immunization evaluation. In preparation for the physician's examination, the medical assistant must ask some questions regarding the patient's current health status and lifestyle. Some medical offices have a standard form the

---

Patient Education

Teaching Wellness and Prevention

The pediatrician's office is a place where the medical assistant can educate caregivers and children on wellness and prevention strategies to promote optimal growth and development for every child. New parents need accurate information regarding nutrition, safety, and prevention of illness and injuries. Even experienced parents need education on new guidelines and prevention strategies.

When providing patient education for a child and her family, the medical assistant should ensure that the discussion takes place in a safe environment where conversation is relaxed and unhurried. The medical assistant must listen carefully to the concerns and questions of pediatric patients and their caregivers. Adolescents may not want a parent present during the examination or history taking. The medical assistant and pediatrician should honor such wishes, and the medical assistant can reassure adolescents that the staff will maintain strict confidentiality.

Here are some important topics to cover when advising patients and caregivers on safety and accident prevention:

- *Infant and child cardiopulmonary resuscitation (CPR)*—The American Red Cross offers courses in infant and child CPR as well as first aid. The medical assistant can direct parents to their community's hospital or fire station for classes.

- *Car seat safety*—The medical assistant can refer parents to the American Academy of Pediatrics for information on car seat installation and safety. Also, some local police or fire stations offer annual car seat safety clinics.

- *Bike helmets*—Head injuries from falls from a bicycle can be devastating, even fatal. The medical assistant can suggest to parents that they can lead by example and wear helmets to cycle with their children.

- *Outlet safety*—The medical assistant should instruct parents or caregivers to cover outlets with a plastic plug cover and avoid leaving exposed electrical cords where children could trip or pull down an appliance such as an iron.

- *Fire safety*—The medical assistant should encourage parents to make sure there are adequate numbers of smoke detectors in the home and ensure that all smoke detectors have working batteries. She can suggest that parents discuss and practice with their children evacuation procedures in case of fire as well as a safe place to meet outside. The well-prepared child is less likely to panic in case of an emergency such as a fire.

- *Accidental poisoning*—The medical assistant should provide the phone number for the Poison Control hotline (at the CDC in Atlanta, Georgia) and instruct parents and caregivers to call if they suspect their child has ingested a poisonous substance. She should tell them to follow instructions from poison control. She should also emphasize that the parent should never induce vomiting before calling poison control. Some poisons are caustic and can cause burning of the esophagus if vomited.

- *Babysitting safety*—The medical assistant can advise parents on general babysitting guidelines, such as leaving a contact number where they can be reached and leaving other emergency numbers, such as the pediatrician's number or a neighbor's number near the phone. In addition, she can explain that many communities offer babysitting certification to teens and adults as well as infant and child CPR, basic first aid, and prevention of injuries and choking.

- *Safe and nutritious snacks*—The medical assistant should advise parents to cut grapes in half, cut hot dogs lengthwise rather than in circles, and ensure that all foods for their infant or toddler are cut into small, bite-sized pieces to prevent choking.

- *Basic first aid*—The medical assistant should advise parents to keep a supply of bandages, gauze pads, and antibiotic creams for administering first aid to children. She should also remind parents to wash wounds and seek medical attention for deep cuts, burns, or suspected broken bones. If a child develops a fever after injury, the parent should bring the child to the office for examination because he could have an infection. The medical assistant should emphasize that a child who suffers a head injury must always undergo examination by a physician.

medical assistant can use as a guide to ask all necessary questions of the parent or caregiver. (See *Well-child examination questions*.)

Well-child examinations should typically occur at 2 or 3 days after birth, 2 weeks, 2 months, 4 months, 6 months, 9 months, 12 months, 15 months, 2 years, then once per year from ages 2 to 5, and then at ages 8 and 10. (See *Neonatal special considerations*.) Some variation can occur with individual pediatricians and the individual needs of the patient.

Apgar Score

The first neonatal examination is done immediately following birth in the hospital. The pediatrician performs a head-to-toe assessment of the neonate 1 minute following birth and then again at 5 minutes following birth. During this examination, the physician uses the Apgar scoring system to evaluate five distinct categories of the neonate:

- muscle tone
- color

Well-child examination questions

At the beginning of the well-child examination, the medical assistant must ask the pediatric patient or caregiver some questions. Some of the most common questions to ask include:

- Is the baby breastfeeding or using formula? If using formula, what brand?
- If the child is older than 6 months, what types of food is he eating?

- What does the child drink?
- How often does the child have a bowel movement?
- What are the child's sleeping habits?

The following form is one example of a standard form used to obtain such information during the well-child examination.

Well-Child Examination

Age in weeks or months: *4 months*

Height: *26¼"*   Weight: *14 lb, 12 oz*   Head circumference: *16¾"*

Nutrition

(Breast milk)   Formula   Solid foods: baby food or table food

Vitamins: *Poly Vi Sol one dropper per day*

Well water or city water: *city*

Bowel movements: *4 x day*

Sleep patterns: *waking to nurse every 2 to 3 hours*

Family/living situation: *stay at home mother, father, 3-year-old sibling*

Siblings: *one brother, 3 years old*

Pets: *cat*

Second-hand smoke: *Father smokes, only outside*

Activities:
Reaches for toys, shakes rattle; studies toys in hand; puts "everything" in mouth; plays with fingers; laughs, giggles; recognizes mom and dad; knows mom is there when out of sight; turns in response to noise; smiles and coos in response to talking; rolls from side to side; pulls head and chest off floor when on stomach; supports head when sitting; kicks legs; focuses clearly on toy and faces

4/28/09; 10:30 a.m. ————————————————————— S. Gonzales, CMA

- respirations
- heart rate
- response to stimuli.

Each of the five categories is given a score of 0, 1, or 2. The Apgar score is expected to increase from the 1-minute exam to the 5-minute exam for healthy neonates. The physician may need to know the Apgar scoring of a neonate, contained in the neonate's hospital medical record, during the follow-up visit when the neonate is several days to several weeks old. (See *Apgar scor.*)

Neonatal special considerations

When seen in the pediatric office, the very young infant requires some special attention to the umbilical cord and circumcision aftercare.

Umbilical Cord Care

During a neonatal examination, the medical assistant should inspect the umbilical cord to ensure that it is shrinking and is not infected. Parents were once instructed to clean the umbilical stump with alcohol or hydrogen peroxide. However, new research suggests that the stump will actually heal faster if left alone. If the area becomes sticky with blood, the MA can instruct the parent to clean the umbilical cord with soap and water. To dry the area, the parent can hold a clean absorbent cloth around the stump and dry the area with a hairdryer on a low setting.

The medical assistant should instruct the parent to alert the pediatrician if there is a foul odor around the cord or if the baby has a fever, as these are signs of infection. The umbilical cord should shrink in size and become progressively dried out until it eventually falls off. Most babies' umbilical cords fall off within the first 3 weeks of life.

Circumcision Care

A **circumcision** is a surgical procedure to remove the foreskin, or *prepuce,* which is the loose fold of skin that covers the penis. It is commonly performed for medical, religious, or cultural reasons. It may be done by a pediatrician a day after the baby's birth or it may be performed by a rabbi in a ceremony known as a bris. The medical assistant may need to instruct parents on cleaning the penis after the procedure. After circumcision, the area should be gently washed daily with soap and water. After cleaning, an antibiotic ointment may be applied to prevent infection. Depending on the surgical technique, there may or may not be a healing incision. If there is an incision, the parents must change the wound dressing with each diaper change. The medical assistant should instruct parents on how to change the dressing. The infant may be fussy while the wound is healing; the pediatrician may prescribe an analgesic ointment for pain control. The penis should heal in 7 to 10 days.

Apgar score

The Apgar score, developed by Dr. Virginia Apgar in 1952, is named after Dr. Apgar; a mnemonic using the letters of her name helps medical professionals remember the five categories assessed in this scoring system:

- **A**ctivity (muscle tone)
- **P**ulse (heart rate)
- **G**rimace (reflex irritability)
- **A**ppearance (color)
- **R**espiration (respiratory effort).

The following table outlines the Apgar score scale used to score a neonate's overall health based on these categories.

Sign	Score		
	0	*1*	*2*
Muscle tone	Flaccid	Some flexion	Active motion of extremities
Heart rate	Not detectable	Below 100	Over 100
Reflex irritability (response to flick on sole)	No response	Grimace, slow motion	Cry
Color	Blue, pale	Body pink, extremities blue	Completely pink
Respiratory effort	Absent	Slow, irregular	Good, crying

Denver Developmental Screening Tool

The pediatrician may also perform a developmental assessment using a test such as the Denver II Developmental Screening Tool (DDST) for children from age 1 month to age 6 years. Although children develop at varying rates, failure to develop or slowed development in one or more of the categories is used to identify developmental delays. Infants and children identified as developmentally delayed can benefit from early diagnosis and treatment. The DDST measures four aspects of development:

- *gross motor skills* to evaluate the child's coordination of large muscle groups. The infant at 3 to 4 months is evaluated for head and neck control and the ability to roll over and bear weight on his legs. The 10-month-old should be able to stand holding on to an object for balance, pull himself to a standing position, and get to a sitting position. The 3-year-old child should be able to balance on one foot for 1 second and do a broad jump.
- *language* to evaluate the child's ability to comprehend language and, later, use language. The 3- to 4-month-old should be able to vocalize "ooh, aah," laugh, or squeal. The 10-month-old should be able to babble with varying syllables and may say "dada" or "mama." At age 3 years, the child should be able to name pictures and an adult should be able to understand at least half of his speech.
- *fine motor skills* to evaluate the child's control of fine motor muscles and hand-eye coordination. The 3- to 4-month-old should be able to follow an object to midline with his eyes and then follow past midline as well as grasp a rattle. The 10-month-old should be able to thumb-finger grasp, bang two blocks held in his hands, and, possibly, put a block into a cup. The 3-year-old can make a tower of 8 blocks, wiggle his thumbs, and, possibly, draw a circle.
- *personal and social skills* to evaluate the child's socialization and self-confidence. The 3- to 4-month-old should smile responsively and begin to smile spontaneously. The 10-month-old can wave good-bye, indicate his needs and wants, and play "pat-a-cake." The 3-year-old will name his friends, wash his hands, and put on clothing.

The cooperation of the child is important for accurate test findings. If abnormal results are obtained, the child should be screened again in 1 to 2 weeks. The parent should be instructed to make sure that the child is fed and well rested for the rescreening.

Sports Physical Examination

Schools and private sports clubs require children to undergo a physical examination before participating. Schools will send an examination form to students for completion by the pediatrician's office. The medical assistant can perform and record results for many of the tests required, including height, weight, vital signs, and urinalysis. The physician will listen to the heart and lungs, palpate the abdomen, and examine the eyes and ears to rule out disorders that would put the athlete in danger, such as a heart murmur, decreased lung function, or organomegaly (enlargement of visceral organs that indicates some form of pathology). The physician will also observe the child's gait (manner and style of walking) to see if he has problems with coordination or injury to the back or lower extremities. She will also ask the patient to bend forward from the waist to rule out scoliosis, a lateral (side) curvature of the spine. If the child has asthma, the physician will determine the severity of the asthma by asking the patient how often he uses his inhaler. If the risk of an exercise-induced asthma attack is severe, the physician cannot clear the child to participate in sports. The medical assistant may be required to record findings while the physician examines the child. The sports physical examination form must be signed by the physician or his agent (medical assistant or nurse) prior to the child's participation in sports. (See *Sports physical season.*)

Sick-Child Examination

Sick children make up about 50% of the pediatrician's office schedule. During cold and flu season, most of the daily schedule may concern sick children. The medical assistant will measure the sick child's vital signs and ask questions regarding the onset and symptoms of the illness. A thorough health history of the current illness is important when a child is ill. The pediatrician will then do a thorough examination, based on the health history and other factors. Some offices have a standard form the medical assistant can fill out for a sick-child examination. (See *Sick-child examination questions.*) The administrative and clinical medical assistants should be aware of the needs of sick children in the examination and reception areas. (See *Comforting sick children in reception*, page 674.)

Front office–Back office connection

Sports Physical Season

In many communities, schools require sports physical examinations prior to the start of the new school year. The administrative medical assistant who schedules appointments should discuss with the physician and clinical staff what the best scheduling strategies might be for this busy time. Offering an evening of only sports physicals or a Saturday sports physical examination clinic may alleviate the burden of working these examinations into busy days.

Sick-child examination questions

At the beginning of the sick-child examination, the medical assistant must ask the pediatric patient or caregiver some questions. Some of the most common questions to ask include:

- How long have you noticed a change or difference in your child?
- Is the child eating and drinking?

- Does the child have diarrhea?
- Has there been a change in the child's sleep patterns?
- Have you given the child any medications?
- Is there anyone else in the household who is ill?

The form shown here is one example of a standard form used to obtain such information during the sick-child examination.

Sick-Child Examination

Child's age in weeks or months: __4 years__

Height: __38"__ Weight: __43 lb__ Head circumference: __NA__

Temperature: __101.8° F__

Eating
What?   When last?
milk, macaroni and cheese, grapes   Last night 5:30 p.m., no breakfast,
                                       he felt too sick, did sip water

Drinking
What?   When last?
water, will only take small sips   9 a.m.
Nausea:
yes, today and last night

Vomiting
How many times?   When last?
2x   1 a.m. this morning
Diarrhea
How many times?   When last?
none   NA

Date of injury or first sign of illness:
Last night 6 p.m., after dinner cried, complained of "tummy hurts"

Sleep pattern:
usually sleeps well, mother reports 8 p.m. to 6 a.m. sleeping is routine.
Last night he was up crying at 10 p.m.; vomited, midnight, crying, 1 a.m.
and vomited again

4/14/08; 9:50 a.m. --- S. Gonzalez, CMA

Reporting Abuse

The Child Abuse Prevention and Treatment Act (CAPTA) of 1996 requires physicians in all 50 states to report suspected child abuse and neglect. The act was originally passed in 1974 and has been amended several times. Every state has a hotline for reporting abuse and neglect that is available to anyone who suspects that a child is in danger. In 2002, 1.8 million cases of child abuse were reported; 896,000 were confirmed as abuse, affecting boys and girls equally. Approximately 1,400 children died in the United States in 2002 as a result of abuse and neglect; of those, 1,000 were under age 4. Approximately 900 of the fatalities were due to neglect. Children from birth to age 3 years are at the highest risk for abuse. Unfortunately, 80% of the abusers are the child's parents, and 58% of all abusers are female.

The presentation of any symptoms of abuse warrants immediate reporting to state authorities. The medical assistant must follow the guidelines of her state. If the pediatrician and medical assistant feel that the child is in imminent danger, they may call social services to the office to remove

Comforting Sick Children in Reception

The administrative medical assistant working at the front desk can offer a sick child and her parents a treatment room or private area of the waiting room for their comfort. Doing so will separate sick children from well children and prevent the spread of infection. Tissues, access to a bathroom, and a cup of water may also comfort the sick child and her caregiver.

The administrative medical assistant should also notify the clinical medical assistants of the sick child so that they can try to obtain a treatment room quickly, make sure the child is comfortable in the room, and keep waiting time for the physician to a minimum.

the child from the abuser immediately. Representatives from child protective services can work with the physician to determine the likelihood of continued abuse and identify the best interests of the child. They may place the child with relatives or in foster care. Alternatively, they may order the abusive family member be removed from the home and, possibly, incarcerated. Protective hospitalization may be required for children with severe injuries.

The medical assistant should be sure to note in the patient's chart any signs or symptoms of abuse and neglect, including signs of physical abuse, sexual abuse, or neglect. She should then notify the physician of these signs.

Physical Abuse

Signs and symptoms of physical abuse include:

- skin lesions that look like they were produced by an object or by a hand slap
- long, bandlike bruises from a belt
- small, round burns from cigarettes
- symmetrical scald burns from being intentionally immersed in hot water
- bite marks
- bald patches on the scalp from hair being pulled
- bone fractures, especially in children who do not yet walk (a sign of throwing the child or hitting him with great force)
- a baby that is comatose or stuporous and, possibly, has retinal hemorrhages (from being vigorously shaken)
- child's excessive fear of the parent or caregiver.

Sexual Abuse

Most commonly, sexually abused children are ashamed of the abuse and are told by the abuser not to tell anyone. This combination of fear and shame makes diagnosis difficult. Behavioral changes can include:

- phobias
- sleep disturbance
- bedwetting
- sexual knowledge inappropriate for the child's age.

Physical signs of sexual abuse include:

- sexually transmitted diseases (STDs)
- bruising
- tearing in the rectum or vagina
- vaginal discharge or pruritis.

Neglect

Signs of neglect include:

- malnutrition
- fatigue
- lethargy
- lack of appropriate clothing
- lack of hygiene
- failure to thrive.

Immunizations

Routine childhood immunizations are state mandated and required for children who attend public schools. When a patient comes to the office for immunizations during a well-child examination, the medical assistant should provide the parent with a recommended immunization schedule and a vaccine information sheet (VIS) for each vaccine administered during that visit. (See *Immunization schedule*.) The VIS explains the safety and efficacy of the vaccine as well as possible adverse reactions and when to contact a physician if the parent is concerned. The pediatrician is obligated by law to provide parents with a VIS statement that outlines the risks and benefits associated with vaccines. (See *VIS*, page 676.) Some states also have informed consent laws that require a parent's signature before administration of a vaccine.

Vaccine Registry

Some states use a database for recording and displaying immunization information for children within that state or region. For example, the Regional Early Childhood Immunization Network (RECIN) is a vaccine database for the northern Wisconsin area. Each child should receive 17 to 18 doses of vaccine by age 2. Because a child may go to different providers to get immunizations, it can be difficult to ensure that the child is getting the proper immunizations at the proper time. A vaccine registry is a way of accessing patient vaccination information outside the pediatric office. The medical assistant should enter vaccination information, including the patient's name, the date of the vaccine, and any reaction to the vaccine into the common database. If the parent brings the child to a different provider, the new office can access the database. This system helps ensure that children do not receive extra doses of the same vaccine or miss a vaccine. The medical assistant should

Immunization schedule

An immunization schedule enables the medical office to inform parents and caregivers of the immunization recommendations of the Centers for Disease Control and Prevention (CDC). The CDC gives specific guidelines for the age at which a child should receive a vaccine as well as how many times he should receive the vaccine. Although the CDC strongly recommends that parents or caregivers follow these guidelines, parents may elect to delay a vaccine for any reason, including illness or allergy. Many pediatricians also routinely delay administration of a vaccine if the child is ill.

The complete immunization schedule includes ranges for catch-up immunizations for children who were incompletely immunized as well as recommendations for high-risk populations. The following table lists the general immunization schedule. Many immunizations are given in several doses over a period of time. Multiple doses are indicated in the table by a number in parentheses.

Age Range	Immunization
Birth	• Hepatitis (Hep) B (1)
1 to 4 months	• Hep B (2)
2 months	• Rotavirus (Rota) (1) • Diphtheria and tetanus toxoids and acellular pertussis (DTaP) (1) • *Haemophilus influenzae* type B conjugate (Hib) (1) • Pneumococcal conjugate vaccine (PCV) (1) • Inactivated poliovirus (IPV) (1)
4 months	• Rota (2) • DTaP (2) • Hib (2) • PCV (2) • IPV (2)
6 months	• Rota (3) • DTap (3) • Hib (3) • PCV (3)
6 to 18 months	• Hep B (3) • IPV (3)
12 to 15 months	• Hib (4) • PCV (4) • Measles, mumps, rubella (MMR) (1) • Varicella (1)
15 to 18 months	• DTaP (4)
12 months to 23 months	• Hep A (1 and 2*)
6 months to 5 years	• Influenza (yearly)
4 to 6 years	• DTaP (5) • IPV (4) • MMR (2) • Varicella (2)
11 to 12 years	• Tetanus and diphtheria toxoids and acellular pertussis (Tdap) • HPV (1, 2, and 3**) • MCV4

*Separated by at least 6 months
** Administered to females only with 2 months separating first and second dose and 6 months separating second and third dose

VIS

The medical assistant must provide a vaccine information sheet (VIS) each time for each vaccine administered at the time of vaccination. Doing so ensures that the parents or caregivers understand the risks and benefits as well as what complications to look for, including a rash and swelling, and when to seek medical attention for a severe reaction.

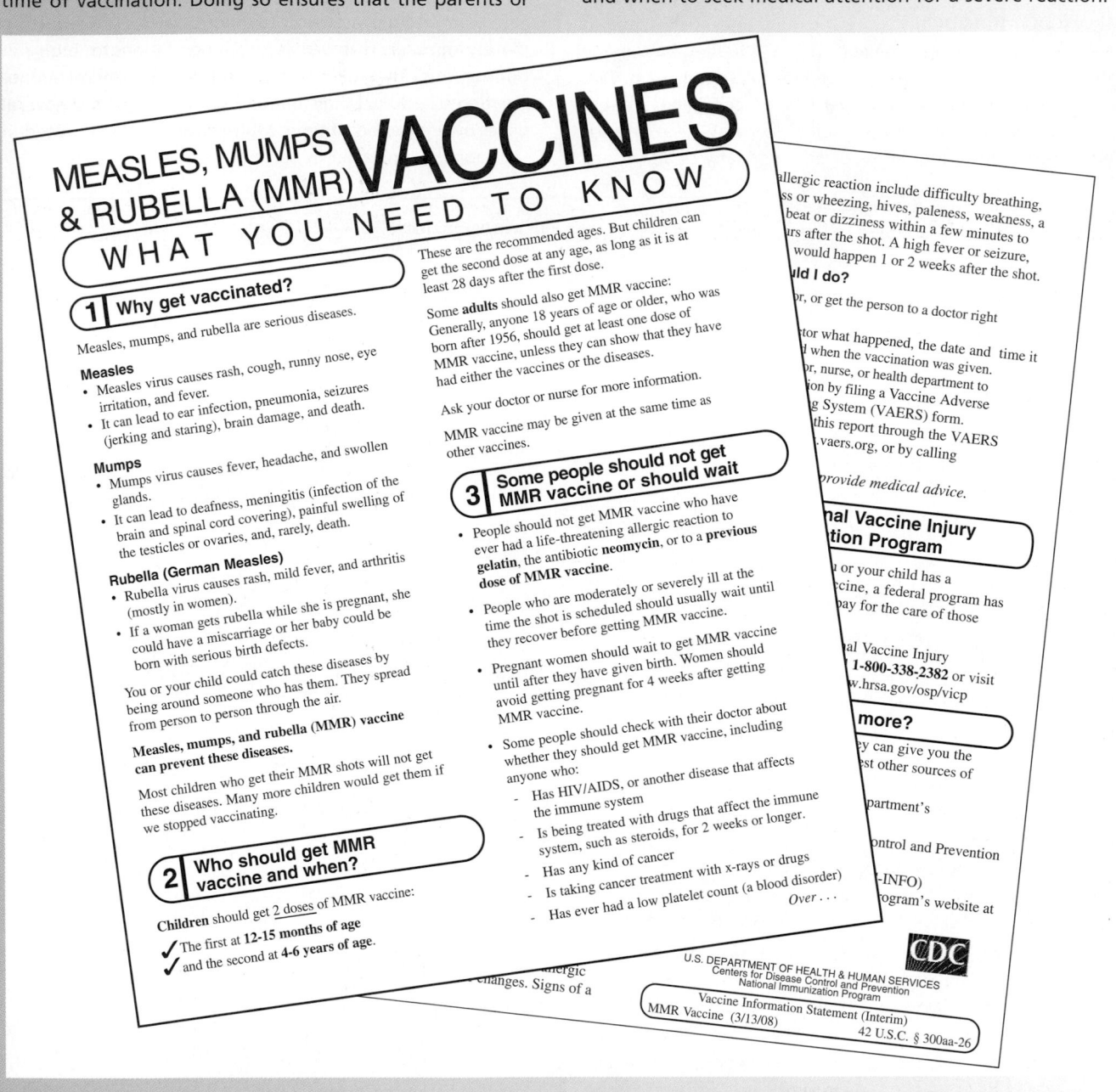

research her local area to see if a common vaccine database is available.

Objections to Vaccination

Some parents or caregivers may have religious, cultural, or medical beliefs that cause them to object to immunizations.

If a parent or caregiver will not allow the child to be vaccinated, the physician has no legal authority to administer the vaccine. In such an instance, the medical assistant should still provide the parent with the vaccine information sheet and tell her that the vaccines are available if she changes her mind.

Pediatric Laboratory Tests

The most common laboratory tests performed in pediatrics are urinalysis, hemoglobin and hematocrit, and rapid *Strep* tests.

Urinalysis

Obtaining a urine sample from a child can be challenging. A child may be uncooperative or unable to urinate. Depending on the age of the patient, the medical assistant can ask the parent or caregiver to go into the bathroom with the child and collect the specimen. She should convey instructions for a clean-catch or midstream urine specimen collection to the parent or child depending on the child's age and maturity level. (For information on specimen collection, see Chapter 44, page xxx.)

If a physician orders a urine sample from an infant who is too young to use the toilet, the medical assistant must obtain the sample using a collection bag. This procedure requires the cooperation of the parent or caregiver. (See *Procedure 33-1: Collecting a urine specimen from an infant.*)

PROCEDURE 33-1

Collecting a urine specimen from an infant

Task
Collect an uncontaminated urine specimen from an infant.

Conditions
- Nonsterile disposable gloves
- Antiseptic wipes
- Sterile water and sterile gauze squares
- Pediatric urine collection bag
- Sterile urine specimen container and label

Standards
In the time specified and within the scoring parameters determined by the instructor, the student will successfully collect a urine specimen from an infant.

Performance Standards
1. Wash your hands to ensure infection control.
2. Assemble the equipment and supplies and check the order in the patient's medical record.
3. Greet the patient and caregiver. Explain the procedure to the caregiver and answer any questions.
4. Apply gloves.
5. Position the infant in the supine position and remove the diaper. Ask the caregiver to position the infant with legs apart.
6. Clean the child's genitalia thoroughly with the antiseptic wipes to prevent contamination of the urine sample.
   a. For a girl, clean the urinary meatus from front to back using a separate wipe for each side. Use a third wipe to clean directly over the urinary meatus, again from front to back to prevent contamination from the anal area. Rinse the area thoroughly with sterile water and a sterile gauze. Dry the area with sterile gauze to enable an airtight seal between the collection bag and the patient's skin.
   b. For a boy who is uncircumcised, retract the foreskin of the penis slightly. Clean the area around the meatus and urethral opening with an antiseptic wipe. Use a fresh antiseptic wipe to clean the scrotum. Rinse the area thoroughly with sterile water and a sterile gauze. Dry the area with sterile gauze to enable an airtight seal between the collection bag and the patient's skin.

7. Prepare the urine collection bag by removing the peel-apart packaging and the paper backing to expose the adhesive strip around the sponge ring of the bag.

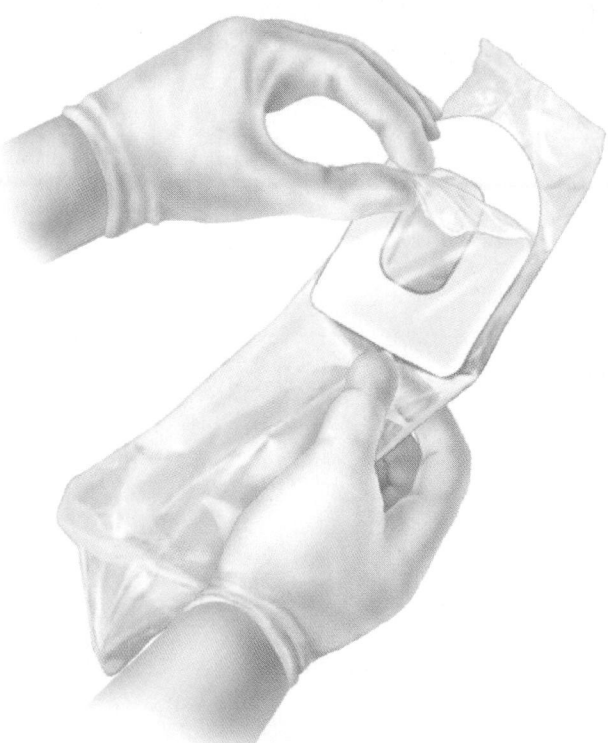

Remove the paper backing to expose the adhesive strip.

Continued

PROCEDURE 33-1—cont'd

8. Attach the collection bag firmly to the infant to prevent leakage and contamination.
   a. For a girl, place the round opening of the bag so as to cover the upper half of the external genitalia, centering the opening of the bag above the urinary meatus.
   b. For a boy, position the bag so that the child's penis and scrotum are projected through the opening of the bag. The loose end of the bag should hang down toward the infant's feet.

9. Place a clean diaper under the child.
10. Offer the caregiver water in the infant's bottle to stimulate urination or ask the mother to breastfeed the infant if he does not take a bottle.
11. Ask the caregiver to stay with the infant until he voids.
12. When the infant has voided a sufficient volume of urine, wash your hands, apply gloves, and gently remove the urine collection bag. Use care in removing the bag to avoid irritating the infant's skin.
13. Clean the genital area with antiseptic wipes and rediaper the child.
14. Pour the urine from the collection bag directly into a sterile urine specimen container.
15. Label the specimen container.
16. Record the procedure in the patient's medical record to ensure a complete, accurate medical record.

Date	
10/15/09: 9:52 a.m.	*Urine collected in pedi bag. -------------S. Gonzales, CMA*

17. Remove gloves and wash your hands.

A

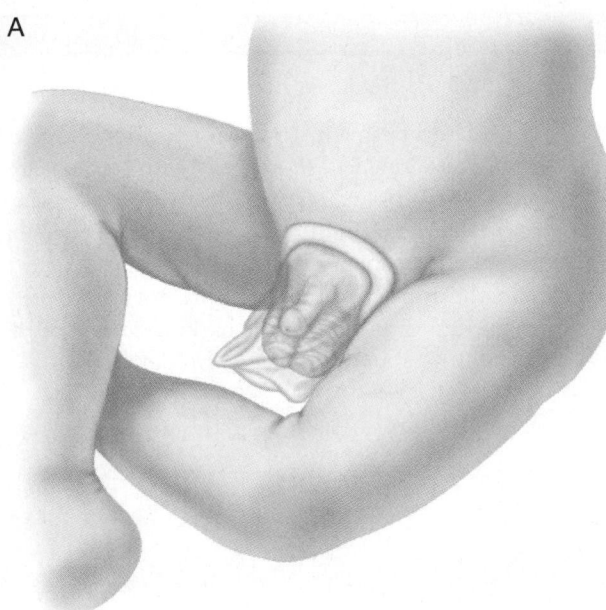

B

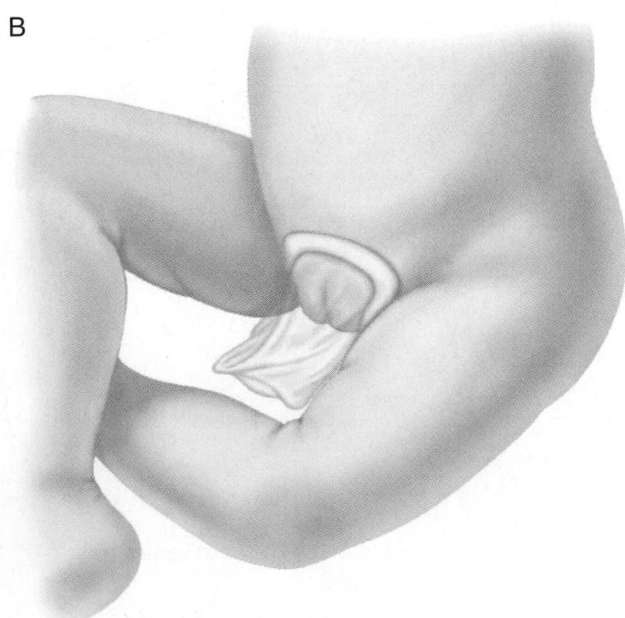

Attach the bag firmly to the infant to collect the urine as the child voids.

Hemoglobin and Hematocrit

The hemoglobin and hematocrit (H&H) test measures values of these substances in the patient's blood. The test, routinely performed to diagnose possible anemia, involves a capillary puncture to obtain a blood specimen. The medical assistant will routinely perform a capillary puncture in the pediatric office, so familiarity with this procedure is essential. (For more information on performing a capillary puncture, see Chapter 41, "Phlebotomy," page 867.)

Because the patient may feel discomfort, or pinching, during a capillary puncture, the patient may cry and want the comfort of his parent or caregiver. The medical assistant can offer the child stickers, a pencil, or a small toy as a reward for good behavior and cooperation. The medical assistant should never offer candy as a reward because it conveys a disregard for proper nutrition and good health.

Rapid *Strep* Test

The rapid *Strep* test determines the presence of the *Streptococcus* pathogen. This test diagnoses *Strep* throat, a common pediatric ailment, and is easily carried out in the pediatric office. Even so, obtaining a throat culture from a child can be a challenge. The patient is most likely in pain and may not want to cooperate with testing. To obtain a sample, the medical assistant must swab the back of the patient's throat, avoiding the teeth and cheeks to prevent contaminating the specimen. Because the results are available quickly, the physician can prescribe the appropriate treatment before the child leaves the office. (For information on obtaining a throat culture for rapid *Strep* testing, see Chapter 45, page 935.)

Nutritional Counseling

In addition to prevention and treatment of illness, the pediatric medical office can offer patients and caregivers information on proper nutrition to support growth and development. Good nutritional habits learned in childhood can promote good health throughout the patient's entire life.

Birth to 6 Months

From birth to age 6 months, an infant should receive breast milk or formula exclusively. Studies have shown that introducing solid foods before 6 months leads to an increased risk of food allergies.

6 Months to 1 Year

From age 6 months to 1 year, breast milk or formula should still make up most of an infant's diet. However, at 6 months, the parent or caregiver can begin introducing solid foods. New foods should be added one at a time for a period of 3 or 4 days for each. In this way, if the child exhibits a sign of allergy, such as a rash, the caregiver can quickly identify the new food as an allergen and eliminate it from the child's diet. Most pediatricians recommend introducing cereals, then vegetables, and then fruits. This progression is gentler for the baby and will not create a dislike for the taste of vegetables in favor of the sweetness of fruits. Common foods added from 6 months on include:

- weeks 1 to 3—cereals, such as rice, oats, and wheat
- weeks 4 to 6—vegetables, such as green beans, peas, sweet potato, and carrots
- weeks 7 to 9—fruits, such as applesauce, strained pears, and peaches.

Age 1

At age 1, the child can transition from breast milk or formula to whole milk. The American Academy of Pediatrics (AAP) strongly urges parents to give children under age 2 whole milk, rather than reduced fat or nonfat milk. The reduction in fat and calories will not meet the caloric requirements of growing babies. At age 1, the child should be eating a variety of nutritious foods, such as:

- whole wheat crackers
- cheese
- applesauce
- bananas
- scrambled or hard-boiled eggs
- mashed potatoes
- variety of bite-sized green, yellow, and orange vegetables
- chicken cut into very small pieces
- crumbled hamburger.

Ages 2 to 5

At ages 2 to 5, the child should be feeding herself and making some food choices. The medical assistant can discuss with parents trying to keep only healthy foods in the home so that the child can make good choices. The preschooler can explore nutritious foods and help in meal preparation. Parents should still be sure to cut food into small pieces to avoid a choking hazard. Foods that are appropriate for this age group include:

- milk, yogurt, cheese
- chicken, eggs, beans, fish, meat
- vegetables of a variety of colors (green, yellow, and orange)
- variety of fruits (such as grapes, apples, oranges, bananas, and pears)
- bread, cereal (unsweetened or with minimal sweeteners) rice, and pasta.

School-Age Children

Parents of school-age children, from ages 5 to 12, should continue offering healthy foods and allowing the child to make good choices. The child may want to explore cuisines from other cultures, add seasonings to foods, and make more of her own food choices. Children can be included in menu planning, the preparation of meals, and cooking with supervision. The child will become increasingly aware of what her peers are eating, so parents should continue to discuss with their child the reasons for making healthy food choices. In addition, parents can use the USDA food pyramid for young children (ages 6 to 11) to help explain healthy food choices. (See Figure 33-9.)

Adolescents

Teenagers, ages 13 to 19, tend to be busy with school and activities and healthy eating habits may decline. The teenager will begin eating more meals outside of the home, and the parent will have less control of her diet. The parent can lead by example, choosing healthy foods for herself and continuing to buy healthy foods to serve at home. Parents can encourage teens to plan and cook meals and invite friends to create healthy meals together.

Vitamin and Mineral Supplements

During infancy, childhood, and adolescence, growth and development require vitamins and minerals to support the many changes in young bodies. Healthy food choices can provide all the essential vitamins and minerals. Thus, education about healthy foods is essential. However, the pediatrician may also recommend a vitamin and mineral supplement to ensure that the child is getting the necessary nutrients. The medical assistant should discuss vitamin and mineral supplementation with children and parents when discussing healthy nutrition. The AAP recommends breastfed infants receive iron supplements at 4 months of age and then supplements or iron-fortified cereal at 6 months of age because iron stores from breast milk are depleted at that age. Iron supplementation can continue until age 1, when the child's diet should contain enough iron for his needs. Many pediatricians also recommend vitamin D supplementation during infancy, especially in northern states where sunlight during the winter is limited. The medical assistant should also document in the patient's chart the name and dosage of any supplements the child is taking. (See *USRDA of vitamins and minerals.*)

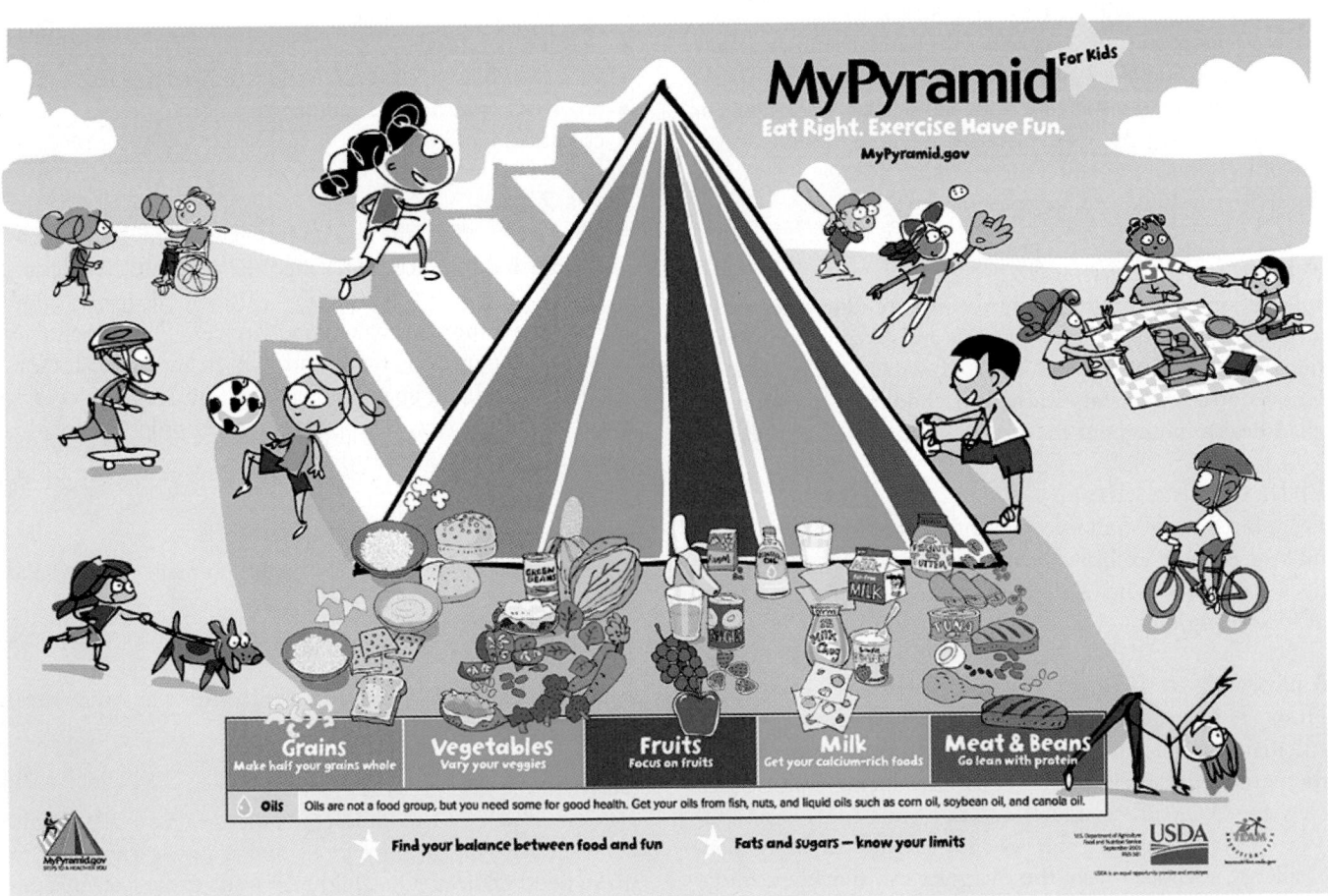

FIG 33-9 USDA food pyramid for young children.

USRDA of vitamins and minerals

While pediatricians should always recommend healthy food choices as the best source of vitamins and minerals, children commonly require supplementation. Many pediatricians recommend a multivitamin and multimineral supplement to ensure that the patient receives the necessary nutrients for good health. Children who refuse to eat a variety of foods, or "picky" eaters, are especially in need of vitamin and mineral supplementation.

Many varieties of vitamin and mineral supplements are available in pharmacies, health food stores, and supermarkets. If the pediatrician recommends supplements for a patient, the medical assistant should record what supplements the patient is taking in the medical record. The following table lists the United States recommended daily allowances (USRDA) of vitamins and minerals for infants, children, and males and females ages 9 to 18.

Vitamin or Mineral	Infants		Children		Males		Females	
	birth to 6 months	*6 to 12 months*	*1 to 3 years*	*4 to 8 years*	*9 to 13 years*	*14 to 18 years*	*9 to 13 years*	*14 to 18 years*
Vitamins								
Thiamine (mg/day)	0.2	0.3	0.5	0.6	0.9	1.2	0.9	1.0
Riboflavin (mg/day)	0.3	0.4	0.5	0.6	0.9	1.3	0.9	1.0
Niacin (mg/day)	2	4	6	8	12	16	12	14
Biotin (mcg/day)	5	6	8	12	20	25	20	25
Pantothenic acid (mg/day)	1.7	1.8	2	3	4	5	4	5
Vitamin B_6 (mg/day)	0.1	0.3	0.5	0.6	1.0	1.3	1.0	1.2
Folate (mcg/day)	65	80	150	200	300	400	300	400
Vitamin B_{12} (mcg/day)	0.4	0.5	0.9	1.2	1.8	2.4	1.8	2.4
Vitamin C (mg/day)	40	50	15	25	45	75	45	65
Vitamin A (mcg/day)	400	500	300	400	600	900	600	700
Vitamin D (mcg/day)	5	5	5	5	5	5	5	5
Vitamin E (mcg/day)	4	5	6	7	11	15	11	15
Vitamin K (mg/day)	2.0	2.5	30	55	60	75	60	75
Minerals								
Sodium (Na) (mg/day)	120	370	1000	1200	1500	1500	1500	1500
Chloride (Cl) (mg/day)	180	570	1500	1900	2300	2300	2300	2300
Potassium (K) (mg/day)	400	700	3000	3800	4500	4700	4500	4700
Calcium (Ca) (mg/day)	210	270	500	800	1300	1300	1300	1300
Phosphorus (P) (mg/day)	100	275	460	500	1250	1250	1250	1250
Magnesium (Mg) (mg/day)	30	75	80	130	240	360	240	360
Iron (Fe) (mg/day)	0.27	11	7	10	8	15	8	15
Zinc (Z) (mg/day)	2	3	3	5	8	9	8	9
Iodine (I) (mcg/day)	110	130	90	90	120	150	120	150
Selenium (Se) (mcg/day)	15	20	20	30	40	55	40	55
Copper (Cu) (mcg/day)	200	220	340	440	700	890	700	890
Manganese (Mn) (mg/day)	0.003	0.6	1.2	1.5	1.6	1.6	1.6	1.6
Fluoride (Fl) (mg/day)	0.01	0.5	0.7	1.0	2	3	2	3
Chromium (Cr) (mcg/day)	0.2	5.5	11	15	21	24	21	24

Chapter Summary

- The medical assistant working in the pediatric office can educate parents and children about health, safety, prevention of illness, transmission of illness, and nutrition.
- Well-baby and well-child visits are an opportunity to monitor the growth and development of infants and children or to diagnose developmental delays as early as possible to start intervention.
- Vision and hearing screening in the pediatric office enables early diagnosis of vision and hearing deficits to initiate treatment as soon as possible.
- Medical assistants and other staff should work together to ensure that sick children do not wait in the reception area if at all possible, to avoid potentially infecting healthy children.
- When children are diagnosed with an illness by the pediatrician, the medical assistant can educate patients and parents in the treatment of their illness.
- Routine childhood immunizations are state mandated and required for children who attend public schools. Immunizations are administered to patients in the pediatric office with the consent and understanding of the vaccines by the parent or guardian.
- Common pediatric laboratory tests include urinalysis, hemoglobin and hematocrit, and rapid *Strep* tests.
- CAPTA requires physicians in all 50 states to report suspected child abuse and neglect. The medical assistant should be sure to note in the patient's chart any signs or symptoms of abuse and neglect, including signs of physical abuse, sexual abuse, or neglect.
- In addition to prevention and treatment of illness, the pediatric medical office can offer patients and caregivers information on proper nutrition to support growth and development.
- While pediatricians should always recommend healthy food choices as the best source of vitamins and minerals, children commonly require supplementation.

Team Work Exercises

1. Divide into groups of four to six students each. Each group should research one of these vaccines: Hib, MMR, Hep B, HPV, or varicella. Each group must create a computerized presentation or a poster that discusses the benefits and risks of the vaccine. Students can role-play the medical assistant and parent discussing a vaccine.
2. Divide into groups of three to five students each. Research and create patient education brochures for a pediatric office, including these topics:

a. bicycle helmet safety and head injury prevention
b. car seat safety, fitting car seats, local resources for getting a car seat fitted properly
c. good nutrition for infants, toddlers, and adolescents.
d. children with ADD and ADHD, including school strategies and so forth
e. drug and alcohol abuse education for adolescents
f. preventing teen pregnancy and sexually transmitted diseases
g. choking hazards for babies and infants, including feeding guidelines as well as infant CPR
h. preventing and responding to poisoning; childproofing the home

Case Studies

1. Yotchi Tanaka is a new mother who has come into the office with a thermometer that she does not know how to use. She has questions regarding the equipment and technique necessary to obtain an accurate temperature for her child. What should the medical assistant do?
2. The medical assistant measures a 3-year-old female patient and plots the measurements on the standardized growth chart. The caregiver of the child notices that the patient's measurements are under all the lines on the chart. She asks the medical assistant what is wrong with her child. How should the medical assistant respond?

Resources

- American Academy of Pediatrics car seat safety guidelines: *www.aap.org/family/carseatguide.htm*
- American Red Cross infant and child CPR and first aid offerings by area: *www.redcross.org/services/hss/courses*
- CDC lead poisoning recommendations: *www.cdc.gov/nceh/lead/ACCLPP/recommend.htm*
- CDC vaccine information statements: *www.cdc.gov/vaccines/*
- Child welfare information for all 50 states: *www.childwelfare.gov/systemwide/laws_policies/state/index.cfm*
- Denver Developmental Materials: *www.denverII.com*
- Ear infection quiz for parents and caregivers: *www.mayoclinic.com/health/ear-infections/QZ00026*
- Immunization schedule from the CDC: *www.cdc.gov/vaccines/recs/schedules/downloads/child/2007/child-schedule-color-print.pdf*
- Information on pediatric health: *www.aap.org*, *www.mayoclinic.com/health/healthy-baby/FL99999*, and *www.mayoclinic.com/health/childrens-health/CC99999*
- Whitney, E.N., and Rolfes, S.R.: *Understanding Nutrition*, 11th ed. Boston: Wadsworth Publishing Company, 2005.
- Wardlaw, G.M., and Smith, A.M.: *Contemporary Nutrition*, 7th ed. New York: McGraw Hill, 2009.

Geriatrics

Learning Objectives

Upon completion of this chapter, the student will be able to:

- define and spell key terms
- describe the impact of an aging population on the American health care system
- list nine myths commonly associated with aging and explain why each is a myth
- discuss the effects of aging on each of the body systems
- differentiate between dementia, delirium, and depression
- identify self-care measures that may be taken to prevent or minimize the risk of developing dementia
- demonstrate in a role-playing scenario the techniques that should be employed when communicating with the patient who has dementia
- identify self-care measures that may be taken to prevent or minimize the risk of developing osteoporosis
- describe a plan for increasing safety and preventing accidents in the home of an elderly individual
- compare and contrast cataracts, glaucoma, and macular degeneration
- describe the medical assistant's role in providing care for elderly patients
- describe why pain management for geriatric patients should be a priority
- list medications commonly used for pain management in the elderly patient and identify specific considerations for each.

CAAHEP Competencies

General Competencies

Professional Communications
  Recognize and respond to verbal communication
  Recognize and respond to nonverbal communication

Legal Concepts
  Identify and respond to issues of confidentiality

Patient Instruction
  Instruct individuals according to their needs
  Provide instruction for health maintenance and disease prevention
  Identify community resources

ABHES Competencies

Professionalism
  Maintain confidentiality at all times

Communication
  Adapt what is said to the recipient's level of comprehension
  Adapt for individualized needs

Administrative Duties
  Locate resources and information for patients and employers

Instruction
  Instruct patients with special needs
  Teach patients methods of health promotion and disease prevention

Chapter Outline

The Aging Population
Ageism
Physiological Changes of Aging
  Integumentary System
  Nervous System
  Cardiovascular System
  Respiratory System
  Digestive System
  Urinary System
  Reproductive System
  Endocrine System
  Musculoskeletal System
  Sensory System
Medical Terminology Related to Geriatrics
Common Geriatric Diseases and Disorders
  Dementia
    Alzheimer disease
  Bone Disorders
    Osteoporosis
    Osteoarthritis
  Sensory Disorders
    Presbyopia
    Cataracts
    Glaucoma
    Macular degeneration
    Presbycusis
Special Needs of the Geriatric Patient
  Communication Strategies
  Safety Promotion
    Mobility aids
    Home safety
  Pain Management
  Extended Care and End-of-Life Issues
    In-home and home health care
    Assisted living
    Nursing center
    Extended care campus
    End-of-life issues
Chapter Summary
Team Work Exercises
Case Studies
Resources

Key Terms

ageism
Form of prejudice and discrimination against individuals because of their age

assisted living
Residential facilities with minimal health care, common dining and social activities, and usually transportation assistance

home health care agency
Private company that employs nursing assistants and nurses who make home visits to provide patients with limited nursing services

hospice care
Program that provides special end-of-life care for terminally ill patients

in-home care
Care provided in the home by spouses, family, close friends, or paid, live-in caregivers

neuritic plaque
Accumulation of bundled fibers surrounding normal and damaged nerve cells in the brain

neurofibrillary tangles
Tangles of neurofibrils that make up part of the nerve cell body

nursing center
Facility in which custodial and nursing care are provided to individuals who need assistance with activities of daily living; also called a *nursing home*

palliative care
Medical care aimed at alleviating disease symptoms, rather than providing a cure

postmenopausal
Period occurring after permanent cessation of menstruation

The Aging Population

Aging is inevitable, but how people age is variable. Everyone ages at a different rate and in a different way, so discussions about the needs of the aging population must take those variables into account. American society has commonly thought of the age of 65 as the start of older adulthood. However, some people look and behave relatively young into their 60s, 70s, or even 80s, and others look and behave old as early as age 40 or 50.

Some factors impacting aging include genetics, lifestyle, diet, activity and exercise, and coping strategies. The effects of aging on a person's health has a huge impact on that person's quality of life.

In general, the U.S. population is aging. In 2000, there were 35 million age 65 or over (12.4% of the population). This number is expected to double to 70 million by the year 2030. In addition, the segment of the population known as the *frail elderly* (over age 85) is also increasing in size. The major reason for this increase is the aging of the "baby boom" generation, which includes those born between 1946 and 1964.

The aging of the U.S. population is having a profound impact on the American health care system. As people age, their need for health care resources also increases. With the total numbers of individuals age 55 and older projected to increase by over 200% in some states by the year 2025, the health care industry can expect to experience ever-increasing demands in the coming years.

Ageism

American culture in general values the qualities of youth and beauty. In fact, some may say that it places too much emphasis on such things, while the experience and wisdom gained from long life is commonly dismissed as unimportant or obsolete. In some situations, the bias toward youth results in **ageism,** a form of prejudice and discrimination against people because of their age. An example of ageism against the elderly is the preferential interviewing, hiring, and promoting of younger workers over equally qualified older workers. Such prejudice is similar to racism, sexism, and other forms of discrimination and is illegal as well as unethical.

Because of the impending impact of an aging population on the American health care system, medical assistants will be increasingly involved in providing health care services to elderly patients. Therefore, the medical assistant should assess her own attitude and potential bias toward elderly patients. She can begin such an assessment by considering myths associated with aging, including the perception that all elderly people end up needing institutional placement. In fact, less than 5% of elderly persons live in institutional settings, and the other 95% live more independently. In some cases, they live in their own residence individually or with a spouse. In other cases, they live semi-independently with family members, friends, or caregivers. (See *Aging myths*.)

Physiological Changes of Aging

As a person ages, his physical body undergoes changes to all systems. Therefore, the health care needs of an aging person change over time. The medical assistant can become more effective in understanding and meeting the needs of aging patients by learning about the changes these patients experience.

Integumentary System

Skin changes create some of the most visible signs of aging. These changes are accelerated by environmental exposure to the sun's ultraviolet rays and pollution. Skin cells reproduce more slowly, causing the skin to thin and become more vulnerable to tearing and other types of injury. Thus, when treating an elderly patient, the medical assistant must take care to use tape, bandages, and other products that are as gentle on the skin as possible. Once injured, the elderly person's skin is slower to heal, especially if he also suffers circulatory or immune system impairment. The skin loses moisture, elasticity, and strength due to changes in elastin fibers, which provide elasticity, and collagen fibers, which provide strength. Age spots develop due to changes in pigmentation and a variety of skin lesions may develop. Most of these lesions are benign; however, cancerous lesions may also occur. Thus, the

Aging myths

This table lists the most common myths and the facts associated with aging

Myth	Truth
All elderly people become senile.	Memory becomes less acute with advancing age and it takes longer for elderly individuals to recall information. However, most continue to have good cognitive function.
All elderly people become incontinent.	Most elderly people maintain control over their bowel and bladder. Incontinence should never be considered a "normal" part of aging.
All elderly people are "set in their ways" and incapable of learning or changing.	Older adults learn more slowly, due to physical limitations affecting vision, hearing, and energy level. They may need more time to process information but are fully capable of learning.
Disease and disability are an unavoidable part of aging.	Elderly people are more vulnerable to some physical ailments; however, most report their health as good or excellent.
Elderly people have no interest in or desire for sex.	A large percentage of elderly people report continued participation and enjoyment in sexual relationships.
Continued interest in sex among elderly people is abnormal and should be discouraged.	Sexuality is not age-dependent and is a healthy dimension of the whole person, regardless of age.
Elderly people are unproductive and a burden on society.	Many people continue paid work well past retirement age. After retirement, most continue contributing time and energies to their families and their communities through a wide variety of activities.
Most elderly people end up living in long-term care institutions.	Less than 5% of the elderly live in institutional settings.
Elderly people have more experience with pain and have, therefore, developed an increased tolerance for pain.	Experience with pain does not create an increased tolerance for pain. Regardless of age, all individuals deserve to have their pain evaluated and managed appropriately.

medical assistant should educate patients about the warning signs of skin cancer. (For more information on skin cancer education, see Chapter 25, "Dermatology," page 411.)

Changes to the dermal layer of the skin include decreased vascularity, which decreases a person's ability to regulate body temperature, resulting in increased vulnerability to heat and cold. An elderly person's skin also has less active sweat and sebaceous glands, which results in dryer skin that is more vulnerable to injury. Fat deposits in the face decrease and increase in the abdomen and thighs of women. Hair on the head begins to thin and turn gray, while hair on the eyebrows, nose, and ears in men becomes longer and coarser. Women may begin to develop more facial hair. Fingernails become more brittle and may split and toenails may thicken.

Nervous System

As aging progresses, the number of neurons in the nervous system decreases and the brain gets smaller. Dendrites begin to shrink, which can slow message transmission. Therefore, an elderly patient may find that information retrieval takes longer, slowing their ability to recall facts or events. Reaction time also slows somewhat. In spite of these changes, loss of brain cells is minimal, and elderly people are still capable of learning new information.

Experts suggest that optimal mental function can be preserved by keeping the brain actively stimulated. Such activities might include reading, taking classes, playing board games and trivia games, and doing crossword puzzles. Some experts believe ingestion of antioxidants, such as vitamin E and ginkgo biloba, has beneficial effects. However, patients should only take such supplements after consultation with a physician, because ginkgo biloba interacts with some medications and too much vitamin E causes toxicity. Other activities that promote cardiovascular health, such as exercise, also positively affect the brain by providing optimal circulation. Avoidance of destructive habits and other risk factors also helps preserve brain health and mental function.

Cardiovascular System

In an aging patient, the cardiovascular system suffers the effects of decreased cardiac output, arteriosclerosis, and atherosclerosis, which combine to contribute to hypertension, cardiovascular disease, and stroke. The aging heart beats less forcefully because it loses strength and mass with age as well as from disease or adverse effects of medication. A less forceful heartbeat results in decreased cardiac output and, therefore, decreased energy and stamina. In addition, the heart tries to compensate for decreased cardiac output by increasing the heart rate. Such an effect is more pronounced during physical exertion, anxiety, or illness. Compounding the problem is the age-related loss in vessel wall elasticity caused by arteriosclerosis. Stiffer vessel walls provide more resistance to blood flow, thus increasing blood pressure and forcing the heart to work even harder. Atherosclerosis (buildup of cholesterol plaques inside of arterial walls), also more common in elderly patients, contributes further to the developing stiffness and narrowing of vessels and results in hypertension, a major contributor to cardiovascular disease, the leading cause of death in the elderly. Over half of elderly patients have some form of hypertension, including systolic hypertension, diastolic hypertension, or both. Hypertension increases the risk of vascular and cardiac events, such as stroke and heart failure.

Respiratory System

Respiratory function in aging adults changes in several ways. The thorax changes shape and loses flexibility due to calcification of ribs and changes in the thoracic vertebrae. Kyphosis, an exaggerated curve of the upper thoracic spine that is sometimes called *hunchback* or *Pott's curvature,* is a common age-related change that affects respiratory function. The development of osteoporosis, a condition characterized by loss of bone mass throughout the skeleton, further contributes to degenerative changes in the vertebrae and thorax. Respiratory muscles also lose strength, resulting in a weaker cough and the need to work harder to cough and even to breathe. Because the cough reflex is an important protective mechanism, a weakening cough reflex puts elderly individuals at increased risk for respiratory problems. In addition, as a person ages, her lung tissue loses elasticity and capacity due to changes in capillaries and alveoli. All of these changes result in less effective movement of the chest wall, an overall decrease in gas exchange, and an increased risk for pneumonia and other respiratory disorders.

Digestive System

In general, elderly persons are at increased risk for gastrointestinal (GI) disorders, such as gastroesophageal reflux disease (GERD), peptic ulcer disease (PUD), and diverticulitis. As individuals age, the digestive system loses some of its muscle tone and elasticity. Thus the digestive tract's smooth muscle wall, which is responsible for peristalsis, becomes less effective. As a result, an elderly person is more vulnerable to constipation. Also, many medications commonly taken by elderly patients also contribute to this problem.

Elderly patients are also more vulnerable to nutritional deficiencies as they experience less tolerance for certain foods. As a result, they are more likely to develop problems with diarrhea and flatulence. As a person ages, the stomach produces less hydrochloric acid, which aids digestion, and less intrinsic factor, which is a compound made in the stomach necessary for vitamin B_{12} absorption. These decreases lead to vitamin deficiencies. Some medications also contribute to nutritional deficiencies by impairing the digestion, absorption, or utilization of certain nutrients. Elderly persons, especially those who live alone, are prone to poor eating habits and, as a result, may be deficient in important vitamins and minerals. Many are hesitant to drink adequate quantities of fluids because of fears of incontinence, nocturia, or being a burden to others. As a result, they are commonly dehydrated, which further contributes to constipation and decreased kidney function and slows waste excretion, which increases the risk of toxicity.

Oral medications may impact elderly persons differently due to changes in GI function. In older patients, liver function decreases, which slows the metabolism of medications and toxins. Oral medications traveling more slowly through the intestines can, in some cases, result in increased absorption of these drugs. In addition, medications may interact with one another, resulting in a decrease or increase in their desired effects. Thus, elderly patients may be at greater risk for drug toxicity.

Urinary System

Elderly men commonly develop benign prostatic hyperplasia (BPH), which is an enlargement of the prostate gland. BPH results in urinary symptoms of frequency, urgency, nocturia, hesitancy, and difficulty maintaining a urine stream. It also increases the risk of urinary retention and incontinence and increased incidence of urinary tract infection (UTI). Incidence of prostate cancer also increases with age and is the second leading cause of cancer death in men over age 50.

In general, bladder capacity decreases as a person ages. This decreased capacity leads to increased urinary frequency during the day and night for men and women. This disrupts sleep patterns and overall quality of sleep. Elderly women sometimes suffer from forms of overactive bladder, including various types of incontinence.

The number of functioning nephrons in the kidneys decreases as a person ages. Thus, kidney function decreases. Decreasing effectiveness of the cardiovascular system also impacts kidney function, because decreased blood flow to the kidneys inhibits their ability to filter and excrete wastes effectively. As a result of these changes, the half-life of some medications may increase, causing a risk of drug toxicity. However, in most cases, the kidneys have a great capacity to continue normal or near normal function late into life.

Reproductive System

In women who are **postmenopausal** (the period after permanent cessation of menstruation), a number of changes develop as a result of decreased estrogen and progesterone levels. The breasts lose underlying muscle mass and tone and the breast tissue loses elasticity and density. These changes result in smaller breasts that tend to droop. The vagina also decreases in size and loses elasticity. The ovaries, uterus, and cervix also decrease in size. Vaginal dryness occurs as secretions decrease.

In men, spermatogenesis (formation of mature functional spermatozoa) continues late into life. However, in addition to an enlarging prostate, men find that erections take longer to develop and may be less firm than in the past. Erectile dysfunction (ED) may develop from various causes, including medication, arthritis, and arteriosclerosis. Gynecomastia (breast enlargement) may develop as a result of adverse effects of medication, obesity, or hormone changes. Men as well as women are at greater risk for breast cancer.

Desire for and participation in sexual activity may continue late into life for women and men. Health care providers should view this behavior as normal and healthy. In some cases, decreased sexual activity may result from illness, disability, adverse effects of medication, loss of a partner, or decreased interest. The medical assistant must be sensitive to such issues and should encourage patients to discuss issues of concern with the physician.

Endocrine System

As individuals age, changes in the level and activity of some hormones may occur. These changes impact each body system regulated by certain hormones. The muscular system is affected by a decreased level of growth hormone, resulting in decreased muscle mass as well as an increased tendency to store fat. Decreased calcitonin and parathyroid hormone levels affect calcium and phosphate levels in the skeletal system, leading to an increased likelihood of osteoporosis. Decreased aldosterone leads to decreased efficiency in salt and water conservation, increasing the risk of dehydration in elderly patients. A decrease in thyroid hormones slows the metabolic rate and increases sensitivity to cold and heat. Decreased insulin production or less effective insulin use leads to hyperglycemia and an increased risk of type 2 diabetes. Decreased glucocorticoid levels lead to a decrease in the ability to deal with stress and a weakened immune system, possibly leading to increased sensitivity to pain and increased vulnerability to infection. A slight decrease in testosterone production in males may lead to diminished libido and changes in erectile function. Decreased estrogen and progesterone in females leads to loss of elasticity and density of breast and vaginal tissue and decreased size of the ovaries, uterus, and cervix.

Musculoskeletal System

A person experiences decreased muscle mass and strength as he ages. Bone mass decreases as bones lose minerals. This decrease is compounded by decreased physical activity, especially weight-bearing activities that stimulate bone growth. Postmenopausal women are at greater risk for loss of bone mass than men (50% over age 50). However, both men and women may develop osteoporosis. Osteoarthritis occurs as joints begin to deteriorate with erosion of cartilage and bone.

Sensory System

A decrease in all five senses is common in aging; however, it is not clear if this effect is due to physiological changes of aging or changes associated with injury, surgery, medications, or chronic disease. Many elderly persons find that, as they age, food does not taste as good. With age, active taste buds decrease in number and lose their sensitivity to salty, sweet, sour, and bitter flavors. This decrease in the sense of taste most commonly begins after age 60. In addition, aging also causes a decrease in the sense of smell, which is a significant part of being able to taste and enjoy food. A decrease in the sense of smell occurs most commonly after the age of 70 and may be due to loss of functional nerve endings in the nose. As a result, some elderly patients tend to oversalt their food in an effort to make it taste better. Others lose interest in eating and, as a result, develop nutritional deficiencies.

Many structures in the body, including skin, muscles, and internal organs, have receptors that detect touch, temperature, pressure, or pain. These receptors send signals to the brain for processing and interpretation. Elderly persons seem to experience decreased perception of such signals. In any case, elderly persons generally experience greater difficulty differentiating temperatures, which may put them at risk for heat- and cold-related injury, such as frostbite and burns. Decreased sensitivity to pressure puts elderly patients at greater risk for developing pressure ulcers. On the other hand, because of their thinning skin, frail elderly patients sometimes notice increased sensitivity to light touch.

One of the most significant challenges in caring for aging patients is communication due to hearing or vision loss.

With advancing age the tympanic membrane in the ears begins to thicken and the delicate structures of the inner ear begin to deteriorate. This may also begin to affect a person's sense of balance, leading to an increased risk of falls. Because many elderly patients suffer some type of hearing or vision loss, the medical assistant must adapt her communication techniques to accommodate these differences. In addition, she must be aware of the impact of these difficulties on the patient's quality of life.

Some adapted communication strategies the medical assistant can use for patients with vision loss include using large print educational materials. In addition, the medical assistant should make sure the reception area, hallways, and examination rooms have good-quality, nonglare lighting. Doing so will help elderly patients with task completion and safe ambulation.

Communication strategies the medical assistant can use for patients with hearing loss include keeping her voice low-pitched and facing the elderly patient so that the patient can read her lips. In addition, the medical assistant should attempt to minimize environmental noise when possible.

Medical Terminology Related to Geriatrics

Terms used in the medical office will include those related to geriatrics, including diseases common to elderly patients and procedures regularly performed as part of regular care for elderly patients. To be effective in her role, a medical assistant must become well versed in the language and vocabulary of geriatrics. The following tables list common medical terminology related to geriatrics.

Table 34.1 | Word Elements

Element	Meaning	Example	Meaning
Combining Forms			
ankyl/o	stiffness; bent, crooked	**ankylosis** (ăng-kĭ-LŌ-sĭs)	Abnormal condition of stiffening or crookedness (of a joint)
ger/o		**geriatric** (jĕr-ē-ĂT-rĭk)	Pertaining to the elderly
geront/o		**gerontologist** (jĕr-ŏn-TŎL-ŏ-jĭst)	Specialist in the study of aging
presby/o	old age	**presbyacusis** (prĕs-bē-ă-KŪ-sĭs)	Age-related hearing loss
rhytid/o	wrinkle	**rhytidoplasty** (RĬT-ĭ-dō-plăs-tē)	Surgical repair (removal) of wrinkles
Prefixes			
a-	without, not	**anacusia** (ăn-ă-KŪ-sē-ă)	Without hearing (total deafness)

Table 34.1 | Word Elements

Element	Meaning	Example	Meaning
brady-	slow	**bradykinesia** (brăd-ē-kĭ-NĒ-sē-ă)	Slow movement
Suffixes			
-asthenia	weakness, debility	**myasthenia** (mī-ăs-THĒ-nē-ă)	Muscle weakness
-penia	decrease, deficiency	**osteopenia** (ŏs-tē-ō-PĒ-nē-ă)	Deficiency of bone mass
-porosis	porous	**osteoporosis** (ŏs-tē-ō-por-Ō-sĭs)	Porous bones
-stenosis	narrowing, stricture	**arteriostenosis** (ăr-tē-rē-ō-stē-NŌ-sĭs)	Narrowing of an artery

Table 34.2 | Pathologic Terms

This table lists some of the most common pathologic terms related to geriatrics with a pronunciation guide and brief definition for each.

Term	Definition
age-related macular degeneration MĂK-ū-lăr dē-gĕn-ĕr-Ā-shŭn	Age-related degeneration of the macula (part of the retina) with resulting loss of central vision
Alzheimer disease ĂLZ-hī-mĕr	Chronic, progressive, degenerative cognitive disorder
anacusis ăn-ă-KŪ-sĭs	Total deafness
cataract KĂT-ă-răkt	Opacity of the lens of the eye as a result of aging, trauma, or disease
dementia dē-MĔN-shē-ă	Progressive, irreversible decline in mental function marked by memory impairment and deficits in reasoning and judgment
glaucoma glaw-KŌ-mă	Group of eye diseases characterized by increased intraocular pressure, resulting in atrophy of the optic nerve
kyphosis kī-FŌ-sĭs	Condition marked by exaggeration of the posterior curve of the thoracic spine; also called *hunchback*
osteoarthritis ŏs-tē-ō-ăr-THRĬ-tĭs	A type of arthritis marked by progressive cartilage deterioration in synovial joints and vertebrae
osteoporosis ŏs-tē-ō-por-Ō-sĭs	Loss of bone mass that occurs throughout the skeleton when more bone is resorbed than laid down
presbyopia prĕz-bē-Ō-pē-ă	Permanent loss of accommodation of the lens of the eye that occurs when people are in their mid-40s
presbycusis prĕz-bĭ-KŪ-sĭs	Progressive loss of hearing with aging
psychosis sī-KŌ-sĭs	Mental disorder marked by loss of contact with reality, evidenced by delusions, hallucinations, disorganized speech patterns, and bizarre or catatonic behaviors

| Table 34.3 | **Abbreviations** |

In geriatrics, as in other areas of health care, abbreviations are commonly used. Abbreviations such as the ones listed in this table save time and effort in documentation and written communications.

Abbreviation	Term
ADLs	activities of daily living
AD	Alzheimer disease
AMD, ARMD	age-related macular degeneration
BMD	bone mineral density
BPH	benign prostatic hyperplasia, benign prostatic hypertrophy
CABG	coronary artery bypass graft
CAD	coronary artery disease
CPAP	continuous positive airway pressure
decub.	decubitus (ulcer); bedsore
DNR	do not resuscitate
ED	erectile dysfunction
HTN	hypertension
LTC	long-term care
OA	osteoarthritis

Common Geriatric Diseases and Disorders

As a person ages, he becomes more vulnerable to certain diseases and disorders. Some of the most common include dementia, bone disorders, and vision disorders.

Dementia

Dementia is a neurological disorder characterized by chronic, progressive, irreversible decline in mental function. It is marked by deficits in reasoning and judgment. It progressively impairs a person's ability to participate in occupational and social activities. About 20% to 40% of those affected by dementia are over age 85. Although there are numerous causes of dementia, Alzheimer disease is responsible for over 60% of dementia cases. The other 40% of dementia causes include Parkinson disease, Huntington disease, stroke, toxicity from excessive alcohol or drug use, severe deficiency of vitamin B_{12} and folate,

brain infection, and head injury. In addition, some other disorders are commonly confused with dementia because the signs and symptoms are similar. (See *Conditions confused with dementia.*)

Alzheimer Disease
ICD-9-CM code: 331.0
Alzheimer disease is the most common form of dementia. It usually occurs in patients over age 65 but may occur as early as age 40. It currently affects approximately 4 million Americans. However, experts estimate that by the year 2050, the number may increase to 14 million. This disorder costs nearly $100 billion each year in direct and indirect health care costs.

The cause of Alzheimer disease is not yet fully understood. However, some contributing factors have been identified, including genetics, some viruses, previous brain injuries from head trauma or minor stroke, and immunologic factors. (See *Preventing Alzheimer disease,* page 692.) Characteristic changes in the brain of those affected by Alzheimer disease include cerebral atrophy and degenerative changes to neurons. These changes include **neuritic plaques**, which are accumulations of bundled fibers surrounding normal and damaged nerve cells in the brain, and **neurofibrillary tangles**, which are a distortion of neurofibrils that make up part of the nerve cell body. Patients with Alzheimer disease also experience a significant decrease in levels of neurotransmitters, such as acetylcholine.

The course of Alzheimer disease has been divided into three stages:

- Stage I is characterized by progressive short-term memory loss.
- Stage II is characterized by deterioration of intellectual ability, personality changes, speech and language problems, impaired judgment, and continued worsening of memory as well as possible paranoia, delusions, hallucinations, seizures, and depression.
- Stage III marks the patient's total dependence on others for care and can also include paranoia, delusions, hallucinations, seizures, and depression.

Diagnosis of Alzheimer disease is made by ruling out other disorders, including delirium and depression. There is no cure for Alzheimer disease. Medications such as donepezil (Aricept) and tacrine (Cognex) temporarily enhance cognitive function by preventing the breakdown of acetylcholine. However, the effects of these medications decrease after several months. Antidepressant and antipsychotic medication may be used when depression and hallucinations are present.

Other treatment measures are the same as for all types of dementia and aim to maximize function and provide safety and comfort. Patients with early dementia may respond to

Conditions confused with dementia

Dementia is sometimes confused with other states, including delirium and depression. Adverse effects of medications are also sometimes mistaken for signs of dementia. Therefore, careful evaluation is necessary to rule out other pathologies and determine an appropriate treatment plan.

By comparing features of delirium and depression, one can differentiate them from dementia. The following table outlines each disorder along with its definition; onset, course, and duration; and its effects on memory, thought processes, perception, psychomotor behaviors, and sleep patterns.

Disorder and Definition	Onset, Course, and Duration	Effects
Dementia Neurological disorder characterized by chronic, progressive, irreversible decline in mental function	• *Onset:* slow • *Course:* long, progressive • *Duration:* years	• *Memory:* short-term memory loss in early stages and remote memory loss in later stage • *Thought processes:* impaired judgment, difficulty with word finding, difficulty performing a familiar task • *Perception:* usually intact • *Psychomotor behaviors:* usually normal in the early stages • *Sleep patterns:* impaired and fragmented
Delirium Acute reversible state of agitated confusion marked by disorientation, hallucinations, or delusions	• *Onset:* sudden • *Course:* short, fluctuates and commonly worsens at night • *Duration:* hours to days, usually less than 1 month	• *Memory:* possible impairment of immediate and recent memory • *Thought processes:* distorted and disorganized, easily distracted from tasks • *Perception:* distorted with delusions and hallucinations • *Psychomotor behaviors:* distorted with delusions and hallucinations • *Sleep patterns:* impaired, with day and night cycles commonly reversed
Depression Mood disorder marked by loss of interest or pleasure in living	• *Onset:* slow • *Course:* slow • *Duration:* weeks to years	• *Memory:* variable effect with episodes of poor memory mixed with clear memory • *Thought processes:* intact with a bleak outlook; ability to focus on task at hand (with some possible impairment); apathetic • *Perception:* usually intact • *Psychomotor behaviors:* usually intact • *Sleep patterns:* impaired; may sleep too little or too much, commonly involving early morning awakenings

efforts to reorient them to time and place. However, this strategy becomes less effective as dementia progresses. Support resources for patients with Alzheimer disease and their families are available, including adult day services, respite care, support groups, and home health care services. In addition, the medical assistant can provide tips on making the home environment safer for the patient with Alzheimer disease or other forms of dementia. (See *Home safety for patients with dementia*, page 692.)

Because a change of routine and environment increases confusion and may increase agitation in the patient with Alzheimer disease, the medical assistant must learn to interact with such patients in a calm, clear, thoughtful manner. She should provide simple instructions one step at time and avoid rushing or forcing the patient. (See *Communicating with patients with dementia*, page 692.) Education and emotional support for family members and caregivers of such patients are also essential.

Patient Education

Preventing Alzheimer Disease

The medical assistant can share these tips with her patients so they can preserve and protect their brain function to help prevent Alzheimer disease:

- Avoid tobacco use.
- Avoid use of illicit drugs.
- Avoid lead exposure.
- Avoid chronically high levels of stress.
- Maintain a healthy blood pressure.
- Manage diabetes effectively.
- Follow all recommended measures to prevent heart disease (which help protect the brain, too).
- Pursue educational or mentally stimulating activities.
- Exercise regularly.
- Participate in social activities.

Patient Education

Home Safety for Patients with Dementia

The medical assistant should share these safety tips with family members and caregivers of patients with Alzheimer disease or other forms of dementia:

- Keep doors and windows locked.
- Install safety latches on cabinets and drawers that contain objects such as knives.
- Install protective gates at the top and bottom of stairs.
- Supervise the ingestion of all medications.
- Keep car keys in a locked cupboard.
- Place nightlights throughout the home, especially in the bedroom and bathroom.
- Keep walkways clear.

Life expectancy for patients with Alzheimer disease is variable but averages 8 to 10 years from the onset of symptoms. Death is not due to Alzheimer disease itself but its complications. These complications most commonly include pneumonia, infection of various types, and injury associated with falls and immobility.

Bone Disorders

Common bone disorders in geriatric patients include osteoporosis and osteoarthritis.

Communicating with patients with dementia

When communicating with patients suffering from Alzheimer disease or other types of dementia, the medical assistant should be sure to learn these important do's and don'ts.

Do's

- Provide for physical discomfort before anything else.
- Physically approach the patient in an unhurried, gentle manner.
- Speak in an unhurried manner using a clear, calm voice.
- Keep sentences short.
- Give instructions one step at time and focus on one subject at a time.
- Allow the patient time to process his response if one is needed.
- Look for cues of increasing anxiety or agitation, such as tensing of the body, or expressions of fear or distress.
- If the patient becomes agitated, move away from him and let the caregiver or family member provide comfort and reassurance.
- Verify important information with the caregiver or family member because the patient's memory and judgment are not reliable.
- If you wish to make conversation, ask about events in the distant past, because the patient is more likely to recall such events.

Don'ts

- Do not ask the patient unnecessary questions.
- Do not remind the patient of his bad memory; simply repeat things as needed.
- Do not argue with the patient.
- Do not try to physically force the patient to do anything.
- Do not overwhelm the patient with too much information or complex instructions.
- Do not expect the patient to remember you from one visit to the next.
- Do not ask or expect the patient to recall recent events (unless the question is being asked to further evaluate the patient's memory).

Osteoporosis

ICD-9-CM code: 733.00

Osteoporosis is a condition characterized by loss of bone mass throughout the skeleton. It affects an estimated 8 million American women and 2 million American men. Those of northern European or Asian descent and those with a family history of osteoporosis are at increased risk. Osteoporosis puts a person at greater risk for vertebral and hip fractures.

Osteoporosis is caused by loss of bone density as more bone is resorbed (removed) than developed. Contributing factors for osteoporosis include a drop in hormone levels after menopause; a diet poor in calcium, magnesium, and vitamin D; immobility and sedentary lifestyle; thyroid hormone excess; corticosteroid use; use of some anticonvulsant medications; and alcohol and tobacco use. Patients with osteoporosis are commonly asymptomatic until bone fractures, such as vertebral and hip fractures, occur. Subsequent immobility exacerbates the condition. Thoracic vertebral changes can cause kyphosis, vertebral compression fractures, or even vertebral collapse with subsequent pain and disability. Loss of bone density in the vertebrae causes changes in posture and decreased height. (See Figure 34-1.)

Diagnosis of osteoporosis usually does not occur until the patient suffers a related injury, such as hip fracture. Diagnosis is based on x-rays, bone scans, CT scans, and dual-energy x-ray absorptiometry (DEXA) scans, all of which reveal decreased bone density.

Treatment is aimed at preventing or minimizing further bone loss and disability. It includes dietary modification, mineral and vitamin supplements, estrogen replacement, weight-bearing exercises, and medications to foster bone density. Medications to treat osteoporosis include calcitonin nasal spray (Miacalcin), raloxifene (Evista), risedronate (Actonel), ibandronate (Boniva), and alendronate (Fosamax). Treatment for injury and disability from osteoporosis includes surgery, physical therapy, and analgesics and muscle relaxants for pain. Even so, the most effective treatment for osteoporosis is prevention. (See *Osteoporosis risk factors and preventive measures.*)

Osteoarthritis

ICD-9-CM Code: 715.90

Osteoarthritis is the most common form of arthritis, a condition of joint inflammation characterized by pain, stiffness, redness, swelling, and deformity. Arthritis affects approximately 43 million Americans and is more common in women than in men. Incidence of arthritis increases with age.

Osteoarthritis is caused by erosion of the joint's cartilage and eventual erosion of the bone surface. The joints most commonly affected are the shoulder, elbow, hip, wrist, finger, knee, ankle, and toe. Bone spurs may develop, causing increased pain with movement. (See Figure 34-2.)

Osteoporosis risk factors and preventive measures

Good self-care, including preventive measures, is the best way to minimize osteoporotic changes. Such preventive measures should begin in childhood. This table contains a list of the most common risk factors for osteoporosis along with preventive measures.

Risk Factor	Prevention
Immobility or sedentary lifestyle	Regular weight-bearing exercise such as walking (30–60 minutes 3–4 times per week) and weight lifting
Diet poor in calcium, magnesium, and vitamin D	Consistent intake of adequate amounts of calcium, magnesium, and vitamin D
Thyroid hormone excess	Timely, appropriate treatment of hyperthyroidism
Decrease in sex hormones	Hormone replacement therapy
Excessive alcohol use	Eliminating or minimizing alcohol consumption
Tobacco use	Eliminating tobacco use
Medications such as corticosteroids and phenytoin (Dilantin)	Determining the smallest therapeutic dose of such medications in consultation with a physician and carefully weighing the risks and benefits

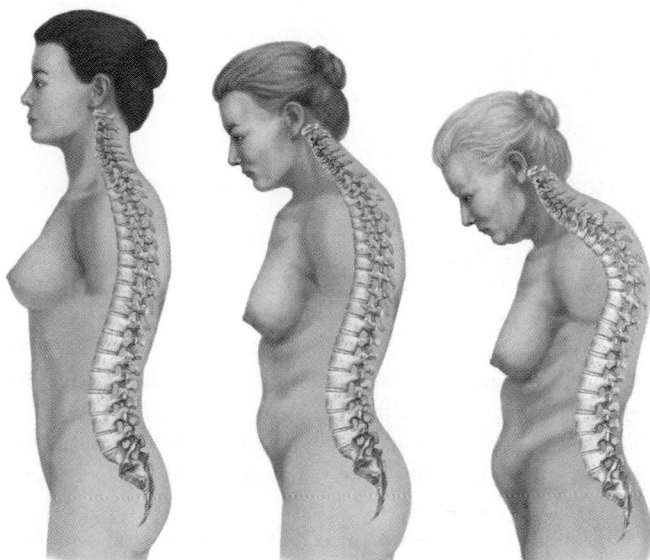

FIG 34-1 Changes in posture and height from osteoporosis.

A

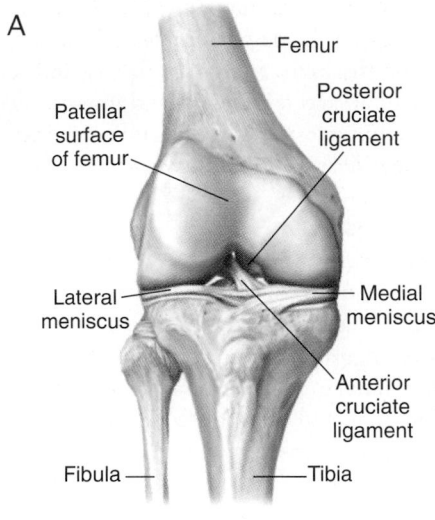

Femur

Posterior
cruciate
ligament

Patellar
surface
of femur

Lateral
meniscus

Medial
meniscus

Anterior
cruciate
ligament

Fibula

Tibia

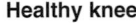

Healthy knee

B

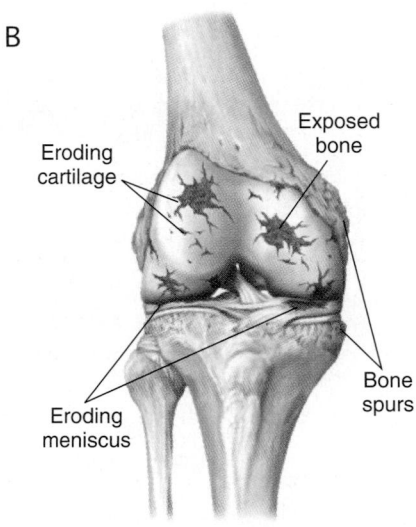

Exposed
bone

Eroding
cartilage

Bone
spurs

Eroding
meniscus

Arthritic knee

FIG 34-2 The degenerative changes of osteoarthritis.

Diagnosis is based on physical examination findings, description of symptoms, and radiological studies. X-rays and, possibly, MRI studies reveal eroded cartilage, narrowing of the joint space, and bone spur formation. Although there is no cure for arthritis, treatment with medication, such as corticosteroids and analgesics, can commonly minimize symptoms and slow disease progression. Other treatment measures include weight loss, joint protection, exercise, and heat or cold application. If joint deterioration is severe, joint replacement surgery may be necessary. Physical and occupational therapy is common with or without surgery. Regardless of the treatment strategy, the goal is to promote function, comfort, and safety.

Osteoarthritis is not life-threatening but commonly impairs quality of life by causing chronic pain and decreasing mobility. For some patients it is a mild annoyance; for others, it may force them to leave work and severely limit everyday activities such as walking.

Sensory Disorders

Common geriatric sensory disorders include presbyopia, cataracts, glaucoma, macular degeneration, and presbycusis.

Presbyopia
ICD-9-CM code: 367.4

Presbyopia is age-related loss of visual acuity. Age-related visual changes occur in nearly everyone as they age and become noticeable around the age of 40. The estimated incidence of presbyopia is extremely high—well over 100 million Americans.

Visual acuity diminishes with age from a variety of factors, including damage to the retina, changes to the lens and cornea, and reduced pupil size. A common symptom of presbyopia is a reduced ability to accommodate for change in distance and, especially, close detail. Other changes include increased sensitivity to light and glare, decreased ability to see in the dark, and decreased ability to discriminate between shades of colors, such as greens and blues, and among pastel colors. Decreased secretions from lacrimal (tear) glands results in drying and irritation of the eye.

Diagnosis is based on the patient's complaint of increased eye fatigue and difficulty focusing on fine print or difficulty with tasks that require visual acuity, such as threading a needle. Standard vision screening tests are used, such as having the patient read text from a card held 14" to 16" away. These tests reveal difficulty focusing on near objects.

Treatment for presbyopia is usually corrective lenses. There is no cure for presbyopia, and it typically progresses to increased vision loss. However, progression is slow and most patients are able to carry out activities of daily living with the use of corrective lenses.

Cataracts
ICD-9-CM code: 366

Cataracts are the gradual clouding of the eye's lens. They are extremely common, affecting more than 40% of people between ages 52 and 64, 60% of those ages 65 to 74, and 91% of those ages 75 to 85. Nearly 6 million Americans are affected by cataracts. In addition, cataracts are the leading cause of blindness worldwide.

Cataracts may be caused by age-related deterioration. Other contributors include traumatic injury, drug toxicity, diabetes, and prolonged, high-dose corticosteroid therapy. Signs and symptoms include blurred vision, halos around lights, blue or yellow tint to the visual field, light sensitivity, and a white-appearing pupil. Diagnosis is based on visual examination of the patient's eyes with an ophthalmoscope, which reveals the milky opacity, or clouding of the lens.

Treatment for cataracts involves surgical removal of the lens and replacement with an artificial lens. There are two types of surgery. The extracapsular cataract extraction (ECCE) involves removal of the lens while leaving most of the lens capsule intact. High-frequency sound waves (phacoemulsification) may be used to break up the lens prior to extraction. Intracapsular (ICCE) surgery is rarely done and involves removal of the entire lens including the capsule. In either case, the lens is removed and replaced by a plastic lens. Because only local anesthetic is required, it can be a day procedure.

Most people (95%) who undergo surgery to treat cataracts recover completely within 3 to 4 weeks and enjoy vastly improved vision. Potential complications include endophthalmitis (inflammation of the intraocular cavities, including the aqueous or vitreous humor), posterior capsular opacification (clouding of the posterior capsule), and retinal detachment.

Glaucoma

ICD-9-CM code: 365.10 (primary or chronic open-angle), 365.2 (acute angle-closure)

Glaucoma is a group of disorders in which increased intraocular pressure (IOP) results in atrophy of the optic nerve, leading to loss of peripheral vision and eventual blindness. There are several types of glaucoma, the most common being chronic (primary open-angle), which develops slowly with no warning signs. Glaucoma is the second most common cause of blindness in the world, with an estimated incidence of 65 million, including between 2 and 3 million Americans. It affects people in all age groups, although the elderly are at increased risk. African Americans have a much higher incidence than Caucasians.

The cause of glaucoma varies with the type. In all types, damage to the optic nerve occurs, usually due to abnormally increased intraocular pressure (IOP). However, there is also a form of glaucoma in which IOP is normal, called *normal tension* or *low tension glaucoma*. The cause of this type of glaucoma is not known. Normally, aqueous humor is produced and circulates through the anterior eye chamber and then drains out through a tiny channel called *Schlemm's canal*. In healthy eyes, the production and flow is continuous and normal pressure is maintained. However, when drainage is impeded, IOP increases, damaging the optic nerve. As the optic nerve degenerates, blind spots develop in the visual field.

The cause of acute (closed-angle) glaucoma is a blockage of outflow of aqueous humor, which causes a rapid increase in IOP. This form is usually associated with a very narrow drainage angle of Schlemm's canal, which makes it prone to blockage. Risk factors for this type of glaucoma are aging

and farsightedness. Triggers for angle closure include anything that causes the pupils to become dilated, including darkness, stress, certain medications, and excitement. Chronic (primary open-angle) glaucoma is caused by aqueous humor draining too slowly, leading to increased IOP, although the exact cause is unclear.

Acute angle-closure glaucoma commonly has a rapid onset, and loss of vision may occur within 1 day. Those with chronic primary open-angle glaucoma are commonly asymptomatic until significant peripheral vision is lost. It affects both eyes, although vision loss may initially progress more rapidly in one eye. The attack may be triggered by darkness. Signs and symptoms include severe eye pain, blurred vision, eye redness, seeing light halos, and nausea and vomiting.

For all types of glaucoma, the physician will carefully examine the eye with an ophthalmoscope for optic nerve damage. The optic disk of the eye is where the nerve fibers join at the back of the eyeball. An optic disk damaged by glaucoma takes on an indented appearance, called *cupping*. Other signs of damage include changes in disk color and contour. The physician also evaluates the eye to detect whether the angle of the eye where drainage occurs is *open, narrow,* or *closed*. Doing so helps determine the diagnosis and appropriate treatment. In primary open-angle glaucoma, ophthalmoscopy reveals an open angle and obvious optic nerve damage. A perimetry (visual field) test reveals peripheral vision loss. IOP measurement with a tonometer will reveal 22 mm Hg or higher, which indicates a high risk for glaucoma. Pachymetry, in which ultrasound waves measure cornea thickness, rules out other disorders that involve a thick cornea, rather than optic nerve damage. Gonioscopy and tonography determine how rapidly fluid drains from the eyes.

Treatment of glaucoma includes reduction of IOP by reducing production of aqueous humor or making the outflow more efficient. Either treatment involves the use of eye drop medication, such as the miotic pilocarpine (Isopto Carpine, Pilocar) and the beta blocker timolol maleate (Timoptic). Other treatments include systemic medications, which also act to decrease production of aqueous humor or increase efficiency of outflow. Laser surgery may be used to open the fluid channel and enhance drainage. If these treatments are not effective, microsurgery may be done to create a drainage hole so that fluid can escape.

Acute angle-closure glaucoma is an emergency in which blindness can develop rapidly. Therefore, emergency treatment includes use of medication to reduce IOP and, typically, iridotomy. In iridotomy, the surgeon uses a laser to create a small hole in the iris to allow aqueous humor to flow into the anterior chamber of the eye where it can then flow out through Schlemm's canal.

There is no cure for glaucoma and any vision loss that develops is permanent. Left untreated, glaucoma causes blindness. Even with treatment, approximately 10% of patients still lose their vision. However, the prognosis for those who get early diagnosis and treatment is very good and further damage can usually be prevented or minimized. Glaucoma is a chronic condition that can change over time. Therefore, ongoing management and regular medical checks are important.

Macular Degeneration
ICD-9-CM code: 362.50

Macular degeneration, sometimes called *age-related macular degeneration* (ARMD), is a disorder involving deterioration of the macula of the retina, located at the back of the eye, resulting in progressive vision loss in the center of the visual field. It is categorized as *atrophic* (dry) or *exudative* (wet). Macular degeneration is a common cause of blindness in persons over age 55. It is more common among Caucasians than other ethnic groups and is more common in women than men.

With atrophic macular degeneration, the macula develops irregular pigmentation but there is no scarring, hemorrhage, or exudates. With exudative macular degeneration, hemorrhage or fluid accumulation occurs and causes elevation of part of the macula and eventual scarring. Contributors include inflammation, injury, or infection. Risk factors include advancing age, genetics, obesity, cigarette smoking, cardiovascular disease, high cholesterol, hypertension, nutritional deficiencies, light eye color, and ultraviolet light exposure.

Atrophic macular degeneration usually manifests slowly and painlessly. The exudative form progresses more quickly, causing rapid vision loss, although color and peripheral vision may remain intact. In either case, vision loss occurs and may develop faster in one eye than the other. Tasks requiring sharp vision become difficult and then impossible. Legal blindness, defined as vision that is less than 20/200 may occur.

Diagnosis is based on inspection of the macula of the retina with an ophthalmoscope (an instrument used to examine the interior of the eye), revealing tiny yellow deposits under the macula called *drusen.* Vision testing identifies vision loss. Other possible tests include angiography, tomography, and funduscopy. Angiography evaluates the blood vessels in the eye for bleeding or evidence of neovascularization (abnormal proliferation of blood vessels beneath the retina).

The optical coherence tomography test helps identify retinal thinning or thickening or abnormal presence of fluid. Funduscopy reveals pigment changes and tiny hemorrhages. Other noted changes may include scarring, atrophy, retinal detachment, and lipid exudates. An Amsler grid may identify visual distortion that occurs rapidly in exudative macular degeneration. Scotomas (central blind spots) may be present in atrophic macular degeneration.

There is no cure for macular degeneration. However, vitamin therapy has been found to slow disease progression.

Recommendations include daily supplements of beta-carotene, vitamin E, vitamin C, zinc oxide, and copper. Patients should consult with their ophthalmologist regarding specific dosage amounts. Treatment of exudative macular degeneration may prevent or delay blindness. In addition to vitamin therapy, a combination of laser and photo therapy may be used. Photodynamic laser therapy (PDT) involves the intravenous injection of the light-activated drug verteporfin (Visudyne), which helps direct a laser to the problematic vessels for destruction. However, it is expensive and may cause scarring. Repeated treatments may also be necessary.

Those who have lost central vision may find adaptive devices helpful, including corrective lenses, magnifiers, telescopic lenses, and use of computer monitors.

Prognosis depends on the type of macular degeneration involved. In most cases, mild to moderate vision loss is experienced over time. Blindness occurs from retinal detachment or scarring in some cases. Ninety percent of such cases involve exudative disease. Atrophic disease causes mild to moderate vision loss but rarely causes blindness.

Presbycusis
ICD-9-CM code: 388.01

Presbycusis is progressive, age-related hearing loss that typically begins after age 55. It usually affects both ears equally and begins with loss of high-pitched sounds. An estimated 4 million Americans currently are deaf or have profound hearing loss. Incidence of hearing loss increases with age and as many as 50% of individuals over age 75 have hearing loss. Internationally, incidence varies widely. However, incidence is higher in westernized countries than in others, possibly due to industrial noise.

Presbycusis is a type of sensorineural hearing loss caused by traumatic injury to tiny hair cells in the inner ear; bacterial or viral infections, such as meningitis or mumps, that damage hair cells or the auditory nerve; and Ménière's disease. Other factors contributing to presbycusis include stress and genetics. Underlying physical disorders that affect circulation to ear structures, including diabetes, hypertension, and atherosclerosis, may also be a factor.

Early hearing loss is usually not detected until family or friends notice the person increasing the volume on the television or radio and requesting them to repeat things they have said. Individuals with presbycusis may complain that others mumble too much or speak too quietly. They have greater difficulty hearing when background noise is present. First lost is the ability to hear high-pitched sounds and *s, sh,* and *ch* consonant sounds. For this reason, they may find a man's lower-pitched voice easier to hear and understand than a woman's voice. They may also complain of tinnitus, which causes abnormal hissing, ringing, or roaring sounds in one or both ears, compounding their hearing difficulties.

Diagnosis is based on otoscopic examination of the ear, a variety of hearing tests and other tests such as CT scan and

MRI, which may rule out structural abnormalities, masses, or lesions that can cause hearing loss. The Weber and Rinne tuning fork tests help differentiate between conductive and sensorineural hearing loss. Presbycusis is diagnosed when other possible causes of hearing loss are ruled out.

Sensorineural hearing loss is permanent; thus, the physician will prescribe hearing aids and other devices to help the person with activities of daily living. A variety of strategies and technological devices are currently available to improve hearing and understanding. Many individuals benefit from hearing aids and amplification devices used with telephones. Some technology makes sounds more clear with or without the use of hearing aids. In addition, some patients may benefit from learning lip reading.

There is currently no cure for presbycusis. However, with appropriate diagnosis and treatment, most patients can maintain a high quality of life using hearing aids or other devices that improve their ability to hear and understand the sounds around them. (See *Hearing loss and confidentiality*.)

Special Needs of the Geriatric Patient

To effectively interact with geriatric patients and their caregivers, the medical assistant must be able to communicate clearly and understand the physical and psychological challenges of the older adult. When asking questions about the patient's health, she should be sure to speak clearly and consider any sensory deficits the patient might have, including vision and hearing loss. She should use various communication strategies to ensure that the patient understands her questions and obtain accurate responses. If the patient suffers from dementia, the medical assistant should try to direct her questions to the patient and caregiver, including them both in the conversation. She should also be alert for opportunities to explain safety promotion for the elderly patient living at home. For patients who are acutely ill or have chronic, degenerative illness, the medical assistant should be alert for signs of caregiver burnout as well as the need for support and assistance, including home health care, assisted living, long-term care, and hospice. In addition, the medical assistant may provide information and referrals regarding nutrition and end-of-life issues.

Communication Strategies
Communication with elderly patients requires patience and sensitivity on the part of the medical assistant. Some elderly individuals are too embarrassed to admit that they don't hear well. Consequently they may not understand what has been said. Health care providers may erroneously assume the older person is confused, forgetful, or suffers from dementia when the real problem is faulty communication. The medical

Front office–Back office connection

Hearing Loss and Confidentiality

Confidentiality is a challenge when the medical assistant communicates with a patient who has moderate to severe hearing loss. Because the medical assistant may have to speak loudly so the patient can hear her questions, she risks violating his confidentiality by enabling others in the office to hear as well. This is an issue for the administrative medical assistant, who may need to confirm information about insurance, address, and telephone number when the patient checks in at the reception desk. It is also an issue for the clinical medical assistant, who must ask questions about symptoms, allergies, and other personal health information. Accurate information is critical, so medical assistants should challenge themselves to be creative in finding confidential ways to obtain it. Here are some suggestions to consider:

- Confirm information, such as insurance, address, and telephone number over the telephone when the appointment is made.
- Show the information in writing (using large print) to the patient for his confirmation or correction.
- Take the patient into a private room where the door may be closed to confirm or obtain information.
- Face the patient so he can see your lips and facial expressions.
- Speak at an adequate volume in a low-pitched voice without shouting.
- Enunciate clearly and speak in an unhurried manner.
- Use visual aids, such as photos or illustrations when appropriate.

assistant can make accommodations for sensory deficits by adjusting the pace and volume of her speech. Clear enunciation will also help the listener hear and understand what she says. She must also allow adequate time for the older patient to process information and formulate a response. Last, but not least, the older patient must be treated with respect and dignity. The medical assistant should refer to the patient by his last name and use the appropriate title, such as Mr., unless the patient instructs her to do otherwise. It is *never* appropriate to refer to the patient with a term of endearment, such as "sweetie" or "honey." Although the medical assistant may do so with good intentions, the message conveyed is one of disrespect and "talking down" to the patient.

Safety Promotion
An important part of the medical assistant's role when providing care for elderly patients is the promotion of

independent function and safety. To help the patient maintain a level of independence, the medical assistant can advise him on the use of tools, including mobility aids and assistive devices (hearing aids and corrective lenses), to compensate for sensory deficits. To help promote the patient's safety, she can provide guidelines for modifying his home environment to reduce hazards and promote safe function. (See *Safety: Everyone's concern.*)

Mobility Aids

Elderly patients commonly use mobility aids, such as canes, walkers, and motorized scooters, on a temporary or permanent basis to compensate for weakness from disease, impairment caused by injury or disability, and general functional decline. The medical assistant may have the responsibility of fitting the patient with a mobility aid and teaching her to use it. (For more information see Chapter 35, "Orthopedics," page 707.)

Crutches are not an appropriate mobility aid for very elderly patients because such patients do not typically have the upper body strength required to use them. Inappropriate use of crutches by a frail older adult increases the risk of further injury. More appropriate choices for such patients include walkers and canes, depending on the level of aid needed, as determined by the physician or therapist. The medical assistant must make sure the device is fitted correctly for the patient and that she knows how to use it safely. After the medical assistant demonstrates correct use, she should ask the patient to perform a return demonstration. Doing so enables the medical assistant to observe the patient and provide feedback and correction as needed.

Home Safety

Home safety is a critical issue for elderly adults because of the risk of injury from falls. An estimated 30% of elderly individuals who live independently in their own homes fall at least once each year. Of those, approximately 5% will suffer a bone fracture. In addition, the risk increases with age.

There are many factors that contribute to the risk of fall-related injury. The medical assistant should review home safety with elderly patients as well as family members or caregivers. General considerations include the patient's degree of mobility, mental status, home setting, and close proximity to potential help. (See *Safety hazards at home.*) In some cases, elderly adults are afforded an extra measure of security by wearing some type of device that allows them to call for help if they fall. Although such a device does not prevent falling or injury, it may help provide more immediate assistance and prevent some complications associated with a delay in treatment.

In addition to injury from falls, elderly patients are at increased risk for adverse effects from medication errors. Because many elderly patients take multiple medications, including prescription and over-the-counter (OTC)

Front office–Back office connection

Safety: Everyone's Concern

Keeping patients safe in the medical office should be the concern of every staff member regardless of her job description. Patients with strength, agility, mobility, and sensory deficits are at significantly higher risk for injury than the general population. Thus, the medical assistant and others must evaluate their work area daily to identify and remove potential hazards and obstacles. Administrative and clinical medical assistants should work together cooperatively on a daily basis to ensure every patient's safety, including following these guidelines:

- Confirm that there are no obstructions in walkways, stairs, and wheelchair ramps.
- Make sure patients have access to entryways and doorways and that patients with disabilities can easily open them.
- Arrange seating in the reception area to facilitate easy navigation by patients with disabilities and those using mobility aids.
- Determine that there is adequate lighting in all rooms.
- Allow patients to sit in chairs or remain in wheelchairs when possible, rather than asking them to climb onto examination tables.
- Safely assist patients onto examination tables if they must do so.
- Never leave a patient with dementia, severe weakness, or disability alone.
- Verify that floors in all areas are clean, dry, and uncluttered.
- Never push, pull, or rush a patient when walking, sitting, standing, or transferring between chairs and examination tables.
- Never "assist" a patient by pulling on her arms or shoulders. Instead, use a second person and a gait belt, if necessary, to help with patient transfers.
- Be willing to interrupt what you are doing to help a patient or coworker with safety issues.

medications, and some suffer from cognitive impairments, a patient can easily become confused regarding when medications should be taken. Such confusion can lead to medication errors and, possibly, illness or death. The medical assistant can help reduce the risk of such complications by providing education to elderly patients about ways to prevent medication errors. (See *Preventing medication problems,* page 700)

Safety hazards at home

In addition to taking safety measures in the medical office, the medical assistant can provide strategies to the elderly patient to decrease the risk of falls and other injuries at home. The following table lists many hazards faced by elderly patients as they deal with sensory deficits, illness, decreased mobility, and increased use of medications as well as solutions to prevent the adverse effects of each.

Hazard	Solution
Vision and hearing impairment	• Referral for vision and hearing evaluation and treatment (corrective lenses and hearing aids) • Keeping corrective lenses accessible at night, such as at the bedside • Ensuring adequate lighting, especially at night
Postural hypotension	• Standing slowly to allow time for blood pressure adjustment
Musculoskeletal disorders, such as arthritis or generalized weakness	• Appropriate evaluation and treatment to maximize function • General self-care measures to maximize energy and functional ability, such as regular exercise and gentle stretching
Altered balance	• Use of cane or other mobility aid for stabilization • Using well-fitting shoes and house slippers with nonskid soles
Impaired bladder function, such as incontinence, nocturia, and urgency	• Evaluation and treatment of the disorder, if possible • Sleeping near a bathroom or keeping a commode at the bedside at night
Medication adverse effects	• Reviewing medications with the health care provider to determine whether adjustments can be made to minimize adverse effects • Learning about prescribed medications to become aware of potential adverse effects, such as sedation and postural hypotension, and using appropriate safety strategies, such as sitting on the bedside for a moment before rising, taking medications at bedtime when possible, and avoiding driving or similar activities
Medication errors	• Labeling medications with large, easy-to-read print • Placing scheduled medications in a daily or weekly organizer, according to day and time
Household hazards, such as throw rugs, stairs, bathtubs, poor lighting, and wet floors	• Evaluating the home environment for potential hazards and rearranging or removing them • Placing nightlights in high-risk areas • Installing handrails in hallways and on stairs • Installing grab bars around the bathtub, shower, and toilet • Keeping emergency numbers posted by the telephone • Replacing the telephone with one that has larger, easy-to-read numbers and a volume adjustment knob
Cognitive impairment	• Educating family members and caregivers about precautions regarding fall prevention, including wearing shoes with nonskid soles, eliminating household hazards, and keeping often needed items, such as reading glasses and tissues, within reach • Reducing environmental hazards, as listed above • Using a bed or chair alarm, which is a device that will emit a loud sound if the individual gets out of his bed or chair unassisted

Patient Education

Preventing Medication Problems

Nearly a quarter of a million elderly patients are hospitalized each year because of the adverse effects of combining prescription medications with over-the-counter (OTC) medications or taking medications improperly. In an effort to prevent or minimize such adverse events, the medical assistant should encourage elderly patients and their caregivers to take these precautions:

- Use nonpharmacologic methods first to try to treat a problem, such as treating pain with heat or cold therapy, insomnia with warm milk or progressive relaxation, or anxiety with relaxation or exercise.

- Talk with your health care provider before using any OTC medications and read the labels of such medications for warnings about interactions.

- Avoid combination OTC products when possible.

- Read and follow instructions on the medication label.

- Avoid using OTC remedies for longer than recommended.

- Consult with your health care provider if a condition does not improve or worsens.

Pain Management

Many elderly patients experience some form of pain on a daily basis due to acute illness or injury or chronic disease. Such pain can severely limit the patient's ability to function socially, maintain independence, obtain good-quality sleep, and enjoy a high quality of life. Unfortunately, health care providers do not always provide adequate pain management for elderly patients. Some reasons for this gap in care include the provider's or patient's fear of adverse effects or "addiction," more appropriately called *psychological* or *physical dependence,* and general misconceptions about pain and pain behaviors. A common yet misguided belief is that elderly patients feel less pain than younger individuals. However, there is little evidence that age impacts pain perception. Elderly patients may have a compromised ability to communicate what they are feeling, which may lead others to mistakenly assume that they feel less pain. In fact, significant evidence indicates that elderly patients suffer from increased pain from illness and injury, including arthritis and various forms of neuropathy. Therefore, all health care providers, including medical assistants, should place a high priority on adequate evaluation and treatment of pain in order to maximize function and quality of life for elderly patients. Health care providers are obligated to do everything possible to relieve suffering and promote the highest quality of life possible to all patients, including elderly patients.

The medical assistant can better understand pain management strategies by learning which medications are most effective for which forms of pain. (See *Medications for managing pain.*) In addition, the medical assistant should be familiar with specific considerations for the elderly patient using these medications. (See *Pharmacokinetic variations in older adults,* page 702.)

Extended Care and End-of-Life Issues

One of the main challenges of the medical assistant working with geriatric patients is to provide correct, timely information on resources for extended care, or care beyond the primary care offered by a medical office, and care at the end of a patient's life. (See *Community resources for elder care,* page 703.) Garnering the support of family, friends, and the community is essential for patients to experience a high quality of life in their elder years. As a person ages and cannot take care of himself without support and aid, he and his spouse or family must consider options for extended care, including in-home care and home health care, assisted living, and nursing centers.

In-Home and Home Health Care

Most elderly persons prefer to remain in their own homes for as long as possible. **In-home care,** or care provided by spouses, family, and close friends who act as caregivers, commonly makes such a preference possible. However, ongoing care can become a hardship for families as a person's care needs increase. Thus, many families eventually choose to enlist the services of a paid in-home caregiver. Some families hire a live-in caregiver who may have some health care training. In these cases, the family usually locates and trains the caregiver on their own and pays them privately or enlists the services of a home care agency that provides the caregivers. However, some families choose to enlist the services of **home health care agencies,** which are located in most communities and are sometimes affiliated with local hospitals. These agencies employ nursing assistants and nurses who make home visits. During these visits, the home health nurse or nursing assistant may provide such nursing services as home infusion of antibiotics and education for patients or family members regarding wound care. However, these agencies do not provide round-the-clock care or assist with all activities of daily living. In addition, because the number of visits and the type of services allowed by insurance or Medicare are limited, long-term use of such services can become extremely expensive for the patient or family.

Assisted Living

If an elderly person is no longer able to live independently and home health care is not possible, she may wish to consider

Medications for managing pain

The following table lists medications used to manage pain in the elderly, along with the form of pain for which they are commonly prescribed as well as any special considerations for geriatric patients.

Medication	Form of Pain	Considerations
analgesics acetaminophen (Tylenol)	Most forms of mild to moderate pain	• Little or no anti-inflammatory property • Nonirritating to the stomach • Should be used cautiously in patients with liver impairment • Possible kidney damage with prolonged use • Additive analgesic effect when coadministered with opiates, possibly allowing a lower opiate dose
salicylates aspirin (Bayer)	Mild to moderate inflammatory pain, such as arthritis	• Should be used cautiously in patients with history of ulcer disease, GI bleeding, alcohol abuse, or kidney or liver impairment • Increased risk of adverse reactions and lower toxicity levels, indicated by tinnitus (ringing in the ears) • Possible adverse interactions with many drugs, including anticoagulants, some anticonvulsants, and antibiotics • Greater risk of allergic reaction in those with asthma • Should be taken with food to minimize gastric irritation, a common adverse effect • Enteric coated form should not be crushed • Additive analgesic effect when coadministered with opiates, possibly allowing a lower opiate dose
Nonsteroidal anti-inflammatory drugs (NSAIDs) ibuprofen (Motrin, Advil) ketorolac (Toradol)	Mild to moderate inflammatory pain, such as arthritis pain	• Should be used cautiously in patients with a history of ulcer disease, GI bleeding, alcohol abuse, or kidney or liver impairment • Commonly causes gastric irritation • Numerous drug interactions possible with such drugs as anticoagulants, digoxin, insulin, and antihyperglycemics • Risk of gastric or duodenal ulceration leading to GI bleeding • Should be started at lower dose because of the higher sensitivity to adverse reactions in geriatric patients • Increased risk of allergic reaction in patients with asthma or aspirin allergies • Should be taken with food to minimize gastric irritation • Additive analgesic effect when coadministered with opiates, possibly allowing a lower opiate dose • Concurrent aspirin or acetaminophen use contraindicated before consulting a health care provider
Opiates acetaminophen and hydrocodone (Vicodin) hydromorphone (Dilaudid) acetaminophen and oxycodone (Percocet) morphine (MS Contin)	Most forms of moderate to severe pain	• May cause constipation (most common adverse effect) • Risk of physical dependence and tolerance when used regularly • Risks of sedation, drowsiness, and respiratory depression with short-term use that lessen with long-term use and development of tolerance • Reduced initial dosage recommended for geriatric patients

Continued

Medications for managing pain—cont'd

Medication	Form of Pain	Considerations
		• Additive depressant effect when combined with other central nervous system (CNS depressants), such as alcohol, sedatives, and opiates
		• Additive analgesic effect when coadministered with nonopioid analgesics, possibly allowing a lower opiate dose
Antidepressants amitriptyline (Elavil) doxepin (Sinequan) imipramine (Tofranil) nortriptyline (Pamelor)	Chronic pain, such as neuropathy caused by diabetes (in low doses)	• Should be used cautiously because of the higher sensitivity to adverse reactions in geriatric patients • Risk of exacerbation of urinary retention in men with benign prostatic hyperplasia (BPH) • Anticholinergic adverse effects (blurred vision, urinary retention, dry eyes, dry mouth, constipation) and drowsiness • Contraindicated for use with or within 2 weeks of use of monoamine oxidase inhibitors (MAOIs) • Additive CNS depressant effects when combined with other CNS depressants • Monitor baseline ECGs in those with a history of heart disease because of risk of irregular heart rhythm • Contraindicated in narrow-angle glaucoma
Anticonvulsants phenytoin (Dilantin) gabapentin (Neurontin)	Chronic pain, such as neuropathy caused by trigeminal neuralgia and peripheral neuropathy	• Risk of drowsiness • Should not be taken within 2 hours of antacids

Pharmacokinetic variations in older adults

This table summarizes the pharmacokinetic variations (absorption, distribution, metabolism, and excretion) of drugs in elderly patients based on route or drug form.

Route and Drug Form	Effect
Oral (tablets, capsules)	• Drier mucous membranes may cause capsules and tablets to adhere to the side or roof of the mouth instead of being swallowed, which impairs absorption and may cause ulceration. • Decreased acid production in the stomach slows absorption of drug.
Rectal, vaginal (suppositories)	• The drug may require more time to melt in this form. • Decreased circulation in rectal and vaginal mucosa may slow absorption. • The patient may expel the drug before it dissolves for many reasons, including sphincter laxity, poor muscle tone or control, or the urge to defecate.
Subcutaneous, intramuscular (injectable solution)	• Loss of skin elasticity may cause medication to leak back out of the injection site. • Decreased circulation may decrease absorption.
Topical (ointments, creams, lotions, powders)	• Skin changes, such as atrophy, scarring, or thinning and loss of subcutaneous tissue may increase or decrease the intended localized effect.
All routes other than topical	• Reduced kidney function extends the half-life.

Community resources for elder care

Medical assistants may need to help their elderly patients identify community resources that can help them with living arrangements, personal care, and other needs. The following resources are available in most communities and can be located by checking the local telephone directory:

- adult care facilities, such as assisted living facilities and nursing homes
- retirement communities for elderly persons with minimal health-related issues
- senior and aging organizations for support and group activities
- chore services for house cleaning and maintenance
- respite services, which provide support to caregivers and patients, by providing resources for caregivers, as well as elder day care, which gives the caregiver some free time and gives the patient social interaction in a safe environment
- senior activity centers for group activities and lifelong learning
- adult protective services for protection from fraud and abuse
- Department of Social and Health Services for legal and social assistance
- housing authority for assistance with housing
- Social Security Administration for financial assistance in retirement and for those with disabilities
- state legislature for help with resources for state aid and other services
- Veterans Administration for help with health care and housing costs for veterans.

an **assisted living** situation. Most assisted living facilities, commonly called *adult family homes*, are privately operated. Many accept only private-pay clients. They are regulated by state agencies, however, and must meet certain criteria for health and safety. Older assisted living facilities are laid out as in a dormitory or hotel, with many small suites with a living space and bedroom, shared bathrooms, and shared dining areas. Newer facilities typically contain more private apartments with small kitchenettes, private bathrooms, and private living areas but still include shared dining areas. Most assisted living facilities offer elderly persons several prepared meals each day as well as many social events and other activities. In addition, they may facilitate transportation to and from shops, supermarkets, doctors' offices, and so on. These facilities commonly allow a person who needs

more intensive care on a short-term basis, such as in a hospital or rehabilitation facility, to return to the facility when that care is complete as long as the person's needs have not increased beyond the scope of the facility.

Nursing Center

A common misconception is that all elderly persons eventually end up in a **nursing center,** formerly called a *skilled nursing facility (SNF)* and commonly referred to as a *nursing home.* In fact, the vast majority of elderly persons are able to maintain a more independent living situation for the duration of their lives. A nursing center provides care for residents who need ongoing medical care on a long-term basis. Staff members include nurses and nursing assistants who meet the residents' health and personal needs, including help with medications, dressing, bathing, toileting, and eating. Other staff members may help with social activities, nutrition, and various therapies. Most nursing centers are designed like hospitals, with private or semiprivate rooms with a bath but no kitchen or living areas.

Extended Care Campus

Facilities that provide various levels of assistance on the same campus are a growing trend in extended care. Such a facility includes retirement apartments, assisted living services, and LTC services. Retirement apartments are available for persons who are able to continue living independently but desire more social interaction with their peers as well as fewer responsibilities for maintaining their own home. These facilities typically offer community dining options to such residents in addition to the kitchen facilities in their private apartment. They also offer the services of a visiting nurse, who can check in on residents from time to time to help with simple tasks, such as organizing weekly medications or blood pressure screening. If a resident experiences a decline in health and needs a greater degree of assistance, she may move to the assisted care facility on the same campus. Because she is able to maintain relationships with those in the larger facility as well as some of the staff, she may more easily transition to the new care setting than she would if moving to a different facility with new caregivers and residents. If, after living in the assisted care facility for a time, her health continues to decline to the point that LTC services are necessary, she can make the transition to the LTC facility on the same campus. This transition, again, may feel less traumatic because she would remain within the same larger community.

End-of-Life Issues

An older person, especially one with chronic illness, may also desire to plan for the eventuality of his death. The medical assistant can help the patient with this planning by providing information about living wills, also called an *advance directive.* In addition, the medical assistant should be aware of any patient who has enacted a living will as well as the content of that will in case it contains instructions regarding treatment that she might administer. For example, if a patient has instructed in a living will that he does not wish anyone to provide lifesaving care, commonly called a *do-not-resuscitate (DNR) order,* she is legally bound to withhold that care. If she provides that treatment, she can be sued for battery. (For more information on legal considerations regarding end-of-life care, see Chapter 6, "Legal Considerations," page 53.)

Hospice

Individuals who are facing a terminal illness may be interested in the services provided by **hospice care.** In its earliest forms, a hospice was a facility designed to provide care to terminally ill individuals. It has evolved into an entire philosophy of care in which death is viewed as the natural and final stage of life. The goal of hospice care is to support patients in maintaining a high-quality, dignified, pain-free life in their last days. It is family-centered and includes the patient and family in decision making. Family members serve as the main hands-on caregivers, supported as needed by the hospice staff. Hospice care may be provided within the home or in a variety of locations, including but not limited to hospice facilities, hospitals, or nursing centers.

Hospice care focuses on **palliative care,** which is medical care aimed at alleviating disease symptoms and enhancing quality of life, rather than curative treatments or quantity of life. Medical and nursing care aim to relieve symptoms and provide physical, emotional, and spiritual comfort as desired by the patient and family. In addition to services by professional health care providers, most hospice organizations also train volunteer staff members to offer respite for family members and a comforting presence for the patient. Although medical assistants do not generally provide hospice care, they should be aware of its purpose and goals so they can answer questions from their elderly patients or family members. (See *Common questions and answers about hospice care.*)

Common questions and answers about hospice care

Medical assistants can answer some of the most common questions asked about hospice care by patients and family members, including:

- **Is hospice care paid for by insurance and when does the patient qualify for care?** Most insurance companies cover hospice care charges. Medicare covers hospice nationwide. Medicaid covers hospice in most states. Patients and family members should always check with their insurance carrier or Medicaid and Medicare representatives to get specific questions answered. Most hospice organizations accept patients who have been determined by their physician as having a life expectancy of 6 months or less.

- **Does hospice provide round-the-clock care?** No. Medicare requires that certified hospices provide a basic level of care but the specific type of services offered by hospice organizations may vary.

- **If a hospice patient makes a physical recovery can she return to regular medical treatment?** Yes. Patients whose disease goes into remission may be discharged from hospice and return to more aggressive therapy or even to their normal daily life.

- **What can the patient expect during the hospice admission process?** Initially, the hospice will contact the patient's physician to verify the appropriateness of hospice care. The hospice will then ask the patient to sign consent and insurance forms similar to those when entering a hospital.

- **Must the patient make changes within her home before hospice care begins?** The hospice provider will evaluate the patient's needs and make recommendations for any necessary equipment. Needs may be minimal initially and increase over time as the patient's disease progresses.

- **Will someone be with the patient at all times?** Initially, the patient may have no need or desire to have someone there continuously. However, as her disease progresses and her needs increase, she may need more care. Hospice will help design and coordinate a plan of care that will meet the patient's needs and involve professional caregivers, volunteers, and family members as needed.

- **What specific services will be provided?** Hospice care is provided by a team of caring individuals, including physicians, nurses, social workers, therapists, clergy, home health aides, and volunteers. Individuals provide help based on their own expertise. Hospice also provides medication, health care supplies, equipment, and other services as needed.

- **Does hospice hasten the dying process?** Hospice does not hasten dying. It views dying as a natural process and seeks to alleviate suffering while enhancing quality of life for the patient as well as family members. It does so by alleviating physical and emotional pain through medication administration, a variety of therapies (physical, occupational, art, music, and so on), dietary counseling, and other measures.

Chapter Summary

- The effects of aging on a person's health have a huge impact on her quality of life. Some of the factors impacting aging include genetics, lifestyle, diet, activity and exercise, and coping strategies.
- Ageism is a form of prejudice and discrimination against individuals because of their age.
- As a person ages, his body undergoes physical changes to all systems. To appropriately meet the health care needs of their aging patients, medical assistants must understand these changes.
- The most common endocrine system disorder that develops secondary to aging is type 2 diabetes, which is commonly not diagnosed until after age 60. Symptoms are commonly atypical but treatment is the same as for younger patients.
- The aging musculoskeletal system decreases in muscle mass and strength as well as bone mass. Osteoarthritis and osteoporosis are significant concerns for both men and women. Osteoporosis is characterized by loss of bone mass throughout the skeleton.
- Dementia is a neurological disorder characterized by chronic, progressive, irreversible decline in mental function and is marked by deficits in reasoning and judgment. It may be confused with delirium, depression, and psychosis.
- Alzheimer disease is the most common form of dementia and most commonly occurs over age 65. Treatment for all types of dementia is aimed at maximizing function and providing safety and comfort.
- Elderly persons are prone to poor eating habits and poor fluid intake. As a result, they may be deficient in vitamins and minerals, are usually dehydrated, and have an overall increased risk of GI disorders, such as GERD, PUD, and diverticulitis.
- Elderly patients commonly must use mobility aids on a temporary or permanent basis due to weakness from disease, impairment caused by injury or disability, and general functional decline.
- Home safety is an issue of critical importance for elderly adults because of the risk of injury from falls.
- Communication with elderly patients requires patience and sensitivity on the part of the medical assistant and she must always treat elderly patients with respect and dignity.
- Many elderly patients experience some form of pain on a daily basis due to acute illness or injury or chronic disease. Such pain can severely limit the patient's ability to function socially, maintain independence, obtain good-quality sleep, and enjoy a high quality of life.

- For an elderly patient who becomes unable to continue living independently, the medical assistant may need to provide information about alternative living arrangements, such as in-home care, services provided by home health care agencies, assisted living facilities, and nursing care centers. In some cases, a range of services may be available on the same extended care campus.
- The medical assistant may provide information to an elderly patient about living wills, which are documents that patients can complete to indicate their wishes regarding life-sustaining measures.
- A person facing a terminal illness may be interested in the services provided by hospice care, which is care centered around the philosophy that death is natural and the final stage of life. Hospice seeks to support patients in maintaining a high-quality, dignified, pain-free life in their last days and focuses on palliative care, rather than curative treatments or quantity of life.

Team Work Exercises

1. Divide into nine teams. Each team must create an educational poster based on a topic listed here. Posters will be graded on accuracy, creativity, professional appearance, and other criteria as indicated by the instructor. After the poster has been approved by the instructor, the team must contact a local organization or facility, such as a senior center, an area agency on aging, nursing home, or church. With permission from the appropriate persons, the team must post and display the poster at the identified facility. Topics include:
   a. home safety, including common hazards and strategies to increase safety
   b. osteoporosis, including the cause, prevention and management strategies, and common medications
   c. dementia, including the cause, risk reduction and management strategies, and common medications
   d. osteoarthritis, including the cause, prevention and management strategies, common medications, and surgical procedures
   f. cataracts, including the cause, prevention and management strategies, common medications, and surgical procedures
   g. macular degeneration, including the cause, prevention and management strategies, and common medications
   h. open-angle glaucoma, including the cause, prevention and management strategies, and common medications
   i. angle-closure glaucoma, including the cause, prevention and management strategies, and common medications.
2. Divide into five teams. Each team must choose a patient from the list provided. For that patient, the team must identify resources available in the community to help the patient meet his or her needs. Then the team must create

a plan that designates what services will be provided by which community resource, including accurate contact information. Finally, the team must describe a safety plan for the patient's home.

a. Mildred Osborne is a 75-year-old woman discharged home after being hospitalized with pneumonia. She was diagnosed with type 2 diabetes in the hospital and must learn more about her disease to be able to do daily glucometer testing and eat an appropriate diet. Mrs. Osborne lives with her 77-year-old husband, who suffers from severe hearing loss but is able to help with minor household chores.

b. Nicholas Stednick is a 68-year-old man who recently suffered a stroke. After several days in the hospital, he spent 2 weeks in a rehabilitation unit and is now preparing to return home. His stroke left him with left-sided weakness and he currently uses a walker. He hopes to be able to transition to using a cane within the next month. He lives in a three-bedroom, one-level house by himself. His grown daughter lives in the same neighborhood and will check on him at least once each day but she has a job and family of her own.

c. Sayoko Oni is a 72-year-old woman recently diagnosed with metastatic lung cancer. She lives at home with her 75-year-old husband and is determined to remain at home for whatever time she has left. Her husband wants to respect her wishes but is concerned that he will be unable to meet her health care needs and does not want her to suffer.

d. Helga Ivarsen is an 88-year-old woman who was recently hospitalized after falling and breaking her hip. She underwent a total hip replacement and spent 3 weeks in a rehabilitation unit. She is now preparing to return home, where she lives with her 66-year-old daughter and 6-year-old great-grandson. She is legally blind and has severe hearing loss but is fiercely independent and wants to be able to provide as much of her own self-care as possible.

e. Hershel Hemminger is a 70-year-old man who has recently been diagnosed with Alzheimer disease. He suffers severe short-term memory loss and is beginning to display impaired judgment. His wife is 65 years old and wants to keep him at home with her for as long as possible. To do this, she needs help keeping him safe and must learn more about Alzheimer disease so that she can anticipate what to expect in the future.

Case Studies

1. Mr. Clancy and his wife Margaret visit the physician's office one morning. Mr. Clancy is concerned about his wife and asks the physician to evaluate her. He states she has been having trouble with her memory lately, her sleep patterns have been "odd," and she sometimes says and does "odd" things. What questions might the medical assistant ask to elicit and clarify important information about Mrs. Clancy's health status and behaviors?

2. Mrs. Halvorson is a 45-year-old woman who is a regular patient at Valley Clinic. She is concerned about the possibility of developing osteoporosis. She is 5' 2" tall, weighs 105 lb, and is currently "perimenopausal." Her elderly mother has severe osteoporosis, suffered a recent hip fracture, and has developed kyphosis. Mrs. Halvorson wants to know what she can do to avoid the same experience. List the type of information that the medical assistant should share with her and describe an effective method of teaching her.

Resources

- Administration on Aging: *www.aoa.dhhs.gov*
- Alzheimer's Association: 1-800-272-3900; *www.alz.org*
- Arthritis Foundation: *www.arthritis.org*
- Glaucoma Research Foundation: *www.glaucoma.org*
- National Council on Aging: *www.ncoa.org*
- National Institute on Aging: *www.nia.nih.gov*
- National Institute on Deafness and Other Communication Disorders: *www.nidcd.nih.gov*
- National Meals-on-Wheels Foundation: *www.mowaa.org*
- National Osteoporosis Foundation: *www.nof.org*

Orthopedics

Learning Objectives

Upon completion of this chapter, the student will be able to:

- define the key terms presented in the glossary
- identify and locate bones of the skeleton and major muscles of the body
- identify and name body movements used in range of motion exercises
- perform procedures outlined in the chapter
- discuss the importance of patient education in the use of assistive devices
- discuss how to comfort and educate a patient with a cast, from application to cast maintenance and removal
- explain how the body reacts to application of heat and cold and their use in soft tissue injuries
- describe the physiological effects of ultrasound, TENS, and massage.

CAAHEP Competencies

Clinical Competencies
Patient Care
Prepare patient for and assist with procedures, treatments, and minor office surgeries

General Competencies
Patient Instruction
Instruct individuals according to their needs
Provide instruction for health maintenance and disease prevention

ABHES Competencies

Clinical Duties
Prepare patients for procedures
Prepare and maintain examination and treatment areas
Prepare patient for and assist physician with routine and specialty examinations and treatments and minor office surgeries

Legal Concepts
Document accurately
Instruction
Instruct patients with special needs
Teach patients methods of health promotion and disease prevention

Procedures

Transferring a patient from a wheelchair to an examination table
Transferring a patient from an examination table to a wheelchair
Performing ROM exercises, upper body
Performing ROM exercises, lower body
Assisting with gait using a gait belt
Assisting a patient in ambulating with a walker
Assisting a patient in ambulating with a cane
Assisting a patient in ambulating with crutches
Assisting with fiberglass cast application
Assisting with cast removal
Applying a triangular arm sling
Administering ultrasound
Teaching a patient to use a TENS unit

Chapter Outline

Structures and Functions of the Musculoskeletal System
　Structures of the Musculoskeletal System
　　Bone
　　Muscle
　　Tendons and ligaments
　Functions of the Musculoskeletal System
　　Bone
　　Muscle
　　Tendons and ligaments
Medical Terminology Related to the Musculoskeletal System
Common Musculoskeletal System Diseases and Disorders
　Injuries to Bones
　　Dislocation

　　Scoliosis
　　Kyphosis
　　Lordosis
　　Gout
　　Osteoarthritis
　　Osteoporosis
　　Rheumatoid arthritis
　　Juvenile rheumatoid arthritis
　Muscle Disorders
　　Fibromyalgia
　　Strain
　　Myasthenia gravis
　　Rotator cuff tear
　　Herniated disk
　Injuries to Tendons and Ligaments
　　Anterior cruciate ligament tear
　　Epicondylitis, medial and lateral
　　Tendinitis Sprain
Orthopedic Procedures
　Assisting with Examination
　Evaluating Muscle Strength and Range of Motion
　　Goniometry
　　Range of motion
　Fitting a Patient with a Walker, Cane, and Crutches
　　Fitting a patient with a walker
　　Fitting a patient with a cane
　　Fitting a patient with crutches
　Casting
　Thermotherapy
　　Moist heat
　　Dry heat
　Cryotherapy
　Ultrasound
　Transcutaneous Electrical Nerve Stimulation
Chapter Summary
Team Work Exercises
Case Studies
Resources

Key Terms

abduction
Motion away from the midline of the body

adduction
Motion toward the midline of the body

ambulation
Action of walking

aponeurosis
Flat, fibrous sheet of connective tissue that attaches muscle to bone or other tissues

articulation
Juncture between two or more bones; also called a *joint*

atrophy
Decrease in mass of a muscle or organ; also called *wasting*

bone
Individual unit of osseous tissue that is part of the framework of the body

circumduction
Circular motion of a body part

contracture
Movement that shortens or tightens a muscle

cryotherapy
Removal of heat from a body part to decrease cellular metabolism and swelling

eversion
Movement of a body part outward

extension
Movement that straightens a body part

fascia
Sheet of fibrous connective tissue that covers, separates, or supports muscle

flexion
Movement that bends a body part

gait
Manner of walking

goniometry
Process of measuring joint movements and angles

hematopoiesis
Production and development of blood cells

hemiplegia
Paralysis of one side of the body

hyperextension
Position of maximum extension, or extending a body part beyond its normal limits

inversion
Movement of a body part inward

ligament
Band or sheet of fibrous tissue that connects two or more bones or cartilage

modality
Method of applying a therapy, usually a physical device

muscle
Tissue made up of contractile fibers that produce movement

muscle testing
Process of evaluating muscle strength and range of motion

myofascia
Tissue consisting of muscle and underlying fascia

pronation
Movement of the arm so the palm is down or movement of the foot outward and up

range of motion
Outer limit of joint movement

reduction
Manual manipulation of a bone to return it to its normal position

rotation
Movement that turns a body part around its axis

supination
Movement of the arm so the palm is up or movement of the foot inward and up

tendon
Band of dense, fibrous tissue that attaches muscle to bone

thermotherapy
Therapeutic application of heat used to treat various muscle injuries

ultrasound
Application of high-frequency sound waves to warm tissues, increasing tissue extensibility and improving local blood flow

vasoconstriction
Decrease in diameter of blood vessels, which decreases blood flow and raises blood pressure

vasodilation
Dilation or enlargement of blood vessels, especially small arteries and arterioles

Structures and Functions of the Musculoskeletal System

The musculoskeletal system consists of muscles, bones, ligaments, and tendons. Together, these structures facilitate movement and protection for internal organs.

Structures of the Musculoskeletal System

The structures of the musculoskeletal system include the bones, muscles, tendons, and ligaments.

Bone

A **bone** is an individual unit of osseous tissue and is part of the framework of the body. Bones are living tissues that are hard in appearance due to their calcium matrix. (See Figure 35-1.)

Muscle

Muscles are tissues made up of contractile fibers. Muscles are covered by a fibrous membrane called a **fascia**. The fascia is connective tissue that is arranged in sheets or bands and covers, separates, and supports muscle. Because the muscle and fascia are connected, these structures are commonly referred to as one structure: **myofascia**—muscle and fascia.

There are three types of muscle tissue:

- skeletal
- smooth
- cardiac. (See Figure 35-2.)

Skeletal Muscle

Striated muscles are found in all skeletal muscles and in the tongue, pharynx, and upper portion of the esophagus. The striations, or "stripes," in this type of muscle are due to the structure of the muscle, which are bundled fibers surrounded by a sheath or connective tissue.

Smooth Muscle

Smooth muscle is found principally in the internal organs of the digestive tract, respiratory passages, urinary bladder, and walls of the blood vessels. No cross striations appear on these muscles. This type of muscle is arranged in sheets or layers.

Cardiac Muscle

The muscles of the heart branch and connect, forming a continuous network. Cardiac muscles are quadrangular in shape and have a single central nucleus. The muscle cells contain striations as in skeletal muscle cells but are arranged in a branching network, not a linear bundle.

Tendons and Ligaments

A **tendon** is fibrous connective tissue structured like a cord or strap and usually attaches to a small area of bone. A tendon that attaches to a larger area of a bone is called an

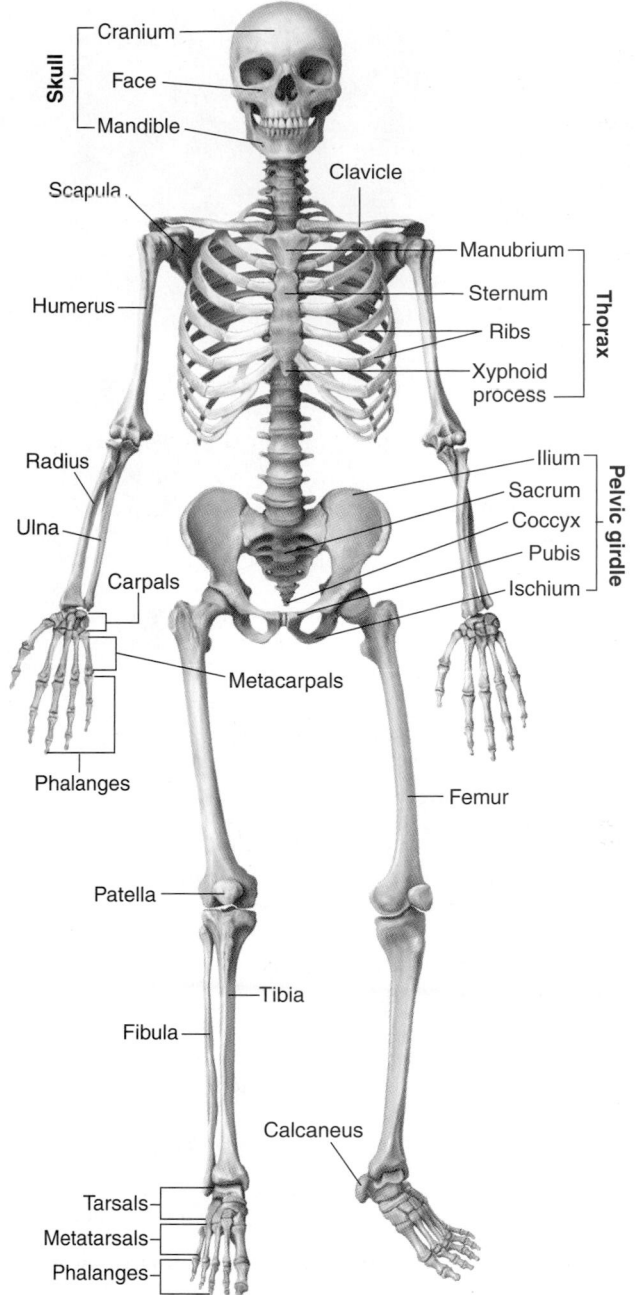

FIG 35-1 Skeletal system.

aponeurosis. This structure is flat or ribbon-like and larger than a typical tendon.

Ligaments are bands or sheets of strong, fibrous connective tissue. This tissue attaches from bone to bone across joints.

Functions of the Musculoskeletal System

The musculoskeletal system, including the bones, muscles, tendons, and ligaments, functions to provide movement, protection, and a framework for the body.

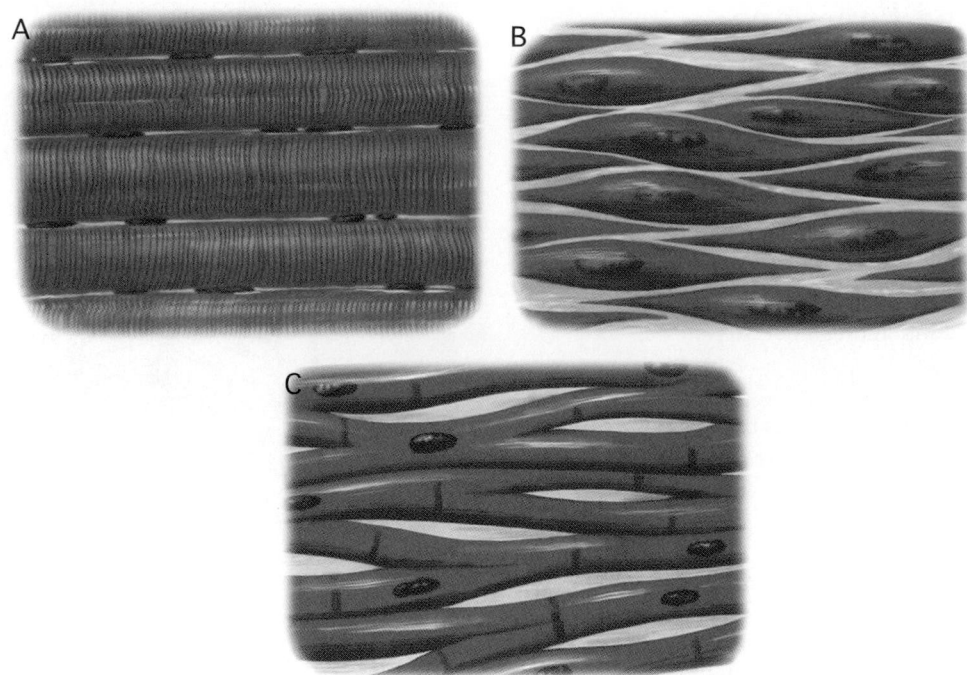

FIG 35-2 Three types of muscle. (A) Skeletal. (B) Smooth. (C) Cardiac.

Bone

Bones provide a framework for the body and protect internal organs. For example, such vital organs as the brain, heart, and lungs are protected by the skull and rib cage.

Bones enable movement at joints through attachments to muscles and tendons. There are three types of bone joint, or **articulation:**

- synarthrosis—immoveable joint, such as the sutures of the skull
- amphiarthrosis—slightly moveable joint, such as a vertebra
- diarthosis—freely moveable joint, such as the knee joint.

Bone marrow within bone performs **hematopoiesis,** or the production of red and white blood cells. Bones also serve to store essential minerals such as calcium and phosphorus. When dietary intake of calcium and phosphorus is inadequate or the need for these minerals increases, as in puberty or pregnancy, the bones release their stores of calcium and phosphorus into the bloodstream for use, leaving the bone vulnerable to deterioration and possibly leading to osteoporosis.

Muscle

The primary function of muscles is to provide movement using contractile cells or fibers. Movement depends on the force of the contraction and the type of muscle.

The muscle fascia supports and separates muscles and subcutaneous tissues, such as fat and the internal organs. The movement of muscles depends on the type of muscle.

Skeletal Muscle

Movement of skeletal muscles is under conscious control (voluntary). Skeletal muscles work with tendons and ligaments to help the body move. Examples of skeletal muscle are those that move bones, the eyeballs, and the tongue. The brain and spinal cord tell muscles to move, or *contract.* Nerves at motor points within the muscle tissue receive these signals from the brain and spinal cord and initiate muscle movement. (See Figure 35-3.) Skeletal muscles are required for such movement as walking. A person's **gait,** or the manner and style in which a person walks, is coordinated by the skeletal muscles of the back, trunk, and legs. Skeletal muscle responds to exercise by increasing in strength, size, and definition. Forceful contraction of a skeletal muscle will cause **vasodilation,** or dilation of blood vessels, increasing blood flow within the muscle tissue to give energy to the muscle. Conversely, if muscles are not used and blood is not directed to blood vessels within the muscle, **vasoconstriction** (a decrease in the diameter of the vessels) occurs. Decreased blood flow to the muscle makes forceful contraction difficult and muscle strength may be lost. If a person does not use his skeletal muscles (for example, in a

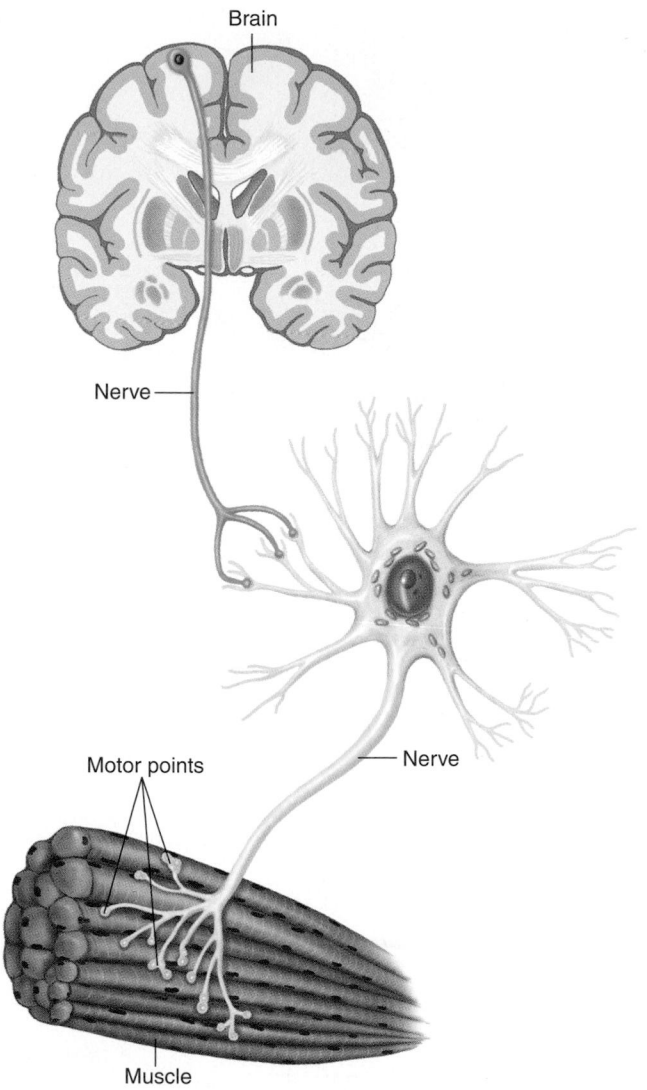

Brain

Nerve

Nerve

Motor points

Muscle

FIG 35-3 Motor point of muscle.

Actions and names of major skeletal muscles

The major movements of the body and the muscles that provide that movement are listed below.

Movement	Skeletal Muscle
Closing of the jaw	Masseter
Closing of the jaw	Temporalis
Flexion and rotation of the head	Sternocleidomastoid
Extension of the head and movement of the scapula	Trapezius
Adduction and flexion of the arm	Pectoralis major
Abduction of the arm	Deltoid
Flexion and supination of the forearm	Biceps
Extension of the forearm	Triceps
Flexion of the forearm	Brachioradialis, Brachialis
Flexion, side bending, and rotation of the trunk	Rectus abdominus, transverse abdominus
Extension of the thigh	Gluteus maximus
Abduction and rotation of the thigh	Gluteus medius
Extension of the leg	Quadriceps femoris
Flexion of the thigh; flexion and rotation of the leg	Sartorius
Flexion of the leg and extension of the thigh	Hamstring
Flexion of the foot	Gastrocnemius

comatose patient), the muscles will **atrophy,** or decrease in size. (See *Actions and names of major skeletal muscles.*)

Smooth Muscle

Smooth muscle is not under conscious control (involuntary) and is found in the internal organs, such as the digestive tract, urinary bladder, gallbladder, and the walls of the blood vessels. In the digestive tract, smooth muscle functions to carry food through the alimentary canal to be broken down for digestion and absorption. In the walls of the blood vessels, smooth muscle moves blood through the vessels to various parts of the body. Smooth muscle structure, arranged in sheets or layers, is determined by its function. Because movement is not directed along a single axis, the structure of this type of muscle must allow for movement in many directions. Unlike skeletal muscle, smooth muscle size and strength

cannot be affected through exercise. The smooth muscles of the alimentary canal do not become stronger with an increase in eating as a skeletal muscle would with increased work, such as weight lifting.

Cardiac Muscle

Cardiac muscle, the muscle of the heart, works to pump blood through the heart and out to the body. The strong contractions of the heart muscle push blood through the circulatory system, supplying blood and oxygen to all the tissues of the body. Blood returns to the heart, which pumps it to the lungs, where it is reoxygenated, and then returns back to the heart. Like skeletal muscles, cardiac muscle efficiency improves with use. Exercise that increases the heart rate increases the efficiency of the cardiac muscle.

Tendons and Ligaments

A tendon attaches muscle to bone. A tendon does not contract or elongate upon movement of the muscle but facilitates the bone's movement. In some places where an aponeurosis attaches muscle to bone, it covers such a large area of bone that it also serves as a protective fascia.

Ligaments attach bone to bone across joints to limit the motion of the joint. Ligaments prevent **hyperextension,** which is the position of maximum extension or extension of a body part beyond its normal limits. They essentially hold the joint together, allowing the attached muscles to move bones upon contraction while preventing the joint from falling apart. (See Figure 35-4.)

Medical Terminology Related to the Musculoskeletal System

Terms used in orthopedic, osteopathic, and chiropractic physician offices will include the names of muscles, bones, and pathologies associated with the musculoskeletal system. Medical assistants in these practice settings will also become familiar with the medications, surgical procedures, and outpatient therapies, or **modalities,** of the various practices. The modalities employed may be therapeutic devices, such as ultrasound and transcutaneous electrical nerve stimulation, or the application of ice or heat. The medical assistant may be required to administer

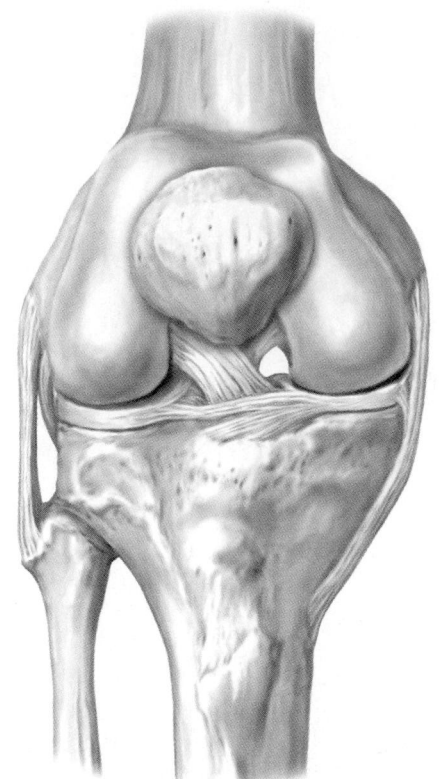

FIG 35-4 Knee joint showing the bones, tendons, and ligaments that prevent this joint from falling apart.

Table 35.1	**Word Elements**		
Element	**Meaning**	**Example**	**Meaning**
Combining forms			
cervic/o	neck	**cervicodynia** (sĕr-vĭ-kō-DĬN-ē-ă)	pain in the neck
chondr/o	cartilage	**chondromalacia** (kŏn-drō-măl-Ā-shē-ă)	softening of cartilage
cleid/o	clavicle	**cleidocostal** (klī-dō-KŎS-tăl)	pertaining to the clavicle and ribs
cost/o	rib	**costophrenic** (kŏs-tō-FRĔN-ĭk)	pertaining to the ribs and diaphragm
crani/o	skull	**craniotomy** (krā-nē-ŎT-ō-mē)	incision through the cranium
cry/o	cold	**cryotherapy** (krī-ō-THĔR-ă-pē)	application of cold to a body part
dors/o, dors/i	back	**dorsiflexion** (dor-sĭ-FLĔK-shŭn)	movement of a part or joint to bend the part toward the back
ili/o	flank	**iliosacral** (ĭl-ē-ō-SĀ-krăl)	concerning the sacrum and ilium

Table 35.1 | **Word Elements—cont'd**

Element	Meaning	Example	Meaning
ischi/o	ischium	**ischium** (ĬS-kē-ŭm)	the lower posterior portion of the hip bone
kines/i, kin/o	movement	**kinesiology** (kĭ-nē-sē-ŎL-ō-jē)	the study of muscles and body movement
kyph/o	humped	**kyphosis** (kī-FŌ-sĭs)	exaggeration of the posterior curve of the thoracic spine
muscul/o, my/o	muscle	**myodynia** (mī-ō-DĬN-ē-ă)	muscle pain
orth/o	straight	**orthodontics** (or-thō-DŎN-tĭks)	area of dentistry concerned with correction of structure
oste/o	bone	**osteopathy** (ŏs-tē-ŎP-ă-thē)	any bone disease
ped/i, ped/o	foot	**podiatry** (pō-DĪ-ă-trē)	diagnosis, treatment. and prevention of conditions of the human feet
phalang/o	bones of the fingers and toes	**phalangitis** (fal-an-JĬ-tis)	inflammation of the fingers and/or toes
poster/o	behind, toward the back	**posterolateral** (pŏs-tĕr-ō-LĂT-ĕr-ăl)	located behind and at side of a part
spondyl/o	vertebra	**spondylolisthesis** (spŏn-dĭ-lō-lĭs-THĒ-sĭs)	forward slipping of a vertebra
stern/o	chest	**sternoclavicular** (stĕr-nō-klă-VĬK-ū-lăr)	pertaining to the sternum and clavicle
tend/o, ten/o	tendon	**tenodesis** (tĕ-NŎD-ē-sĭs)	surgical reattachment of tendon to bone
therm/o	hot; heat	**thermotherapy** (thĕr-mō-THĔR-ă-pē)	therapeutic application of heat to the body
thorac/i, thorac/o	chest	**thoracentesis** (thō-ră-sĕn-TĒ-sĭs)	inserting a needle into the chest wall
vertebr/o	vertebra	**vertebroplasty** (VĔR-tē-brō-plăs-tē)	surgical repair of a vertebra
Prefixes			
a-	without, not	**atrophy** (ĂT-rō-fē)	wasting; decrease in size of an organ or tissue
hyper-	above, excessive	**hyperkinesia** (hī-pĕr-kĭn-Ē-zē-ă)	excessive movement
hypo-	under, below	**hypoesthesia** (hī-pō-ĕs-THĒ-zē-ă)	dulled sensitivity to touch
subing-	under, below	**suboccipital** (sŭb-ŏk-SĬP-ĭ-tăl)	situated below the occiput
supra-	above, excessive	**supraclavicular** (soo-pră-klă-VĬK-ū-lăr)	located above the clavicle
syn-	union, together, with	**syndesis** (sĭn-DĒ-sĭs)	surgical fixation or ankylosis of a joint
Suffixes			
-asthenia	weakness, debility	**myasthenia** (mī-ăs-THĒ-nē-ă)	muscle weakness and fatigue
-blast	embryonic cell	**osteoblast** (ŎS-tē-ō-blăst)	cell of mesodermal origin concerned with the formation of bone
-clast	to break, surgical fracture	**osteoclast** (ŎS-tē-ō-klăst)	device used to fracture a bone to correct deformity; large multinuclear cell formed in the bone marrow of growing bones
-desis	binding, fixation	**arthrodesis** (ăr-thrō-DĒ-sĭs)	binding together of a joint
-malacia	softening	**osteomalacia** (ŏs-tē-ō-măl-Ā-shē-ă)	softening of bone
-plegia	paralysis, stroke	**hemiplegia** (hĕm-ē-PLĒ-jē-ă)	paralysis of one side of the body

Table 35.2 | Bone fractures

Bone fractures are common, especially to the clavicle, wrist, and ankle. The medical assistant should become familiar with the various types of bone fractures. This table lists fracture types along with a description and example of each.

Fracture Type	Description	Example
closed or simple	Bone fractured without external wound	
Comminuted	Bone broken into pieces	
greenstick	Bone bent and partially broken (common fracture in children)	

Table 35.2 | Bone fractures—cont'd

Fracture Type	Description	Example
impacted	Bone broken with one end wedged into the interior of the other (crushed into the fracture)	
incomplete	Line of fracture that does not continue through entire bone	
oblique	Bone with slanted fracture of the shaft on its long axis	

Continued

Table 35.2 | Bone fractures—cont'd

Fracture Type	Description	Example
open or compound	Broken bone sticking out of an open wound or fragments of bone seen through the skin	

Table 35.3 | Musculoskeletal Abbreviations

In orthopedics, as with other areas of health care, abbreviations are commonly used. Abbreviations such as the ones listed below save time and effort in documentation and written communications.

Abbreviation	Term	Abbreviation	Term
ACL	anterior cruciate ligament	MVA	motor vehicle accident
ADL	activities of daily living	NSAID	nonsteroidal anti-inflammatory drug
AK	above the knee	ORIF	open reduction and internal fixation
ALS	amyotrophic lateral sclerosis	OT	occupational therapy
AS	ankylosing spondylitis	PT	physical therapy
BK	below the knee	RA	rheumatoid arthritis
DJD	degenerative joint disease	RLE	right lower extremity
DTR	deep tendon reflex	ROM	range of motion
JRA	juvenile rheumatoid arthritis	RUE	right upper extremity
LLE	left lower extremity	TENS	transcutaneous electrical nerve stimulation
LP	lumbar puncture	TMJ	temporomandibular joint
LUE	left upper extremity	US	ultrasound
MD	muscular dystrophy	WNL	within normal limits

various modalities under the direction of the physician. To be effective in her role, a medical assistant must become well versed in the language and vocabulary that pertain to the musculoskeletal system. The following tables list common medical terminology related to the musculoskeletal system.

Common Musculoskeletal System Diseases and Disorders

There are innumerable diseases and disorders of the musculoskeletal system. In addition to bone fractures, some of the most common diseases and disorders include dislocation, arthritis, osteoporosis, curvature of the spine, torn ligaments and tendons in the knees or shoulders as a result of sports injuries, and injuries to the intervertebral disks of the lower back, affecting the sciatic nerve. Damage to bones, muscles, or tendons and ligaments can result in loss of function to the musculoskeletal system. Treatments are aimed at regaining normal function and controlling pain.

Injuries to Bones

In addition to bone fractures, bone pathologies can include dislocations, various forms of arthritis, osteoporosis, and abnormal curvatures of the spine. The medical assistant can offer information on treatments to reduce pain in chronic bone conditions and safety strategies to prevent bone injuries.

Dislocation

ICD-9-CM code: 830–839 (code by specific site)

Dislocation is the displacement of a bone from its normal articulation. Dislocation is evident upon visual inspection. An x-ray confirms the diagnosis. Treatment for dislocation includes manual repositioning by the physician in the office or, if anesthesia is required, in the operating room.

Scoliosis

ICD-9-CM code: 737.43

Scoliosis is an abnormal lateral curvature of the spine. Scoliosis is more common in adolescents because the adolescent spine is still developing. Symptoms include lateral spinal deformity with back pain. Mild scoliosis generally causes no problems and is usually not noticeable. Severe scoliosis can cause significant back pain and, possibly, heart or lung problems because of the decreased space in the thoracic cavity on one side. Diagnosis is based on a physical examination and radiographic studies. Treatment includes bracing and asymmetrical exercise to correct muscle imbalances where one side is stronger than the other. In severe cases, surgical correction is necessary. (See Figure 35-5.)

Kyphosis

ICD-9-CM code: 737.0 (adolescent); 737.1 (acquired)

Kyphosis is an outward curvature of the thoracic region of the spine. Kyphosis may be due to a congenital anomaly, disease (tuberculosis, syphilis), a malignancy, or a compression fracture. Kyphosis is most common in older women. A symptom of kyphosis is a stooped posture. Diagnosis depends on an x-ray of the spine, which reveals a curvature. Treatment includes supplemental calcium; vitamin D; medications to slow the progression of bone loss, such as Boniva and Fosimax; and pain management in the form of analgesics, massage, and acupuncture.

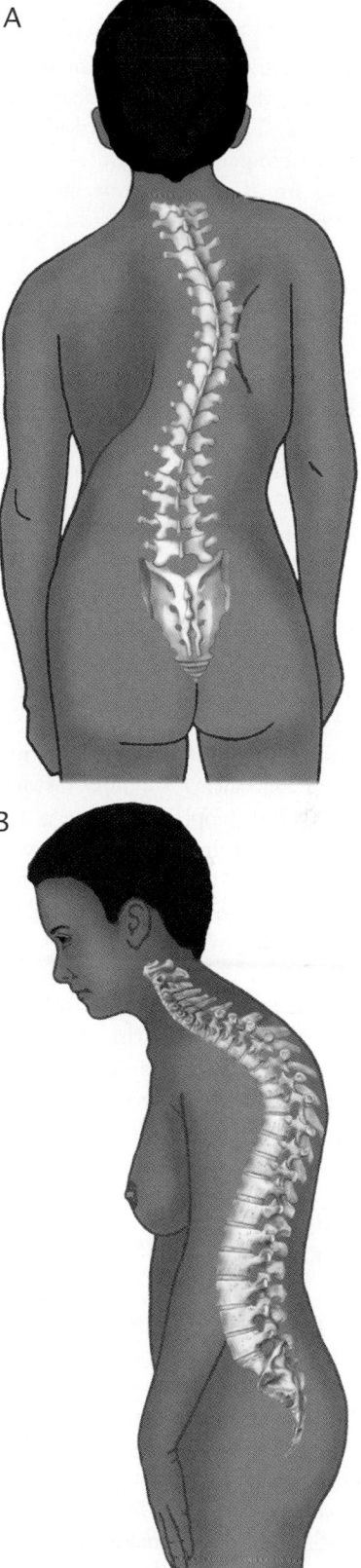

FIG 35-5 (A) Scoliosis, or lateral curvature of the spine. (B) Kyphosis, or increased curvature of the thoracic spine.

Lordosis

ICD-9-CM code: 737.20 (acquired); 754.2 (congenital)

Lordosis is excessive curvature in the lumbar portion of the spine, which gives a swayback appearance and prominence of the buttocks. The cause of lordosis is unknown but is thought to be congenital or associated with poor posture, back surgery, hip dysplasia, or overtraining in gymnastics. Lordosis is most commonly diagnosed in childhood; school nurses will commonly screen students for lordosis. Lordosis is an asymptomatic condition. Children complaining of back pain, pain down the legs, and changes in bowel and bladder habits should be evaluated for other conditions. Diagnosis is obtained by x-ray of the lumbar spine and physical examination, including observing the patient's standing posture. Early detection and treatment prevents injury to lumbar discs and the paraspinal musculature. The goal of treatment is to stop the progression of the abnormal curve and prevent deformity. Exercises conducted at home or with a physical therapist correct postural abnormalities. If underlying hip abnormalities are the cause of lordosis, correction of hip pathology will help decrease abnormal curvature.

Gout

ICD-9-CM code:274.0 (acute)

Gout is a disease caused by a congenital or acquired disorder of uric acid metabolism. A family history of the disease is present in 20% of people who have gout. Risk factors for acquiring the disease include obesity; excessive alcohol consumption; diet high in purines and protein, including such foods as cream, anchovies, meats, and fish; exposure to lead; and such underlying medical conditions as renal insufficiency, high blood pressure, and hypothyroidism. Medications that can cause gout in some people include diuretics, salicylate-containing drugs such as aspirin, niacin, and cyclosporins. In the disorder, the body is unable to clear uric acid from the bloodstream and uric acid crystals deposit in the articular cartilage of joints. The knee and great toe are the joints most commonly affected. The deposits provoke an inflammatory response in the affected joints, causing pain and restriction of the degree of movement, or **range of motion (ROM)**, of the joint. The deposits commonly increase in size and burst through the skin, causing a chalky white material to appear. Affected joints will also appear red, swollen, and painful to the touch and the patient may have a fever during an acute episode. Gout is commonly chronic with episodes of acute attacks. It is most prevalent among African American males, in whom the incidence is twice that of Whites.

Diagnosis is made using physical examination, patient history, and blood uric acid levels greater than 7.0 mg/dl in males and 6.0 mg/dl in females (hyperuricemia). Treatment is directed at pain relief with nonsteroidal anti-inflammatory drugs (NSAIDs) and intra-articular glucocortoids to reduce inflammation. Aspirin should never be used for pain relief because it can exacerbate the condition. Patients with a history of gout can elect to take allopurinol, a medication that directly reduces the production of uric acid. Allopurinol is a lifelong medication and cannot be initiated during an attack because it will make the acute gout worse. The medical assistant should educate the patient about dietary changes that can prevent further attacks. (See *Foods and gout*.)

Osteoarthritis

ICD-9-CM code: 715.9 (use 5th digit to code site)

Osteoarthritis is an inflammation of the joints, which causes pain, swelling, redness, warmth, and limited ROM. These afflictions affect the weight-bearing joints in the body. Osteoarthritis usually affects elderly patients and may be due to angina, obesity, overuse or abuse of joints in sports or strenuous occupations, and trauma. Patients with osteoarthritis complain of gradually increasing joint pain and gradually decreasing ROM in the affected joint. Diagnosis is based on x-rays, which show increasing changes in the joint surfaces and narrowing joint space. Treatment includes rest, heat, massage, acupuncture, weight reduction (if necessary), and analgesics. The main goals for treatment are relieving pain, gaining normal ROM for the joint, and preventing the osteoarthritis from getting worse.

Osteoporosis

ICD-9-CM code: 733.00 (generalized)

Osteoporosis is a loss of bone mass throughout the skeleton. It is most common in postmenopausal women but can be associated with parathyroid abnormalities that result in loss of calcium to the bone matrix. Osteoporosis may be due to increased age; immobilization; thyroid hormone excess; use of corticosteroids and some anticonvulsant drugs; consumption of alcohol, tobacco, or caffeine; and menopause. Symptoms of osteoporosis include frequent fractures, exaggerated thoracic kyphosis, decreased height, and back pain. Diagnostic blood tests for osteoporosis are serum calcium, alkaline phosphatase, estrogen level, total protein, and creatinine. A bone scan can be performed as a definitive diagnostic test. Treatment includes supplemental calcium, regular weight-bearing exercise, and bisphosphate drugs. Estrogen supplementation may also be used (for women only) but there may be some risks involved that should be assessed.

Rheumatoid Arthritis

ICD-9-CM code: 714.0

Rheumatoid arthritis is a chronic systemic inflammation of the joints and synovial membranes that also involves elevated serum rheumatoid factor levels. Researchers believe that rheumatoid arthritis is triggered by an infection in people with an inherited susceptibility to the disease. Symptoms of rheumatoid arthritis include severe joint pain and joint deformity. Diagnostic blood tests for rheumatoid arthritis are

Patient Education

Foods and Gout

The medical assistant should make sure the patient suffering from gout receives nutritional counseling about foods that will help ease gout and those to be avoided.

Good for gout

These foods will help reduce uric acid production and should be recommended for the patient with gout:

- mushrooms
- spinach
- asparagus
- cauliflower
- cherries
- strawberries.

Bad for gout

These foods contain elements, such as purine, that should be limited or avoided in the patient with gout:

- alcohol
- cream
- meat
- fish
- pinto, kidney, and red beans.

---

rheumatoid factor, antinuclear antibody (ANA) test, and erythrocyte sedimentation rate (ESR). Treatment includes disease-modifying antirheumatic drugs (DMARDs), such as hydroxychloroquine and methotrexate. Immunosuppressive agents, such as cyclosporine and azathioprine, may also be used for treatment. Gold compounds are sometimes used; however, they are usually not as effective.

Juvenile Rheumatoid Arthritis
ICD-9-CM code: 714.30

Juvenile rheumatoid arthritis (JRA) is a chronic systemic inflammation of the joints and synovial membranes, which usually involves elevated ANA. The onset of juvenile rheumatoid arthritis is usually more acute than in the adult form. Systemic effects are typically more noticeable; however, the rheumatoid nodules are absent. The systemic form of JRA, called *Still's disease,* forms with fever, rash, lymphadenopathy, and hepatomegaly as well as joint involvement. The second form of JRA causes polyarticular inflammation similar to the adult form. The third form involves four or less joints but causes uveitis (inflammation of the iris). Treatment of all forms of JRA includes DMARDs, such as hydroxychloroquine and methotrexate. Immunosuppressive agents, such as cyclosporine and azathioprine, may also be used as well as gold compounds, although they are less effective.

Muscle Disorders

Injury or disease to the muscular system can be acute or chronic and associated with underlying disease or trauma. The most common of these disorders is fibromyalgia. Other common disorders include muscle strains from exercise and muscle weakness in the paraspinal musculature leading to a herniated disk. Loss of strength or ROM may be an indication of neurologic pathology. Skeletal muscle strength and ROM can be assessed manually by **muscle testing,** where a

physician or physical therapist will assess the strength and ROM of specific muscle groups. Severe loss of muscle function can cause paralysis. For example, a stroke can cause **hemiplegia,** paralysis of half of the body due to injury in the brain on the opposite side.

Fibromyalgia
ICD-9-CM code: 729.1

Fibromyalgia is chronic pain in the muscles and soft tissues due to various causes. Fibromyalgia can be found in people of all ages and is more common in women than men. Associated conditions can include sleep disorders, irritable bowel syndrome, chronic headaches, temporomandibular joint (TMJ) problems, increased chemical sensitivity, and other musculoskeletal complaints. Fibromyalgia can be triggered by an automobile accident, bacterial or viral infection, or an underlying medical condition, such as rheumatoid arthritis (RA), lupus, or hypothyroidism. Fibromyalgia is aggravated by changes in monthly hormonal variations, weather or temperature, stress, anxiety, and depression. Symptoms of fibromyalgia include diffuse aches and pains all over the body. Diagnosis is made by eliminating any other cause for the symptoms and finding 11 of 18 specific points to be extremely tender to touch. Treatment includes anti-inflammatories, trigger point injections, nutritional and herbal support, exercise, and massage. There is no known cure for fibromyalgia. (See Figure 35-6.)

Strain
ICD-9-CM code: 840-848 (code by site)

A strain is trauma to a muscle and, sometimes, a tendon due to violent contraction or excessive forcible stretching. Symptoms can be moderate to severe and include pain, heat, discoloration, and localized swelling in the affected area. An x-ray rules out an avulsion fracture of the ligament's

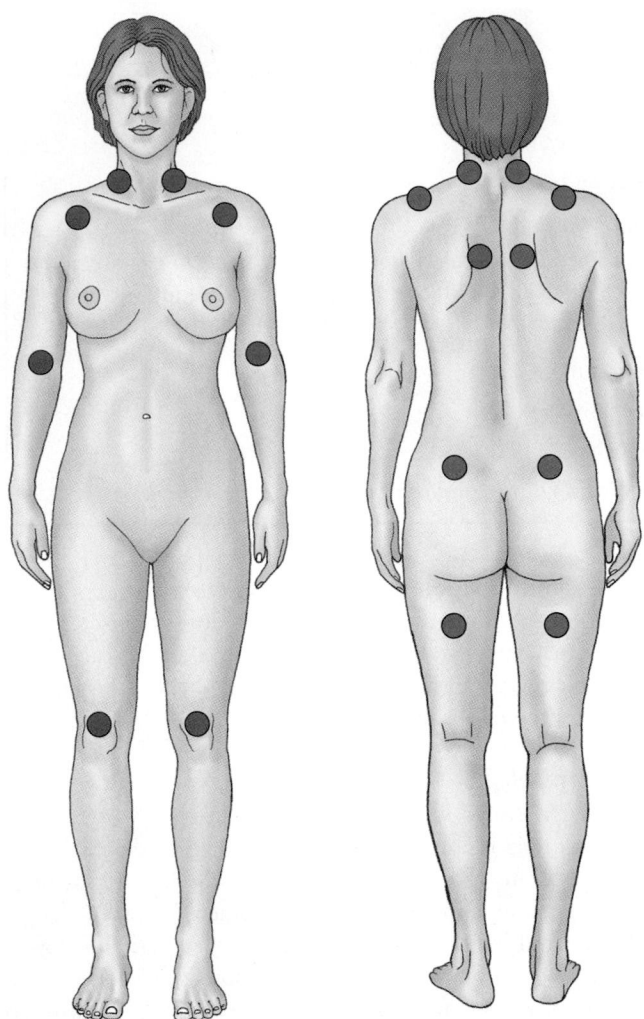

FIG 35-6 Fibromyalgia tender points.

attachment. Treatment includes ice, rest, compression, elevation, massage, ultrasound, electrical muscle stimulation, and analgesics.

Myasthenia Gravis
ICD-9-CM code: 358.0
Myasthenia gravis (MG) is a neuromuscular disorder characterized by muscle weakness and muscle fatigue. The disease results from an abnormal immune reaction in which antibodies inappropriately attack and gradually destroy certain receptors in muscles that receive nerve impulses. The cause of myasthenia gravis is unknown but, in some cases, it is associated with tumors of the thymus gland. Patients with other immune disorders such as rheumatoid arthritis and systemic lupus erythematosus are at increased risk. Although the disorder usually becomes apparent during adulthood, symptom onset may occur at any age. The condition may be generalized, involving multiple muscle groups, or restricted to certain muscle groups, particularly those of the eyes

(called *ocular myasthenia gravis*). Most individuals with myasthenia gravis develop drooping of the eyelids (ptosis); weakness of eye muscles; inability to maintain a steady gaze, resulting in double vision (diplopia); extreme muscle fatigue following activity; and weakness of facial muscles. Difficulty speaking (dysphasia), difficulty swallowing (dysphagia), and weakness of the upper arms and legs are also common. Patients will have difficulty climbing stairs and lifting heavy objects due to muscle weakness. In about 10% of cases, affected individuals may develop potentially life-threatening complications due to severe involvement of muscles used during breathing, causing *myasthenic crisis.*

Diagnosis is made by physical examination, including muscle strength assessment. As the disease progresses, muscle strength decreases and can progressively involve more muscle groups. A test using edrophonium (Tensilon), a medication that blocks the action of enzymes that break down the neurotransmitter acetylcholine, can be used to make a definitive diagnosis of MG. Temporary improvement of muscle function after administration of edrophonium confirms the diagnosis of MG. There is no known cure for MG; treatment is directed at reducing symptoms of muscle weakness and fatigue. The medical assistant should advise patients to avoid stress and exposure to heat, because they can exacerbate symptoms. The patient may want to wear an eye patch if diplopia is problematic. Some medications, such as neostigmine (Prostigmin) and pyridostigmine (Mestinon), can improve communication between nerves and muscles and decrease weakness. Surgical removal of the thymus may cause permanent remission or decrease the need for medication.

Rotator Cuff Tear
ICD-9-CM code: 840.4 (traumatic); 726.10 (degenerative)
The rotator cuff is made up of four muscles and their tendons that wrap around the front, back, and top of the shoulder joint. Together, the rotator cuff muscles help guide the shoulder through many motions and provide stability to the joint. At the ends of the rotator cuff muscles, tendons attach to the humerus. A rotator cuff tear is seen in patients of all ages; however, they are more common in older patients. As a person ages, the muscles and tendons of the rotator cuff lose some elasticity, causing an increased susceptibility to tears. Around 30% of 70-year-olds have some degree of rotator cuff tear, although not all of these people experience symptoms. In younger patients, usually a traumatic injury or excessive use of the shoulder (as seen in athletes) is the cause of a tear in the rotator cuff. The most common symptom of a rotator cuff tear is generalized pain exacerbated by shoulder movement. Depending on the severity of the tear, loss of motion and decreased strength may also occur. Diagnosis of a rotator cuff tear is based on patient history and physical examination, which will reveal loss of strength and ROM.

Diagnosis is confirmed by an arthrogram with contrast dye injection into the joint capsule. If a tear is present, the dye will leak out of the joint capsule, confirming the diagnosis. Treatment for rotator cuff tear includes physical therapy to strengthen the muscles and maintain normal function. Anti-inflammatory medications and cortisone injections decrease inflammation and pain. If conservative measures are ineffective, surgical repair will be necessary.

Herniated Disk

ICD-9-CM code: 722 (code by specific site and conditions)
A herniated disk is a prolapse of the nucleus pulposus of a ruptured disk into the spinal canal. Patients with a herniated disk complain of back pain and extremity pain or weakness. The most common symptom of a herniated disk is sciatica, a compression of the sciatic nerve. The compression on the nerve causes irritation of the nerve and can produce pain radiating down the back of the leg as far as the ankle. The pain can be sharp and stabbing or the patient may complain of numbness and weakness in the leg. Procedures used to diagnose a herniated disk include computed tomography (CT) and magnetic resonance imaging (MRI). Treatment for a herniated disk is a laminectomy, a surgical excision of the vertebral posterior arch to remove the herniated disk or lesion. Conservative treatment may include anti-inflammatories, chiropractic adjustment, physical therapy, traction, and acupuncture. Such treatments are palliative, not curative, and may offer the patient some pain relief. (See Figure 35-7.)

Injuries to Tendons and Ligaments

Tendons and ligaments, the tissues that hold joints together and attach muscle to bone, are commonly injured in sports-related accidents. Injuries can occur as the result of collision with another player or can be due to a chronic overuse of the joint. The medical assistant can provide information on injury prevention in athletics. (See *Preventing musculoskeletal injuries*, page 722.) Common injuries to the tendons and ligaments include anterior cruciate ligament (ACL) tear, tendinitis at various sites, and sprains of various ligaments.

Anterior Cruciate Ligament Tear

ICD-9-CM code: 717.83
The anterior cruciate ligament (ACL) is the ligament of the knee that originates on the anterior portion of the femur in the intercondylar notch, which can tear from a twisting motion. This injury is most common in athletes, especially those in basketball and skiing. It is also more common in females. Symptoms include severe pain and an inability to bear weight on the leg. Diagnosis is usually based on pain and functional instability of the knee and is confirmed by MRI or CT scan. Treatment includes surgical reattachment

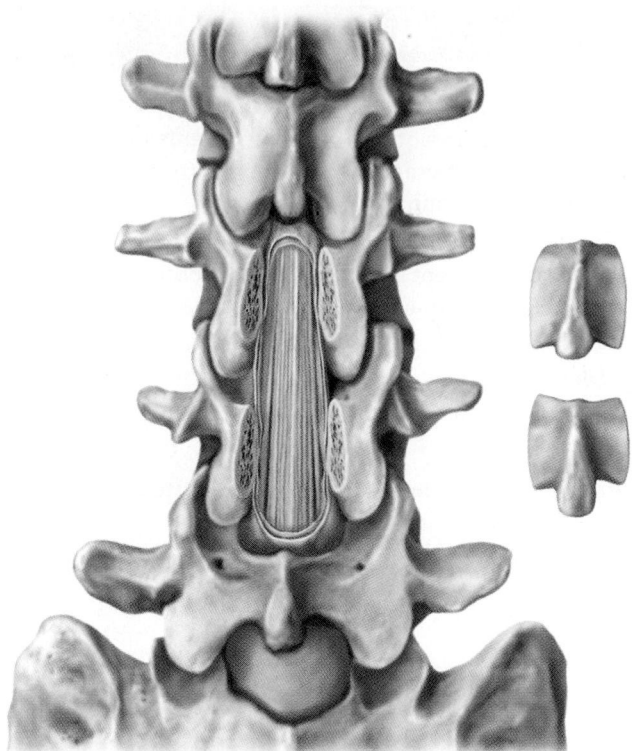

FIG 35-7 Laminectomy.

of the ligament followed by rest and physical therapy to strengthen and stabilize the knee joint. Knee bracing for return to contact sports is commonly utilized.

Epicondylitis, Medial and Lateral

ICD-9-CM code: 726.32 (lateral epicondylitis); 726.31 (medial epicondylitis)
Tennis elbow is trauma or overuse of the elbow, which causes inflammation along the medial side of the joint, specifically to the epicondyle. Tennis elbow is common in sports such as tennis and weight lifting. A similar condition, lateral epicondylitis, is the same injury except that it affects the lateral side of the joint. Lateral epicondylitis is also called *golfer's elbow* because the repeated motion of driving the golf club is the most common cause. Symptoms of both conditions include tenderness, stiffness, inflammation, and pain around the elbow. Diagnosis is determined mainly through symptoms and palpation of the elbow, which is inflamed and tender on palpation. Treatment includes immobilization with a splint, strapping (strap positioned around the arm 2" to 3" below the elbow joint to take pressure off the wrist extensor tendons), ultrasound, friction massage, acupuncture, ice, NSAIDs, and muscle relaxants. Cortisone injections may be administered if the injury does not respond to other treatments.

Preventing Musculoskeletal Injuries

The medical assistant can help her patients prevent injury by providing information on safety in their environment and while exercising.

Creating an injury-proof environment

People can prevent injury by injury-proofing their home and using safe behaviors, including:

- Making sure carpets are not loose, which could cause trips and falls.
- Making sure electrical cords are not in walk areas, to prevent trips.
- Never standing on a chair; using a step stool to change light bulbs or dust ceiling fans.
- Removing snow, ice, and wet leaves to prevent falls.
- Providing adequate lighting in all areas of the home to prevent injury.

Exercise and behaviors

The risk of injury increases during exercise. The medical assistant can advise her patient to prevent injury by including these instructions:

- Get proper sleep (to prevent tripping and falling).
- Reduce emotional stress.
- Stop smoking (which contributes to back injuries).
- Stretch muscles before working out to prevent cramping or pulling ligaments and tendons.
- Exercise within reason. Do not go from "couch potato" to marathon runner in 1 week.
- Apply ice to sore muscles after exercise.
- Eat a balanced diet to fuel muscles for exercise.

Tendinitis

ICD-9-CM code: 726 (4th and 5th digit code by site)

Tendinitis is inflammation of a tendon due to overuse. Symptoms can be moderate to severe and include pain with decreased ROM in the affected area. X-rays rule out the possibility of a fracture. Treatment includes moist heat, ultrasound, electrical muscle stimulation, and strengthening ROM exercises. Corticosteroid injections may be administered if these more conservative treatments yield a poor response.

Sprain

ICD-9-CM code: 840–848 (code by site)

A sprain is a stretched or torn ligament, which causes pain and immobility. Sprains are most common in the ankle joint. Symptoms can be moderate to severe and include pain, heat, discoloration, and localized swelling in the affected area. An x-ray rules out an avulsion fracture of the ligament's attachment. Treatment includes ice to reduce swelling, circumferential compression and support with a bandage, rest and elevation, stretching exercises, ultrasounds, electrical muscle stimulation, analgesics, and anti-inflammatories. (See *Treating sprains at home*.)

Orthopedic Procedures

Orthopedics is the medical specialty that focuses on the study and treatment of the musculoskeletal system. Many

Treating Sprains at Home

The medical assistant can encourage patients to start treatment for a suspected sprain right away. She can advise her patients to come to the office, but start with *RICE*:

- **R:** rest
- **I:** ice
- **C:** compression
- **E:** elevation.

health care providers, including chiropractors, osteopaths, and general practitioners, will treat disorders of the musculoskeletal system with conservative therapies and refer patients to an orthopedic surgeon for surgical correction. Orthopedic procedures conducted by various providers are directed at diagnosing and treating musculoskeletal disorders to restore normal function. Because each patient is unique, the provider and medical assistant must work with each one to attain optimal function.

Assisting with Examination

People suffer injuries to the musculoskeletal system every day. To reach an accurate diagnosis, the physician must obtain a medical history, including a description of the accident or injury, and the signs and symptoms of the injury. A sports injury, car accident, fall, or other trauma can result in partial or total loss of the use of an extremity. Stroke and head or spinal cord injury can leave a patient unable to perform independent tasks. Such patients can receive care from an orthopedic surgeon, chiropractor, osteopath, physical or occupational therapist, and speech pathologist. The goal of treatment for these patients can vary but is generally focused on reestablishing normal function, strength, and movement of the affected body areas.

In an examination, the medical assistant must prepare the patient by checking vital signs and obtaining a health history. She should then assist the physician as needed with undressing and positioning, remembering to take care, as the patient may be in pain or unable to move. For example, a patient with a herniated disk will need her assistance to climb onto the examination table and may be in considerable discomfort. (See *Procedure 35-1:*

Transferring a patient from a wheelchair to an examination table.) The clinical medical assistant can play a vital role in the care of these patients in various ambulatory and inpatient settings.

During the patient examination, the physician may ask the medical assistant to help position the patient, support the patient, and document examination findings. The medical assistant should be attentive to the needs and physical limitations of the patient. (See *Procedure 35-2: Transferring a patient from an examination table to a wheelchair*, page 724.)

Patients using crutches, canes, or walkers to ambulate may require assistance to transfer to and from examination tables. Offer help as needed, being sure to use your knees and hips for bending and not bending from the lower back. Depending on the injury, the patient may require help getting from the waiting room to the treatment room. Offering to perform simple tasks such as carrying a purse or bag can show the patient that the medical assistant is receptive to their needs.

PROCEDURE 35-1

Transferring a patient from a wheelchair to an examination table

Task
Move a patient from a wheelchair to an examination table safely.

Conditions
- Gait belt
- Stool with rubber tips and a handle for gripping

Standards
In the time specified and within the scoring parameters determined by the instructor, the student will successfully transfer a patient from a wheelchair to an examination table.

Performance Standards
1. Wash your hands.
2. Introduce yourself and address the patient by name. Explain to the patient that you will help him onto the examination table to promote patient cooperation and understanding.
3. Place the wheelchair next to the examination table and lock the brakes. Place the patient with his stronger side (if applicable) closest to the examination table to allow him to balance on that leg during transfer.
4. Place the gait belt securely (but not too tightly) around the patient's waist to provide support and

comfort. Tuck in the ends of the gait belt so that it does not interfere with assisting the patient.

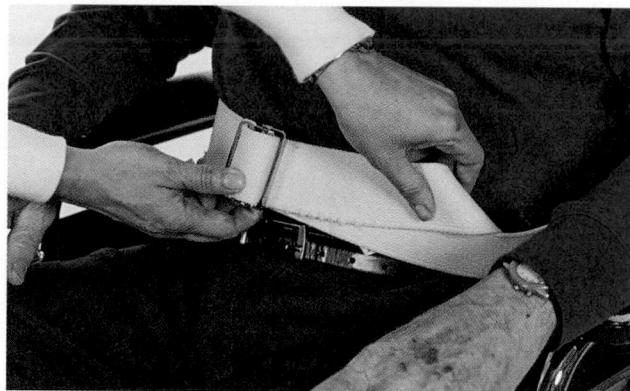

Tuck in the ends of the gait belt so that it does not interfere with assisting the patient.

5. Move the footrests up and out of the way, and ask the patient to place his feet on the floor.
6. Position the stool in front of the examination table as close to the wheelchair as possible so that the patient does not have to take any additional steps.
7. Ask the patient to move to the front edge of the wheelchair.

Continued

PROCEDURE 35-1—cont'd

8. Stand directly in front of the patient with your feet hip-width apart for a strong base. Bending at the hips and knees (to avoid straining your lower back), grasp the gait belt on both sides. Instruct the patient to use the arm-rests of the wheelchair to push upward if he is able. Proper body positioning while assisting a patient from the wheelchair prevents injury to you and the patient.

9. Give the patient a signal to push off with his arms and good leg while you lift the gait belt so that you and he work at the same time.

10. Tell the patient to allow you and the gait belt to support him while he moves his stronger foot to step onto the stool. Do NOT let go of the gait belt.

11. Tell the patient to pivot his back to the examination table to sit. Make sure that the patient's buttocks are high enough to get onto the table. Support the patient's weaker, outer leg.

12. Instruct the patient to grasp the stool handle and place the other hand on the examination table.

13. Help the patient adjust his position on the examination table as necessary; make sure that the patient is balanced and comfortable.

14. Move the wheelchair out of the way to provide room for the physician to examine the patient.

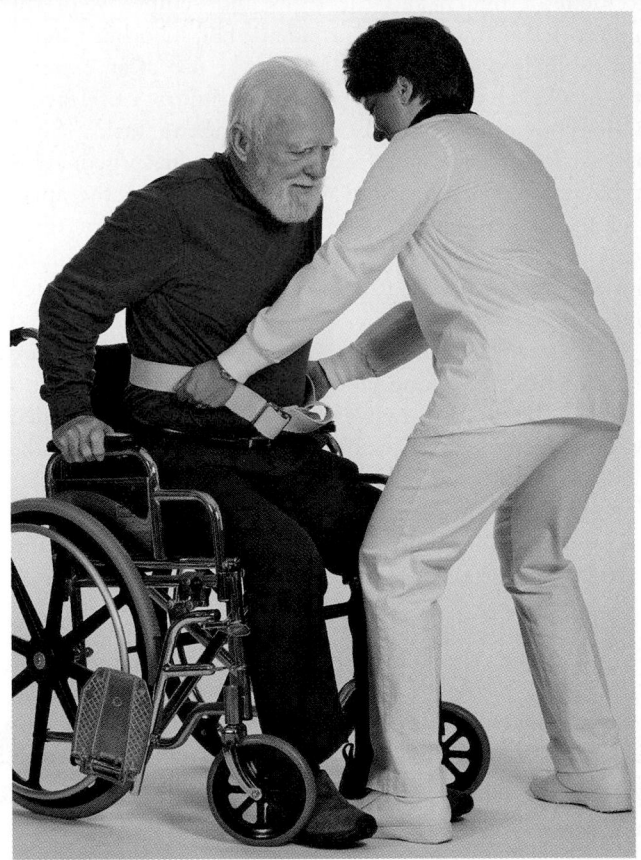

Proper body positioning while assisting a patient from the wheelchair prevents injury to you and the patient.

PROCEDURE 35-2

Transferring a patient from an examination table to a wheelchair

Task
Move a patient from an examination table to a wheelchair safely.

Conditions
- Gait belt
- Stool with rubber tips and a handle for gripping

Standards
In the time specified and within the scoring parameters determined by the instructor, the student will successfully transfer a patient from an examination table to a wheelchair.

Performance Standards
1. Wash your hands.
2. Introduce yourself (if you were not assisting the patient previously) and address the patient by name. Explain to the patient that you will help him back to his wheelchair.
3. Position the wheelchair next to the examination table and lock the brakes. The chair should be positioned closest to the patient's stronger side so that he can transfer weight onto his stronger foot on the way down.
4. Position the stool next to the examination table.
5. Assist the patient into a sitting position (if not sitting already) and put the gait belt on the patient. The belt should be snug but not tight, and the excess belt should be tucked in the back.
6. Place one arm under the patient's arm and around his shoulders and the other arm under the patient's knees. Pivot the patient so that his legs dangle over the edge of the examination table.

7. Position your body directly in front of the patient without removing your hand from the patient. You should always make the patient feel secure.

8. Grasp the patient by the gait belt on both sides. You should position your feet apart with your knees bent for a strong base of support.

9. Instruct the patient that when you give him a signal, he should push off of the examination table and grasp the stool handle for support. Give the patient the signal as you pull him slightly towards you so his feet come down onto the stool.

10. Keeping both hands on the gait belt, ask the patient to step onto the floor with his strong leg. Pivot the patient so that his back is to the wheelchair.

11. Ask the patient to grasp the armrests of the wheelchair and assist him to a seated position in the wheelchair.

12. Lower the footrests and place his feet on them.

13. Remove the gait belt.

In addition to helping patients in the office, the medical assistant can offer her patient and caregivers strategies to promote independent function without compromising safety. (See *Independent function strategies*.)

Evaluating Muscle Strength and Range of Motion

The orthopedic, osteopathic, or chiropractic physician or a licensed physical therapist will evaluate the patient's muscle strength in the upper or lower extremities and back or neck region as necessary to help in the diagnosis and treatment of the patient. The role of the medical assistant may also be to record ROM and strength results or position and comfort the patient during the physical examination. (See *Muscle strength scale*.)

Goniometry

Measurement of the degree of movement, or *range of motion*, of a joint is called **goniometry**. Goniometry is performed using a device called a *goniometer*, which is a protractor with a moveable pointer. If the joint only moves in a single direction, such as the elbow, the measurement is *flexion* (bending) or *extension* (straightening). If a joint allows for more than one axis of movement, the measurement is more complex.

Patient Education

Independent Function Strategies

Disabled or elderly patients may need accommodations to help them function as independently as possible. Caregivers can promote independence by:

• adding side rails to a bed or bathtub to ease patient transfer

• using a bathtub seat and handheld shower nozzle to help patients with disabilities or decreased range of motion bathe themselves

• placing items in cupboards or shelves that are accessible without reaching too far

• using ramps and wide hallways to accommodate wheelchairs or walkers as needed

• buying clothing that the patient can put on and remove herself such as elastic waistbands and pullover tops.

• ensuring that banisters on stairways are secure and can provide support while the patient is on the stairs.

Muscle strength scale

The following table shows the scale used for evaluating muscle strength, including the response to resistance, its rating, and what this response and rating mean.

Muscle Response	Rating	Meaning
No response	0	Paralysis
Slight contraction of muscle	1	Severe weakness
Passive range of motion (ROM) when resistance is removed	2	Moderate weakness
Active ROM against gravity or light resistance	3 or 4	Mild weakness
Active ROM against heavy resistance	5	Normal strength

(See Figure 35-8.) A goniometer can measure 10 movements, including:

- **abduction**—moving away from the midline of the body, such as moving a straightened leg outward at the hip joint
- **adduction**—moving toward the midline of the body, such as moving a straightened leg inward at the hip joint
- **eversion**—turning outward, such as moving the ankle so that the sole of the foot turns outward
- **inversion**—turning inward, such as moving the ankle so that the sole of the foot turns inward

- **flexion**—bending, such as moving the hand up to the shoulder by flexing at the elbow
- **extension**—straightening, such as moving the hand away from the shoulder by elongating or extending the elbow joint
- **pronation**—twisting to face downward, such as turning the wrist so the palm faces down
- **supination**—twisting to face upward, such as turning the wrist so the palm faces up
- **rotation**—moving along an axis, such as turning the head by looking left and right

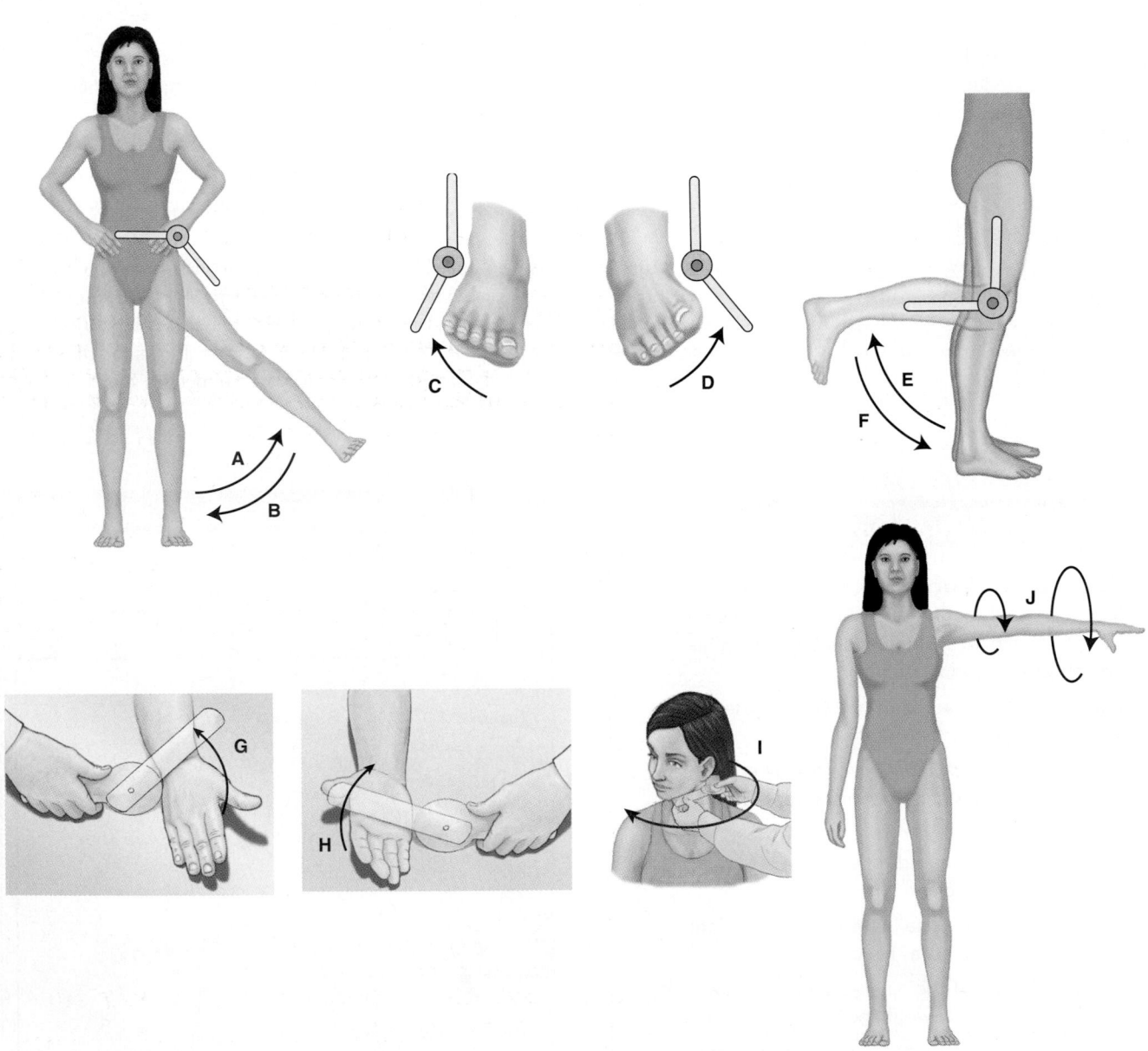

FIG 35-8 Goniometer measurements. (A) Abduction. (B) Adduction. (C) Eversion. (D) Inversion. (E) Flexion. (F) Extension. (G) Pronation. (H) Supination. (I) Rotation. (J) Circumduction.

- **circumduction**—moving in a circle, thus including multiple directions, such as the shoulder or hip joint. (Due to its complexity, circumduction requires a specialized goniometer.) (See *Documenting goniometer measurements*.)

Range of Motion

Range of motion (ROM) of any joint will decrease without movement. Hospitalized or bedridden patients must move extremities to avoid **contracture,** a loss of range of motion due to lack of movement. A patient can perform ROM exercises passively; that is, the patient does not move the extremities, the medical assistant gently moves the extremities for the patient. These exercises will not only prevent contracture but also promote adequate blood flow and prevent pressure ulcers. (See *Procedure 35-3: Performing ROM exercises, upper body*, page 728, and *Procedure 35-4: Performing ROM exercises, lower body*, page 730.)

Fitting a Patient with a Walker, Cane, and Crutches

Ambulation, or walking, may be compromised due to injury, stroke, or weakness. (See *Procedure 35-5: Assisting with gait using a gait belt*, page 731.) Patients can use assistive devices for ambulation, such as walkers, canes, and crutches, to enjoy the freedom associated with mobility. Proper fitting and instruction in the use of assistive devices promotes safety and stability and prevents reinjury.

Fitting a Patient with a Walker

Most walkers are adjustable to accommodate various heights. The medical assistant fitting a walker to a patient should adjust the walker height so that the top of the walker is just below the patient's waist, at the top of the femur. (See Figure 35-9.) After adjusting the height of the walker, the medical assistant should make sure that screws are secure so that the walker will not collapse when the weight of thepatient is applied. The patient should be able to stand with elbows bent at approximately 30 degrees when touching the hand grips. After fitting the walker, the medical assistant should instruct the patient about its use and assist him in trying to use it. (See *Procedure 35-6: Assisting a patient in ambulating with a walker*, page 733.)

Fitting a Patient with a Cane

A patient should use a cane when he has one weak side. It is useful to patients that have generalized but minor weakness and may be used on an "as needed" basis by

Documenting goniometer measurements

These goniometers are measuring a patient's elbow at extension and flexion.

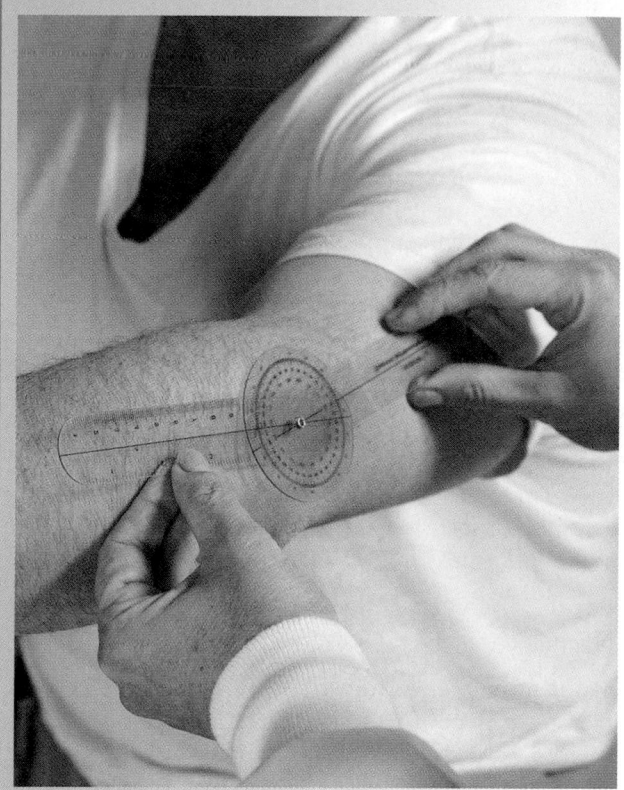

Extension

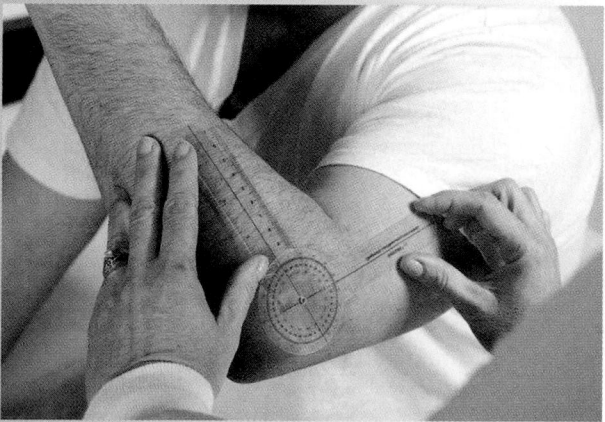

Flexion

Here is an example of how these measurements should be documented.

Date	
11/22/08; 9:30 a.m.	ROM about the left elbow: Extension 170 degrees. Flexion, 25 degrees. ———————————————— J. Morgan, CMA

the patient. For example, some patients may feel comfortable at home without the cane but rely on the cane in public for extra support and to act as a deterrent to other people who may inadvertently bump into the person. Patients with poor balance may also benefit from the use of a cane.

Canes can be made of wood or lighter-weight aluminum and come in three basic types:

- The *standard cane* has a single tip and a simple curved handle or a bent grip handle.
- A *quad cane* is a four-legged cane that adds extra support by its increased contact with the floor. It provides more

stability to patients who may suffer from severe walking difficulties.

- A *walk cane* is similar to a walker; it has four legs and a handlebar, but is unilateral and can be used by hemiplegic patients. (See Figure 35-10.)

Because canes are the most portable assistive device, patients may ask for canes rather than wheelchairs, walkers, or crutches. The physician must prescribe the appropriate assistive device for each patient. After fitting the patient with a cane, the medical assistant should assist and instruct the patient in its use. (See *Procedure 35-7: Assisting a patient in ambulating with a cane*, page 734.)

PROCEDURE 35-3

Performing ROM exercises, upper body

Task
Use passive range-of-motion (ROM) exercises to maintain and increase joint mobility in the upper extremities to prevent contracture.

Conditions
None.

Standards
In the time specified and within the scoring parameters determined by the instructor, the student will successfully use passive ROM exercises.

Performance standards
1. Wash your hands.
2. Introduce yourself and address the patient by name. Explain to the patient that you will be gently moving his arms, within pain tolerance and flexibility of the limb, to assure him that the ROM exercises will not hurt.

Shoulder flexion
1. Keeping the patient's arm straight and holding the arm at the wrist and elbow, lift the patient's arm straight over his head until it rests flat on the bed or to range-of-motion (ROM) tolerance to attain end range of motion without discomfort.
2. Bring the arm back to the patient's side. Repeat according to the physician's instructions.

Shoulder abduction and adduction
1. Keeping the patient's arm straight by his side with the palm facing up, bring the arm out straight away from the patient's body. Be sure to support the arm at the wrist and elbow for his safety and comfort.

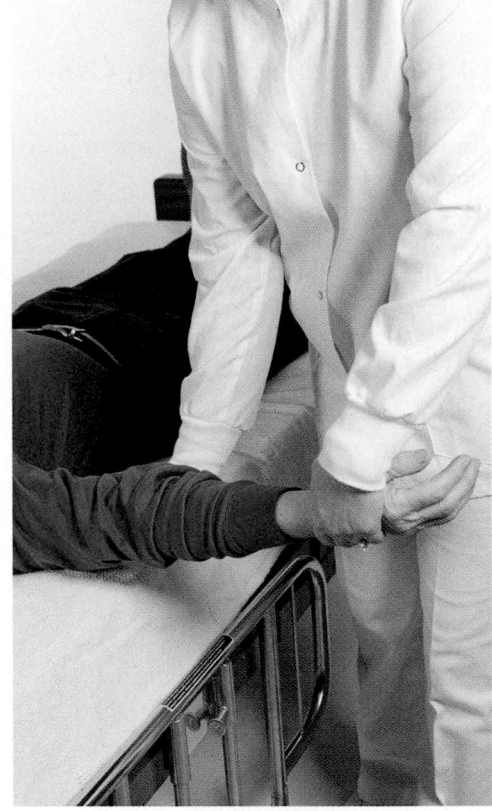

For the patient's safety and comfort, be sure to support his wrist and elbow during the ROM exercise.

2. Return the patient's arm to his side and bring it across his body (adduction) to adduct the shoulder to a comfortable end range.
3. Return the patient's arm to his side. Repeat according to the physician's instructions.

PROCEDURE 35-3—cont'd

External and internal shoulder rotation

1. Bring the patient's arm out at a right angle from his body.
2. Bend the elbow at a right angle, keeping the upper arm on the bed, and the hand straight up to ensure rotation of the shoulder.
3. Keeping the patient's elbow bent at 90 degrees, gently press down on his shoulder with one hand while holding up his hand with your other hand to stabilize the shoulder and facilitate rotation of the joint. Observe his facial expression to ensure his comfort.

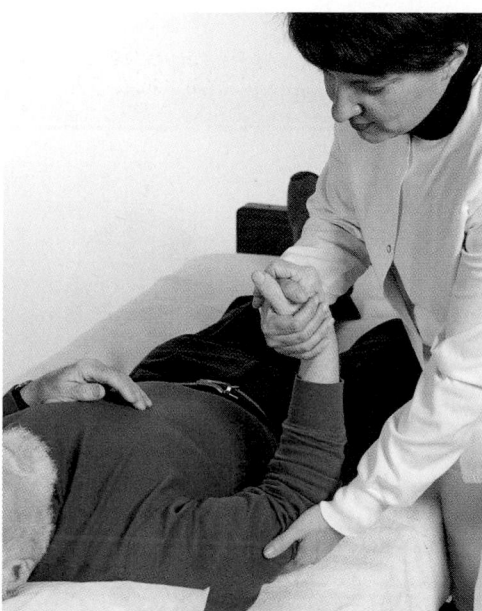

Be sure to stabilize the patient's shoulder with your hand while rotating the shoulder joint. Observe his facial expression to ensure his comfort.

4. Move the patient's hand gently back until it touches the bed next to his head.
5. Bring his hand back down until the palm of his hand touches the bed. Repeat as necessary.

Elbow flexion and extension

1. With the patient's arm by his side and his palm up, flex and extend the elbow to comfortably reach end range of flexion and extension. Repeat as necessary.

Wrist extension and flexion

1. Supporting the patient's arm above the wrist, hold the palm of the hand and extend and flex the wrist to comfortably reach end range of wrist flexion and extension.

Wrist inversion and eversion

1. Grasp the patient's wrist with one hand and grasp her hand with the other to stabilize the hand and wrist.

2. Slowly bend the patient's hand toward her body, then away to comfortably reach end range of wrist inversion and eversion.

Wrist supination and pronation

1. Grasp the patient's wrist with one hand and his hand with the other to stabilize the hand and wrist.
2. Slowly turn the patient's hand toward his feet, then toward his head to comfortably reach end range of supination and pronation.

Finger flexion and extension

1. Support the patient's wrist with one hand.
2. Cover his fingers with the other hand and curl them over to make a fist to comfortably reach full flexion.
3. Uncurl the patient's fingers and straighten them to comfortably reach full extension. Note the patient's reaction and ask him if he is comfortable to identify the extent of comfortable extension and avoid moving the fingers past a comfortable ROM.

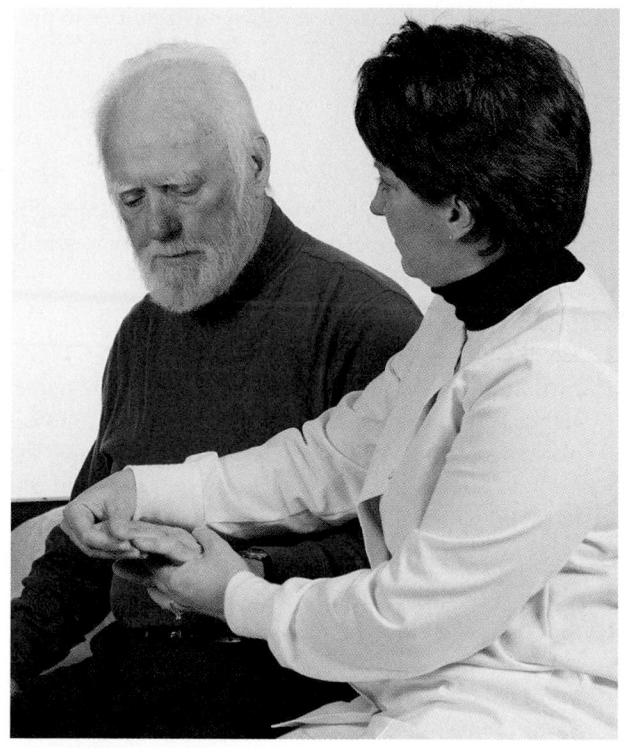

Extend the fingers, noting the patient's reaction.

Documentation

1. Document the procedure, noting the patient's reaction.

Date	
10/18/08; 10:30 a.m.	ROM exercises to upper body performed. Movements all within normal limits, patient does not report pain in any movement. ———————————— J. Morgan, CMA

Fitting a Patient with Crutches

Crutches can be used in pairs or one crutch can be used to assist gait. Most crutches are made of aluminum but some axillary crutches are wooden. There are three basic types of crutches:

- *Axillary crutches* are fitted to the patient's armpit height. Because upper body strength and balance is needed for axillary crutch use, they are best utilized by stronger patients, children, and patients with minor injuries. (See Figure 35-11.)
- *Forearm, or Lofstrand, crutches* are fixed with a plastic cuff around the forearm and a handlebar for each hand. The height of the crutch is shorter than the axillary crutch and provides less stability. The forearm crutch height should accommodate the patient's hand and forearm in a slightly bent position, with approximately 10 degrees of elbow flexion.
- *Platform crutches* are preferred for patients who cannot bear weight in the upper arm or hand. The top of the platform crutch should reach the forearm with the elbow bent at 90 degrees. (See *Procedure 35–8: Assisting a patient in ambulating with crutches,* page 736.)

Casting

Casts are applied to immobilize a fracture and allow the bone to heal itself. The cast protects the body from reinjury

---

PROCEDURE 35-4

Performing ROM exercises, lower body

Task

Use passive range-of-motion (ROM) exercises to maintain and increase joint mobility in the lower extremities to prevent contracture.

Conditions

None.

Standards

In the time specified and within the scoring parameters determined by the instructor, the student will successfully perform passive ROM exercises.

Performance Standards

1. Wash your hands.
2. Introduce yourself and address the patient by name. Explain to the patient that you will be gently moving his legs, within pain tolerance and flexibility of the limb, to assure him that the ROM exercises will not hurt.

Hip abduction and adduction

1. Support the patient's knee and ankle to ensure proper movement of the hip. Keep your hand under the patient's knee and hold the ankle to support the leg during abduction and adduction.
2. Keep the patient's leg straight, while moving the entire leg away from his body to comfortably reach full abduction.
3. Move the patient's leg back toward the midline of the body to comfortably reach full adduction.

Hip and knee flexion and extension

1. Support the patient's knee and ankle to ensure proper knee and hip movement.

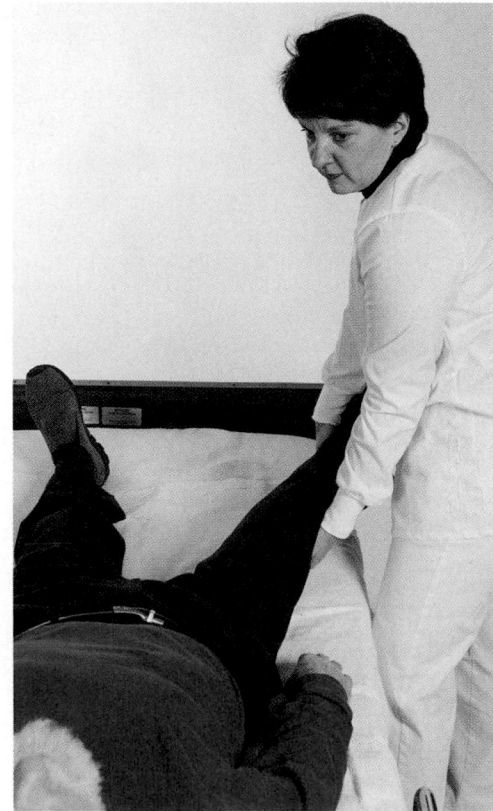

Keep your hand under the patient's knee and hold the ankle to support the leg during abduction and adduction.

PROCEDURE 35-4—cont'd

2. Bend the patient's knee and raise it as far toward the patient's chest as tolerated with comfort to comfortably reach full hip flexion.
3. Lower and straighten the patient's leg to comfortably reach full hip extension.

Hip rotation
1. Support the patient's leg at the knee and ankle to ensure proper hip movement.
2. Roll the patient's leg in a circular motion, away from the body to comfortably reach full external rotation.
3. Roll the patient's leg in a circular motion, toward the body to comfortably reach full internal rotation.

Ankle and dorsiflexion and plantar flexion
1. Keeping the patient's leg flat on the bed. Grasp the ankle with one hand and the heel of the foot with the other to stabilize the ankle.
2. While holding the heel with the one hand, flex the patient's foot and rest the bottom of the foot against your forearm.
3. Dorsiflex the ankle by pushing the foot toward the patient's head to comfortably reach full dorsiflexion.
4. Keep your hand on the patient's ankle and plantar flex the foot by pushing the foot down toward the foot of the bed to comfortably reach full plantar flexion.

Foot inversion and eversion
1. Grasp the patient's ankle with one hand and the arch of his foot with the other.
2. Gently turn the patient's foot inward.
3. Return the foot to midline, then gently turn it outward.

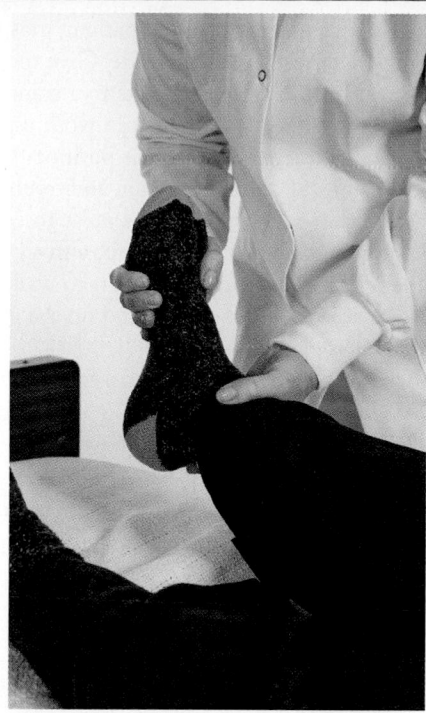

Stabilize the patient's ankle while performing range-of-motion exercises.

Documentation
1. Document the procedure, noting the patient's reaction.

Date	
10/18/08; 11:10 a.m.	ROM exercises to lower body performed. Patient reports some pain and stiffness upon extension of the left knee. All other movements within normal limits and pain free. ———————————————————————— J. Morgan, CMA

PROCEDURE 35-5

Assisting with gait using a gait belt

Task
Help the patient ambulate safely using a gait belt.

Conditions
■ Gait belt

Standards
In the time specified and within the scoring parameters determined by the instructor, the student will successfully assist with gait using a gait belt.

Performance Standards
1. Wash your hands.
2. Introduce yourself and address the patient by name. Explain to the patient that you will assist him in standing and walking.
3. Lock the brakes on the wheelchair; place the patient's feet on the floor, and move the foot plates out of the way.
4. Place the gait belt around the patient's waist. The belt should be snug but not tight for comfort and support. Any excess belt should be tucked in the back and out of the way.

Continued

PROCEDURE 35-5—cont'd

5. Standing directly in front of the patient, grasp the gait belt from underneath on either side. Give the patient a signal to push up on the arm rests to a standing position so that you and the patient can work together.

6. Steady the patient in the standing position. Check the patient for signs of dizziness, pallor, and trouble balancing. If necessary, take the patient's pulse to ensure that he is able to walk and to prevent injury from fainting.

7. If the patient looks steady and wants to walk, move to the patient's side, keeping one hand on the gait belt at all times for support.

8. Place one hand on the patient's arm for support. Make sure that your hand is on the gait belt with fingers underneath, palm upward, and elbow bent.

9. Starting with the same foot as the patient, keep in step with the patient. Allow the patient to control the pace and ask how he is feeling during walking for his safety.

10. Document the procedure, including the date, time, duration of ambulation, patient's response, and instructions given in the patient's medical record.

Modification: Two-person assist with ambulation

1. Perform the preceding steps 1 thru 5.

2. Have an assistant stand on either side of the patient. Grasp the gait belt from underneath with one hand, and place the other hand on the patient's back for support.

3. During ambulation, a person should be on either side of the patient. Both assistants should be slightly behind the patient to stabilize him and catch him if necessary. As in a one-person assist, allow the patient to set the pace.

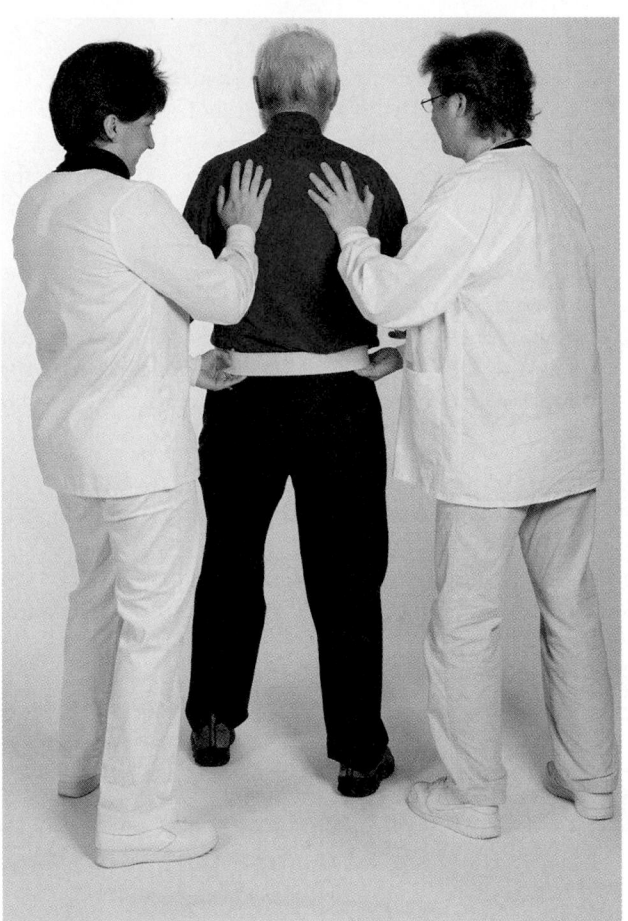

Two-person assistance with a gait belt.

4. Document the procedure as above.

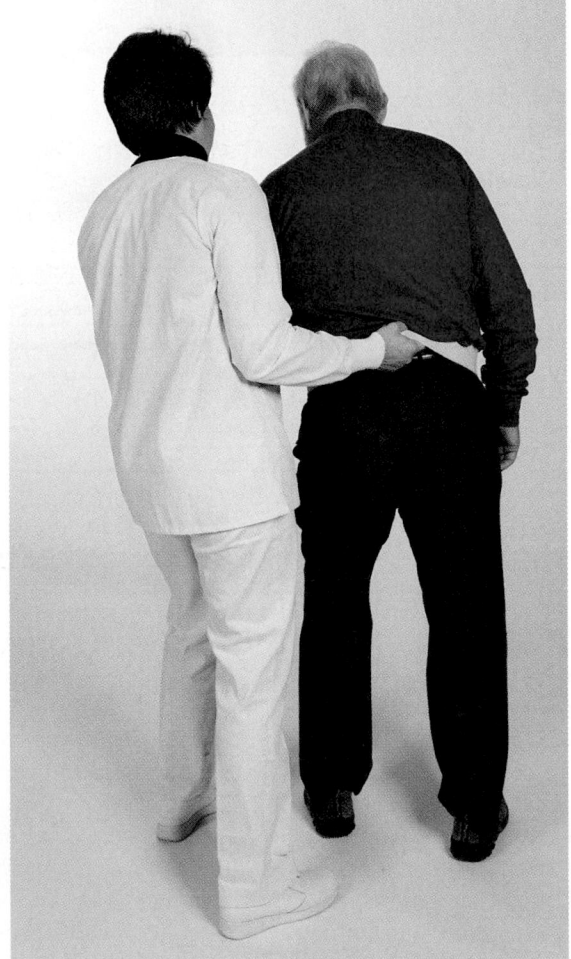

Proper positioning for holding a gait belt.

Date	
10/18/08; 12:20 p.m.	Patient assisted from wheelchair to walking with use of gait belt. He walked across the room and reported no dizziness. ------------------------------- C. Smith, CMA

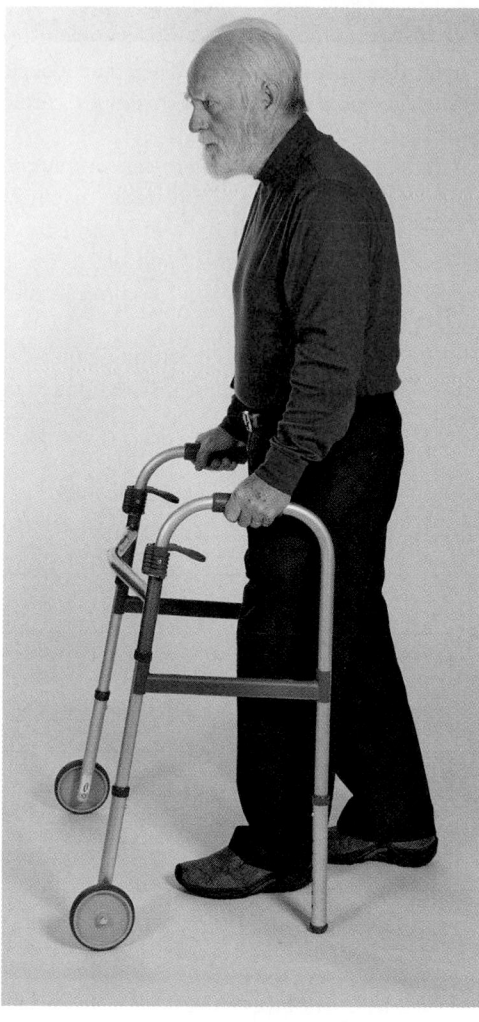

FIG 35-9 Patient properly fit for height to a walker.

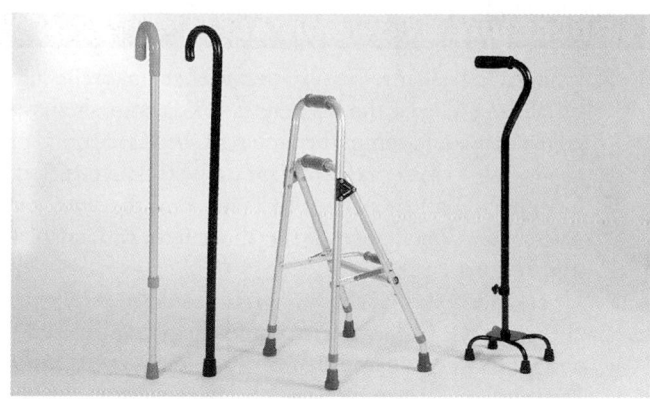

FIG 35-10 Standard canes and a walk cane.

and movement that would prevent the fractured bone from healing. Casting material can include plaster of Paris, fiberglass, or an air cast. Plaster of Paris is the oldest form of casting material and is seldom used. An air cast can be used if some mobility is allowed, because the patient can remove the air cast to bathe. If no mobility is desired, the patient will be fitted with a fiberglass cast, the most common type of cast. The material is durable and easy to care for. (See *Proper cast care*, page 738.)

Bone fractures must be reduced before casting. **Reduction** of a fracture is placing the fractured bone in a position conducive to healing in the proper position. Reduction of fractures is performed by the orthopedist in the office or in the operating room. A closed reduction is a reduction of a fracture that does not involve an incision and can be performed in the office by the orthopedist with or without the use

---

PROCEDURE 35-6

Assisting a patient in ambulating with a walker

Task
Teach a patient how to ambulate with a walker independently and safely.

Conditions
- Walker
- Gait belt

Standard
In the time specified and within the scoring parameters determined by the instructor, the student will successfully assist a patient in ambulating with a walker.

Performance Standards
1. Wash your hands.
2. Introduce yourself and address the patient by name. Explain to the patient that you will assist him to standing and walking with the aid of a walker.
3. Lock the brakes on the wheelchair, place the patient's feet on the floor, and move the foot plates out of the way.
4. Place the gait belt around the patient's waist. The belt should be snug but not tight. Any excess belt should be tucked in the back and out of the way.

Continued

PROCEDURE 35-6—cont'd

5. Check the walker to be sure that rubber tips are secure on all legs. Check the hand rests for damage or sharp edges that could injure the patient. Check the joints of the walker to make sure they are in the locked position.

6. Check the patient's shoes to make sure that any ties are secure. Check to see if the shoes have rubber soles and are not slippery.

7. Check the height of the walker. It should be level with the tip of the patient's femur, and the patient's elbows should be flexed at approximately 30 degrees for comfort and support to prevent the patient from falling and decrease the risk of fatigue.

8. Position the patient inside the walker.

9. Have the patient lift the walker and place all four legs of the walker in front of him so that the back legs of the walker are even with his toes to ensure that he does not move too far away from the walker and risk falling.

10. Instruct the patient to lean forward and transfer some of his weight to his arms while stepping with his stronger foot first. Then follow with a step with the weaker leg.

11. Hold on to the back of the gait belt and check the patient for signs of fatigue. Be ready to catch the patient if he falls.

12. If the walker has rollers, the patient can simply roll the walker in front of him at a comfortable distance and pace. If the walker does not have rollers, instruct the patient to lift the walker slightly and place it in front of him. Allow the patient to find a comfortable distance to move at each step.

13. Document the date, time, and duration of ambulation, the response of the patient, and instructions given to him. Initial the report.

Date	
12/22/08: 1:05 p.m.	Patient assisted in use of walker. He was assisted out of his wheelchair and he walked across the room with a walker. He reported feeling dizzy and was returned to his wheelchair. ------------------------- J. Morgan, CMA

PROCEDURE 35-7

Assisting a patient in ambulating with a cane

Task
Teach a patient how to ambulate with a cane independently and safely.

Conditions
■ Cane

Standards
In the time specified and within the scoring parameters determined by the instructor, the student will successfully assist a patient in ambulating with a cane.

Performance Standards
1. Wash your hands.
2. Introduce yourself and address the patient by name. Explain to the patient that you will assist him in walking with a cane.
3. Check the cane to make sure that the bottom has a rubber tip, the handle is not broken, and no sharp edges are present that could injure the patient.
4. Apply the gait belt snugly (but not too tightly) around the patient's waist. Tuck in any excess belt in the back of the belt so that the gait belt does not interfere with your contact and support of the patient.
5. Assist the patient to a standing position. Look for signs of dizziness to prevent the patient from falling.
6. Place the cane in the patient's hand on the side of the strong leg. The cane should be adjusted so that the handle is at hip joint level. The cane on the strong side provides extra support to the weak side during gait.
7. During weight-bearing, the patient's elbow should be flexed at 20 to 30 degrees to promote the patient's using the arm for balance.
8. Have the patient move the cane forward 10" to 18" ahead of him, depending on his ability and size.
9. Have the patient move his weak leg forward while transferring his weight to the cane. Transferring weight to the cane and not the weak leg will prevent pain to the affected leg and stabilize the gait.
10. Have the patient move his strong leg forward past the cane. Keep your hand on the gait belt and look for signs of fatigue or dizziness to ensure patient safety.
11. Follow along behind the patient on his weak side to be able to catch the patient in case he falls. Allow the patient to set the pace.

Follow along behind the patient and allow him to set the pace.

12. Document the date, time, duration of ambulation, patient's response, and instructions given in the patient's medical record.

Date	
12/30/08; 1:05 p.m.	Patient assisted in use of cane. He was helped out of his wheelchair using a gait belt and instructed on using the cane. He was able to take 5 steps but reported pain in the left knee. He was returned to the wheelchair. The left knee was inspected and found to be slightly swollen. An ice pack was applied to the knee. The patient was told to tell Dr. Rodriguez of the knee pain at his office visit tomorrow. ------------------------------ J. Morgan, CMA

of local anesthesia as necessary. If the bone fracture is more complicated, such as a compound, comminuted, or impacted fracture, reduction may be performed in asurgical setting. Surgical reduction of a fracture is referred to as *open reduction with internal fixation*. After a reduction is carried out, a cast is generally applied. (See *Procedure 35-9: Assisting with fiberglass cast application*, page 739, and *Procedure 35-10: Assisting with cast removal*, page 739.)

An arm sling provides support to an injured shoulder or arm. The sling helps the patient keep the arm in the appropriate position so that healing can occur properly. The arm sling also alerts people around the patient to his injury so they will avoid bumping into his arm. (See *Procedure 35-11: Applying a triangular arm sling*, page 740.)

Thermotherapy

The quantity of blood within the vessels of the muscle can be manipulated by **thermotherapy,** the therapeutic application of heat used to treat various muscle injuries. The application of heat to an injury promotes blood flow and comforts the injured patient. Heat should only be applied to an injury 24 hours after trauma to avoid excess swelling. When the time of injury is not certain, ice is applied.

Moist Heat

The application of moist heat to an injury will promote increased blood flow to the affected area and, therefore, promote healing. Most patients find moist heat to be soothing to an injury. To administer moist heat, a

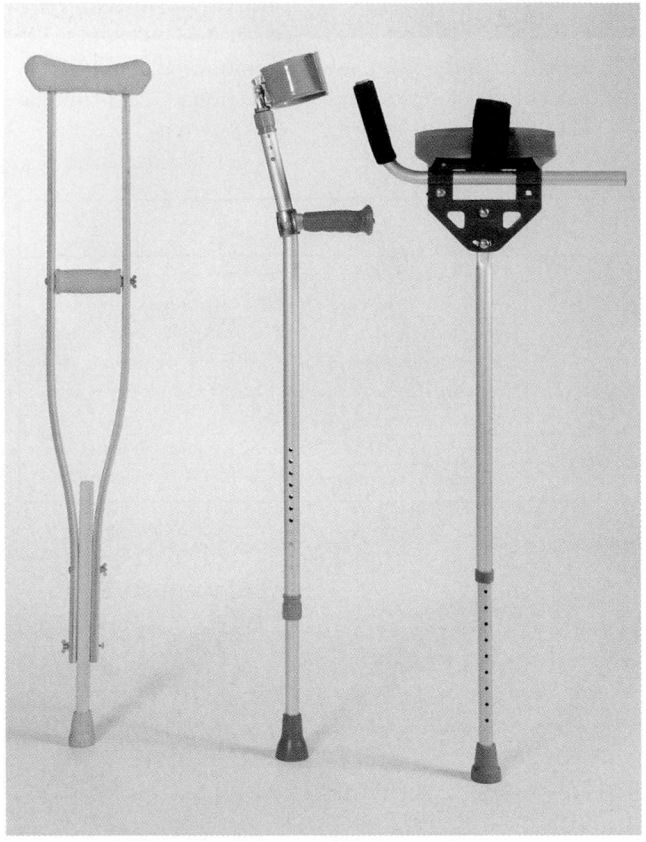

FIG 35-11 Axillary, forearm, and platform crutches.

hydrocollator is used. A hydrocollator is a thick, cloth sleeve filled with a porous clay that will retain water and heat. It is put in hot water to soak and placed in a terry cloth holder to place on the patient. For home use, patients can buy hydrocollators and covers at many pharmacies. (See Figure 35-12.)

When placing the hydrocollator on a patient, observe the following safety precautions:

- Place the unit *on* the patient. The patient should never lie on top of a heating unit because the weight of the patient will cause too much contact with the heat and could result in burns to the patient.
- After placing the unit on a patient, stay in the room for a few minutes. Ask the patient if the heat is too hot.
- Use extra towels wrapped around the hydrocollator cover when putting heat on an elderly patient. Decreased circulation in the elderly may cause them to fail to feel a burn forming.

Application of Warm, Moist Compresses

A warm, moist compress is applied by soaking and wringing gauze or a washcloth in warm water. Because warm (not hot) water is used, the compress can be placed directly on the skin. Patients can easily use warm compresses at home. Instruct patients to use warm compresses, not hot, to avoid burns.

■ PROCEDURE 35-8

Assisting a patient in ambulating with crutches

Task
Teach a patient how to ambulate with crutches independently and safely.

Conditions
- Crutches

Standards
In the time specified and within the scoring parameters determined by the instructor, the student will successfully assist a patient in ambulating with crutches.

Performance Standards
1. Wash your hands.
2. Introduce yourself and address the patient by name. Explain to the patient that you will assist him in crutch walking.
3. Assemble and fit the axillary crutches to the patient. Be sure that the joints of the crutches are secure; the rubber tips are on the ends, axillary pads, and hand rests; and the hand rests are in good shape (for example, no tears, missing pieces, or cracks in the wood).

4. Apply the gait belt and assist the patient to stand; place the crutches under his armpits.
5. Instruct the patient to carry his weight completely on his hands and not on his armpits to prevent injury to the shoulder joints.
6. Have the patient put all of his weight on the strong leg and bend his weak leg slightly so it will not drag on the floor to prevent stubbing his toe on the injured foot or scraping the cast or boot.
7. Assist the patient with the appropriate gait pattern.
8. Document the date, time, duration of ambulation, and instructions given in the patient's medical record.

Date	
10/20/08: 12:05 p.m.	*Crutches were fitted to the patient and he was instructed on their use. He was able to walk across the room with crutches. He was able to maintain balance and reports no pain. ———————————— J. Morgan, CMA*

PROCEDURE 35-8—cont'd

Non-weight-bearing to injured leg (2 crutches)

1. Instruct the patient to transfer all his weight to his hands and step with the strong leg.
2. Tell him to bring the crutches forward and then swing his injured leg through without putting any weight on the injured leg to prevent transferring weight to the injured leg. Have him repeat these steps.

Non-weight-bearing, 2 crutches

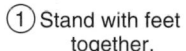
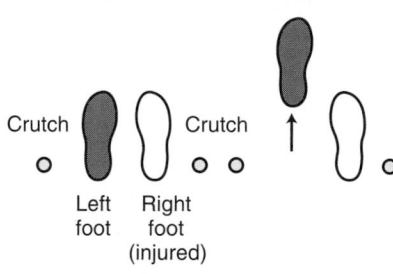
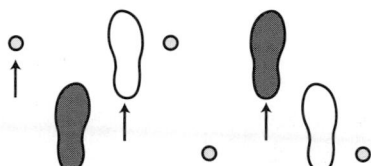

Non-weight-bearing, two crutches. (1) Stand with feet together. (2) Bring the strong leg forward. (3) Bring crutches forward and swing the weak leg through. (4) Bring the strong leg forward.

Weight-bearing to injured leg with support of crutches (2 crutches)

1. Tell the patient to transfer all his weight to his hands and step with his strong leg. Instruct him to use the crutches and step with his injured leg at the same time. Explain that the patient can put some weight on his injured leg, but only when he transfers some of the weight to his hands for support and balance. Ask him to repeat the steps.

Weight-bearing, 2 crutches

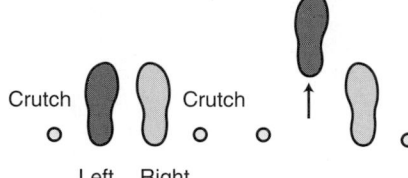
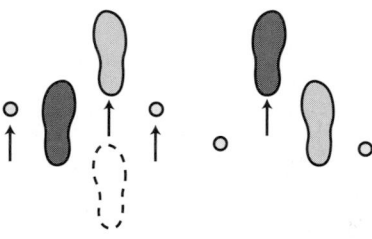

Weight-bearing, two crutches. (1) Stand with feet together. (2) Bring the strong leg forward. (3) Bring crutches and the weak leg forward, applying limited pressure to the weak leg. (4) Bring the strong leg forward.

Weight–bearing to injured leg with support of one crutch

1. Explain to the patient that one crutch can be used on his strong side to assist his weak side.
2. Instruct the patient to step with his strong leg and then move the weak leg and the crutch forward at the same time for support to the injured leg.
3. Tell the patient to gauge the amount of weight to put on his weak leg according to his comfort level to prevent straining the injured leg and causing reinjury.

PROCEDURE 35-8—cont'd

Weight-bearing, 1 crutch

① Stand with feet together.

② Bring strong leg forward.

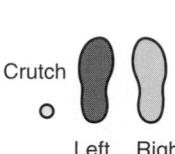

Crutch

Left foot   Right foot (injured)

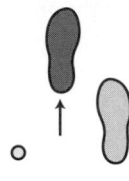

③ Bring weak leg and crutch forward.

④ Bring strong leg forward.

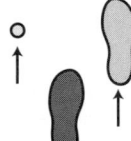

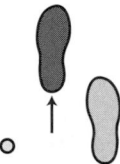

Weight-bearing, one crutch. (1) Stand with feet together. (2) Bring the strong leg forward. (3) Bring the weak leg and crutch forward at the same time. (4) Bring the strong leg forward.

Patient Education

Proper Cast Care

After assisting with cast application, be sure to explain proper cast care to the patient, including:

• Showing the patient how to cover the cast while bathing.

• Keeping the cast dry and exposed to air as much as possible. A wet cast can remodel and cause tissue damage to the affected body part.

• Elevating the casted extremity as much as possible. This will help reduce swelling and pain.

• Observing fingers or toes for changes in color, temperature, or decreased sensation. This could indicate that the cast is too tight. The patient should call the office immediately.

• Calling the office if any bad odor, loss of sensation, numbness, tingling, bleeding about the cast is noted.

• Not sticking anything down the cast to itch the skin—this could cause infection.

• Cleaning the cast with a damp cloth; decorating the cast with magic markers or paints, but not cutting or puncturing the cast for any reason.

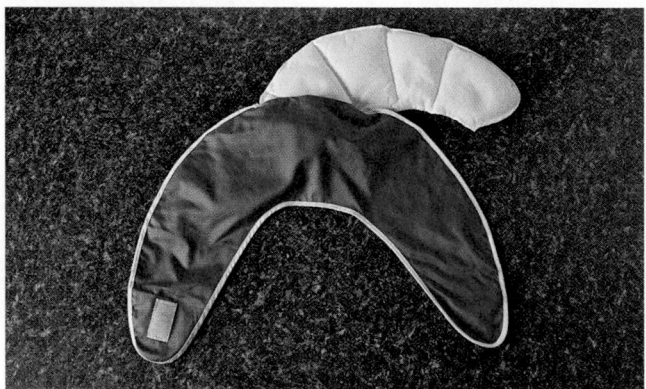

FIG 35-12 Hydrocollator and cover.

Dry Heat

Application of dry heat affects superficial tissues, not deep tissues. It is used to improve circulation, relieve swelling, promote wound healing, and relax muscle spasm. Dry heat is most commonly applied using an electric heating pad. As with a hydrocollator, the heating pad should never be placed directly on the skin. Heating pads should be used for 15 to 20 minutes at a time, because prolonged heating could cause

PROCEDURE 35-9

Assisting with fiberglass cast application

Task
Assist the physician in applying a fiberglass cast.

Conditions
- Fiberglass casting material
- Basin of warm water
- Stockinette
- Webril padding rolls
- Bandage scissors
- Rubber gloves
- Sponge rubber (for padding)

Standards
In the time specified and within the scoring parameters determined by the instructor, the student will successfully assist with a fiberglass cast application.

Performance Standards
1. Wash your hands.
2. Explain the procedure to the patient. Tell him that the fiberglass cast will feel wet and cool as it is applied and that it dries and hardens quickly. Explain that it will be completely hardened and protect the body part within 30 minutes so that he understands not to move the body part during the procedure. Answer any questions about the procedure or the patient's injury to promote patient understanding and cooperation.
3. Prepare the stockinette by cutting to a length appropriate for the cast. Assist the physician in placing the stockinette directly on the skin under the cast to prevent the cast material from adhering to body hair or causing skin irritation.
4. Assist the physician in wrapping the cast padding (Webril) around the stockinette to protect the patient's skin when the cast is removed and to cushion bony areas under the cast.
5. Assist the physician as required.
6. Minimize patient discomfort by supporting the affected area.
7. Provide cast care instructions to the patient and answer any questions he may have.
8. Document the procedure in the patient's chart.

Date	
11/10/08; 2:15 p.m.	Fiberglass cast applied to right forearm and wrist. Patient given instructions on cast care and told to report any discoloration of fingers or numbness to any part of the arm or hand. ------------------------------------- J. Morgan, CMA

PROCEDURE 35-10

Assisting with cast removal

Task
Assist the physician in the removal of a cast.

Conditions
- Cast cutter
- Cast spreader
- Bandage scissors
- Bag or container for disposing of cast materials
- Basin, soap, and water

Standards
In the time specified and within the scoring parameters determined by the instructor, the student will successfully assist with cast removal.

Performance Standards
1. Wash your hands.
2. Explain the procedure to the patient. Tell him that the cutter vibrates but does not spin. Explain to the patient that he may feel some pressure and warmth but his skin will not be cut by the cast cutter to allay the fears of the patient so that he will not move or jump during the procedure.
3. Tell the patient that when he sees the limb without the cast, it will appear small and the color may be gray so that the patient is not afraid of the appearance of the limb. Reassure the patient that color and muscle tone will improve with therapy and exercise.
4. After the procedure, give the patient written instructions and answer any questions.
5. Gently wash the extremity with soap and water and apply skin lotion to remove any debris and prevent skin dryness.
6. Clean the equipment to prevent contamination to the next patient.
7. Wash your hands.

Continued

PROCEDURE 35-10—cont'd

8. Document the cast removal and the appearance of the body part. Record that written instructions were given to the patient.

Date	
12/19/08; 3:25 p.m.	Cast removed from patient's right forearm and hand. Skin is intact. Skin was washed with soap and water and lotion applied. Patient is able to move the wrist slightly. He was instructed to begin physical therapy tomorrow and not to grip or lift with the right hand until evaluation tomorrow with the therapist. ------------------------J. Morgan, CMA

PROCEDURE 35-11

Applying a triangular arm sling

Task
Apply a triangular arm sling.

Conditions
- Sling

Standards
In the time specified and within the scoring parameters determined by the instructor, the student will successfully assist with triangular arm sling application.

Performance Standards
1. Wash your hands.
2. Introduce yourself and address the patient by name.
3. Place the patient's elbow in a 90-degree position against her chest. The patient can hold her injured arm with her opposite hand to avoid holding up the injured arm, which would cause pain.
4. Place one point of the triangle at the patient's good shoulder and one point towards the affected elbow.
5. Slide the sling under the injured arm. Ask the patient to steady the injured arm with her other hand. Look for signs of pain and discomfort to ensure that the sling is comfortable.
6. Pull the bottom of the triangle up and around the injured arm next to the neck.
7. Tie the ends of the sling at the side of the neck because tying a knot at the back of the neck causes pain and interferes with mobility.
8. Make sure that the patient holds her injured arm at approximately 90 degrees so the arm is supported and blood flow is not compromised.
9. Use a safety pin to secure the elbow end of the sling.
10. Wash your hands and document the procedure.

Date	
10/14/08; 10:30 a.m.	Sling applied to left arm; patient instructed to remove the sling for bathing. ------------------------J. Morgan, CMA

burns. Place a towel, cloth, or blanket between the patient and the heating pad. Heating pads can also be purchased at most pharmacies.

Cryotherapy
Cryotherapy, the application of ice to an injury, is commonly used to reduce swelling and decrease pain. Ice is applied to injuries in the first 24 to 48 hours. Ice constricts blood vessels to decrease swelling, reduces bleeding, and numbs pain sensation by acting as a topical anesthetic. Ice can safely be applied for up to 20 minutes; if ice is left on the skin too long, it could damage tissues. "Chemical ice" is commonly used in physician offices as well as at sporting events, in school nurses' offices, and in other settings. The medical assistant can activate the bag of chemical ice by popping an internal bag that mixes two liquids within the bag. When these two chemicals mix, they cause an endothermic reaction, and the bag gets cold. The medical assistant should apply the ice directly to the skin or wrapped in a towel for comfort. Gel packs are also used to apply cold to the body. Gel packs are stored in a freezer and retain cold for approximately 30 to 45 minutes after

application. A gel pack should not contact the skin directly because it could adhere to the skin and cause discomfort. (See Figure 35-13.)

Ultrasound

Ultrasound can be used to administer heat to an injured body area. With ultrasound, high-frequency sound waves enter the musculature, creating friction in the tissues. This friction produces heat. The ultrasound can heat tissues more deeply than applying heat to the skin's surface. (See *Procedure 35-12: Administering ultrasound.*)

Transcutaneous Electrical Nerve Stimulation

Pain management for chronic conditions can be aided by the use of a transcutaneous electric nerve stimulation (TENS) unit. The unit delivers an electrical current to the painful area and disrupts the pain signal from the body to the brain. The units are portable and inexpensive and can be self-administered after proper instruction. The medical assistant can provide instruction in the use and care of the unit. (See *Procedure 35-13: Teaching a patient to use a TENS unit,* page 742.)

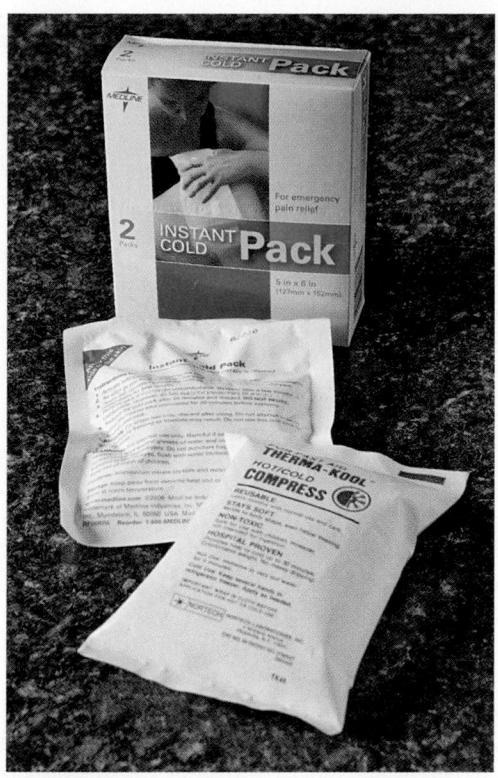

FIG 35-13 Typical cold packs.

PROCEDURE 35-12

Administering ultrasound

Task
To administer ultrasound to a body area of a patient.

Conditions
- Ultrasound
- Aqueous-based gel

Standards
In the time specified and within the scoring parameters determined by the instructor, the student will successfully administer an ultrasound.

Performance Standards
1. Wash your hands.
2. Introduce yourself and address the patient by name.
3. Explain the procedure to the patient.
4. Ask the patient if she has any metal inside her body, such as surgical pins or screws. Ultrasound **cannot** be performed over metal because it will heat the metal inside the patient's body, resulting in severe injury to the patient's tissues.
5. Apply gel to the skin of the affected area. The gel should be kept at room temperature.

6. Touch the wand of the ultrasound to the gel on the skin. Move the wand around to the entire area to be examined to ensure that the entire area is treated.
7. Turn the timer on the machine to the appropriate time. Slowly turn up the intensity of the ultrasound from zero and ask the patient when she feels warmth or tingling to ensure that the patient is comfortable with the prescribed wattage. Turn the machine up to the prescribed wattage.
8. While turning up the machine, always keep the wand moving. Stopping the wand can cause burning inside the tissues.
9. When the time expires, remove the wand and clean it with a dry cloth or towel. Clean the patient's skin with a separate dry cloth or towel.
10. Wash your hands and document the procedure.

Date	
11/12/08:	Ultrasound applied for 10 minutes to lumbar paraspinals.
10:30 a.m.	Patient reports warming sensation. ------J. Morgan, CMA

PROCEDURE 35-13

Teaching a patient to use a TENS unit

Task
Apply a transcutaneous electrical nerve stimulation (TENS) unit to a patient and teach him how to apply and regulate the TENS unit for home use.

Conditions
- TENS unit
- Disposable sticky pads

Standards
In the time specified and within the scoring parameters determined by the instructor, the student will successfully teach a patient to use a TENS unit.

Performance Standards
1. Wash your hands.
2. Introduce yourself and address the patient by name.
3. Wash the patient's skin with alcohol to remove any lotion that may cause the pads to fail to adhere to the skin.
4. Make sure that the sticky pads are in good condition and that wires are safe (without exposed, frayed ends). Frayed ends may shock the patient, causing discomfort.
5. Apply the sticky pads to the patient's skin on designated body areas, as directed by the physician, to ensure that the proper body area is stimulated.

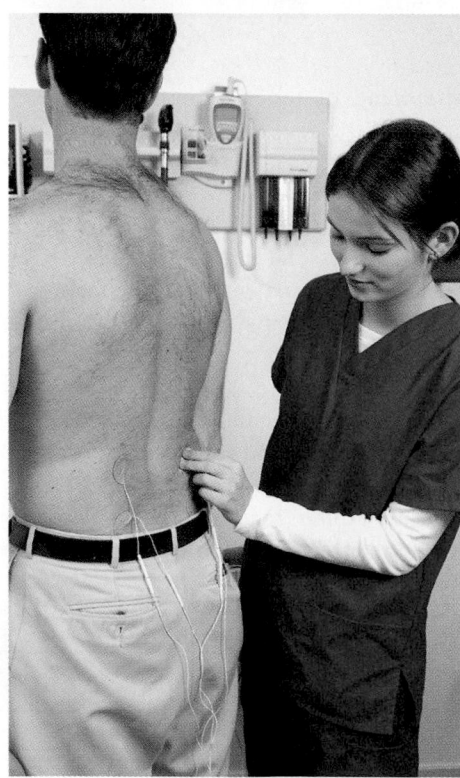

Apply the pads to the patient's skin as directed by the physician.

6. Make sure that the wires that connect to the TENS unit are secure. Turn on the TENS unit slowly to avoid startling the patient with the sensation.
7. Ask the patient when he first feels stimulation. Turn the machine up to a comfortable tolerance to promote stimulation without discomfort.
8. Explain to the patient that tolerance will increase and that he can turn the unit up or down as needed to promote therapeutic value along with comfort.

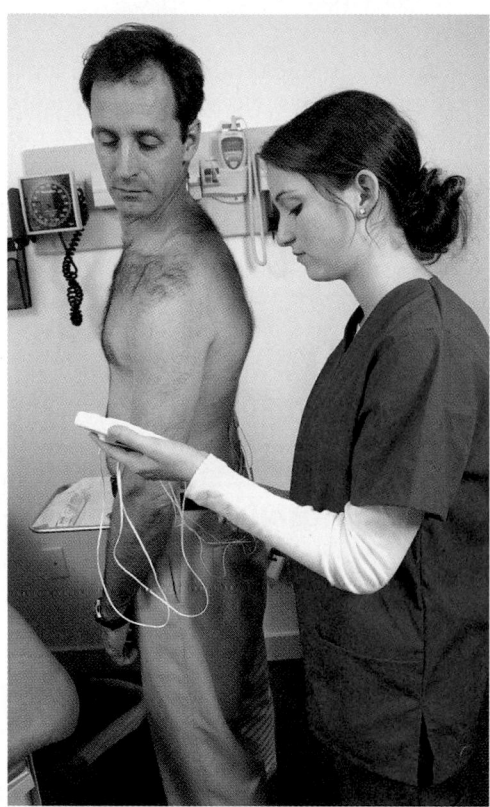

Explain to the patient that he can control the unit as needed.

9. Show the patient that he can wear the unit on his belt or clip it to his pocket and he can turn it on or off at any time.
10. Answer any questions, wash your hands, and document the procedure.

Date	
10/18/08; 9:30 a.m.	*Applied TENS unit to lower thoracic and lumbar paraspinals. Patient instructed on use of TENS device. He was also advised to call the office if lower back pain increases.*
	-- C. Smith, CMA

Chapter Summary

- The musculoskeletal system functions to provide movement and framework to the body.
- Musculoskeletal injuries are treated with therapy that restores physical function and educates patients to prevent reinjury.
- Modalities to treat musculoskeletal injuries range from application of ice packs to surgical correction.
- Because injury severity can vary greatly, rehabilitation can be very short for minor injuries or lengthy in the case of severe injuries that require surgery, immobilization, and casting.
- The medical assistant's role in rehabilitation of musculoskeletal injuries is to help patients ambulate; provide care for wounds, sprains, and strains; and teach strategies for independent function.
- Using such modalities as ultrasound, TENS, and range-of-motion exercises, the medical assistant can promote healing and pain control.
- The medical assistant is responsible for maintaining assistive devices, such as wheelchairs, crutches, canes, and walkers.

Team Work Exercises

1. Split into groups of three to four students. Role-play various patient transfers with classmates, asking a classmate to play the part of a paraplegic patient. Use rooms on your campus, such as the cafeteria, classroom, and restroom. Discuss with the group the challenges that you encountered.

2. Practice gait training with the gait belt. Create a course through which fellow students must guide the patient using the gait belt. Make the course simulate the hazards that a patient may face.

Case Studies

1. Mike Jones, a patient well known to the office, comes in appearing to be in a great deal of pain. His gait is very guarded and he doesn't put any weight on his right foot. He is unable to sit and prefers to stand leaning on the reception desk. What assistance should you offer to Mike? What assistance might he need during the physician examination? What questions should you ask Mike before the physician comes into the examination room? Why?

2. Hannah Morales is a 7-year-old with a broken forearm. She came to the office last week and was casted for the injury. Mrs. Morales calls the office and tells you that Hannah will not use her hand. She says that making a fist or moving the hand causes shooting pain in the hand and up the arm. She notices that the hand is slightly discolored. What should you do?

Resources

- About Orthopedics: *orthopedics.about.com*
- HealthWeb Orthopedic Associations: *www.healthweb.org/orthopedics*
- Musculoskeletal injuries: *healthweb.org/browse.cfm?categoryid=2955*
- Rotator cuff tear: *orthopedics.about.com/cs/rotatorcuff/a/rotatorcuff_3.htm*

Ophthalmology and Otolaryngology

Key Terms

accommodation
Ability of the eye to see objects in the distance and then adjust to a close object

astigmatism
Abnormality of the eye in which the refraction of a ray of light is spread over a diffuse area rather than sharply focused on the retina

audiometer
Instrument used to measure hearing

cataract
Opacity (clouding) of the lens of the eye

cerumen
Yellow or brown waxy substance produced in the ceruminous glands of the ear

color deficiency
Genetic or acquired abnormality in color perception

conjunctivitis
Inflammation of the conjunctiva caused by bacteria or virus

corneal abrasion
Injury to the translucent anterior structure of the eye

equilibrium
State of balance, which is controlled by structures of the inner ear

glaucoma
Disorder that involves increased intraocular pressure, resulting in atrophy of the optic nerve and, possibly, blindness

gustation
Sense of taste

hyperopia
Error of refraction in which affected individuals can see distant objects clearly but cannot see near objects; also called *farsightedness*

Ménière disease
Syndrome characterized by recurring episodes of hearing loss, tinnitus, and vertigo that can progressively lead to deafness

myopia
Error of refraction in which light rays are focused in front of the retina, enabling the person to see distinctly for only a short distance; also called *nearsightedness*

olfaction
Sense of smell

ophthalmoscope
Handheld instrument used to view the internal structures of the eye, including the retina, optic nerve, and blood vessels

otitis
Inflammation of the ear

otoscope
Handheld instrument used to visualize the internal structures of the ear, ear canal, and ear drum

presbyopia
Permanent loss of accommodation of the crystalline lens that occurs in people over age 40

sinusitis
Inflammation of the sinuses, which can be caused by a virus, bacteria, or an allergy

tinnitus
Ringing in the ears

visual acuity
Ability to see at different distances

Structures and Functions of the Eyes, Ears, Mouth, Nose, and Throat

The eyes, ears, mouth, nose, and throat are the structures that provide the special senses. These special senses include vision, hearing, balance, taste, and smell.

Structures of the Eyes, Ears, Mouth, Nose, and Throat

The eyes, ears, mouth, nose, and throat are made up of several structures, including the sclera, cornea, and retina of the eye; the auricle, tympanic membrane, and cochlea of the ear; the teeth, gums, tongue, and papillae of the mouth; the nares and olfactory neurons of the nose; and the nasopharynx, oropharynx, and laryngopharynx of the throat.

Eyes
The eye is a globe-shaped organ that consists of three layers, or *tunics:*

- sclera, the outer portion
- middle choroid, the middle portion
- retina, the inner portion. (See Figure 36-1.)

Sclera and Cornea
The outermost layer of the eye includes the sclera and cornea. The sclera is opaque and has a distinctive white color. At the front of the eye, the sclera bulges forward to become the cornea, which is transparent. A thin mucous membrane called the *conjunctiva* covers the outer surface of the eye and lines the eyelids.

Choroid
The middle layer of the eyeball is the choroid. The choroid is a dark blue vascular layer between the sclera and retina. The optic nerve, also called the *second cranial nerve,* is attached to the retina at one end and the diencephalon of the brain at the other. An opening in the choroid allows the optic nerve to enter the inside of the eyeball. Other structures in the choroid include the iris, ciliary body, lens, and suspensory ligaments. The iris is a colored structure that surrounds the pupil, which is a "hole" in the iris. The ciliary body is a circular muscle that lies posterior to the iris. The ciliary body is attached to a capsular bag that contains the lens (a clear, hard, transparent disk) and suspensory ligaments.

Retina
The innermost layer of the eye is the retina. (See Figure 36-2.) The retina is further divided into two layers. The thin outer layer is red due to blood flow from its main central artery. This outer layer lies next to the choroid. The thicker inner

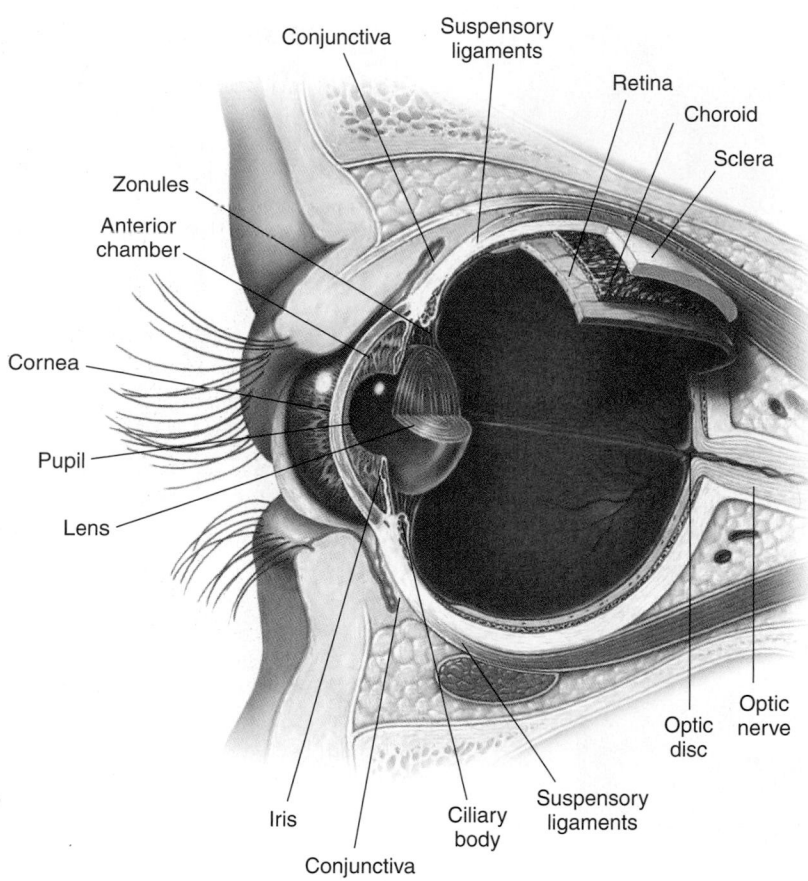

FIG 36-1 Structures of the eye.

layer is the visual portion and contains two types of visual receptors, called *rods* and *cones*. Rods and cones are elongated nerve cells that are lined up along the posterior portion of the retina. (See Figure 36-3.) They contain photopigments that undergo chemical changes when light strikes them.

Other structures

The eye contains two fluids, or *humors*. Aqueous humor is found in the posterior and anterior chambers. Aqueous humor drains through a small opening called the *Canal of Schlemm*. The posterior chamber contains aqueous humor and vitreous humor. Vitreous humor is a jellylike substance that fills the posterior chamber.

Lacrimal glands are located on the medial side of the eye and open through the lacrimal duct at the inner corner of the eye next to the nose. The lacrimal gland is connected to the nose through the nasolacrimal duct and drains into the nasal cavity.

Ears

The ear consists of three major sections: the outer, or external, ear; the middle ear, which consists of the tympanic

membrane and tympanic cavity; and the innermost section, called the *inner ear* or *labyrinth*. (See Figure 36-4.)

External Ear

The external ear consists of the auricle, or *pinna*. It is made up of cartilage covered with skin and sits visibly outside of the head. The auricle cannot be moved by voluntary or involuntary muscles to focus sound from a given direction, and the shape of the auricle does not contribute to hearing. The auricle is connected to the external auditory canal, which is a slender tube that leads to the middle ear. The canal is lined with modified sweat glands called *ceruminous glands*.

Middle Ear

At the inner end of the external auditory canal is the tympanic membrane, which is a flat, membranous structure. The tympanic membrane is connected to the first of three tiny ossicles (bones) of the middle ear. These bones are, in order, the *malleus* (hammer), *incus* (anvil), and *stapes* (stirrups). These tiny articulating bones are located in the tympanic cavity.

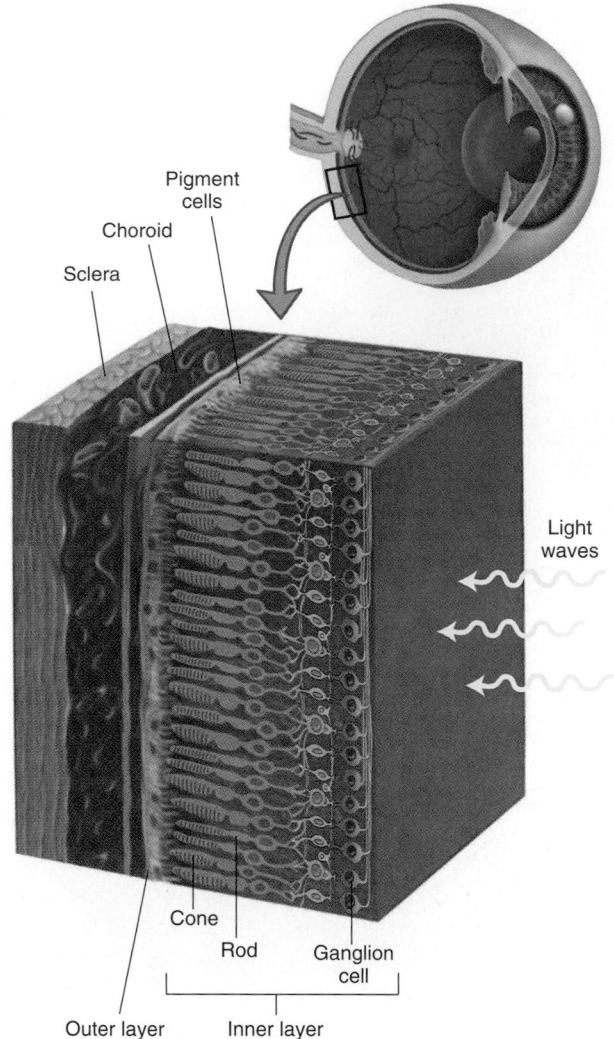

FIG 36-2 Microscopic structures of the retina.

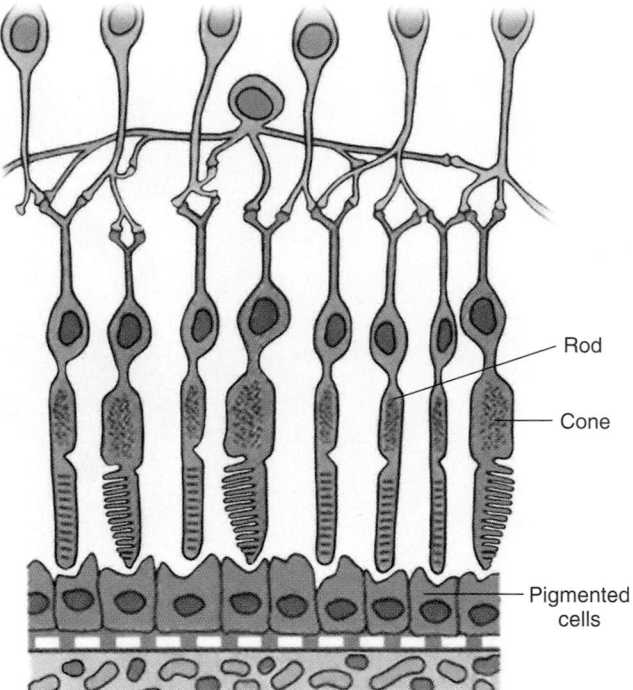

FIG 36-3 Rods and cones.

Inner Ear

The first structure of the inner ear is the cochlea, a snail-shaped structure filled with a fluid called *perilymph*. The inner surface of the cochlea is lined with a highly sensitive hearing structure called the *organ of Corti*. The organ of Corti contains nerve endings called *hair cells*, which are long, hairlike projections. The hair cells transmit impulses to the auditory nerve, located behind the ossicles.

The last of the three ossicles, the stapes, fits into an opening on the cochlea called the *oval window*. The round window is an opening in the lower part of the temporal bone and is covered with a thin membrane. The semicircular canals, located behind the ossicles and two windows, contains perilymph and endolymph, a pale, transparent fluid. Together with the cochlea, these structures make up the vestibular system. The tympanic cavity has a connecting downward canal called the *eustachian tube*. The eustachian tube connects the middle ear to the pharynx.

Mouth

The mouth, or *oral cavity*, contains the teeth, gums, and the tongue. (See Figure 36-5.) The tongue is a muscular organ that lies partly in the floor of the mouth and partly in the pharynx. The surface of the tongue contains papillae, which contain the taste buds on their surface.

Nose and Throat

The nose is a triangular structure made up of bone and cartilage. (See Figure 36-6.) It is covered with skin and lined with a mucous membrane. It contains two openings, called *nares* (nostrils), which are separated by a cartilage portion called the *nasal septum*. The nasal cavity is two cavities, right and left, separated by the septum. Behind and above the nasal cavity are the sinuses, which are hollow, mucus-lined cavities. The sinuses are grouped by their location into the *frontal sinuses* (above the eyebrows in the frontal bone of the skull), *maxillary sinuses* (which are the largest sinuses and are located on either side of the nose), *sphenoid sinuses* (located in the sphenoid bone), and *ethmoid sinuses* (located between the nose and eyes in the ethmoid bone). Olfactory neurons are located among the epithelial cells of the nasal cavity. The receptors are located higher in the nasal cavity than air is normally inhaled.

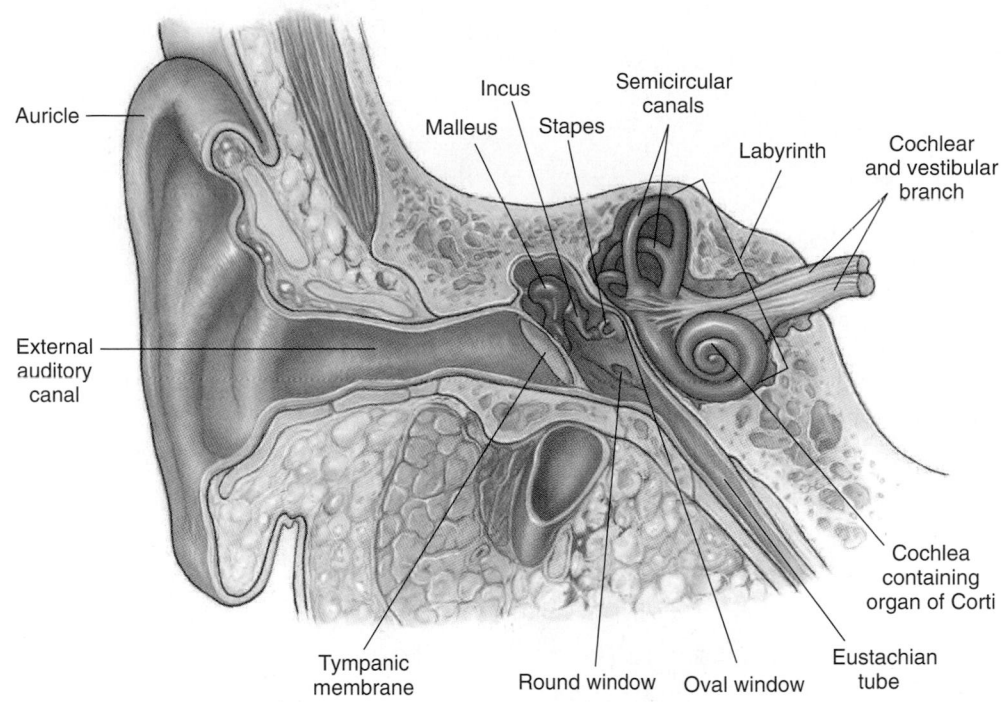

FIG 36-4 Structures of the ear.

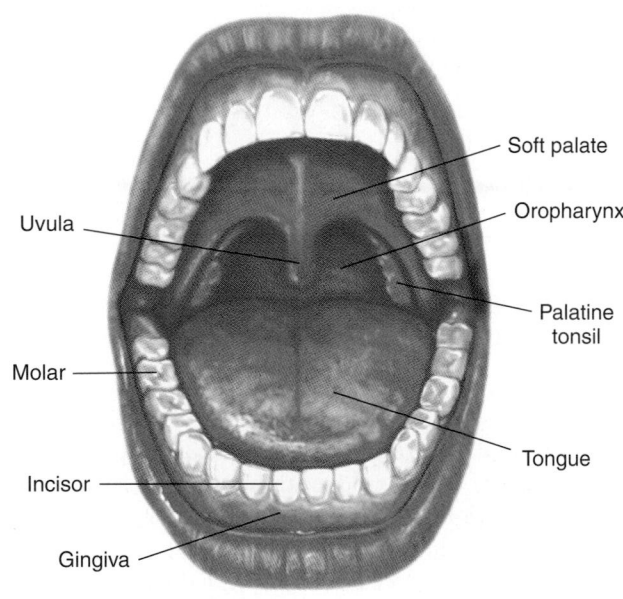

FIG 36-5 Structures of the mouth.

The nasal cavity is connected to a muscular tube called the *pharynx*, or *throat*, which is divided into three sections: the *nasopharynx*, *oropharynx*, and *laryngopharynx*. The nasopharynx, the first portion of the pharynx, is a rigid muscular tube that is open to the eustachian tube on either side. The top and sides of the nasopharynx also contain the adenoids, also called *pharyngeal tonsils*, which are lymphatic tissues. The nasopharynx continues inferiorly and becomes the oropharynx, which is softer than nasopharynx. It begins at the level of the soft palate and ends at the epiglottis. Located on either side of the oropharynx are the palatine tonsils, a collection of lymphatic tissue. Inferior to the oropharynx is the laryngopharynx, the lowest portion of the pharynx. It begins at the base of the tongue and is also made up of soft tissue. The inferior end of the laryngopharynx is connected to the larynx. The larynx further divides into the esophagus, which leads to the stomach, and trachea, which leads to the lungs.

Functions of the Eyes, Ears, Mouth, Nose, and Throat

The eyes, ears, mouth, nose, and throat serve several important functions in the body, including providing the special senses of vision, hearing, taste, and smell as well as balance and protection against injury.

Eyes

The eyes are the sensory organ responsible for sight. Each of the layers of the eye functions to protect the eye, provide vision, or communicate that vision to the brain.

Sclera and Cornea

On the outer layer of the eye, the sclera, or "white of the eye," provides the strength, structure, and shape of the eye.

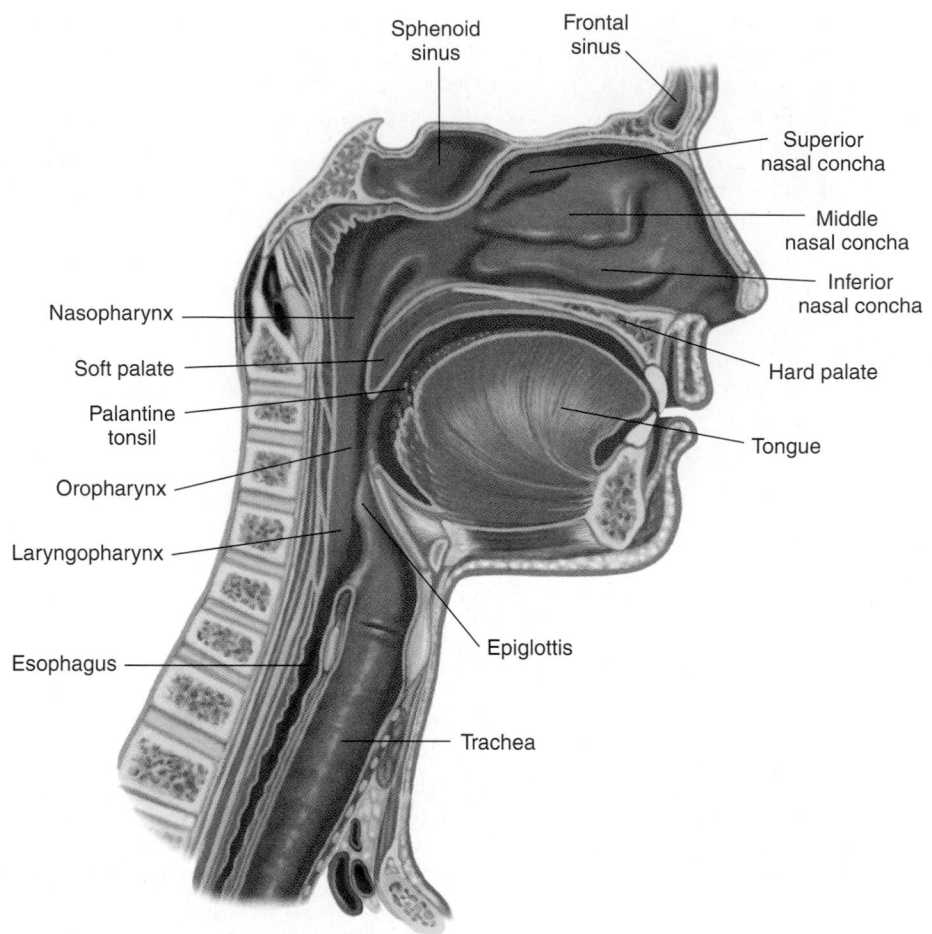

FIG 36-6 Structures of the nose and throat.

The transparency of the cornea allows light into the eye. The conjunctiva protects the cornea from dust and debris. Blinking, which normally occurs 12 to 20 times per minute, helps to protect the cornea against microscopic injury.

Choroid

In the middle layer of the eyeball, the vascular choroid supplies blood to the entire eye. The colored iris surrounding the pupil expands and contracts to modify the quantity of light entering the pupil. When light is low, the pupil dilates (or the iris expands), appearing bigger to allow more light into the eye. If a bright light is then turned on, the iris expands causing the pupil to constrict, limiting the light entering the eye. The ciliary body produces aqueous humor and changes the shape of the lens to accommodate near and far sight. For near vision, the ciliary muscles contract, causing increased rounding of the lens; for far vision, the ciliary muscles expand, causing flattening of the lens. This process of adjusting the thickness of the lens to see near and far

objects is called **accommodation**. The suspensory ligaments function to attach the ciliary body to the lens and keep the lens in place.

Retina

The innermost tunic of the eye, the retina, is responsible for the reception of visual impulses through the lens and transmission of these impulses to the brain. The retina has two layers with individual functions. The thin, outer layer contains pigment that protects the choroid and sclera from light at the back of the eye. The thick, inner layer of the retina contains rods and cones. Rods detect the presence of light. They function in dim light and produce images that are black and white only. Cones function in bright light and detect color. A deficiency of cones results in **color deficiency**, a genetic or acquired inability to distinguish colors. (See *Color deficiency*.) As light waves from the anterior portion of the eye hit the retina, they stimulate the rods and cones. The visual information from the rods and cones is directed to the optic nerve fibers located on the inner surface of the thick inner layer of the retina. The optic nerve fibers transmit visual information via ganglion neurons, which converge at the optic disc. The optic disc contains no rods or cones and is commonly called the *blind spot*. The optic nerve gathers visual stimuli from the ganglion neurons and then transmits the visual information to the brain for interpretation.

Other Structures

Aqueous humor in the anterior chamber provides nourishment for the lens and cornea. Vitreous humor in the posterior cavity gives shape to the eye. The aqueous humor, vitreous humor, and lens are all refractory structures; they bend light rays to focus them sharply onto the retina. Lacrimal glands keep the eye moist by producing tears that bathe and lubricate the eye. The anterior mucous membrane, the conjunctiva, produces a clear, watery mucus that allows the eyelid to slide over the eye without scraping when a person blinks. **Corneal abrasion**, a scrape to the anterior surface of the eye, can occur if the conjunctiva did not produce adequate amounts of mucus or if an object, such as a hairbrush, came in contact with the cornea.

Ears

The structures in the three major sections of the ear function together to protect internal structures and provide hearing.

External Ear

The auricle of the external ear collects sound waves traveling through the air and channels them into the external auditory canal. Ceruminous glands that line the canal secrete **cerumen**, a yellow or brown waxy substance that traps tiny foreign particles and prevents them from entering the deeper structures.

Middle Ear

In the middle ear, the tympanic membrane vibrates when sound waves hit it. Vibration of the tympanic membrane causes movement of the ossicles. Sound, in the form of vibration, is transmitted from the tympanic membrane to the malleus, then incus, then stapes and then to the cochlea of the inner ear.

Inner Ear

The cochlea receives vibration from the stapes through the oval window. Vibration from the stapes causes a disturbance of the perilymph, which disturbs the hair cells on the organ of Corti. The hair cells transmit impulses to the auditory nerve, where they are interpreted as sound.

Because the eustachian tube connects the middle ear to the pharynx, it equalizes pressure on the outer and inner surfaces of the tympanic membrane. It allows air pressure in the middle ear to equalize with air pressure in the mouth and, therefore, outside of the body. (See *Under pressure*.)

The inner ear also functions to provide **equilibrium**, which is the sense of balance. *Static equilibrium* is feeling a sense of balance when at rest; *dynamic equilibrium* refers to the sense of balance when in motion. The vestibular system controls both forms of equilibrium. Endolymph, the pale, transparent fluid within the membranous labyrinth, responds to changes in body position based on gravity. The vestibulocochlear nerve transmits this information to the brain and the brain interprets the body's position in space.

Mouth

The mouth contains the teeth, gums, and tongue. The teeth are used for chewing food, or *mastication*. The anterior teeth, the incisors, tear food, and the posterior teeth, the molars, grind food. The gums anchor the teeth in place. Gustation,

---

Color deficiency

Color deficiency, formerly called *color blindness,* is the inability to distinguish colors. This disorder is a genetic or acquired abnormality. Complete color deficiency, also called *achromatopsia,* is rare. Patients with achromatopsia may have no cones or malformed cones in the retina. The most common deficiency, called *Daltonism* after chemist John Dalton, is the inability to distinguish red from green. Daltonism is caused by a recessive sex-linked genetic trait. Mothers pass the deficiency on to daughters and sons; however, only sons will have the deficiency. Approximately 8% of males have some degree of Daltonism.

A patient may also acquire color deficiency as a result of damage to the retina, optic nerve, or higher brain areas. This type of acquired color deficiency can affect the perception of one or more colors. Deficiencies in the ability to distinguish one color are:

- *protanopia*—the inability to see red
- *deuteranopia*—the inability to see green
- *tritanopia*—the inability to see blue.

Under pressure

When pressure changes suddenly, such as in an airplane, pressure can be equalized by deliberate swallowing. Many people chew gum because it causes jaw movement and simulates swallowing.

The medical assistant can advise patients who are planning to travel by airplane to bring chewing gum, especially for children, because the anatomy of the head and eustachian tubes can cause pain when external pressure changes. Babies can be bottle or breastfed on an airplane to equalize pressure and prevent pain in the ears.

the sense of taste, is a function of the tongue. The tongue contains papillae, or taste buds, which detect the flavors of sweet, salty, sour, and bitter. The muscular nature of the tongue also aids in swallowing food after chewing. (For more information on the digestive processes associated with the teeth, gums, and tongue, see Chapter 30, "Gastroenterology," page 537.)

Nose and Throat

Hairs just inside of the nostrils of the nose block the entrance of dust and small insects into the nasal cavity. The nasal cavity filters, moistens, and warms inspired air to prepare the air for entrance to the lungs. Olfactory neurons function as receptors for the sense of smell, or *olfaction*. Because the receptors are located higher in the nasal passage than air is normally inhaled, weak scents must be inhaled deeply for identification. The sinuses, located behind and around the nose, drain secretions from the nasal cavity and equalize pressure inside the head to match the surrounding air pressure. **Sinusitis**, inflamed and infected sinuses, can occur from allergies, flu viruses, or the common cold.

After air is inspired, filtered, moistened, and warmed, it enters the pharynx. The pharynx serves as a passageway for air, food, and liquids. The adenoids in the nasopharynx produce white blood cells to fight infection in the throat and will grow in size if the throat is infected. The lower sections of the pharynx, the oropharynx and the laryngopharynx, are muscular and push food down into the esophagus when a food bolus is pushed backward by the tongue during swallowing. The palatine tonsils protect the opening to the respiratory tract from microscopic organisms that may cause infection.

Medical Terminology Related to the Eyes, Ears, Mouth, Nose, and Throat

Disorders of the eyes, ears, mouth, nose, and throat are among the most common problems that lead people to seek medical care. Whether they work in family practice offices, in pediatrics, in urgent care centers, in ophthalmology offices, with audiologists, or in plastic surgery centers, medical assistants play an important role in the provision of health care to these patients. To be effective in their role, medical assistants must become well versed in the language and vocabulary that pertain to the eyes, ears, nose, and throat. The following tables list common medical terminology related to the eyes, ears, nose, and throat.

Table 36.1 | Word Elements

This table contains combining forms, prefixes, and suffixes related to the eyes, ears, mouth, nose, and throat, along with examples of terms that use the word element, a pronunciation guide, and a definition for each.

Word Element	Meaning	Example	Meaning
Combining Forms			
acous/o	hearing	**acoustic** (ă-KOOS-tĭk)	Pertaining to hearing
audi/o	hearing	**audiometry** (aw-dē-ŎM-ĕ-trē)	Measurement of hearing
blephar/o	eyelid	**blepharitis** (blĕf-ă-RĪ-tĭs)	Infection and inflammation of the eyelid
corne/o	cornea	**corneous** (KOR-nē-ŭs)	Pertaining to the cornea
dipl/o	double	**diplopia** (dĭp-LŌ-pē-ă)	Two images of an object seen at the same time
irid/o	iris	**iridesis** (ī-RĬD-ĕ-sĭs)	Surgical repositioning of the pupil by bringing a portion of the iris through an incision in the cornea
kerat/o	cornea (or hard substance)	**keratocele** (kĕr-ĂT-ō-sēl)	Herniation of the cornea
myring/o	tympanic membrane	**myringoplasty** (mĭr-ĬN-gō-plăs-tē)	Surgical repair of the tympanic membrane
nas/o	nose	**nasopharyngeal** (nă-zō-făr-ĬN-jē-ăl)	Pertaining to the nose and pharynx
ocul/o	eye	**oculomycosis** (ŏk-ū-lō-mī-KŌ-sĭs)	Any disease of the eye caused by fungus

Table 36.1 | Word Elements—cont'd

Word Element	Meaning	Example	Meaning
ophthalm/o	eye	ophthalmalgia (ŏf-thăl-MĂL-jē-ă)	Pain in the eye
or/o	mouth	orofacial (or-ō-FĀ-shē-ăl)	Concerning the mouth and face
ot/o	ear	otorrhea (ō-tō-RĒ-ă)	Flow or discharge from the ear
phac/o	lens	phacomalacia (făk-ō-mă-LĀ-shē-ă)	Softening of the lens, usually as a result of a cataract
pharyng/o	pharynx	pharyngoparalysis (făr-ĭn-gō-păr-ĂL-ĭ-sĭs)	Paralysis of the muscles of the pharynx
presby/o	old age	presbyopia (prĕz-bē-Ō-pē-ă)	Age-related loss of lens accommodation
retin/o	retina	retinopathy (rĕt-ĭ-NŎP-ă-thē)	Any disorder of the retina
rhin/o	nose	rhinoplasty (RĪ-nō-plăs-tē)	Plastic surgery of the nose
scler/o	sclera, hardening	sclerectasia (sklĕ-rĕk-TĀ-zē-ă)	Protrusion of the sclera
stomat/o	mouth	stomatosis (stō-mă-TŌ-sĭs)	Any disease of the mouth
tympan/o	tympanic membrane	tympanosclerosis (tĭm-păn-ō-sklĕ-RŌ-sĭs)	Hardening of the tympanic membrane
Prefixes			
diplo-	double, twin	diplopia (dĭp-LŌ-pē-ă)	Double vision
ex-	out, away from	exophthalmia (ĕks-ŏf-THĂL-mē-ă)	Abnormal protrusion of the eyeball
hyper-	excessive	hyperacusis (hī-pĕr-ă-KŪ-sĭs)	Abnormal sensitivity to sound
Suffixes			
-opia	vision	myopia (mī-Ō-pē-ă)	Nearsightedness
-plegia	paralysis, stroke	ophthalmoplegia (ŏf-thăl-mō-PLĒ-jē-ă)	Paralysis of ocular muscles
-ptosis	prolapse downward	blepharoptosis (blĕf-ă-rō-TŌ-sĭs)	Drooping or prolapse of the eyelid
-scope	instrument for viewing	ophthalmoscope (ŏf-THĂL-mō-skōp)	Instrument used for the examination of the interior of the eye
-tropia	turning	exotropia (ĕks-ō-TRŌ-pē-ă)	Abnormal outward turning of one or both eyes

Table 36.2 | Pathologic Terms

This table lists some of the most common pathologic terms related to the eyes, ears, mouth, nose, and throat with a brief definition for each.

Term	Definition
anacusis ăn-ă-KŪ-sĭs	Total deafness
Chalazion kă-LĀ-zē-ŏn	Benign hard tumor of the eyelid
retinal detachment RĔT-ĭ-năl	Separation of the inner visual layer of the retina from the outer pigment layer

Continued

Table 36.2 | **Pathologic Terms—cont'd**

Term	Definition
epistaxis ĕp-ĭ-STĂK-sĭs	Nosebleed
gingivitis jĭn-jĭ-VĪ-tĭs	Inflammation, swelling, and redness of the gums
glossoplegia glŏs-ō-PLĒ-jē-ă	Paralysis of the tongue due to injury of 12th cranial nerve (commonly from a stroke)
hordeolum hor-DĒ-ō-lŭm	Localized swelling of one or more glands of the eyelid; also called *stye*
nyctalopia nĭk-tă-LŌ-pē-ă	Inability to see in low light or at night
nystagmus nĭs-TĂG-mŭs	Involuntary eye movement that may be back and forth or circular
otosclerosis ō-tō-sklē-RŌ-sĭs	Hardening of the oval window causing progressive deafness
pharyngitis făr-ĭn-JĪ-tĭs	Inflammation of the mucous membranes and lymphoid tissues of the pharynx

Table 36.3 | **Abbreviations**

In ophthalmology and otolaryngology, as with other areas of health care, abbreviations are commonly used. Abbreviations such as the ones listed below save time and effort in documentation and written communications.

Abbreviation	Term	Abbreviation	Term
Ophthalmology		*Otolaryngology*	
ARMD	age-related macular degeneration	**AC**	air conduction
CK	conductive keratoplasty	***AD**	right ear
EOM	extraocular movement	***AS**	left ear
IOL	intraocular lens	***AU**	both ears
IOP	intraocular pressure	**BC**	bone conduction
LASIK	laser-assisted keratomileusis (surgical correction to the lens)	**BOM**	bilateral otitis media
		EAC	external auditory canal
LTK	laser thermal keratoplasty	**ENT**	ears, nose, and throat
***OD**	right eye	**HEENT**	head, eyes, ears, nose, and throat
***OS**	left eye	**NIHL**	noise-induced hearing loss
***OU**	both eyes together	**PND**	post nasal drip (or drainage)
PERRLA	pupils equal, round, and reactive to light and accommodation	**PE tube**	pressure-equalizing tube (placed in the eardrum)
RK	radial keratotomy	**SOM**	serous otitis media
ROP	retinopathy of prematurity	**T&A**	tonsillectomy and adenoidectomy
RP	retinitis pigmentosa	**TM**	tympanic membrane
VA	visual acuity	**TMJ**	temporomandibular joint
VF	visual field		

* The Joint Commission has determined that these abbreviations create confusion and error in charting and providing care. Although the medical assistant should refrain from using these abbreviations, she must know their meanings in order to correctly interpret medical records.

Common Diseases and Disorders of the Eyes, Ears, Mouth, Nose, and Throat

There are many diseases and disorders that involve the eyes, ears, mouth, nose, and throat. Some of the most common include errors of refraction, bacterial infection, hearing deficits, and structural abnormalities of the nose and throat that cause snoring or obstructed breathing.

Eyes

Common disorders of the eyes include astigmatism, blepharitis, conjunctivitis, exophthalmos, myopia, hyperopia, presbyopia, photophobia, cataracts, glaucoma, and macular degeneration.

Astigmatism
ICD-9-CM code: 367.20

In **astigmatism**, the cornea or lens has a defective curvature so that light rays diffuse over a large area on the retina. This diffusion causes the light coming into the eye to be focused on more than one point on the retina. The patient will not see a sharply focused image and may see more than one image. The exact cause of astigmatism is unknown and may be hereditary. Diagnosis is determined using an astigmatometer, a device that measures the degree of astigmatism. Treatment involves corrective lens surgery if the degree of astigmatism is limited. Severe defects to the cornea or lens can be treated with corrective lenses only, either glasses or contacts.

Blepharitis
ICD-9-CM code: 373.0

Blepharitis is an inflammation of the hair follicles and glands along the edges of the eyelids. This inflammation may develop from bacteria and excess secretions on the eyelid hair follicles. Blepharitis may also develop from pediculosis (infestation with lice) of the eyebrows and lashes. Symptoms include itching and burning sensations, constant rubbing and itching of the eyes, red-rimmed eyelid margins, greasy scales, and sticky, crusted eyelids. Ulcerated lid margins, loss of lashes, and presence of lice eggs with pediculosis may be seen. Diagnosis is determined by visual inspection. Treatment includes warm saline compresses and antibiotic ointments applied to the lid margins.

Conjunctivitis
ICD-9-CM code: Acute 372.0; Chronic 372.1

Conjunctivitis, also called *pinkeye*, is a viral or bacterial inflammation of the conjunctiva, the mucous membrane of the anterior eye. Conjunctivitis is usually caused by bacteria (*Streptococcus* or *Staphylococcus*) or a virus (herpes simplex). Symptoms include redness and a "bloodshot" appearance in the eyes, pain, swelling, and, sometimes, a yellow discharge from the eyes. Diagnosis is determined by visual inspection. Treatment includes antibiotic eyedrops and proper hand washing. (See *Hands off the eye!*)

Diabetic Retinopathy
ICD-9-CM code: 362.01

Diabetes, when poorly controlled, can cause progressive damage to the retina by prolonged dilation of blood vessels. The chronic dilation of the retinal blood vessels can cause hemorrhage and macular edema. As the dilated blood vessels leak, they form exudates of dried fluid deposits that float on the retina and can cause blindness. Nearly all patients who have had diabetes for 15 years or longer have some retinal damage. Damage to the retina is irreversible, but strict control of diabetes prevents further damage and preserves vision. Regular ophthalmological screening is recommended for patients with diabetes to detect retinopathy before irreversible damage occurs. (See Figure 36-7.)

Hypertensive Retinopathy
ICD-9-CM code: 362.11

The retina can be damaged by chronic hypertension in which increased blood pressure pushes more blood into the vessels of the retina. The chronic dilation of the retinal blood vessels causes the same damage as seen in diabetic retinopathy. Increased blood volume and pressure cause leakage of fluid and cellular debris from blood vessels into the retina, which then dries, forming deposits on the retina. Conditions that lead to hypertension include toxemia of pregnancy, glomerulonephritis, and coronary artery disease. Treatment for hypertension will prevent further damage to the retina but, as with diabetic retinopathy, the damage is irreversible. Regular ophthalmological screening is recommended to detect damage; monitoring of blood pressure and adjusting antihypertensive medication to maintain healthy blood pressure will prevent further damage. (See Figure 36-8.)

Patient Education

Hands Off the Eye!
Conjunctivitis is commonly spread from one eye to the other when the patient rubs the affected eye to try to ease itching. The medical assistant should instruct the patient with conjunctivitis to avoid touching the affected eye and, if he does, to wash his hands immediately to prevent the spread of infection to the unaffected eye.

The medical assistant should also explain that conjunctivitis is extremely contagious. To prevent the spread of conjunctivitis to others, the patient should not share bath towels, face cloths, pillowcases, or sunglasses with others.

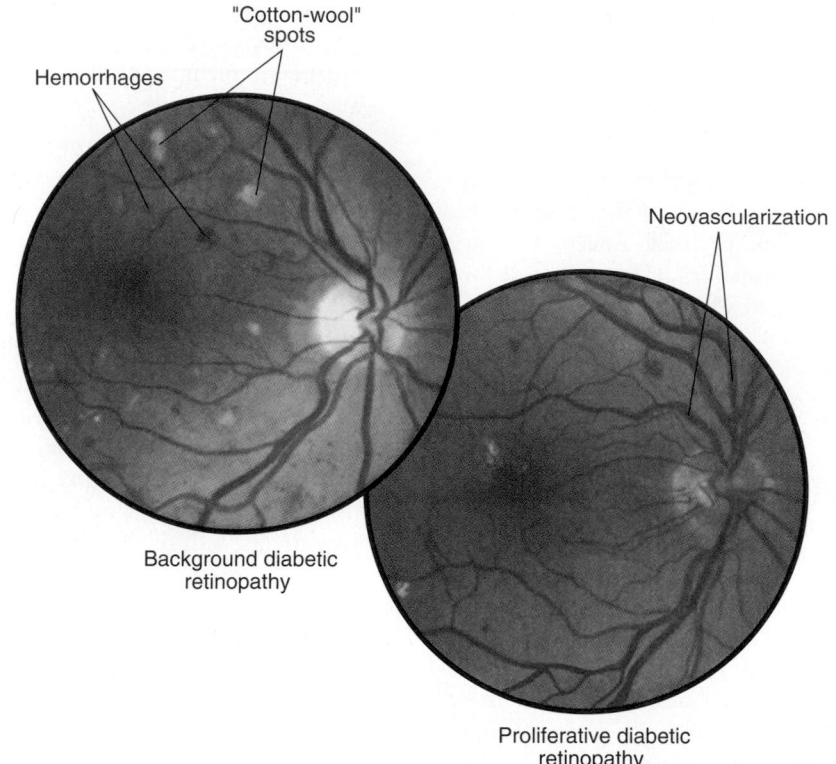

FIG 36-7 Diabetic retinopathy.

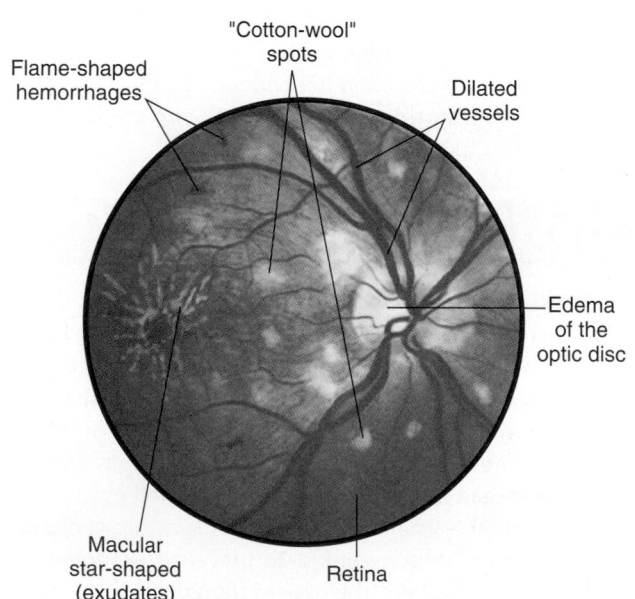

FIG 36-8 Retinal changes due to hypertension.

Exophthalmos
ICD-9-CM code: 376.30

Exophthalmos is a protrusion of one or both eyeballs. Possible causes include a hyperactive thyroid, a tumor, orbital cellulites, leukemia, an aneurysm, or trauma. Symptoms include protrusion of the eyeball and other symptoms, depending on the cause, such as tachycardia and increased systolic blood pressure (hyperthyroidism); weight loss, fatigue, and, possibly, facial deformity (tumor); inflammation and erythema (orbital cellulites); decreased white blood cell count (leukemia); and intracranial bleeding (aneurysm and trauma). Diagnosis is determined by visual inspection. Treatment is directed at the cause of exophthalmia, such as thyroid hormone rebalancing, tumor resection, antibiotics for orbital cellulites, chemotherapy for leukemia, surgical repair for aneurysm, and reconstruction in the case of trauma.

Myopia
ICD-9-CM code: 367.1

Myopia, also called *nearsightedness,* is an error of refraction that causes light rays to focus in front of the retina. This refraction error limits clear vision to only a short distance. The main cause of myopia is a misshapen eyeball. Symptoms are blurred vision when the patient is looking at objects beyond immediate surroundings. Errors of refraction that are related to the shape of the eyeball are generally hereditary.

Diagnosis is established using a vision test. Treatment includes a negative, or concave, lens of the proper strength to counter the effect of the defect and cause sharp focus at far distances. Radial keratotomy, a surgical procedure to correct the shape of the lens, will correct the problem.

Hyperopia
ICD-9-CM code: 367.0

Hyperopia, also called *farsightedness,* is a defect in vision in which parallel light rays come into focus behind the retina. This refraction error limits clear vision to objects at a long distance. Symptoms include ocular fatigue and poor vision. Errors of refraction that are related to the shape of the eyeball are generally hereditary. Diagnosis is established using a vision test. Treatment includes a positive, or convex, lens of the proper strength to counter the effect of the defect or radial keratotomy to correct the shape of the lens. (See Figure 36-9.)

Presbyopia
ICD-9-CM code: 367.4

Presbyopia is permanent loss of accommodation of the crystalline lens of the eye and usually occurs in people in their mid-40s. This disorder causes an inability to maintain focus on objects held near to the eye. Symptoms include an inability to read small print without straining and the use of bright light. As the illness advances, all normal-sized print is out of focus at a normal reading distance. Diagnosis is established using a vision test and considering age. Treatment is usually glasses or contact lens for reading.

Photophobia
ICD-9-CM code: 368.13

Photophobia is an unusual intolerance to light that occurs in patients suffering from measles, mumps, rubella, meningitis,

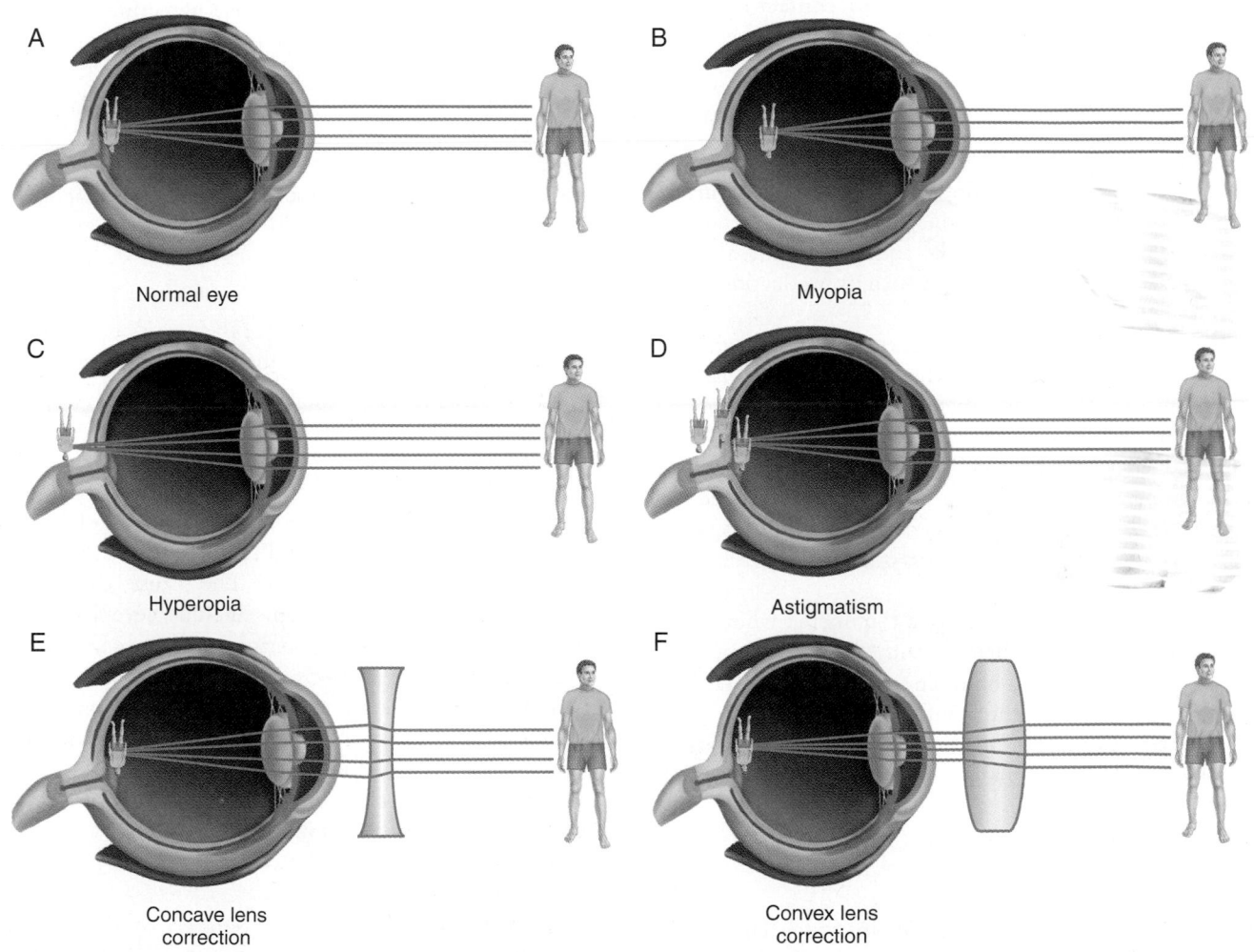

FIG 36-9 Eyeball shape affects where the image is projected. (A) Normal—on the retina. (B) Myopia—in front of the retina. (C) Hyperopia—behind the retina. (D) Astigmatism—multiple images on the retina. (E) Concave lens correction for myopia. (F) Convex lens correction for hyperopia.

or eye inflammation. The major symptom is sensitivity to light. Diagnosis is determined by visual inspection and patient history. Treatment is directed at the cause of photophobia (specific infectious agent).

Cataracts
ICD-9-CM code: 366- (use 4th and 5th digit)

Cataracts are opacities of the lens of the eye and usually occur with age, trauma, endocrine or metabolic disease, or intraocular disease. Cataracts are the leading cause of blindness in adults worldwide. After the age of 65, 90% of adults have some cataract formation. Symptoms include gradual blurring, loss of **visual acuity** (sharpness of vision at varying distances), and a milky-white pupil. People with cataracts complain of seeing halos around lights and being blinded at night by oncoming automobile headlights. Diagnosis is determined by visual examination (in advanced cases) and a vision test. Treatment is surgical removal of the lens. Wearing sunglasses, contact lenses, or glasses can improve vision; however, these are not curative measures.

Glaucoma
ICD-9-CM code: 365- (use 4th and 5th digit)

Glaucoma is an increased intraocular pressure resulting in atrophy of the optic nerve, which can lead to blindness. Glaucoma may be caused by the aqueous humor draining from the eye too slowly to keep up with its production in the anterior chamber.

There are two types of glaucoma: acute (narrow-angle) and chronic (open-angle). Because the progression of narrow-angle glaucoma is rapid, diagnosis can be determined quickly; the disease will cause extreme ocular pain, blurred vision, redness of the eye, and dilation of the pupil. Nausea and vomiting can accompany eye symptoms and blindness can occur in 2 to 5 days. Open-angle glaucoma may produce no symptoms except the gradual loss of peripheral vision over a period of several years.

Diagnosis is determined using a tonometer, which takes measurements of intraocular pressure (IOP). The normal IOP range for adults and children is 14 to 16 mm Hg. An IOP of 22 mm Hg or higher confirms the diagnosis of glaucoma. Treatment includes medication with miotics (eserine and pilocarpine), timolol maleate, intravenous mannitol, and parenteral acetazolamide.

Macular Degeneration
ICD-9-CM code: 362.50

Macular degeneration is a disorder in which changes in the pigmented cells of the retina and macula lead to progressive loss of fine vision. The maculae are the most sensitive cells of the retina and are responsible for central vision. Macular degeneration is incurable and one of the leading causes of blindness in people over 55 years of age. Risk factors, besides age, include cigarette smoking, family history, cardiovascular disease, elevated blood cholesterol levels, light eye color, and excessive sun exposure.

Macular degeneration can occur from inflammation and infection or injury. However, most macular degeneration is related to age, referred to as *age-related macular degeneration (ARMD)*. There are two types of ARMD: wet and dry. Dry ARMD is the more common type and accounts for 90% of cases of ARMD. Symptoms include small yellow deposits (drusen) that form under the macula and interfere with central vision. The drusen are dried retinal pigment cells, which is why this type is called *dry ARMD*. Dry ARMD causes some loss of vision but rarely leads to total blindness. Wet ARMD affects 10% of patients and is much more severe. In this type, new blood vessels form under the macula, which is why the alternative name for this type is *neovascular ARMD*. Blood and vitreous fluids can leak from these cells, destroying central vision cells and leading to permanent blindness. Diagnosis of all forms of macular degeneration is established by inspecting the maculae with an **ophthalmoscope** (an instrument used to examine the interior of the eye). Treatment includes laser therapy to delay or prevent blindness.

Ears

Common diseases and disorders of the ears include Ménière disease, **otitis** (inflammation of the ear) externa, otitis media, labyrinthitis, tinnitus, and vertigo.

Ménière Disease
ICD-9-CM code: 386.0

Ménière disease involves recurring episodes of hearing loss, tinnitus, vertigo, and aural fullness, which commonly result in progressive deafness. The cause of Ménière disease is unknown. Symptoms include severe dizziness (vertigo), ringing in the ears (tinnitus), nausea, vomiting, perspiration, and periodic loss of balance. Diagnosis is established by physical examination, which may reveal nystagmus and hearing loss, and patient history, which may reveal a feeling of fullness and pain in the ear. Treatment includes bed rest for acute attacks, antihistamines, sedatives, smoking cessation, low-salt diet, and, possibly, diuretics.

Otitis Externa
ICD-9-CM code: 380.10

Otitis externa, also called *swimmer's ear,* is an infection or inflammation of the external auditory canal. Contact allergy, acute bacterial infection, or fungi can cause otitis externa. Children are most commonly affected. Symptoms include pain and temporary hearing loss. Diagnosis is established using physical examination, which reveals a red, inflamed, tender outer ear as well as narrowing of tissues in the ear canal due to swelling. Treatment includes antibiotic ear drops, pain medication, and thorough ear cleaning. (See *Handling swimmer's ear.*)

Patient Education

Handling Swimmer's Ear

Because otitis externa (swimmer's ear) is common in children, the medical assistant can teach patients and parents how to deal with the symptoms as well as prevent the occurrence or recurrence of the condition. The medical assistant should advise patients to:

- use a clean towel to dry the ear canals after swimming while refraining from pushing anything into the ear canal (because doing so can cause irritation or injury)

- place a warm heating pad (not hot) on top of the ear or warm the ear gently with a hair dryer to reduce the pain of an existing infection

- use earplugs while swimming, diving, or waterskiing to prevent recurrence (then remove the earplugs after swimming and dry the ear canals properly).

Otitis Media

ICD-9-CM code: Acute nonsuppurative 381.0; Acute suppurative 382.0

Otitis media is the presence of fluid in the middle ear and is commonly associated with respiratory infections. Otitis media usually occurs from an organism that has caused a sore throat or cold. Small children are most commonly affected because the eustachian tubes are positioned horizontally during growth and development of the head. In addition, small children may not yet have the ability to clear their noses properly. Symptoms include severe pain, fever, and temporary hearing loss. The tympanic membrane may be red and inflamed and can rupture. (See *Tympanic membrane in otitis media.*) Diagnosis is established from visual examination of the tympanic membrane and patient history. Treatment includes nasal decongestants or antibiotics for the inflammation or infection and acetaminophen or ibuprofen for pain.

Labyrinthitis

ICD-9-CM code: 386.30

Labyrinthitis, also called *otitis interna*, is an inflammation of the labyrinth. It is caused by a viral or bacterial infection or head trauma. Symptoms include vertigo, vomiting, and nystagmus. Diagnosis is determined using the patient history of symptoms. Treatment is directed at the cause: antibiotics for infection or treatment of the head trauma.

Tinnitus

ICD-9-CM code: 388.3

Tinnitus is a subjective ringing, buzzing, tinkling, or hissing sound in the ear. Tinnitus may be caused by impacted cerumen,

Tympanic membrane in otitis media

Inspection of the tympanic membrane is used to diagnose otitis media, commonly seen in children. The healthy tympanic membrane is gray and shiny. The infected tympanic membrane is red or pink, possibly with a visible discharge.

Children get otitis media or middle ear infections more commonly than adults because the eustachian tube in a child is parallel to the pharynx. The infection may be caused by a virus but is most commonly caused by *Streptococcus pneumoniae*. Around 12,000,000 cases of otitis media occur every year in the United States.

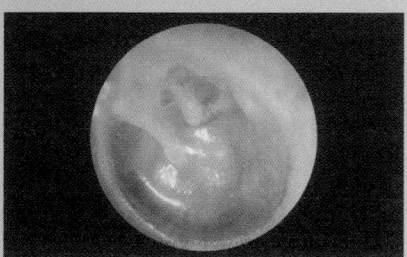

Healthy tympanic membrane

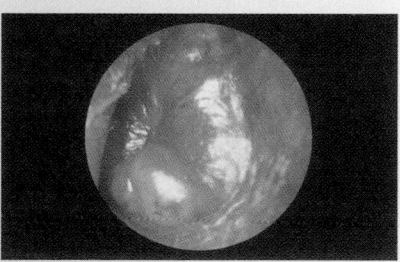

Infected tympanic membrane

myringitis, otitis media, otosclerosis, or drug toxicities (salicylates and quinine). Symptoms include difficulty hearing conversational speech and difficulty sleeping due to the continuous sensation of ringing in the ears. Diagnosis is established taking a detailed patient history. Treatment is directed at the cause of tinnitus, including irrigating impacted cerumen, antibiotics for infection, or cessation of ototoxic medication.

Vertigo
ICD-9-CM code: 386.2

Vertigo is the sensation of moving around in space or having objects move around the person. Vertigo may be caused by middle ear disease, salicylate toxicity, alcohol, streptomycin administration, sunstroke, postural hypotension, or toxemia due to food poisoning. Symptoms include dizziness, sensation of faintness, or inability to maintain normal balance. Diagnosis is established by taking a detailed patient history. Treatment is directed at removing the cause of vertigo and may include medication, cessation of medication, reducing body temperature and administering IV fluids, or eliminating alcohol from the diet. (See *Preventing injury from an inner ear disturbance*.)

Mouth

Common diseases and disorders of the mouth include oral herpes, oral thrush, cleft lip, and cleft palate.

Oral Herpes
ICD-9-CM code: 054.9

Oral herpes, also called a *cold sore*, is a vesicular eruption caused by herpes virus. It is transmitted by contact with infected saliva. The major symptom is lesions inside the mouth. Diagnosis is established by visual inspection and confirmed by wound culture. Treatment includes oral acyclovir to treat the outbreak and recurrences. The medical assistant should instruct the patient to avoid touching lesions, because the virus can spread via contact. The medical assistant can discuss hygiene habits with the patient to prevent spread to family members.

Oral Thrush
ICD-9-CM code: 112.0 (newborn 771.7)

Oral thrush, also called *candidiasis,* is an infection of the skin or mucous membrane with any species of *Candida*, but mainly *Candida albicans*. Oral thrush is caused by a disruption in the composition of normal flora or a change in host defenses. Patients with suppressed immune systems, such as those with human immunodeficiency virus (HIV) or patients being treated with chemotherapy or immunosuppressive drugs, are at higher risk. Neonates are sometimes born with oral thrush because normal flora in the mouth has not yet been established. Symptoms include oral lesions; white patches on the mucosa and tongue; a red, irritated surface of the tongue; and lesions on other parts of the body, including the groin and abdomen, and under pendulous breasts. Diagnosis is established using visual inspection. Treatment includes fluconazole, clotrimazole lozenges, or nystatin oral solution.

Cleft Lip
ICD-9-CM code: 749.10

Cleft lip is a common developmental abnormality that occurs between 4 to 8 weeks of fetal development. Incidence

---

⬛ Patient Education

Preventing Injury from an Inner Ear Disturbance

Various inner ear disturbances can cause dizziness and loss of balance. The medical assistant can advise patients and caregivers on certain measures to prevent injury from dizziness.

Ride the rails

The medical assistant should urge patients and caregivers to use side rails on beds and railings on stairs for added stability. Bathtubs can be equipped with seats, railings, and handheld shower heads for safer bathing. Patients who suffer from severe symptoms of vertigo should not bathe independently if safety is compromised.

Other measures

In addition to using railings, the medical assistant should encourage patients to rise slowly from sitting and avoid rushing to walk or change positions. Sudden movement can exacerbate vertigo.

Also, alcohol consumption disturbs the vestibulocochlear nerve and its ability to transmit information about balance and body position to the brain. It can cause uncoordinated movements and delayed reactions. The medical assistant should advise patients to refrain from drinking alcohol if they experience dizziness or nausea, as in Ménière disease, labyrinthitis, and vertigo, because alcohol will exacerbate the symptoms.

of cleft lip is approximately 1 in 700 births. The cleft, or opening, results from a failure of the maxillary processes to fuse and can be unilateral or bilateral. The length of the opening can range from a small notch to a cleft that extends into the base of the nostril. The infant will have feeding problems because the lips cannot completely close around a nipple to create suction. Treatment with plastic surgery is effective in correcting the defect and appearance.

Cleft Palate
ICD-9-CM code: 749.00
Cleft palate is the failure of the soft and hard palates to fuse in the 7th to 12th week of fetal development. The opening between the oral and nasal cavities greatly increases the risk of aspirating fluid into the lungs. Incidence of cleft palate, as with cleft lip, are 1 in 700. An infant may be born with either disorder or a combination of both. The infant with cleft palate will have feeding difficulty due to a lack of pressure created in the mouth for swallowing. Prior to surgical correction, a special nipple may be used to close the opening to the nasal cavity while feeding the infant. Plastic surgery corrects the defect and appearance. Speech therapy is commonly needed later in life, as is orthodontic care. The risk of a baby being born with either cleft lip or palate increases with the number of affected relatives and the severity of the clefts. Environmental factors that increase risk for both disorders include cigarette smoking, alcohol, phenytoin, and methotrexate.

Nose and Throat
Common diseases and disorders of the nose and throat include rhinitis and tonsillitis.

Rhinitis
ICD-9-CM code: 477 (use 4th digit)
Rhinitis is inflammation of the nasal mucosa. This inflammation can occur seasonally or year-round. Allergic rhinitis is a reaction to airborne allergens. Symptoms include sneezing, profuse watery discharge, itching of the eyes and nose, conjunctivitis, and tearing. Diagnosis is established using visual inspection and patient history. Treatment includes rest, adequate fluids, and a well-balanced diet. Avoidance of allergens is also recommended if possible. Analgesics and antipyretics may be administered for comfort.

Tonsillitis
ICD-9-CM code: 463
Tonsillitis is inflammation and infection of the tonsils. It causes pain upon swallowing. Many infectious agents can cause tonsillitis; however, the most common is *Streptococcus*. Symptoms include intense pain in the throat for a short period of time, fever, and general malaise. Diagnosis is established by patient history and visual inspection, which reveals a red, inflamed throat and, commonly, white pustules. The causative organism is determined by throat culture. Treatment may include a tonsillectomy for chronic infection, antibiotic treatment, bed rest, liquid-to-soft diet, and analgesic throat spray.

Ophthalmology and Otolaryngology Procedures

Ophthalmology is a medical specialty that focuses on the study and treatment of disorders of the eye. Otolaryngology is a medical specialty that focuses on the study and treatment of disorders of the ear, mouth, nose, and throat. Physicians that specialize in these areas of the body include:

- ophthalmologist—medical doctor who diagnoses and treats disorders and diseases of the eye and can perform eye surgery
- optometrist—doctor of optometry who prescribes corrective eyewear and diagnoses and treats disorders and diseases of the eye
- optician—specialist who fills prescriptions for corrective lenses for eyeglasses and contact lenses (not a medical doctor)
- otorhinolaryngologists—medical doctor who diagnoses and treats diseases and disorders of the ear, nose, and throat as well as the mouth as it pertains to the structural needs of eating and breathing (also called an *ENT*).

Family physicians, pediatricians, internists, and school nurses may also evaluate the function of eyes and ears in annual screenings or school examinations. They will refer patients with vision or hearing deficits to a specialist for treatment. The medical assistant working for a specialist or a general practice may be required to assist in the evaluation or treatment of the eyes, ears, mouth, nose, and throat.

Assisting with Ophthalmic Examination
The physician examines the interior of the eye with an ophthalmoscope. The ophthalmoscope is a handheld instrument that shows the condition of the retina, optic nerve, and the blood vessels of the eye. The physician may administer mydriatic drops to dilate the pupil and view it

with the ophthalmoscope. (See *Mydriatics and patient safety and comfort*.) The medical assistant must keep the ophthalmoscope's bulbs and batteries in working order and the instrument must be sanitized with an alcohol wipe.

Assessing the patient's visual acuity and ability to see color begins with manual vision testing. The medical assistant or physician may ask a patient to read a chart to assess the patient's vision. The most common chart used in this type of examination is the Snellen chart. (See *Procedure 36-1: Measuring distance and visual acuity using the Snellen chart*.) She may also measure near visual acuity using a near-vision acuity card, such as the Jaeger card. (See *Procedure 36-2: Measuring near visual acuity*, page 764.) The medical assistant may also test a patient's ability to distinguish color using the Ishihara color vision test. (See *Procedure 36-3: Measuring visual acuity using the Ishihara color vision test*, page 765.) Under the direction of a physician, the medical assistant can perform these screenings independently. If visual deficiencies associated with errors of refraction are noted, the physician will then conduct further testing to prescribe corrective lenses if necessary.

Assisting with Ophthalmic Irrigation and Instillation

The eye can become irritated and inflamed by irritants that get into the conjunctiva or by infection, most commonly caused by bacteria. The medical assistant can irrigate the patient's eye to remove irritants and cleanse the eye of pus formed by the infection process. (See *Procedure 36-4: Irrigating the eye*, page 766.)

The medical assistant can also instill medications into the eye that soothe the eye or kill pathogenic bacteria. (See *Procedure 36-5: Instilling eyedrops*, page 768.) While instilling eyedrops, the medical assistant should teach her patient or caregiver the proper techniques for medication instillation into the eye. (See *Instilling eyedrops*, page 769.)

Assisting with Otic Examination

The physician examines the ears with an **otoscope**, which is a handheld instrument with a light used to examine

(Text continues on page 770)

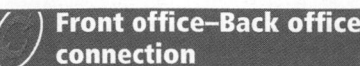

Mydriatics and Patient Safety and Comfort

In the ophthalmologist's office, the physician may dilate the pupils for examination or treatment with a medication called a mydriatic. Mydriatics dilate the pupil and prevent constriction of the pupil when light enters the eye. Because dilating the pupils causes an increased amount of light to enter the eye, the patient's eyes will be sensitive to this added light.

The administrative medical assistant who is making an appointment for an ophthalmic examination or treatment that requires mydriatics should advise the patient to bring sunglasses and explain why. The clinical medical assistant can turn off the lights in the examination room for the patient's comfort.

The patient may not be able to drive himself after administration of the mydriatic. The effects of the mydriatic wear off in a few hours, so the medical assistant should tell the patient not to read or watch TV until the effects have worn off.

PROCEDURE 36-1

Measuring distance and visual acuity using the Snellen chart

Task

Accurately measure visual acuity using a Snellen eye chart. Document the procedure in the patient's medical record.

Conditions

- Snellen eye chart
- Eye occluder
- Floor mark at 20 feet from the eye chart
- Patient's medical record
- Pen

Standards

In the time specified and within the scoring parameters determined by the instructor, the student will accurately measure visual acuity using a Snellen eye chart.

Performance Standards

1. Wash hands.
2. Ensure that the examination room is well lit.
3. Assemble equipment and supplies, including sanitizing the occluder and allowing it to dry completely to ensure that it is not contaminated.

PROCEDURE 36-1—cont'd

4. Introduce yourself and address the patient by name.
5. Explain the procedure to the patient and answer any questions she may have. Tell the patient that she will be asked to read lines of letters, objects, or a rotating "E." Explain to the patient that she should not squint during the examination, because squinting changes the results of the test. Make sure that the patient does not have an opportunity to memorize the chart to ensure that her vision, not her memory, is assessed.
6. Ask the patient if she is wearing contact lenses and observe for eyeglasses. Because the test is a screening test, confirm with the physician if the patient should keep corrective eyewear on during the examination to ensure that the procedure is correctly charted with or without corrective lenses.
7. Ask the patient to stand (or sit if standing is difficult) on the floor mark, 20 feet from the Snellen chart to ensure accurate results.
8. Select the appropriate Snellen chart for the patient. Use an object chart for preschoolers who may not know the letters of the alphabet. Use a rotating "E" chart for adult patients who speak a foreign language, because they may not know the correct English names for the letters. Be sure to explain the procedure through an interpreter or through hand motions, if necessary. Confirm that the patient understands the procedure. (See step 5.)
9. Position the center of the Snellen eye chart at the patient's eye level so that the patient doesn't need to look up or down to see the chart. Stand to the side of the chart during the procedure so you do not obstruct the patient's view of the chart.
10. Ask the patient to cover her left eye with the occluder and to keep her left eye open. Keeping the left eye open makes it harder to squint with the right eye, which would increase visual acuity and change test results. Preschoolers may not know their right and left, so assist them as necessary.

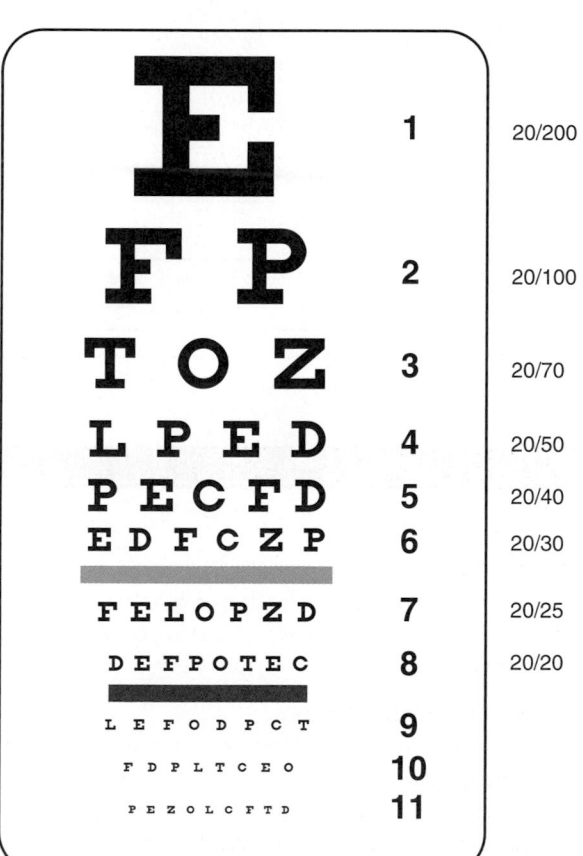

Snellen chart with Letters

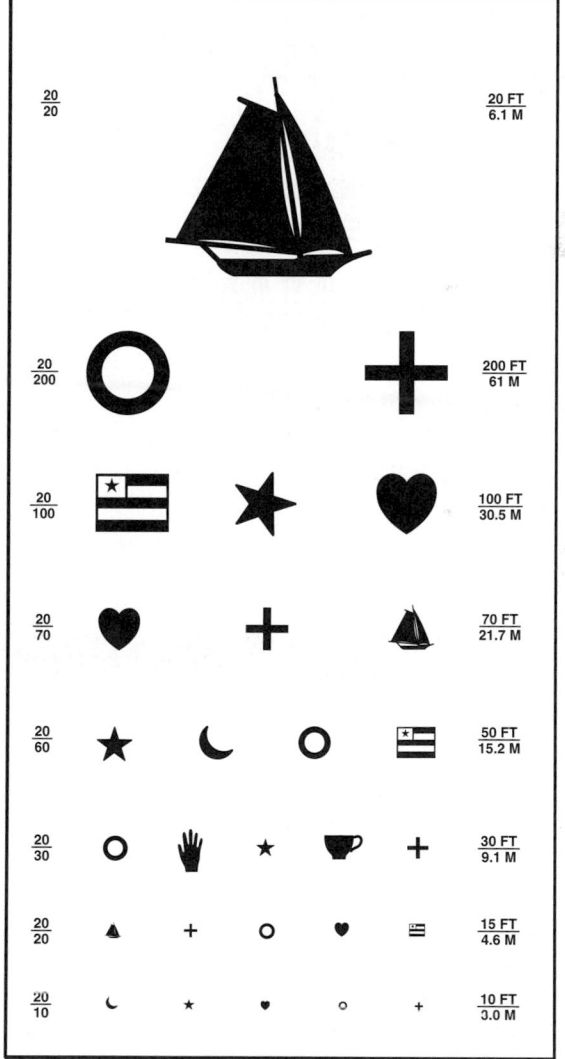

Object Snellen chart

Continued

PROCEDURE 36-1—cont'd

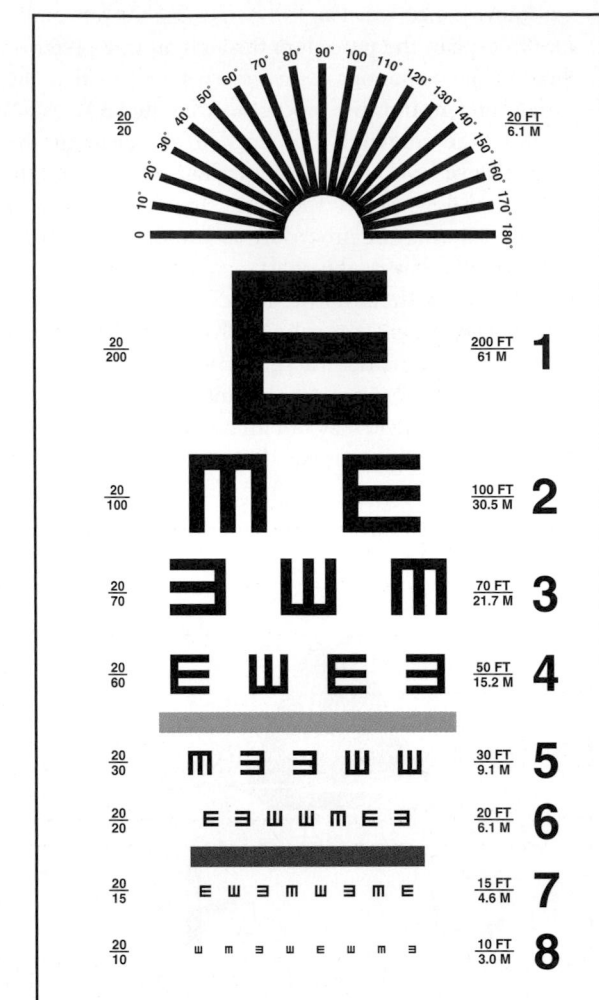

Rotating "E" Snellen chart

11. Measure the visual acuity of the right eye. Always starting with the right eye creates a routine and makes charting consistent, which can reduce errors.

12. Ask the patient to identify each letter, object, or direction of the "E" verbally or with a hand motion (whichever is preferred by the patient) as you point to it. Start at the 20/70 line. Starting at a line that is above the 20/20 line gives the patient an opportunity to become familiar with the test and gain confidence in the procedure.

13. Proceed up or down the chart as necessary.

14. If the patient is able to read the 20/70 line, proceed down the chart asking her to read the 20/50 line, 20/40, 20/30, 20/20, and further if possible.

15. If the patient is unable to read the 20/70 line, proceed up the chart to the 20/100 line. If the patient is unable to read this line, ask them to read the 20/200 line.

16. Chart the results of the right eye. Record the smallest line that the patient can read with one or no errors. If the patient makes two or more errors on a line, the patient may be guessing, which is not a true assessment of vision. (*Note:* Observe the patient for squinting, leaning, tilting the head, or eyes watering. These signs indicate that the patient is having difficulty reading the chart.)

17. Repeat the procedure for the left eye. Ask the patient to place the occluder in front of her right eye. Remind the patient to keep her right eye open.

Date	
02/18/08; 10:00 a.m.	*Snellen test: Right eye 20/30 -1, left eye 20/20 ——————— ————————————————————————————— C. Smith, CMA*

PROCEDURE 36-2

Measuring near visual acuity

Task
Accurately measure near visual acuity using the Jaeger near-vision acuity card. Document the procedure in the patient's medical record.

Conditions
- Jaeger card
- Eye occluder
- 18-inch ruler or tape
- Patient's medical record
- Pen

Standards
In the time specified and within the scoring parameters determined by the instructor, the student will accurately measure near visual acuity.

Performance Standards
1. Make sure the examination room is well lit and wash your hands.
2. Assemble the equipment and supplies. Sanitize the occluder and allow it to dry completely to prevent contamination.

PROCEDURE 36-2—cont'd

3. Introduce yourself and address the patient by name.

4. Explain the procedure to the patient; answer any questions he may have to promote cooperation and understanding.

5. Have the patient sit in a comfortable position.

6. Hand the patient the Jaeger card. Ask him to hold the card 14" to 16" away from his eyes and measure the distance to promote accurate results.

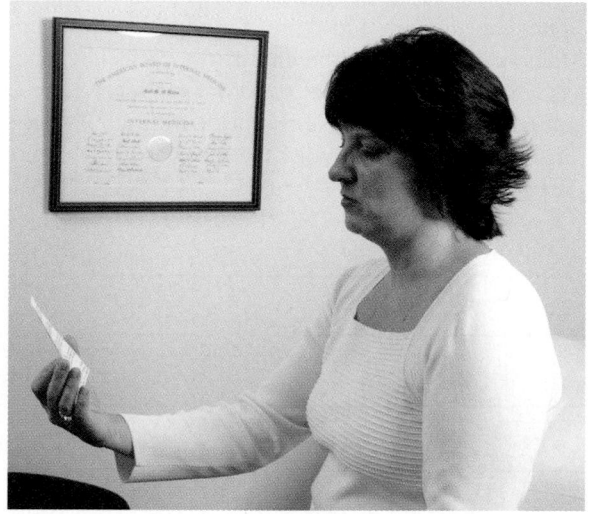

Ask the patient to hold the Jaeger card 14" to 16" away from his eyes.

7. Ask the patient to cover his left eye with the occluder. Instruct him not to close his left eye to prevent squinting.

8. Ask the patient to read the paragraphs on the card out loud. The patient should start reading at the top of the card (largest print) and continue reading until he cannot read the smaller print. Starting with the large print ensures that the patient understands the procedure and will continue to read until he is unable to distinguish the letters.

9. Record the results of the right eye in the medical record.

10. Ask the patient to cover his right eye with the occluder and repeat the test for the left eye.

11. Record the results of the left eye in the medical record.

12. Ask the patient to read the card without the occluder, testing vision in both eyes.

13. Record the results of both eyes in the medical record.

Date	
02/18/08; 10:30 a.m.	*Jaeger card: Right eye - successfully read no. 6 (1.25M)*
	without glasses; left eye - successfully read no. 7 (1.50M)
	without glasses. Both eyes successfully read no. 6 (1.25M)
	without glasses. ------------------------------ C. Smith, CMA

PROCEDURE 36-3

Measuring visual acuity using the Ishihara color vision test

Task

Accurately measure color visual acuity using the Ishihara color vision test. Document the procedure in the patient's medical record.

Conditions

- Ishihara color plate book
- Cotton swab
- Watch with second hand
- Patient's medical record
- Pen

Standards

In the time specified and within the scoring parameters determined by the instructor, the student will accurately measure visual acuity using the Ishihara color vision test.

Performance Standards

1. Wash your hands and ensure that the examination room is well lit with natural light if possible. Natural daylight is most accurate; artificial light may change the appearance of the test plates.

2. Assemble the equipment and supplies.

3. Introduce yourself and address the patient by name.

4. Explain the procedure to the patient to promote accurate results.

5. Use the first plate in the book to explain the procedure to the patient. Tell the patient that he will have 3 seconds to identify numbers verbally or trace a winding path formed by the colored dots on the card. The patient should keep both eyes open during the procedure. The first plate is highly contrasted and is designed so that it can be read correctly by everyone. The medical assistant can ensure that the patient understands the procedure.

Continued

PROCEDURE 36-3—cont'd

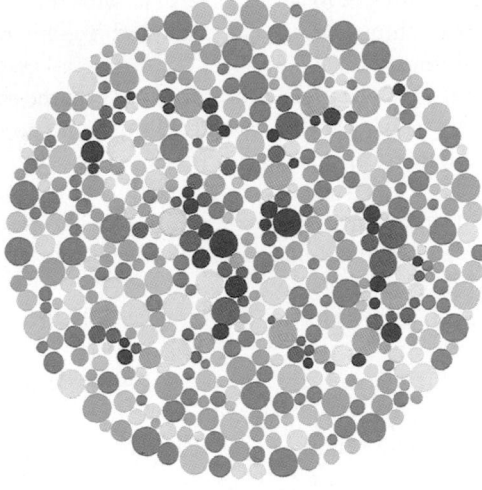

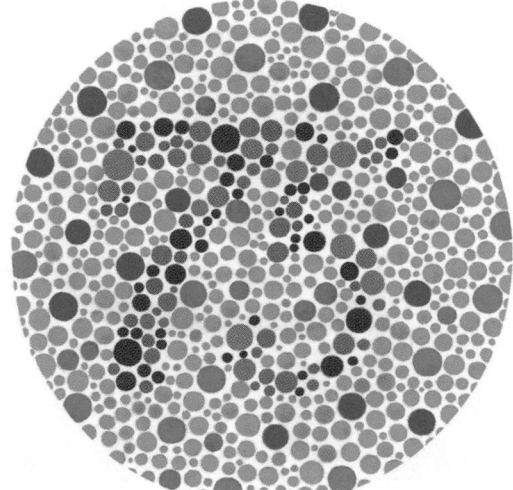

Ishihara color vision test plates

7. Ask the patient to identify the number on the plate or, using a cotton-tipped swab, trace the winding path. Sometimes require the patient to trace the number. Tracing ensures that the number was not memorized and that the patient can truly distinguish the colors.

8. Record the results of each plate on a piece of paper. After all 11 plates have been tested, record the results in the patient's medical record. Writing in the medical record and performing the test simultaneously may cause you to rush and write sloppily. Take your time and record results at the end of the procedure. Indicate the plates that the patient read incorrectly by recording the number of the plate with an X next to it. Alternatively, simply list the numbers of the plates read incorrectly.

Date	
02/19/08; 10:30 a.m.	Ishihara test: Plates 8X, 9X. ---------------- C. Smith, CMA

Date	
02/19/08; 10:30 a.m.	Ishihara test: Pt. unable to identify plates 8 & 9. ------------ --- C. Smith, CMA

Date	
02/19/08; 10:30 a.m.	Ishihara test: vision on all plates normal. - C. Smith, CMA

6. Hold the color plate 30" from the patient at a right angle to the patient's line of sight to ensure that the patient can see the plate.

PROCEDURE 36-4

Irrigating the eye

Task
Irrigate the patient's affected eye to cleanse it of a foreign object, cleanse a discharge, cleanse chemicals, apply antiseptic, or apply heat.

Conditions
- Sterile irrigation solution
- Sterile bulb syringe (rubber)
- Kidney-shaped basin to catch irrigation solution
- Sterile cotton balls
- Sterile gloves
- Biohazard waste container
- Patient's medical record
- Pen

PROCEDURE 36-4—cont'd

Standards

In the time specified and within the scoring parameters determined by the instructor, the student will successfully irrigate the patient's eye.

Performance Standards

1. Wash hands.
2. Assemble equipment and supplies. Use separate equipment if both eyes are to be irrigated to prevent cross-contamination.
3. Introduce yourself and address the patient by name.
4. Explain the procedure to the patient and answer any questions she may have to promote patient understanding and cooperation.
5. Position the patient in the supine position to aid the entrance of the solution into the eye.
6. Check the expiration date on the solution bottle. Expired solution may be harmful to the eye.
7. Check the label for the right medication three times to be sure to use the correct solution for irrigation.
8. Warm the solution to body temperature to ensure patient comfort.
9. Tilt the patient's head toward the affected eye and place a towel on the patient's shoulder to avoid cross-contamination of the affected eye by allowing the solution to flow laterally away from the unaffected eye.
10. Place the basin next to the affected eye as shown.

11. Put on sterile gloves to prevent contamination.
12. Moisten two or three cotton balls with the irrigation solution and clean the eyelids and eyelashes of the affected eye from the inner to the outer canthus to protect the unaffected eye from cross-contamination. Discard the cotton ball after each wipe.

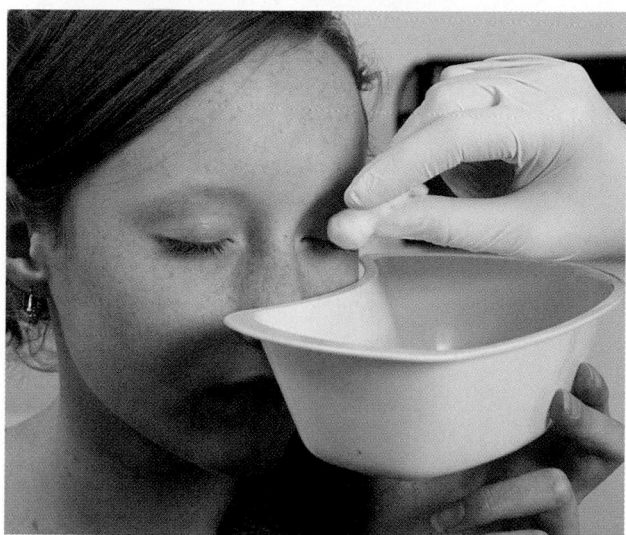

Direct the flow of solution from the inner canthus to the outer canthus to prevent the solution from entering the other eye.

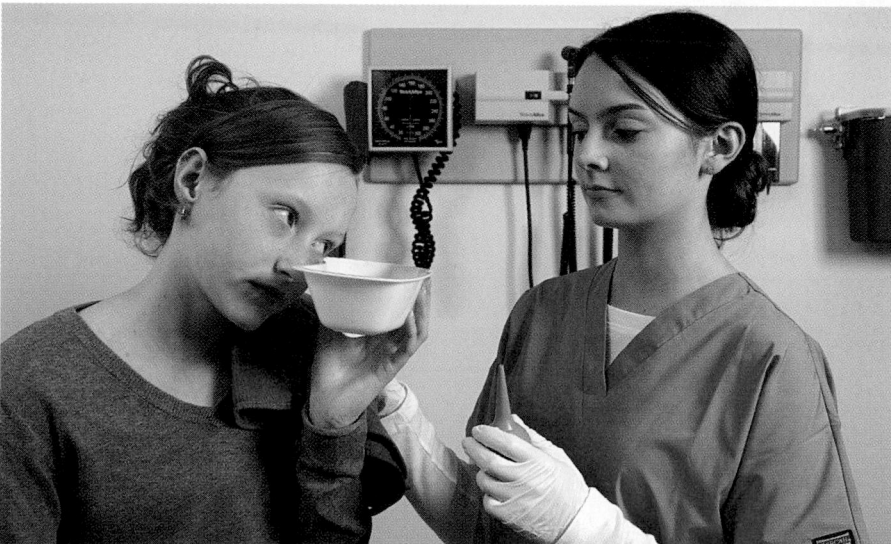

Ask the patient to hold the basin next to her eye and to remain still.

Continued

PROCEDURE 36-4—cont'd

13. Expose the lower conjunctiva by separating the eyelid with your index finger and thumb, as shown, making sure that the flow of irrigation solution is away from the unaffected eye.

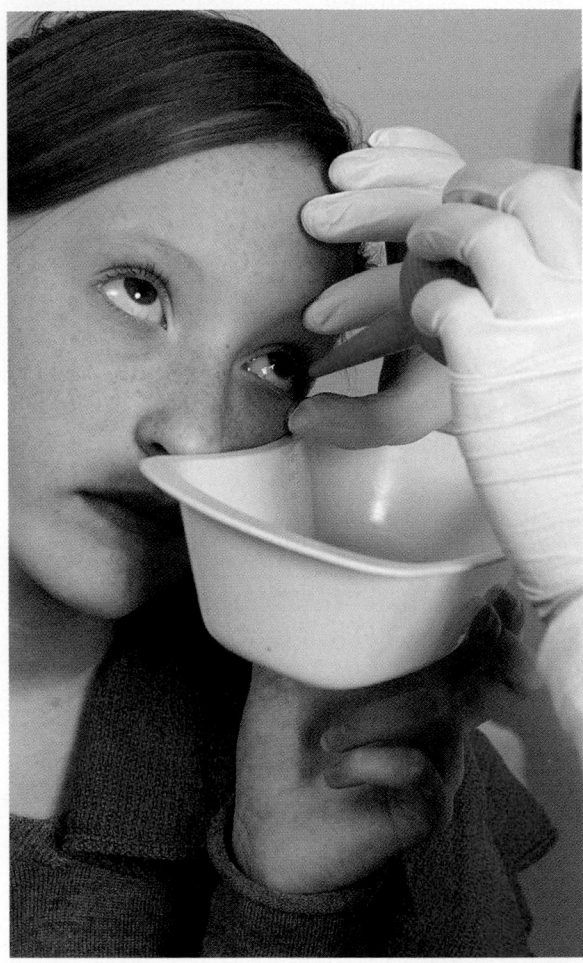

Separate the eyelid with your index finger and thumb.

14. Ask the patient to stare at a fixed spot to decrease the reflex to close the eye. *Note:* You will still need to keep the eye open with your fingers during irrigation. The patient's reflex is to shut the eye.

15. Irrigate the affected eye with sterile solution by resting the bulb on the bridge of the patient's nose. Be careful not to touch the tip of the bulb syringe to any part of the patient's face to avoid contaminating the sterile bulb syringe and solution.

16. Allow the stream to flow from the inner canthus to the outer canthus, as seen below.

17. After irrigation, dry the eyelid and eyelashes with sterile cotton balls to prevent contamination of the eye.

18. Discard supplies in a biohazard container if discharge or exudate is present because bodily fluids are considered biohazard waste.

19. Remove your gloves.

20. Wash your hands and document the procedure.

Date	
02/20/08; 11:15 a.m.	*Left eye irrigation, small amount of particle irritants removed. --- C. Smith, CMA*

21. Repeat the procedure on the other eye if a bilateral procedure is indicated.

PROCEDURE 36-5

Instilling eyedrops

Task
Instill eyedrops to treat eye infections, soothe irritation, anesthetize the eye, or dilate pupils.

Conditions
- Sterile eye dropper
- Sterile ophthalmic medication as ordered by the physician
- Sterile cotton balls
- Sterile gloves
- Biohazard waste container
- Patient's medical record
- Pen

Standards
In the time specified and within the scoring parameters determined by the instructor, the student will successfully instill eyedrops.

PROCEDURE 36-5—cont'd

Performance Standards

1. Wash your hands.
2. Assemble the necessary equipment and supplies.
3. Introduce yourself and address the patient by name.
4. Explain the procedure to the patient and answer any questions that she may have to promote patient cooperation. Tell the patient that the instillation may temporarily blur her vision. If the medication is to dilate the pupil for examination, explain to the patient that the eye will be very sensitive to light.
5. Check the medication label carefully against the physician's orders. Note the name of the medication and the expiration date. Check the label three times to avoid instilling the wrong medication or expired medication that may harm the eye.
6. Position the patient in a sitting or supine position to ensure that all of the medication enters the eye.
7. Ask the patient to stare at a fixed spot up on the ceiling to decrease the reflex to close the eye.
8. Hold the eye open by placing a tissue under the eye and gently pulling down on the skin below the eye to ensure all of the medication enters the eye. Use the patient's forehead as a rest for your hand, as shown.
9. Place the number of drops ordered in the lower conjunctival sac or a thin line of ointment in the lower surface of the eyelid. Be careful not to touch the tip of the eye dropper to any portion of the patient's eye to avoid contaminating the dropper and medication.
10. Ask the patient to close her eye and roll her eyeball to distribute the medication evenly.
11. Document the procedure in the patient's chart.

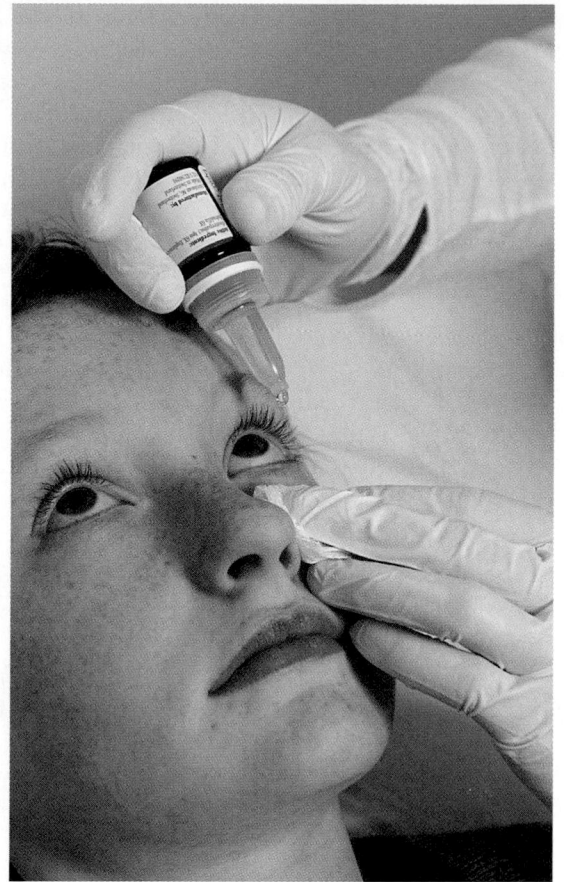

Use the patient's forehead as a rest for your hand.

Date	
02/20/08; 11:30 a.m.	3 drops Alphagan P in left eye. ----------- C. Smith, CMA

📓 Patient Education

Instilling Eyedrops

When the medical assistant instills eyedrops in the medical office she can teach the patient or caregiver how to instill them at home. While administering the drops, the medical assistant should mention these points:

• Wash your hands before and after administering drops.

• Do not touch the tip of the dropper to the eye or any object because it is sterile.

• Avoid contaminating the eyedrops to prevent reinfection.

• Store eyedrops as directed on the label, usually at room temperature in the sealed container.

• Remember that prescription eyedrops are a medication and should be used only by the patient for whom it was prescribed.

• Never share eyedrops because they may be contraindicated for some patients.

the ear. The physician is able to check the appearance of the ear canal and the tympanic membrane, or eardrum. To straighten the canal, the physician will pull the adult's auricle upward and backward and a child's auricle downward and backward (up to age 3). The otoscope uses a speculum that fits into the external ear canal and must be disposable or sanitized for reuse. The medical assistant is responsible for maintaining the otoscope and charging and changing the batteries as necessary. She should follow the manufacturer's guidelines for cleaning and maintenance. (See Figure 36-10.)

Tuning Fork Test

Testing hearing acuity with a tuning fork can detect both conduction defects and nerve impairment. There are two basic tests: the Weber and Rinne tests. The physician may perform these tests or train the medical assistant to do so.

Weber Test

In the Weber test, the medical assistant should hold the tuning fork at the base and strike it against her palm to cause the tuning fork to vibrate. She should then hold the fork on the center of the patient's head. If the patient hears the sound equally in both ears, the test result is normal. If the patient has a conductive hearing loss, the sound will be stronger in the problem ear. A sensorineural hearing loss will cause the sound to be heard faintly or not at all in the affected ear. (See Figure 36-11.)

Rinne test

In the Rinne test, the medical assistant should place the base of the vibrating tuning fork on the patient's mastoid bone. She should then ask the patient to report when he can no longer hear the sound. The medical assistant should then

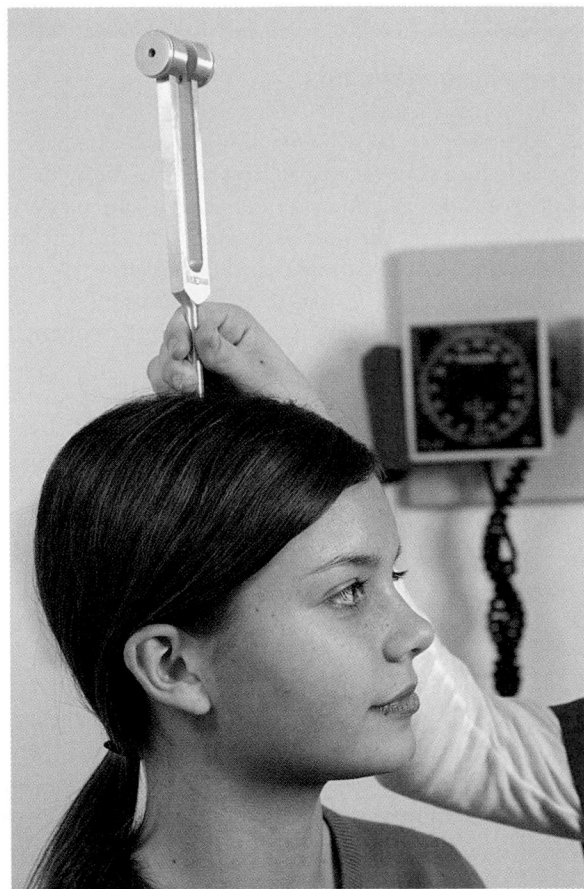

FIG 36-11 Weber test for sensorineural hearing loss.

hold the tuning fork beside the patient's ear (without touching the patient's head) and ask the patient if he can hear it. If the patient hears the tuning fork, the test result is normal, because air conduction hearing should be greater than bone conduction hearing. Conductive hearing loss will cause the patient to hear the sound longer through bone conduction, so when the tuning fork is then placed next to the ear, no sound is heard. If the patient has a sensorineural hearing loss, the sound will be reduced. The patient will hear the sound longer through air conduction than bone conduction but not twice as long. (See Figure 36-12.)

Audiometric Testing

Hearing tests can be administered through the use of an **audiometer**, an instrument used to test a patient's hearing by determining hearing thresholds of pure tones at varying frequencies. The manufacturer's specific guidelines should be followed when administering the test. If hearing deficits are recognized, the patient can be referred to an audiologist for hearing aids or other assistive therapies. (See *Procedure 36-6: Testing hearing using an audiometer.*)

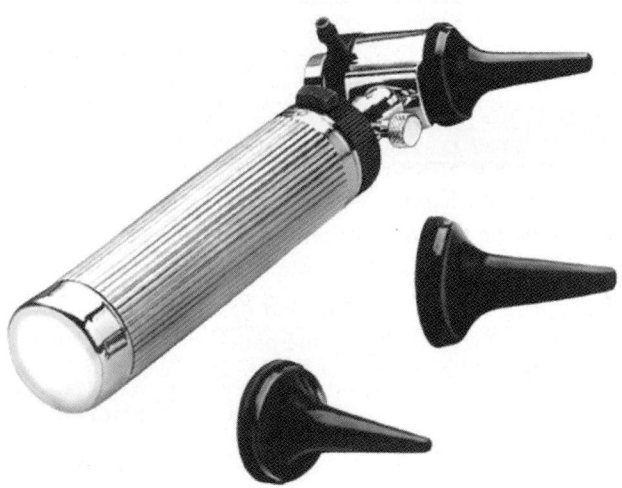

FIG 36-10 Otoscope.

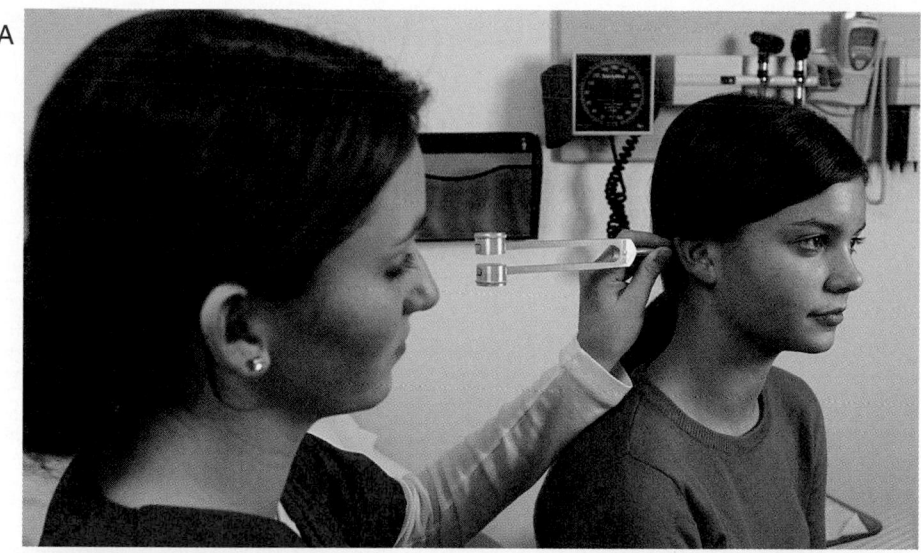

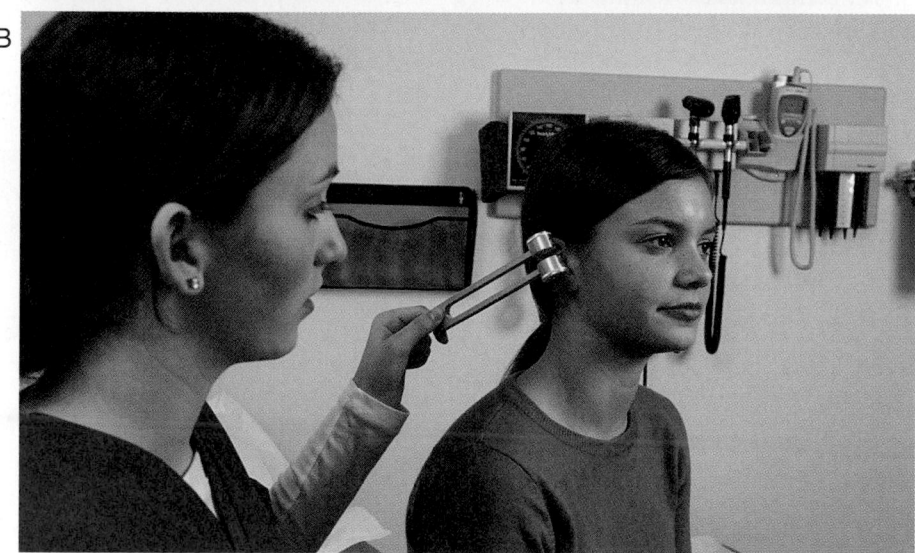

FIG 36-12 Rinne test. (A) On the mastoid bone. (B) Beside the patient's ear.

PROCEDURE 36-6

Testing hearing using an audiometer

Task
Use an audiometer to test a patient's hearing.

Conditions
- Audiometer
- Headphones
- Enclosed area (such as a small room or cubicle)

Standards
In the time specified and within the scoring parameters determined by the instructor, the student will successfully test hearing using an audiometer.

Performance Standards
1. Wash your hands.
2. Assemble the equipment and supplies.
3. Introduce yourself and address the patient by name.
4. Explain the procedure to the patient and establish a signal for the patient to give when she hears the tone (such as holding up a hand or finger on the same side as she hears the tone) to ensure that the patient gives the signal corresponding to each ear.
5. Make sure that the patient is comfortably seated and place headphones over one of her ears.

Continued

PROCEDURE 36-6—cont'd

6. Begin with a low frequency and watch the patient for an indication that she hears the sound. Push the button to record the results. Beginning the test with sounds that are more commonly heard ensures that the patient is performing the test correctly.
7. Gradually increase frequency until you complete the test for the first ear.
8. Repeat the procedure for the other ear.

9. Document results in the patient's medical record.
10. Clean the equipment as directed by manufacturer's instructions to prevent contaminating the next patient.

Date	
02/21/08: 10:30 a.m.	Audiometry test administered in both ears. No hearing deficits observed. ———————————— C. Smith, CMA

Assisting with Otic Irrigation and Instillation

The ear may require a cleaning procedure known as *irrigation*. The medical assistant can perform an ear irrigation to dislodge a foreign object or clear the ear of impacted cerumen. (See *Procedure 36-7: Irrigating the ear*.) The medical assistant may also be required to instill medication into the ear to combat infection or soften dried cerumen. (See *Procedure 36-8: Instilling eardrops*, page 774.) In each procedure,

the medical assistant must take care to observe the patient. Many patients with inner ear disturbances may need assistance because of feelings of dizziness, nausea, or pain.

Assisting with Examination of the Mouth, Nose, and Throat

The physician will examine the mouth, nose, and throat during routine examinations or if the patient complains of pain or an inability to breathe, swallow, or speak easily. The

PROCEDURE 36-7

Irrigating the ear

Task
Irrigate the patient's affected ear to relieve inflammation or cleanse it of cerumen, a foreign object, or discharge.

Conditions
- Irrigation solution, as ordered by the physician, warmed to body temperature (98.6°F)
- Ear syringe
- Kidney-shaped basin to catch irrigation solution
- Basin for warmed solution
- Towel
- Cotton balls
- Gloves
- Patient's medical record
- Pen

Standards
In the time specified and within the scoring parameters determined by the instructor, the student will successfully irrigate the ear.

Performance Standards
1. Wash your hands.
2. Assemble the equipment and supplies.
3. Introduce yourself and address the patient by name.
4. Explain the procedure to the patient and inform her that she may experience minimal dizziness or discomfort during the procedure when the solution comes into

contact with the tympanic membrane. Answer any questions that the patient may have to promote patient understanding and cooperation.
5. Check the label of the solution three times and check the expiration date to ensure that you are not instilling the wrong or expired medication, which may harm the ear.
6. Warm the bottle of solution under running water. The solution should be close to body temperature (98.6°F) for the comfort of the patient.
7. Pour the solution into a basin and fill the syringe with the warmed irrigation solution as prescribed by the physician. Use approximately 30 to 50 ml of solution at a time to promote patient comfort.
8. Position the patient in the sitting position, with her head tilted toward the affected ear so that the solution will enter the ear and then wash out of it.
9. Place a towel on the patient's shoulder and the ear basin under the affected ear. Ask the patient to hold the basin in place to retain the fluid washed from the ear.
10. Clean the outer ear with a wet cotton ball moistened with irrigation solution to ensure that the material collected in the basin is only from inside the ear.
11. Gently pull the auricle upward and backward to straighten the ear canal (downward and backward if the patient is 3 years old or younger) to straighten the ear canal and allow the fluid to enter it.

PROCEDURE 36-7—cont'd

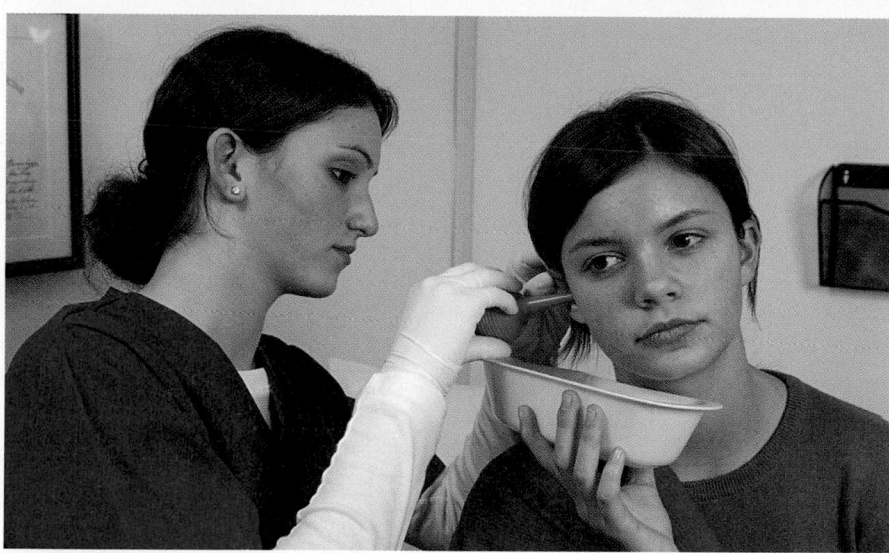

Ask the patient to hold the basin.

12. Expel air from the syringe and gently insert the syringe tip into the affected ear. Be careful not to insert the syringe too deeply. Direct the solution upward toward the roof of the canal to allow the solution to flow downward, cleansing the entire canal. Be careful to avoid occluding the external auditory canal because complete occlusion of the canal can cause increased pressure and, possibly, a ruptured tympanic membrane.

13. Note in the medical record any material that is irrigated, such as impacted cerumen, objects, dirt, and small particles of metal.

14. Refill the syringe with more clean, warmed solution from the other basin.

15. Repeat the irrigation, allowing the solution to drain from the ear. Ask the patient how she feels. Stop the procedure if the patient is too uncomfortable to prevent dizziness and possible fainting.

16. Dry the outer ear and inspect the canal with the otoscope to verify the procedure has removed the foreign body. If the foreign material is still in the canal, repeat the procedure.

17. After you complete the procedure, dry the patient's ear and face and remove the towel and basin. Have the patient lie on her affected side on the examination table so that the ear can continue to drain. If you are performing a bilateral procedure, allow the patient to rest before performing the second irrigation to prevent dizziness or fainting.

18. Give cotton balls to the patient to wipe any further drainage. Ask the patient how she feels.

19. Dispose of supplies.

20. Wash your hands.

21. Document the procedure, noting the return and amount.

22. Provide postcare instructions to the patient. Be sure to tell the patient to call the office and speak to the physician if she feels pain or continued dizziness. Also emphasize to the patient that she should not insert a cotton applicator or any other object into the ear canal.

Date	
02/21/08; 10:30 a.m.	*Right ear irrigation. impacted cerumen dislodged. Patient reports tinnitus has stopped. hearing "seems louder." ------- -- C. Smith, CMA*

medical assistant can provide tongue depressors and the otoscope light to the physician to use to inspect the inside of the nose and view the back of the throat. If the throat appears inflamed, the physician may direct the medical assistant to perform a throat culture.

Many patients get sore throats from a bacterial infection. *Streptococcus* is one bacteria that causes a sore throat, commonly called *"Strep" throat*, which can be treated with antibiotics. However, many patients have a sore throat that is caused by a virus, an allergic reaction, or overuse (for example, singing or yelling). The medical assistant can provide patient education on the use of antibiotics to help patients choose the appropriate treatment for their sore throat. (See *Antibiotic overuse*, page 775.)

PROCEDURE 36-8

Instilling eardrops

Task

Instill eardrops to soften impacted cerumen, fight infection locally with antibiotic drops, or administer analgesics to relieve pain.

Conditions

- Otic medication as prescribed by the physician
- Sterile eardropper
- Cotton balls
- Gloves
- Drape or paper towel
- Patient's medical record
- Pen

Standards

In the time specified and within the scoring parameters determined by the instructor, the student will successfully instill eardrops.

Performance Standards

1. Wash your hands.
2. Assemble equipment and supplies.
3. Introduce yourself and address the patient by name.
4. Explain the procedure to the patient to promote patient cooperation.
5. Check the label of the medication three times for correct medication and expiration date because expired medication or the wrong drug can cause harm to the patient.
6. Warm the ear drops under running warm water for patient comfort.
7. Position the patient to lie on her unaffected side or in a sitting position with her head tilted toward her unaffected ear so that the medication will flow into her ear and will not run down her neck.
8. Provide the patient with a paper towel or nonsterile drape for her shoulder to protect her clothing from staining by the medication.
9. Draw up the prescribed amount of medication into the sterile eardropper.
10. Gently pull the top of the auricle up and back (for adults) or pull the earlobe down and back (for children ages 3 and under) so that the medication will flow into the ear and will not run out.
11. Squeeze the rubber bulb to instill the prescribed dose of medication into the affected ear.
12. Ask the patient to maintain the position for about 5 minutes after instillation so that the ear will retain the medication.

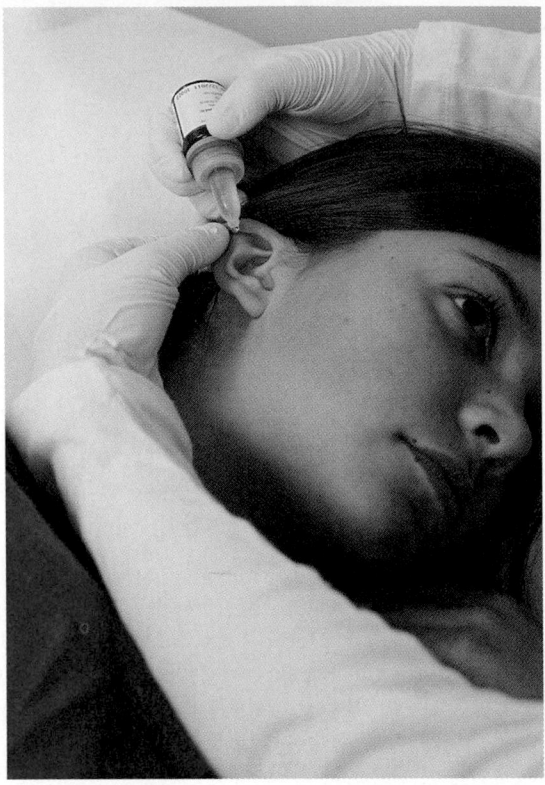

Squeeze the rubber bulb to instill the prescribed dose into the affected ear.

13. If instructed by the physician, insert a moistened cotton ball into the external ear canal for 15 minutes because moistened cotton will not absorb the medication and will help retain the medication in the ear.
14. Wash your hands.
15. Document the procedure in the patient's medical record.

Date	
02/21/08: 10:35 a.m.	4 drops Ciprodex administered to right ear. —————————— ——————————————————————————————— C. Smith, CMA

16. Repeat the procedure with the other ear if a bilateral procedure is ordered.
17. Teach the patient or caregiver how to instill the drops, stressing the importance of handwashing before and after instillation. As with eyedrops, make sure the patient understands that she should avoid touching the tip of the dropper to her ear or any object.

Patient Education

Antibiotic Overuse

Before or after taking a throat culture is a great time for the medical assistant to educate her patient about the difference between a viral infection and a bacterial infection. A patient may view antibiotics as a "magic pill" or cure-all. Some patients may be quite insistent that they need an antibiotic even though no bacterial infection is found.

The physician or the medical assistant can explain that viruses and bacteria are different organisms and that antibiotics are unable to kill a virus. The medical assistant should make sure the patient knows that, in fact, overuse of antibiotics will actually strengthen the bacteria's defenses and make them harder to kill when bacterial infection is present. The medical assistant should emphasize proper handwashing techniques as a means of preventing future infection.

Chapter Summary

- The medical assistant assisting with examination and treatment of the eyes, ears, mouth, nose, and throat must have an understanding of the anatomy and physiology of these areas.
- Proper patient education during vision and hearing assessment will ensure that accurate test results are obtained.
- When performing irrigation or instillation of medication to the eye or ear, the medical assistant must answer patient questions and inform the patient of the procedure as it occurs.
- Because the patient or caregiver will probably need to administer the medication at home, the medical assistant should teach the proper sterile technique during the procedure and answer any questions as they arise.
- Educating patients on the benefits of frequent handwashing will prevent infection of the eye, ear, mouth, nose, and throat.

Team Work Exercises

1. Ask a local school nurse if you can assist or observe Snellen, Jaeger, or Ishihara eye testing of students. Ask the nurse what follow-up procedures are in place for children with visual impairments, referrals to specialists, and so forth. What resources are available for eyewear for students who cannot afford glasses or contact lenses?

2. Discuss what signs and symptoms parents should be aware of that may indicate a vision or hearing impairment in their child. Create a brochure to give to parents of infants, toddlers, and preschoolers that includes anatomical diagrams of the eye, ear, mouth, nose, and throat and warning signs of problems.

Case Studies

1. Wendy Howard brings her 7-year-old son Devin to the office because he has an earache. Devin has had several colds this winter and has missed several days of school. He appears tired and lethargic. Upon examination, the physician diagnoses Devin with otitis media and prescribes oral antibiotics and eardrops. In addition to treating the present infection, what can you tell Wendy and Devin to do to prevent future infections?

2. Mr. McDaniels is a 67-year-old patient who has been coming to the office for several years. He exercises often, eats right, and is very fit. You notice lately that he asks you to repeat questions and you and the other staff members need to speak more loudly for him to hear you. Mr. McDaniels doesn't acknowledge that his hearing is gradually diminishing. Discuss with the group how to approach the patient without insulting him.

Resources

- Anatomy of the ear: *ctl.augie.edu/perry/ear/hearmech.htm*
- Anatomy of the eye: *www.emedicinehealth.com/anatomy_of_the_eye/article_em.htm* and *www.discoveryfund.org/anatomyoftheeye.html*
- Diabetic retinopathy: *www.allaboutvision.com/faq/diabetic.htm*
- *Digital Journal of Ophthalmology: www.djo.harvard.edu*
- Information on diagnosis and treatment of streptococcal throat infection:*www.emedicinehealth.com/strep_throat/article_em.htm*
- Macular degeneration: *www.blindness.org/Macular Degeneration/*
- Otitis media in children: *www.kidsource.com/ASHA/otitis.html*
- Scanlon, V.C., and Sanders, T.: *Essentials of Anatomy and Physiology*, 5th ed. Philadelphia: F.A. Davis Co., 2007.
- Swimmer's ear self-care: *www.mayoclinic.com/health/swimmers-ear/DS00473/DSECTION=10*

Nutrition

Learning Objectives

Upon completion of this chapter, the student will be able to:

- define the key terms presented in the glossary
- define energy and nonenergy nutrients
- discuss how a balanced diet promotes good health
- discuss the dangers of overnutrition and obesity
- define nutrient density
- name and give a food source for water-soluble and fat-soluble vitamins
- name and give a food source for the major minerals
- name a deficiency symptom of two vitamins and two minerals
- discuss syndrome X and its health implications
- define anorexia and bulimia and some of their signs and symptoms.

CAAHEP Competencies

General Competencies

Patient Instruction

Instruct individuals according to their needs

Provide instruction for health maintenance and disease prevention

Identify community resources

ABHES Competencies

Instruction

Instruct patients with special needs

Teach patients methods of health promotion and disease prevention

Understanding Nutrition

Finding a diet that is nutritionally balanced, satisfies taste, and fits a busy lifestyle is an ongoing struggle for many Americans. Because food choices and quantity of food eaten impact all aspects of health, the medical assistant can play an important role in educating patients to make good food choices and control portions. In addition, the successful health care educator leads by example and benefits from practicing healthy eating and exercise habits.

A **nutrient** is a chemical substance obtained from food and used in the body to provide energy, build structural materials, support growth and maintenance, or repair body tissues. Nutrients also reduce the risk of disease by promoting proper function of organs and tissues. Nutrients can be divided into two main categories: macronutrients and micronutrients.

Macronutrients

Energy in the body is defined as the capacity to do work. The human body needs energy to do physical and chemical work. The sum of these physical and chemical processes that enable the body to meet the demands of living is called **metabolism**. The body uses the energy in foods to create body heat, move muscles, conduct nervous signals, produce hormones, regulate functions such as heart rate, and repair damaged tissues. Energy taken into the body is measured in calories. A **calorie** is a unit of measure that represents the amount of heat energy needed to raise 1 g of water 1° Celsius. Because a calorie is such a tiny measure of energy, food energy is expressed in Kilocalories, which is equal to 1000 calories. Kilocalories are more commonly known as *Calories* (with a capital C). Thus, calorie values on food labels are always capitalized to denote the kilocalorie. Nutrients that are measured in Calories (kcal) and, thus, contain energy include:

- carbohydrates
- fats
- proteins.

Carbohydrate

Carbohydrates are the main source of fuel for humans and should comprise 45% to 55% of total calorie intake. (See *Economics of proper nutrition.*) They are molecules made up of carbon, hydrogen, and oxygen. Carbohydrates are categorized as *simple* or *complex,* depending on the amount of energy needed to digest them.

Economics of proper nutrition

Carbohydrates are the most abundant and cheapest food source and represent the bulk of caloric consumption worldwide. Because most sources of protein and fat come from animals in the form of meats, milk, and cheese, these foods are more expensive to produce. Thus, people in developing countries may only have carbohydrate sources of foods. This lack of adequate dietary protein can cause nutritional disorders, especially in children.

Although sources of protein in the United States and other developed countries are abundant, they are expensive. Patients with a limited income are, thus, restricted in the variety of food in their diet due to cost. If a patient is unable to buy enough food, the medical assistant can help identify local social service agencies, such as food banks, food stamps, and meal services.

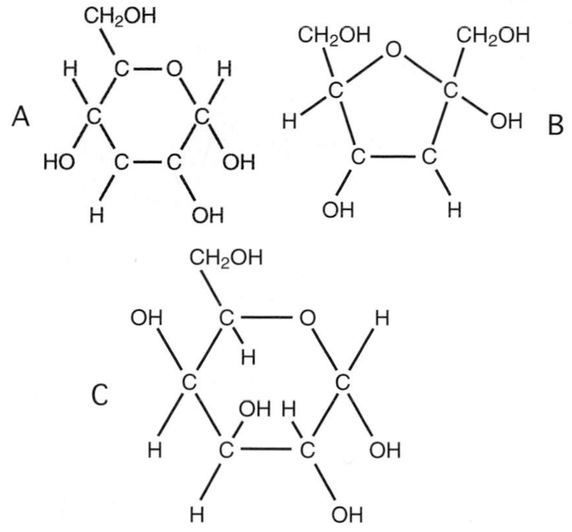

FIG 37-1 Chemical structures of monosaccharides. (A) Glucose. (B) Fructose. (C) Galactose.

Simple Carbohydrates

Simple carbohydrates are commonly referred to as *simple sugars*. Because of their uncomplicated chemical structure, they require little time for digestion by the body. There are two types of simple carbohydrate:

- monosaccharides
- disaccharides.

Monosaccharides

All carbohydrates are made up of **monosaccharides**, which are single units of sugar. Although there are many monosaccharides, including xylose, mannose, and sorbose, three are more common in the human diet:

- **glucose**
- fructose
- galactose. (See Figure 37-1.)

Other than fructose, which is present naturally in fruit and added to processed foods as *crystalline fructose* or *high fructose corn sweetener*, monosaccharides are not present in foods. More commonly, they are chemically bonded together in various combinations of two monosaccharides to form a **disaccharide**.

Disaccharides

Three disaccharides constitute the main dietary sources of sugar for humans:

- sucrose, a combination of glucose and fructose and found in such foods as granulated sugar, sugar beets, honey, and maple syrup
- lactose, made up of glucose and galactose and found in milk and dairy products
- maltose, made up of two molecules of glucose and found in beer. (See Figure 37-2.)

When a person ingests disaccharides, his body must break them down into usable forms of energy. First, it breaks disaccharides down into their separate monosaccharide units. Thus, sucrose breaks down into glucose and fructose, lactose into glucose and galactose, and maltose into the two glucose molecules. Then the body rearranges fructose and galactose into glucose in the liver for energy needs. The body uses glucose as its main source of fuel. Glucose circulates in the bloodstream, which delivers it to all of the organs and tissues of the body. An anaerobic reaction in tissues converts glucose to lactic acid. In the conversion process, each glucose molecule yields two molecules of **adenosine triphosphate** (ATP). ATP is the fuel that cells use to perform their necessary functions. A similar reaction in the presence of oxygen (aerobic) changes glucose to pyruvate and then, in a multistep reaction called the *Kreb cycle*, also yields two ATP molecules.

Complex Carbohydrates

Complex carbohydrates, also known as polysaccharides, are made up of many units of monosaccharides, the simple sugars. There are three types of complex carbohydrates:

- starch
- glycogen
- fiber.

Unlike simple sugars, complex carbohydrates have more complicated chemical structures. Thus, they require more time in digestion to break the chemical bonds between the sugar units to make them usable by the body. The sugar units in polysaccharides are linked together by chemical bonds in straight chains, which take more time to break down, or branching arrangements, which break down more readily. (See Figure 37-3.)

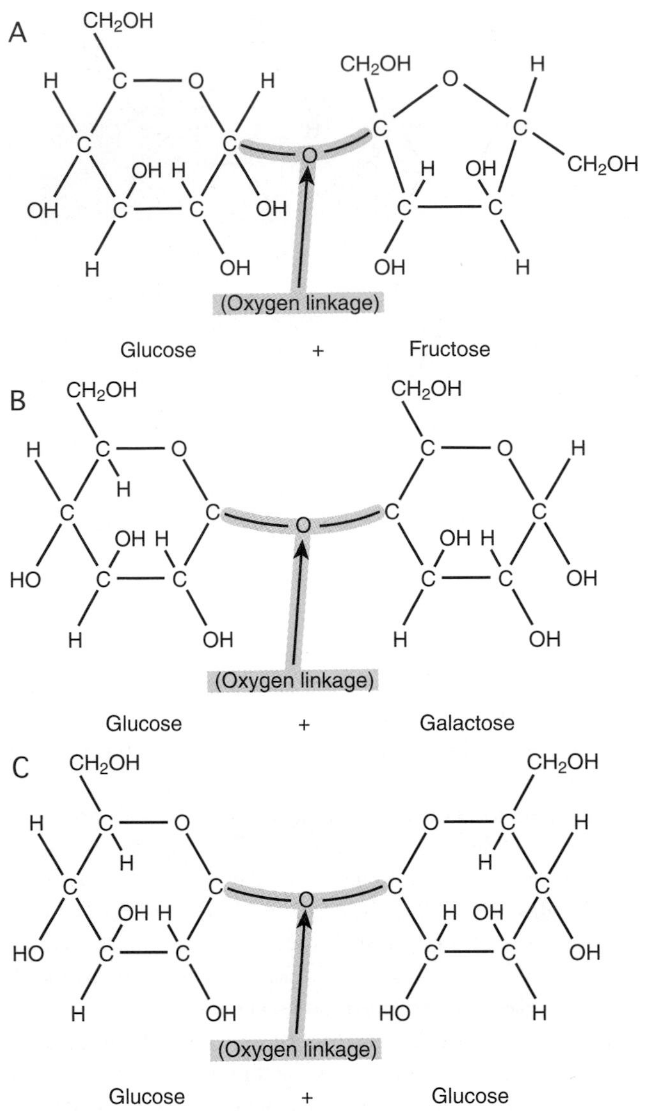

FIG 37-2 Chemical structures of disaccharides. (A) Sucrose. (B) Lactose. (C) Maltose.

Starch

Starch is found in plants. There are two kinds of starch molecules: *amylose* and *amylopectin*. Amylose is a straight chain of glucose units. Amylopectin is a mostly linear molecule of glucose units with some branching. Although their chemical structures differ, both types of molecules have alpha bonds, which are the links between the simple sugar units. Salivary and later pancreatic enzymes break down the alpha bonds that link the sugar units, enabling the bloodstream to absorb the sugar. Starch is the main type of digestible complex carbohydrate. Examples of food sources of starch include wheat, rice, potatoes, and legumes, such as beans and peas.

Glycogen

By contrast, the complexity of the branching chains of the glycogen molecule enables enzymes to break down glycogen molecules more quickly in the body. The body uses glycogen as a storage form of energy. It is the primary source of glucose (in storage) and releases glucose into the bloodstream to raise blood glucose in times of fasting, such as during sleep. The primary storage site for glycogen is the liver and muscles. Although meats contain glycogen, they are not a significant dietary source.

Fiber

Although fiber is a kind of complex carbohydrate, most dietary fiber is not digestible. Thus, it does not contribute energy to the diet. However, although we do not digest fiber, it is important because it provides bulk to feces and promotes intestinal motility (movement of feces through the intestines). There are two main types of fiber:

- insoluble
- soluble.

Insoluble Fiber

Fiber that does not break down in water is classified as *insoluble*. There are three types of **insoluble fiber:** cellulose, hemicellulose, and lignin. These fibers are the structural components of plants. Although cellulose is made up of a straight chain of glucose molecules, similar to amylose, the molecules are linked together by beta bonds, which human enzymes cannot break down. Hemicellulose is made up of glucose but also galactose, xylose, and other monosaccharides. As with cellulose, human enzymes cannot break the bonds of the hemicellulose molecule; thus, it is also indigestible. Cellulose and hemicellulose are found in such foods as whole wheat breads, bran, oatmeal, lentils, and black beans. Lignin does not contain glucose; it is made up of alcohols and acids and is the woody fiber found in wheat bran and the seeds of many fruits and vegetables.

Soluble Fiber

There are three kinds of **soluble fiber:**

- pectin
- gum
- mucilage.

Human enzymes cannot break down any of these types of fiber either. However, they are an essential food source for bacteria in the large intestines of the body. Thus, soluble fiber is important in maintaining normal bacteria in the intestine. (See *Fiber and colorectal health*, page 782.) Pectin and gums are more common in the American diet than mucilage. Pectin is found in citrus fruits, strawberries, apples, carrots, jams, and jellies. Gums are found in oats, legumes, and barley. Mucilage is found in flaxseed and kelp. All three types are made up of various combinations of monosaccharides and acids.

A

Amylose
- Straight chains of glucose
- 500 to 20,000 glucose units

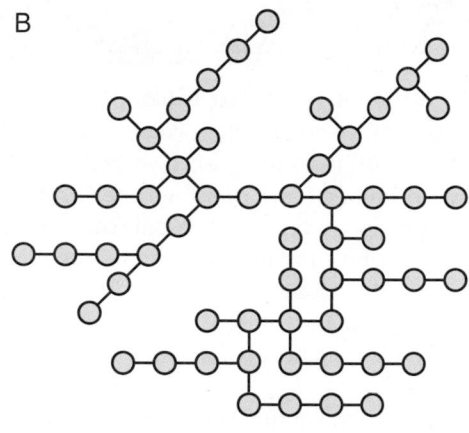

B

Amylopectin
- Amylose chains connected in branches
- Up to 30 amylose branches

Glycogen
- Many more branches than amylopectin
- Approximately 60,000 glucose molecules

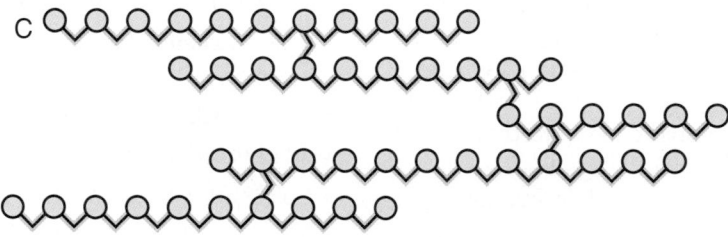

C

Fiber
- Linked by indigestible beta bonds

FIG 37-3 Chemical structures of polysaccharides. (A) Starches. (B) Glycogen. (C) Fiber.

Carbohydrate Digestion

The process of carbohydrate digestion begins in the mouth with the release of salivary enzymes. Salivary amylase mixes with food products and breaks some starches into smaller units. Then the carbohydrates reach the stomach, where the acidic environment of the stomach inactivates the amylase. The carbohydrates then pass through the stomach and into the small intestine, where most digestion and absorption occurs. The pancreas and walls of the small intestine secrete digestive enzymes. The enzyme pancreatic amylase breaks starch into disaccharides and small polysaccharides. Enzymes from the cells of the intestinal wall break down the remaining polysaccharides and disaccharides into their monosaccharide components (glucose, fructose, and galactose). Then the cells of the small intestines absorb these monosaccharides. After absorption, the monosaccharides travel to the liver, where the liver converts fructose and galactose into glucose molecules. Then the liver releases glucose into the bloodstream or links the molecules together to form glycogen for storage. Dietary fiber is not digested and passes into the colon unchanged, providing bulk to form stools.

Regulation of Blood Glucose

Carbohydrates are the main food source of glucose, stored in the liver and muscles as glycogen. Storage of a large amount of glucose enables blood glucose regulation when a person is not eating. How quickly different types of food deliver glucose to the bloodstream is indicated in the **glycemic index**, which rates foods on a scale from slowest to fastest delivery of glucose to the bloodstream. (See *Glycemic index*, pages 784 and 785.) Carbohydrates that are "slower" are recommended for inclusion in the diet, especially for people trying to lose weight. Slower carbohydrates take longer to affect blood glucose levels. Therefore, they create less of an insulin response, resulting in a longer period before a person becomes hungry again. (See Figure 37-4.)

Proteins

Proteins are amino acids linked together in chains and branching arrangements by peptide bonds. A protein consists of these long peptide chains that can range from 50 amino acids to thousands. Peptide bonds break down spontaneously in water, although slowly. Digestive enzymes, called *proteases*, help speed up the process somewhat; however, the breakdown

Patient Education

Fiber and Colorectal Health

Most patients who develop colon cancer, diverticulitis (weakening of the intestine), diverticulosis (infection of weakened areas of the intestine), hemorrhoids, fistulae, and fissures have a history of chronic constipation or irregular bowel habits. The most common cause of chronic constipation is inadequate dietary fiber. The medical assistant can educate patients on the need for adequate dietary fiber by explaining how it functions to preserve colorectal health.

For optimal bowel function, a person must ingest 25 to 30 g of fiber each day. After the body digests food, the colon receives approximately 1 pint of liquid stool along with the undigested fiber. Normally, the colon gradually removes the remaining water, and forms a shaped stool. The fiber in the stool retains some water, making the stool soft and bulky, enabling it to move easily toward the rectum for elimination. When dietary fiber is scarce, the stool becomes hard, dry, and small and requires more force to move through the colon for elimination.

Because the patient must strain to defecate, he causes damage to the intestinal wall. The straining produces pressure on the walls of the colon, creating diverticulitis and diverticulosis. Hemorrhoids and anal fistulae and fissures can also be caused by damage to the tissues from straining. Colorectal cancers can be caused by hard, dry stool remaining in the colon too long, resulting in reabsorption of carcinogens into the surface of the colon. Also, because straining to defecate is painful, many patients may take over-the-counter stool softeners or laxatives. Long-term use of these products can render the colon unable to eliminate feces without the help of a laxative or stool softener (dependence).

The medical assistant should educate her patient that he should use laxatives only for a short-term correction of bowel health to avoid becoming dependent on them. She should recommend that the patient use laxatives only with the physician's consent. She should also encourage the patient to correct the dietary fiber inadequacy to achieve normal bowel movements. She can suggest incorporating the following foods into the diet to increase fiber intake:

- beans, including baked, kidney, pinto, black, and lima beans
- bran cereals, whole wheat breads, and pastas
- dried fruits, including apricots, prunes, and raisins
- fruits, including raspberries, blackberries, cherries, strawberries, plums, pears, and apples
- vegetables, including broccoli, spinach, collard greens, and peas

---

of peptide bonds is slow compared to that of alpha and beta bonds. In addition, proteins are found in numerous body tissues in the form of cellular components, enzymes, and hormones. The human body contains over 10,000 different types of these proteins, called *body proteins.*

Protein is an important component of a healthy diet. Although proteins are energy-yielding nutrients, their main function is to provide amino acids to build various body tissues. Because the body does not store amino acids as it does carbohydrates, it needs adequate supplies of protein in the diet every day. The Institute of Medicine recommends that adults get a minimum of 0.8 g of protein per day for every 20 lb of body weight. The body uses this amount of protein to maintain body tissues and ensure that the body is not breaking down its own tissues for fuel. (See *Food sources of protein,* pages 785 and 786.)

Essential and Nonessential

There are 20 different amino acids that make up proteins. The name *amino acid* is derived from the structure of an amino acid molecule. At one end, the molecule has an amine group (containing nitrogen) and at the other end, an acid group (containing carboxylic acid). The two ends are connected to a central carbon atom. The type of amino acid is determined by the side group, or molecule attached to the central carbon atom, including hydrogen (forming the amino acid glycine), a methyl group (forming the amino acid alanine), or a larger heterocyclic group (forming the amino acid tryptophan). (See Figure 37-5.)

Amino acids are categorized as *essential* or *nonessential.* Essential amino acids are those that the body cannot synthesize (or create on its own) to build necessary body tissues. Thus, dietary sources of these amino acids are necessary (essential) for health. An adult's diet has eight essential amino acids. Another four amino acids are essential in a child's diet because a child's body has not yet developed the metabolic pathways to synthesize these amino acids. Nonessential amino acids may be synthesized by the body or supplied in dietary sources.

Amino acid structure

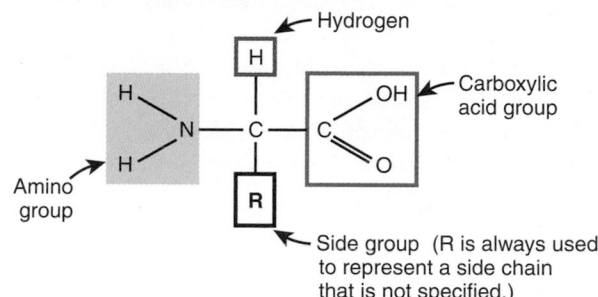

FIG 37-5 Amino acid structure with side group (R).

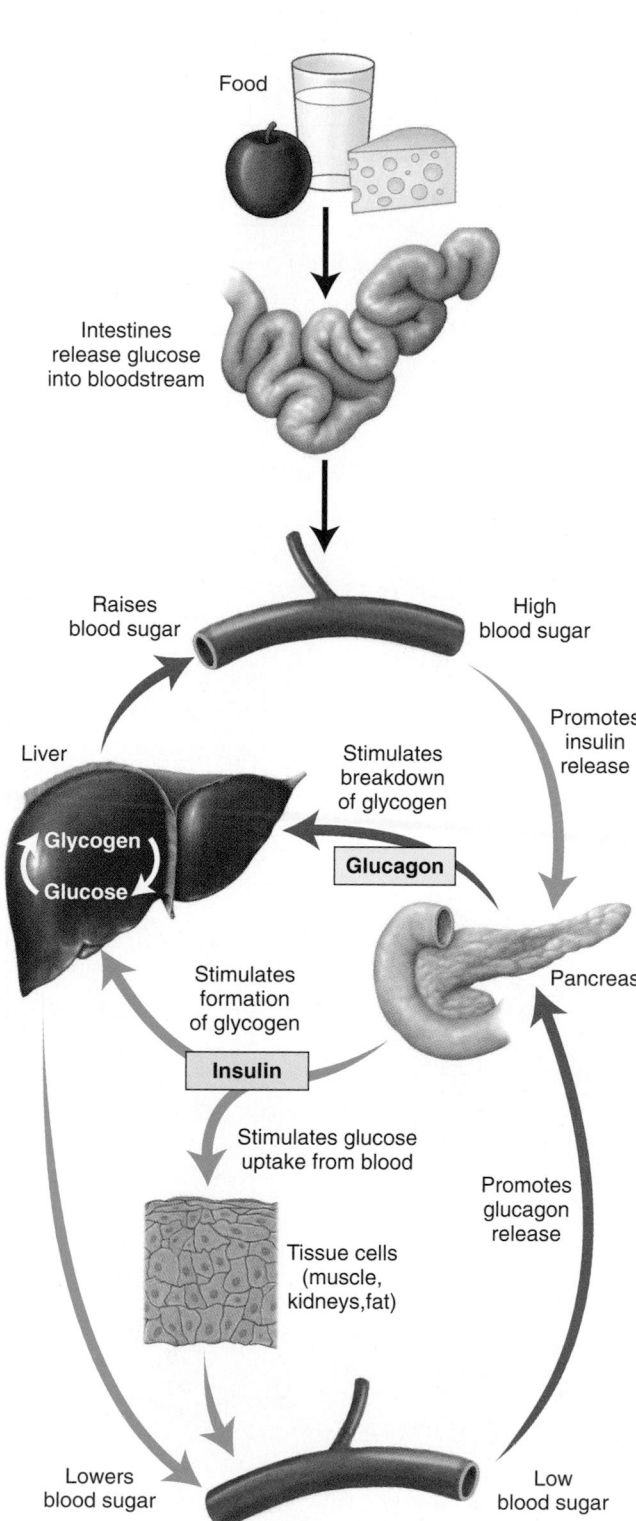

FIG 37-4 Blood glucose regulation in the body.

The eight essential amino acids adults need are:

- isoleucine
- leucine
- lysine
- methionine
- phenylalanine
- threonine
- tryptophan
- valine.

The nonessential amino acids are:

- alanine
- arginine (essential in children)
- asparagine
- aspartate
- cysteine (essential in children)
- glutamate
- glutamine
- glycine
- histidine (essential in children)
- proline
- serine
- tyrosine (essential in children).

Protein Digestion

The first phase of protein digestion takes place in the stomach. Stomach acid begins to break down some of the protein molecules into amino acids. Then pepsin, an enzyme secreted in the stomach, begins to digest those amino acids. However, only a few protein molecules break down into amino acids in the stomach; most remain connected together. In the duodenum (first segment of the small intestine), the pancreas secretes the enzymes trypsin and chymotrypsin. Like pepsin, these enzymes break the bonds between individual amino acids through a process called *hydrolysis,* because it requires a water molecule to unlink the amino acids. When amino acids are not linked, they are small enough to pass through the

Glycemic index

The glycemic index (GI) is a scale that rates foods based on how fast they raise blood glucose levels. Pure glucose is given the value of 100, and the index compares how fast each food delivers glucose to the bloodstream compared to pure glucose. For example, carbohydrates that break down quickly during digestion have a high GI of 70 or more. Carbohydrates that break down slowly have a low GI of 55 or less. Medium GI range is 56 to 69.

The following table lists a sampling of foods and their glycemic index.

Food	Glycemic Index		
	Low	Medium	High
Vegetables			
Artichoke, asparagus, broccoli, cauliflower, celery, cucumber, eggplant, onion, spinach	15		
Lima beans, chick peas, kidney beans, lentils	30		
Carrots, fresh or boiled	49		
Sweet corn		56	
Beets, peas		65	
Fruit			
Prunes	15		
Cherries	22		
Apple, plum, pears, strawberries	38		
Orange, peach, grapes	43		
Kiwi	52		
Mango, bananas, fruit cocktail (in syrup)	55		
Pear, papaya, apricots		58	
Raisins, cantaloupe		64	
Pineapple		66	
Watermelon			72
Dates			103
Dairy Products			
Plain yogurt	14		
Whole milk	30		
Skim milk	32		
Chocolate milk	35		
Yogurt (fruit flavored)	36		
Ice cream, vanilla		60	
Grains, Breads, and Pastas			
Fettuccine	32		
Spaghetti	40		
Linguini, rye bread, multigrain bread	49		
Pita bread, brown rice		56	
White rice		58	
Wheat bread, taco shells		68	
White bread			70
Plain bagel			72
Saltine crackers			74
Prepared Foods and Snacks			
Peanuts, walnuts	15		
Cashews	22		

Glycemic index—cont'd

Food	Glycemic Index		
	Low	*Medium*	*High*
Peanut M&Ms	32		
Fish sticks	38		
Chocolate chip cookies, sponge cake	44		
Cheese tortellini, strawberry jam, chocolate bar	50		
Snickers bar, popcorn (light), potato chips, oatmeal cookies	55		
Cheese pizza		60	
Macaroni and cheese, corn chips		64	
Angel food cake, croissant		67	
French fries, doughnuts, graham crackers, waffles			75
Rice cakes, jelly beans			80
Pretzels			83
Tofu frozen dessert			115
Beverages			
Tomato juice	38		
Apple juice	41		
Pineapple juice, carrot juice	46		
Grapefruit juice	48		
Orange juice	52		
Cola		65	
Cranberry juice cocktail		68	
Gatorade			78

intestinal wall into the capillaries that surround the intestines, which distribute them via the bloodstream. Amino acids in the bloodstream are used to build many body proteins.

Body Protein Manufacturing

After amino acid distribution in the body, cells link amino acids back together again in different arrangements to make specific proteins for their needs. Examples of proteins that the body manufactures include:

- *insulin*, a protein made by the pancreas to deliver glucose to cells
- *ferritin*, a protein made in the intestinal mucosa through the union of iron with the protein apoferritin (Ferritin stores iron and will release it as needed by the body.)
- *hemoglobin*, a protein made in red bone marrow and used by red blood cells to deliver oxygen to cells
- *myoglobin*, an iron-containing protein found in muscle cells that stores oxygen for use in cell respiration

Food sources of protein

Cells synthesize proteins according to their specific needs. Adequate dietary protein delivers the amino acids necessary to build complex proteins with a variety of functions. Foods high in protein include meats, dairy, eggs, nuts, and seeds. The following table lists some of these foods along with a typical serving size and the quantity of protein it contains.

Food Source	Serving Size	Quantity of Protein
pecans	¼ cup	2.5 g
cashews	¼ cup	5 g
chicken wings (2)	4 oz	6 g
egg	1 large	6 g
sunflower seeds	¼ cup	6 g
almonds	¼ cup	8 g

Continued

Food sources of protein—cont'd

Food Source	Serving Size	Quantity of Protein
beans (black, pinto, lentils)	½ cup	8 g
milk	1 cup	8 g
peanut butter	2 Tbs	8 g
soy milk	1 cup	8 g
swiss or Cheddar cheese	1 oz	8 g
peanuts	¼ cup	9 g
chicken thigh	3 oz	10 g
parmesan cheese	1 oz	10 g
yogurt	1 cup	10 g
chicken drumstick	one drumstick, average size	11 g
cottage cheese	½ cup	15 g
ham	3 oz	19 g
tofu	½ cup	20 g
turkey (white meat)	3 oz	21 g
fish fillet (cod, haddock) or salmon steak	3.5 oz	22 g
pork chop	one, average size	22 g
hamburger patty	4 oz	28 g
roast beef	3.5 oz	28 g
steak	4 oz	28 g
pork tenderloin	4 oz	29 g
chicken breast	3.5 oz	30 g
canned tuna	6 oz	40 g

- *antibodies*, giant protein molecules manufactured to combat invaders (pathogens) in the blood
- *bone sialoprotein*, *osteocalcin*, and *osteonectin*, used, among other functions, to keep calcium in bone matrix, contributing to its strength. (See *Protein and bone health*.)

Fats

Although fat is commonly associated with obesity and thought to be a "bad" component of food, fats, or **lipids**, perform important functions as part of a balanced diet. Structurally, lipids look different from carbohydrates. They are chains or branched chains of carbons or contain four rings (as in cholesterol). There are four types of lipids:

- fatty acids
- triglycerides
- phospholipids
- sterols.

Patient Education

Protein and Bone Health

In the past, health care providers and others thought that high-protein diets increased urinary output of calcium and, therefore, were detrimental to bone health. However, recent studies now show that patients who habitually consume low-protein diets demonstrate decreases in bone density and increases in bone loss.

Thus, the medical assistant must educate her patients on this new information to combat misconceptions about protein's effects on bone health. The medical assistant should explain to patients that to build and repair bone, the body needs protein to create the matrix that will be mineralized by calcium, phosphorus, magnesium, and fluoride. Without adequate protein, the body is unable to utilize the minerals for bone maintenance, so calcium supplements or bone-density-enhancing drugs such as Fosamax will not increase bone mineralization.

Fatty Acids

A **fatty acid** is an organic acid made up of a chain of carbon atoms with hydrogen atoms attached and an acid group at one end. Fatty acids can be saturated or unsaturated based on the number of hydrogen atoms attached to the carbon atoms on the chain. A saturated molecule has as many hydrogen atoms as it can hold. Unsaturated molecules are missing hydrogen atoms. If a hydrogen atom is missing between two carbon atoms, a double bond is created between those carbon atoms. This double bond is a site where there is no saturation, and the fatty acid is considered *monounsaturated*. If more than one double bond occurs in a fatty acid, it is *polyunsaturated*. (See Figure 37-6.)

Polyunsaturated fats are better sources of dietary fat because their consumption reduces the incidence of coronary artery disease and cholesterol levels in the blood. Although the exact mechanisms are unclear, the body can use polyunsaturated fat molecules to make cell membranes. Saturated fat molecules, which contain only single bonds, are not flexible enough to be incorporated into cell membranes. In addition, saturated fat molecules are larger and less dense because they have more hydrogen attached. Therefore, they can lodge in arteries, contributing to coronary artery disease.

Fatty acids are necessary components of the structural portion of cells. They also participate in the immune response to injury and help regulate blood pressure as well as many other functions. The body is able to synthesize all fatty acids except two, which are called *essential fatty acids*. The essential fatty acids are linoleic acid and linolenic acid. Inclusion of food sources of the essential fatty acids or

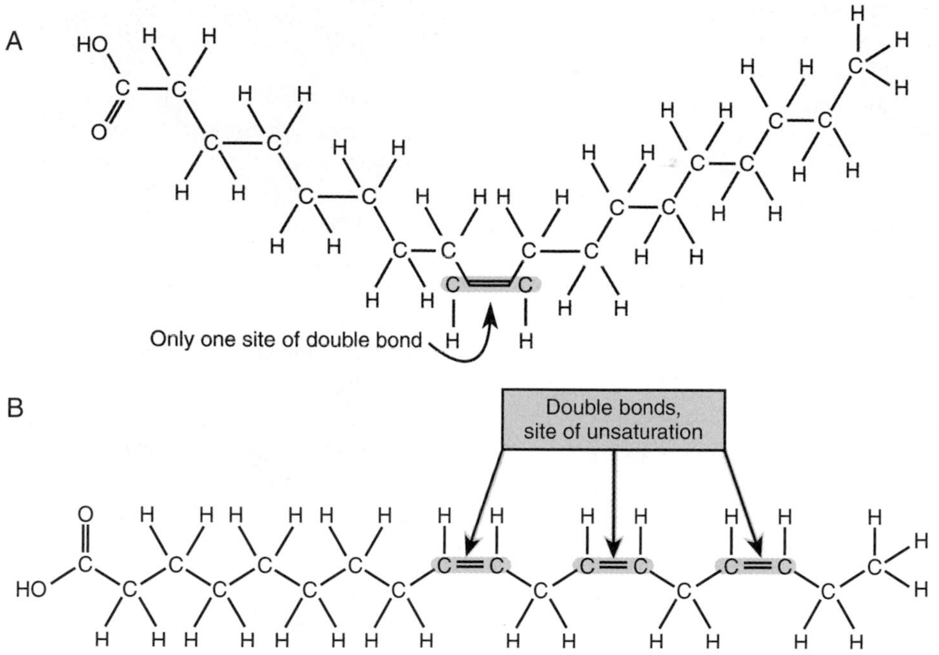

FIG 37-6 Fatty acids. (A) Monounsaturated (oleic acid). (B) Polyunsaturated (linolenic acid).

supplements containing them is vital to a complete diet. (See *Food sources of essential fatty acids*.)

Triglycerides

Most foods do not contain single fatty acids, called *free fatty acids*. More commonly, they contain triglycerides, which are three fatty acid chains attached to one glycerol unit. (The glycerol converts to glucose for energy needs.) Triglycerides, the most common form of fat in the diet, are the major storage form of fat in the body. Triglycerides are used by the body as a source of energy and as insulation in their storage form as body fat. Because a triglyceride molecule contains three fatty acid chains, it is a larger molecule than a free fatty acid. The degree of unsaturation on the fatty acids also impacts the use of the triglyceride in the body and, therefore, health. The more saturated the molecule, the larger it is and the more likely it will contribute to stagnation in the bloodstream and the formation of fatty streaks.

Phospholipids

Phospholipids are structurally similar to triglycerides; however, instead of three fatty acids, there are two fatty acids and a phosphate group. The phosphate group on the phospholipids makes the molecule soluble in water; the fatty acid component makes it soluble in fat. This dual solubility is unique in the body and allows the molecule to create cell membranes. Without phospholipids in the diet, cell membrane integrity suffers. This dysfunction can lead to structural damage within the body and promote the likelihood of cancer and other disorders.

Because the cell membrane structure is water and fat soluble, it can help lipids move in and out of cell membranes into the watery fluid on both sides. Thus, hormones and fat-soluble vitamins can pass into the cell as needed. Phospholipids can also keep fat-soluble substances suspended in a watery media by a process called **emulsification**. Emulsified fats are broken down into components that are small enough

---

Food sources of essential fatty acids

Because the body is unable to synthesize linoleic and linolenic acids, the healthy diet must include sources of these fatty acids.

Linoleic Acid
- Corn oil
- Safflower oil
- Soybean oil
- Chicken fat
- Turkey fat

Linolenic Acid
- Flaxseed oil
- Canola oil
- Soybean oil
- Soybeans
- Walnuts

to become suspended in water. They are not dissolved in water but are suspended in the watery media. An excess of fat in the diet will cause the emulsified fat to be transported to adipose cells (fat cells). For most people, the number of cells does not increase; however, the size of the cells does. Thus, as a person increases intake of fatty foods, the amount of fat stored in the adipose cells also increases, causing weight gain and increased body size. Some research indicates that, in cases of morbid obesity (body weight 50% greater than normal or higher), the total number of fat cells will increase as well as the size of the cells.

Sterols

Sterols are lipids that contain a sterol group, which is a four-ring carbon structure. Bile acids found in the liver and gallbladder, vitamin D, and sex hormones are all made from sterols. The most well known sterol is cholesterol.

Cholesterol

Although people commonly talk about "good cholesterol" and "bad cholesterol," there is only one chemical known as **cholesterol**. The compounds mistaken for cholesterol are actually lipoproteins, which are compounds made of lipids and proteins. High-density lipoproteins (HDLs) are helpful blood constituents that carry cholesterol to the liver for breakdown and excretion. Low-density lipoproteins (LDLs) circulate in the bloodstream and transport cholesterol and triglycerides from the liver to the peripheral tissues. Thus, too much LDL in the blood enables too much cholesterol and too many triglycerides to reach body tissues. The ratio of HDL to LDL dictates how much cholesterol is excreted and how much is stored. Chylomicrons (large lipoproteins) and very-low-density lipoproteins (VLDLs) contain even more cholesterol than LDLs.

Cholesterol is derived only from animal sources, such as eggs, meats, fish, and poultry. Plant food sources may contain sterols, but not cholesterol. Surprisingly, most cholesterol is synthesized in the liver, not found in the diet. Cholesterol becomes harmful when it forms deposits of fatty streaks and fibrous plaques along artery walls. (See Figure 37-7.) High levels of LDLs, which contain a large percentage of cholesterol, are associated with obesity and overeating. Excessive intake of *any food* can cause obesity and higher levels of the more dangerous lipoproteins. (See *Food and cholesterol.*

Digestion of Fat

Digestion of fat begins in the stomach, where stomach acid breaks some short-chain triglycerides into glycerol and fatty acids. The longer-chain triglycerides are more abundant in the diet and are broken down in the small intestine (by bile acids manufactured in the liver and lipases manufactured in the pancreas) and delivered to the duodenum by the gallbladder. Bile acids emulsify triglycerides into individual fatty acids and monoglycerides so that the molecules are small

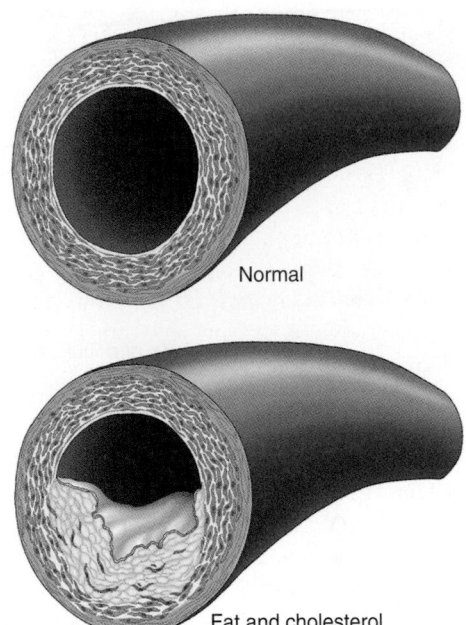

Normal

Fat and cholesterol
accumulate

FIG 37-7 Build-up of cholesterol along artery walls.

enough to be absorbed through the walls of the intestines. After they are absorbed into the bloodstream, they reassemble into triglycerides. Chylomicrons then carry them through the lymph system to the liver. The liver uses cholesterol to manufacture bile acids and bile salts. Various tissues also use cholesterol and other sterols to produce hormones.

Cholesterol and other sterols ingested in foods do not provide any calories in adults and children. Only about 25% of the cholesterol in food is absorbed and even fewer amounts of sterols. Infants absorb more cholesterol because their bodies are building more tissues, especially in the brain and central nervous system. Fat digestion in infancy is quite different than in children and adults, especially if the infant is ingesting breast milk. Digestion of fat in breast milk begins in the infant's mouth with enzymes that are only present in the mammary gland and are delivered with the milk.

Micronutrients

Vitamins and minerals are also essential components of a complete diet. Because these substances do not contribute calories (energy), they are called **micronutrients**. They are essential to body functions in various ways. Vitamins facilitate the release of energy from carbohydrate, fat, and protein; minerals provide building materials for body structures and influence blood and pH. Water provides the environment for body processes to occur, acts as a transport medium for materials in and out of cells, and keeps organs and tissues lubricated and pliable.

Patient Education

Food and Cholesterol

Patients can reduce high levels of low-density lipoproteins (LDLs), commonly known as the "bad cholesterol," with diet modification, exercise, and weight reduction. Although lipid-lowering medications are available (statins), the patient should attempt to correct a poor diet before adding medication. Patients may not realize that their poor food choices and sedentary lifestyle not only contribute to high LDL levels but also to cardiovascular disease, onset of diabetes, orthopedic injuries due to obesity, and lack of muscle mass.

Carbohydrates that have a low glycemic index and are high in fiber can reduce serum cholesterol by inhibiting the intestinal absorption of cholesterol in foods. The medical assistant can advise her patients to include oats, bran, and apples in their diets. In addition, telling them to substitute polyunsaturated fats for saturated fats will help to lower their serum cholesterol levels as well. Polyunsaturated fats are found in safflower, corn, soybean, sesame, and sunflower oils and can be used for cooking in place of saturated fats, such as butter. Saturated fat is concentrated in the white streaks of fat in meats. The medical assistant can advise patients to choose lean cuts of meat and trim fat or drain fat while cooking to reduce saturated fat in the diet. They should also avoid oils that are "hydrogenated," which means that the polyunsaturated fat has been converted to a saturated fat to increase its shelf life and stability. Foods to avoid include egg yolk, organ meats, whole milk, and ice cream.

Vitamins

Vitamins are complex organic molecules that contain carbon and several different elements needed by the body to support chemical reactions. They are essential for health because they facilitate the release of energy from macronutrients. Vitamins are present in many food sources, sometimes in an inactive form, such as in vitamin B_{12} and vitamin D, that the body must convert to an active form. Many vitamins work together in complex chemical reactions in the body. Thus, a deficiency of one vitamin can negatively impact the absorption of another vitamin. For example, an insufficient intake of vitamin B_{12} causes a deficiency of folate, which depends on vitamin B_{12} to facilitate its absorption. Also, adequate intake of vitamin C aids reactivation of oxidized vitamin E so it can serve as an antioxidant. Paying close attention to inclusion of all vitamins in a balanced, healthy diet promotes proper function of organs and tissues, production of hormones and neurotransmitters, and healthy growth, maintenance, and repair. (See *Vitamin functions and food sources.*)

Minerals

Minerals are inorganic elements that do not contain carbon as vitamins do. They are made up of only themselves and are very small in relation to vitamins, carbohydrates, fats, and proteins. Minerals are commonly divided into two groups:

- major minerals, which appear in the body in amounts greater than 5 g
- trace minerals, which are in smaller quantities.

Although the body only needs small amounts of trace minerals, a deficiency in these minerals can cause health

Vitamin functions and food sources

The table shown here lists vitamins along with their major functions and common food sources.

Vitamin	Function	Source
Vitamin A**	• Promotes vision • Participates in protein synthesis • Supports growth	• Fortified milk, cheese, eggs, beef liver, spinach, broccoli, apricots, carrots, cantaloupe, sweet potatoes, squash, pumpkin
B Vitamins		
• Thiamine* (B_1)	• Assists in energy metabolism	• Peas, tomato juice, watermelon, acorn squash, soy milk, pork chops, ham
• Riboflavin* (B_2)	• Coenzyme needed for release of energy from nutrients in body cells	• Spinach, broccoli, mushrooms, milk, yogurt, eggs, beef liver, clams

Continued

Vitamin functions and food sources—cont'd

Vitamin	Function	Source
• Niacin* (B_3)	• Two major coenzymes that enable energy transfer in cells	• Peas, corn, potatoes, peanut butter, shrimp, chicken, ham, tuna, liver, halibut
• Biotin* (B_7)	• Coenzyme of the citric acid cycle, involved in gluconeogenesis and fatty acid synthesis	• Egg yolks (cooked), soybeans, fish, beef liver, whole grains (also produced by GI bacteria)
• Pantothenic acid* (B_5)	• Synthesis of lipids, neurotransmitters, steroid hormones, and hemoglobin	• Mushrooms, avocado, broccoli, beef liver, whole grains
• Vitamin B_6*	• Amino acid metabolism, synthesis of heme, nucleic acids and lecithin	• Meat, fish, chicken, potatoes, legumes, fortified cereals, liver, soy milk
• Folate* (B_9)	• Coenzyme complex that helps to synthesize DNA	• Spinach, broccoli, pinto and kidney beans, asparagus, lentils
• Vitamin B_{12}*	• Part of coenzyme system that synthesizes new cells, maintains nerve cells, and breaks down some fatty acids and amino acids	• Meat, fish, chicken, shellfish, milk, cheese, eggs, fortified cereals
Vitamin C*	• Collagen synthesis • Provides matrix for bone growth • Antioxidant • Thyroxin synthesis • Amino acid metabolism • Strengthens resistance to infection • Aids in the absorption of iron	• Citrus fruits, spinach, broccoli, cantaloupe, strawberries, tomatoes, papaya, mangoes
Vitamin D**	• Aids in the mineralization of bone	• Fortified milk, cereals, veal, beef, egg yolks, salmon, sardines, fish oils (also synthesized in the body with the help of sunlight)
Vitamin E**	• Antioxidant that stabilizes cell membranes • Inhibits oxidation reactions that can cause cellular damage	• Spinach, broccoli, wheat germ, whole grains, beef liver, eggs, nuts, seeds
Vitamin K**	• Aids in synthesis of blood-clotting proteins	• Beef liver, spinach, broccoli, cabbage, milk (also synthesized by GI bacteria)

* Water-soluble vitamins
** Fat-soluble vitamins

problems. Eating a variety of whole foods that include vegetables, meats, and whole grains will probably supply adequate quantities of major and trace minerals. In addition, intake of a multimineral supplement may ensure that all minerals are present in adequate amounts; however, such supplements should not replace healthy food choices. Vitamin and mineral supplements are safe when taken in amounts that do not exceed toxicity levels and can be used as a guarantee of vitamin and mineral intake. The medical assistant should urge her patients to tell the physician what supplements they are taking because some supplements can affect prescribed medications or blood testing results. (See *Minerals and their functions.*)

Water

Water is an essential non-energy-yielding nutrient. Water is the most abundant molecule in the body and makes up 65% of body weight in males and 55% in females. Without adequate water intake, the body cannot survive for long. Water is a component of intracellular fluids that allow chemical reactions to occur within cells and of extracellular fluids that allow transport of nutrients to cells.

Minerals and their functions

The following table lists minerals along with their function, minimum dietary requirements, major food sources, and symptoms of deficiency.

Mineral	Major Functions	Minimum Requirements	Major Food Sources	Deficiency Symptoms
Calcium (Ca)	• Mineralization of bones and teeth • Muscle contraction and relaxation • Nerve function • Blood clotting • Blood pressure maintenance	• Adults: 1000 mg/day • Adolescents: 1300 mg/day	Milk, yogurt, cheese, tofu, sardines, spinach, broccoli	Osteoporosis in adults, rickets in children
Phosphorus (P)	• Mineralization of bones and teeth • Part of phospholipids (which is important to each cell of the body) • Used in energy transfer and buffer system (acid-base balance)	• Adults: 700 mg/day	Beef, eggs, fish, chicken, turkey	Weakness, bone pain
Potassium (K)	• Fluid and electrolyte balance • Assistance with nerve impulses and muscle contractions	• Adults: 2000 mg/day	Bananas, potatoes, sweet potatoes, avocado, acorn squash, soybeans, chicken, beef	Muscle weakness, paralysis, confusion
Sulfur (S)	• Part of proteins (creates disulfide bridges that stabilize protein structures)	• No requirement alone (part of B vitamins)	All protein-containing foods, including meats, eggs, cheese, legumes, and nuts	No known deficiency (because severe protein deficiency would occur first)
Chloride (Cl)	• Fluid and electrolyte balance • Part of stomach acid	• Adults: 750 mg/day	Table salt, soy salt, meats, eggs, processed food	No known deficiency (because of its abundance in foods)
Magnesium (Mg)	• Mineralization of bones and teeth • Muscle contraction • Nerve transmission • Immune system function	• Adults: 350 mg/day	Nuts, legumes, whole grains, dark vegetables, seafood, chocolate	Weakness, confusion, convulsions, eye and facial muscle twitching, hallucinations, dysphagia, lack of growth in children
Iron (Fe)	• Part of hemoglobin protein that carries oxygen to tissues • Part of myoglobin protein in muscles	• Men: 8 mg/day • Women: 18 mg/day (ages 19 to 50); 8 mg/day (ages 51 and over)	Red meats, fish, chicken, shellfish, eggs, legumes	Reduced immune system function, poor wound healing, impaired cognitive function in children, lethargy, fatigue, itchy skin, inability to regulate body temperature

Continued

Minerals and their functions—cont'd

Mineral	Major Functions	Minimum Requirements	Major Food Sources	Deficiency Symptoms
Zinc (Zn)	• Part of many enzymes • Involved in making proteins • Necessary for taste perception • Transport of vitamin A • Normal fetal development	• Men: 11 mg/day • Women: 8 mg/day	Meat, fish, chicken, turkey, whole grains, vegetables	Growth retardation in children, weak sense of smell and taste, night blindness, decreased appetite, hair loss, slow wound healing, rough, dry skin
Copper (Cu)	• Necessary for absorption and use of iron • Part of many enzymes	• Adults: 900 mcg/day	Seafood, nuts, whole grains, legumes	Bone loss, anemia
Manganese (Mn)	• Necessary for building various enzymes	• Men: 2.3 mg/day • Women: 1.8 mg/day	Nuts, whole grains, broccoli, spinach	Poor growth, neurological symptoms, inability to reproduce (adults)
Iodine (I)	• Component of thyroid hormones, which regulate growth, development, and metabolic rate	• Adults: 150 mcg/day	Iodized salt, seafood, bread, dairy foods	Goiter, cretinism
Selenium (Se)	• Antioxidant • Regulation of thyroid hormones	• Adults: 55 mcg/day	Seafood, meat, whole grains	Heart disease, increased risk of cancer

Water in the body is responsible for:

• carrying nutrients and waste products in the body
• aiding in the regulation of body temperature through sweat and thirst mechanisms
• maintaining the structure of large molecules, such as proteins and glycogen
• participating in metabolic reactions within cells
• maintaining blood volume and blood pressure
• acting as a lubricant in eyes, joint capsules, the spinal cord, and the amniotic sac in pregnancy
• serving as a solvent for vitamins, minerals, amino acids, and glucose in the blood, cells, and extracellular fluid.

Intake of water is principally driven by thirst. The body derives water from liquids and solid foods, such as vegetables, fruits, and, to a lesser degree, meats and grains. **Dehydration**, when water output exceeds water intake, may occur rapidly and can result in death if not treated immediately. Symptoms of dehydration start with thirst, fatigue, loss of appetite, dry mouth, and reduced urine output and progress to include irritability, sleepiness, and, later, dizziness, loss of balance, muscle spasms, delirium, and collapse. Dehydration is a complication of infections that cause diarrhea, where water loss exceeds

water intake. Infants and toddlers are susceptible to dehydration when they have diarrhea. Treatment with electrolyte-based drinks or intravenous fluids will correct water loss. Hot weather can cause dehydration if a person does not continue to drink water in the heat. Avoiding diuretic drinks, such as those containing alcohol or caffeine, will help avoid dehydration.

Planning for Good Nutrition

Adequate calories from healthy food sources promote healthy body weight, growth in children, maintenance and repair of injured tissues, and overall good health. A diet that supplies the necessary nutrients in adequate amounts requires planning. References, such as the food pyramid, can guide a person in making good food choices. The number of servings in the food pyramid refers to portions of each food. Balancing amounts of nutrients is just as essential as including necessary nutrients. The food pyramid provides adequate intake of macronutrients and micronutrients for good health and weight control. It also recommends *whole* grains to include adequate fiber and varying colors of vegetables to ensure a variety of vitamins in vegetable selections. It recommends primarily fresh fruit to include fiber from fruits. Canned, dried, and frozen fruits, while better than no fruit, are a secondary option. Dairy recommendations specify low-fat and nonfat products, which will add calcium to the diet without adding unnecessary fats. Meat and bean recommendations specify low-fat, lean meats and poultry, and the inclusion of beans, nuts, and legumes for protein to limit, once again, unnecessary fat in the diet. The pyramid also recommends cooking methods that do not add fat to foods, such as broiling and baking, rather than frying. The new pyramid also includes recommendations for exercise practices that not only promote weight control but also contribute, along with fiber intake, to intestinal motility. (See Figure 37-8.)

In addition, restaurants and people cooking at home commonly serve portions that are equal to two to three times the recommendation for a serving or portion. The medical assistant should counsel patients on portion control to maintain their ideal weight. (See *Portion control and eating out*.) Finally,

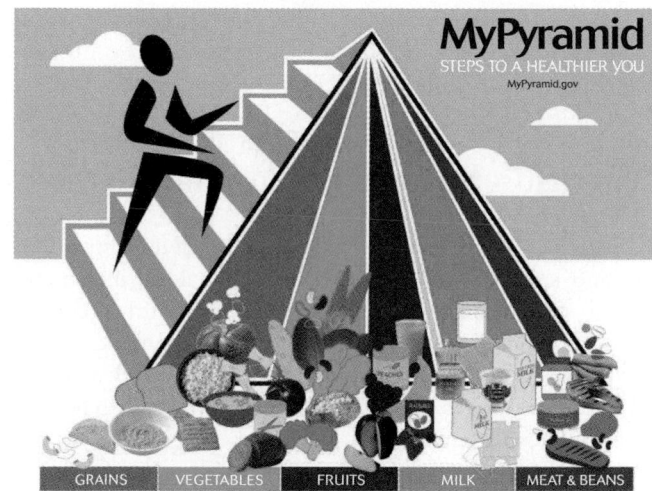

FIG 37-8 USDA food pyramid.

📖 Patient Education

Portion Control and Eating Out

Although some patients eat healthy foods, they commonly eat a larger portion than is healthy. The medical assistant should explain the amount of food that the patient should eat, based on these averages:

- fruit—approximate size of a tennis ball
- vegetables—1 cup cooked (approximately the size of a closed fist)
- meat—3 oz (about the size of a deck of cards)

- cheese—1 oz (about the size of four dice)
- ice cream—½ cup (half the size of a closed fist).

In addition, the medical assistant should advise a patient to use his bread plate to put aside excess food when eating in a restaurant. She should tell the patient to eat a healthy serving of each food, based on appropriate portion sizes, and then ask the server to wrap the leftover food to bring home. Finally, the medical assistant should encourage patients to avoid restaurants that do not offer healthy food choices.

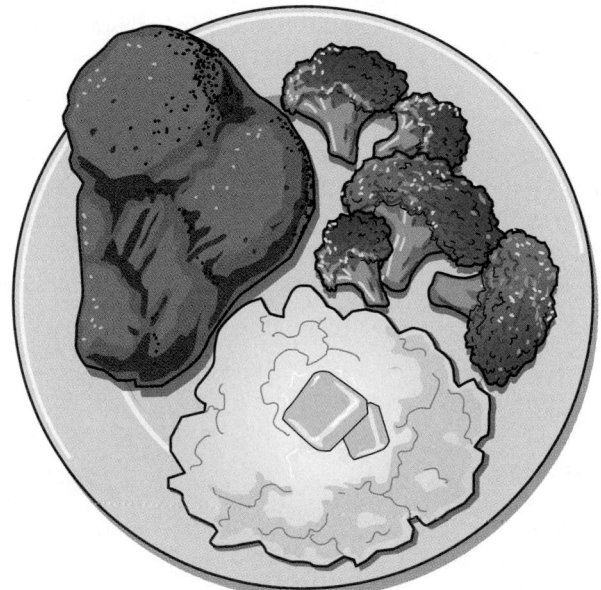

Unhealthy portions

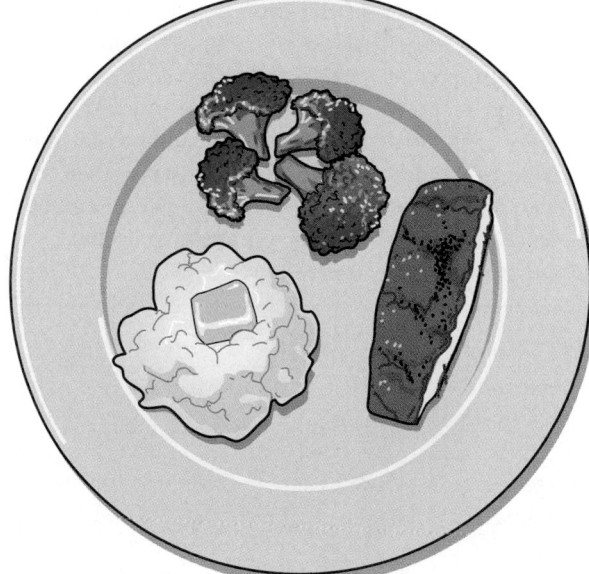

Healthy portions

the medical assistant can caution her patients about choosing foods that contribute calories to their diet without contributing many necessary nutrients. (See *Making calories count*.)

Nutrition for Special Populations

Nutritional needs vary for people in different stages of life and are impacted by health status. Calorie intake and specific demands for vitamins, minerals, and protein change based on health, need for growth and development, weight reduction measures, and activity levels. Such changes or adjustments are common for pregnant women, children from infancy through adolescence, and older adults.

Pregnancy

During the second and third trimesters of pregnancy calorie needs increase by approximately 300 kcal per day. Pregnant teenagers and underweight women may require even more of an increase. Extra calories should be nutrient-dense foods with an emphasis on increasing levels of nutrients needed for fetal growth and development. (See *Dietary needs during pregnancy*.)

The medical assistant should advise pregnant women to limit processed foods, because nutrients are less available in those foods than in whole foods. Problems associated with pregnancy can include nausea and constipation. The pregnant woman can lessen nausea by eating small, frequent meals; eating dry toast or crackers; and avoiding foods with strong odors. She can lessen constipation by eating high-fiber foods, such as cereals and fruits; drinking plenty of water; and exercising daily.

Children

From infancy through adolescence, children's nutritional needs change. The medical assistant must have an understanding of a child's nutritional status in relation to overall nutritional health in the developing child. A child's nutritional needs can be summarized in three basic phases: infancy, age 2 to 12, and adolescence.

Infancy to Age 2

From birth to age 6 months, an infant should receive breast milk or formula exclusively. Studies have shown that introducing solid foods before 6 months leads to an increased risk of food allergies. From age 6 months to 1 year, breast milk or formula should still make up most of an infant's diet. However, at 6 months, the parent or caregiver can begin introducing solid foods, such as cereals, vegetables, and fruit. By age 1, the child can transition from breast milk or formula to whole milk and partake of an expanded diet that includes whole wheat crackers, cheese, applesauce, bananas, scrambled or hard boiled eggs, vegetables, fruits, and meats.

▨ Patient Education

Make Calories Count

Some food choices are "empty calories"; they are foods that contain many calories but little or no fiber, vitamins, minerals, or other essential nutrients. "Junk" foods, such as candy, processed meats, potato chips, and soda commonly contain large amounts of sodium or saturated fat. The medical assistant should explain to her patient that these empty calories should be a very small part of his diet.

For example, the table shown here comparing an apple and a cupcake as a snack shows the apple to be the nutrient-dense, lower-calorie, low-fat choice.

	Apple	**Cupcake**
Calories	125 kcal	154 kcal
Fiber	6 g (0.048/kcal)	1 g (0.006/kcal)
Potassium	244 mg (1.95/kcal)	84 mg (0.55/kcal)
Sodium	0 mg (0/kcal)	140 mg (0.91/kcal)
Fat	0 g (0/kcal)	5 g (0.03/kcal)

Per calorie, the apple supplies eight times the fiber, three and one-half times the potassium, and no sodium. The cupcake contains 140 mg of sodium (0.91/kcal). The apple has no fat, while the cupcake has 5 g of fat. The apple represents a more *nutrient-dense* choice for a snack.

Educating patients in healthy diet and exercise habits will improve their overall health. The healthy medical assistant is not only an educator but leads by example. Encouraging and praising patients as they lose weight or begin an exercise regimen will help them stay focused on improving their overall health.

Dietary needs during pregnancy

The following table lists dietary components of which a woman should increase her intake during pregnancy, along with the amount of the increase and the function of each.

Dietary Component	Increase	Function
Dairy foods for added calcium and vitamin D	To 600 mg/day (calcium); to 5 mcg/day (vitamin D)	Fetal bone and tooth development
Protein	Additional 10 g/day	Development of fetal muscles, hemoglobin, and brain
Essential fatty acids	To 1.4 g/day	Fetal brain development
Folate	To 600 mcg/day	Prevention of neural tube defects
Iron	To 30 mg/day	Hemoglobin synthesis; prevention of reduced maternal stores of iron
Vitamin B$_{12}$	To 26 mcg/day	Activation of folate; assistance with digestion

Ages 2 to 12

Starting at age 2, the child's diet should include a variety of dairy products, meats, beans, vegetables, fruits, bread, pasta, and cereals. As the child ages and tastes vary, the diet can grow to include more seasonings and varied flavors. Portion sizes will increase as the child grows, requiring more calories. (For more information, see Chapter 33, page 641.)

Adolescence

Adolescents experience periods of rapid growth, such as the onset of puberty, that require more energy. The appetite of teenagers varies but should always include healthy foods, not empty calories that offer limited nutritional value. The medical assistant can advise her young patients to drink milk to build strong bones and to avoid soda, which adds unnecessary sugar to the diet. She can also advise adolescent female patients that additional iron in the diet is necessary to replace iron lost in menstrual blood; this additional dietary iron may help symptoms of fatigue during menses.

Older Adults

As a person ages, he may become less active. A decrease in activity slows metabolism and, thus, decreases the need for calories. If eating habits of early adulthood do not change, weight gain will ensue. A decrease in activity is commonly due to painful arthritis or other medical complications. The medical assistant should encourage patients to exercise within their ability in order to decrease weight gain and promote good health. Special nutritional concerns of the aging adult include:

- *dentition*—Patients with ill-fitting dentures may have trouble chewing and swallowing. High-nutrition soft

foods (such as yogurt or soft cheese) provide the needed calcium.
- *income*—Patients on a fixed income are sometimes forced to reduce food expenditures to afford prescription medications or rent. Because carbohydrates are cheap, they may not get the protein and fresh fruits and vegetables needed for good health. The medical assistant can investigate government assistance (such as food stamps) for patients in need.
- *sense of taste*—As a person ages, sense of taste decreases. Because the sweet taste is strongest for elderly patients, they may crave sweets. Thus, the medical assistant must emphasize to patients the importance of balancing sweets in the diet.
- *digestive disorders*—Digestive enzymes and stomach acids decrease as a person ages. These changes may create symptoms of heartburn, gas, and acid reflux that can discourage eating. Treatment for digestive disorders will allow more balanced food choices.

Medical Conditions

In addition to the various stages of life, medical conditions can change nutrient needs and tolerance. Dietary adjustments are commonly necessary for patients who have HIV or AIDS, cancer, or diabetes or have a restricted diet, such as a diet that is soft, bland, sodium-restricted, or aimed at weight loss.

HIV and AIDS

Patients with human immunodeficiency virus (HIV) or acquired immune deficiency syndrome (AIDS) should have a high-protein diet. Protein, along with adequate vitamins and minerals (especially vitamins A, B$_{12}$, and C;

zinc; and copper), will help the patient support the compromised immune system. Because a reduced appetite is common, due to infection or medication, patients with HIV and AIDS commonly experience malnutrition and wasting. Thus, the patient should consume frequent, small meals consisting of nutrient-dense foods to minimize weight loss.

Cancer

Chemotherapy causes many adverse effects, including nausea and loss of appetite, which can lead to malnutrition and wasting as seen in patients with AIDS. Small, frequent meals can help the patient consume sufficient calories and prevent weight loss. Such patients should also avoid fatty foods, spices, and strong odors, because these foods are not well tolerated when the patient feels nauseous.

Diabetes

The physician will prescribe a diabetic diet to a patient with diabetes, whether the patient is using oral or injectable insulin. The focus of the diet is to eat frequent, small meals that will decrease fluctuations in blood glucose levels. The diet also emphasizes foods with a lower glycemic index. Foods to avoid include candy, donuts, cakes, syrups, and alcohol. The physician may prescribe exercise along with a special diet for weight loss (if needed). The medical assistant can suggest that patients contact the American Diabetes Association to learn about their disease and get information on healthy eating habits.

Soft Diet

Foods in a soft diet produce low residue and are easy to digest. The soft diet is commonly prescribed for GI problems to reduce strain on the GI tract. The diet consists of dairy products such as milk, yogurt, and soft cheeses; cooked and pureed vegetables and fruits; pastas; and ground beef or chicken. The diet excludes any foods that require a lot of chewing and produce a large residue, such as raw fruits and vegetables and fried foods.

Bland Diet

The bland diet is used for patients with irritation to the digestive tract such as ulcers and colitis. It includes foods that are low in fiber, dairy products, eggs, cooked vegetables, pasta, and boiled chicken. In addition, the diet prohibits adding spices or salt to foods to decrease irritation.

Sodium-Restricted Diet

Patients with kidney disease, high blood pressure, edema, or cardiovascular disease may benefit from a sodium-restricted diet. Because many processed foods contain a lot of sodium, the diet consists of natural foods and no addition of table salt. Although there are low-sodium processed foods available, such as tomato sauces, soups, and pretzels, patients must read labels and understand the sodium per serving that is included in the food. High-sodium condiments include ketchup, pickles, mustard, mayonnaise, and salad dressing. Patients must pay close attention to the salt content of any condiments they may use. Spices can be added to foods to enhance flavor as long as no sodium is added.

Weight-Loss Diets

Weight-loss diets are abundant and can vary in composition. Low-fat or low-carbohydrate diets can yield weight loss; however, patients may tolerate them differently. A healthy weight-loss diet does not promise dramatic weight loss in a short period of time and does not compromise nutrient supply. Patients seeking weight loss should be educated in balancing nutrition and exercise to lose weight safely and keep weight off in the future. (See *Fad diet hazards*.)

Common Nutritional Diseases and Disorders

Deficiencies in energy-yielding and non-energy-yielding nutrients can lead to disease and dysfunction. Although clinical symptoms may appear slowly, inadequate nutrition always compromises health.

Macronutrient Disorders

Macronutrients supply the calories that the body needs to perform functions. Growth, maintenance, and repair of tissues depend on adequate calories from food sources. If dietary sources provide insufficient calories, called **undernutrition**, the body goes through a process called **catabolism**, in which it breaks down its own tissues to perform necessary functions. In catabolism, the body destroys complex structures to convert them to simpler structures, which usually releases energy. **Malnutrition** is a condition caused by insufficient intake of nutrients, even if the amount of food eaten is adequate. Poor food choices leave the body lacking key nutrients, such as protein, vitamins, and minerals. Undernutrition and malnutrition lead to diseases of catabolism, such as kwashiorkor and marasmus. These two conditions are referred to as *protein energy malnutrition* (PEM).

Undernutrition is a less prevalent problem in the United States. Conversely, overnutrition is a big problem in the United States, as shown by the growing number of obese children, teens, and adults in the country. **Overnutrition** is a condition caused by excess intake of food in general, nutrients, or both. Interestingly, an overfed person can also be lacking in specific vitamins and minerals and be malnourished.

Patient Education

Fad Diet Hazards

Weight loss in the United States is a multibillion-dollar industry. Many people are overweight or obese and are seeking ways to lose weight. Unfortunately, many diet strategies are unsafe. Although they yield initial weight loss, they commonly promote weight gain after the diet ends. Revising eating habits to control portions, limiting empty fat and sugar calories, and incorporating exercise into the patient's lifestyle are the best ways to lose weight.

In general, people should be wary of:

- diets that promise rapid weight loss of more than 2 lb per week
- weight-loss pills that contain large amounts of caffeine, which can cause diuresis and affect the kidneys and heart
- unbalanced diets that limit calories or carbohydrates to very low levels
- diets that require purchasing special foods, which will not teach the patient how to eat after the diet
- use of junk-science terms such as *starch blockers* or *fat burners*
- programs that require a large amount of money to sign up (Most reputable weight-loss clinics earn the bulk of the fee after the weight loss.)
- use of liquid diets, which can cause diarrhea or constipation, lack of motility, and rarely include all the nutrients needed for health.

Intake of a sufficient quantity of food or too much food does not guarantee adequate nutrient intake. Excess calorie intake causes weight gain. Lack of exercise commonly accompanies poor eating habits and adds more weight gain.

Kwashiorkor
ICD-9-CM code: 260

Kwashiorkor is a severe protein deficiency seen in young children in developing countries. Approximately 13 million children worldwide suffer from severe acute malnutrition—either kwashiorkor (protein deficiency) or general calorie deficiency, known as *marasmus*. Of these 13 million victims, 10 million die each year, approximately 4 million from kwashiorkor. Kwashiorkor occurs after the child is weaned from breastfeeding, commonly after the birth of another sibling. The change in diet from protein-rich breast milk to starchy cereal causes lethargy, apathy, irritability, and failure to thrive. It usually affects children ages 1 to 4 years, although it can occur in older children and adults. Adult patients in nursing homes may develop kwashiorkor due to neglect or lack of appetite.

Symptoms of kwashiorkor include a swollen abdomen, alternating bands of light and dark hair, weight loss, dermatitis, and depigmented skin. Because antibodies that fight infection are made of protein, the child with kwashiorkor is at high risk for infection. Additionally, children with kwashiorkor fail to produce antibodies after vaccination against diphtheria and typhoid. Lack of protein carriers that transport fat out of the liver cause the liver to become fatty, and the abdomen swells.

Diagnosis is based on physical examination, which shows an enlarged liver and generalized edema in the abdomen. Urinalysis shows decreased renal function with an increase in specific gravity due to poor urinary output. Complete blood count (CBC) shows anemia, reduced blood urea nitrogen (BUN), serum creatinine and hypoalbuminemia (less than 2.8 g/dl).

Treatment is directed at feeding the patient increased calories in the form of carbohydrates, sugars, and fats. When calorie sources have provided adequate energy, protein may be added to the diet and then vitamin and mineral supplementation after protein.

Prognosis is based on how long the child has been without adequate protein. Early intervention can produce good results with no permanent complications. Children with more advanced kwashiorkor may suffer permanent physical and intellectual disabilities or death.

Marasmus
ICD-9-CM code: 261

Marasmus is severe muscle wasting and loss of subcutaneous fat associated with lack of calorie intake. It occurs most commonly in children ages 6 to 18 months who are living in overpopulated urban conditions. The World Health Organization estimates that deaths attributable to marasmus approach 50% of the more than 10 million deaths of children under age 5 who die of nutritional deficiencies.

Signs and symptoms include emaciated appearance and reduced body weight that may be lower than 80% of the normal weight for that height. Adipose tissue normally found on the buttock and thighs is absent. The child is irritable and voraciously hungry. Marasmus most commonly occurs prior to age 1, whereas kwashiorkor occurs after age 18 months. The diet of such children commonly is diluted cereals, which do not provide enough protein, vitamins, minerals, and calories to sustain life and promote proper growth and development.

Treatment consists of feeding the child at least 150 kcal/kg/day. Children with marasmus are commonly dehydrated and require oral rehydration therapy. Micronutrient deficiencies are addressed after establishment of adequate calories. As with kwashiorkor, calories initially must come from carbohydrates, sugars, and fats. When calorie sources have provided adequate energy, protein is added to the diet. Repeat immunizations may be necessary if malnutrition prevented the child from manufacturing antibodies to previously immunized infections.

Early intervention with feeding will prevent death, but patients with marasmus most commonly have permanent physical and intellectual disabilities. If marasmus is not treated early enough, the body will have lost the ability to synthesize necessary proteins and, even with food or protein, the patient will die. Marasmus is uncommon in the United States, except in cases of severe child neglect.

Morbid Obesity
ICD-9-CM code: 278.01

Morbid obesity is a condition in which the person has a body mass index (BMI) of 40 or greater. The normal BMI range for healthy adults is 18.5 to 24.9. (See *Calculating BMI*.) Obesity increases such health risks as cardiovascular disease, development of type II diabetes, orthopedic injuries to stressed knee and hip joints, sleep apnea, and osteoarthritis.

Obesity in the United States is generally caused by sedentary lifestyle and an abundance of high-calorie food. Certain medications can contribute to weight gain, such as antidepressants, anticonvulsants, and corticosteroids. Genetic factors may include a deficiency of leptin, a neurotransmitter in the brain that tells the person to stop eating.

Treatment for obesity includes a decreased intake of calories and increased exercise. For patients who are morbidly obese, diet and exercise may not be enough to lose weight. Surgical procedures, such as gastric bypass, can dramatically decrease food intake and, therefore, body weight. The medical assistant may be required to educate a gastric bypass patient on eating after the procedure. Compliance with reduced consumption of food is vital for the long-term success of the procedure. (See *Gastric bypass surgery*.)

Syndrome X
Insulin resistance—ICD-9-CM code: 277.7
Hypertension—ICD-9-CM code: 401 to 405 (code specific conditions)
Hyperlipidemia—ICD-9-CM code: 414 (use 4th digit for specific conditions)
Obesity—ICD-9-CM code: 278.00 (nutritional obesity)

When poor dietary habits and lack of exercise lead to obesity, a multitude of health risks accompany that weight gain. Obese people are more likely to suffer from diabetes, hypertension, cardiovascular disease, sleep apnea, osteoarthritis, some forms of cancer, gallbladder disease, and respiratory problems.

Calculating BMI

A body mass index (BMI) of 18.5 to 24.9 is considered healthy. A BMI of 25 to 29.9 is considered overweight, and 30 or greater is considered obese. To calculate a person's BMI, the medical assistant should use this formula:

$$\frac{\text{Body weight in pounds}}{\text{Height in inches}^2} \times 703$$

The BMI formula and values are constant across all patient populations. However, the medical assistant may advise patients differently, depending on their age group.

Adults
To calculate BMI on an adult, the medical assistant must use the BMI formula. Thus, the BMI for a man who is 6' 1" tall and weighs 226 lb would be:

$$\frac{216}{73^2} \times 703 = 28.5$$

The medical assistant can advise the patient that his BMI of 28.5, while not an indication of obesity, does indicate that he is overweight. She should also discuss healthy weight loss strategies with the patient.

Pediatric Patients
A boy who weighs 65 lb and is 48 inches tall would have a BMI of 19.8, as shown below:

$$\frac{65}{48^2} \times 703 = 19.8$$

After calculating the child's BMI, the medical assistant can chart his progress on a BMI growth chart. These charts are used for patients ages 2 and over and are different for girls and boys. Each chart indicates the percentile of growth for that population.

Syndrome X, or *metabolic syndrome*, is a combination of risk factors that greatly increase a person's risk of developing heart disease. Syndrome X includes four conditions:

- *Insulin resistance*. Insulin is produced in the pancreas. Its release is triggered by increased blood levels of glucose. With insulin resistance, the insulin is unable to deliver the glucose to the cells of the body because the cells have become resistant to the insulin. Thus, body tissues do not get the needed glucose for energy. Consequently, the person feels tired and hungry. Polyphagia, or overeating, results adding to the problem of weight gain.
- *Hypertension*. Hypertension (increased blood pressure) accompanies obesity and insulin resistance or diabetes. Higher than normal pressure in artery walls can cause damage to the lining of the arteries. In an effort to heal

Patient Education

Gastric Bypass Surgery

The gastrointestinal system is responsible for getting vital nutrients into the body. People who eat too much food will store the excess calories as fat and compromise good health. Exercise and healthy eating habits are recommended for all people, but sometimes more aggressive treatment is necessary for weight loss.

Patients who are morbidly obese (with a BMI of 40 or greater) may choose gastric bypass surgery to achieve major weight loss. Physicians perform this procedure to treat severe obesity in adults. However, some physicians are also performing the procedure on teenagers. The gastric bypass procedure greatly reduces the size of the stomach

and prevents the patient from eating a lot of food. Weight loss after gastric bypass surgery is usually dramatic, with most patients losing 50% of their body weight. The patient's ability to keep the weight off in the long term depends on her ability to comply with the dietary restrictions. If the patient overeats, her stomach can stretch, allowing her to consume more food.

The long-term safety of the gastric bypass procedure is not yet established. Gastric bypass patients who eat too much may suffer from dumping syndrome, where food is forcefully vomited.

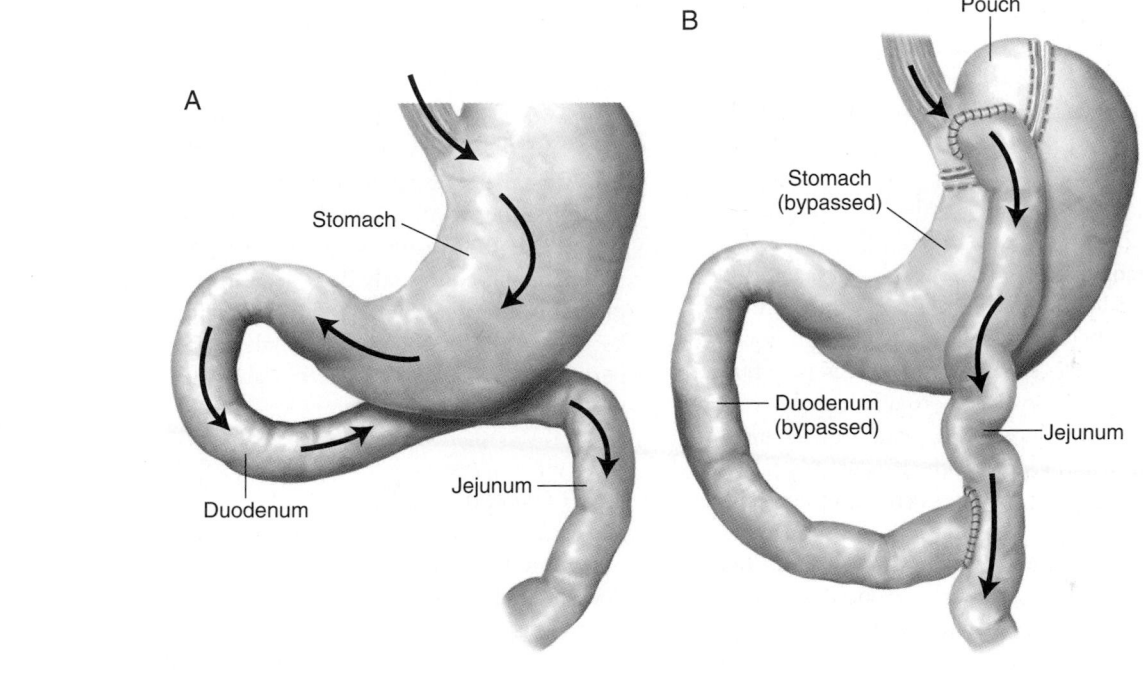

itself, the artery wall will line itself with a fatty plaque, as if it were a bandage. This plaque leads to atherosclerosis (fatty accumulations of plaque that clog the arteries).

- *Hyperlipidemia.* Hyperlipidemia (increased levels of lipids in the blood) occurs in response to arteries damaged by chronic hypertension. High levels of LDLs and VLDLs are associated with increased risk of coronary artery disease.
- *Obesity.* Having a BMI of 30 or higher is considered obese. Obesity in combination with the other three factors in syndrome X greatly increases the risk of coronary artery disease.

A weight-loss program for the patient with syndrome X should include a well-balanced diet, an exercise program, and supervision by a physician. Insulin resistance, hypertension, and hyperlipidemia will decrease with weight loss. Medication to reduce blood pressure and blood lipids may be necessary; however, the loss of body weight will offer the most beneficial results. Dietary changes should include lowering fat and sugar intake, and patients should avoid artificial sweeteners. (See *Artificial sweeteners and weight loss,* page 800.) The medical assistant can educate her patients to take charge of their health using weight reduction and exercise.

Micronutrient Disorders

Diets that lack adequate vitamins or minerals result in various disorders. These vitamin and mineral deficiencies will eventually lead to a diagnosed disorder; however, signs and symptoms of mild deficiency will be present prior to the full illness. Such diseases include rickets, scurvy, pellagra, and beriberi.

Rickets
ICD-9-CM code: 268

Rickets is a weakening and softening of bone caused by a lack of vitamin D, calcium, or phosphate. It is uncommon in developed countries because calcium and phosphorous are found in milk and green vegetables. Rickets is very rare in the United States and is most likely to affect children during periods of rapid growth, when demand for calcium and phosphorous for new bone development is at its peak. It is uncommon in neonates but may be seen in young children ages 6 to 24 months.

When the body is deficient in vitamin D, it is unable to control calcium and phosphate levels. Proper levels of calcium and phosphate are necessary to keep the heartbeat regular. If blood levels of calcium and phosphate get too low, the body will remove calcium and phosphate from bone to replenish blood levels. Vitamin D is found in foods and is also produced by the skin upon exposure to sunlight. Lack of vitamin D and lack of sunlight can lead to a deficiency and, eventually, the patient will develop rickets. In addition, because vitamin D is fat soluble, digestive disorders that reduce the body's ability to absorb fats can cause a deficiency, even if the patient is eating adequate amounts of foods rich in vitamin D. For example, vegetarians who do not drink milk products due to lactose intolerance or a strict policy of no animal products in the diet are at an increased risk for rickets. Rarely, rickets is due to a hereditary disorder, in which the kidneys are unable to retain phosphorous, or disorders of the liver, in which the patient cannot convert vitamin D to its active form.

Symptoms of rickets include bone pain and tenderness in the arms, legs, spine, or pelvis. Skeletal deformities are common, including bowed legs ("bowleg"), a forward-projecting breastbone ("pigeon chest"), an odd-shaped skull, and such spinal deformities as scoliosis or kyphosis. The patient may have multiple bone fractures due to demineralization, causing bone weakening. Delays in formation of teeth and defects in the structure of teeth, including increased cavities and holes in the enamel, are common. Decreased muscle tone and strength are also present.

Diagnosis is based on physical examination, which reveals tenderness and pain in the bones rather than joints or muscles. Blood testing will show low serum calcium and serum phosphorous. Serum alkaline phosphatase may be elevated. X-rays will show bone loss and changes in the shape and structure of bones. Treatment with replacement calcium, phosphorous, and vitamin D will eliminate most symptoms. A combination of foods rich in these substances and supplemental vitamins and minerals will correct early signs of rickets. If rickets is caused by metabolic abnormalities, a prescription for a high dose of vitamin D is necessary to overcome the body's inability to utilize the vitamin.

With treatment, laboratory values and x-ray findings will begin to improve after 1 week. If rickets is corrected early, no permanent abnormalities are observed. Skeletal deformities diminish and commonly disappear with time. Severe skeletal deformities may be treated with bracing or corrective surgery. If rickets is not corrected when the child is growing, permanent skeletal deformities and stunted height may result. (See Figure 37-9.)

Scurvy
ICD-9-CM code: 267

Scurvy is a deficiency disease caused by an insufficient intake of vitamin C. Scurvy is rare in the United States, with a few documented cases due to poor dietary choices. Historically, scurvy was common in sailors and pirates, who were unable to store fruits and vegetables aboard ships for extended periods of time.

Vitamin C is necessary for collagen synthesis. A diet deficient in vitamin C will take 4 to 8 months to develop clinical signs. Signs and symptoms of scurvy include formation of dark purple spots on the skin and bleeding from the gums and the nose. The patient looks pale, may be depressed, and lacks energy. In advanced scurvy, there are open wounds and loss of teeth. Pasteurization destroys vitamin C, so babies fed with ordinary bottled milk sometimes suffer from scurvy if they are not provided with adequate vitamin supplements. All commercially available baby formulas contain added vitamin C for this reason. Human breast milk contains sufficient vitamin C if the mother has an adequate intake. The medical assistant can inform parents to give infants breast milk or baby formula and to never feed an infant under age 1 cow's milk.

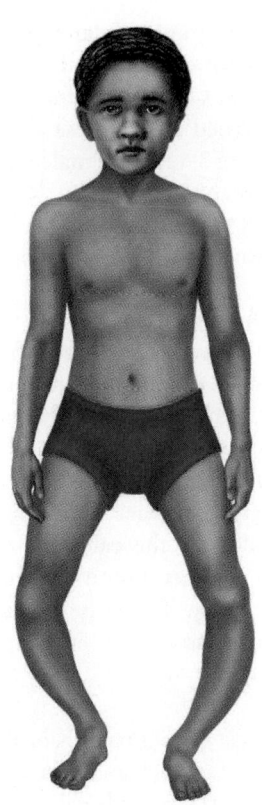

FIG 37-9 Rickets.

A person can easily prevent developing scurvy by including foods rich in vitamin C, such as oranges, lemons, tomatoes, strawberries, carrots, broccoli, and spinach. Because vitamin C is destroyed by cooking and canning, fresh raw fruit is the best source of vitamin C. Vitamin C is so abundant, it is even found in some candy. Need for vitamin C increases after injury, surgery, and burns due to the need to repair tissues and build collagen. People who smoke, women who take oral contraceptives, and people who live in cities with high carbon monoxide levels require extra vitamin C. If left untreated, scurvy is always fatal due to bleeding and infection.

Pellagra

ICD-9-CM code: 265.2

Pellagra is a vitamin-deficiency disease caused by a lack of niacin (vitamin B_3). The deficiency may be caused by a diet that lacks niacin or a diet low in protein, especially the essential amino acid tryptophan, which can be converted into niacin in the body. Foods that contain tryptophan but not niacin, such as milk, can prevent pellagra. However, if the dietary tryptophan is used for protein production (its primary function), the niacin deficiency will still be present. Pellagra is commonly seen in Africa, Mexico, Indonesia, and China among the very poor who do not have adequate food resources. In the United States, pellagra is commonly seen in poor persons who do not have access to adequate nutrients, in psychiatric patients who refuse food, and as a secondary condition related to alcoholism.

Symptoms of the disorder include redness and swelling of the mouth and tongue, diarrhea, skin rash, and memory loss. Early symptoms will begin as a light rash, which over time makes the skin grow thicker and more pigmented and, possibly, slough off. The skin also becomes prone to bacterial infection. Abdominal bloating occurs and abdominal symptoms progress to nausea, vomiting, and bloody diarrhea. Initially, mental changes present as insomnia, fatigue, and apathy. Later, these mental changes progress to memory loss, depression, confusion, and hallucinations. Severe progression of pellagra includes stiffness in the arms and legs and involuntary sucking and grasping motions called *encephalopathic syndrome*. Pellagra symptoms can be summarized as the "four Ds": dermatitis, diarrhea, dementia, and, finally, death. Diagnosis of pellagra is based on the patient's symptoms and appearance. There are no blood or chemical tests to confirm the diagnosis.

Treatment of pellagra is feeding the patient niacin supplements and niacin-rich foods, such as liver, meat, fish, whole-grain cereals and breads, and legumes. The frequency and amount of niacin administered depends on the degree to which the condition has progressed. Dietary requirements for niacin depend on the age, sex, size, and activity level of the patient. Niacin requirements range from 5 mg in infants up to 20 mg in adults with diseases that compromise niacin uptake. Untreated, the disease can be fatal within 4 or 5 years.

Beriberi

ICD-9-CM code: 265.0

Beriberi is a disease caused by a lack of dietary thiamine (vitamin B_1). It is seen in areas of the world where the main staple is white rice, such as poor regions of China. White rice is very low in thiamine because the thiamine-rich husk of the grain has been removed. Beriberi is now rare in the United States because most foods are vitamin-enriched. However, it may be seen in chronic alcoholism, which decreases the absorption of thiamine. It is also seen as an adverse effect of gastric bypass surgery and in patients on dialysis or receiving high doses of diuretics. Infants breast-fed from a mother with beriberi may also develop beriberi. Rarely, beriberi is an inherited genetic disorder where absorption of thiamine is impaired.

Symptoms of beriberi include weight loss, impaired sensory perception, edema, emotional disturbances, weakness, and pain in the limbs. Diagnosis of beriberi is based on physical examination, which reveals swelling of the legs, fluid in the lungs, rapid heart rate, and difficulty breathing. Late-stage beriberi will include memory loss, delusions, and decreased vibratory sense. Decreased reflexes and gait changes are common. Chemistry testing will reveal decreased thiamine levels in the blood and urine. Genetic beriberi progresses slowly and is not symptomatic until adulthood. It is commonly misdiagnosed because it is rare in adults who are not alcoholics.

Treatment involves oral or IM administration of thiamine hydrochloride. A rapid, dramatic recovery is typical within hours of administration. Heart damage is usually not permanent and a regular heartbeat returns within hours of administration. Nervous system damage is also reversible if treated early; memory loss with early treatment is minimal. Food sources of thiamine include unrefined cereals, meats, legumes, green vegetables, fruit, and milk. If left untreated, heart and neurological deficits are permanent and eventually beriberi is fatal.

Chapter Summary

- Nutrients can be divided into macronutrients (carbohydrates, proteins, and fats) and micronutrients (vitamins, minerals, and water).
- Digestion of nutrients occurs in the mouth, stomach, and small intestines with the aid of digestive enzymes and acids.
- Inclusion of all of the vital dietary nutrients will promote good health and prevent disease.
- Because weight management is a lifelong commitment, the medical assistant can help patients of all ages maintain a sensible diet that promotes health by including all of the nutrients needed for their age and physical condition.
- Patients with specific health concerns may require diet modification.
- Although deficiency diseases are rare in the United States, the medical assistant should have an understanding of these conditions and be able to educate her patients to avoid nutrient deficiency.
- Diet aids that promise quick results are potentially dangerous; educating patients on the hazards of junk science can help them make good nutritional choices.

Team Work Exercises

1. Separate into groups of four to six students each. Each team must create two dinners consisting of the same basic foods: a meat or protein source, a starch, and a vegetable. One meal is healthy, with a balance of carbohydrate, protein, and fat and includes vitamins and minerals. The other meal is high in saturated fat and low in vital nutrients. Create a poster or computer presentation comparing the two meals. Calculate the calories from carbohydrates, fat, and protein and determine the vitamin and mineral content of each meal.

2. Separate into groups of three or four students each. Each team will be assigned one of these patients:
   a. morbidly obese 53-year-old male with type II diabetes
   b. pregnant 16-year-old girl
   c. 7-year-old boy with type I diabetes
   d. 42-year-old woman who is receiving chemotherapy for breast cancer
   e. 31-year-old AIDS patient
   f. 74-year-old widower who lives alone
   g. 20-year-old male college student on a limited budget
   h. 20-year-old female college student on a limited budget.

Each team must create a 7-day diet for their patient. Include specific food choices and estimate the cost of the week's food. Calculate the calories from carbohydrates, fat, and protein and determine the vitamin and mineral content for each day. Then the team must present its findings to the class as a poster or computer presentation.

Case Studies

1. Mr. Rodriquez has been a patient in the office for many years. He is 52 years old and has gained considerable weight in the last 10 years. He tells the medical assistant that he has been fatigued, thirsty, and experiencing lower back pain. What blood and urine tests will the doctor order? What should the medical assistant expect the results to show? How can the medical assistant educate Mr. Rodriquez to achieve a healthier lifestyle and weight loss?

2. Monica Durdan is a 14-year-old who comes in for her yearly physical. Although Monica has grown 1" since her last visit, she has also gained 27 lb. She does not participate in sports and talks to the medical assistant about her interest in online games. She states that she hates physical education class at school and usually goes to the nurse's office to avoid class. She tells the medical assistant that by the end of the school day, she is so tired that she comes home and takes a nap or watches television. She wants to lose weight, but because her mom and dad both work late, she snacks and rarely eats dinner. What strategies can the medical assistant give to Monica to help her lose weight and increase energy?

Resources

- American Diabetes Association: *www.diabetes.org*
- American Dietetic Association: *www.eatright.org*
- FDA information on cholesterol: *www.fda.gov/fdac/features/1999/199_chol.html*
- General nutrition information: *www.nlm.nih.gov/medlineplus/nutrition.html*

- Guidelines for a healthy diet during pregnancy: *www.pregnancyfoodguide.org*
- Healthy food choices for diabetics: *www.diabetes.org/nutrition-and-recipes/nutrition/healthyfoodchoices.jsp*
- Healthy People 2010: *www.health.gov/healthypeople*
- Information on vitamins: *www.nlm.nih.gov/medlineplus/vitamins.html*
- WHO diet and exercise guidelines for preventing obesity: *www.who.int/dietphysicalactivity/diet/en/index.html*

- Bales, C.W., and Ritchie, C.S. (eds.): *Handbook of Clinical Nutrition on Aging.* New York: Springer-Verlag, 2008.
- Borushek, A.: *Calorie, Fat, and Carbohydrate Counter,* 20th ed. Costa Mesa, CA: Allan Borushek and Associates, Inc., 2007.
- Holzmeister, L.A.: *The Diabetes Carbohydrate and Fat Gram Guide.* New York: McGraw Hill, 2006.

Introduction to Pharmacology

Learning Objectives

Upon completion of this chapter, the student will be able to:

- define, spell, and pronounce terminology related to pharmacology
- identify the role of the medical assistant in pharmacology
- understand government regulation of drugs
- identify proper disposal of drugs
- differentiate between over-the-counter (OTC) and prescription drugs
- identify controlled substances
- utilize drug reference books
- differentiate chemical, generic, and trade names for drugs
- list major sources of drugs
- identify medical uses of drugs
- identify effects of drugs
- identify classifications of drugs
- differentiate various drug forms
- identify special considerations for geriatric and pediatric patients
- safeguard against drug abuse
- identify patient education regarding drug therapy.

CAAHEP Competencies

Clinical Competencies

Fundamental Principles
  Dispose of biohazardous materials
Patient Care
  Apply pharmacology principles to prepare and administer oral and parenteral (excluding IV) medications

General Competencies

Legal Concepts
  Document appropriately
  Demonstrate knowledge of federal and state health care legislation and regulations

Patient Instruction
  Instruct individuals according to their needs

ABHES Competencies

Communication
  Adapt what is said to the recipient's level of comprehension
  Serve as a liaison between the physician and others
Legal Concepts
  Dispose of controlled substances in compliance with government regulations
  Monitor legislation related to current health care issues and practices
Instruction
  Teach patients methods of health promotion and disease prevention

Chapter Outline

Pharmacology and the Medical Assistant
  Drug Forms
  Drug Categories
    Prescription
    Over the counter
    Natural
  Drug Sources
    Plants
    Animals
    Minerals
    Laboratories
Drug Action and Uses
  Pharmacokinetics
    Absorption
    Distribution
    Metabolism
    Excretion
  Pharmacodynamics
  Pharmacotherapeutics
    Cure
    Treatment
    Diagnosis
    Prevention
    Replacement

Drug Names
  Chemical Name
  Generic Name
  Trade Name
Drug Classifications
Drug Effects
  Therapeutic Effect
  Adverse Effects and Reactions
    Allergic reaction
    Idiosyncratic effect
    Cumulative effect
    Toxic effect
    Tolerance
Drug Interactions
  Synergism
    Antagonism
    Potentiation
  Contraindications
Drug Regulation
  Drug Enforcement Agency
    DEA registration
    Controlled substances
    Record keeping
  Food and Drug Administration
    OTC drugs
Drug Safety
  Drug Disposal
  Drug References
    United States Pharmacopeia-National Formulary
    Physician's Desk Reference
    Drug handbooks
    Package inserts
    Patient prescription information
Teaching Patients About Drugs
Special Considerations
  Geriatrics
  Pediatrics
Chapter Summary
Team Work Exercises
Case Studies
Resources

Key Terms

absorption
Passage of a drug into the body's bloodstream through the digestive system, mucous membranes, or skin

action
Ability of a drug to act on body processes at the cellular level

administer
To give a medication to a patient as directed by a physician

adverse effect
Result of taking a drug that is not therapeutic and may be unpleasant or harmful

allergy
Immune response to a medication that results in inflammation and organ dysfunction

anaphylaxis
Severe allergic reaction

contraindication
Condition under which a drug should never be used

cumulative medication action
Action of repeated doses of a medication that are not immediately eliminated from the body

dispense
To prepare or deliver medicines

distribution
Transport of a drug to body fluids, tissues, and cells

dosage
Physician's indication of how much and how often a patient should take a drug

dose
Amount of a drug a patient takes each time

drug
Any substance that, when taken into a living organism, may modify one or more of its functions

drug class
Grouping of drugs by their therapeutic effect, the body system affected, or their action

efficacy
Ability of a medication to produce a desired effect

excretion
Elimination of waste products from the body

indication
Approved use of a drug, as approved by the Food and Drug Administration

interaction
Effect in the body as the result of a combination of a drug with food or another drug

local effect
Impact of a medication that is specific only to a certain part of the body

metabolism
Change to a medication by the body, which converts it to an inactive water-soluble compound for excretion

opiate
Class of analgesic drugs that depress the central nervous system; also called *narcotic*

over-the-counter
Type of drug that can be obtained without a prescription

pharmacodynamics
Study of the body's biochemical and physiological response to drugs

pharmacokinetics
Study of the action of drugs as they move through the body, including absorption, distribution, metabolism, and excretion

pharmacology
Study of drugs and their origin, nature, properties, and effects on living organisms

pharmacotherapeutics
Study of the use and effect of drugs in the treatment and prevention of disease

polypharmacy
High-risk situation in which a patient is taking multiple medications, thus increasing the risk of adverse effects

prescribe
To indicate a drug to be administered

systemic effect
Impact of a medication throughout the body

teratogenic effect
Adverse effect of a drug on a developing embryo or fetus

therapeutic effect
Desired response in the body from a prescribed drug

tolerance
Need for increased dose of a drug to produce the same effect

toxic
Poisonous or harmful

Pharmacology and the Medical Assistant

Pharmacology is the study of drugs and their origin, nature, properties, and effects on living organisms. A **drug** is any substance that, when taken into a living organism, may modify one or more of its functions. Drugs are used to treat, prevent, diagnose, and cure disease. A health care provider will **prescribe**, or indicate, a drug to be **administered**, or given to a patient. The prescription indicates the drug's **dosage**, which is the **dose** (amount of the drug to be taken each time) and the number of times the drug should be taken (such as *twice per day* or *once per week*). The medical assistant is responsible for understanding the various drugs that can be prescribed as well as the drug dispensing laws in the state where she practices. She must also have the skills to prepare and administer medications to patients safely. For more information on preparing and administering drugs, see Chapter 39, "Dosage Calculation and Medication Administration," page 825.)

Drug Forms

There are two basic forms of drugs: solids and liquids. Some forms are actually semisolid but are placed in the solids category. Categories are based on how easily the medication dissolves. Solids include tablets, chewable tablets, sublingual tablets, enteric-coated tablets, capsules, sustained-release capsules, caplets, lozenges, creams, ointments, suppositories, and the transdermal patches.

Liquids include elixirs, emulsions, liniments, lotions, solutions, spirits, sprays, suspensions, aerosol suspensions, syrups, and tinctures. Tinctures and elixirs are preparations that contain alcohol. The medical assistant must explain to a patient recovering from substance abuse that alcohol is present in such preparations and that an alternate preparation may be indicated.

Drug Categories

There are three categories of drugs:

- prescription
- over the counter
- natural.

All drugs affect the body in some way, regardless of how patients purchase them. The medical assistant must ask her patient what drugs, including herbal remedies and vitamin or mineral supplements, they currently use. The physician must have this information to properly diagnose and treat the patient.

Prescription

Prescription drugs are drugs that are only distributed to persons who have the permission of a physician, usually in the form of a written prescription. In order to obtain a prescription, the person must consult with a physician, who deems the drug necessary and safe for that person to use. Prescription drugs vary in their use and safety; however, all require monitoring by a physician. Examples of prescription drugs include oral contraceptives, antibiotics, **opiates** (narcotics), and medications for hypertension.

Over the Counter

Drugs that a person can purchase without a prescription are called **over-the-counter** (OTC) drugs. An OTC drug does not require a physician to monitor its use. Examples of OTC drugs include acetaminophen (Tylenol), ibuprofen (Motrin), antacids (Tums, Rolaids), and diphenhydramine (Benadryl Allergy).

Natural

Natural products are those such as herbal remedies and vitamin or mineral supplements. Natural products are also sold without a prescription and do not require the monitoring of a physician. Examples include red yeast rice (monascus purpurea) and aspalathus linearis (Rooibos) to lower cholesterol and white willow (salix alba) for headaches.

Drug Sources

The active chemicals found in drugs are from four main sources: plants, minerals, animals, or synthetic drugs developed in laboratories. Drugs that are prescribed by a physician, over-the-counter (OTC) preparations, and herbal supplements all contain active ingredients that allow the drug or supplement to create a physiological change in the body.

Plants

The chemicals that make up drugs can develop naturally in plants and can be found in the roots, leaves, or flowers of the plant. For example, the drug digitalis is found in the foxglove plant and is used to treat certain heart conditions. Morphine and codeine, opiates that can be used to treat moderate to severe pain, originate from the poppy plant.

Animals

Some drugs come from animals. In the past, insulin was obtained from the pancreas of cows and pigs. Today most insulin is made synthetically in laboratories. Cod liver oil is obtained from codfish liver and is rich in vitamins A and D. Heparin, a drug used to slow the clotting process, is obtained from the intestines of cattle and pigs.

Minerals

Drugs are also derived from minerals. Examples of minerals with pharmaceutical properties include iron, potassium, calcium, magnesium, and gold. A patient who has low levels of iron, a mineral necessary for the formation of red blood cells, may have to take an iron supplement. Calcium, found in milk and dairy products, is another common mineral supplement.

Laboratories

Most drugs today are developed synthetically in the laboratory. New drugs are made using biotechnology and genetics. An example of a synthetic drug is co-trimoxazole (Bactrim), which is used to treat bacterial infections such as urinary tract infections. Pharmaceutical companies spend a great deal of time and money on drug research, development, and marketing. As a result, new medications frequently become available, making it essential for medical assistants to continually educate themselves regarding new medications.

Drug Action and Uses

A drug's **action** is the ability of the drug to act on body processes at the cellular level. A drug's *use* is the therapeutic effect it has on a person's body. Drugs can stimulate (speed up) cellular function or depress it (slow it down). Some drugs can destroy cells or replace substances. However, drugs cannot make a cell function in a new or different way. It is important for medical assistants to understand the action of a drug from the time it enters the patient's body until the time that it is excreted from the body. A drug's action and use can be broken down into three main categories:

- pharmacokinetics
- pharmacodynamics
- pharmacotherapeutics.

Pharmacokinetics

Pharmacokinetics is the study of the action of drugs as they move through the body. These actions include absorption, distribution, metabolism, and excretion.

Absorption

Absorption is the passage of medication through some surface or opening of the body at the site of administration of the drug into the body's bloodstream. Key factors that affect absorption include:

- type of drug (For example, adequate absorption of the beta-blocker propranolol depends on normal blood circulation through the liver. Thus, absorption of propranolol in patients with liver disease will be decreased, while absorption of other drugs in such patients will not be impaired.)

- amount of drug (For example, a physician will commonly prescribe a "loading" dose, or large initial dose, of penicillin for a patient with an infection in order to establish therapeutic penicillin levels more quickly in the bloodstream.)
- route of administration (For example, the body will absorb more slowly a medication given by mouth than one that is injected because it must go through the digestive system before it is absorbed into the bloodstream.)
- bioavailability of the drug, or a percentage that expresses the amount of the drug that reaches the bloodstream and the length of time needed to reach it (For example, fluoxetine hydrochloride (Prozac) has a high bioavailability of 72% with a peak concentration in the bloodstream within 6 to 8 hours of administration.)

Distribution

After absorption of the drug into the bloodstream, the circulatory system distributes it into body fluids, tissues, and cells, carrying it to the intended site of action. **Distribution** of the drug may be slow or fast, depending on the patient's size and the amount of the drug given. Circulation impairment can also affect the ability of the medication to be distributed to the intended site.

Metabolism

After the body uses the drug, it must inactivate it (or break it down chemically) in order to eliminate it. Such a process is called **metabolism**, or *biotransformation*. Chemical reactions break down the drug into different substances that the body can easily use and excrete. If these substances are harmful to the body, the body must also detoxify the substances before elimination. The liver is the major organ involved in drug metabolism. Several factors can affect metabolism, including age, the presence of liver disease, and characteristics of the drug.

Excretion

Excretion is how the body eliminates a drug. Similar to food, after the body has used the drug, it must be eliminated. Most drugs are excreted in urine; thus, the kidneys are the major organs involved in drug excretion. However, the body may also excrete drugs via feces, hair, lungs, breast milk, and skin.

Pharmacodynamics

Pharmacodynamics is the study of the body's biochemical and physiological response to a drug. In other words, pharmacodynamics studies what the drug does to a person's body and how that effect is achieved. Many factors affect pharmacodynamics, or the drug's action in a person's body, including the patient's size, age, and genetic makeup. (See *Factors that affect drug action*.)

Factors that affect drug action

Because each patient is different, the medical assistant must have a sound knowledge of factors that can affect the action of drugs prescribed for her patients. These factors include:

- *age*—Infants and young children require smaller doses of a drug because of their smaller body mass as well as their immature body systems. Older adults may suffer from declining liver function, which makes them vulnerable to drug toxicity. Thus, they may also require smaller drug doses.

- *body mass (weight)*—The average adult dosage is based on an approximate body mass of 150 lb. Patients who are less than 100 lb or more than 300 lb will require a dosage adjustment.

- *sex*—Men and women have different proportions of body fat and water, which are factors that affect drug absorption and action.

- *pregnancy*—Most drugs are contraindicated during pregnancy because of their potential for causing birth defects (teratogenic).

- *environment*—Extremes of heat or cold will affect circulation and, therefore, the distribution of medication. High-stress environments such as a patient's workplace or a stressful home life will affect digestion and, therefore, drug absorption.

- *food*—The presence of food in the digestive tract will decrease absorption of most drugs but may enhance the absorption of some. Patients may need to take some drugs with food because they cannot tolerate the drug on an empty stomach.

- *fluids*—Insufficient fluid intake may delay the breakdown of oral drugs in tablet or capsule form.

- *pathological states*—Diseases that affect digestion, circulation, or renal function will decrease absorption, distribution, or excretion. Intense pain will decrease the effect of opioid analgesics. Thus, patients with underlying disease states may require adjustment of drug dosages.

- *genetic factors*—Enzyme deficiencies that inhibit drug metabolism are commonly genetic and will cause idiosyncratic effects. Asking a patient if a family member has had an adverse or unusual reaction to a medication before its administration may avoid adverse reactions.

- *psychological factors*—Some patients' strong belief in the **efficacy** of a drug therapy will cause the placebo effect, in which ingestion of a placebo yields a positive benefit. Other patients may distrust drugs or the physician to the extent that the drug is less effective. In addition, heightened emotional states affect adrenalin levels, which will impact a drug's action. Understanding a patient's emotional or psychological status is important when selecting the proper course of treatment. If the physician suspects that the patient will not be able to comply with a drug regimen that involves four daily doses, she may select a drug that only requires two daily doses.

Pharmacotherapeutics

Pharmacotherapeutics is the study of the use and effect of drugs in the treatment and prevention of disease. (See *Kinetics, dynamics, or therapeutics?* page 810.) The medical reasons physicians and other health professionals prescribe drugs are:

- to cure disease
- to treat symptoms of a disease
- to diagnose disorders and diseases
- to replace a deficiency
- to prevent disease.

Cure

Some drugs can cure disease. When a patient has been diagnosed with a disease or disorder and the physician prescribes a drug to eliminate the disease, the patient is cured of that disease. For example, a bacterial throat infection known as *Strep throat* can be cured by taking an antibiotic, such as penicillin. Also, after a full course of an antifungal drug for a diagnosis of ringworm, a fungal infection, the patient is cured and no longer has the infection.

Treatment

Drugs used to treat a disease without curing it seek to relieve or alleviate symptoms of that disease. This type of treatment is sometimes called *palliative care*. For example, at present, there is no cure for arthritis. However, the physician may prescribe an anti-inflammatory drug to reduce the inflammation caused by arthritis, thereby decreasing pain. Although the patient's pain decreases, she still has arthritis. Also, an antihistamine will not cure allergies but will reduce and relieve some symptoms associated with allergies.

Diagnosis

Drugs can help diagnose a disease or disorder. For example, a radiopaque dye, also called a *contrast medium*, is injected into patients for certain tests. The dye aids visualization of glands and organs, helping the physician make a diagnosis.

Kinetics, dynamics, or therapeutics?

Pharmacokinetics, pharmacodynamics, and *pharmacotherapeutics* may be confusing terms at first. However, the medical assistant can use some clues to help remember the meaning of each.

Pharmacokinetics

To remember the meaning of *pharmacokinetics,* the medical assistant can remember that the word *kinetic* means *movement.* Pharmacokinetics describes the movement of the drug through the body, or how the body processes the drug. The body absorbs and eliminates drugs in the same way that it absorbs and eliminates food.

For example, an antibiotic drug acts to kill pathogenic (harmful) bacteria in the body. The pharmacokinetic action of the drug is oral ingestion of the drug, absorption of the drug into the bloodstream in the intestinal tract, its distribution throughout the body via the bloodstream, and excretion of its by-products in urine.

Pharmacodynamics

To help remember the meaning of *pharmacodynamics,* the medical assistant can remember the *D* in <u>d</u>ynamics stands for what the drug <u>d</u>oes to the body. *Pharmacodynamics* describes what the drug does to the body, or how the drug can speed up or slow down a body process.

In the same example of an antibiotic drug, the pharmacodynamic action of the drug is to target the bacteria and destroy the wall of the bacteria, killing the organism.

Pharmacotherapeutics

Unlike pharmacokinetics and pharmacodynamics, pharmacotherapeutics does not describe a drug's action. Rather, pharmacotherapeutics describes the use of a drug for treating a disorder. Thus, the medical assistant can remember *pharmacotherapeutics* contains the word *therapeutic,* or *therapy,* which is a treatment for disease.

Thus, in the example of an antibiotic drug, the *pharmacotherapeutic* effect of the drug is to cure the infection by eradicating the harmful bacteria from the body.

Prevention

Drugs can help prevent conditions and diseases. Such drugs are commonly called *prophylactic drugs.* For example, oral contraceptives help prevent pregnancy and vaccinations prevent tetanus, diphtheria, measles, mumps, rubella, hepatitis B, and chickenpox.

Replacement

Drugs can replace a deficient substance in the body. For example, diabetic patients, whose pancreas lacks the ability to produce adequate insulin, may take replacement insulin by injection. Calcium supplements help achieve adequate levels of calcium when the patient's diet does not contain a sufficient amount. Patients with hypothyroidism (low thyroid hormone production) can take Synthroid, a synthetic form of thyroid hormone.

Drug Names

All drugs have a chemical name, a generic name, and a trade (or brand) name. The medical assistant must know the many names each drug has to avoid confusion, especially if two drugs have similar names. Additionally, the medical assistant's experience with medical terminology helps her understand some of the drug names. For example, the trade name *Cardizem* has the word root *cardi,* which means "heart."

Chemical Name

The chemical name of a drug indicates the chemical composition of the drug. For example, *butanoic acid* is the chemical name for the drug known as *lovastatin.* Such information is included in the *Physician's Desk Reference* (PDR) or in the package insert. Medical assistants will not use the chemical names of drugs.

Generic Name

The generic name of a drug, also called the *official* or *nonproprietary name,* is not protected by a trademark. It usually is not capitalized and is much easier to pronounce than the chemical name. For example, *lovastatin* is the generic name for *butanoic acid.* Generic forms of drugs may be cheaper than trade name products. Most drug directories or handbooks list drugs by their generic name.

Trade Name

A drug's trade name, or *brand name,* is the name developed and marketed by a pharmaceutical company under a registered trademark. Although a medication has only one chemical name and one generic name, it may have several trade names. The trade name of a drug is indicated with a capital letter at the beginning. For example, the trade names for lovastatin include *Mevacor, Advicor, Altocor, Altoprev,* and *Statosan.*

When a company trademarks a drug, it has exclusive rights to manufacture and sell that drug for 17 years. Within that time period, no other company can develop the drug. After 17 years, other companies can market the same drug using the generic name or another trade name. Because some trade name forms of drugs are so commonly used, that name enjoys the same type of brand recognition as Band-Aids or Coca-Cola. For these drugs, people do not recognize the generic name as readily as the trade name. For example, *Coumadin* is the trade name for the anticoagulant *warfarin sodium*, which is used to prevent and treat embolism, venous thrombosis, and recurrent myocardial infarction (MI). Use of Coumadin is so common, many physicians and nurses simply call the drug *Coumadin*, rather than *warfarin sodium*. Thus, medical assistants must become familiar with a drug's generic and trade names, including correct spelling and pronunciation.

The pharmacologic class of a drug groups drugs by their chemical characteristics and describes what the drug does to the body. For example, the drug Prozac is grouped in the pharmacologic class *serotonin-reuptake inhibitors*. Prozac increases the quantity of serotonin in the brain, which alleviates symptoms of depression. The therapeutic class of a drug groups drugs by their therapeutic effect, or use. For example, the same drug, Prozac, is grouped in the therapeutic class *antidepressants* because it is used to treat depression.

It is essential for the medical assistant to learn and understand the therapeutic drug classes in order to care for and educate patients about why the patient is taking the drug and how it will affect him. (See *Common drug classes*.) Although remembering all the drug classes and their effects may seem challenging, the new medical assistant can sometimes use the drug's name as a clue to its effects. (See *Drug classification clues*, page 814.)

Drug Classifications

Drugs are categorized by two classification systems, or **classes:**

- pharmacologic class
- therapeutic class.

Drug Effects

A drug's effect is the biological, physical, and psychological impact that it has on the body. Drug effects include therapeutic (beneficial) effects as well as adverse (harmful) effects.

Common drug classes

The following table lists common therapeutic drug classes grouped by body system and includes examples and their therapeutic effect.

Class and Examples	Therapeutic Effect
Cardiovascular System Drugs	
Antiarrhythmics propranolol (Inderal), procainamide (Procanbid, Promine)	Promote regular heart rhythm
Anticoagulants warfarin (Coumadin), heparin	Increase clotting time
Antihypertensives enalapril (Vasotec), captopril (Capoten)	Prevent high blood pressure
Antiplatelet drugs ticlopidine (Ticlid), clopidogrel (Plavix)	Inhibit platelet aggregation
Cardiac glycosides digoxin (Lanoxin)	Strengthen and slow heartbeat
Electrolytes and replacement solutions potassium chloride (K-Dur), calcium (Caltrate, Rolaids), zinc	Replace minerals or electrolytes

Continued

Common drug classes—cont'd

Class and Examples	Therapeutic Effect
Lipid-lowering drugs lovastatin (Lescol), simvastatin (Zocor, Pravachol), fluvastatin (Lipitor), niacin (Niacor, Niaspan), gemfibrozil (Lopid, Tricor)	Decrease blood cholesterol
Thrombolytics streptokinase (Streptase), urokinase (Abbokinase)	Dissolve clots
Vasoconstrictors norepinephrine (Levophed)	Constrict blood vessels
Vasodilators nitroglycerine (NitroBid)	Dilate blood vessels
Respiratory System Drugs	
Antihistamines diphenhydramine (Benadryl)	Block effect of histamine
Bronchodilators albuterol (Proventil), epinephrine	Dilate the bronchi
Gastrointestinal System Drugs	
Antacids calcium carbonate (Tums), simethicone (Mylanta), milk of Magnesia (MOM)	Neutralize stomach acid
Antidiarrheal diphenoxylate and atropine (Lomotil), kaolin-pectin	Slow intestinal motility
Antiemetic prochlorperazine (Compazine)	Inhibit nausea and vomiting
Antiulcers omeprazole (Prilosec), cimetidine (Tagamet), ranitidine (Zantac)	Decrease acid secretion
Laxatives psyllium (Fiberall, Metamucil), bisacodyl (Bisco-Lax), docusate (Kaopectate)	Induce bowel movement
Central Nervous System Drugs	
Antianxiety drugs alprazolam (Xanax), diazepam (Valium), lorazepam (Ativan)	Produce generalized central nervous system (CNS) depression
Anticonvulsants phenobarbital, valproic acid (Depakene), phenytoin (Dilantin)	Decrease incidence and severity of seizures
Antidepressants sertraline (Zoloft), fluoxetine (Prozac), amitriptyline (Elavil)	Prevent or relieve depression
Antiparkinson drugs carbidopa-levodopa (Sinemet)	Treat Parkinson disease
CNS stimulants amphetamine mixtures (Adderall), methylphenidate (Ritalin)	Produce general CNS stimulation

Common drug classes—cont'd

Class and Examples	Therapeutic Effect
Nonopiate analgesics and antipyretics aspirin (Bayer, St. Joseph), acetaminophen (Tylenol), ibuprofen (Motrin, Advil)	Reduce fever and decrease pain sensation without causing drowsiness
Opiate analgesics codeine-APAP (Tylenol with codeine), meperidine (Demerol), hydrocodone-APAP (Vicodin), oxycodone-ASA (Percodan)	Alter pain perception
Endocrine System Drugs	
Antidiabetic agents (hypoglycemics) insulin (injectable), glipizide (oral)	Lower blood glucose levels
Hormones estrogen (Estradiol), progesterone (Endometrin), somatropin (Posilac), testosterone (Nilvear), insulin (Humulin), glucagon	Replace hormones
Urinary System Drugs	
Diuretics furosemide (Lasix), hydrochlorothiazide (Microzide, Capozide), spironolactone (Aldactone)	Increase urine excretion
Musculoskeletal System Drugs	
Skeletal muscle relaxants diazepam (Valium), cyclobenzaprine (Flexeril)	Relax skeletal muscle
Multisystem Drugs	
Anesthetics lidocaine (Xylocaine), novocaine (Novocain)	Produce loss of pain sensation (local)
Antibiotics (anti-infectives) amoxicillin (Amoxil), azithromycin (Zithromax), cephalexin (Keflex)	Kill or inhibit growth of bacteria
Antifungals nystatin (Mycostatin), fluconazole (Diflucan), miconazole (Monistat)	Kill or stop growth of fungi
Antineoplastics tamoxifen (Nolvadex), methotrexate (Amethopterin)	Kill or destroy malignant cells
Antivirals acyclovir (Zovirax)	Inhibit viral replication
Corticosteroids prednisone (Pediapred, Prelone), hydrocortisone (Colocort, Cortef)	Suppress inflammation
Immunosuppressants cyclosporine (Gengraf, Neoral), methotrexate (Folex)	Suppress the immune response
Nonsteroidal anti-inflammatory drugs (NSAIDs) naproxen (Aleve), ibuprofen (Motrin, Advil)	Reduce inflammation

Drug classification clues

The ending of a drug name can give the medical assistant a clue to its class. The table shown here lists common drug classes along with a drug name ending that is commonly used in that class and an example of each.

Drug Class	Common Ending	Examples
Antihypertensives	-olol	propanolol
	-pril	benazepril
Antianxiety drugs	-lam	diazepam
	-pam	alprazolam
Antibiotics	-cillin	penicillin
	-cycline	tetracycline
	-micin	gentamicin
	-mycin	erythromycin
	-oxacin	ciprofloxacin
Antilipemics	-statin	lovastatin
Antivirals	-vir	acyclovir
Diuretics	-mide	furosemide
	-zide	hydrochloro-thiazide
Local anesthetics	-caine	novocaine, lido-caine
Opioid analgesics	-done	primidone
	-phone	hydromorphone
Oral contraceptives	-diol	estradiol
Steroids	-sone	cortisone

Therapeutic Effect

Physicians prescribe drugs for their **therapeutic**, or desired, **effect**. The therapeutic effect is the predicted effect that the drug will have in the body. It is also sometimes called a drug's **indication**. Therapeutic effect can be further classified as a **systemic effect**, such as a drug given for generalized pain, or **local effect**, such as a drug used to numb an area of the mouth. Whether the drug has a local or systemic effect depends largely on the route of administration. For example, oral drugs almost always have a systemic effect. If a patient takes a pain reliever for a headache and then stubs her toe, the pain reliever will also help to alleviate pain from the toe injury. However, a topical drug, such as Flexall 454 or trolamine salicylate (Aspercreme) rubbed on the skin only affects the local area. Thus, if a patient rubbed the cream on an injured knee, it would not alleviate the pain of her stubbed toe.

Adverse Effects and Reactions

Unfortunately, even if a prescribed drug provides the desired therapeutic effect, it can also produce other effects. **Adverse effects**, or *side effects*, of drug therapy are effects other than the therapeutic or desired effect. For many drugs, their adverse effects are well known, and a physician will take into account such adverse effects before prescribing a drug. Most adverse effects are merely a nuisance; however, some may be harmful and even life-threatening. The medical assistant should encourage patients to report unexpected or severe adverse effects to the physician immediately so that she can determine if a change is required. Common adverse effects include nausea, vomiting, diarrhea, headache, dry mouth, and constipation.

An adverse reaction is an unexpected, usually dangerous, response to a drug. Adverse reactions can occur as a result of a patient's health status, the number of drugs the patient is taking, or the length of time he has been taking them. Such reactions can be classified as allergic reaction, idiosyncratic effect, cumulative effect, toxic effect, and tolerance.

Allergic Reaction

An **allergic** reaction is an immune response to a drug that results in inflammation and organ dysfunction. Reactions can occur immediately or even days later. Reactions range from itching, sneezing, and a mild rash to life-threatening symptoms. In a severe allergic reaction, called **anaphylaxis**, the patient will experience swelling of the face and throat, shortness of breath, or an inability to breathe. Anaphylaxis can occur within minutes of drug administration. A patient who is exhibiting symptoms of anaphylaxis requires emergency treatment.

Idiosyncratic Effect

An idiosyncratic effect is an abnormal drug response in a patient with a peculiar defect in his body chemistry. Because of the defect, administration of the drug causes effects that are totally unrelated to the drug's normal pharmacological action. Unlike an allergy, the chemical defect of the patient is not part of a hypersensitivity reaction. The drug will have the same idiosyncratic effect when administered at another time. Because body chemistry errors are commonly hereditary, the medical assistant should ask the patient if any relatives have had an unusual reaction to drugs. In addition, she should instruct patients to report unusual drug effects to the physician immediately. (See *Neuroleptic malignant syndrome*.)

Cumulative Effect

Sometimes the body cannot metabolize and properly excrete a drug, causing a **cumulative** drug action. The drug stays in

Neuroleptic malignant syndrome

Neuroleptic malignant syndrome (NMS) is a rare, sometimes fatal idiosyncratic reaction to administration of neuroleptic (antipsychotic) drugs. The features of the reaction include extreme hyperthermia, with body temperature rising up to 104°F; marked muscle rigidity; coma; and, sometimes, death. About 5% to 11% of all patients with neuroleptic syndrome die from the disorder. Drugs that can induce this syndrome include haloperidol (Haldol), levodopa-carbidopa (Sinemet), and chlorpromazine (Thorazine).

the body and when the patient takes subsequent doses, the drug level in the blood rises, becoming unsafe for the patient and causing symptoms of overdose. For example, preparations containing lead, silver, and mercury tend to accumulate in the body and can produce symptoms of poisoning. Also, patients with impaired kidney and liver function and some elderly patients may have cumulative effects of drug therapy because of an impairment in their ability to clear drugs from the body. These patients require smaller or less frequent dosages.

Toxic Effect

Some drug therapy can cause toxic effects that are so harmful that the patient must discontinue use of the drug immediately. Some drugs are inherently **toxic**, such as chemotherapeutic drugs, which cause the death of healthy tissue and may cause heart attack and brain inflammation. Other drugs, while not inherently toxic, can cause toxic effects even when used as directed. For example, antidepressants increase the patient's risk of suicide, cancer, diabetes, and osteoporosis. Nonsteroidal anti-inflammatory drugs (NSAIDs) can also increase the risk of heart attack. The physician must monitor the dosage closely and look for signs and symptoms of toxicity to avoid causing a toxic effect. In addition, some patients, whether knowingly or not, may take too much of any drug (overdose). The medical assistant must educate patients regarding the signs and symptoms of drug overdose, toxicity, or poisoning. The occurrence of toxic effects may be a medical emergency.

Tolerance

When a patient has taken a drug for an extended period of time, the desired effect may lessen or will not occur at all. This effect is called **tolerance**. Because the body of a patient who has developed a tolerance is accustomed to the drug, the physician may have to increase the dose to achieve the desired effect or change drugs completely. Tolerance is a common reaction in patients with Parkinson disease, who

develop a tolerance over time to the drugs carbidopa-levodopa (Sinemet) and amantadine hydrochloride (Symmetrel) used to treat the disease. Because of the risk of tolerance with these drugs, physicians will commonly counsel their patients to take a "drug holiday," which is a temporary discontinuance of the drugs, so that when they resume administration, the drugs will have a renewed effect. However, developing a tolerance to some drugs can actually be beneficial. For example, some patients who take antihistamines for allergies develop less sleepiness when taking the drug after using it for 5 to 6 days.

Drug Interactions

A drug **interaction** happens when the combination of a drug with food or other drugs creates an effect in the body. (See *Drug interactions with foods,* page 816.) When patients take more than one drug, the combination of drugs can affect the actions of the drugs in harmful or beneficial ways. The combination of two or more drugs can cause three different effects:

- synergism
- antagonism
- potentiation.

Synergism

Synergism, or a synergistic drug effect, occurs when two drugs taken together have a greater therapeutic effect together than the expected effects of each drug. Thus, the effect of the drugs is *enhanced* by their concurrent administration. For example, a physician may begin treating a patient with hypertension (high blood pressure) by prescribing hydrochlorothiazide (Hydrodiuril) to lower his blood pressure. However, to achieve better results, the physician may add a prescription for enalapril (Vasotec), another drug for treating high blood pressure. When taken together, these drugs lower the patient's blood pressure to a greater degree than a higher dosage of one of the drugs taken alone.

Because taking two drugs for the same indication increases the effect, the medical assistant should remind the patient to tell the physician what medications she is currently taking to avoid an unintended synergistic effect of drugs from different prescribers. For example, a patient taking eszopiclone (Lunesta) prescribed by one physician for her insomnia should not take zolpidem tartrate (Ambien) prescribed by a second physician. The combined effect of two sleep aids will cause dangerous central nervous system (CNS) depression.

Antagonism

Antagonism, or an antagonistic effect, happens when drugs work in opposition to one another. For example, antibiotics negate the effects of most oral contraceptives. When the

Drug interactions with foods

A patient's diet can affect a drug's therapeutic effect. The physician and medical assistant may need to advise a patient to alter his diet during the course of drug therapy.

Doing so will ensure the drug's proper absorption and intended effects. The following table shows common interactions between drugs and food.

Drug	Food	Interaction
• acetaminophen (Tylenol)	High-pectin foods	Delayed absorption
• amoxicillin • ampicillin • aspirin • erythromycin • levodopa • methotrexate • phenobarbital • tetracycline	Any food	Decreased absorption
• warfarin (Coumadin)	Diets rich in vitamin K (for example, broccoli, liver, beans, rice, pork, and fish)	Decreases the effect of the drug (antagonistic effect)
• cyclosporine • caffeine • warfarin (Coumadin)	Grapefruit juice	Increases absorption, prolongs caffeine half-life, delays excretion of the metabolized form of warfarin
• diazepam • phenytoin	Dietary fats	Increases absorption
• digoxin • lovastatin	High-fiber meals	Decreases absorption
• digoxin • warfarin (Coumadin)	High-fat meals	Reduces absorption
• levodopa	High-protein diet	Decreases absorption
• lovastatin	Grapefruit juice	Increases lovastatin and delays excretion of metabolized form of lovastatin
• methyldopa	Iron	Decreases absorption
• quinidine	Grapefruit juice	Delays absorption, inhibits metabolism of quinidine

physician prescribes antibiotics to a patient taking oral contraceptives, the medical assistant should advise the patient to use an alternative form of birth control during the course of antibiotic therapy. In addition, many stomach acid reducers inhibit drug absorption as well as absorption of nutrients from food. Even so, an antagonistic effect is not always harmful. Physicians can use this same effect to save the life of a patient who is suffering from a drug overdose. For example, the physician can give sedatives to a patient who is suffering a cocaine overdose to control his rapid heart rate and help return blood pressure and pulse to normal levels to avoid heart attack and stroke.

Potentiation

Potentiation is an interaction between two drugs that enhances the effect of either drug, producing a heightened response similar to an overdose. Unlike synergism, in potentiation, the two drugs are taken for different conditions. For example, a patient taking the anticoagulant warfarin (Coumadin) for MI may wish to take aspirin for a headache. However, because aspirin potentiates the anticoagulant effect of warfarin to dangerous levels, the patient risks internal bleeding if he takes the two drugs together.

The physician must adjust drug dosages when a patient is taking more than one drug with a risk of potentiation.

Potentiation may be so severe in some drug combinations that the physician should always avoid the combination, as in the case of aspirin and warfarin. The medical assistant should instruct patients who have been prescribed more than one drug to report an increased effect of either drug to the physician immediately. Although potentiation can be dangerous, it can also be beneficial in such cases as the treatment of headache. Caffeine, when taken with aspirin, will potentiate the analgesic effect of the aspirin.

Contraindications

An indication is the reason why a physician might prescribe a drug; a **contraindication** is a condition under which a drug should never be used. Contraindications identify for a physician situations in which she must never prescribe a certain drug to a certain patient. For example, patients with liver disease should never receive a prescription for lipid-lowering drugs because the mechanism of such drugs is to prevent formation of cholesterol in the liver, which stresses the liver, making it harder for the liver to manufacture bile, metabolize amino acids, and detoxify the blood. Also, patients with glaucoma cannot take some drugs that affect the urinary system because antidiuretics that decrease urinary output can increase fluid retention in the eye, raising intraocular pressure.

In addition, many drugs are contraindicated in patients who are pregnant because they can cause birth defects. These drugs are described as **teratogenic**, or causing defects to the developing embryo or fetus. Drugs known to cause severe birth defects include CNS stimulants and depressants and alcohol in any form. Because many drugs are contraindicated during pregnancy, the medical assistant should ask the female patient if she might be pregnant before the physician prescribes a drug.

Drug Regulation

The United States government regulates all drugs approved for patient use, including OTC and prescription drugs. Two government agencies that work together to ensure our safety are the Drug Enforcement Agency and the Food and Drug Administration.

Drug Enforcement Agency

The purpose of the Drug Enforcement Agency (DEA) is to enforce drug laws. The DEA was formed under the Department of Justice in 1973. Physicians and pharmacists are licensed by each state to practice but must register with the DEA to receive a number if they prescribe (indicate a drug to be administered) or **dispense** (prepare or deliver a drug) controlled substances. The physician has the lawful right to

indicate a prescription (drug to be administered) after she has registered and obtained a DEA number. A physician's DEA number is listed on her blank prescription pads. A licensed pharmacist can prepare drugs prescribed by physicians, and patients can purchase them at a pharmacy. The physician's office may also give samples of drugs to patients at no cost. Without a DEA license, prescribing, dispensing, or selling drugs is illegal. The DEA is responsible for prosecuting drug possession and distribution offenses. Many states have mandatory prison sentences for drug offenses.

DEA Registration

Physicians must register with the DEA by filling out Form 224, which is available online. The DEA assigns the physician a number that must be printed on each prescription the physician writes. This registration must be renewed every 3 years.

Controlled Substances

The Controlled Substances Act of 1990 identifies five schedules, or *categories*, of drugs that have potential for abuse and illegal use. Thus, when a physician prescribes opiates for severe pain, he must do so thoughtfully and cautiously. (See *Drug abuse*.) The legislation provides regulations for prescribing, refilling, dispensing, and medical use of these drugs. The drugs have mood-altering effects and the potential for physical dependence; therefore, they have the potential for abuse. For example, although physicians can prescribe opiates for severe pain, they must take care to avoid overprescribing them and causing addiction in the patient. (See *Controlled substance schedules*, page 818.)

⬛ Patient Education

Drug Abuse

Drug abuse, also called *substance abuse,* is the misuse of alcohol and other drugs. Abuse of drugs may involve legal or illegal medications and can occur suddenly or develop over time. Psychological dependence (when a person merely thinks he needs the drug) can turn into physical dependence (when a person's body needs the drug to prevent adverse effects, including death). Commonly abused drugs include alcohol, marijuana, nicotine, central nervous system stimulants (such as Ritalin), and central nervous system depressants (such as opiates). The medical assistant can direct a patient who abuses drugs to a treatment facility or a support group, such as Alcoholics Anonymous or Narcotics Anonymous.

Controlled substance schedules

The full schedules of controlled substances in the Controlled Substances Act of 1990 describe the medical uses, potential abuse level, prescription requirements, and safety of each group of drugs. The table shown here lists each schedule number along with a description of the drugs' uses and potential for abuse and examples of the drugs included in that schedule.

Schedule	Description	Examples
I	• No currently accepted medical use in the United States • High potential for abuse	• heroin • lysergic acid diethylamide (LSD) • MDMA (ecstasy) • marijuana* • mescaline • peyote
II	• Currently accepted medical use in United States with severe restrictions • High potential for abuse • Written prescription must be provided to pharmacist within 7 days • No refills allowed for a prescription	• cocaine • hydromorphone (Dilaudid) • meperidine (Demerol) • methylphenidate (Ritalin) • morphine (MS Contin) • oxycodone (OxyContin)
III	• Currently accepted medical use in the United States • Potential for abuse is less than for Schedules I and II • Telephone orders allowed • Can be refilled 5 times within 6 months of prescription date	• acetaminophen (Tylenol) with codeine • acetaminophen and hydrocodone (Vicodin) • anabolic steroids, such as oxandrolone (Oxandrin)
IV	• Potential for abuse is less than for Schedule III • Telephone orders allowed • Can be refilled 5 times within 6 months of prescription date	• diazepam (Valium) • alprazolam (Xanax) • zolpidem (Ambien) • phentermine (Fastin)
V	• Potential for abuse is less than Schedule IV • Telephone orders allowed • Number of refills determined by physician	• cough suppressants with restricted amounts of codeine • diphenoxylate and atropine (Lomotil)

* Some states have adopted a Schedule VI, which includes only marijuana that is prescribed for limited medicinal purposes, such as to alleviate nausea from chemotherapy treatment.

Record Keeping

In addition to obtaining a DEA registration number, physicians who prescribe controlled substances must keep records for 2 years of drugs dispensed, including the patient's full name and address, date prescribed, dosage (amount to be taken), route of administration, and the reason the drug was given. The physician must also maintain proper security for these records, which are subject to inspection by the DEA. In addition, the medical office must keep a progress note in the patient's medical record that includes the prescription.

Controlled Substances Inventory

If a physician's office keeps a supply of controlled substances, the staff must conduct a controlled substances inventory at the date of DEA registration and every 2 years thereafter. In addition, the office must keep a separate inventory record for Schedule II drugs. With the inventories, the office must include the name of the physician or practice, address of the medical office, DEA number, date and time of inventories, and the signature of the person checking the inventories. The office must keep these inventory records on file for

2 years. The office must keep controlled substances in a locked cabinet, separate from other drugs, such as samples and OTC drugs. Because the inventory must be complete and accurate, the medical assistant and other staff members should log the administration of a controlled substance in the inventory log at the time of administration to avoid forgetting to log the drugs. If an opioid analgesic is accidentally broken or spilled, two staff members must witness the disposal and sign the inventory log. The office must report any theft of a controlled substance to local police and the DEA and complete a police report and Form DEA-116.

Food and Drug Administration

Through testing, labeling, and enforcing laws regarding the sale and distribution of drugs, the FDA, a department of Health and Human Services, is responsible for ensuring the safety and efficacy of all new drugs, regardless of the source of the drug (plant, mineral, animal, or synthetic). The Pure Food and Drug Act of 1906 prohibits mislabeling of food and drugs. Thus, the FDA must test and verify that a drug whose label claims to relieve pain does have analgesic (pain-relieving) effects before the manufacturer can sell the drug as a pain reliever. In addition, the act mandates that labels on drugs and food are accurate and that all ingredients are listed. Such information is important for people with severe food or drug allergies. In 1938, this law was extended to include cosmetics and to mandate drug testing before granting permission to market a drug.

OTC Drugs

Over-the-counter (OTC) drugs are available without a prescription in the United States. The FDA tests these drugs for safety and regulates the marketing and sale of these drugs, including accurate labeling. The consumer must read the label, decide if the drug is right for her needs, and follow the directions for use. Although the consumer does not need a prescription, she could suffer harm from an OTC drug if she misuses it. Patients commonly call the physician's office for information regarding OTC drugs. Because patients will have varied drug regimens and health histories, the medical assistant should check with the physician or nurse before answering questions about OTC drugs. (See *Buying drugs outside the country*.)

Drug Safety

Although the DEA and FDA have created laws to protect consumers, the administration of drugs to individual patients is made safe by medical personnel adhering to rules for drug administration. Because drugs modify body functions, the medical assistant and others must use extreme care

---

▮ Patient Education

Buying Drugs Outside the Country

Because of the rising costs of prescription drugs in the United States, many patients—especially elderly patients—seek to obtain prescription drugs from other countries in which drug costs are significantly lower. In addition, drugs sold only by prescription in the states, such as antibiotics, are sold over the counter (OTC) in other countries.

However, because the Food and Drug Administration (FDA) can only ensure the purity of drugs manufactured and sold in the United States, patients seeking drugs from abroad are at greater risk for suffering adverse effects as well as fraud. Enforcement of laws that ensure purity and proper labeling and drug dosages can vary greatly from country to country. The medical assistant should encourage a patient who is considering purchasing medication from another country to talk to the physician or a pharmacist about the safety and efficacy of the specific drug in the country of purchase.

In addition, the medical assistant should explain to the patient that many generic drugs are available at a lower price. Patients without prescription drug coverage can save a lot of money by asking for generic drugs. Even for patients who have drug coverage, the copayment for the generic drugs is commonly lower than for trade name drugs. The medical assistant should tell the patient to ask the physician if a drug with a lower cost might be available.

---

in preparing and administering them. Serious harm or death can occur if a health care provider administers a drug incorrectly. To safely administer a drug, the medical assistant must have a basic understanding of pharmacology and follow the instructions of the physician. She must read the drug label three times prior to administration to ensure the proper drug is prepared. In addition, she must always follow the "seven rights" of drug administration:

- right drug
- right dose
- right time
- right route
- right patient
- right technique
- right documentation.

If the medical assistant closely follows each of these steps every time she administers a drug, she can eliminate medication errors. Even when the medical assistant becomes familiar with common drugs, she must follow the seven rights to ensure drug accuracy and patient safety.

Drug Disposal

The medical office must dispose of expired drugs in a safe manner. Specific laws for drug disposal vary from state to state and each medical office must establish a procedure for disposing of drugs and include it in its policies and procedures manual. For disposal of an expired controlled substance or a portion of a prefilled syringe with a controlled substance, a staff member must discard the drug and a second staff member must witness the procedure. Disposal of expired samples of such drugs as antibiotics, nonopiate analgesics, and OTC medications does not require a witness unless specified by office policy.

Drug References

The medical assistant can never memorize all there is to know about every drug, as pharmaceutical companies release new drugs almost daily. Therefore, the medical assistant must learn to use drug references as a resource for important information about drugs. Drug references contain such vital information as drug names, classifications, indications, action, dosages, adverse effects, contraindications, and drug interactions.

Some books are large, heavy, and sometimes difficult to use. There are several smaller pocket guides that are easier to use and understand. Publishers of drug references update them annually and supply information regarding the most commonly used drugs. Most references are also available in software form and the medical assistant can download them onto a handheld computer or data organizer.

United States Pharmacopeia-National Formulary

The *United States Pharmacopeia-National Formulary (USP/NF)* is the official source of drug standards in the United States. This reference book lists by their official (generic) name all the medications approved for dispensing. It lists only drugs that have been tested and certified as having met established standards of quality, purity, and potency. The *USP/NF* is issued every 5 years by the Council on Pharmacology of the American Medical Association, with periodic supplements. It is prepared under the supervision of a national committee of pharmacists, pharmacologists, physicians, chemists, biologists, and allied personnel.

Physician's Desk Reference

The *Physician's Desk Reference (PDR)* is an annual publication concerning prescription medications and diagnostic products. The information listed is generally the same information the manufacturer includes in the labeling or package insert as required by the Food and Drug Administration

(FDA), including a drug's indication, action, dosage, administration, warnings, hazards, contraindications, drug interactions, adverse effects, and precautions. The *PDR* is divided into six sections, which are color-coded for ease of use. In addition, it contains an alphabetical product identification guide that includes actual-size color photos of tablets and capsules by manufacturer. Most medical offices keep a current *PDR*. A *PDR* for OTC drugs is also available. (See Figure 38-1.)

Drug Handbooks

Drug handbooks, such as *Davis's Drug Guide for Nurses,* is a handy reference that provides much of the same information as the *PDR,* yet is smaller and easier to use. It is written for the nonphysician provider (nurse or medical assistant) and omits such data as chemical structure and a manufacturer's index. It can be used as a quick reference when administering a drug for the first time or to answer a patient's question.

Package Inserts

Package inserts are also quick sources of information. These inserts are provided in drug samples that a manufacturer provides to physicians to give to patients. Information in the package insert includes generic and trade name of the medication, drug class, clinical studies conducted, contraindications, common adverse reactions that the patient should report to the physician, how the medication should be taken, other drugs to avoid, and adverse effects.

Patient Prescription Information

Because patients need direct, written information about their prescription drugs, pharmacies attach patient prescription information sheets to the drug container when the patient fills the prescription at the pharmacy. Many pharmacy personnel will ask the patient to sign for his prescription and will ask him, "Do you need to speak to the pharmacist?" The pharmacy should make an effort to inform patients about their prescriptions. The medical assistant, in turn, should encourage the patient to read patient prescription information when filling their prescriptions. (See Figure 38-2.)

Teaching Patients About Drugs

An important part of preparing and administering drugs is educating the patient about the drug prescribed for them. Physicians prescribe a certain dosage to best treat the patient's problem. Patients must be sure to take the correct dose at the correct time to achieve the beneficial effects of the drug. If a patient understands why and how the drug works, he is more apt to take it correctly, enabling him to succeed in his recovery. Patient education regarding drug

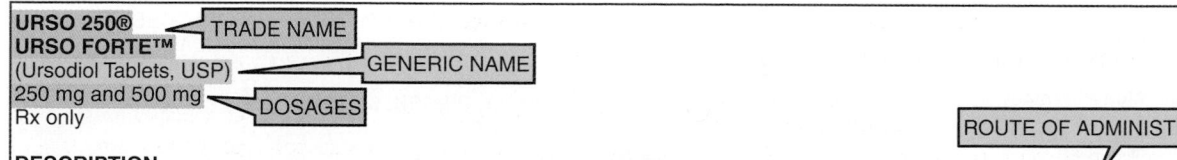

URSO 250® TRADE NAME
URSO FORTE™ GENERIC NAME
(Ursodiol Tablets, USP)
250 mg and 500 mg DOSAGES
Rx only

℞

ROUTE OF ADMINISTRATION

DESCRIPTION
URSO 250® (ursodiol, 250 mg) and **URSO Forte™** (ursodiol, 500 mg) are available as film-coated tablets for oral administration. Ursodiol (ursodeoxycholic acid, UDCA) is a naturally occurring bile acid found in small quantities in normal human bile and in larger quantities in the biles of certain species of bears. It is a bitter-tasting white powder consisting of crystalline particles freely soluble in ethanol and glacial acetic acid, slightly soluble in chloroform, sparingly soluble in ether, and practically insoluble in water. The chemical name of ursodiol is 3α, 7β-dihydroxy-5β-cholan-24-oic ($C_{24}H_{40}O_4$). Ursodiol has a molecular weight of 392.56. Its structure is shown below.

CHEMICAL FORMULA

H₃C
CH₃
COOH
CH₃
HO
H
OH

MECHANISM OF ACTION

Inactive ingredients: microcrystalline cellulose, povidone, sodium starch glycolate, magnesium stearate, ethylcellulose, dibutyl sebacate, carnauba wax, hydroxypropyl methylcellulose, PEG 3350, PEG 8000, cetyl alcohol, sodium lauryl sulfate and hydrogen peroxide.

CLINICAL PHARMACOLOGY
Ursodiol (UDCA) is normally present as a minor fraction of the total bile acids in humans (about 5%). Following oral administration, the majority of ursodiol is absorbed by passive diffusion and its absorption is incomplete. Once absorbed, ursodiol undergoes hepatic extraction to the extent of about 50% in the absence of liver disease. As the severity of liver disease increases, the extent of extraction decreases. In the liver, ursodiol is conjugated with glycine or taurine, then secreted into bile. These conjugates of ursodiol are absorbed in the small intestine by passive and active mechanisms. The conjugates can also be deconjugated in the ileum by intestinal enzymes, leading to the formation of free ursodiol that can be reabsorbed and reconjugated in the liver. Nonabsorbed ursodiol passes into the colon where it is...

CLINICAL STUDIES
A U.S., multicenter, randomized, double-blind, placebo-controlled study was conducted to evaluate the efficacy of ursodeoxycholic acid at a dose of 13 to 15 mg/kg/day, administered in 3 or 4 divided doses in 180 patients with PBC (78% received QID dosage). Upon completion of the double-blind portion, all patients entered an open-label active treatment extension phase.

INDICATIONS AND USAGE

INDICATIONS AND USAGE
URSO 250® and **URSO Forte™** (ursodiol) tablets are indicated for the treatment of patients with primary biliary cirrhosis.

CONTRAINDICATIONS
Hypersensitivity or intolerance to ursodiol or any of the components of the formulation. CONTRAINDICATIONS

PRECAUTIONS
Patients with variceal bleeding, hepatic encephalopathy, ascites or in need of an urgent liver transplant, should receive appropriate specific treatment.

Drug Interactions
Bile acid sequestering agents such as cholestyramine and colestipol may interfere with the action of **URSO 250®** and...

ADVERSE EVENTS (AEs) ADVERSE REACTIONS
The following table summarizes the AEs observed in the two placebo-controlled clinical trials.

ADVERSE EVENTS	VISIT AT 12 MONTHS		VISIT AT 24 MONTHS	
	UDCA n (%)	Placebo n (%)	UDCA n (%)	Placebo n (%)
Diarrhea	—	—	1 (1.32)	—
Elevated creatinine	—	—	1 (1.32)	—
Elevated blood glucose	1 (1.18)	—	1 (1.32)	—
Leukopenia	—	—	2 (2.63)	—
Peptic ulcer	—	—	1 (1.32)	—
Skin rash	—	—	2 (2.63)	—

DOSAGE AND ADMINISTRATION
The recommended adult dosage for **URSO 250®** and **URSO Forte™** in the treatment of PBC is 13–15 mg/kg/day administered in two to four divided doses with food. Dosing regimen should be adjusted according to each patient's need at the discretion of the physician.

FIG 38-1 Example entry from the *Physician's Desk Reference.*

PATIENT PRESCRIPTION

IF YOU HAVE ANY QUESTIONS AB
MEDICATION, PLEASE CONTACT
PROUST, MARK, RPH

#0785 Ph:860.487-2034   **HARTVEIL, SADIE**
                          7 LINECREST ROAD   11-05-09
Mall Pharmacy   WILLBURGTON, CT 06665   **Prscbr: PIECEK, SHARON**
604 REEDY TURNPIKE   PH: 860.123.3245   Refills: 0
BLUEVILLE, CT
06010–0000

IBUPROFEN 600 MG TABLET CPL

CLAY-PARK LABS.

TAKE 1 TABLET EVERY 6 HOURS AS NEEDED

This is a WHITE, ELLIPTICAL-shaped, TABLET imprinted with L167 on the front.
IBUPROFEN - ORAL (eye-byou-PRO-fen)
COMMON BRAND NAME(S): Advil, Motrin, Nuprin

PRECAUTIONS	**WARNING:** This drug may infrequently cause serious (rarely fatal) bleeding from the stomach or intestines. Also, related strokes. This medication might also rarely cause similar problems. Talk to your doctor or pharmacist about the benefi you notice any of the following rare but very serious side effects, stop taking ibuprofen and seek immediate medical atten coffee grounds, chest pain, weakness on one side of the body, sudden vision changes, slurred speech.
INDICATIONS	**USES:** Ibuprofen is a nonsteroidal anti-inflammatory drug (NSAID), which relieves pain and swelling (inflammation). It is u cramps, arthritis, or athletic injuries. This medication is also used to reduce fever and to relieve minor aches a enzyme in your body that makes prostaglandins. Decreasing prostaglandins helps to reduce pain, swelling, and fever.
HOW TO USE	**HOW TO USE:** Read the Medication Guide provided by your pharmacist before you start using ibuprofen and each time y your doctor or pharmacist. Take this medication by mouth with a full glass (8 oz or 240 ml) of water unless your doctor di this drug. If stomach upset occurs while taking this medication, take it with food, milk, or an antacid. The dosage is based needed, they are usually given 6 or 8 hours apart; or as directed by your doctor. When ibuprofen is used in children, the the appropriate dose for your child's weight. Consult the pharmacist or doctor if you have questions or if you need help in arthritis), it may take up to two weeks, taken regularly, before the full benefits of this drug take effect. If you are taking thi that pain medications work best if they are used as the first signs of pain occur. If you wait until the pain has significantly for migraine headache, and the pain is not relieved or worsens after the first dose, tell your doctor immediately. For medication to a child for undiagnosed fever or pain, consult the doctor immediately if symptoms do not improve within 24 reduce your risk of stomach bleeding and other side effects, take this medication at the lowest effective dose for the sho take it for a longer time than prescribed. Do not take the over-the-counter product for more than 10 days unless otherwise
SIDE (ADVERSE) EFFECTS	**SIDE EFFECTS:** Upset stomach, nausea, vomiting, heartburn, headache, diarrhea, constipation, drowsiness, and dizzin pharmacist promptly. If your doctor has directed you to use this medication, remember that he or she has judged that t cation do not have serious side effects. Tell your doctor immediately if any of these serious side effects occur: st in, ringing in the ears (tinnitus). Tell your doctor immediately if any of these unlikely but serious side effects occur: visio
DRUG INTERACTIONS	**DRUG INTERACTIONS:** Ibuprofen is associated with several suspected or probable interactions that can affect the action of other drugs. Ibuprofen may increase the blood levels of lithium (Eskalith) by reducing the excretion of lithium by the kidn ased levels of lithium may lead to lithium toxicity. Ibuprofen may reduce the blood pressure-lowering effects of drugs t given to reduce blood pressure. This may occur because prostaglandins play a role in the regulation of blood pressure. When ibuprofen is used in combination with aminoglycosides (for example, gentamicin [Garamycin]) the blood levels of th aminoglycoside may increase, presumably becasue the elimination of aminoglycosides from the body is reduced. This ma lead to aminoglycoside-related side effects. Individuals taking oral blood thinners or anticoagulants (for example, warfarin [Coumadin]) should avoid ibuprofen because ibuprofen also thins the blood, and excessive blood thinning may lead to ble

FIG 38-2 Patient prescription information insert.

administration is an important responsibility of the medical assistant. The medical assistant should share all considerations about the drug with the patient, such as important adverse effects or special instructions on when and how to take the drug. For example, a patient should take some drugs on an empty stomach to aid absorption. Other drugs cause photosensitivity, so the medical assistant must advise the patient to avoid the sun. The medical assistant should use drug references as needed to provide information to the patient that will help him with his drug therapy. Key teaching points include:

- generic and trade name of drug
- how, when, and how many times per day to take the drug
- adverse effects and what to report to the physician
- possible drug interactions and food-drug interactions

- importance of taking all of the prescription, even after feeling better
- importance of using a back-up contraceptive method in addition to oral contraceptives, if appropriate
- importance of using sunscreen if drug causes photosensitivity
- determining the female patient's pregnancy status before prescribing a drug.

Special Considerations

Some groups of patients require special consideration for drug administration. Two of the major groups requiring special consideration include elderly patients and children because they do not necessarily respond to a drug in the same way an adult patient would. Patients who are extremely small (under 100 lb) or large (over 300 lb) will also require different dosages to achieve the desired effect of the prescribed drug.

Geriatrics

Patients ages 65 and older are categorized as *geriatric*. The physician must give special consideration to drugs prescribed to geriatric patients for several reasons. First, as the body ages, body processes slow down. These changes in the body effect a change in the pharmacokinetics of a drug, including its absorption, distribution, metabolism, and excretion. In addition, cumulative effects may occur if drugs are not dosed properly (usually lower than in adults) or eliminated effectively. Second, the medical assistant should ask the patient if he has dysphagia (difficulty swallowing), because the physician may need to indicate that the pharmacy should provide an oral drug in liquid form. Third, many geriatric patients are taking multiple medications, a situation called **polypharmacy**, which increases the risk of drug interactions and adverse effects. As a patient's hearing and vision decrease, the pharmacy or medical assistant should provide information in large print and speak clearly and slowly, asking the patient to repeat the information to ensure accurate understanding of the instructions. In addition, the patient may need help from a family member to administer drugs correctly. The medical assistant should recommend that the patient use a pill container, which separates pills into individual compartments by day or time, to ensure that he is taking the required drugs at the appropriate time and dosage. If the patient can put a week's worth of drugs into a marked container, he will more easily remember to take them on time. (See Figure 38-3.) The medical assistant should also encourage patients to rotate injection sites and use mapping for daily injection therapy to avoid scarring and infection. Finally, the medical assistant should take

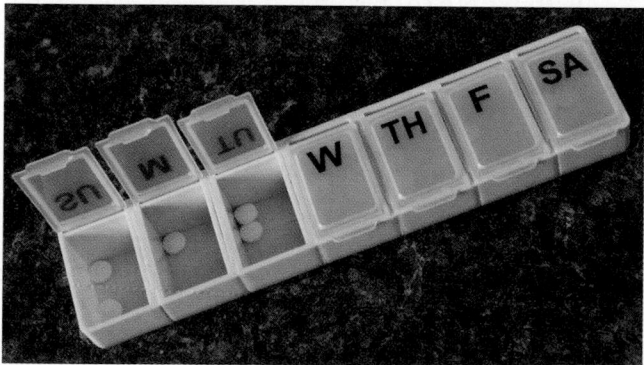

FIG 38-3 Pill container with drugs separated by days of the week.

extra time with geriatric patients to explain drug therapy and answer any questions they may have.

Pediatrics

Pediatric patients include neonates, infants, and children up to about age 18. This group requires special consideration because medications are based on body weight or body mass. A pediatric patient's body weight and body mass are lower than average for regular drug dosages, so the medical assistant should take care to properly weigh and measure pediatric patients and record their vital signs. The pediatrician or medical assistant must calculate pediatric dosages by milligrams per kilogram of body weight. When calculating pediatric dosages, the medical assistant should double-check her results and ask the physician or other allied health professionals for assistance, if needed. (For more information on calculating pediatric dosages, see Chapter 39, "Dosage Calculation and Medication Administration," page 825.) In addition, some children have trouble swallowing tablets or capsules. If doing so is difficult or impossible, the physician may need to prescribe the drug in a liquid form. Finally, the medical assistant should provide clear instructions to parents or caregivers and speak at the child's level of understanding when explaining drug therapy. She should emphasize that a drug is not candy, even if it tastes good, and that only a parent or caregiver, school nurse, medical assistant, or physician in the office should give drugs to the child.

Chapter Summary
- The role of the medical assistant in pharmacology is to safely and accurately prepare and administer medications as directed by a physician.
- Drug sources include plants, animals, minerals, and laboratories.
- Drugs come in basically two forms: solids and liquids.
- The medical assistant must have an understanding of the pharmacotherapeutics, pharmacodynamics, and pharmacokinetics of drugs to educate her patients and understand how the body uses drugs.
- Medical uses of drugs include to cure, treat, prevent, and diagnose disease or replace a substance that is missing or lost.
- Prescription drugs are obtained when the physician writes a prescription for that specific medication. Over-the-counter medications are available without a prescription. Natural products are also OTC products and include vitamins, minerals, and herbal supplements.
- Many factors influence drug action, including age, body mass, sex, environment, presence of food in the digestive tract, and genetics.

- Drugs have an official name, a chemical name, a brand or trade name, and a generic name.
- Drugs can be classified according to their pharmacologic action or therapeutic effect.
- Drug effects include therapeutic effect, adverse effect, cumulative effect, tolerance, and toxic effect.
- Drug reference materials include *USP/NF, PDR,* nursing drug handbooks, package inserts, and software. These materials provide vital information for medical assistants and patients.
- Government regulation of drugs is overseen by the DEA and FDA.
- Controlled substances are listed in five schedules, categorized according to abuse potential.
- The medical assistant must be familiar with drug storage and proper drug disposal.
- Patient education is an important part of drug therapy. The medical assistant is a source of information for patients, so she must provide safe, accurate, up-to-date information regarding drugs and drug therapy.
- Geriatric and pediatric patients metabolize drugs differently, so the medical assistant must consider adjustments in dosages and choices of drugs.

Team Work Exercises

1. Divide into groups of two to three students. The instructor will provide each group with a drug class. Each group must research various drugs within the class and create a poster about the drug that includes:
   a. generic names of drugs
   b. trade names of drugs
   c. uses for each drug (such as disease, body system, and so on)
   d. actions of each drug
   e. adverse effects and adverse reactions of each drug
   f. contraindications for each drug.
2. Divide into groups of two to three students. Each group must research and report to the class on one of the following topics, as assigned by the instructor:
   a. Doctor of Pharmacy Program—Look at programs in the area and provide a list of colleges that offer the program and the requirements.
   b. Pharmaceutical Manufacturer—Research one pharmaceutical company and provide a list of the drugs they manufacture. Does this company have a program that provides medications to patients free of charge? If so, describe the program.
   c. Federal Drug Enforcement Agency—Log onto the DEA website and read and report on the current press releases.
   d. Food and Drug Administration—log onto the FDA website and report on the recalls and safety alerts posted, any current job opportunities, and information on medical devices.

Case Studies

1. Ricardo is a 34-year-old male patient who complains of nausea whenever he takes his medication. He tells the medical assistant that he just started this new medication a couple of days ago. What type of effect is Ricardo describing? What will the physician likely talk to Ricardo about?
2. Mary, a 10-year-old female patient, has *Strep* throat. The physician treated her the day before with penicillin. After the first dose, Mary's mother noticed a red rash on her neck and chest. Mary does not complain of itching, but her mother thought she should call the physician anyway. Did Mary's mother do the right thing? What is the likely cause of Mary's rash?

Resources

- DEA forms: *www.dea.gov*
- Information on clinical drug trials and substance abuse: *www.nih.gov*
- Information on vaccines, drug-resistant antibiotics, and methadone dispensing: *www.cdc.gov*
- U.S. Food and Drug Administration: *www.fda.gov*
- Deglin, J.H., and Vallerand, A.H.: *Davis's Drug Guide for Nurses,* 11th ed. Philadelphia: F.A. Davis Company, 2008.
- Katzung, B.G.: *Basic and Clinical Pharmacology,* 10th ed. New York: McGraw-Hill Co., 2006.
- *Physician's Desk Reference* online: *www.pdr.net*
- Ritter, J.M., et al.: *Textbook of Clinical Pharmacology and Therapeutics,* 5th ed. New York: Oxford University Press, USA, 2008.
- Swanson, T.A., and Kim, S.I.: *Pharmacology Flash Cards.* Philadelphia: Lippincott Williams & Wilkins, 2004.

Dosage Calculation and Medication Administration

Learning Objectives

Upon completion of this chapter, the student will be able to:

- define and spell terms related to dosage calculation and medication administration
- identify the role of the medical assistant in medication administration
- understand state laws and guidelines for medication administration
- identify systems of measurement
- identify common conversions between systems
- calculate drug dosages
- practice safety in dosage calculation and medication administration
- identify routes of administration
- identify parts of a prescription
- accurately use accepted abbreviations associated with prescriptions and medication administration
- refill telephone prescriptions per a physician's order
- identify special considerations in dosage calculation and medication administration
- differentiate between types of medication orders
- identify supplies used in medication administration
- educate the patient regarding medication administration.

CAAHEP Competencies

Clinical Competencies

Patient Care

Apply pharmacology principles to prepare and administer oral and parenteral (excluding IV) medications

Maintain medication and immunization records

General Competencies

Legal Concepts

Perform within legal and ethical boundaries

Document appropriately

Demonstrate knowledge of federal and state health care legislation and regulations

Patient Instruction

Instruct individuals according to their needs

ABHES Competencies

Professionalism

Evidence a responsible attitude

Conduct work within scope of education, training, and ability

Communication

Adapt what is said to the recipient's level of comprehension

Serve as a liaison between the physician and others

Clinical Duties

Apply principles of aseptic techniques and infection control

Prepare and administer oral and parenteral medications as directed by the physician

Dispose of biohazardous materials

Practice standard precautions

Legal Concepts

Dispose of controlled substances in compliance with government regulations

Procedures

Administering an oral medication

Preparing a parenteral medication from a vial

Preparing a parenteral medication from an ampule

Administering a subcutaneous injection

Administering an intradermal injection

Administering an intramuscular injection

Administering a transdermal patch

Chapter Outline

Dosage Calculation

Systems of Measurement

Metric system

Apothecary and household systems

Calculation Methods

Dose on hand

Ratio and proportion

Fractional equation

Using conversions

Calculating infant and child dosages

Medication Administration

Parts of a Prescription

Routes of Medication Administration

Oral

Parenteral

Chapter Summary

Team Work Exercises

Case Studies

Resources

Key Terms

apothecary
System of weights and measures based on the yard

buccal
Route of administration that involves placement of a drug between the cheek and gum

capsule
Special container made of gelatin sized to contain a single dose of an oral medication

enteric-coated
Drug formulation in which tablets or capsules are coated with a compound that does not dissolve until exposed to the fluids of the small intestine

household
System of volume measurement using the teaspoon and tablespoon

intradermal
Route of administration that involves injection of a drug just under the epidermis

intramuscular
Route of administration that involves injection of a drug into the muscle

intravenous
Route of administration that involves injection of a drug into a vein

meniscus
Curved upper surface of a liquid in a container

metric
System of weights and measures based on the meter

oral route
Route of administration of a medication through the mouth and into the GI tract

route of administration
Way in which medication is introduced into the body

subcutaneous
Route of administration that involves injection of a drug into the fatty layer under the skin

sublingual
Route of administration that involves placement of a drug under the tongue

suspension
Solid particles mixed in a liquid but not dissolved

syrup
Concentrated solution of sugar and water to which medicine is added and taken orally

tablet
Small, disklike mass of medicine in compressed powder form taken orally

Z-track injection
Intramuscular injection technique where the skin is pulled to one side to prevent medication from leaking into the subcutaneous tissues

Dosage Calculation

When a physician orders a medication, the medical assistant must administer the correct amount of the medication. Because the dosage ordered will not always match the available doses, the medical assistant must calculate the proper dosage for her patient.

Systems of Measurement

In order to accurately calculate dosages, the medical assistant must have an understanding of the metric, household, and apothecary systems of measurement. No matter what system is used, medications dispensed to patients are measured in quantities of liquid (volume) or solid (weight).

Metric System

The **metric** system is a system of weights and measures based on the meter. It is the most commonly used system for drug dosages. Within that system, the milliliter (ml), sometimes called a cubic centimeter (cc), is used for liquid medications and milligram (mg) is used for solid medications. (See *How to remember metric fix unequal word/units.*)

Apothecary and Household Systems

Although the metric units of milligrams and milliliters are most common in medication dosages, the apothecary and household systems are sometimes used. The **apothecary** system is a system of measurement based on the yard. The units of weight in this system include grain and ounce. Volume measures in the apothecary system include minim, fluidram, pint, and quart. The **household** system measures for liquids are drop, teaspoon, tablespoon, fluid ounce, pint, cup, and quart. Household measures for weight are ounce and pound. Some of the units of measure for apothecary and household units are the same, which can cause confusion. In addition, teaspoon and tablespoon containers are commonly poorly calibrated; thus, the patient may get too much or too little of the medication. In addition, these units of measure are used to measure liquid and dry ingredients, adding more confusion. For these reasons, medications are most commonly ordered in metric doses and should be calculated in metric doses. In addition, household measures do not provide precise measurement of smaller quantities of prescribed drugs. For example, 60 mg of a drug would equal less than 1/4 teaspoon, the smallest unit in the household system. If the medical assistant must convert from apothecary or household to metric, she must pay careful attention to the conversions to avoid overmedicating or undermedicating her patient. (See *Converting to metric.*)

How to remember metric units

To help remember the metric units of measure, the medical assistant can use this mnemonic:
King Henry Died While Drinking Chocolate Milk:

King	Henry	Died	While	Drinking	Chocolate	Milk
Kilo	Hecto	Deca	Whole	Deci	Centi	Milli
1000	100	10	1	0.1	0.01	0.001

Calculation Methods

To administer the correct amount of medication to the patient, the medical assistant must calculate the correct dose. There are several methods for calculating the dose. For example, the medication order reads *Dilantin 50 mg PO t.i.d.* The drug available is *Dilantin 125 mg/5 ml.* Methods for calculating the dosage include:

- dose on hand method
- ratio and proportion method
- fractional equation method.

Converting to metric

The following table provides conversions from apothecary and household units into metric units. The medical assistant can use a table such as this to quickly convert measurements, aiding timely, accurate dosage calculations.

Household	Apothecary	Metric
Dry		
—	1 gr	60 milligrams (mg)
¼ teaspoon (tsp)	15 grains (gr)	1 gram (g)
1 tablespoon (Tbs)	4 drams (dr)	15 g
(3 tsp)		
1 ounce (oz)	1 oz	30 g
2.2 pounds (lb)		1 kilogram (kg)
		(1000 mg)
Liquid		
1 drop (gt)	1 minim (m)	
15 drops (gtt)	15 m	1 milliliter (ml)
1 tsp	1 fldr (fluidram)	5 ml (5 cubic
		centimeters)
1 Tbs	4 fldr	15 ml
1 fluid ounce	1 oz (8 fldr)	30 ml
(fl oz) (2 Tbs)		
1 pint (pt) or	1 pint (pt)	480 ml
2 cups (c)		
4 c (1 quart)	1 quart (qt) (2 pt)	960 ml

For each method, the medical assistant must remember a formula containing these elements:

- dose ordered or desired dose (D)
- dose on container label or dose on hand (H)
- form and amount in which the drug is available, such as tablet, capsule, or liquid (V)
- amount to give (A).

Dose on Hand

To calculate the dose using the dose on hand method, the medical assistant must remember this formula:

$$\frac{D \times V}{H} = A$$

$$\frac{50 \text{ mg} \times 5 \text{ ml}}{125 \text{ mg}} = A$$

$$\frac{250 \text{ ml}}{125} = 2 \text{ ml}$$

Ratio and Proportion

To calculate the dose using the ratio and proportion method, the medical assistant must remember this formula:

$$HA = DV$$
$$125 \text{ mg} \times A = 50 \text{ mg} \times 5 \text{ ml}$$
$$125 \text{ mg} \times A = 250 \text{ mg/ml}$$
$$A = \frac{250 \text{ mg/ml}}{125 \text{ mg}}$$
$$A = 2 \text{ ml}$$

Fractional Equation

To calculate the dose using the ratio and proportion method, the medical assistant must remember this formula:

$$\frac{H}{V} = \frac{D}{A}$$

$$\frac{125 \text{ mg}}{5 \text{ ml}} = \frac{50 \text{ mg}}{A}$$

$$125 \text{ mg} \times A = 50 \text{ mg} \times 5 \text{ ml}$$

$$A = \frac{50 \text{ mg} \times 5 \text{ ml}}{125 \text{ mg}}$$

$$A = 2 \text{ ml}$$

Using Conversions

If the dose on hand and the dose ordered are measured with different systems, the medical assistant must perform some conversions before she can calculate the correct dose. For example, if the order contains the dosage *Nitrostat gr 1/400 prn for angina pain* and the dose on hand is *Nitrostat 0.3-mg tablets*, the medical assistant must first convert grains to milligrams. Using the conversion table, the medical assistant will know that 1 grain equals 60 mg. Using this conversion, the medical assistant can calculate the dose using the dose on hand method:

$$1 \text{ grain} = 60 \text{ mg}$$

$$\frac{\text{gr } 1}{400} = \frac{60 \text{ mg}}{400} = \frac{3 \text{ mg}}{20} = 0.15 \text{ mg}$$

$$\frac{0.15 \text{ mg}}{0.3 \text{ mg}} = 0.5 \text{ tablet}$$

Also, some doses are measured with the same system but with different units within the system. The medical assistant must also perform conversions in this case. For example, if the order says *0.5 g amoxicillin* and the dose on hand is *250-mg tablets*, the medical assistant must first convert grams to milligrams. Using the conversion table, the medical assistant will know that 0.5 g equals 500 mg. Using this conversion, the medical assistant can calculate the dose:

$$\frac{500 \text{ mg}}{250 \text{ mg}} = 2 \text{ tablets}$$

Calculating Infant and Child Dosages

The medical assistant must calculate dosages for pediatric patients according to their body size. Administering an adult dose of a medication to an infant or child would increase the risk of overdose and would not be therapeutic. Two main methods of calculating pediatric dosages include the weight method and the body surface area method.

Weight Method

The medical assistant can calculate infant and child dosages according to the patient's weight. Because most dosages are expressed using kilograms (kg), the medical assistant must also convert pounds to kilograms in order to calculate accurately. For example, the medical assistant is calculating a dosage for a 6-year-old patient who weighs 55 lb. The physician's order reads *lidocaine 1 mg/kg*. In order to provide the accurate dose, the medical assistant must convert 55 lb into equivalent kilograms. Using the conversion table, she will know that 1 kg equals 2.2 lb. Using this conversion, the medical assistant can calculate the dose:

$$55 \div 2.2 \text{ kg} = 25 \text{ kg}$$
$$25 \times 1 \text{ mg} = 25 \text{ mg}$$

Body Surface Area Method

The medical assistant can also use the body surface area (BSA) of the infant or child to calculate an accurate dose for a pediatric patient. In order to calculate BSA, the medical assistant must use a chart called a *nomogram*. On the chart, the medical assistant enters the height and weight of the child. Then she must draw a straight line from the point on the chart where the height is plotted to the point where the weight is plotted. The intersection of that line on the BSA line is the body surface in square meters. (See Figure 39-1.) For example, if the child's height is 45" and his weight is 38 lb, his BSA equals 0.74. Thus, if the adult dose of the medication is 500 mg, the medical assistant can calculate the desired dose by using this formula:

$$(BSA^2 \div 1.7) \times \text{adult dose} = \text{desired dose}$$
$$(0.74^2 \div 1.7) \times 500 \text{ mg}$$
$$(0.55 \div 1.7) \times 500 \text{ mg}$$
$$0.32 \times 500 \text{ mg} = 160 \text{ mg}$$

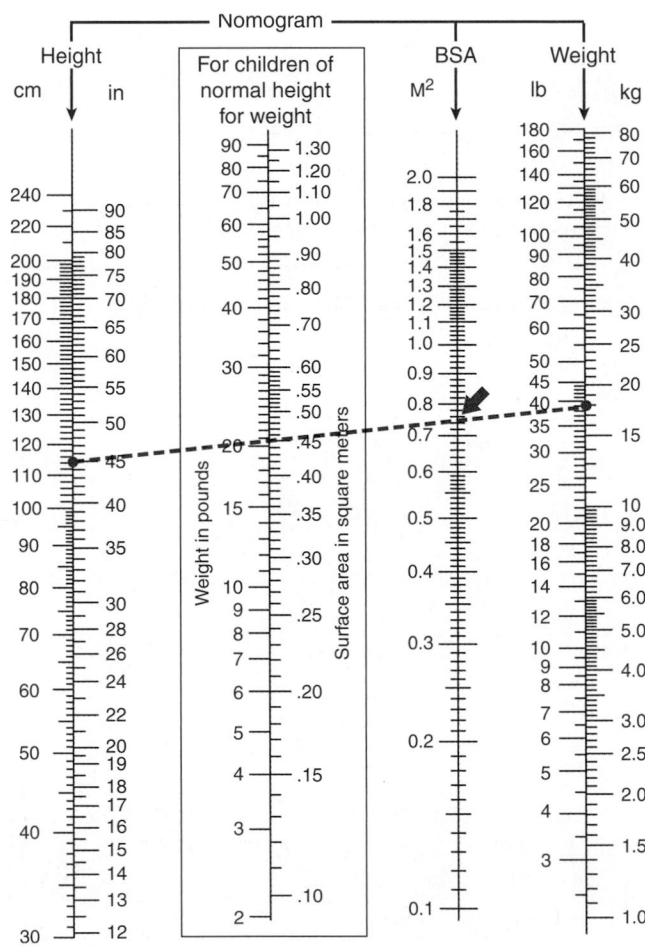

FIG 39-1 Nomogram plotting BSA of a child.

Medication Administration

Administering medication to patients must be done carefully and properly. Medication errors can harm patients, so great care must be taken to administer medications correctly and educate patients on the correct self-administration techniques when necessary.

Parts of a Prescription

A medical assistant may fill out a written prescription. However, it must be signed by the ordering physician. The prescription must be accurate, complete, and legible. Some abbreviations are commonly used on prescription pads; the medical assistant must ask the prescriber if she cannot interpret the abbreviations. (See *Common abbreviations in medication orders,* page 830.) The medical office may transmit the prescription to the pharmacy by telephone or the patient may present the written prescription at the pharmacy. However, the patient must present prescriptions for opiates in person. (The pharmacy will not accept telephone orders for such drugs.) The medical assistant must indicate refills for prescriptions on the original prescription. (See Figure 39-2.) In addition, the physician should always keep

her prescription pad in her pocket, not in a patient treatment room. Easy access to prescription pads may tempt some patients to use them in order to obtain opiates or barbiturates fraudulently.

Routes of Medication Administration

The **route of administration** is the way in which medication is introduced into the patient's body. The route of administration is chosen according to the speed of absorption desired and the site of drug action. For example, a physician may choose the oral route for a drug so it can be absorbed through the GI tract, which happens at a relatively slow rate. Conversely, the patient cannot take some medications orally, such as insulin, because gastric secretions will destroy them. In addition, administering medication by injection enables faster delivery of the drug to the patient's system and is the more appropriate route if the effect of the medication must be immediate. For example, epinephrine, used to counteract an extreme allergic response, is delivered via an injection. The respiratory route, involving inhalation of medication, is also effective in emergencies, such as in bronchial spasm to open airways within seconds.

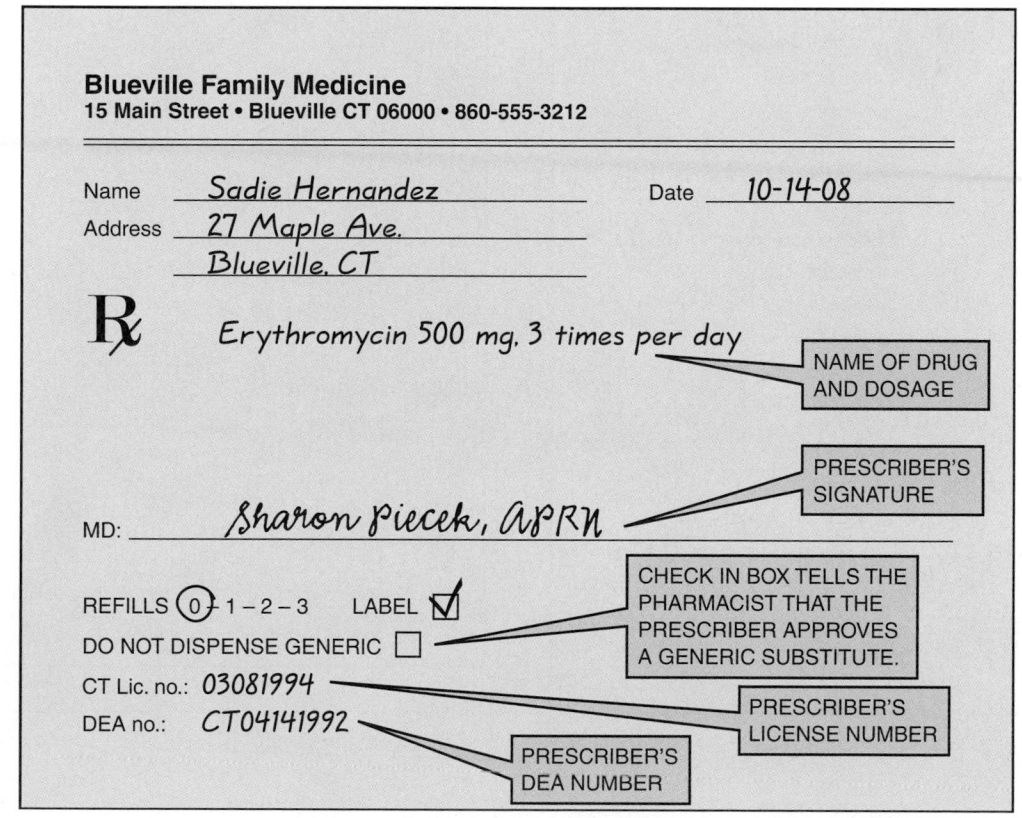

FIG 39-2 Sample prescription.

Common abbreviations in medication orders

The following table lists common abbreviations used in medication orders along with their meanings. Although these abbreviations are common, many health care professional organizations, such as the American Association of Medical Transcriptionists, recommend writing out medication orders to avoid mistakes. Many of these abbreviations may appear in patients' records from previous years when abbreviations were more common, thus the well-prepared medical assistant should be aware of the abbreviated and fully written form of medication orders.

Abbreviation	Meaning
a	before
ac	before meals
ad lib	as desired
aq	water
bid	twice a day
c̄	with
cap	capsule
cc*	cubic centimeter
cm	centimeter
DC, disc, dc	discontinue
EC	enteric-coated
fl, fld	fluid
gr	grain
g, G, Gm	gram
gtt	drop
h, hr	hour
hs, HS*	at bedtime, at hour of sleep
IM	intramuscularly
IU*	International Unit
IVPB	intravenous piggyback
kg, Kg	kilogram
L	liter
mEq	milliequivalent
µg*, mcg	microgram
mg	milligram
ml, mL	milliliter
mm	millimeter
NaCl	sodium chloride
noc, noct, n	night
NPO, npo	nothing by mouth (*nil per os*)
OD*	right eye (*oculus dexter*), overdose
OS*	left eye (*oculus sinister*)
os	mouth
OTC	over the counter
OU*	both eyes (*oculus uterque*)
oz	ounce

Abbreviation	Meaning
pc	after meals
PM, pm	afternoon
Po, PO	by mouth, orally (*per os*)
PRN, prn	whenever necessary (*pro re nata*)
qd*	every day
qh	every hour
q2h	every 2 hours
q3h	every 3 hours
qid	four times a day
QNS	quantity not sufficient
qod*	every other day
qs	quantity sufficient
R	rectal
Rx	prescription
SC, subcu, subq	subcutaneously
SL	sublingual
sol	solution
SR	sustained release
stat	immediately
supp	suppository
syr	syrup
T	temperature
tab	tablet
Tbsp, T, Tbs	tablespoon
tid	three times a day
tinct, tr	tincture
TO	telephone order
TPR	temperature, pulse, respiration
Tsp, t, tsp	teaspoon
U*	unit
ung	ointment
vag	vaginal
VO	verbal orders

* The Joint Commission has identified these abbreviations as the cause of many errors and much confusion. Thus, they strongly recommend their discontinuance.

There are two main routes of medication administration: oral and parenteral.

Oral

The **oral route**, or ingestion through the mouth and into the GI tract, is the most common route of medication administration. It is safe and convenient and most patients are able to take medications in this manner. In addition, it requires no special equipment. However, a patient with dysphagia (difficulty swallowing) should not take oral medications because of the risk of aspirating an oral medication into the respiratory tract. Oral drug forms include:

- **tablets**, which are compressed, disklike masses of medication manufactured from a powder form and require the patient to drink enough liquid so that the tablet does not stick in his throat
- **capsules**, which are medication surrounded by a gelatin container that will not dissolve until it reaches the acidic environment of the stomach, thus preventing the patient from tasting the medication
- **syrups**, which are concentrated solutions of sugar, water, and the medication that make it easier for the patient to tolerate swallowing drugs with a bitter flavor
- **suspensions**, which are solid particles mixed in a liquid but not dissolved and require shaking before use because the medication will not be equally dispersed in the liquid due to settling.

Physicians commonly prescribe syrups and suspensions to young children because they may not be able to swallow tablets or capsules. When a liquid medication is poured into a container, the surface of the liquid, called the **meniscus**, will curve slightly due to surface tension with the sides of the container. When measuring a liquid dose, the medical assistant must be at eye level with the meniscus to ensure accurate dosing. (See Figure 39-3.)

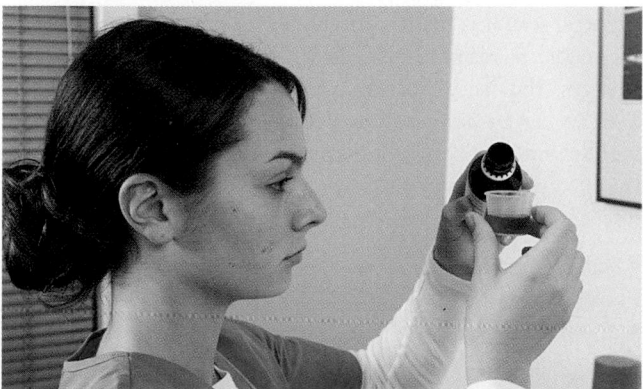

FIG 39-3 Measuring liquid medication at eye level.

The stomach or small intestine digests and absorbs an oral drug. The rate of absorption for oral drugs is fairly slow, approximately 20 minutes. Other factors may cause acceleration or delay of oral drug action, including food in the stomach, the patient's emotions, or physical activity. In addition, some oral medications are safe to administer with food, while others are not. The medical assistant must pay careful attention to recommendations regarding food with oral medications. Whenever administering drugs, the medical assistant must always confirm the "seven rights." (See *Seven rights of medication administration*.)

Some oral drugs can be irritating to the stomach, causing nausea or heartburn. **Enteric-coated** capsules or tablets are coated with a compound that does not dissolve until exposed to the fluids of the small intestine. The medication passes through the stomach into the intestines without causing irritation to the upper GI tract. Thus, the medical assistant

Seven rights of medication administration

The medical assistant can ensure proper medication administration by always following the "seven rights," including:

1. *Right Patient*—The medical assistant can make errors in dispensing medications when the patient is unfamiliar to her. Thus, she should be sure to confirm the patient's name on the medication order with the patient in front of her. If the patient is unable to identify himself, as with infants and patients with a language barrier or confusion, she can ask a caregiver to identify the patient. She must be extremely careful when administering medications to patients with the same or similar names. In such a case, the medical assistant should ask each patient for his date of birth or address.

2. *Right Drug*—Because drug names may sound similar or be spelled similarly, the medical assistant must check the spelling and read the label three times before administering the drug to a patient. She should do her first check before removing the drug from storage, her second check before preparing the medication, and her third check before returning the drug to storage.

3. *Right Dose*—Medication dosages are based on body weight, age, sex, general state of health, and previous known reactions to medications. The medical assistant may need to calculate the dosage of the medication ordered. Because medications come in various dosages, she must be sure to calculate the proper dose to be administered to the patient.

Continued

4. *Right Route*—Because the route of administration of a medication affects its effectiveness and rate of absorption, the medical assistant must take care to administer medication via the right route. For example, because absorption in the gastrointestinal route is slow, oral medication administration would not be an appropriate route for an emergency dose of epinephrine. The medical assistant should check the package or medication order to ensure the right route.

5. *Right Time*—The medical assistant must administer medications at proper intervals in order to maintain proper blood levels of the medication and avoid exceeding the therapeutic dosage. For example, some oral medications must be taken on an empty stomach (between mealtimes) and others are better tolerated with food (at mealtimes).

6. *Right Documentation*—The medical assistant must properly document medication administration in the patient's medical record. She should do so immediately after administering the medication and include the date, time, route, dosage, lot number (if applicable), and the patient's reaction to the medication.

7. *Right Technique*—The medical assistant may administer medication via an injection. There are many routes for administering an injection, including subcutaneously, intradermally, and intramuscularly. The medical assistant must ensure that she performs the correct injection technique for the desired route, such as inserting the needle at the proper angle so that the medication will be delivered to the intended site. For example, if the medical assistant must administer an injection into the dermal area of the skin but uses a 45-degree angle to insert the needle, she will not deliver the medication into the dermal layer of the skin, which will most likely lessen or nullify the drug's therapeutic effect.

must never cut an enteric-coated tablet or capsule or the medication could produce irritation and change the intended site of absorption. (See *Procedure 39-1: Administering an oral medication.*)

Parenteral

Any route other than the oral, or *enteral*, route is considered a *parenteral* route. Parenteral routes of administration include:

- sublingual
- buccal
- inhalation
- injection
- topical
- vaginal
- rectal.

Sublingual and Buccal

Sublingual (under the tongue) and **buccal** (between the cheek and gum) administration of drugs involves placing the medication in the patient's mouth without his swallowing it. Unlike oral drugs, sublingual and buccal medications do not travel to the GI tract for absorption. Instead, the mucous membranes in the interior of the mouth absorb it and deliver it to the bloodstream. Thus, absorption through these routes is more immediate. For example, nitroglycerine, a strong vasodilator, is commonly administered sublingually for patients experiencing acute angina pectoris. Opiate analgesics are commonly administered buccally for severe breakthrough pain in cancer patients.

Inhalation

Patients can inhale medications for delivery to the respiratory tract using a *nebulizer*, a machine that mixes room air with a medication. The nebulizer uses an atomizer to mix the medication with water to create a vapor that the patient can inhale. The patient can sleep or sit quietly in the room with the nebulizer and breathe in the medication with the humidified air. Patients with asthma or emphysema can also use portable metered-dose inhalers (MDIs) for immediate relief of respiratory distress.

Injection

For a parenteral administration via injection, the medical assistant must first measure the correct amount of the drug by drawing it into a syringe. She may draw the medication from a vial or an ampule. A vial is a relatively small glass bottle used to store liquid medication. It has a metal or rubber removable cap to allow the medical assistant to push a needle through the rubber top and draw out the drug. (See *Procedure 39-2: Preparing a parenteral medication from a vial*, pages 834 and 835.) An ampule is made of glass like a vial. However, it has no rubber or metal seal; it is made entirely of glass. To open the ampule, the medical assistant must break the glass neck of the ampule to access the drug. (See *Procedure 39-3: Preparing a parenteral medication from an ampule*, pages 836 and 837.) In addition to withdrawing the correct amount of medication into a syringe, the medical assistant must have an understanding of the different methods of injection, of which there are four:

- subcutaneous
- intradermal
- intramuscular (IM)
- intravenous (IV).

The medical assistant must also develop skill in performing subcutaneous, intradermal, and IM injections. However,

PROCEDURE 39-1

Administering an oral medication

Task
Properly interpret a physician's order and apply pharmacological principles to prepare and administer an oral medication.

Conditions
- Medication ordered by the physician
- Medication cup (for liquid administration)
- Water, when appropriate
- Patient's medical record

Standards
In the time specified and within the scoring parameters determined by the instructor, the student will successfully read the medication order and prepare and administer an oral medication to a patient.

Performance Standards
1. Wash your hands to ensure infection control.
2. Review the "seven rights" of medication administration.
3. Assemble equipment and supplies and read the medication order to check the written order for clarification of the oral route and to determine if enough time has passed since the last dose, if appropriate. If in doubt, check with the physician.
4. Select the right drug and check the medication label. If the medication is unfamiliar, read the package insert or use a drug reference—the first of three checks to ensure that you are administering the correct medication.
5. Check the expiration date of the medication because administering expired medication could be hazardous.
6. Read the dosage information on the label and calculate the correct dose. For example, if the physician orders 50 mg and 25-mg tablets are on hand, calculate the dose using the formula:

$$\frac{\text{Dose ordered}}{\text{Dose on hand}} = \text{amount to give}$$

$$\frac{50 \text{ mg}}{25 \text{ mg}} = 2 \text{ tablets}$$

7. Check the medication label again for the second of three checks for the right medication.
8. Prepare the dose needed.
   a. For solids, such as capsules and tablets, pour the medication from the bottle into the bottle cap and then transfer it to a medication cup. Do not touch the medication or the inside of the cup with your hands to ensure infection control.
   b. For liquids, pour syrups and mix suspensions as directed on the bottle. Pour the medication into the medication cup, measuring the meniscus to ensure an accurate measurement.
9. Check the medication label a third and final time before returning it to the cabinet.
10. Carry the medication to the treatment room taking care not to spill it and using a tray if needed.
11. Administer the medication to the patient, being sure to confirm the "right" patient once more.
12. Offer the patient some water, as appropriate, to help him swallow solid oral medication.
13. Remain with the patient until he swallows the medication.
14. Wash your hands to ensure infection control.
15. Document the procedure in the patient's medical record.

Date	
09/23/08: 9:25 a.m.	Two 200-mg ibuprofen tablets administered to patient for pain. ———————————————————— C. Chapin, CMA

medical assistants are not legally permitted to perform IV injections.

Subcutaneous
When administering a **subcutaneous** injection, the medical assistant injects the drug into the subcutaneous layer of the integument (skin), which is the fatty layer beneath the dermis and above the muscle tissue. Because the fatty layer is less vascular than muscle, the drug absorption rate is moderate with this type of injection. However, the site of subcutaneous injection can affect the rate of absorption. (See Figure 39-4.) For example, injection of a drug in the abdomen or arm offers quicker absorption than one in the thigh or upper buttocks. Subcutaneous injection sites are in areas where a substantial amount of connective tissue is present between the muscle and skin to absorb the medication without hitting nerves, muscle, bone, or blood vessels. (See *Procedure 39-4: Administering a subcutaneous injection,* page 839.)

■ **PROCEDURE 39-2**

Preparing a parenteral medication from a vial

Task
Measure the correct amount of medication from a vial into a 3-ml hypodermic syringe for injection.

Conditions
- Vial of medication ordered by physician
- 70% isopropyl alcohol wipes
- Appropriate syringe for ordered dose
- Needle with safety device appropriate for site injection
- 2" × 2" sterile gauze pads
- Sharps container
- Patient's medical record

Standards
In the time specified and within the scoring parameters determined by the instructor, the student will successfully measure the correct medication dose from a vial into a syringe for injection.

Performance Standards
1. Wash your hands.
2. Assemble the equipment and supplies and verify the order.
3. Check the expiration date of the medication to avoid using expired medication, which may cause injury.
4. Follow the "seven rights" of medication administration.
5. Check the medication against the physician's order to perform the first of three checks.
6. Check the patient's medical record for allergies or conditions that may contraindicate the medication.
7. Calculate the correct dose to be given (if not already provided).
8. Check the medication against the physician's written order to perform the second of three checks.
9. If the vial is new, remove the hard plastic or metal cover. If it is a multidose vial that has already been used, wipe the top of the vial with an alcohol wipe to ensure infection control.
10. Allow the top of the vial to dry before withdrawing the medication to avoid contaminating the medication with alcohol.
11. If the medication needs mixing, rotate the vial between the palms of your hands.
12. To prepare the needle and syringe, open the peel-apart sterile packaging around the syringe and needle and assemble the needle and syringe.

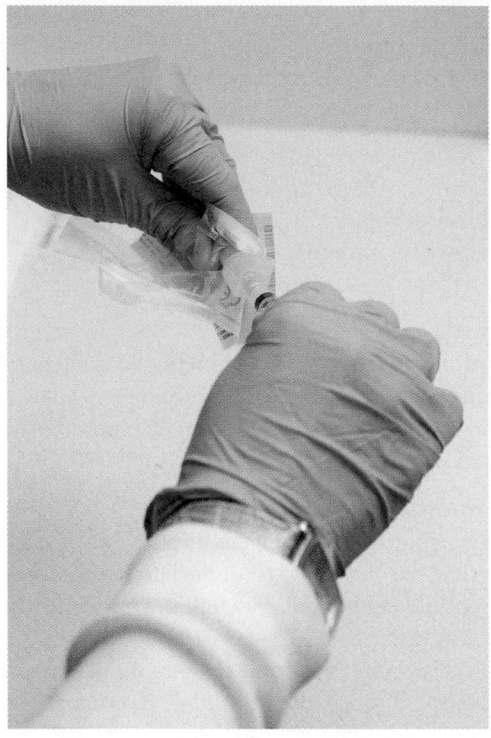

Open the sterile packaging and assemble the needle and syringe.

13. If the needle and syringe are packaged separately, open both packages using sterile technique, remove the small plastic cap covering the Luer-Lok on the syringe, and attach the needle by twisting it securely to the Luer-Lok.
14. Do not allow the hub of the needle to touch anything other than the Luer-Lok to avoid contaminating the needle.

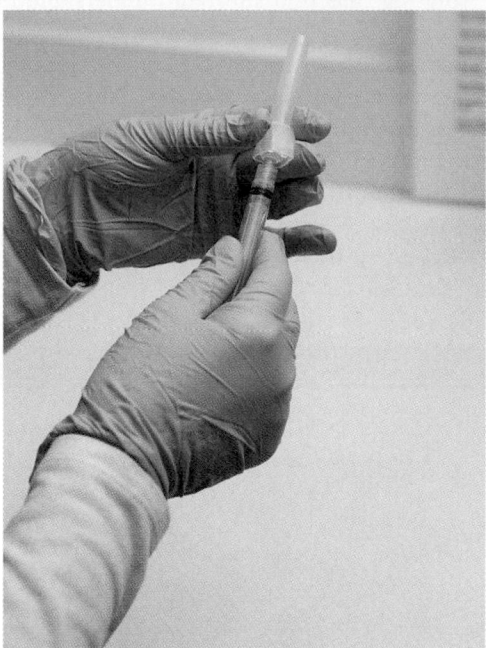

Do not allow the needle hub to touch anything other than the Luer-Lok.

15. Remove the cover from the needle. Hold the barrel of the syringe with one hand and carefully remove the cover with the other hand. Place the needle cover on the counter.

16. Closely inspect the needle at eye level and discard if any burrs are present on the tip or the shaft of the needle.

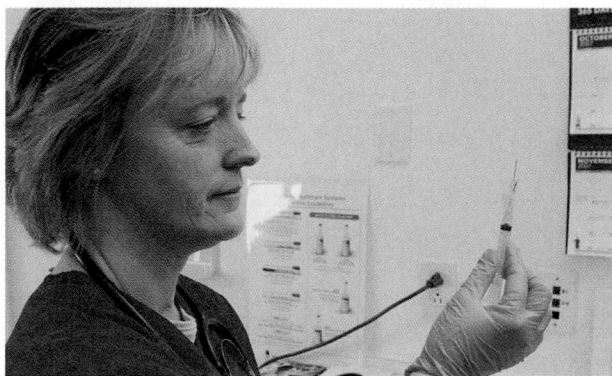

Closely inspect the needle at eye level for burrs.

17. Draw air into the syringe. With the needle cover over the needle, draw an amount of air equal to the volume of medication to administer.

18. Insert the needle into the vial. Place the vial on the counter without holding it. This will prevent an accidental needle stick to your hand. Hold the barrel of the syringe with one hand guiding the needle into the rubber stopper. Once the needle has penetrated the stopper, use the other hand to hold the vial. Inject the air into the vial.

19. To fill the syringe, invert the vial and syringe so that the tip of the needle is immersed in the medication. Withdraw a little more than the required volume of medication from the vial to ensure that you have enough medication in case of an air bubble within the volume drawn.

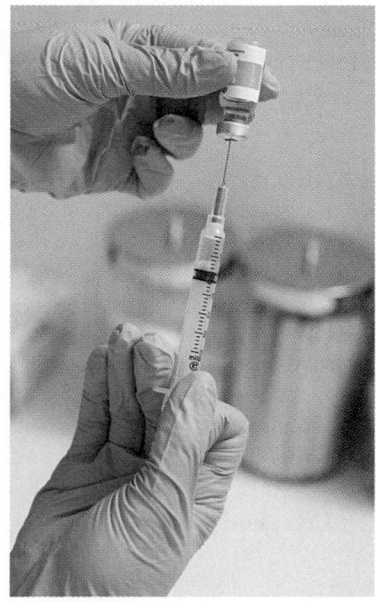

Invert the vial and syringe and withdraw the medication.

20. If air bubbles have formed in the syringe, invert the syringe and tap the barrel with your finger or fingernail until the air bubble rises to the top of the liquid. Advance the plunger to express the air out of the syringe. When you have expelled the air, measure the exact dose needed by advancing the plunger to the required mark on the barrel.

21. Remove the needle from the vial stopper by pulling your hands away from each other. Be careful not to touch the needle because doing so will contaminate it and put you at risk for a needlestick.

22. If necessary, recap the needle by placing the needle cap on a clean dry surface (such as the countertop), holding the syringe in one hand, and carefully guide the exposed needle into the cap without touching the needle to the cap. When the cap is on the needle, secure it with your hand, touching only the cap, not the needle.

23. If preparing the needle in a different room than the patient, cap and carry the needle on a tray to avoid contamination and accidental needlesticks.

Insulin is an example of a subcutaneously injected drug. Because patients or caregivers commonly administer subcutaneous insulin injections daily, they must rotate injection sites to prevent lipodystrophy (atrophy or hypertrophy of fat tissue), bruising, swelling, or infection. Thus, the medical assistant may need to instruct the patient with diabetes about administration of insulin by subcutaneous injection. The patient must be able to inspect and choose administration sites, clean the site, and properly inject herself with insulin. In addition to performing the procedure, the medical assistant must educate the patient about monitoring her blood glucose level, properly storing her insulin, rotating injection sites, and understanding variations in absorption rates of these sites. The medical assistant should ask the patient to return-demonstrate the self-injection technique and ask her questions to ensure that she has an understanding of her disease and medication. (See Figure 39-5.) The medical assistant should also give the patient written instructions and tell her to call the office if she has any questions. She should always be sure to document such demonstration and instruction in the patient's medical record.

PROCEDURE 39-3

Preparing a parenteral medication from an ampule

Task
Measure the correct amount of medication from an ampule into a 3-ml hypodermic syringe for injection.

Conditions
- Ampule of medication ordered by physician
- 70% isopropyl alcohol wipes
- Appropriate syringe for ordered dose
- Needle with safety device appropriate for injection site
- Filter needle (for ampule)
- 2" × 2" sterile gauze pads
- Sharps container
- Patient's medical record

Standards
In the time specified and within the scoring parameters determined by the instructor, the student will successfully measure the correct medication dose from an ampule into a syringe for injection.

Performance Standards
1. Wash your hands.
2. Assemble the equipment and supplies and verify the order.
3. Check the expiration date of the medication to avoid using expired medication, which may cause injury.
4. Follow the "seven rights" of medication administration.
5. Check the medication against the physician's order to perform the first of three checks.
6. Check the patient's medical record for allergies or conditions that may contraindicate the medication.
7. Calculate the correct dose to be given (if not already provided).
8. Check the medication against the physician's written order to perform the second of three checks.
9. Clean the ampule with an alcohol wipe and allow it to air dry before withdrawing the medication to avoid contaminating the medication with alcohol.

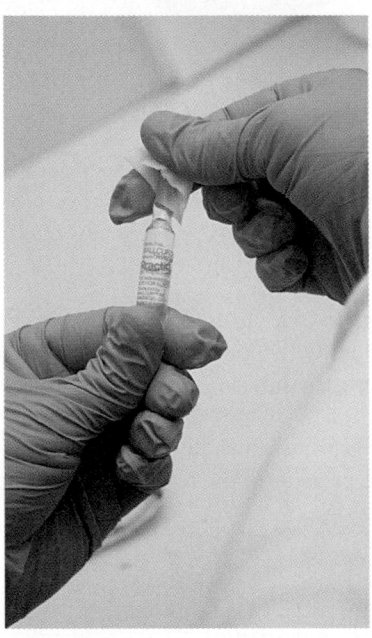

Clean the ampule with an alcohol wipe.

10. Using an ampule breaker or a piece of gauze wrapped around the top of the ampule, break off the top of the ampule. Be sure to do so in the direction away from your body to prevent injury. Discard the ampule top in the sharps container.

PROCEDURE 39-3—cont'd

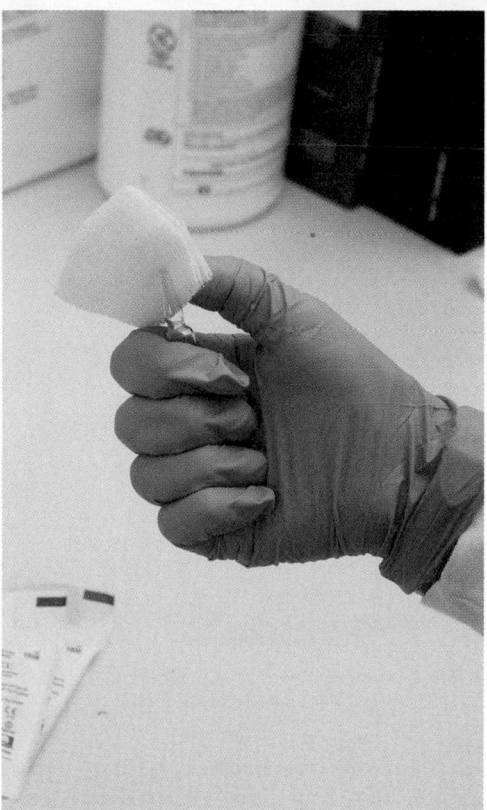

Break off the top of the ampule in a direction away from your body.

11. Hold the barrel of the filter needle syringe with one hand and carefully remove the needle cover with the other hand. Place the needle cover on its side on the counter.

12. Inspect the needle and discard if any burrs are present on the tip or the shaft of the needle.

13. Insert the filter needle into the ampule. Placing the ampule on the countertop, hold the barrel of the syringe with one hand and carefully lower the needle into the ampule so that the bevel of the needle is below the surface of the liquid.

14. Do not inject air into the ampule and do not touch the broken edge of the ampule with the needle or your fingers to avoid contamination and injury.

15. Withdraw the entire amount of medication, if ordered, to ensure that you have enough medication in case of an air bubble within the volume drawn. Keep the bevel of the needle under the surface of the liquid as you withdraw the medication to avoid introducing excess air into the syringe.

16. Using sterile technique, exchange the filter needle for an injection needle with a safety device. Inspect the injection needle for defects and discard if found. Do not touch the end of the hub of the needle or the tip of the barrel of the syringe.

17. Remove the cover of the new needle. If air bubbles have formed in the syringe, invert the syringe and tap the barrel with your finger or fingernail until the air bubble rises to the top of the liquid. Advance the plunger to express the air out of the syringe. When any air has been expelled, measure the exact dose needed by advancing the plunger to the required mark on the barrel.

18. Recap the needle if necessary. Place the needle cap on a clean dry surface (such as the countertop) and, holding the syringe in one hand, carefully guide the exposed needle into the cap without touching it. When the cap is on the needle, secure it with your hand, touching only the cap, not the needle.

19. If you are preparing the needle in a different room than the patient, cap and carry the needle on a tray to avoid contamination and accidental needlesticks.

20. Check the medication label to perform the third of three checks and discard the ampule in the sharps container.

21. Wash your hands.

Intradermal

The medical assistant administers **intradermal** injections into the dermis, the layer of skin under the epidermis (surface of the skin). The intradermal route is most common in performing allergy testing or tuberculosis (TB) testing. Common intradermal injection sites are the upper arms for TB screening and the upper back for allergy testing. The quantity of medication given intradermally is small because the medication is not intended to be absorbed beyond the local site but should remain just under the surface for the patient's body to react to the allergen or TB test. The physician then reads the reaction on the surface of the skin. (See *Procedure 39-5: Administering an intradermal injection,* pages 840 and 841.)

Intramuscular

When the medical assistant administers an **intramuscular** (IM) injection, she injects the drug directly into the muscle. Absorption happens quickly in the rich blood supply of the muscle. The muscle can be injected with much more

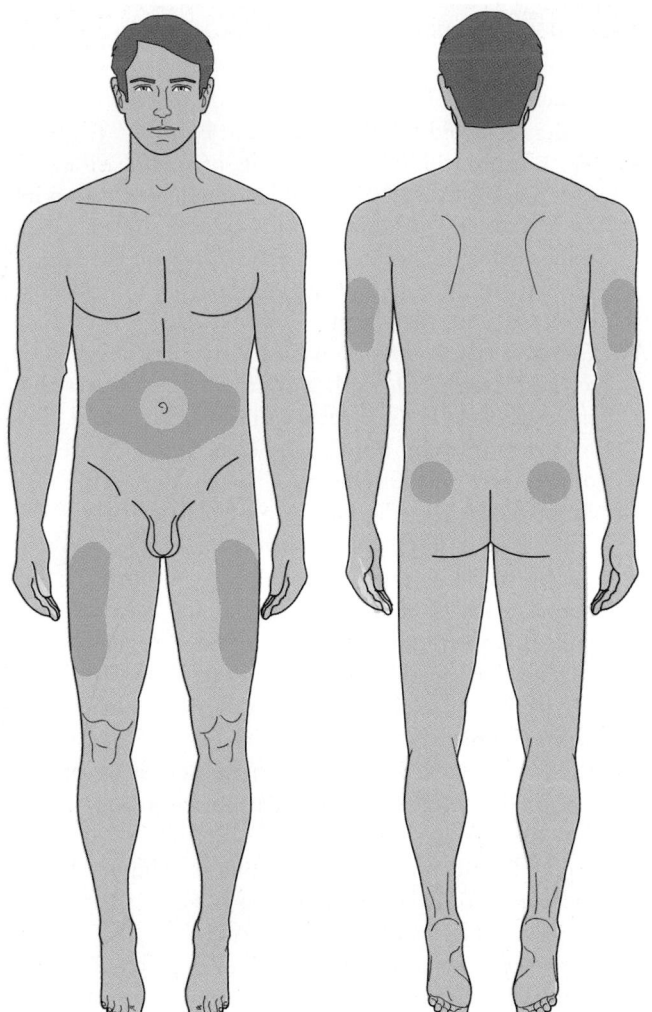

FIG 39-4 Subcutaneous injection sites.

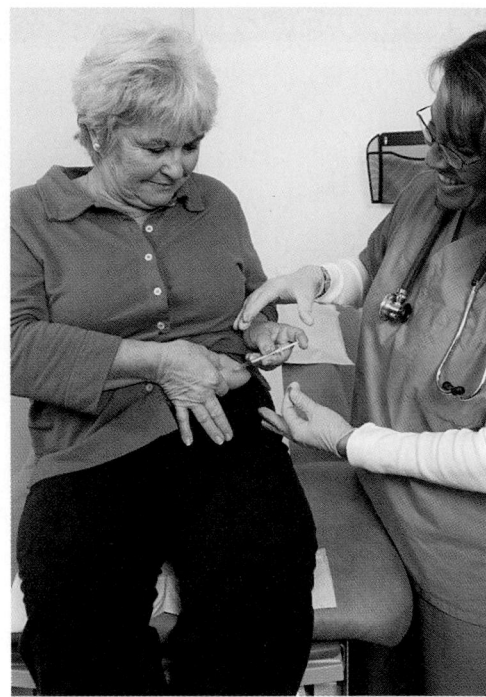

FIG 39-5 Return-demonstration of subcutaneous injection technique.

medication than in the intradermal or subcutaneous methods because the muscle is capable of retaining more liquid. Careful measurement of medications into syringes is necessary to ensure proper dosage. Common IM sites of administration include the ventrogluteal, deltoid, and vastus lateralis muscles. (See Figure 39-6.)

The most common injection site for neonates and infants less than age 7 months is the rectus femoris. The dorsogluteal site was one of the most common administration sites in the past; however, it is no longer recommended. Recent studies reveal that the ventrogluteal site is the best choice for adults and children over age 7 months. The ventrogluteal site, located on the lateral hip, is located away from major blood vessels and nerves, limiting the risk of hitting a nerve or blood vessel and causing nerve damage or damaging an artery. This site is also less painful than the dorsogluteal and rectus femoris sites.

The **Z-track injection** method is a modification of IM injection technique. To use the Z-track method, the medical assistant must pull the skin to one side and hold it while inserting the needle at a 90-degree angle. She should then follow regular procedure for injecting the medication. After administering the medication, she must wait 10 seconds and then withdraw the needle and release the skin. This technique leaves a zigzag needle track from the surface of the skin to the muscular layer, which stops the medication from leaking out into the subcutaneous tissue and onto the skin surface. The preferred sites for the Z-track method are the vastus lateralis and ventrogluteal muscles. This method is used for medications that may discolor or irritate subcutaneous tissues. (See Figure 39-7.)

Medications administered IM include antibiotics, vaccines, and drugs to treat a severe allergic reaction. When the medical assistant must administer multiple IM injections, she should use sites on both hips, arms, and legs to avoid excessive soreness in one area. (See *Procedure 39-6: Administering an intramuscular injection,* pages 843 and 845.)

Patients with severe allergies to such foods as peanuts, tree nuts, or shellfish may need to carry an EpiPen, which is a device that delivers an IM injection of a premeasured amount of epinephrine to counteract the effects of a severe allergic reaction. Because the medical assistant cannot ask the patient to actually demonstrate injecting himself with epinephrine, she should ask him to "role-play" what to do if he accidentally comes in contact with the allergen. The

PROCEDURE 39-4

Administering a subcutaneous injection

Task
Select the proper site and properly administer a subcutaneous injection.

Conditions
- Nonsterile disposable gloves
- Medication ordered by the physician
- Appropriate syringe for the ordered dose
- Needle with a safety device
- 2" × 2" sterile gauze pads
- 70% isopropyl alcohol wipes
- Sharps container
- Biohazardous waste container
- Patient's medical record

Standards
In the time specified and within the scoring parameters determined by the instructor, the student will successfully select the proper site and properly administer a subcutaneous injection.

Performance Standards
1. Wash your hands to ensure infection control.
2. Assemble the equipment and supplies and verify the order.
3. Check the expiration date of the medication.
4. Follow the "seven rights" of medication administration.
5. Check the medication against the physician's written order to perform the first of three checks.
6. Check the patient's medical record for allergies or conditions that may contraindicate the medication.
7. Calculate the correct dose to be given, if necessary.
8. Prepare the syringe with the ordered dose to ensure that the patient receives the correct dose.
9. Follow the procedure for drawing medication into the syringe.
10. Greet and identify the patient to ensure that you administer the medication to the right patient.
11. Explain the procedure to the patient to ensure patient understanding and compliance.
12. Select the appropriate injection site and position the patient.
13. Expose the injection site and inspect the site for scars and inflammation. If scarring or inflammation is present, choose a different site because scarred, broken, or inflamed skin will decrease absorption of the drug. Be sure to explain to the patient why you must change the site.
14. Put on gloves.
15. Recheck the medication against the physician's written order to perform the second of three checks.

16. Prepare the injection site by cleaning it with an alcohol wipe, beginning at the center and working in an outward circular motion. Allow the site to air dry. Do not touch the site or allow the patient to touch the site to avoid contaminating the site.
17. Remove the cover from the needle.
18. Recheck the medication against the physician's written orders to perform the third of three checks.
19. Secure the skin at the injection site. Grasp a generous portion of skin around the injection site between the thumb and forefinger of your nondominant hand. Hold the syringe at a 45-degree, upward angle.
20. Puncture the skin with the needle in a quick, smooth motion.
21. Check to see if blood aspirates into the syringe. If it does, withdraw the syringe from the site because blood in the syringe is a sign that the needle has pierced a blood vessel. Then begin the procedure again with a new needle.
22. If blood does not aspirate into the syringe, release your grasp of the skin and pull back on the plunger. **NOTE:** Do not aspirate with heparin or insulin because it may cause tissue damage.
23. If blood does not aspirate into the syringe when pulling the plunger, inject the medication slowly.
24. Place a gauze pad over the injection site and quickly withdraw the needle from the site at the same 45-degree angle.
25. Use a 2" × 2" sterile gauze pad to massage the injection site gently but firmly to help distribute the medication into body tissues. **NOTE:** Do not massage the injection site of heparin or insulin because it may cause tissue damage.
26. Discard the syringe and needle in the sharps container, remove your gloves and discard them in the biohazardous waste container, and wash your hands to ensure infection control.
27. Check on the patient. Ask the patient how she feels and observe her for any signs of immediate emergency reaction, such as dizziness, lightheadedness, or fainting.
28. Document the procedure, including the date, time, lot number of the medication, dose given, and injection site used. Chart any reactions you observe.

Date	
10/15/08; 4:15 p.m.	Egg allergy injection, 0.20 cc, Lot # GY4453, exp date 12/30/2009 subcutaneous right upper arm. Arm check 15 minutes after injection - no reaction noted. Patient in no distress; verbal and written follow-up instructions given. ———————————————— C. Chapin, CMA

■ **PROCEDURE 39-5**

Administering an intradermal injection

Task
Select the proper site and properly administer an intradermal injection.

Conditions
- Nonsterile disposable gloves
- Medication ordered by the physician
- Appropriate syringe for ordered dose (tuberculin syringe)
- Needle with safety device (26G or 27G, $3/8$" to $1/2$")
- 2" × 2" sterile gauze pads
- 70% isopropyl alcohol wipes
- Written patient instructions for post-testing
- Sharps container
- Biohazardous waste container
- Patient's medical record

Standards
In the time specified and within the scoring parameters determined by the instructor, the student will successfully select the proper site and properly administer an intradermal injection.

Performance Standards
1. Wash your hands to ensure infection control.
2. Assemble the equipment and supplies and verify the order.
3. Check the expiration date of the medication.
4. Follow the "seven rights" of medication administration.
5. Check the medication against the physician's written order to perform the first of three checks.
6. Check the patient's medical record for allergies or conditions that may contraindicate the medication.
7. Calculate the correct dose to be given, if necessary.
8. Prepare the syringe with the correct dose to ensure the patient receives the correct dose.
9. Follow the procedure for drawing medication into the syringe.
10. Greet and identify the patient to ensure that you administer the medication to the right patient.
11. Explain the procedure to the patient to ensure patient understanding and compliance.
12. Select the appropriate injection site and position the patient.
13. Recheck the medication against the physician's written orders to perform the second of three checks.
14. Expose the injection site and inspect the site for scars and inflammation. If scarring or inflammation is present, choose a different site because scarred, broken, or inflamed skin will prevent an accurate reading of the injection site. Be sure to explain to the patient why you must change the site.
15. Put on gloves.
16. Prepare the injection site by cleaning it with an alcohol wipe, beginning at the center and working in an outward circular motion. Allow the site to air dry. Do not touch the site or allow the patient to touch the site to avoid contaminating the site.
17. Recheck the medication against the physician's written orders to perform the third of three checks.
18. Remove the cover without touching the needle. Visually inspect the injection site to be sure that the alcohol has dried before you inject to avoid contaminating the drug with alcohol.
19. Secure the skin at the injection site. Pull the skin at the injection site taut with the thumb and forefinger of the nondominant hand. Position the needle almost parallel to the skin at an angle of 10 to 15 degrees.
20. Insert the needle until the bevel barely penetrates the skin. Be sure that the entire bevel is below the surface of the skin so that you inject the liquid under the skin layer and not on top of the skin.
21. Release your grasp on the forearm skin and use your nondominant hand to inject the medication slowly. Keep a slow, steady pressure on the plunger until all of the liquid is injected and a wheal forms. The wheal should be 6 to 10 mm in diameter.

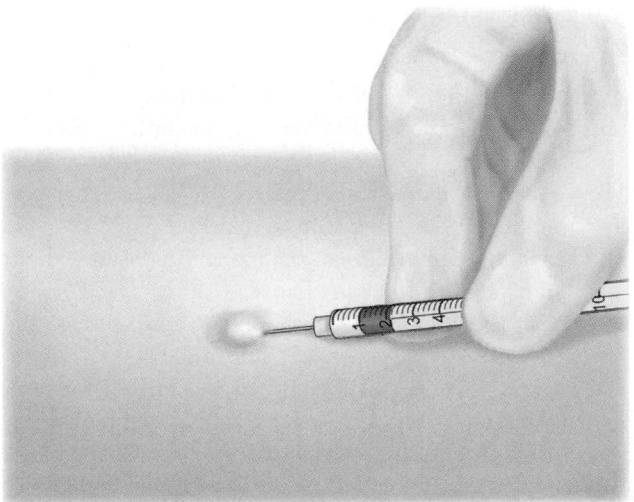

Observe the formation of a wheal as you inject.

PROCEDURE 39-5—cont'd

22. If no wheal forms, notify the physician immediately because the injection was too deep and the reaction to the medication will not be visible at the skin's surface.

23. Withdraw the needle from the injection site at the same angle (10 to 15 degrees) and activate the safety device to cover the needle.

24. Dab the area with a gauze pad. Do not apply pressure to the wheal because doing so could push the liquid away from the injection site.

25. Discard the needle in the sharps container and wash your hands to ensure infection control.

26. Ask the patient how he feels and observe him for any signs of an immediate emergency reaction, such as dizziness, lightheadedness, or fainting.

27. Discuss the monitoring of test results with the patient. Based on the type of test and the office policy, you may be required to:

  a. Read the test result in the office. Using inspection (looking) and palpation (feeling) at the site of the injection, determine the presence of a reaction and the amount of induration.

  b. Inform the patient of a date and time to return to the office to have the physician read the results of the injection.

  c. Instruct the patient on reading and interpreting the injection site at home. Give him a card with various levels of induration for comparison. Instruct the patient to call the office with the test results.

  d. Be sure to explain the importance of reading the site at the correct date and time. Checking the site too soon or too late could result in a false-negative result and delay treatment.

28. Document the procedure in the patient's chart.

Date	
10/15/08: 2:20 p.m.	Mantoux tuberculin test, 0.10 ml, intradermal, Lot #XB4432, exp date 12/30/2009, right anterior forearm. Gave patient verbal and written instructions on inspecting the site and to return on 10/18/2008 to have results read. ———————————— ———————————————————————————————— C. Chapin, CMA

patient can show the medical assistant how he would take the cap off of the EpiPen and inject himself. She should also provide written instructions to the patient. In the case of children, the medical assistant should show the parents or caregivers how to administer the medication and how to look for signs of severe allergy.

Intravenous

Intravenous medication administration is the fastest route of absorption because the medication is injected into a vein and, thus, enters the bloodstream directly. Although a medical assistant cannot legally administer IV medications, she must have an understanding of IV medication administration and fluid replacement therapy.

Patients receive IV solutions to:

- replace lost fluids and electrolytes
- correct an acid-base imbalance
- administer medications quickly
- maintain ready access to venous circulation
- administer essential nutrients
- administer blood products or replacement products.

The most common IV solutions are combinations of salt, glucose, sterile water, and other electrolytes to rebalance fluid loss. The four basic types are:

- *hypotonic solutions* used to rehydrate the body or to prevent dehydration

- *isotonic solutions* used to replace cellular fluids lost through blood loss or vomiting (The salt, or *sodium chloride*, concentration of an isotonic solution is the same as that in the patient's body.)
- *maintenance solutions*, including isotonic solutions and others, used to replace electrolytes in the case of severe diarrhea and vomiting (Minerals and, sometimes, vitamins in the solution replace what is lost.)
- *hypertonic solutions* used to treat overhydration.

Topical

The medical assistant can administer medication by placing it on top of the skin, enabling absorption into the bloodstream via the skin. Examples of topical medications include creams and ointments. Cleaning the skin with soap and water enhances absorption of topical creams and ointments. Another method of topical medication administration is the transdermal method, which involves placing a patch made of a semipermeable membrane that releases the medication into the skin. (See *Procedure 39-7: Administering a transdermal patch*, pages 845 and 846.) Transdermal medication is absorbed more slowly, over a period of 12 to 24 hours. Examples of transdermal medications include nicotine smoking cessation patches, nitroglycerine patches for angina, and patches for contraception.

Vaginal

The medical assistant may administer medications vaginally by inserting them into the vaginal cavity in the form of a

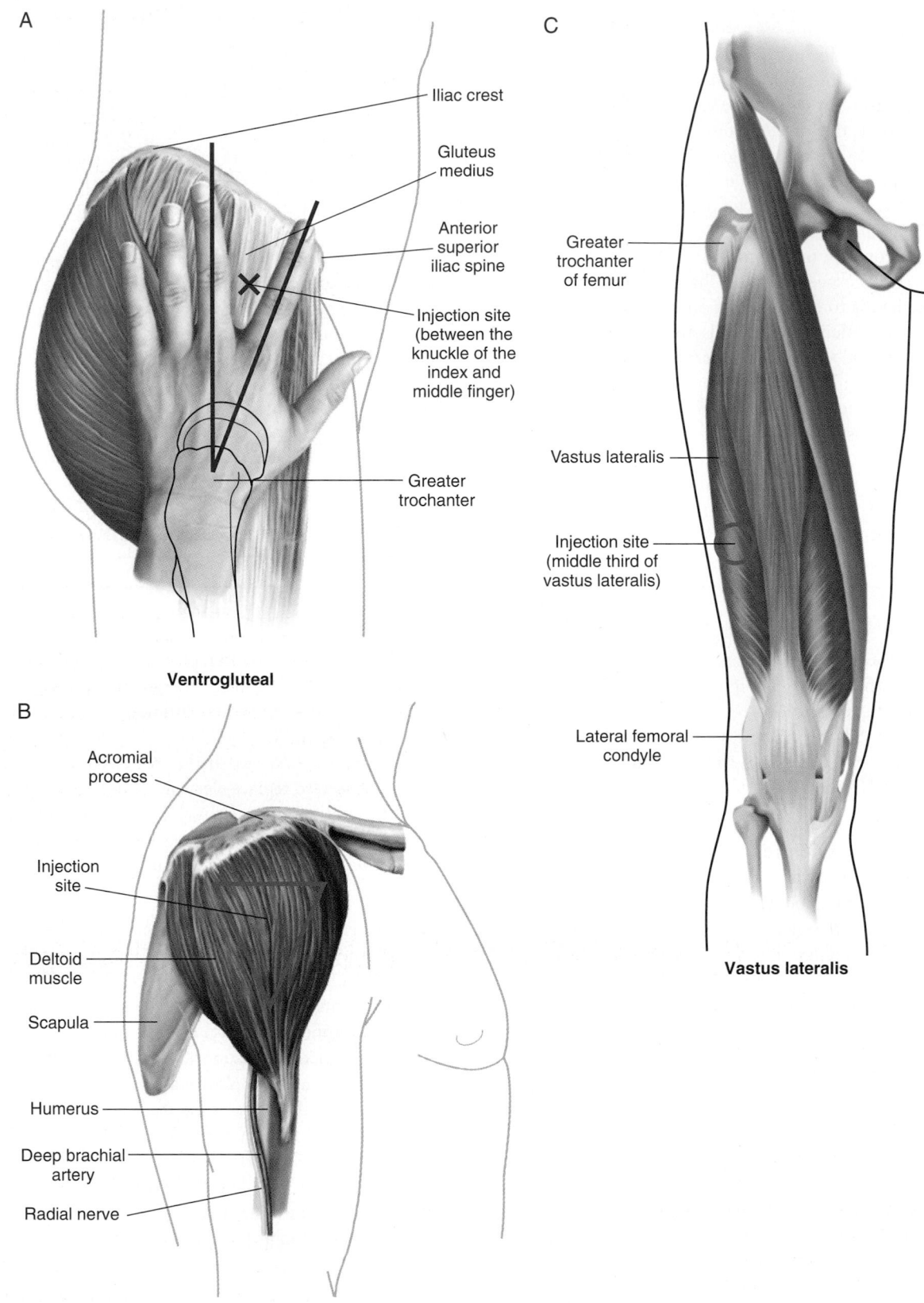

A

Iliac crest

Gluteus medius

Anterior superior iliac spine

Injection site (between the knuckle of the index and middle finger)

Greater trochanter

Ventrogluteal

B

Acromial process

Injection site

Deltoid muscle

Scapula

Humerus

Deep brachial artery

Radial nerve

Deltoid

C

Greater trochanter of femur

Vastus lateralis

Injection site (middle third of vastus lateralis)

Lateral femoral condyle

Vastus lateralis

FIG 39-6 Intramuscular injection sites.

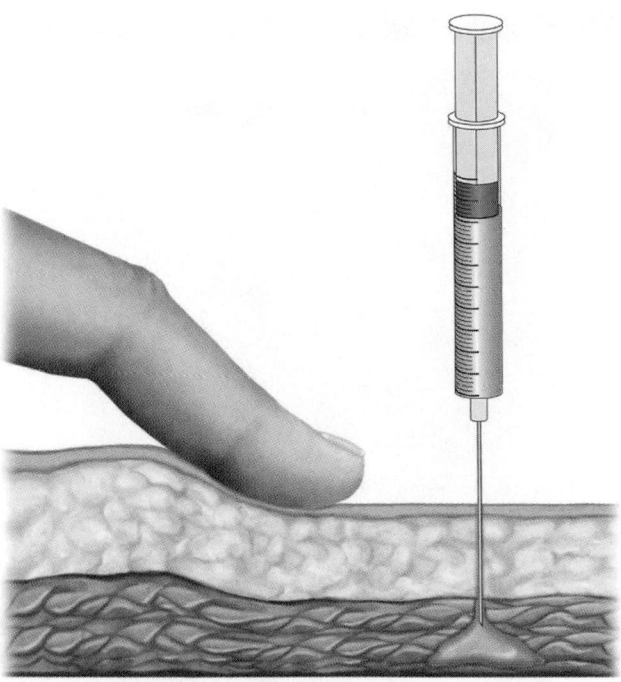

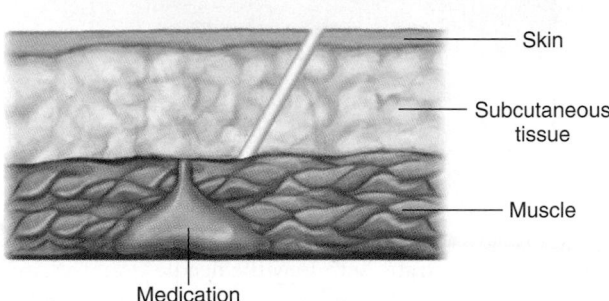

— Skin

— Subcutaneous tissue

— Muscle

Medication

FIG 39-7 Z-track injection method.

cream, foam, or suppository. Patients may need specific instructions on inserting the medication. Administration of foams and creams involves insertion with an applicator. The medical assistant should be sure to give the patient the written instructions that accompany the medication. Insertion of suppositories, which are hard, is similar to that of a tampon. The patient's warm body temperature melts the suppository so that the medication can be absorbed through the mucosa. The patient may need to lie in a recumbent position after inserting the medication to ensure absorption. Thus, physicians commonly order vaginal medication administration at bedtime. Examples of vaginal medications are antifungal creams and estrogen replacement therapy.

Rectal

The medical assistant may administer medications rectally by inserting them into the rectum for localized or systemic action. Rectal medications are in suppository form, which melt from the patient's body heat. Rectal administration is common for medications to treat nausea and vomiting, when the patient cannot tolerate anything taken orally. Pain relievers and fever reducers are also available in suppository form.

If the patient or caregiver must administer the suppository at home, the medical assistant should instruct the patient on proper insertion. She should explain that the patient should remove the foil wrapper and apply a small amount of water soluble lubricant to the suppository. She should instruct the patient or caregiver to insert the suppository past the internal anal sphincter to enable absorption and avoid expulsion of the drug from the body. Rectal drug action takes 15 to 30 minutes after insertion, so the patient should lie quietly for this time period. The medical assistant should always provide written instructions to the patient and

---

■ PROCEDURE 39-6

Administering an intramuscular injection

Task
Select the proper site and properly administer an intramuscular injection.

Conditions
- Nonsterile disposable gloves
- Medication ordered by the physician
- Appropriate syringe for ordered dose
- Needle with safety device
- 2" × 2" sterile gauze pads
- 70% isopropyl alcohol wipes
- Sharps container

- Biohazardous waste container
- Patient's medical record

Standards
In the time specified and within the scoring parameters determined by the instructor, the student will successfully select the proper site and properly administer an intramuscular injection.

Performance Standards
1. Wash your hands to ensure infection control.
2. Assemble the equipment and supplies and verify the order.

Continued

PROCEDURE 39-6—cont'd

3. Check the expiration date of the medication.

4. Follow the "seven rights" of medication administration.

5. Check the medication against the physician's written order to perform the first of three checks.

6. Check the patient's medical record for allergies or conditions that may contraindicate the medication.

7. Calculate the correct dose to be given, if necessary.

8. Prepare the syringe with the ordered dose of the medication to ensure that the patient receives the correct dose.

9. Follow the procedure for drawing medication into the syringe.

10. Greet and identify the patient to ensure that you administer the medication to the right patient.

11. Explain the procedure to the patient to ensure patient understanding and compliance.

12. Select the appropriate injection site and position the patient.

13. Recheck the medication against the physician's written orders to perform the second of three checks.

14. Expose the injection site and inspect the site for scars and inflammation. If scarring or inflammation is present, choose a different site because scarred, broken, or inflamed skin will decrease absorption of the drug. Be sure to explain to the patient why you must change the site.

15. Put on gloves.

16. If the patient is a child, you may need to ask the parent or caregiver to help restrain the child to avoid injury to you or the patient. If the parent or guardian is unable to assist you, obtain assistance from a second health care professional. Restrain the patient only when necessary. You should not restrain a child who is willing to cooperate.

17. Prepare the injection site by cleaning it with an alcohol wipe, beginning at the center and working in an outward circular motion. Allow the site to air dry. Do not touch the site or allow the patient to touch the site to avoid contaminating the site.

18. Recheck the medication against the physician's written orders to perform the third of three checks.

19. Remove the cover without touching the needle. Visually inspect the injection site to be sure that the alcohol has dried before you inject.

20. Secure the skin at the injection site by spreading the skin around the injection site taut with the thumb and forefinger of your nondominant hand to ensure that the muscle tissue is injected and not the subcutaneous layer.

21. Puncture the skin quickly at a 90-degree angle and insert the entire needle up to the hub.

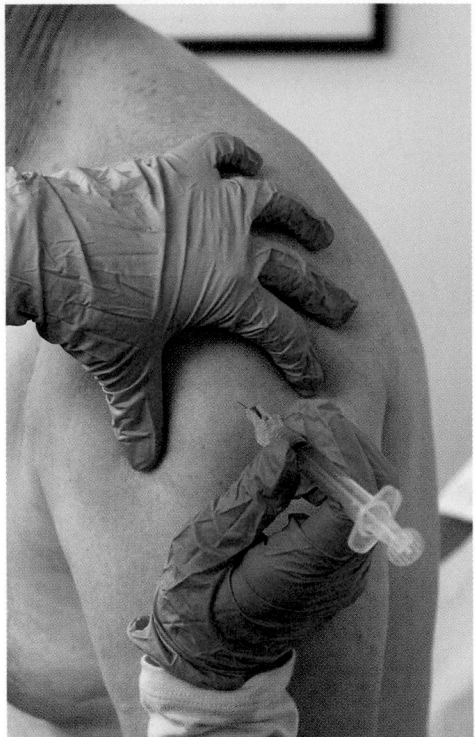

Spread the skin taut and puncture it at a 90-degree angle.

22. Check to see if blood aspirates into the syringe by releasing your grasp of the tissues and pulling back on the plunger a little with your nondominant hand. If blood does aspirate, withdraw the needle from the site because blood in the syringe is a sign that the needle has pierced a blood vessel. Then begin the procedure again with a new needle.

23. If blood does not aspirate into the syringe, push the plunger of the syringe slowly and steadily into the intramuscular tissue. Be careful to hold the needle still while administering the medication to avoid bruising the skin.

24. Place a gauze pad over the injection site and withdraw the needle from the site at the same 90-degree angle.

25. Use a 2" × 2" sterile gauze pad to massage the injection site gently but firmly to help distribute the medication into body tissues. **NOTE:** Do not massage the injection site of heparin or insulin because it may cause tissue damage.

25. Discard the syringe and needle in the sharps container, remove your gloves and discard them in the biohazardous waste container, and wash your hands to ensure infection control.

26. Check on the patient. Ask the patient how she feels and observe her for any signs of immediate emergency reaction, such as dizziness, lightheadedness, or fainting.

PROCEDURE 39-6—cont'd

27. Document the procedure, including the date, time, lot number of the medication, dose given, and injection site used. Chart any reactions you observe.

Date	
10/20/08; 10:45 a.m.	Hep B, first series, Lot #44776, exp date 12/30/2009, IM left deltoid. Pt. instructed to return in 1 month for second shot in series. Injection well tolerated, no adverse effects noted.
	--- C. Chapin, CMA

PROCEDURE 39-7

Administering a transdermal patch

Task
Apply a transdermal patch to the appropriate site.

Conditions
- Medicated transdermal patch
- Nonsterile disposable gloves
- Patient education-instruction sheet
- Patient's medical record

Standards
In the time specified and within the scoring parameters determined by the instructor, the student will successfully apply a transdermal patch to the appropriate site.

Performance Standards
1. Wash your hands to ensure infection control.
2. Assemble the equipment and supplies and verify the order.
3. Check the expiration date of the medication.
4. Follow the "seven rights" of medication administration.
5. Check the medication against the physician's written order to perform the first of three checks.
6. Check the patient's medical record for allergies or conditions that may contraindicate the medication.
7. Calculate the correct dose to be given, if necessary.
8. Check the medication against the written order again to perform the second of three checks.
9. Greet and identify the patient to ensure that you a dminister the medication to the right patient.
10. Explain the procedure to the patient and discuss any possible adverse effects, contraindications, and reactions listed on the package. Give the patient an education-instruction sheet. Confirm that the patient understands the instructions by asking him to repeat the directions to you.
11. Expose the patient's skin in an area that is relatively free from hair, such as the chest, upper back, or upper arm.
12. Clean the skin if needed with mild soap and water to ensure that the area is clean and free from lotions or oils. If you must remove hair, clip it close to the skin, rather than shaving it because shaving may cause nicks in the skin that cause the medication to be absorbed incorrectly.
13. Instruct the patient to rotate subsequent patches to different sites for each application to prevent skin irritation. Discuss the need for hair removal and skin cleaning.
14. Put on gloves and open the patch packaging. Peel away the protective cover from one side of the patch and stick the patch to the patient's skin. Smooth the edges of the patch for full skin contact.

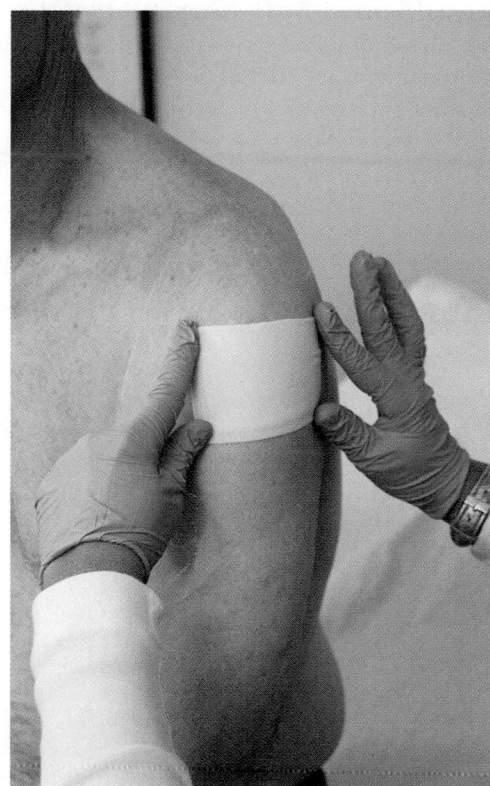

Apply the patch and smooth the edges.

Continued

PROCEDURE 39-7—cont'd

15. Provide further patient education, including:
    a. information on removal of the patch and proper disposal
    b. emphasis on removing the patch himself, if possible, and instructing anyone else who removes the patch to wear gloves to avoid transdermal effects of the medication being absorbed into the skin
    c. information on application of a patch and remembering to rotate application sites
    d. reminder to wash and dry his hands after applying the patch and that the medication may get onto his hands and so transmission to others is possible
    e. written instruction-direction sheet
    f. encouragement for the patient to share any questions he has
16. Dispose of waste materials.
17. Remove your gloves and wash your hands.
18. Document the application of the patch in the patient's medical record as well as patient education conducted.

Date	
10/22/08; 3:10 p.m.	Nicoderm 0.5 mg/patch applied to upper left arm. Patient given instructions on removal and application of daily patch and site rotation. Pt. given verbal and written instructions. Pt. understood and repeated instructions. ————————— ————————————————————————— C. Chapin, CMA

instruct the patient to call the office if further questions arise. In addition, she should advise the patient to store the medication in a cool, dry place to avoid melting before administration. (See *Teaching about self-administration*.)

Patient Education

Teaching About Self-Administration

The medical assistant plays a vital role in educating patients in the proper self-administration of their medications. Because a patient may take many prescription medications on a daily basis, he must self-medicate. The medical assistant should ensure that the patient is aware of signs of allergy to his medication and what medications or foods he should avoid consuming with his medication.

One of the most powerful forms of educating patients about their medications is the medication insert. These inserts include information for prescription and over-the-counter medications that can help patients understand their medications. The intended effects, adverse effects, contraindications, and dosage information are all listed on the medication insert, sometimes called a *package insert*. The medical assistant should remind patients to read the inserts, ask the pharmacist, or call the office if they have questions.

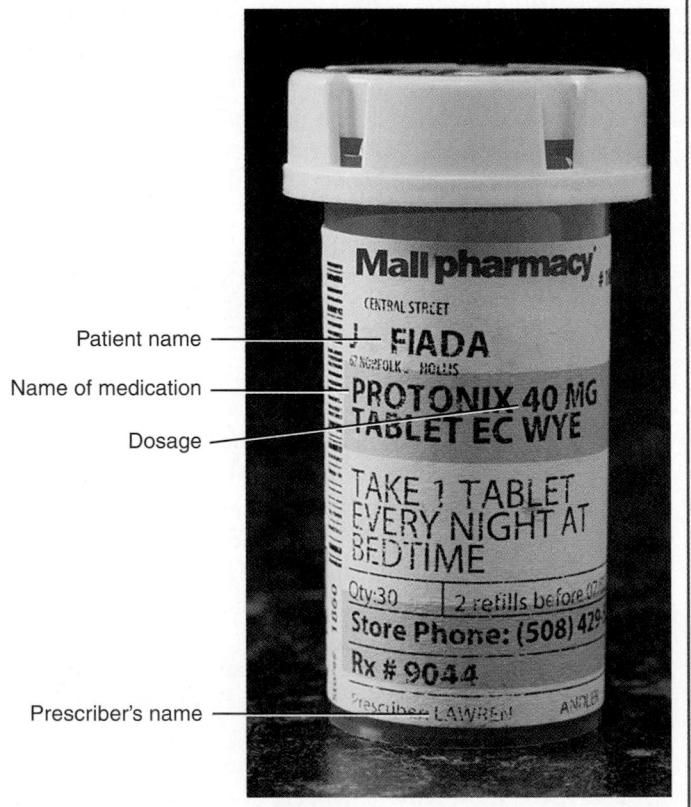

Patient name — FIADA

Name of medication — PROTONIX 40 MG TABLET EC WYE

Dosage

Prescriber's name

Chapter Summary

- The medical assistant must calculate the proper dosage of medications to be administered to her patient based on the amount ordered and what she has available (on hand).
- The medical assistant can calculate dosages for children using the BSA method and a nomogram.
- The medical assistant must administer medication to patients carefully and properly, following the "seven rights" of medication administration.
- There are several routes of administration. The major routes are oral and parenteral. The oral route is the most common route of medication administration.
- Parenteral routes of administration include inhalation, injection, topical, vaginal, and rectal routes.
- Routes of administration are based on how quickly the drug reaches the bloodstream and the ease of administration.
- When administering medications, the medical assistant must check the medication against the order three times to prevent errors.
- The medical assistant can use three types of injections to administer medications: subcutaneous, intradermal, and intramuscular.
- A subcutaneous injection is administered into the fatty layer beneath the dermis. An intradermal injection is administered by injecting the medication into the dermis. An intramuscular injection is administered into the muscle.
- Administering medications intravenously is the fastest absorbing route since the medication enters the bloodstream directly.
- Although a medical assistant cannot legally administer IV medications, she must have an understanding of IV medication administration and fluid replacement therapy.
- Patients can inhale medications through the respiratory tract for immediate absorption. Bronchodilators are an example of an inhaled medication that has an immediate action.
- Medication placed on top of the skin and absorbed into the bloodstream via the skin is called *transdermal*. The medication absorbs more slowly, over a period of 12 to 24 hours.
- Rectal administration of medications may be indicated if a patient is unable to tolerate medications orally.
- Vaginal administration of medications treat local infection or administer hormone therapy.
- The medical assistant must educate patients in administering medications orally, by use of an inhaler, injection, vaginally, and rectally. Her effective communication with the patient is vital.

Team Work Exercises

1. Divide into groups of three to five students. Each group must research a drug classification and create a poster or computer presentation that describes the therapeutic effects of the drugs in the classification. How does the drug work in the body? What disorders does it treat? What patients or concurrent conditions would contraindicate use of the medication? Each group should provide three examples of medications in the classification. Based on the work of each group, the class should determine if one of the meds is a better choice. If so, why? Consider issues of price, safety, adverse effects, and concurrent conditions.

2. Divide into groups of two to three students. Each group must create a practice examination with 10 dosage calculation questions for classmates to complete. Be sure to include a pediatric patient in one of the examples. Correct each other's examinations and give feedback on performance.

Case Studies

1. Logan Shaw is a newly diagnosed diabetic. He is 60 years old and depressed about his weight and diabetes. The medical assistant is instructing him on the use of the glucometer and injecting insulin. He seems distracted and uninterested in learning to inject himself. How should the medical assistant engage him in recording his blood glucose and injecting his insulin?

2. Mrs. Czarnecki comes to the office with her granddaughter. She is 78 years old and taking several medications. Her blood pressure pill, lipid-lowering medication, arthritis medication, and calcium tablets look very similar. She tells the medical assistant that she is afraid she will get confused and forget to take medications or take too much. How can the medical assistant work with Mrs. Czarnecki and her granddaughter to form a strategy for ensuring that she takes her medications properly each day?

Resources

- Body surface area calculator: *www.halls.md/body-surface-area /bsa.htm*
- Injection sites for insulin administration: *www.dlife.com /dLife/do/ShowContent/type1_information/treatment /insulin.page1*
- Intramuscular and subcutaneous injection sites and technique guides: *www.drugguide.com/intraInjectNew.asp* and *www.healthinfotranslations.com/pdfDocs/Subcutaneous -Injection-Sites.pdf*
- Joint Commission's Do-Not-Use Abbreviation List: *www.jointcommission.org/PatientSafety/DoNotUseList/*
- Review of dosage calculations: *www.classes.kumc.edu/son /nurs420/clinical/basic_review.htm* and *www.nursesaregreat .com/articles/drugcal.htm*

Introduction to the Clinical Laboratory

Learning Objectives

Upon completion of this chapter, the student will be able to:

- define the key terms in the glossary
- describe the functions of the clinical laboratory
- explain the purposes of performing laboratory tests
- identify the different departments within the clinical laboratory
- identify various tests performed in each laboratory department
- demonstrate an understanding of the physician's office laboratory and its relationship with the clinical laboratory
- explain the purpose of CLIA '88 and identify the various categories of testing within the CLIA '88 regulations
- explain the concepts of quality control and quality assurance as they relate to the clinical laboratory
- discuss the purpose and importance of the laboratory requisition
- discuss the importance of proper patient preparation and education as it relates to specimen collection
- explain proper procedures for collecting, handling, and transporting specimens
- list and describe various types of laboratory equipment and properly use the equipment
- perform proper maintenance on various types of laboratory equipment.

CAAHEP Competencies

Clinical Competencies

Fundamental Principles
Dispose of biohazardous materials
Practice standard precautions

Specimen Collection
Obtain specimens for microbiological testing

Diagnostic Testing
CLIA-waived tests
Perform urinalysis
Perform hematology testing
Perform chemistry testing
Perform immunology testing
Perform microbiology testing

Patient Care
Screen and follow up test results

General Competencies

Legal Concepts
Document appropriately

Operational Functions
Perform routine maintenance of administrative and clinical equipment
Use methods of quality control

ABHES Competencies

Clinical Duties

Use quality control
Collect and process specimens
Perform selected CLIA-waived tests that assist with diagnosis and treatment
Screen and follow up patient test results

Chapter Outline

Key Terms

analyzer
Automated instrument used to test blood and other body fluids for various substances

anatomical laboratory
Section of the laboratory that includes histology and cytology

automated method
Laboratory test performed on an automated instrument or machine

biopsy
Removal and microscopic observation of a small piece of living tissue

clinical diagnosis
Diagnosis based on actual observations, diagnostic results, and symptoms

manual method
Test method in which the steps of testing are done by hand instead of by an automated instrument

normal range
Range of values in which a test result should fall for most healthy individuals

panel
Group of blood tests that evaluate the function of a particular body system; also called *profile*

physician's office laboratory (POL)
Laboratory within the medical office

proficiency testing
Tests on unknown specimens provided by an external monitoring agency, such as the state health department and the College of American Pathologists, to meet quality control requirements

qualitative result
Laboratory result that is descriptive, rather than providing a numerical value

quality control
Methods used to monitor the accuracy of laboratory results

quantitative result
Laboratory result that includes a numerical value

reagent
Substance used in a chemical reaction

reference laboratory
Independent laboratory used by POLs and hospital laboratories to perform specialized testing

requisition slip
Form used to order laboratory tests

routine test
Laboratory test ordered as part of a regular office visit

specimen
Blood, other body fluid, or body tissue submitted for laboratory analysis

Purpose of the Clinical Laboratory

Health care providers request laboratory tests for many reasons. These tests can be used to diagnose a disease or condition, to monitor or manage a patient's condition, or to assess a patient's health status. A patient's test results in conjunction with his overall physical assessment are important factors in maintaining proper health.

The clinical laboratory is an integral part of the health care system. Most hospitals, medical centers, and HMOs contain full-service laboratories. **Reference laboratories**, such as Quest Diagnostics, are independent clinical laboratories that offer various services to medical offices and other health care facilities.

Physicians' offices request laboratory analysis on **specimens**, which are small portions of a patient's blood, body fluids (including secretions, such as urine and lower respiratory fluid), or tissue (such as skin scrapings and tumors). The medical assistant may collect these specimens and then process them to be sent to the laboratory for analysis.

Laboratory Tests

When a patient comes to the office with a chief complaint of fever and sore throat, the physician will conduct a physical examination and may then ask the medical assistant to obtain a throat culture to be sent to the clinical laboratory. A throat culture is one of many laboratory tests that can be ordered for a patient. (See *Abbreviations for common laboratory tests.*)

In other cases, the diagnosis may not be so straightforward and the physician may need to order a series of laboratory tests to assess the patient's current condition. The medical assistant's responsibility in both of these situations would consist of understanding the process, beginning with the physician's order and ending with the laboratory report received by the office. (See *Life cycle of a laboratory test.*)

Panel

A physician can order a single laboratory test, such as a blood glucose level or a cholesterol level. The physician may also order a group of laboratory tests, called a **panel** or, sometimes, a *profile*. All the tests included in the panel relate to the specific organ of the body or a particular disease state. For example, a *hepatic panel* is used to assess liver function and assist in diagnosis or evaluation of a pathogenic condition that affects the liver. The medical assistant should know the names of common panels listed on the laboratory requisition slip and the tests generally contained in each.

Abbreviations for common laboratory tests

A physician may order any of thousands of laboratory tests. Many of these tests are known mainly by their abbreviation. The following table lists some common laboratory tests known by their abbreviation, along with the normal values for those tests.

Abbreviation	Laboratory Test
ALT	alanine aminotransferase
AST	aspartate aminotransferase
BUN	blood urea nitrogen
C&S	culture and sensitivity
CBC	complete blood count
ESR	erythrocyte sedimentation rate; also known as *sed rate*
FBS	fasting blood sugar
H&H	hemoglobin and hematocrit
Lytes	electrolytes
PTT	partial thromboplastin time
TSH	thyroid stimulating hormone

Manual or Automated

Laboratory tests can also be classified as manual or automated. **Manual methods** of laboratory testing involve performing the series of testing steps by hand rather than using an automated system of instruments. Performing a rapid Strep test, for example, is done manually using the proper testing kit. **Automated methods** involve, for example, testing a blood specimen on a complex **analyzer** (an automated instrument used to test blood and other body fluids for various substances) or on a smaller testing instrument such as a glucose meter. Automated methods take less time and have greater accuracy than manual methods if all the necessary quality controls and instrument maintenance practices have been established.

Purpose of Laboratory Tests

There are many reasons why a physician may order a laboratory test, including:

- health assessment—for example, evaluation of electrolytes, such as sodium ($Na+$), chloride ($Cl-$), potassium ($K+$), and carbon dioxide (CO_2) to assess a person's electrolyte balance
- disease detection—for example, test for prostate specific antigen (PSA) to screen for prostate cancer

Life cycle of a laboratory test

The following illustration shows the typical life cycle of a laboratory test, from the physician's order through the laboratory report that is filed in the patient's chart.

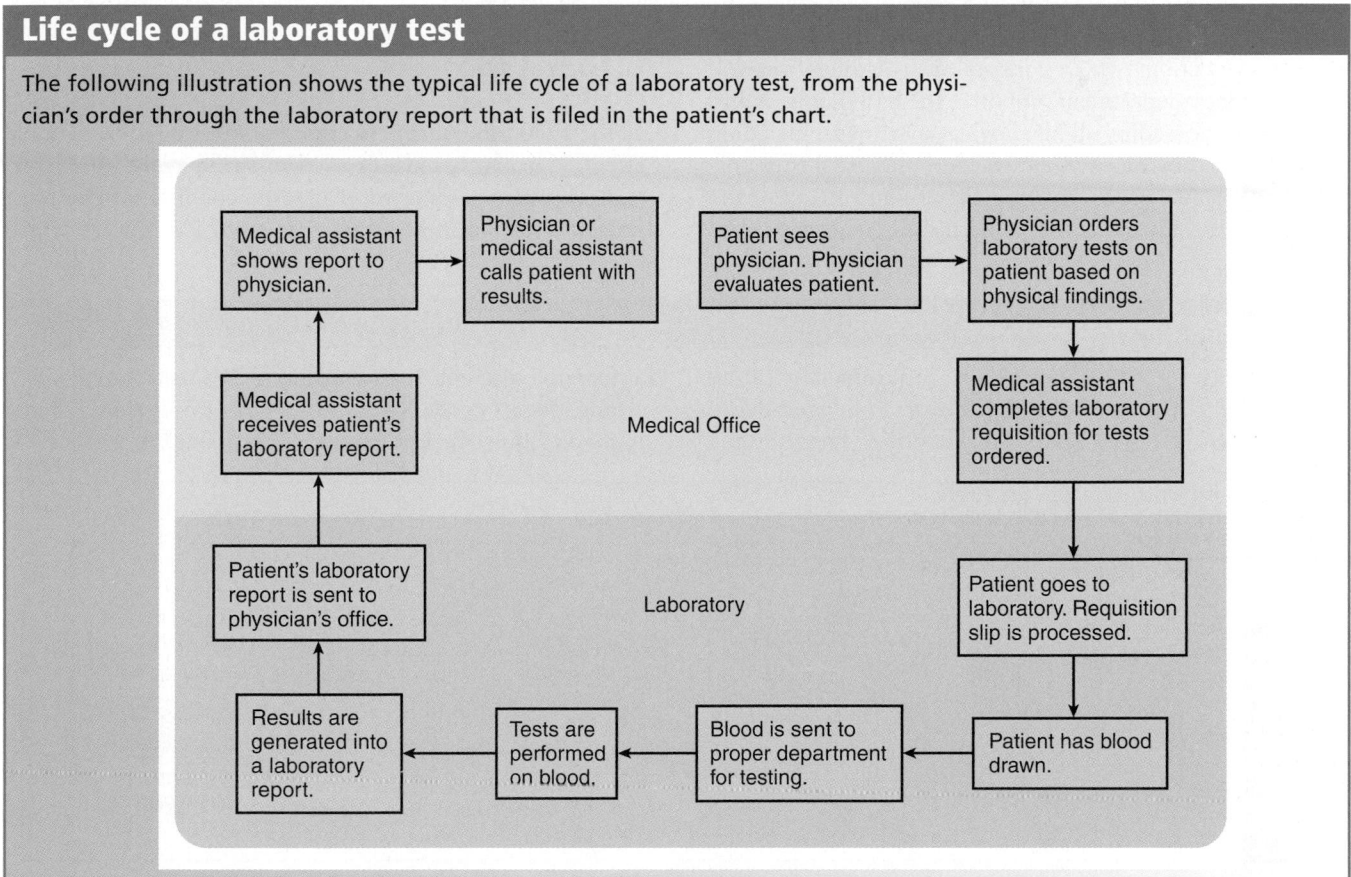

- diagnosis—for example, a rapid *Strep* test to diagnose a streptococcal throat infection
- monitor treatment or disease progression—for example, measuring levels of thyroid stimulating hormone to monitor treatment for hypothyroidism
- disease prevention—for example, a Papanicolaou (Pap) smear to detect certain viral infections and other cancer-causing conditions.

Quantitative or Qualitative Results

Results obtained from laboratory tests can be classified as *quantitative* or *qualitative*. A **quantitative result** is a numerical value, such as 87 mg/dl for a glucose level. A **qualitative result** is a result that describes a condition, rather than providing a numerical value as in a quantitative result. An example of a qualitative result would be "throat culture: positive for Beta Strep Group A."

Laboratory Profession

The clinical laboratory employs many health care professionals in many departments. (See *Laboratory departments*.) The director of the laboratory is usually the pathologist. A *pathologist* is a medical doctor who oversees all diagnostic operations of the laboratory. If there is an **anatomical laboratory** section (which consists of a histology department, cytology department, or both), the pathologist is also responsible for reading all histological specimens, including those obtained by **biopsy** (removal and microscopic examination of a small piece of living tissue), and many of the cytological specimens, as well as performing autopsies. The *laboratory manager,* who is typically a medical technologist and holds a bachelor's and master's degree, is responsible for such daily operations as scheduling, purchasing, and budgets. Each department usually has a department supervisor, also called a *section head,* who is a medical technologist and may have an advanced degree or certification. The department supervisor oversees the daily tasks of her assigned department and supervises the technologists and technicians within that department. Each department has technologists and technicians who perform the tests within that department. (See *MTs and MLTs,* page 854.) Many medical technologists and technicians may be *generalists,* which means they are able to perform testing throughout two or more departments instead of specializing in just one department.

The laboratory may also employ various support staff. A *phlebotomist* collects blood and other body specimens and may also carry out specimen processing duties. He collects specimens from the inpatient floors, the emergency room, and the outpatient laboratory. Some phlebotomists collect specimens from homebound and nursing home patients. The laboratory may also employ a medical secretary. Her duties include reception, receiving specimens, filing, transcribing pathology reports, and sending laboratory reports.

CLIA 1988

In the 1980s, the quality of laboratory testing drew national attention in part because of an increase in patient complaints and lawsuits regarding misdiagnosed conditions. The most notable situation involved misreading of Pap smears, which

Laboratory departments

The physician's office may have different laboratory departments that perform routine testing procedures. Some departments perform their laboratory tests by the automated method. The following table lists common laboratory departments, along with a description of each and routine tests performed in each department.

Department	Description	Routine Tests
Blood bank	Section of the laboratory where blood is collected, stored, and prepared for transfusion	• Blood typing • Type and screen
Chemistry	Most automated area of the laboratory, where instruments are computerized and designed to perform single and multiple tests from a small specimen	• Basic metabolic panel • Blood urea nitrogen (BUN) • Calcium (Ca) • Cholesterol • Creatine kinase (CK) • Creatine kinase-MB (CK-MB) • Creatinine

Laboratory departments—cont'd

Department	Description	Routine Tests
		• Electrolytes • Glucose (blood sugar) • Liver function panel • Thyroid stimulating hormone (TSH) • Troponin
Coagulation	Usually a subsection of the Hematology Department that evaluates the overall process of hemostasis	• Bleeding time (BT) • Partial thromboplastin time (PTT) • Platelet count • Prothrombin time with INR
Cytology	Anatomic section of laboratory that deals with the study of cells.	• Papanicolaou (Pap) smear • Urine cytology • Sputum cytology
Hematology	Study of the formed (cellular) elements of the blood	• Complete blood count (CBC) • Erythrocyte sedimentation rate (ESR) • Hematocrit • Hemoglobin
Histology	Some physicians perform biopsies or routine excisions in the office and submit the specimen to a histology laboratory or reference laboratory for processing	• Biopsy
Microbiology	Responsible for identification of pathogenic microorganisms and hospital infection control	• Rapid *Streptococcus* A test • Throat culture • Urine culture • Wound culture
Mycology	Responsible for the collection and isolation of fungi	• Fungal culture
Parasitology	Responsible for microscopic examination of stool specimens for the presence of parasites, ova, or larvae	• Ova and parasite test (O&P)
Serology	Responsible for evaluating the body's immune responses	• Infectious mononucleosis test • Rheumatic factor test • Syphilis tests, such as rapid plasma reagin (RPR) or fluorescent treponemal antibody (FTA-ABS)
Urinalysis	Possibly a separate section or part of the hematology or chemistry section where routine screening procedures are performed to detect disorders and infections of the kidney	• Complete urinalysis • Urine pregnancy test

resulted in the death of patients in some cases. In 1988, Congress passed the Clinical Laboratory Improvement Amendment (CLIA 1988) to improve the quality of laboratory testing in the United States. CLIA 1988, which became effective in 1992, mandates that all laboratories must be regulated using the same standards, regardless of their location, type, or size. This law requires every clinical laboratory facility in the country to obtain a certificate from the federal government to help reassure customers that the laboratory testing performed at the facility is reliable and accurate. CLIA regulations cover testing categories, qualifications of personnel performing the testing, and standards

MTs and MLTs

Medical technologists (MTs) and medical laboratory technicians (MLTs) work together in a clinical laboratory. However, they have different education and certification requirements, credentials, duties, and salary ranges, as outlined here.

	MT	MLT
Education	Bachelor of Science degree in medical technology, clinical laboratory science, or biotechnology (4- to 5-year program)	Associate of Science degree for a medical laboratory technician (2- to 3-year program)
Certification	Examination taken through the American Association of Clinical Pathologists (ASCP)	Examination taken through the ASCP
Credentials	MT (ASCP)	MLT (ASCP)
Duties	Laboratory manager, department supervisor, specialist, or generalist technologist	Generalist technician in all laboratory departments
Annual salary	$41,000 to $52,000	$31,000 to $41,000

of testing, as well as quality control and proficiency testing protocols.

Laboratory Testing Categories

The CLIA testing category for an individual laboratory is determined by the complexity of testing done at the facility. The four categories of laboratory testing established by CLIA regulations include waived tests, moderate-complexity tests, high-complexity tests, and provider-performed microscopy procedures.

Waived Tests

Waived tests are simple procedures and include many the patient can perform at home. The majority of testing performed in a physician's office will be of this type. Many of the more stringent CLIA requirements do not apply to waived tests. In order to be exempt from the CLIA requirements for moderate- or high-complexity tests, a laboratory that performs only waived tests must apply for and be granted a certificate of waiver from the Health Care Financing Administration (HCFA). (See Figure 40-1.) It is important to note that if a laboratory performs only one test and it is a waived test (for example, a rapid *Strep* test), the laboratory must still apply for and be granted a waiver or be held to the more stringent requirements. Here are some examples of waived tests:

- dipstick reagent urinalysis
- fecal occult blood testing
- urine pregnancy tests

- hemoglobin determinations using a CLIA-waived analyzer such as the HemoCue
- blood glucose determination using an FDA-approved blood glucose analyzer such as One Touch glucometer
- rapid *Streptococcus* testing such as BD Strep Link Group A Rapid test.

Moderate-Complexity Tests

Tests in the *moderate-complexity* category are more difficult to perform than waived tests and require documentation of the technologist or technician's training in testing principles, instrument calibration, quality control, and proficiency testing. **Proficiency testing** consists of testing unknown specimens provided by an external monitoring agency, such as the state health department and the College of American Pathologists, to meet quality control requirements. Examples of moderate-complexity tests performed in the medical office include hematology and blood chemistry tests performed on automated blood analyzers that are not CLIA-waived.

High-Complexity Tests

High-complexity tests require sophisticated instrumentation and a high degree of interpretation by the testing personnel. Personnel performing within this category must have a formal education with a degree in laboratory medicine. High-complexity tests also require documentation of the technologist's training in testing principles, instrument calibration, quality control, and proficiency testing. Examples of high-complexity tests are performed in microbiology,

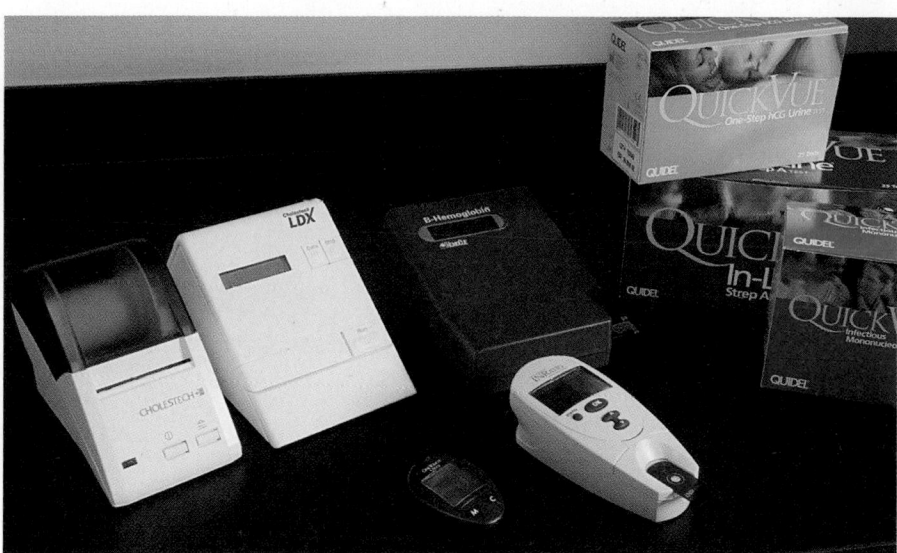

FIG 40-1 CLIA-waived test kits and analyzers.

immunology, immunohematology, and cytology departments and include cultures, type and screens, and Pap smears.

Provider-Performed Microscopy Procedures

Provider-performed microscopy (PPM) procedures are tests classified as moderate complexity. These tests involve direct visual examination of specimens using a microscope. Persons authorized to conduct these tests include physicians, mid-level practitioners such as physician's assistants, and dentists. A physician's office that performs PPM must apply for a Certificate of Provider-Performed Microscopy and follow the same requirements as listed in the moderate-complexity category. Examples of PPM procedures include direct wet mounts for the presence of bacteria, fungus, parasites, and human elements; potassium hydroxide (KOH) preparations; pinworm examinations; urine sediment examinations; and nasal smears for eosinophils.

Quality Control

Understanding and following **quality control** (QC) procedures is an essential component of laboratory testing. QC consists of methods and procedures that are used to monitor the accuracy and reliability of laboratory results. QC testing includes testing samples of known values (controls) to ensure the proper function of the machine and the technical process, as well as any **reagents** (substances used in a chemical reaction) that may be used in the procedure.

Prior to testing patient samples, control samples must be tested and the results must be documented. For most laboratory analyzers, testing control samples might include using control reagents designed to obtain high, normal, or low results. Many commercial testing kits, such as the rapid *Streptococcus* test or mono test, contain an internal control with each patient test cassette or strip as well as a positive and negative external control reagent. (See Figure 40-2.)

The manufacturer of the control samples provides a range of values that each control must fall within in order to ensure the accuracy of the method being used. If a control result falls outside the acceptable range, corrective action must be taken. Under no circumstances should the patient sample be tested until all control sample results are within acceptable ranges. If results don't fall within acceptable ranges, corrective steps include:

- repeating the control (If the repeated test results fall within the acceptable range, the technician may proceed with patient testing.)
- checking the control sample's expiration date (The technician should never use control samples that have expired.)
- checking the expiration date of all testing reagents (The technician should discard the reagent if it's outdated.)
- checking to make sure the instrument is calibrated correctly and functioning properly.

The process of quality control also includes proper documentation of the procedures performed. As with most medical procedures, the statement "not documented, not done" applies to the laboratory. The medical office puts policies and procedures in place, as required by CLIA or other laboratory accreditation agencies, to include documentation. (See Figure 40-3.) Examples of documentation include recording:

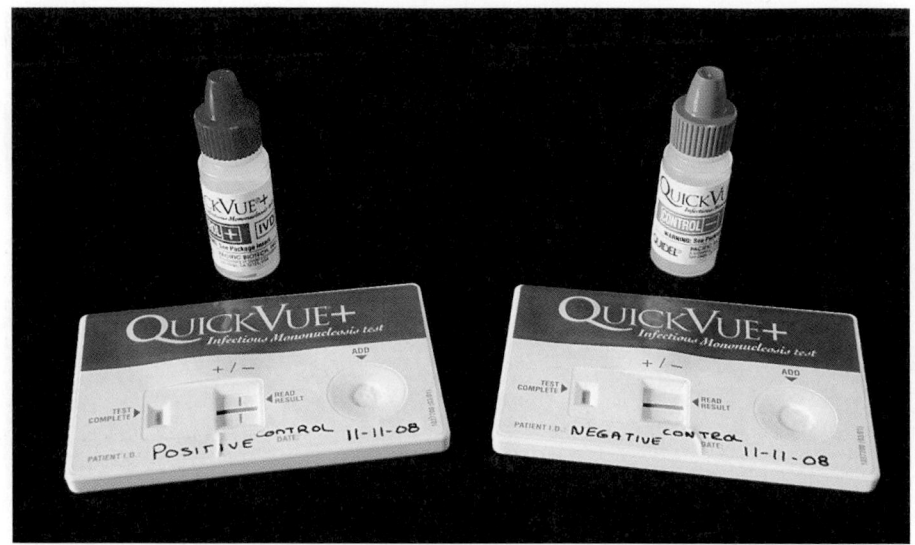

FIG 40-2 Quality control results from a mono test kit.

- all control sample results and corrective action that may have been taken
- daily temperatures of laboratory refrigerators, incubators, freezers, and instruments as well as room temperature
- preventive maintenance performed on an analyzer or instrument
- instrument calibrations that may have been performed.

Physician's Office Laboratory

Because the patient will find it more convenient to undergo testing at the physician's office, a **routine test**, which is a laboratory test ordered as part of a regular office visit, may be performed in the **physician's office laboratory** (POL). Examples of routine tests that are commonly performed include fasting blood sugar and urinalysis. The medical assistant is most commonly the person in charge of the POL or the one who performs most of the patient testing. The medical assistant must familiarize herself with the types of tests that are performed in the office. For the most part, the most common type of test performed in the POL is the CLIA-waived test. As mentioned, the medical assistant should follow testing, quality control, and reporting guidelines when performing any patient testing.

Tests that are considered time-consuming, highly sophisticated, expensive, or complex are referred to an outside laboratory, such as a hospital laboratory or privately owned commercial laboratory. The outside laboratory provides the POL with a laboratory directory that serves as a valuable reference guide for the proper collection, handling, and transport of clinical specimens. Although directories vary among organizations, they generally include:

- comprehensive list of test procedures in alphabetical order
- method used for each test
- current procedural terminology (CPT) code
- patient preparation necessary for each test

CHOLESTECH QUALITY CONTROL LOG SHEET

Date	Optics check results	QC range	QC results	Initials/comments
02/06/07	94 96 95 98	130-210	183	OK cg
02/07/07	94 96 95 98	130-210	186	OK cg
02/08/07	94 96 95 98	130-210	181	OK cg

FIG 40-3 Proper documentation of a QC log sheet.

- amount and type of specimen required
- proper storage and handling for the specimen
- transport instructions for the specimen.

The medical assistant should familiarize herself with the individual laboratory directory as well as the services offered by each outside laboratory used. If she is unable to find in the directory the answer to a specimen collection question, she should call the reference laboratory prior to collecting the specimen.

Laboratory Requisitions and Reports

In the life cycle of a laboratory test, the requisition (order) for the test is the first step. The medical assistant must familiarize herself with each requisition slip she may complete. Some laboratories will have a separate requisition slip for clinical laboratory tests, Pap smear specimens, and histological specimens. The medical assistant or other office staff should be sure to stock each examination room, the POL area, and the front office area with sufficient quantities of each type of laboratory requisition slip for easy access. In addition, a POL may use the services of a hospital laboratory as well as a reference or private laboratory, so the staff may be dealing with more than one type of laboratory requisition form. Upon testing the patient's specimen, the laboratory will generate a formal report of the patient's test results. The laboratory report will include much of the patient's demographic information found on the requisition slip, as well as the results to the tests ordered.

Laboratory Requisition Slip

A laboratory **requisition slip** is a printed form that contains a list of the most frequently ordered laboratory tests, some of which are grouped into panels. The medical assistant should know about each of the tests listed on the requisition slip. (See Figure 40-4.) Specific information required on the laboratory requisition slip includes:

- *name of the hospital or laboratory where the form was issued,* which usually appears on the top portion of the requisition form with the laboratory's complete address, telephone number, and fax number
- *type of test,* such as STAT, fasting, nonfasting, and routine, with a clear indication from the physician (by checking the appropriate box) about how the specimen should be handled and the test conducted (For example, the laboratory technician performs tests that are marked STAT as soon as possible, telephones the results to the physician, documents the results, and then faxes the results to the physician.)
- *priority,* which tells the laboratory exactly how soon the physician needs the results (For example, if *routine* is checked, the test will be performed with the daily work. If

the physician needs the results immediately, *STAT* will be checked and the laboratory will perform the test immediately and call the results directly to the physician. If *ASAP,* or *as soon as possible,* is checked, the laboratory will give the test a higher priority than a routine order, but not as immediate as a STAT order.)

- *patient's name and address,* listing the patient's last name first, followed by the first name and middle initial (required by most hospitals), and including the city, state, and zip code in the address for billing purposes
- *physician's name and address* to facilitate the reporting of tests results
- *patient's age and gender* because these factors may determine whether results fall in the **normal range,** which is a range of values in which a test result should fall for most healthy individuals (For example, the normal range for a hemoglobin determination for a female is 12 to 16 g/dl, while the normal hemoglobin range for a male is 14 to 18 g/dl.)
- *date of the specimen collection* to indicate to the laboratory the freshness of the specimen, and the time of collection, which is critical because the significance of some test results depend on whether the specimen is collected in the morning versus the afternoon or evening
- *laboratory tests requested,* usually indicated by checking boxes next to those tests on the list
- *microbiological specimen type* (such as "sputum sample") and, possibly, *location from which the specimen was taken* (such as "infected abdominal incision" or "discharge from right eye") to aid the laboratory in identifying the presence of possible pathogens
- *physician's* **clinical diagnosis** (also known as a *tentative diagnosis*), established by evaluating the patient's health history and the physical examination without conducting laboratory or diagnostic tests (The clinical diagnosis confirms the laboratory test results, alerts laboratory personnel to potentially dangerous pathogens, and is required for insurance billing information.)
- *medications,* some of which may interfere with the accuracy and validity of test results. (The medical assistant should note on the requisition slip all medications the patient is taking, regardless of their ability to interfere with results.)

Laboratory Report

A laboratory report, which is usually a computer printout, is used to communicate test results to the physician. A laboratory report includes:

- name, address, telephone, and fax number of the laboratory
- physician's name and address
- patient's name, age, and gender
- patient's accession number, which is assigned to each specimen received by the laboratory (Most laboratories

HARTELL MEMORIAL HOSPITAL LABORATORY

LAB REQUISITION

☐ STAT ☒ FASTING ☐ NON FASTING
☐ CALL RESULTS ☒ ROUTINE

NAME: *Jacqueline Garrett*

ADDRESS: *25 Hilltop Drive, Presley, CT* D.O.B.: *12/30/65*

PHONE: *(860) 555-2345* DR. *Greer* DATE & TIME DRAWN: *7/17/08; 7:00 a.m.*

DX: *Annual physical* SYMPTOM: *n/a*

BILL TO: (CIRCLE ONE) Medicare Medex (BCBS) Patient Other

Policy #: *RS7650M20* Subscriber's name: *Jacqueline Garrett*

CHEMISTRY PANELS	CC	
ELECTROLYTES	R/G	
BASIC METABOLIC	SS	
COMP METABOLIC	SS	
RENAL	SS	
HEPATIC	SS	
ACUTE HEPATITIS	R	
X LIPID	SS	
OBSTETRICAL	R	
CARDIAC *	R	
THYROID SCREEN	SS	
THYR CASCADE *	R	
S DRUGS ABUSE	R	
U DRUGS ABUSE	U	
CHEMISTRY		
ALB	SS	
ALK PHOS	SS	
ALT (SGPT)	SS	
ALT (SGOT)	SS	
AMYLASE	SS	
T BILI	SS	
D BILI	SS	
BUN	SS	
CALCIUM	SS	
CHOL	SS	
CREAT	SS	
CK	SS	
X GLUC	SS	
GLUC TOLERANCE	SS	
GLUC 1 HR	SS	
HDL	SS	
LDH	SS	
LDL (Quant)	SS	
PHOS	SS	
NA	SS	
K	SS	
CHLORIDE	SS	
CO₂	SS	
T PROTEIN	SS	
TRIG	SS	
URIC ACID	SS	
ACETAMINOPHEN	SS	
ALCOHOL	SS	
B-HCG (Quant)	R	
B-HCG TUMOR	R	
CARBAMAZEPINE	R	
CEA	R	
DIGOXIN	SS	
DILANTIN	SS	
GENTA TROUGH	SS	
GENTA PEAK	SS	
GLYCOHEM	L	
FERRITIN	R	
FOLIC ACID	R	
IRON	R	
IBC	R	

CHEMISTRY	CC	
MAGNESIUM	SS	
PHENOBARB	R	
PSA	R	
RUBELLA	R	
SALICYLATE	SS	
T3 UPTAKE	SS	
T4	SS	
F4 FREE	R	
TSH	SS	
VALPROIC ACID	LG	
VITAMIN B₁₂	R	
COAGULATION		
PRO TIME-INR	B	
PRO TIME	B	
PTT	B	
FIBRINOGEN	B	
BLEEDING TIME	B	
HEMATOLOGY		
X CBC w DIFF, PLTS	L	
CBC wo DIFF	L	
HCT	L	
HGB	L	
HCT/HGB	L	
PLATELET COUNT	L	
RETIC CT	L	
SED RATE	L	
WBC	L	
WBC/DIFF	L	
SEROLOGY		
ANA	R	
ASO	R	
CMV IgG	SS	
CMV IgGM	SS	
CRP RH.	R	
PYLORI ab	R	
Mono	R	
RA/RF	R	
RPR	SS	
RUBELLA	SS	
OTHER		
STOOL ANALYSIS		
OCCULT BLOOD	S	
FECAL FAT (Quant)	S	
FECAL WBC	S	
C. DIFFICILE	S	
OVA & PARASITES	PK	
URINALYSIS		
X URINALYSIS	U	
24 HR. URINE	U	
HCG-SERUM	R	
HCG-URINE	U	
MICROALBUMIN	U	

FLUIDS	CC	
SOURCE		
FLUID CELL CT	F	
FLUID DIFF	F	
FLUID GLUCOSE	F	
FLUID PROTEIN	F	
FLUID LDH	F	
FLUID CHLORINE	F	
FLUID CULTURE	F	
FLUID CRYSTALS	F	
FLUID PH	F	
POST VAS SPERM	F	
MICROBIOLOGY		
AFB STAIN		
AFB CULTURE		
ANAEROBIC CULTURE		
BLOOD CULTURE		
CHLAMYDIA/GC PROBE		
EAR CULTURE		
R L		
FLUID CULTURE		
SOURCE		
FUNGAL CULTURE		
GC CULTURE		
GRAM STAIN		
SOURCE		
KOH PREP		
NOSE CULTURE		
RAPID STREP		
RAPID UREASE		
SPUTUM CULTURE		
STOOL CULTURE		
THROAT CULTURE		
URINE CULTURE		
VAGINAL CULTURE		
VIRAL CULTURE		
SOURCE		
WOUND CULTURE		
SOURCE		
VAGINAL VP3		

BLOOD BANK	CC	
ABO/RH BLOOD TYPE	R	
DIRECT COOMBS	L	
TYPE & SCREEN	R	
TYPE & CROSS 1U	R	
TYPE & CROSS 2U	R	
TYPE & CROSS 3U	R	
TYPE & CROSS 4U	R	
OTHER TESTS	CC	
AFP	SS	
CA 125	SS	
CLOZARIL	R	
CORTISOL AM	SS	
CORTISOL PM	SS	
CYCLOSPORINE	L	
ESTROGEN	SS	
FSH	SS	
LH	SS	
HEP BE Ag	SS	
HEP BE Ab	SS	
HEP Bs Ag	SS	
HEP Bs Ab	SS	
HEP C	SS	
HIV 1.2 MASTERTUBE	SS	
LEAD	L	
RUBEOLA	SS	
ADDITIONAL TESTS		

COLLECTION CODES			
B	Blue	U	Urine
R	Red	SS	SST
G	Green	F	Fluid
L	Lavender		
S	Stool		

PHYSICIAN ACKNOWLEDGMENT The undersigned physician certifies for the laboratory: 1) the tests ordered on this requisition are medically necessary for the diagnosis and treatment of the patient; the physician is treating the patient in connection with the diagnosis or symptoms listed on this requisition; and the medical necessity of each test ordered on the requisition is appropriately documented in the patient's medical record. 2) tests ordered using customized panels may result in denial of payment by Medicare and, 3) the physician believes the tests ordered are appropriate for patient care, and payment may be denied by Medicare for reasons explained to the patient, who has agreed to pay for the tests personally by signing an Advanced Beneficiary Notice (ABN).

Robert Greer
SIGNATURE

7/15/08
DATE

FIG 40-4 Example of a completed laboratory requisition slip.

have computerized systems that assign a specific bar code for the automated instrument to identify when it is processing the specimen.)

- date the specimen was received by the laboratory
- date the results were reported by the laboratory
- names of the tests performed or panels requested
- results of the tests performed
- normal range for each test performed because the normal range, or *reference range*, of each test varies slightly among laboratories, depending on the test method, equipment, and reagents used to perform the test (See Figure 40-5.)

Whenever the physician orders laboratory tests that are to be performed in a laboratory other than the POL, the medical assistant must complete the laboratory requisition slip completely and legibly. Even if blood or other specimens are collected in the office but sent to an outside laboratory for testing, the laboratory requisition slip must accompany the specimen. If a laboratory receives a patient specimen without a laboratory requisition slip, it will not accept the specimen and the patient may have to come back for a repeat collection, which may delay diagnosis and treatment. When the medical assistant has completed the slip, she must stamp it with the physician's signature and then document the order (and specimen collection if any) in the patient's chart. In addition to documenting the order, some medical office procedures require the medical assistant to put a copy of the completed laboratory slip in the patient's chart.

Completed reports are hand-delivered, faxed, sent electronically to the physician's office computer, or mailed to the medical office by the laboratory. Abnormal results that are critical and indicate a threat to the patient's health or reports on requisitions that are marked STAT are telephoned immediately, documented in the computer system, and then faxed to the medical office. A hard copy of the report will also be generated and sent to the office via mail or computer network printer. The medical assistant should review each laboratory report, compare the patient's results to the normal ranges, and then immediately notify the physician of an abnormal result. When the physician has reviewed and initialed the laboratory report, the medical assistant may be responsible for calling the patient with the results, scheduling a follow-up visit with the patient, and filing the patient's results.

Patient Preparation

It is the responsibility of the medical assistant to instruct the patient about preparation for testing because such factors as food consumption, medications, activity, and the time of day could affect or invalidate certain laboratory results. A patient who is not instructed properly may have to come back to the laboratory for a repeat test. The medical assistant must explain the reasons for the advanced preparation so that the patient will be more likely to comply with the instructions. After she has explained the instructions, the medical assistant should determine if the patient completely understands the instructions and answer any questions the patient has. The medical assistant should also provide the patient with written instructions to serve as a reference if the patient forgets some of the information after leaving the office. The medical assistant should go slowly when providing instructions and always reinforce those instructions by repeating the procedure and have the patient repeat the instructions back to her. She should always remember that the quality of laboratory rest results can only be as good as the quality of the specimen collected.

Fasting

Certain laboratory tests require the patient to fast prior to collection. Fasting is sometimes necessary because the composition of blood and, thus, the laboratory test may be altered by the consumption of food. Examples of tests affected by fasting include blood glucose and triglycerides. Fasting requires that the patient abstain from eating and drinking (except water) for a specific amount of time before the specimen is collected. The most common fasting time is 12 to 14 hours.

Medication Restrictions

The physician determines whether a patient should abstain from her medication prior to laboratory testing. The medical assistant is responsible for ensuring that the patient understands medication restriction instructions and recording her medications, including the dosage, on the laboratory request form. If the physician determines that the patient cannot stop taking her medication, the medical assistant should also document this information on the laboratory request form.

Specimen Collection, Handling, and Transport

Proper specimen collection, handling, and transport are critical to the accuracy of test results. Such circumstances as a delay in transport or unsterile specimen collection could seriously affect a laboratory result and lead to improper treatment of the patient. (See *Specimen collection tips,* page 861.)

PATIENT LABORATORY REPORT

HARTELL MEMORIAL HOSPITAL LABORATORY

Name: Seth Banas   Sex: M
M/R#: 032608
D.O.B.: 05/02/63   Age: 45
Physician: Greer, R.
Location: Outpatient

Date ordered: 08/30/2008
Date collected: 08/30/2008
Time collected: 0
Date tested: 08/30/2008
Time tester: 21:41
Accession Number: 0007413225

HEMATOLOGY

<<<<<<<<<<COMPLETE BLOOD COUNT>>>>>>>>>>

ELECTROLYTES	RESULT	REFERENCE	UNITS
WBC	6.0	3.80–10.80	10^3
RBC	5.0	4.70–6.10	10^6
Hemoglobin	14.4	14–18	g/dl
Hematocrit	42.3	42–52	%
MCV	85	77–104	FL
MCH	29	27–34	PG
MCHC	34.0	31–37	g/dl
RDW	11	11–16	%
PLT CT	237	150–400	10^3
MPV	10	6–14	FL
Neutrophils	61	44–80	%
Lymphocytes	28	14–44	%
Monocytes	8	4–12	%
Eosinophils	2	0–5	%
Basophils	1	0–2	%
ABS NEU CT	4		

Manual diff	Not indicated
RBC morph	Not indicated

CHEMISTRY

<<<<<<<<<<BASIC METABOLIC PANEL>>>>>>>>>>

		REFERENCE	UNITS
Glucose	94	70–110	mg/dl
Sodium	141	136–145	mmol/L
Potassium	4.7	3.50–5.10	mmol/L
Chloride	105	98–107	mmol/L
CO_2	27	22–29	mmol/L
Anion gap	9		
BUN	19.0 H	7–18	mg/dl
Creatinine	1.3	0.60–1.30	mg/dl
BUN/creat	15		
Calcium	9.1	8.5–10.10	mg/dl

FIG 40-5 Example of a typical patient laboratory report.

Specimen collection tips

When collecting a specimen for a laboratory test, remember these tips:

1. Collect specimens before antibiotic therapy whenever possible.
2. Collect material from where the suspected organism will most likely be found.
3. Observe asepsis in collection of all specimens.
4. Consider the stage of disease.
5. Instruct the patient clearly, giving him written instructions whenever possible.
6. Use proper containers and transport media.
7. Deliver specimens promptly.
8. Provide sufficient information to the laboratory.

Guidelines for Specimen Collection

Specific guidelines should be followed for the collection, handling, and transport of specimens:

- Always follow OSHA guidelines on standard precautions during specimen collection.
- Follow requirements of collection and handling for the specific specimen—for example, the correct type of blood tube for plasma versus serum, the proper amount of specimen, if the specimen should be delivered on ice or protected from light. (See Figure 40-6.)
- Use proper equipment and supplies. Use only the appropriate specimen containers or equipment for specimen

collection as specified by the laboratory or medical office. Specimens submitted in an inappropriate container can affect the test results. Microbiological specimens should be submitted in a sterile container or sterile swab. The medical assistant should check each container or swab before use for cracked, chipped, or otherwise damaged equipment.

- Properly identify the patient and provide clear instructions. The medical assistant must properly identify the patient before specimen collection. An explanation of the procedure helps relax and reassure the patient and gains his confidence and cooperation. The medical assistant should determine whether the patient complied with pre-collection instructions. For example, if the patient did not fast for a fasting blood glucose (FBG) and lipid panel and the tests were performed, the results could be falsely elevated. If the patient has not prepared properly, notify the physician prior to collection. The physician may want the patient to return or she may tell the medical assistant to proceed with collection but to document on the laboratory requisition slip and laboratory report that the patient was not fasting at the time of collection. (See *Specimen collection*, page 862.)
- Collect the specimen using the proper techniques. Specimen collection involves a combination of medical and surgical aseptic techniques. When collecting specimens for microbiological studies, the medical assistant must ensure that the culture medium used is protected from contamination. She must also be sure to collect the proper type of specimen for each test ordered. For example, the collection of a random urine specimen when a clean-catch midstream (CCMS) specimen is required

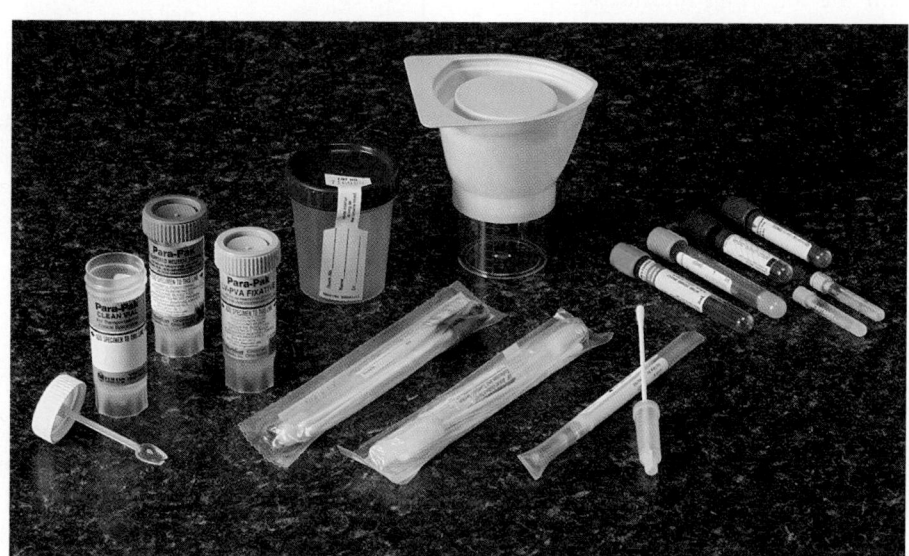

FIG 40-6 Various specimen collection containers.

Patient Education

Specimen Collection

As a medical assistant, you may instruct patients about how to properly collect specimens. When providing patient instructions, it is important to remember the following:

• Speak slowly and clearly.

• Ask the patient to repeat the instructions back to you.

• Provide written instructions whenever possible, especially if the patient is to collect the specimen at home.

• Provide written instructions in other languages native to the community.

• Emphasize the importance of following these instructions fully, to avoid requiring the patient to repeat the procedure.

• Repeating procedures is not only costly but also delays the diagnosis and treatment.

Date	
01/2/08 2:10 p.m.	Collected sputum specimen for C&S. Sent to Lewis Laboratory Services for processing. ------- C. Chapin, CMA

FIG 40-7 Sample of charting for specimen collection.

Specimen collection manual

All hospital and reference laboratories follow specific specimen collection and handling protocols. These written protocols make up a specimen collection procedure manual. A typical specimen collection procedure manual includes:

• required supplies, such as a sterile specimen container or specimen collection swab

• patient preparation instructions, if any

• step-by-step instructions for collection

• storage requirements (room temperature, refrigeration, freezer)

• transportation requirements

• time restrictions, such as "specimen must be processed within 1 hour of collection"

• reasons for specimen rejection, such as "quantity not sufficient" (QNS), an unsterile container, and so forth

• miscellaneous instructions or special considerations.

If the medical assistant has any questions about the proper procedure when collecting a specimen, she should call the laboratory prior to collecting the specimen. The laboratory will fax the instructions for collection or explain them over the phone.

Most physician office laboratories have their own specimen collection manual for commonly collected procedures, such as urinalysis, urine culture, throat culture, sputum culture, wound culture, and Papanicolaou smear. Such a procedure manual is a useful tool and reference for newly hired medical assistants.

will affect the accuracy of results. The medical assistant must know the correct amount to collect for a given test, depending on the specimen type and the number of laboratory tests ordered. If she fails to collect the specified amount, the laboratory may not be able to perform the test and the laboratory report will be marked as *quantity not sufficient* (QNS). Such a result would require the patient to come back for another specimen collection. After the medical assistant has collected the specimen, she should document the following information in the patient's chart:

a. date and time of collection

b. laboratory test ordered

c. type of specimen collected

d. special instructions for correct transport of the specimen (such as refrigerated, room temperature, or frozen)

e. medical assistant's initials. (See Figure 40-7.)

• Conduct proper specimen handling and storage. Whenever possible, laboratory tests are best performed with fresh specimens because they yield the most reliable test results. When transporting a specimen to an outside laboratory, the medical assistant must follow the guidelines set by the outside laboratory regarding storing and packaging the specimen until it is picked up by the courier service. (See *Specimen collection manual*.)

Laboratory Equipment

The physician's office laboratory should have the most up-to-date equipment needed for proper specimen processing and testing. (See Figure 40-8.) Most offices performing laboratory tests will have the following equipment:

• microscope (See *Parts of a microscope*, page 864.)

• centrifuge

- microcentrifuge
- 37°C incubator
- laboratory refrigerator
- various automated analyzers
  - HemoCue
  - Cholestech
  - One Step glucometer
  - automated urine dipstick reader.

Proper Equipment Maintenance

The medical assistant may be responsible for the setup, operation, and maintenance of all laboratory equipment. Upon purchase of laboratory equipment, the manufacturer's specific instructions for assembly and operation as well as recommendations for proper maintenance and troubleshooting should be followed. The operation manual should be stored in an area that is accessible to anyone who needs to operate the equipment. Daily, monthly, and yearly maintenance should be documented as well as any troubleshooting procedures that may be required. (See *Common equipment maintenance procedures,* page 865.)

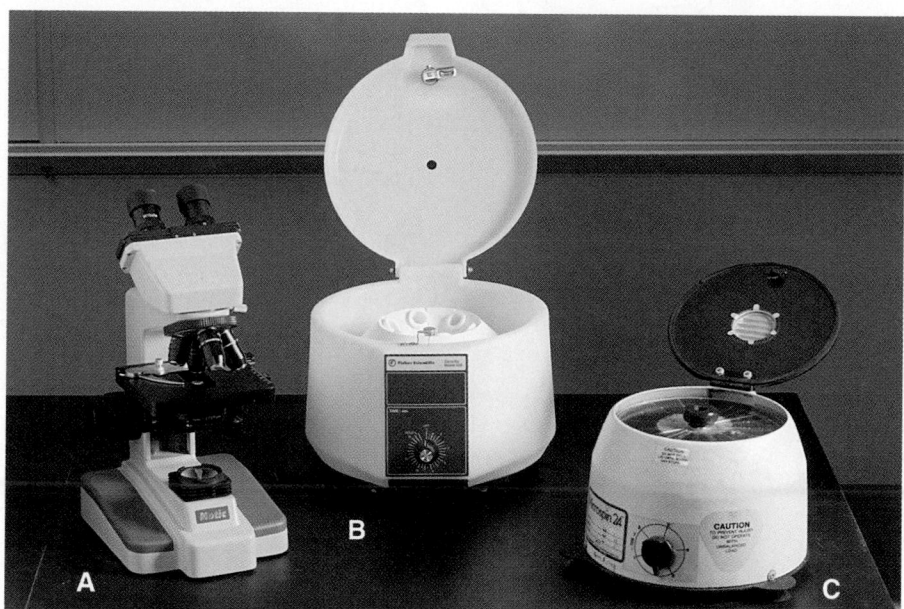

FIG 40-8 Various equipment used in a medical office. (A) Microscope. (B) Centrifuge. (C) Microhematocrit centrifuge.

Parts of a microscope

The microscope shown here is one of the most commonly used pieces of laboratory equipment in the physician's office. Understanding the function and use of each part of a microscope will help the medical assistant use this equipment properly.

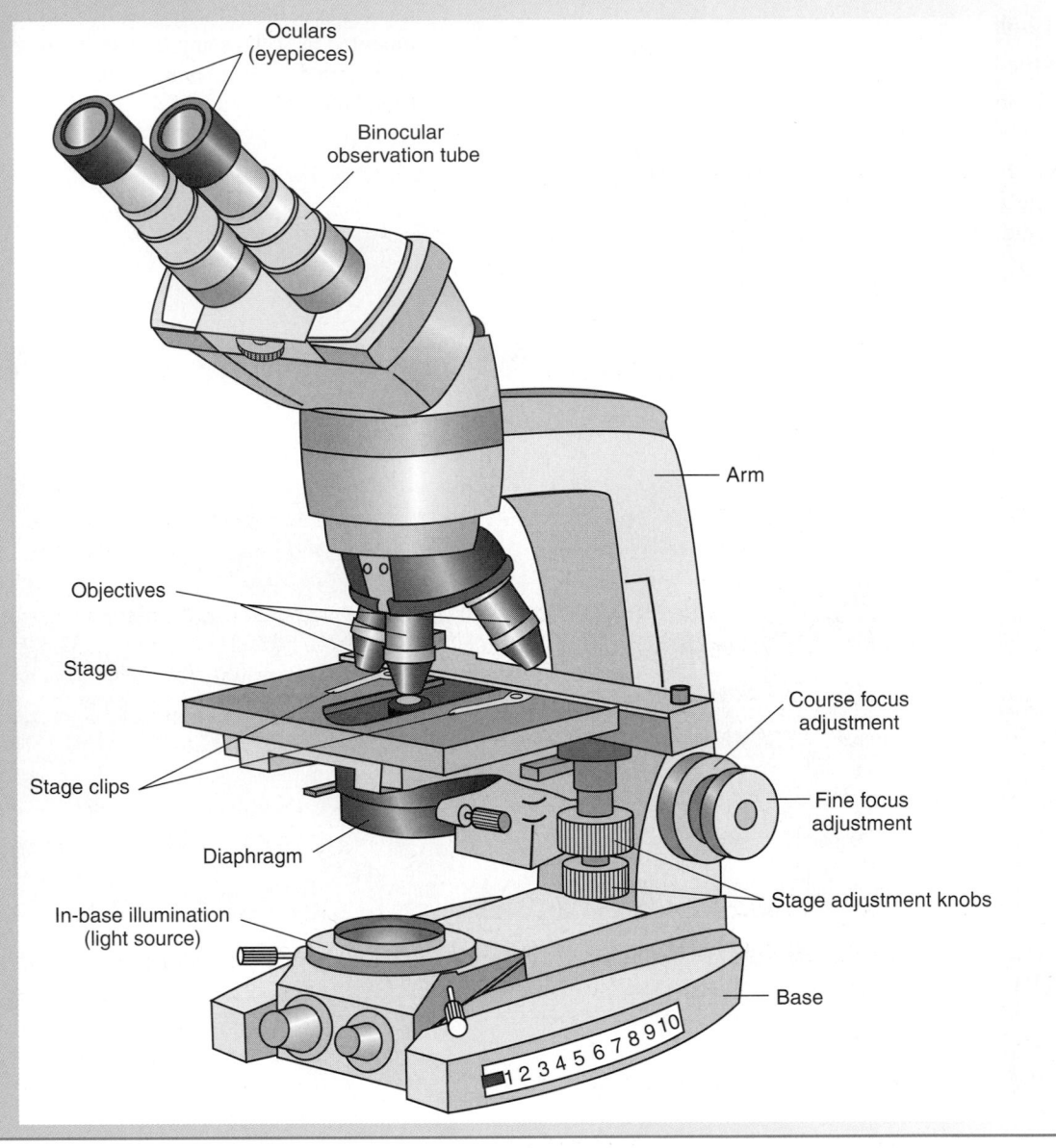

Oculars (eyepieces)

Binocular observation tube

Arm

Objectives

Stage

Course focus adjustment

Fine focus adjustment

Stage clips

Diaphragm

Stage adjustment knobs

In-base illumination (light source)

Base

1 2 3 4 5 6 7 8 9 10

Common equipment maintenance procedures

The following table lists common laboratory equipment along with maintenance procedures for each.

Equipment	Maintenance
Microscope	• Clean eyepieces and objectives daily with approved cleaner. • Ensure that a yearly professional cleaning is conducted. (The office may have a service contract with the manufacturer or another company.)
Centrifuge/microcentrifuge	• Clean the inside of the centrifuge using a 10% bleach solution as needed. • Change brushes as needed. • Check rotation speed with a tachometer yearly. (The office may have a service contract with the manufacturer or another company.)
Incubator	• Check temperature daily.
Refrigerator	• Check temperature daily.

Chapter Summary

- The clinical laboratory is an integral part of the health care team.
- Members of the laboratory team are responsible for proper specimen collection and testing to ensure that all patient results are reported in a timely and accurate manner.
- The medical assistant must be knowledgeable about the different areas of the clinical laboratory and the various tests performed in each department.
- The medical assistant may be responsible for the overall direction and operation of the physician's office laboratory.
- The medical assistant must know CLIA regulations as well as the proper documentation required for CLIA.
- Quality control procedures are essential for reliable and accurate patient results.
- The physician's office laboratory may perform many laboratory tests.
- The medical assistant may also need to know how to properly use and maintain the equipment in the laboratory.

Team Work Exercises

1. Gather in groups of two or three people. Obtain a microscope. Your instructor will supply you with various types of prepared slides (blood smears, bacteria smears, or tissue slides). First, take turns identifying the parts of the microscope. Then, put a slide on the stage and try to get the slide in focus. Each student should take turns getting a slide into focus.

2. The list of waived tests is continually updated by the federal government. Log onto the CLIA website (*http://www.cms.hhs.gov/clia/*) and, in groups of two to three people, select a topic from the following list (or your instructor will assign each group a topic) to research. Give a report to the class on what you found in your research.

   a. applying for a certificate of waiver
   b. categorization of tests
   c. proficiency testing
   d. CLIA regulations and federal registry documents
   e. interpretive guidelines for laboratories

Case Studies

1. Mr. McGregor comes to the medical office for a complete physical examination. Dr. Manuel orders a fasting glucose and a lipid panel. Jack Brown, CMA, explains to Mr. McGregor what patient preparation is necessary for the test. Mr. McGregor returns the next morning to have the blood tests. At that time, Jack notices that Mr. McGregor is chewing gum. What type of questions should Jack ask prior to collecting Mr. McGregor's blood sample?

2. Jennifer performs a rapid group A *Streptococcus* test in the office laboratory. What are the proper steps Jennifer will take when collecting the specimen? What are some of the various test kits that are on the market for the rapid diagnosis of Strep throat?

Resources

- Brassington, C., and Goretti, C.: *MA Notes: Medical Assistant's Pocket Guide.* Philadelphia: F.A. Davis, 2006.
- Sacher, R.A.: *Widmann's Clinical Interpretation of Laboratory Tests*, 11th ed. Philadelphia: F.A. Davis, 2000.
- Strasinger, S.K., and DiLorenzo, M.S.: *The Phlebotomy Workbook,* 2nd ed. Philadelphia: F.A. Davis, 2003.
- American Society for Clinical Pathology: *www.ascp.org*
- Clinical Laboratory Improvement Amendments at the U.S. Department of Health and Human Services: *www.cms.hhs.gov/clia*
- Lab Tests Online: *www.labtestsonline.org*
- Laboratory Corporation of America: *www.labcorp.com*

Phlebotomy

Learning Objectives

Upon completion of this chapter, the student will be able to:

- define the key terms in the glossary
- describe the composition and function of blood
- identify and explain various equipment and supplies used in phlebotomy
- explain the evacuated tube system
- identify the proper tube selection according to the tests being ordered
- discuss proper patient preparation procedures prior to performing phlebotomy
- discuss various patient considerations when performing phlebotomy
- perform venipuncture procedures accurately
- perform capillary puncture procedures accurately
- explain the proper standard precautions when performing phlebotomy
- describe patient education regarding phlebotomy.

CAAHEP Competencies

Clinical Competencies
Fundamental Principles
  Dispose of biohazardous materials
  Practice standard precautions
Specimen Collection
  Perform venipuncture
  Perform capillary puncture
General Competencies
Legal Concepts
  Document appropriately

ABHES Competencies

Clinical Duties
  Apply principles of aseptic techniques and infection control
  Use quality control
  Collect and process specimens
  Screen and follow up patient test results
  Perform sterilization techniques
  Practice standard precautions
  Perform venipuncture
  Perform capillary puncture
  Perform hematology
Communication
  Recognize and respond to verbal and nonverbal communication

Procedures

  Performing a venipuncture
  Performing a venipuncture using a winged infusion set
  Performing a capillary puncture

Chapter Outline

  Types of Phlebotomy Procedures
  Venipuncture
    Composition of Blood
    Venipuncture Equipment
      Tubes
      Plastic adapters
      Needles
      Syringes
      Winged infusion sets
      Tourniquet
      Gloves
    Proper Site Selection for Venipuncture
    Patient Preparation for Venipuncture
    Venipuncture Procedure
  Capillary Puncture
    Composition of Capillary Blood
    Capillary Puncture Equipment
      Capillary puncture devices
      Capillary puncture collection containers

    Proper Site Selection for Capillary Puncture
    Patient Preparation for Capillary Puncture
    Capillary Puncture Procedure
  Special Phlebotomy Considerations
    Fainting
    Failing to Obtain Blood
    Dealing with Problem Specimens
  Chapter Summary
  Team Work Exercises
  Case Studies
  Resources

Key Terms

additive
Substance, such as an anticoagulant or preservative, that may be added to an evacuated blood collection tube

antecubital space
Space inside the arm at the bend of the elbow that is the best site for routine venipuncture

anticoagulant
Substance that inhibits blood clotting

buffy coat
Middle layer of a whole blood tube that has been allowed to settle or has been centrifuged and contains leukocytes and platelets

capillary puncture
Process of performing a skin puncture to obtain blood

erythrocyte
Red blood cell responsible for carrying oxygen to all cells and tissues in the body

evacuated tube
Plastic tube that contains a vacuum, which draws blood from the vein into the tube through a dual needle system

hematoma
Discoloration of the area around a puncture site caused by an accumulation of blood around the site; also called *bruise*

hemoconcentration
Accumulation of blood caused by leaving the tourniquet on the venipuncture arm longer than 1 minute, causing an increase in red blood cells and a decrease in plasma volume

hemolysis
Destruction of red blood cells, causing a red tinge in serum

lancet
Capillary puncture device that usually contains a retractable blade

leukocytes
White blood cells responsible for fighting off infection and producing antibodies

phlebotomy
Process of collecting blood for analysis

plasma
Liquid portion of blood that contains clotting factors

serum
Liquid portion of blood without the cells and clotting factors

thrombocytes
Platelets responsible for clot formation

tourniquet
Device used to aid vein protrusion

venipuncture
Process of puncturing a vein with a needle to obtain blood

whole blood
Blood composed of formed elements (cells) and plasma

Types of Phlebotomy Procedures

Although the term **phlebotomy** refers specifically to inserting a needle into a vein for the purpose of obtaining a blood sample for analysis, it is used in the health care field to refer to *venipuncture*, the process of puncturing a vein with a needle to obtain blood, or **capillary puncture**, the process of performing a skin puncture to obtain blood. Blood is composed of various components that, when tested, can tell a physician a lot about what is going on with a patient. Phlebotomy is an extremely important skill for a medical assistant to possess. The medical assistant will employ venipuncture or capillary puncture when obtaining blood from patients. The medical assistant who can understand and perform venipuncture and capillary puncture properly and efficiently will help win her patient's confidence.

Venipuncture

Venipuncture is defined as the process of piercing a vein with a needle to withdraw blood. However, the actual process involves more than the definition describes. In addition to piercing a vein, the venipuncture procedure consists of proper patient preparation, an understanding of the blood tests being ordered, and proper selection of supplies. The first step in properly performing this technical process is understanding the composition of blood.

Composition of Blood

Whole blood is composed of formed elements, or blood cells, and plasma. (See Figure 41-1.) The formed elements consist of:

- **erythrocytes** (red blood cells), which are responsible for transporting oxygen to all cells in the body and removing carbon dioxide, the waste product of cellular activity, to the lungs for elimination via the respiratory system
- **leukocytes** (white blood cells), which are an important part of the immune system because they protect against infection and disease
- **thrombocytes** (platelets which are fragments of larger cells and are responsible for clot formation. (For more information on blood cells and their function, see Chapter 42, "Hematology and Coagulation Procedures," page 889.)

The formed elements are suspended in **plasma**, the liquid portion of blood. (See Figure 41-2.) Plasma makes up about 55% of blood volume and is approximately 90% water. Plasma also contains clotting factors (such as fibrinogen), gases, carbohydrates, electrolytes, and various other substances. (See *Substances found in plasma*.) If a tube of

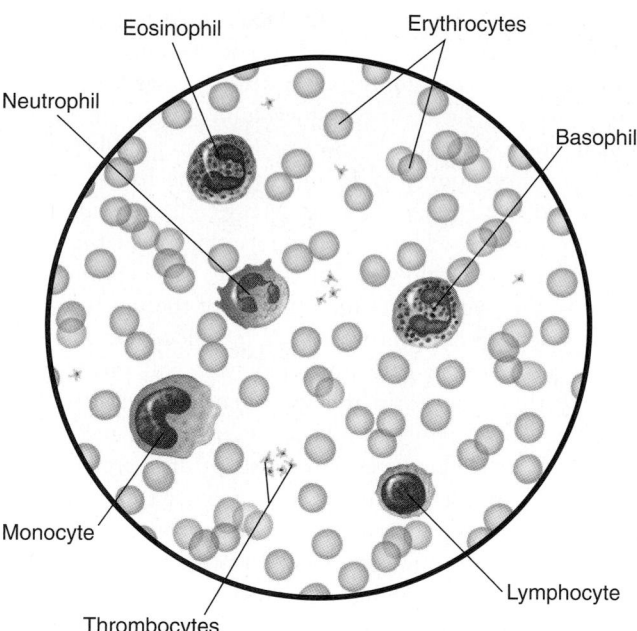

FIG 41-1 Various types of blood cells found in whole blood.

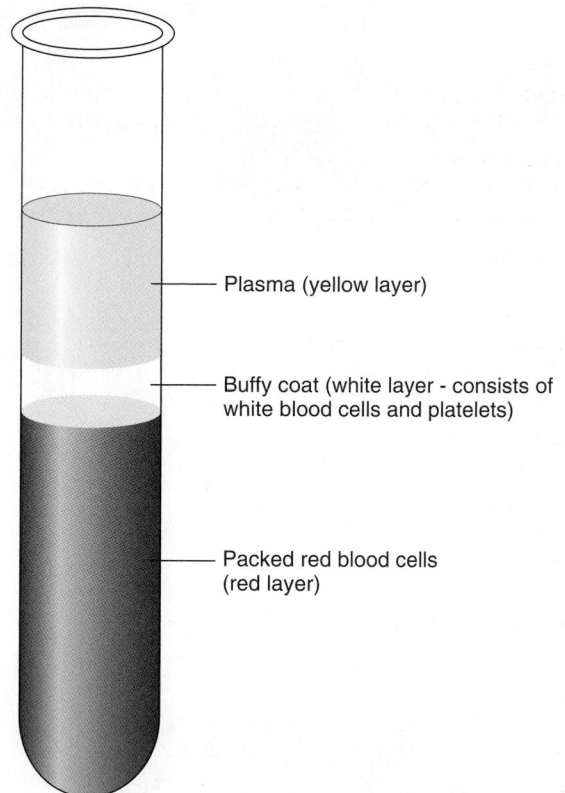

FIG 41-2 Buffy coat (layers of uncoagulated blood that form when a blood tube is left standing or centrifuged).

uncoagulated whole blood is allowed to stand straight up for a period of time, the tube will develop three layers:

- plasma, which is the top layer and appears as a cloudy yellowish color
- **buffy coat**, which sits atop the layer of red blood cells and consists of the white blood cells and the platelets
- red blood cells, which will separate out and settle to the bottom of the tube.

Serum is the liquid portion of blood that does not contain fibrinogen or blood cells. Serum contains all of the same substances found in plasma. If a tube of clotted blood were spun in a centrifuge, it would separate into serum and clotted cells. (See Figure 41-3.) Serum is the most common portion of blood that is analyzed for medical testing. A medical assistant selects the type of tube based on whether serum or plasma is required for the test.

Venipuncture Equipment

When performing phlebotomy, the medical assistant must be sure to select the proper equipment for the procedure. She must decide on the proper tube for the tests being ordered and the size and type of needle to use, as well as proper site-cleaning solution.

Tubes

The blood collection tubes used in venipucture use the evacuated system. **Evacuated tubes** are plastic tubes that contain a vacuum, which draws blood from the vein and collects the

Substances found in plasma

Plasma contains many substances that can be measured by a blood test:

- glucose
- hormones, such as thyroid stimulating hormone (TSH), follicle-stimulating hormone (FSH), growth hormone (GH), and human chorionic gonadotropin (HCG)
- cholesterol
- medications
- drugs of abuse
- protein
- albumin
- calcium
- carbon dioxide
- clotting factors.

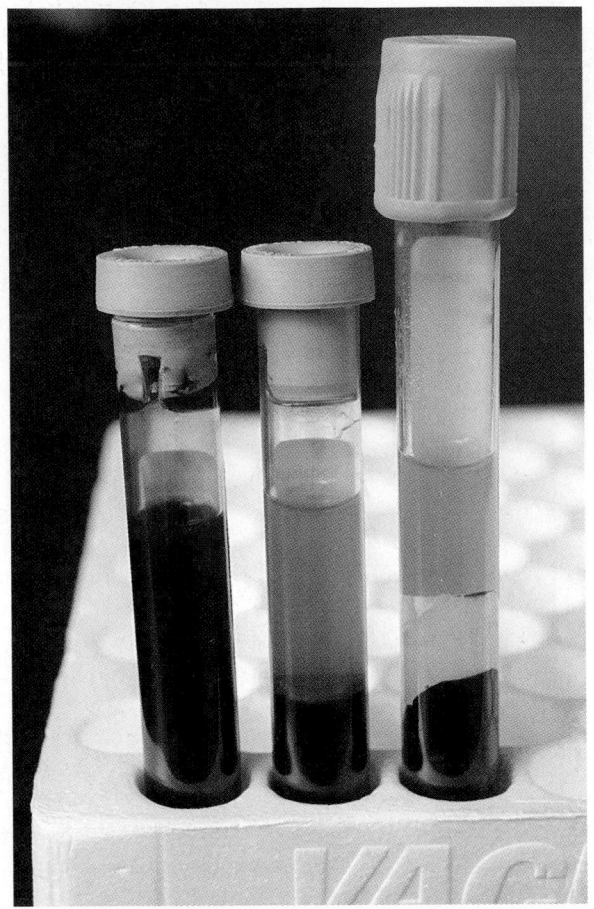

FIG 41-3 The first lavender top tube shows whole blood before centrifugation. The second lavender top tube shows plasma sitting on top of a layer of blood cells after centrifugation. The SST (gold top) tube shows serum sitting on top of clotted blood cells.

blood directly into the tube through a dual needle system. These tubes come in glass and plastic versions, but plastic tubes are more commonly used because they are safer. Tubes are available in different sizes by volume, depending on how much blood is needed or how fragile a vein is. Tube volume size can vary from 2 to 15 ml. Each tube has a different color-coded stopper, or *tube top*. Many collection tubes contain an **additive**, which is a substance that will act upon the specimen in a certain way. For example, a preservative is an additive that will protect the integrity of the specimen. Because glucose is easily broken down in a blood specimen, the preservative in the gray-stoppered tube will preserve any glucose that may be in the specimen, protecting it from breaking down, which would cause erroneous test results. Each color-coded stopper correlates with the type of additive that is inside the tube. Other tubes have an additive that, rather than preserving a specimen, acts on it to yield a whole blood or serum specimen. For instance, a tube with a lavender stopper contains ethylenediaminetetraacetic acid (EDTA), an **anticoagulant**, which is a substance that does not allow the blood to clot. Blood collected in this type of tube remains in the whole blood state. In contrast, blood drawn in a red-topped tube containing a clot activator will coagulate and yield serum upon centrifugation. (See *What tube colors mean*.)

To select the proper tube size for venipuncture, the medical assistant must consider:

- amount of blood needed for the tests ordered—If the tube selected is too small, it may not yield enough blood for the tests being ordered. The patient may be called to return to the laboratory or office to have the sample redrawn.

What tube colors mean

This table provides a complete listing of tube colors, along with the additive contained in the tube, the specimen type it yields, and common tests drawn using the tube.

Tube Color	Additive	Specimen	Common Tests
Yellow	Sodium polyanethol sulfonate (SPS)	Whole blood	• Blood cultures

What tube colors mean—cont'd

Tube Color	Additive	Specimen	Common Tests
Light blue	Sodium citrate	Whole blood or plasma	• Prothrombin time (PT-INR) • Partial thromboplastin time (PTT)
Serum-separator tube (SST)	Thixotropic separator gel	Serum	• Fasting blood glucose (FBG) • Blood urea nitrogen (BUN) • Creatinine • Electrolytes • Thyroid stimulating hormone (TSH) • Lipid panel • Cardiac panel
Plain red	No additive	Serum	• ABO/RH • Type and screen • Most serological tests
Green	Sodium heparin	Whole blood or plasma	• Ammonia • Electrolytes (STAT orders)

Continued

What tube colors mean—cont'd

Tube Color	Additive	Specimen	Common Tests
Lavender	Ethylenediaminetetraacetic acid (EDTA)	Whole blood or plasma	• Complete blood count (CBC) • Hemoglobin and hematocrit (H&H) • Platelet count • White blood cell count • Red blood cell count • Erythrocyte sedimentation rate (ESR)
Gray	• Sodium fluoride with Na$_2$ EDTA • Sodium fluoride • Potassium oxalate and sodium fluoride	Whole blood or plasma	• FBG • Glucose tolerance test (GTT)

- needle size—If a needle that has a small opening is used with a large-volume tube, then the force of the blood coming through that opening may destroy the red blood cells in the specimen, a process called **hemolysis**. Hemolysis of a specimen is indicated by a red tinge to the serum.
- type of vein—If a large tube, which has a more forceful vacuum, is used on a small or fragile vein, the vein could collapse and the medical assistant may have to redraw the sample, causing additional discomfort to the patient.

Plastic Adapters

A venipuncture adapter is made of clear, rigid plastic that holds the needle and the collection tube. The needle is screwed into one end and the blood tube is inserted into the barrel of the holder. The Occupational Safety and Health Administration (OSHA) requires all personnel to discard the adapter with the used needle. The medical assistant should refer to her facility's procedure manual for the needle-adapter disposal protocol. (See Figure 41-4.)

Needles

Needles used in evacuated tube venipuncture are double-pointed and consist of an anterior needle and a posterior

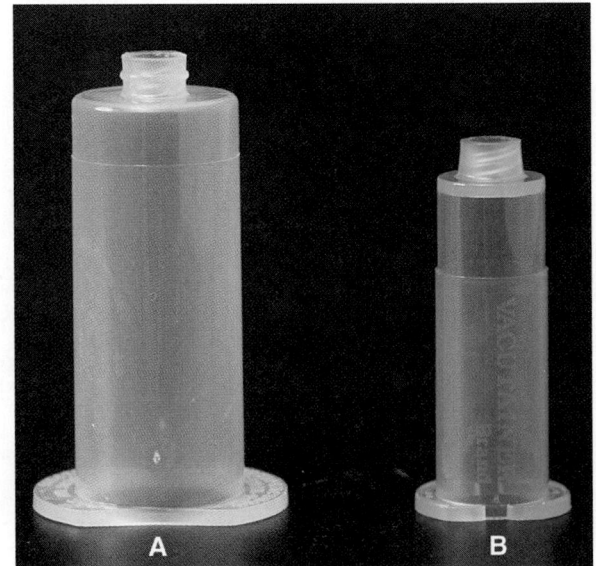

FIG 41-4 Blood tube adapters. (A) Adult. (B) Pediatric.

needle. The anterior needle is longer (1" to 1 ¹/₂" long) with a beveled point for easy entry into the skin and the vein. The posterior needle is shorter and covered by a rubber sheath. The needle screws into the top of the tube adaptor and the posterior end of the needle enters the inside of the adaptor. When the tube is inserted into the adaptor, it goes into the back of the needle. At the same time, the tube pushes the sheath back. When the medical assistant removes the tube from the adaptor, the sheath rolls forward into place to prevent blood from leaking out.

The size of the needle opening is called the *gauge.* Needles come in various gauge sizes ranging from 16G to 25G. Needles with a larger opening have a smaller gauge number. A medical assistant may use a 16G needle on a patient donating blood because a large amount of blood is required in a shorter period of time; the typical gauge for an adult venipuncture is 20G to 21G. A medical assistant would use a smaller-gauge needle, such as 23G, on the elderly and children, who typically have fragile or smaller veins. (See Figure 41-5.)

Regardless of the size, all phlebotomy needles are for one use only. After using a needle, the medical assistant should dispose of it in the proper puncture-resistant biohazard container. (See Figure 41-6.)

Safety Needles

To increase needle safety and prevent needlestick injuries, the Needlestick Prevention and Safety Act mandates the use of safety needle devices. (See *Accidental needlestick: What to do,* page 874.) Devices such as the Punctur-Guard needle and the Vacutainer Eclipse blood collection needle are just a

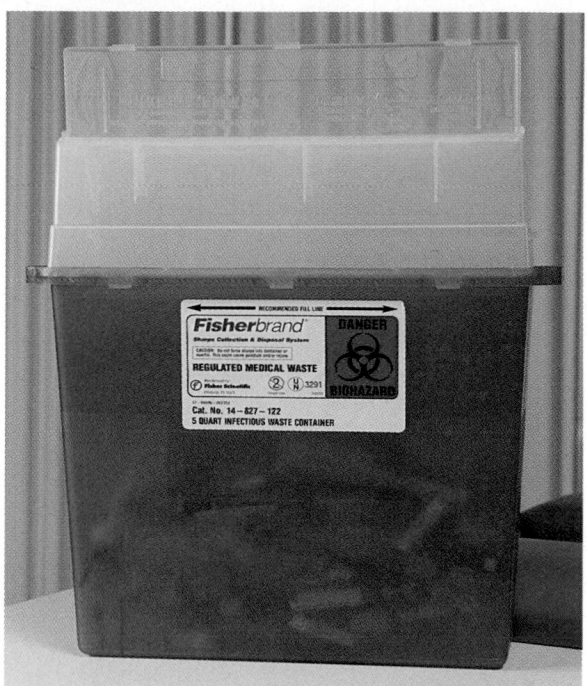

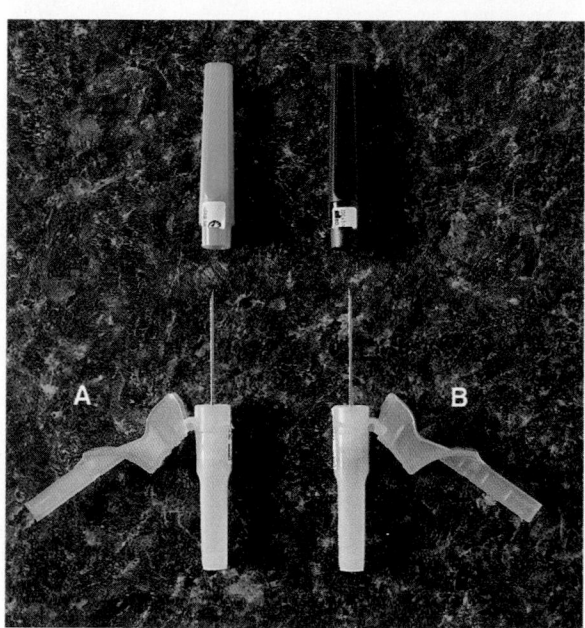

FIG 41-5 Needles used during venipuncture. (A) A 21-gauge needle. (B) A 22-gauge needle.

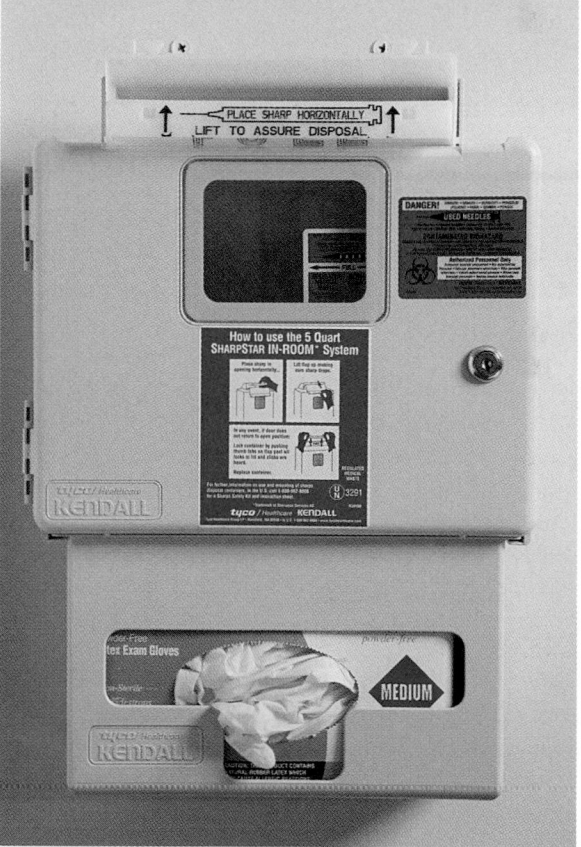

FIG 41-6 Different types of puncture-proof needle-disposal containers.

few of the many types of safety needles available. In addition, some devices are adaptors in which the safety feature is attached to the adaptor and, when engaged, covers the needle to prevent an accidental needlestick. (See Figure 41-7.)

Syringes

Syringes are sometimes used when collecting blood for analysis. Some situations in which a medical assistant might select a syringe for venipuncture include patients with fragile or small veins or when drawing from a hand vein. Syringes are preferred in these instances because the medical assistant is able to control the suction pressure in the vein to prevent the veins from collapsing. (See Figure 41-8.) If the medical assistant draws blood in a syringe, she should immediately transfer the blood to the appropriate evacuated tubes to prevent clot formation.

Winged Infusion Sets

A winged infusion set, commonly called a *butterfly needle*, consists of a needle that is attached to plastic tubing. The winged infusion set is used when encountering a small or fragile vein, which is common in children and elderly patients. (See Figure 41-9.) Using a winged infusion set puts less pressure on the vein when the vacuum tube is attached to the tubing. It is preferred over a syringe because the risks of specimen contamination and accidental needlestick are lower than with a syringe. A winged infusion set used for phlebotomy is usually 21G, 23G, or 25G with lengths of

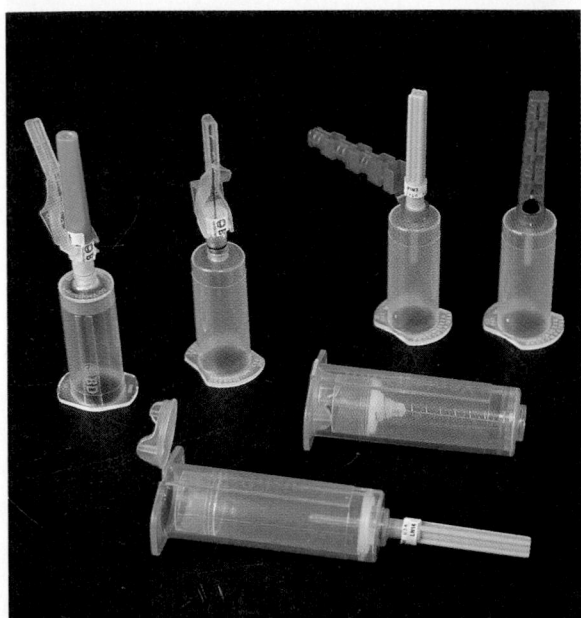

FIG 41-7 Safety needles and safety adapters.

Accidental needlestick: What to do

Medical assistants should strictly adhere to standard precautions and proper safety procedures when performing phlebotomy. However, regardless of these procedures, accidental needlesticks do happen. In the event of an accidental needlestick, the medical assistant should:

1. remove her gloves immediately and wash the puncture site with soap and water (If she has punctured her finger, she should press on the finger to help the site bleed out slightly, while still washing the site.)

2. dry the punctured area and bandage it

3. notify the supervisor of the incident

4. have the patient stay until the supervisor arrives and determines a course of action

5. follow the procedure outlined by the supervisor and the formal needlestick exposure protocol for obtaining immediate medical attention

6. document the incident.

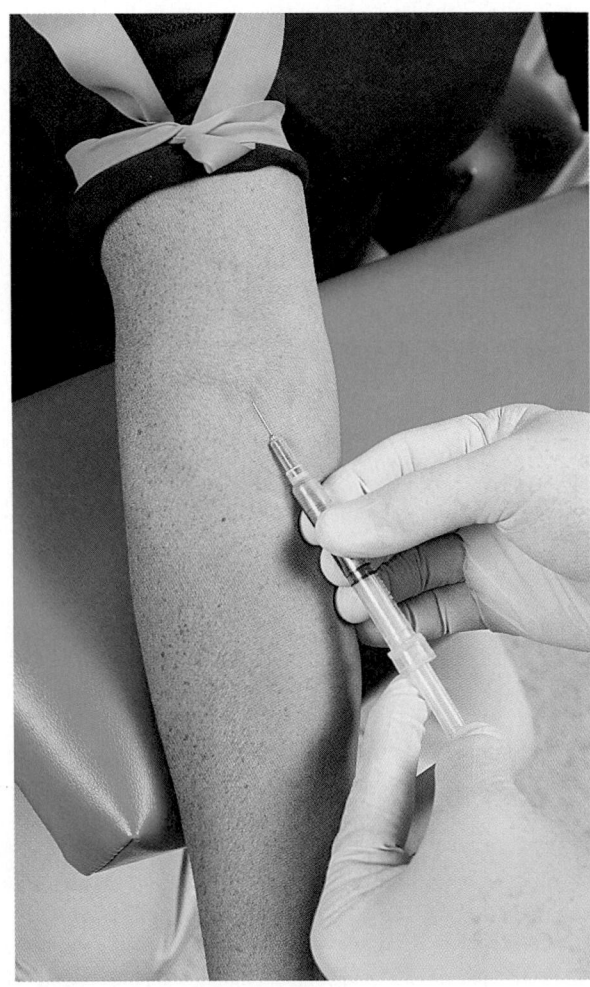

FIG 41-8 Venipuncture procedure using the syringe method.

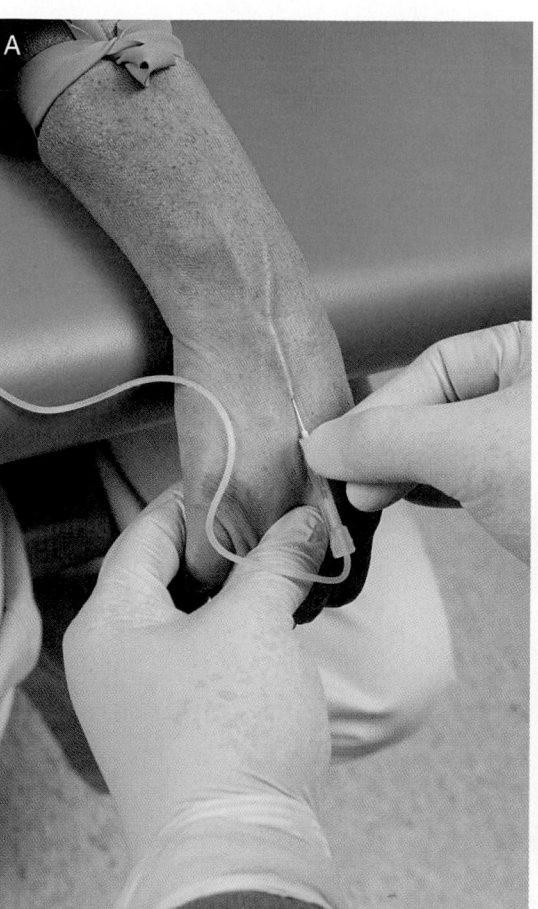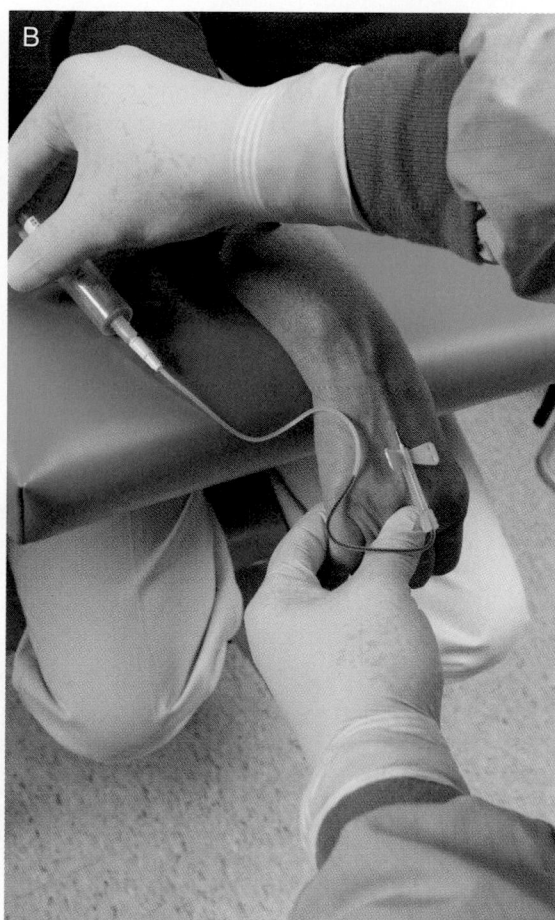

FIG 41-9 Venipuncture procedure using a winged infusion set. (A) Insertion of a winged infusion set. (B) Insertion of the tubes into the adapter.

$^1/_2$" to $^3/_4$". The medical assistant should learn the proper technique for activating the safety feature of the winged infusion set to avoid accidental needlesticks.

Tourniquet

A **tourniquet** is a flat, soft elastic band approximately 1" wide and 18" long. It is used to locate patient veins by impeding venous but not arterial blood flow. Tourniquets are inexpensive and can be disposed of if they become contaminated or soiled. Nonlatex tourniquets are available for phlebotomists and patients who are allergic to latex.

Tourniquet placement is a key step in successful venipuncture. The medical assistant should place the tourniquet approximately 3" to 4" above the bend of the patient's elbow. She should take care to avoid tying the tourniquet too tightly or keeping it on too long. Otherwise, hemoconcentration in the area can occur. **Hemoconcentration** is the accumulation of blood with increased levels of red blood cells and decreased plasma volume. It can cause the breakdown of red blood cells (hemolysis) in the specimen.

Hemoconcentration or hemolysis could cause inaccurate results or specimen rejection, which would require another venipuncture and more patient discomfort. Additionally, if a tourniquet is kept on the arm longer than 1 minute, it may cause a **hematoma**, which is a discoloration of the area around a puncture site caused by an accumulation of blood. Not only can a hematoma be painful to the patient, it can also cause the vein to be rendered useless for subsequent venipunctures because the blood from the old hematoma may seep into the needle and contaminate the venous blood.

Gloves

Latex allergy is increasing among health care workers. As mandated by OSHA, gloves must be worn when performing venipuncture and must be changed after each patient. Gloves are available in powdered or powder-free latex and nonlatex (vinyl or nitrile). The medical assistant should ask the patient if he has a latex allergy and, if so, be sure to use nonlatex gloves when performing the venipuncture. (See *Additional venipuncture supplies,* page 876.)

Additional venipuncture supplies

In addition to tubes, needles, adaptors, syringes, winged infusion sets, tourniquets, and gloves, a medical assistant will need additional supplies in order to perform a proper venipuncture. These supplies include:

- alcohol cleansing pads (70% isopropyl alcohol)
- sterile 2 × 2 gauze pads
- adhesive bandage or surgical tape
- ammonia inhalant
- puncture-proof biohazard disposal container.

Most physician's office laboratories (POLs) will have a separate area for blood drawing called a *blood drawing*

station. The medical assistant should make sure that venipuncture supplies are readily available and within reach. In some POLs, the medical assistant will draw blood in an examination room. In that case, the medical assistant will bring a phlebotomy tray to the examination room in order to draw the patient's blood. Regardless of where she draws the blood, the medical assistant should routinely keep the blood drawing station and phlebotomy tray stocked, preferably on a daily basis.

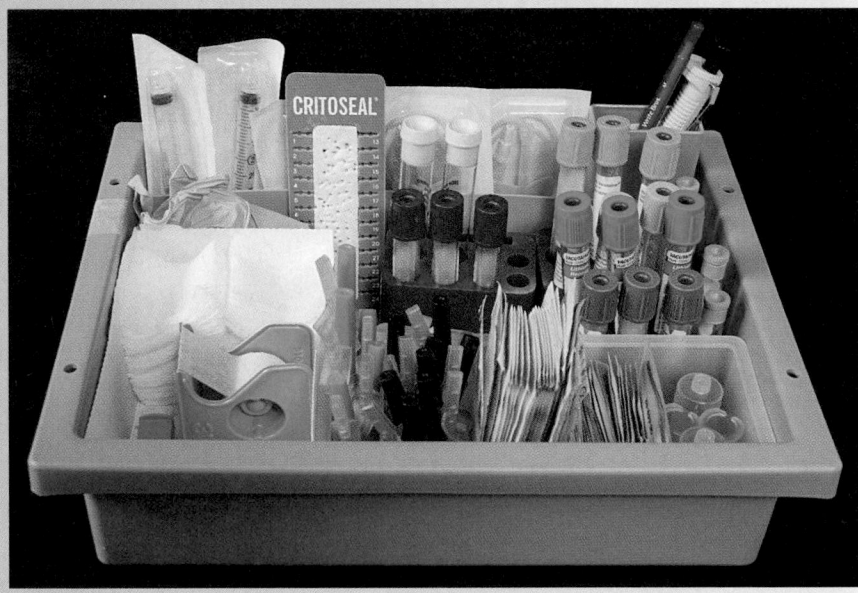

Typical set-up for a phlebotomy tray

Proper Site Selection for Venipuncture

After proper identification of the patient, the first thing the medical assistant must do is select the proper site for venipuncture. The **antecubital space**, which is located at the surface of the arm anterior to the elbow, is the preferred site for routine venipuncture. (See Figure 41-10.)

The three major veins located in this area are the median cubital, cephalic, and basilic veins. For a routine venipuncture, the median cubital vein should be the medical assistant's vein of choice because it is close to the skin's surface and, thus, is not as likely to move or roll to the side when a needle is inserted. The cephalic or basilic veins should be the second choice because they tend to be smaller and may move during puncturing. Regardless of the vein used, the medical assistant must properly anchor the vein prior to puncture so

the vein does not move or roll. Movement of a vein during venipuncture can cause the needle to enter through the vein or miss the vein altogether, requiring a repeat puncture and additional patient discomfort. (See *Sites to avoid in venipuncture.*)

Sites to avoid in venipuncture

Avoid these sites when performing a venipuncture:

- scarred, bruised, or edematous areas
- sites above an IV
- arm side of a mastectomy
- sites containing fistulas or vascular grafts.

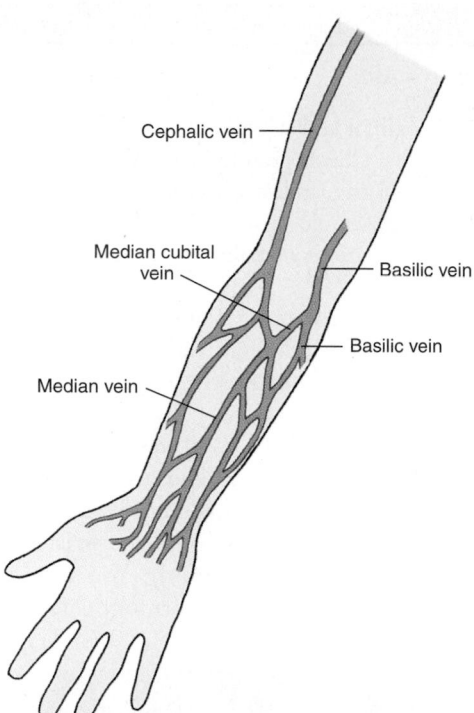

FIG 41-10 Antecubital area of arm showing proper veins for venipuncture.

Patient Preparation for Venipuncture

The medical assistant should demonstrate confidence in her ability to perform phlebotomy. Upon greeting the patient with a smile and professional tone, the medical assistant should seat the patient comfortably and put him at ease. She should briefly explain the procedure to the patient, verify that he followed pretesting preparation, such as fasting, and ask him if he is allergic to latex. In addition, the medical assistant should ask the patient if he has ever had a problem with venipuncture. She can be better prepared to assist the patient if she knows that he may experience faintness or other problems.(See *Blood test desk check*.)

Next, the medical assistant should review the laboratory requisition slip to see which tests have been ordered. Knowing which tests are ordered will determine the proper tube color to select. (See *Order of the draw*.)

Venipuncture Procedure

The medical assistant should be familiar with the proper procedure for selecting a vein. Palpation enables her to feel around for the vein rather than simply looking at the vein. The medical assistant should use the index finger of her nondominant hand to palpate the area and determine the

Front office–Back office connection

Blood Test Desk Check

The front office medical assistant may be responsible for asking a patient coming to the office for blood work if he has conformed to pretesting requirements. "When was the last time you ate or drank anything?" or "Did you take your medication today?" are important questions to ask the patient when he is checking in at the front desk. The medical assistant should document in the patient's chart any information that may be helpful to the clinical medical assistant before the patient's blood is drawn.

Order of the draw

When drawing blood, the medical assistant must follow the proper order of the draw, because some tube anticoagulants may contaminate other tubes being drawn or sterile specimens may become contaminated. Here is the proper order of the draw:

- yellow-top tube or culture bottles
- light blue
- plain red
- SST
- green
- lavender
- gray.

direction, depth, and size of the vein. Determining these vein characteristics will allow the medical assistant to select the proper size needle and collection tube. In addition, the medical assistant should visually inspect both arms and notice scars or moles, which are areas she should stay away from because they may interfere with the venipuncture procedure. (See *Procedure 41-1: Performing a venipuncture*, page 878, and *Procedure 41-2: Performing a venipuncture using a winged infusion set*, page 883.)

Capillary Puncture

While venipuncture is the most commonly performed phlebotomy procedure, there are certain circumstances in which a medical assistant may be required to perform a capillary puncture, also called a *dermal puncture*. Such circumstances include drawing blood from an infant, a burned or scarred

PROCEDURE 41-1

Performing a venipuncture

Task
Perform a venipuncture.

Conditions
- Requisition slip
- Blood tubes
- Needles
- Gauze
- Alcohol cleansing pad
- Tourniquet
- Adaptor
- Adhesive bandage or surgical tape
- Biohazard sharps container

Standards
In the time specified and within the scoring parameters determined by the instructor, the student will successfully perform a venipuncture.

Performance Standards

1. Examine the requisition slip to identify the tests ordered and, therefore, to select the proper tubes to use for collection.

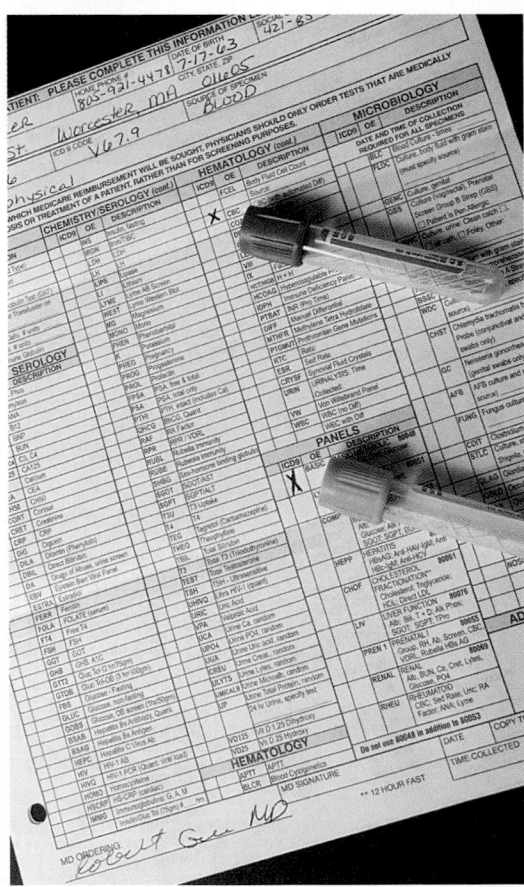

Completed requisition slip showing correct tubes selected for tests ordered

2. Greet the patient and ask him to state his full name and date of birth. Check pretesting requirements, such as fasting, nonfasting, and medication restrictions to avoid rendering the sample unacceptable due to misidentification of the patient or failure to adhere to pretesting specifications.

3. Reassure the patient and explain the procedure.

4. Select the correct equipment and tubes for the procedure. Have extra tubes handy in case the first tube does not work.

5. Wash your hands and put on gloves.

6. Position the patient's arm. The arm with the vein selected for venipuncture should be extended and in a straight line from the shoulder to the wrist with the antecubital veins facing anteriorly. You may need a towel to support the arm if the armrest is too low.

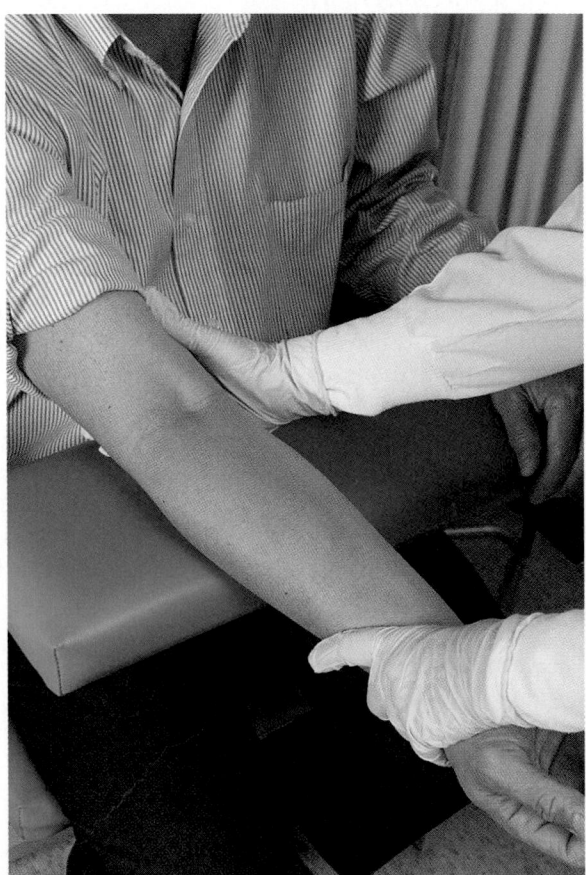

Correct positioning of patient's arm

PROCEDURE 41-1—cont'd

7. Apply a tourniquet 3" to 4" above the antecubital area of the patient's arm and ask the patient to clench his fist.

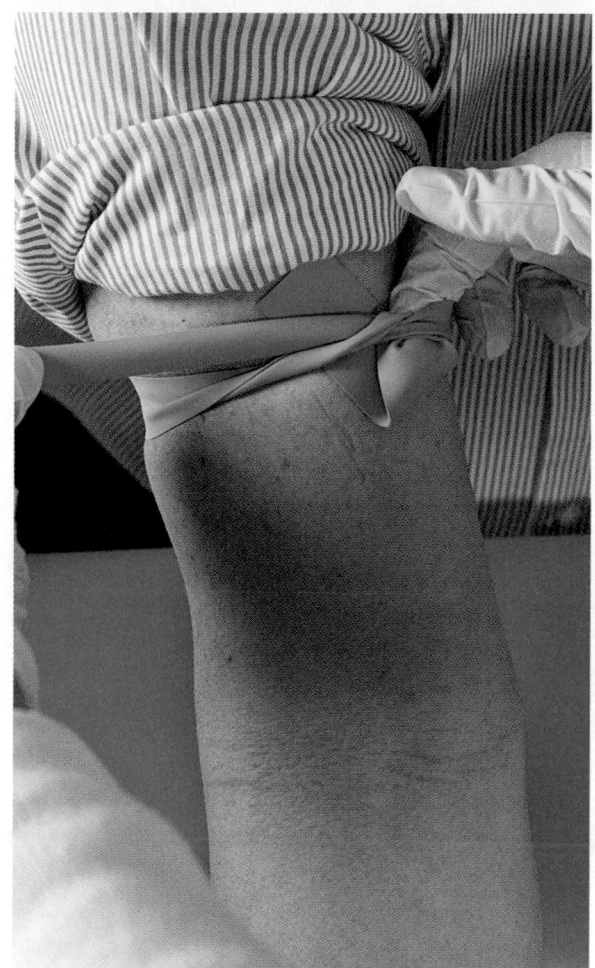

Tourniquet properly applied 3" to 4" above the antecubital area

8. Identify the vein of choice by palpation.

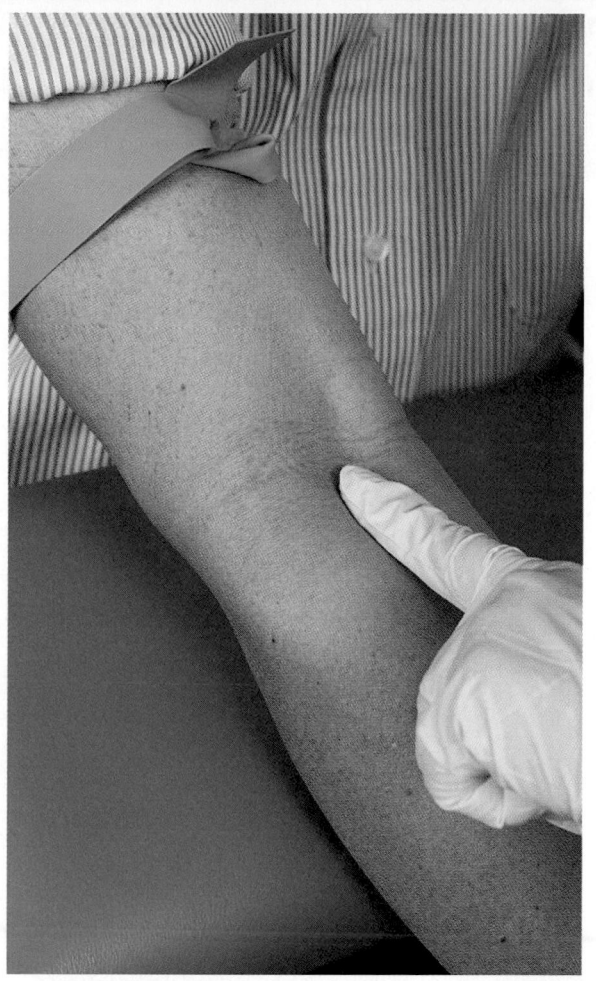

Palpating a vein for venipuncture

9. Release the tourniquet to avoid patient discomfort and altered test results, which can occur if the tourniquet is left on for more than 1 minute.

10. Clean the site and allow it to air dry. Cleaning should be done in a circular motion starting from the inside and moving away from the puncture site to allow the site to dry because a wet injection site can cause a stinging sensation and contaminate the sample, leading to inaccurate test results.

11. Assemble the equipment. Screw the needle into the adaptor and select the first tube to be drawn. Position within reach all items to be used during the procedure. Rest the tube in the back of the adaptor without pushing it into the back of the needle to avoid having to reach for the tube, which may cause the needle to move in the patient's arm.

12. Reapply the tourniquet, positioning it 3" to 4" above the antecubital space and making it snug but not tight.

Continued

PROCEDURE 41-1—cont'd

13. Do not touch the puncture site to avoid contaminating the area after cleaning the site.

14. Anchor the vein below the puncture site. Then grasp the patient's arm with your nondominant hand, placing your thumb 1" to 2" below the puncture site. Using your thumb, draw the skin over the vein in the direction of the patient's hand.

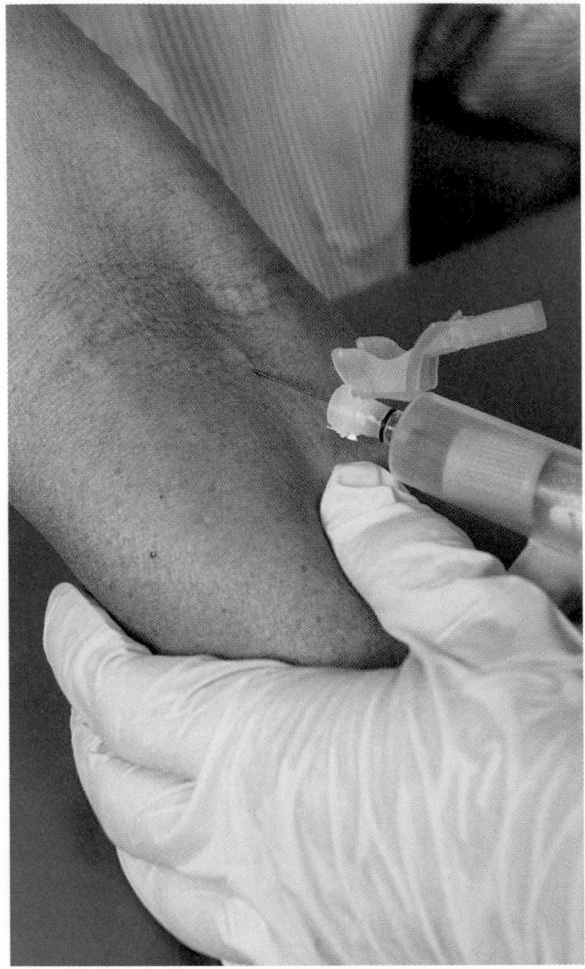

Nondominant hand anchoring the vein and dominant hand holding the venipuncture equipment

15. When the vein is securely anchored, align the needle with the vein and insert the needle, bevel up, at an angle of 15 to 30 degrees, depending on the depth of the vein.

16. Once you are in the vein, push the tube into the back of the needle; blood should start flowing into the tube.

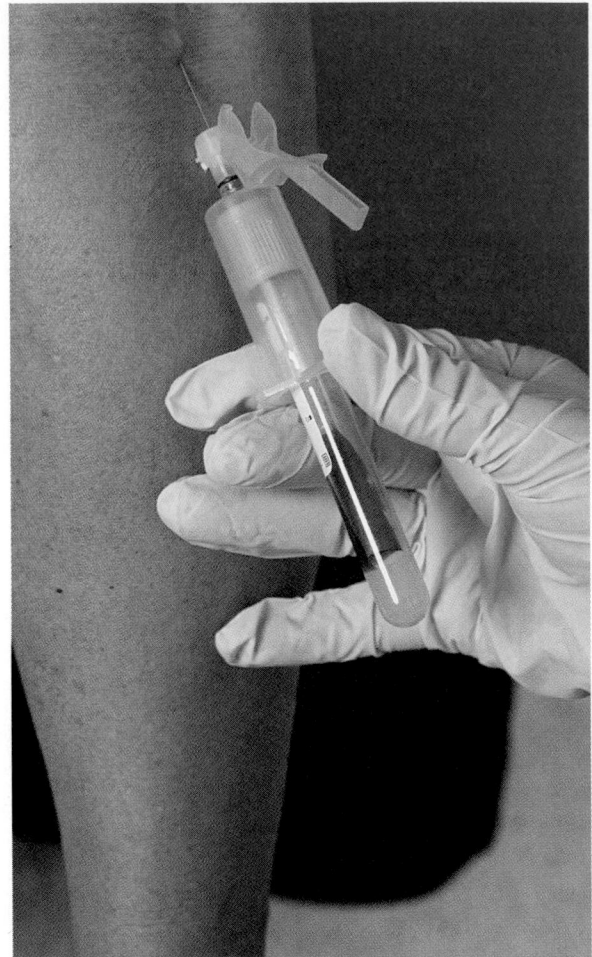

Inserting the needle at a 20-degree angle and blood flowing into the tube

17. Do not move the needle when changing tubes. The hand used to hold the needle assembly should remain braced on the patient's arm when tubes are inserted or removed from the adaptor to avoid movement that could cause patient discomfort and the needle to come out of the vein, thus losing the vacuum in the tube.

18. Use tubes in the correct order to follow the correct order of draw and prevent cross-contamination.

19. Make certain to mix tubes gently and promptly. Rotate the tube eight to ten times to mix it with the anticoagulant to avoid a delay that may allow the specimen time to clot, which will make it unacceptable for testing.

20. Make certain that each evacuated tube is filled to the level appropriate for that tube. Tubes that are not filled to the correct level may be rejected for testing.

PROCEDURE 41-1—cont'd

21. Release the tourniquet after inserting the last tube to avoid patient discomfort and altered test results, which can occur if the tourniquet is left on for more than 1 minute.
22. Be sure to remove the last tube from the adaptor to prevent blood from dripping out of the tip of the needle.
23. Place a sterile gauze pad over the needle and quickly withdraw the needle. Do not apply pressure to the puncture site until the needle is completely removed to avoid patient discomfort and scratching the patient's skin.

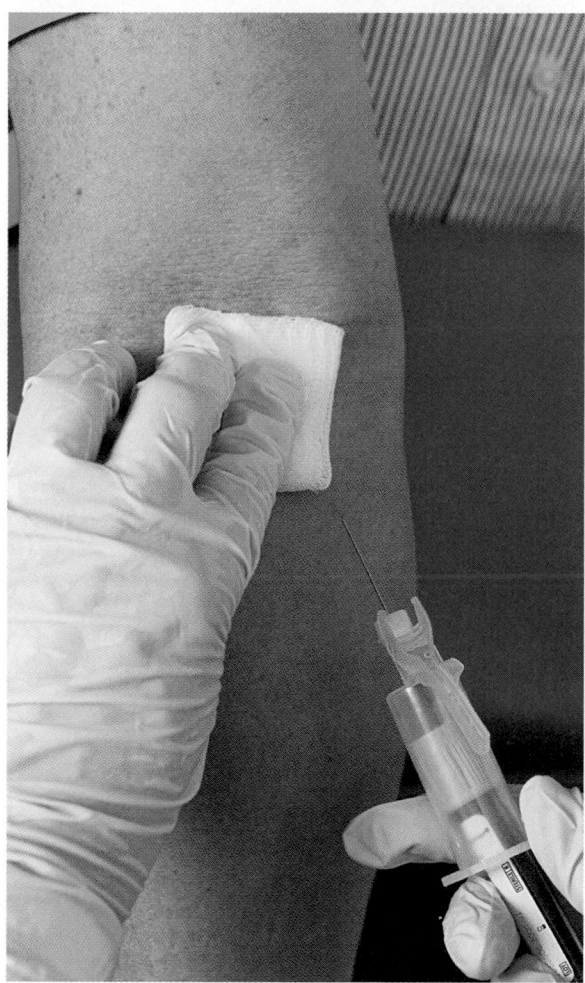

Removing the needle from the arm and placing gauze over the puncture site

24. Activate the safety needle.

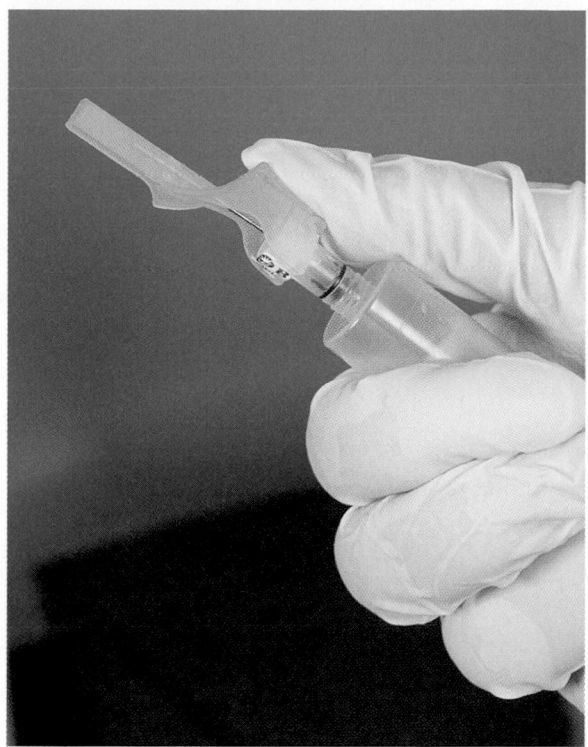

Safety needle activation

25. Apply pressure with the gauze pad for 1 to 2 minutes or longer for a patient on anticoagulation therapy.
26. Dispose of the needle and holder in a biohazard sharps container.

Continued

PROCEDURE 41-1—cont'd

27. Label the tubes containing the samples.

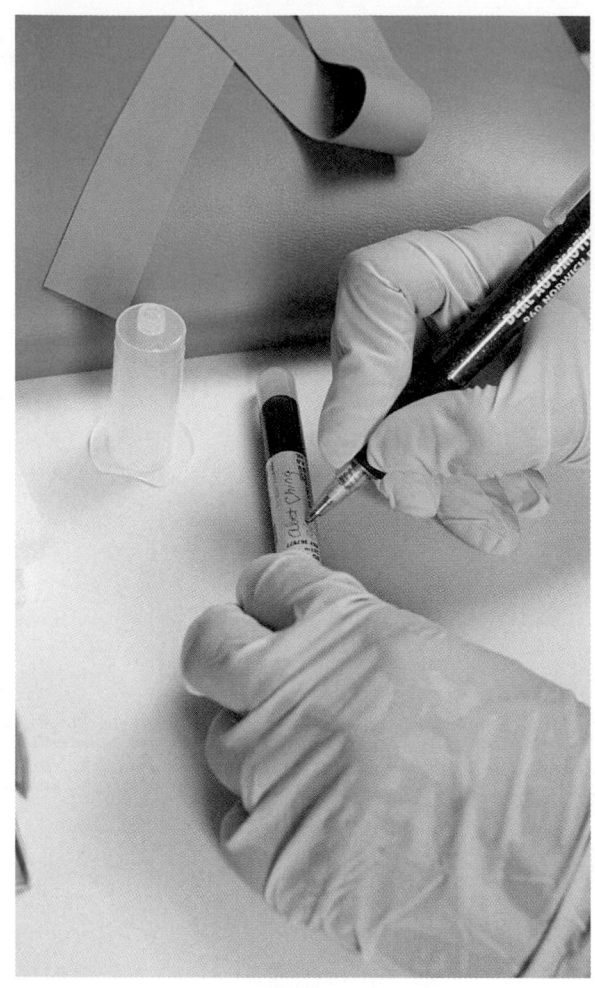

Labeling a blood tube

28. Examine the puncture site for bleeding.
29. Apply a bandage over the puncture site.

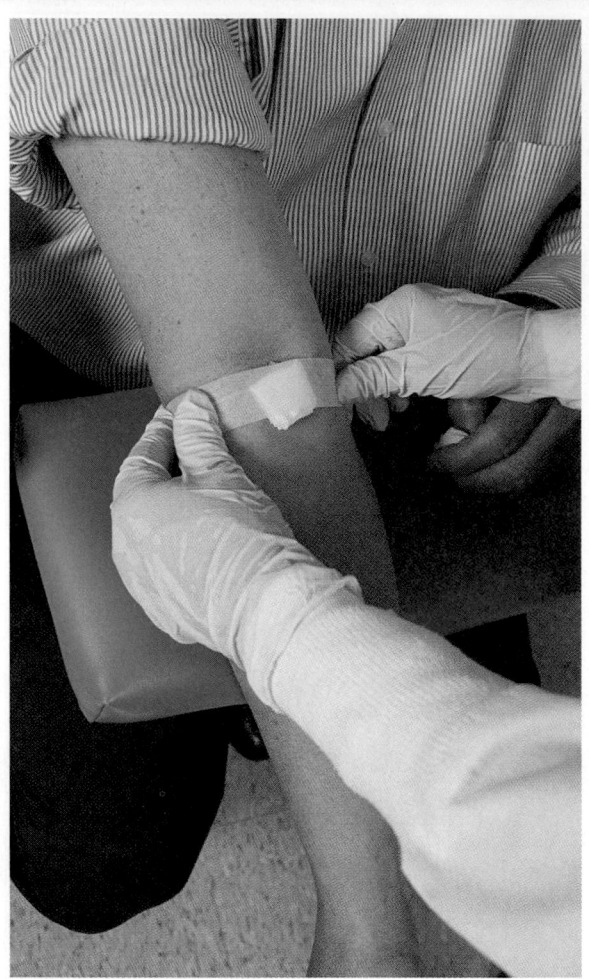

Applying a bandage to the venipuncture site

30. Dispose of all used supplies in appropriate containers.
31. Remove your gloves and wash your hands.
32. Document the procedure in the patient's chart.

Date	
07/17/08; 7:09 a.m.	Labs drawn for CBC and FBG. tubes sent to hospital laboratory. ————————————————— C. Chapin. CMA

patient, a patient with fragile or inaccessible veins, and a patient who only requires point-of-care testing (such as a glucose or hemoglobin determination).

Composition of Capillary Blood

Blood collected by capillary puncture contains a mixture of blood from arterioles, venules, capillaries, and interstitial (tissue) fluid. The medical assistant must warm the puncture site to increase blood flow to the area. She should also avoid squeezing the puncture site, because doing so may cause more tissue fluid to mix with the blood, thus interfering with the test results.

The medical assistant must understand the difference between blood obtained by venipuncture and blood obtained by capillary puncture. For example, glucose levels in blood obtained from a capillary puncture may be higher than

PROCEDURE 41-2

Performing a venipuncture using a winged infusion set

Task
Properly perform a venipuncture using a winged infusion set or butterfly system.

Conditions
- Winged infusion set with push-button needle activation
- Requisition form
- Blood tubes
- Alcohol wipe
- Gauze
- Tourniquet
- Adaptor
- Adhesive bandage or surgical tape
- Biohazard disposable container

Standards
In the time specified and within the scoring parameters determined by the instructor, the student will successfully perform a venipuncture using a winged infusion set.

Performance Standards
1. Examine the requisition slip to identify the tests ordered and, therefore, to select the proper tubes for collection.
2. Greet the patient and ask him to state his full name and date of birth to avoid drawing blood from the wrong patient. Check pretesting requirements, such as fasting, nonfasting, and medication restrictions, to avoid rendering the sample unacceptable because of failure to adhere to pretesting specifications.
3. Reassure the patient and explain the procedure.
4. Select the correct equipment and tubes for the procedure.
5. Wash your hands and put on gloves.
6. Position the patient's arm. The arm with the vein selected for venipuncture should be extended and in a straight line from the shoulder to the wrist with the antecubital veins facing anteriorly. The arm should also be supported on the armrest by a towel.
7. Apply a tourniquet and identify the vein of choice by palpation.
8. Release the tourniquet to avoid patient discomfort and altered test results, which can occur if the tourniquet is left on for more than 1 minute.
9. Clean the site and allow it to air dry. Cleaning should be done in a circular motion starting from the inside and moving away from the puncture site to allow the site to dry. A wet injection site can cause a stinging sensation and contaminate the sample, leading to inaccurate test results.

10. Assemble the winged infusion set. Peel back the packaging at the arrows so that the back of the winged infusion set is exposed. Grasp the rear barrel of the set and remove it from the package. If the winged infusion set has a button, be careful not to activate the button when removing the set from the package. If the button is pushed, the needle will retract into the winged infusion set, rendering it useless.
11. Attach the adaptor to the multiple sample Luer adaptor at the end of the tubing.
12. Assemble additional supplies and position all of the items to be used during the procedure within reach.
13. Reapply the tourniquet 3" to 4" (7.5 to 10 cm) above the antecubital space, making it snug but not tight.
14. Do not touch the puncture site to avoid contaminating the area after cleaning the site.
15. Anchor the vein below the puncture site. Then grasp the patient's arm with your nondominant hand, placing your thumb 1" to 2" (2.5 to 5 cm) below the puncture site. Using your thumb, draw the skin over the vein in the direction of the patient's hand.
16. When the vein is securely anchored, grasp the wings together with your thumb and index finger and insert the needle into the vein at a 15- to 20-degree angle. (You can also hold the body of the device instead of the wings during insertion if you prefer.) Inserting the needle to deep or too shallow may cause it to miss the vein.
17. You should see a flash of blood enter the tubing, which indicates successful entrance into the vein.
18. Attach the proper blood collection tube to the adaptor and watch as blood enters the tube.
19. Make certain to mix tubes with anticoagulant promptly because a delay in mixing may allow the specimen to clot, which will make it unacceptable for testing.
20. Make certain that each evacuated tube is completely full because tubes that are not completely full may be rejected for testing.
21. After inserting the last tube, release the tourniquet to avoid patient discomfort and altered test results, which can occur if the tourniquet is left on for more than 1 minute. Remove the last tube from the adaptor before removing the needle.
22. After blood collection is complete, place a gauze pad over the venipuncture site and, while the needle is still in the vein, grasp the body of the infusion set with your thumb and middle finger and activate the button, if available, with the tip of your index finger to retract the needle into the winged infusion system, decreasing the chance of an accidental needlestick.

Continued

PROCEDURE 41-2—cont'd

23. Remove the needle from the patient's arm and apply pressure to the venipuncture site with gauze.
24. Dispose of the winged infusion set in a biohazard sharps container.
25. Label the tubes containing samples.
26. Examine the puncture site for bleeding. Patients on anticoagulant therapy may bleed for a longer time than other patients.
27. Apply a bandage over the puncture site and dismiss the patient.

28. Dispose of all used supplies in the appropriate containers.
29. Remove your gloves and wash your hands.
30. Document the procedure in the patient's chart.

Date	
05/26/08: 9:45 a.m.	CBC and glucose drawn using winged infusion set. ———— ————————————————————— S. Gonzales, CMA

levels in blood obtained from a venipuncture. Therefore, the medical assistant must document in the patient's chart (on the laboratory report) if the sample was obtained from a capillary puncture.

Capillary Puncture Equipment

When performing capillary puncture, the medical assistant must be sure to select the proper capillary puncture device and puncture site as well as the proper microcollection container to collect the sample.

Capillary Puncture Devices

Most capillary puncture devices are manual or semiautomatic lancets. A **lancet** is a device with a sterile, sharp-pointed blade used to puncture the skin to obtain blood. Many disposable lancets are available in various depths and widths. But, regardless of the device, the puncture must not penetrate deeper than 3.0 mm on adults and 2.0 mm on infants and children. (See Figure 41-11.)

Capillary Puncture Collection Containers

The types of collection containers used to collect blood from a capillary puncture include:

- capillary tubes—available as plain or coated with heparin and typically used for microhematocrit determinations
- microcollection tubes—plastic tubes, available with or without additives, that are preferred when larger amounts of blood are needed. (See Figure 41-12.)

Proper Site Selection for Capillary Puncture

The medical assistant must take care when selecting a site for capillary puncture. (See Figure 41-13.) Acceptable sites include:

- plantar surface of the heel—preferred site for infants from birth to 1 year
- plantar surface of the big toe—acceptable for infants

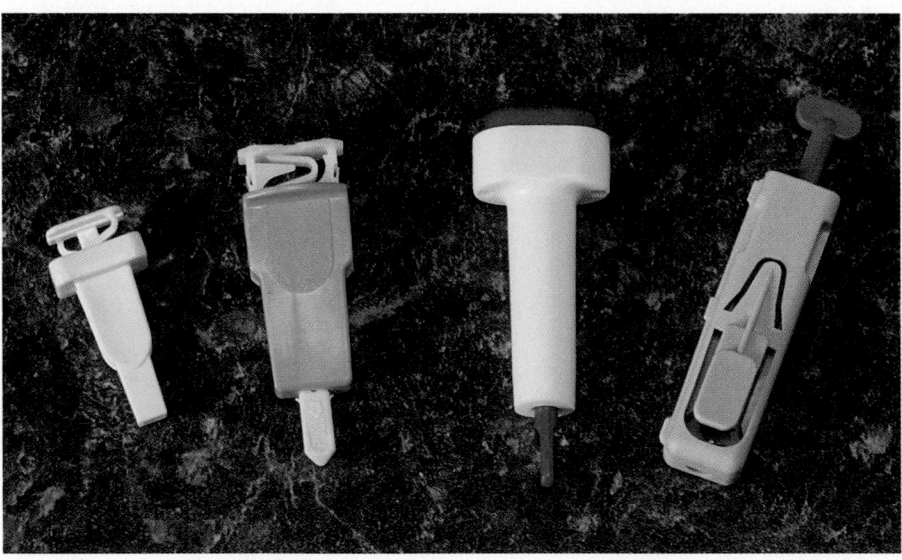

FIG 41-11 Different types of capillary puncture devices available.

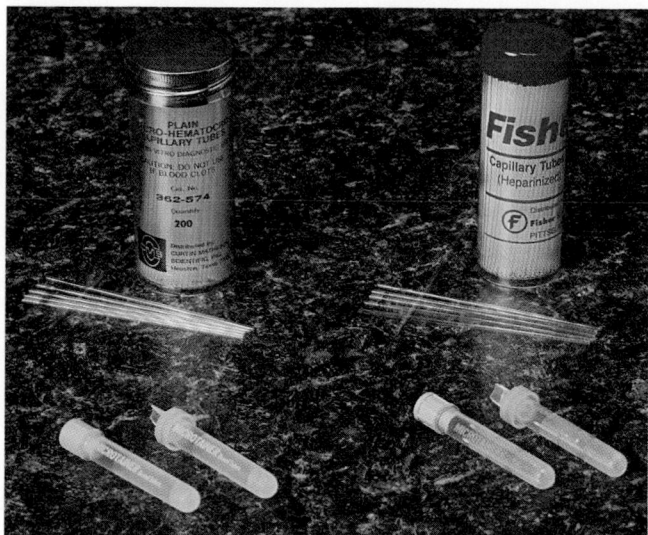

FIG 41-12 Various types of microcollection containers that can be used during a capillary puncture.

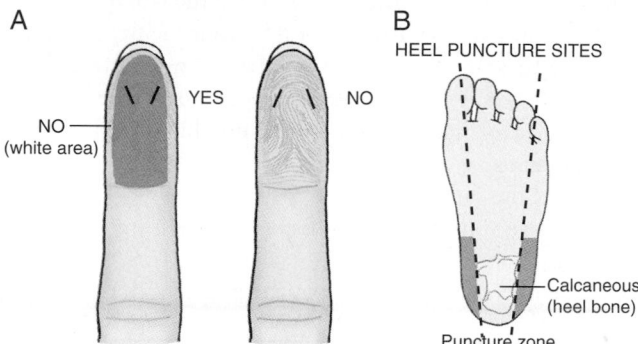

FIG 41-13 The ring and middle fingers as well as the plantar surface of a heel or big toe are acceptable sites for a capillary puncture. . (from Brassington/Goretti: MA Notes. FA Davis, Philadelphia, 2005, p 90, with permission)

- lateral fleshy area of third or fourth finger—preferred site for adults and children over 1 year of age.

  Sites to avoid include:

- bruised, scarred, calloused, or previously punctured areas
- toes other than the big toe
- thumb, index, or pinky fingers
- back area of heel—too close to calcaneus bone
- arch of the foot.

Patient Preparation for Capillary Puncture

The patient preparation procedure for a capillary puncture is similar to that used for a venipuncture, with the exception of warming the site. As mentioned earlier, it is always a good idea to warm the puncture site prior to performing the procedure in order to increase the blood flow to the area. Commercial heel warmers are available; however, the same effect can be obtained by running a towel under warm water and then placing it on the heel or fingertip for a few seconds. In addition, the medical assistant must remember to document on the requisition slip when a sample is collected by capillary puncture. (See *Capillary puncture*.)

Capillary Puncture Procedure

When performing capillary puncture, the medical assistant must identify the patient, following the same procedures as for venipuncture (patient requisition slip and verbal identification or identification band). The medical assistant must remember to let the alcohol dry on the site or the blood will be runny, a rounded drop of blood will not form, and the drop of blood may contain alcohol, interfering with the test results. After puncturing, the medical assistant must wipe away the first drop of blood using a sterile pad, because the first drop could be contaminated with interstitial fluid. She must also be careful not to squeeze the site, or the sample will also become contaminated with interstitial fluid or may be hemolyzed, rendering the sample inadequate. (See *Procedure 41-3: Performing a capillary puncture*, page 886.) In addition to obtaining the proper type of blood specimen, the medical assistant should be sure to collect the appropriate amount of blood in order to maintain the proper ratio of blood to anticoagulant.

Patient Education

Capillary Puncture

When performing a capillary puncture on a patient, the medical assistant should understand that this procedure may be new to the patient and the patient may ask how this differs from a typical venipuncture. The main differences include:

- use of a lancet to make the puncture instead of a needle
- various sites used, including the ring or middle finger and the plantar surface of the heel
- preparation of the site, which may include warming the site prior to puncture to increase the blood flow to the area.

  It is important for the medical assistant to provide proper patient education prior to performing the procedure.

Performing a capillary puncture

Task
Perform a capillary puncture.

Conditions
- Gauze
- Alcohol cleansing pad
- Adhesive bandage or surgical tape
- Lancets
- Microcollection tubes or capillary tubes
- Biohazard sharps container

Standards
In the time specified and within the scoring parameters determined by the instructor, the student will successfully perform a capillary puncture.

Performance Standards
1. Examine the requisition slip to identify the tests ordered and, therefore, to select the proper tubes to use.
2. Greet the patient and ask him to state his full name and date of birth to avoid rendering the sample unacceptable due to patient misidentification. Check pretest requirements, such as fasting, nonfasting, and medication restrictions to avoid rendering the sample unacceptable because of failure to adhere to pretesting specifications.
3. Reassure the patient and explain the procedure.
4. Select the correct equipment and tubes for the procedure.
5. Wash your hands and put on gloves.
6. Select the puncture site.
7. Warm the puncture site if necessary to increase blood flow to the area and promote bleeding from the puncture site.

8. Clean the site and allow it to air dry. Cleaning should be done in a circular motion starting from the inside and moving away from the puncture site to allow the site to dry, because a wet injection site can cause a stinging sensation and contaminate the sample, leading to inaccurate test results.
9. Assemble the equipment. Position within reach all items that will be used during the procedure.
10. Perform the puncture using the proper lancet.
11. Wipe away the first drop of blood to avoid contaminating the sample, because the first drop of blood is diluted with tissue fluid and, possibly, alcohol, both of which could interfere with testing.
12. Collect the sample using the proper collection tubes.
13. Mix the sample if necessary.
14. If you must do point-of-care testing, perform the test according to the manufacturer's specifications.
15. Apply pressure to the site. Examine the site for bleeding and bandage it according to your facility's policy, because some health care facilities do not allow adhesive bandages to be applied to babies or children.
16. Dispose of the puncture device in a biohazard sharps container.
17. Label the sample.
18. Remove your gloves and dispose of them properly.
19. Wash your hands.
20. Document the procedure in the patient's chart.

Date	
10/04/08: 9:45 a.m.	*Hemoglobin determination performed via capillary puncture.* ------------------------------ *S. Gonzales, CMA*

Special Phlebotomy Considerations

The medical assistant may encounter difficult situations while performing a venipuncture or a capillary puncture. She must be aware of such situations in order to prevent them or handle them properly as they happen. Such situations may include fainting and failing to obtain blood. In addition, the medical assistant may have to field calls from outside laboratories regarding problems with a specimen that her office submitted to the laboratory for analysis.

Fainting
When performing venipuncture or capillary puncture, the medical assistant may encounter a patient who faints. A patient may faint at the sight of the needle or blood or after the blood collection procedure. Symptoms a person may exhibit prior to fainting include becoming pale, sweating, and feeling dizzy or lightheaded. As part of the initial patient questioning, the medical assistant should ask the patient if he has ever had adverse affects to needles or his blood being drawn. If he has, the medical assistant should request that the patient lie down on an examination table while she is drawing his blood.

If the patient faints while the blood is being drawn, the medical assistant should pull the needle out immediately and help the patient lie down. Applying a cold compress to his forehead or the back of his neck may help him. She should keep smelling salts handy to help awaken the patient. She should never allow the patient to leave the office if she feels he is in danger of fainting again.

Failing to Obtain Blood

Another challenging situation when performing venipuncture is the failure to obtain blood. There are many reasons why blood may not be obtainable, including:

- missing the vein with the needle
- vein rolling away from the needle
- vein collapsing
- needle going through the vein.

Whatever the reason, the medical assistant should try again. However, if the second attempt is unsuccessful, she should ask another member of the health care team for assistance. In any event, the patient always has the right to refuse to have blood drawn again. If the patient does refuse, tell the physician immediately and document the occurrence in the patient's chart.

Dealing with Problem Specimens

A hospital or reference laboratory may contact a physician's office regarding problems with a specimen. (See *Taking phone calls from an outside laboratory*.) They may even reject the specimen outright. The major reasons for specimen rejection include:

- unlabeled or mislabeled sample
- inadequate volume
- collection in the wrong tube
- grossly hemolyzed sample
- clotted blood in an anticoagulant tube
- improper handling during transport, such as not chilling the sample and not protecting it from light
- samples without a requisition slip
- contaminated specimen containers.

Front office–Back office connection

Taking Phone Calls from an Outside Laboratory

The front office medical assistant may field calls from the outside laboratory the office uses for patients' blood specimens. The laboratory may call the medical office because incorrect blood tubes were drawn. Because the laboratory cannot process the tubes that were drawn, the front office medical assistant must notify the physician of the delay in results, let the clinical medical assistant know of the error, and call the patient to return to the office or medical laboratory to get his blood tests redrawn.

Chapter Summary

- Major components of blood include formed elements, such as erythrocytes, leukocytes, and platelets.
- Substances found in plasma include hormones, glucose, cholesterol, calcium, electrolytes, and fibrinogen.
- Selection of the proper site and equipment is essential when performing a venipuncture or capillary puncture.
- Tube selection is based on the tests ordered and the type of sample required for testing.
- Needle selection is based on the size and depth of the patient's vein.
- Pretesting criteria must be met by the patient before blood can be drawn.

Team Work Exercises

1. Divide into teams of two to three persons. Each group should select a type of safety needle currently in use (or your instructor will assign each group a type). Research the assigned type. Discuss the advantages and disadvantages of your type and present the information to the class.
2. Divide into teams of two to three persons. Practice applying a tourniquet to each other's arm. The person who is having the tourniquet applied should tell the student if it is too tight, too loose, or not positioned correctly. After the tourniquet is applied, take turns palpating the veins, pointing out the median cephalic, basilic, and cephalic veins.

Case Studies

1. Tim is a medical assistant working as a phlebotomist in a hospital laboratory. He is sent to the emergency room to collect an EDTA sample for a STAT hemoglobin and hematocrit (H&H). He properly identifies the patient and is in the process of filling the lavender-top tube when an ER nurse tells him that the ER physician wants to add coagulation studies to the test order. He finishes filling the lavender top tube and grabs a light blue-top tube. After completing the draw, he takes the sample to the laboratory for immediate processing.
   a. Which one of the samples collected is compromised and why?
   b. How could this situation be avoided?
2. Rachel, a medical assistant working in a family medicine practice, is asked to collect a complete blood count (CBC) on a 2-year-old patient. Neither arm has a palpable vein, so Rachel decides to perform a skin puncture on the middle finger of the child's right hand. She has not performed many skin punctures. Although the child is uncooperative, Rachel is able to puncture the site. However, the blood did not form a rounded drop. Instead, the

blood runs down the child's finger. The child keeps pulling away and Rachel has to grab and squeeze the finger forcefully. Rachel is able to fill the container to the minimum level. When the sample is tested, the platelet count is low. What factors may have contributed to this result and why?

Resources
- American Society for Clinical Laboratory Science (ASCLS): *www.ascls.org*
- American Society for Clinical Pathology (ASCP): *www.ascp.org*
- American Society of Phlebotomy Technicians (ASPT): *www.aspt.org*
- Becton, Dickinson and Company: *www.bd.com*
- National Phlebotomy Association (NPA): *www.nationalphlebotomy.org*
- Strasinger, S.K., and Di Lorenzo, M.S.: *The Phlebotomy Workbook*, 2nd ed. Philadelphia: F.A. Davis Company, 2003.

Hematology and Coagulation Procedures

Learning Objectives

Upon completion of this chapter, the student will be able to:

- define the key terms in the glossary
- list the components and functions of blood
- list the tests included in a complete blood count
- describe the different cellular elements and their roles
- describe the components of hemoglobin and hematocrit and their functions
- describe the different leukocytes and their functions
- state the normal range for the different hematological tests
- state the importance of a differential cell count
- list the tests associated with a coagulation determination
- describe the importance of knowing the patient's International Normalized Ratio in relation to prothrombin time.

CAAHEP Competencies

Clinical Competencies
  Diagnostic Testing
    CLIA-waived tests
      Perform hematology testing
General Competencies
  Operational Functions
    Use methods of quality control

ABHES Competencies

Clinical Duties
  Use quality control
  Collect and process specimens
  Perform hematology testing

Procedures

  Measuring hemoglobin using the hemoCue analyzer
  Measuring hematocrit using a microhematocrit centrifuge
  Measuring prothrombin time using a CLIA-waived analyzer

Chapter Outline

  Hematology and Coagulation Overview

Hematology and Coagulation Overview

Hematology is the study of the formed or cellular elements of the blood. Hematology testing includes the morphologic appearance and function of blood cells as well as diseases associated with blood and blood-forming tissues. Through the interpretation of various hematological results, a physician is able to diagnose such disorders as **anemia** and infection. **Coagulation** is usually a subsection of the hematology department that evaluates the overall process of **hemostasis**, which is the blood clotting process. Medical assistants should have an understanding of the many tests performed in the hematology and coagulation departments of the clinical laboratory because they may be required to review patient results and refer them to the appropriate health care professional.

Whole Blood, Plasma, and Serum

Blood is responsible for transporting nutrients, gases, medications, wastes, and other substances throughout the entire body. The average adult body contains approximately 5 to 6 L of blood. Depending on the collection method, a blood sample can be in the form of:

- whole blood
- plasma
- serum.

Whole Blood

Whole blood is a mixture of blood cells and plasma. Whole blood is obtained by using a collection tube with an anticoagulant to prevent blood clotting. Most tests performed in the hematology section of the laboratory require whole blood.

Plasma

The liquid portion of blood is called **plasma**. Plasma is obtained when a tube of whole blood undergoes centrifugation. Upon centrifugation, the blood in the tube will separate into three layers; plasma is the first layer. Similarly, if a tube of whole blood is left to stand in a test tube rack, the contents of the tube will settle into different layers. (For more information on these layers, see Chapter 41, "Phlebotomy," page 867.) Plasma is clear and straw-yellow in color. It consists of 90% water and 10% solutes and makes up approximately 55% of the body's total blood volume. Substances found in plasma include hormones, nutrients, and plasma proteins. Plasma also contains the blood's clotting factors.

Serum

Blood that is allowed to clot and then centrifuged is called *serum*. Serum, a clear yellow fluid that results from centrifuging clotted blood, is the most commonly used specimen in the clinical chemistry department. Serum contains such substances as nutrients, hormones, and antibodies but does not contain clotting factors. (See Figure 42-1.)

Blood Cells and Their Functions

Blood is the body's main fluid. It functions to transport gases (such as oxygen from the lungs to the tissues and carbon dioxide from the tissues to the lungs), antibodies and white blood cells (for defense against pathogenic microorganisms), nutrients (such as glucose and vitamins), and waste products (such as urea). In addition to transporting nutrients, blood assists in regulating body temperature, acid-base balance, fluid and electrolyte balance, and hemostasis.

Blood cells, or formed elements, constitute 45% of the total volume of blood. These cells include:

- red blood cells (RBCs), or erythrocytes, which make up 99% of total blood volume
- white blood cells (WBCs), or leukocytes
- platelets, or thrombocytes, which, combined with WBCs, constitute the other 1% of blood volume. (See Figure 42-2.)

Hematopoiesis, or the process of blood formation, occurs in bone marrow. In the bone marrow, all blood cells go

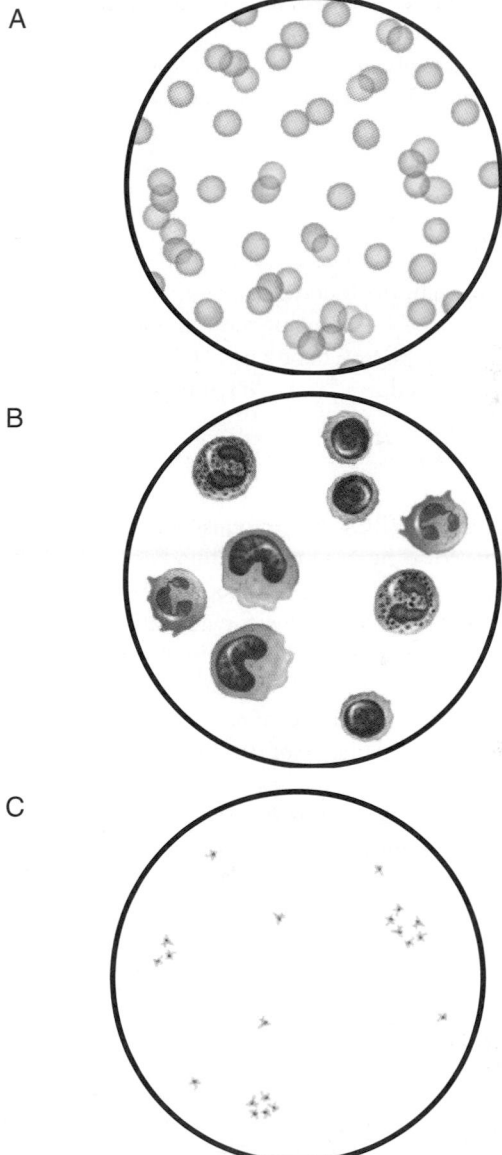

A

B

C

FIG 42-2 Blood cell types. (A) Red blood cells. (B) White blood cells. (C) Platelets.

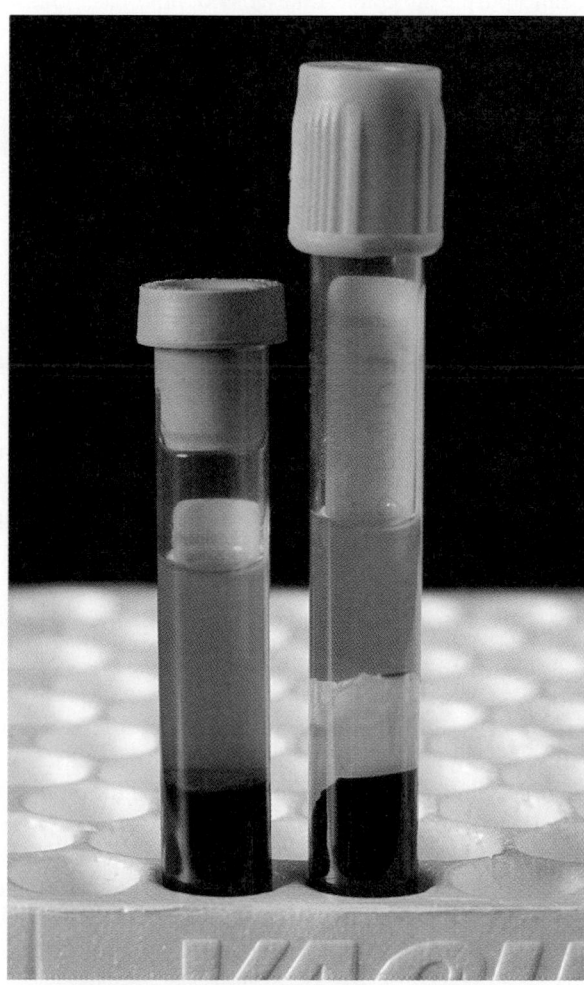

FIG 42-1 The lavender top tube shows plasma and the SST (gold top) tube shows serum.

through a maturation process before being released into the bloodstream. Normally, the bone marrow releases only mature, functional blood cells into the circulating bloodstream. Thus, release of immature blood cells into the bloodstream could indicate a hematological disorder or a reaction to a severe infection or hemorrhage.

RBCs

Red blood cells (RBCs) contain the protein **hemoglobin**, an iron-containing protein. Hemoglobin is responsible for transporting oxygen and carbon dioxide. Oxygen molecules attach to the hemoglobin on the RBC and are transported throughout the body. RBCs are formed in the bone marrow and, once mature, are released into the bloodstream. The normal life span for an RBC is 120 days. Old RBCs are destroyed by **macrophages**, which are known as *tissue cells* because they are a type of WBC that leaves the bloodstream and resides in the body's organs and tissues. Macrophages that reside in the spleen and liver are responsible for destroying cellular debris such as old red blood cells. Low levels of RBCs in a patient could indicate a loss of blood, which may be due to trauma or a chronic condition.

RBCs also contain the blood group antigens. These antigens are located on the surface of the cell and determine a person's blood type. (See Chapter 43, "Clinical Chemistry and Serological Procedures," page 903, for more information on blood typing.)

WBCs

White blood cells (WBCs) are responsible for fighting off infection. They do so by producing antibodies or through a process in which specialized white blood cells (phagocytes) engulf and destroy microorganisms, foreign antigens, and cellular debris or other foreign substances. Produced in the bone marrow, the life span of a WBC ranges from 1 day to 1 year, depending on the type. An increase or decrease in the WBC count can indicate a wide range of diseases and conditions.

WBCs are classified as *granulocytes* or *agranulocytes*. Granulocytes contain granules in their cytoplasm; agranulocytes do not. In addition, granulocytes contain smaller, segmented nuclei, and agranulocytes contain very large nuclei. Within these two classifications, there are five types of leukocytes.

Granulocytes

There are three types of granulocytes:

- neutrophils
- eosinophils
- basophils

Neutrophils

Neutrophils are the most numerous of the types of WBC and are responsible for phagocytosis of pathogens, particularly bacteria. Their granules are purple in color and they contain a segmented nucleus. They are also known as *segmenters* or *polymorphonuclearcytes* because of their segmented nucleus. An increase in neutrophils is commonly seen in bacterial infections. The normal range for neutrophils is 40% to 60%.

Eosinophils

Eosinophils assists with the inflammatory response by releasing histamine and they are also phagocytic. The number of these cells increases during allergic reactions, skin infections, and parasitic infections. Their granules are bright orange-pink in color. Eosinophils are rarely seen in a patient's blood; thus, their normal range is 0% to 4%.

Basophils

Basophils are the least common of all types of WBC. They assist with the inflammatory response by releasing histamines and are also phagocytic. They also release heparin to prevent abnormal blood clotting. Their granules are very dark blue-purple in color. Like eosinophils, basophils are rarely seen in a patient's blood and have a normal range of 0% to 1%.

Agranulocytes

There are two types of agranulocytes:

- lymphocytes
- monocytes.

Lymphocytes

Lymphocytes are the second most numerous type of WBC and are responsible for producing antibodies. Lymphocyte levels increase during viral infections such as infectious mononucleosis. Lymphocytes can be further differentiated into B-cell lymphocytes (which produce antibodies) and T-cell lymphocytes (which aid the immune system.) Lymphocytes have a large, round, bluish-purple nucleus that tends to take up the entire cell. The normal range for lymphocytes in the blood is 20% to 40%.

Monocytes

Monocytes are the largest circulating WBC. They are responsible for phagocytosis and are effective against chronic infection such as tuberculosis (TB). A monocyte is a large cell that contains vacuoles, or holes, in its cytoplasm and has a large, blue, slightly indented nucleus. The monocyte quickly leaves the bloodstream and travels to tissues (where it becomes a macrophage) to aid in phagocytosis within the tissues. The normal range for monocytes is 3% to 8%. (See Figure 42-3.)

Platelets

Platelets are small, irregularly shaped disks that are fragments of a larger cell called a *megakaryocyte,* which is formed

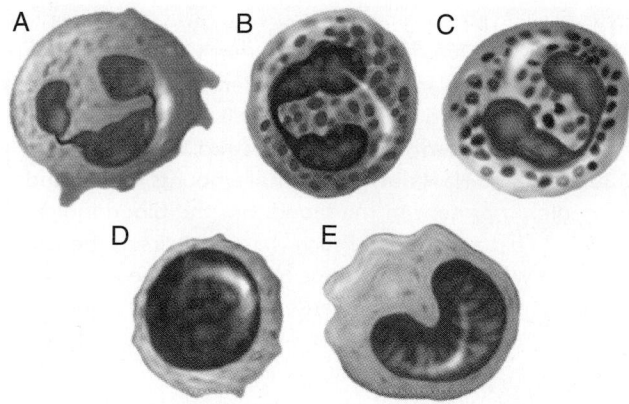

FIG 42-3 White blood cells. (A) Neutrophils. (B) Eosinophils. (C) Basophils. (D) Lymphocytes. (E) Monocytes.

in the bone marrow. A platelet's life span is 9 to 12 days. Platelets are responsible for blood clotting and are important in all stages of the coagulation process. An increase in platelet count can cause a person to suffer from a blood clot; a decrease could hinder the ability to stop bleeding from a minor cut.

Tests and Procedures Associated with Hematology

Tests and procedures associated with hematology include a hemoglobin and hematocrit test (H&H), complete blood count (CBC), erythrocyte sedimentation rate, and reticulocyte count.

Hemoglobin and Hematocrit

Hemoglobin (Hgb) and hematocrit (HCT) values, also known as *H&H*, are important indicators of the RBCs' ability to carry oxygen. **Hematocrit** is the percentage of the volume occupied by RBCs compared to the volume of whole blood. (See *Common hematology and coagulation tests*.) The H&H and RBC count tests are commonly performed together and the physician evaluates them to determine if a patient is anemic or is suffering from a severe loss of blood. Patient results that the analyzer flags as critical values must receive immediate attention from the medical assistant, who should notify the physician without delay. (See *Reporting critical values*, page 894.)

Complete Blood Count

The most commonly ordered hematological test is the complete blood count (CBC). A CBC can be considered a

---

Common hematology and coagulation tests

The following table lists common hematology and coagulation tests along with their normal values.

Test	Normal Range
Red blood cells (RBCs)	
• Male	• 4.7 to 6.1 $\times$ 10^6 cells/microliter
• Female	• 4.2 to 5.4 $\times$ 10^6 cells/microliter
Hemoglobin (Hgb)	
• Male	• 14.0 to 18.0 g/dl
• Female	• 12 to 16 g/dl
Hematocrit (HCT)	
• Male	• 42% to 52%
• Female	• 37% to 47%
WBC (total)	4.8 to 10.8 $\times$ 10^3
Differential	
• Neutrophils	• 40% to 60%
• Lymphocytes	• 20% to 40%
• Monocytes	• 3% to 8%
• Eosinophils	• 0% to 4%
• Basophils	• 0% to 1%
Platelets	130,000 to 400,000/microliter
Erythrocyte sedimentation rate (ESR)	
• Male	• < 15 mm/hr
• Female	• < 20 mm/hr
Prothrombin time (PT)	11.0 to 14.5 seconds
Partial thromboplastin time (PTT)	24 to 36 seconds
International Normalized Ratio (INR)	2.0 to 3.0
Bleeding time	Up to 10 minutes

---

panel because it is composed of numerous individual blood counts, calculations, and microscopic evaluations of blood cells. However, other than an H&H, a physician would rarely order one test within the CBC, because the hematological instruments used to perform a CBC will not test just one component. When the instrument tests the blood specimen, it will perform a test for and report on all of the components within the CBC. In the case where an H&H is ordered, the technologist will make sure to report only

Front office–Back office connection

Reporting Critical Values

The administrative medical assistant working in the front office may frequently receive laboratory results for a patient. A critical value, one that is out of the normal range, may indicate a threat to a patient's health. Thus, it is important for the administrative medical assistant as much as the clinical medical assistant to know the normal ranges for values. For example, if an administrative medical assistant receives results of a patient's complete blood count (CBC) that reveal a white blood cell (WBC) count below 4.0 or higher than 13.0, she must know that such a result may indicate a critical condition for the patient. Hemoglobin levels below 11 g/dl or hematocrit above 35% may indicate blood loss and possibly the need for a blood transfusion. Any of these results would require immediate attention from the physician. The administrative medical assistant should be able to recognize these abnormal results and respond appropriately based on the procedure set by the office.

Blood cell indices

Blood cell indices are calculations used to determine the average size of red blood cells as well as the amount of hemoglobin present in the average red blood cell. The RBC count and H&H determine total amounts of cells and hemoglobin present in the blood, but the blood indices provide a better picture of such characteristics as the volume and weight of RBCs. These results help the physician understand the potential causes of a patient's anemia and, thus, better assess his condition and prescribe treatment. Blood cell indices include:

- mean corpuscular hemoglobin (MCH), which measures the average amount of hemoglobin within RBCs

- mean corpuscular hemoglobin concentration (MCHC), which measures the concentration of hemoglobin in an average red blood cell and compares it with the size of the cell.

- mean corpuscular volume (MCV), which measures the size of RBCs

- red cell distribution width (RDW), which measures the variations in size of RBCs.

the H&H results from the CBC. Components of a CBC include:

- WBC count, which measures the number of circulating WBCs
- RBC count, which measures the number of circulating RBCs
- hemoglobin (Hgb), which measures the oxygen-carrying capacity of RBCs
- hematocrit (HCT), which measures the volume of packed RBCs
- blood cell indices, which provide additional information on RBCs (See *Blood cell indices.*)
- platelet count, which measures the number of platelets in the circulating blood
- differential count, which measures the percentage of different types of WBCs (neutrophils, eosinophils, basophils, lymphocytes, and monocytes) and evaluates the size, shape, and appearance of WBCs, RBCs, and platelets. (See *CBC with differential.*)

CLIA-Waived Hematological Tests

Although a clinical laboratory will use an automated hematology analyzer to perform a CBC, a POL may use less sophisticated technology to obtain some hematological results. A medical assistant may perform CLIA-waived hematological tests in the physician's office. Tests such as hemoglobin and hematocrit measurements are quick, easy procedures to perform and are convenient for the patient. Many offices use the

HemoCue B-Hemoglobin Test System to test a patient's hemoglobin. The test system consists of the B-Hemoglobin Analyzer and disposable microcuvettes. (See Figure 42-4.) Results are measured in 1 minute and require a drop of blood from a dermal puncture. (See *Procedure 42-1: Measuring hemoglobin using the HemoCue analyzer,* page 896.)

The hematocrit test is another test commonly performed in the POL and is used to evaluate anemia, blood loss, hemolytic anemia, and **polycythemia**. This test requires a special microhematocrit centrifuge and heparinized capillary collection tubes. (See Figure 42-5.) The medical assistant must prepare the patient for a capillary puncture and blood collection and fill as required two heparinized capillary tubes. Upon sealing each tube, she processes the tubes in the microhematocrit centrifuge and then determines the percentage of packed RBCs that are contained in the centrifuge tubes. The hematocrit result is expressed as a percentage. (See *Procedure 42-2: Measuring hematocrit using a microhematocrit centrifuge,* pages 897 and 898.)

Although the medical assistant can perform a hemoglobin and hematocrit test in a POL, in offices that do not perform these tests, the medical assistant may be required to draw blood from a patient and send the specimen to a hospital or reference laboratory for testing. The medical assistant should know not only which tube to draw for the specimen (lavender) but should also be familiar with the testing abbreviations used on the various laboratory requisitions forms. (See *Understanding hematological abbreviations,* page 898.)

CBC with differential

On some laboratory requisition slips, the complete blood count (CBC) order may say *CBC w/Diff* (differential), rather than just *CBC*. This phrasing is a holdover from the past, before more advanced hematology analyzers were available. Back then, the differential was always a manually performed part of the complete blood count and some laboratories considered the differential to be a separate procedure.

In the past, when a CBC was ordered the technologist would put the blood tube through the hematology analyzer for the cell counts. The hematology technologist would then take a drop of blood and smear it onto a microscope slide, let it dry, and then stain the slide with Wright's stain. Then the technologist would look at the smear under the microscope and count the first 100 white blood cells observed. As she counted, she would identify, or differentiate, each type. For example, if she identified 34 neutrophils, 61 lymphocytes, 3 monocytes, and 2 eosinophils out of the first 100 white blood cells seen, she would report out *34% neutrophils, 61% lymphocytes, 3% monocytes, 2% eosinophils*. She would then inspect the red blood cells and platelets for their size, shape, and appearance and report her visual findings. The completed CBC report would include the automated cell counts as well as the manual differential results.

Hematology analyzers today are capable of performing the differential. Thus, unless the analyzer flags a result that requires a subsequent manual differential, the entire CBC testing is done automatically.

PATIENT LABORATORY REPORT

HARTELL MEMORIAL HOSPITAL LABORATORY

Name: Seth Banas   Sex: M
M/R#: 032608
D.O.B.: 05/02/63   45
Physician: Greer, R.
Location: Outpatient

Date ordered: 08/30/2008
Date collected: 08/30/2008
Time collected: 0
Date tested: 08/30/2008
Time tester: 21:41
Accession Number: 0007413225

HEMATOLOGY   <<<<<<<<<<COMPLETE BLOOD COUNT>>>>>>>>>>

Electrolytes	Result	Reference	Units
WBC	6.0	3.80-10.80	10^3
RBC	5.0	4.70-6.10	10^6
Hemoglobin	14.4	14-18	g/dl
Hemotocrit	42.3	42-52	%
MCV	85	77-104	FL
MCH	29	27-34	PG
MCHC	34.0	31-37	g/dl
RDW	11	11-16	%
PLT CT	237	150-400	10^3
MPV	10	6-14	FL
Differential			
Neutrophils	61	44-80	%
Lymphocytes	28	14-44	%
Monocytes	8	4-12	%
Eosinophils	2	0-5	%
Basophils	1	0-2	%
ABS NEU CT	4		
Manual diff	Not indicated		
RBC morph	Not indicated		

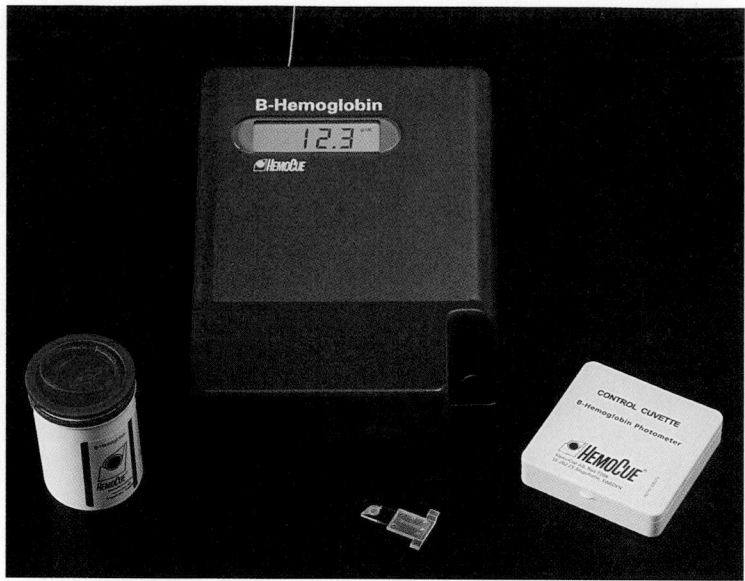

FIG 42-4 HemoCue test system.

PROCEDURE 42-1

Measuring hemoglobin using the HemoCue analyzer

Task
Measure hemoglobin using the HemoCue analyzer.

Conditions
- HemoCue analyzer
- Calibrator cuvette
- Quality control sample
- Testing cuvettes
- Lancet
- Alcohol preparation
- Gauze
- Gloves
- Manufacturer's manual
- Biohazard waste container

Standards
In the time specified and within the scoring parameters determined by the instructor, the student will successfully measure hemoglobin using a HemoCue analyzer.

Performance Standards
1. Wash or sanitize your hands and put on gloves and other personal protective equipment (PPE) as designated by your facility.
2. Assemble the supplies.
3. To ensure proper functioning, calibrate the analyzer by putting the calibrator cuvette into the machine.
4. Perform the necessary quality control procedures and record the results. You must run quality control to ensure accurate results and achieve results within the normal range prior to patient testing.
5. Greet and identify your patient and introduce yourself. Explain the procedure.
6. Perform a capillary puncture on the patient using the proper procedure.
7. Using a testing cuvette, collect the appropriate specimen from the capillary puncture.
8. Wipe off the end of the cuvette in the proper manner to avoid erroneous results.
9. Placed the cuvette in the machine.
10. Read the results.
11. Record the results in the patient's chart.

Date	
05/26/08; 9:45 a.m.	Hgb: 13.4 g/dl. -------------------------------- S. Gonzales, CMA

12. Dispose of the cuvette in the biohazard waste container.
13. Disinfect the equipment if indicated to avoid erroneous results from a dirty or contaminated machine.
14. Dispose of the gloves and wash or sanitize your hands.

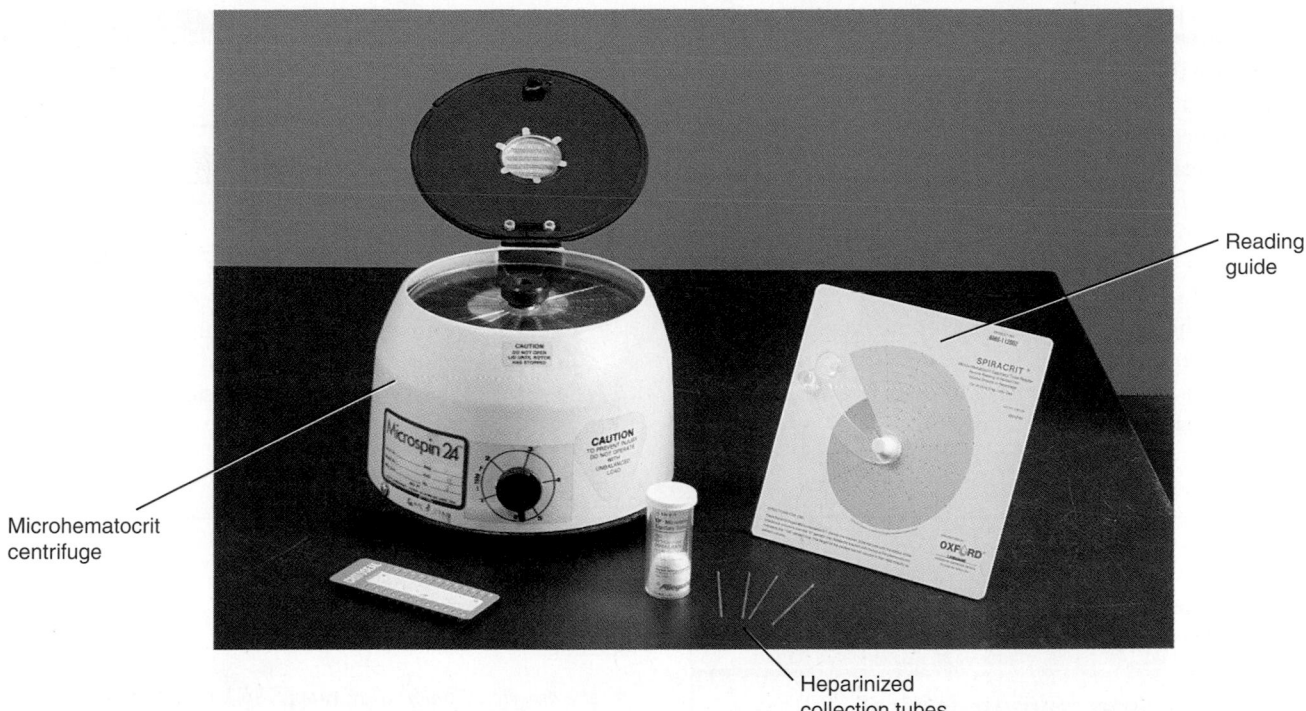

FIG 42-5 Microhematocrit centrifuge, heparinized collection tubes, and reading guide.

Reading guide

Microhematocrit centrifuge

Heparinized collection tubes

PROCEDURE 42-2

Measuring hematocrit using a microhematocrit centrifuge

Task
Measuring hematocrit using a microhematocrit centrifuge.

Conditions
- Microhematocrit centrifuge
- Heparinized capillary tubes
- Lancet
- Gloves
- Hematocrit reader grid
- Sealing clay
- Alcohol preparation
- Gauze
- Biohazard sharps container

Standards
In the time specified and within the scoring parameters determined by the instructor, the student will successfully measure hematocrit.

Performance Standards
1. Wash or sanitize your hands and put on gloves and other personal protective equipment (PPE) as designated by your facility.
2. Assemble the supplies.

3. Greet and identify your patient and introduce yourself. Explain the procedure.
4. Perform a capillary puncture on the patient using the proper procedure.
5. Collect the appropriate specimen from the capillary puncture using the heparinized capillary tubes. Using nonheparinized capillary tubes will cause the specimen to clot and render the test inaccurate.
6. Fill both tubes as required. Two tubes are required to balance the centrifuge correctly and to ensure a sufficient sample if one tube breaks during the procedure.
8. Seal both tubes by gently pushing the end of one tube into the clay two to three times. Unsealed tubes will cause the blood to leak out of the tube and render the specimen unacceptable.
9. Place both tubes in the microhematocrit centrifuge, making sure the tubes are placed directly across from each other (also called *balanced*). Unbalanced tubes will cause the tubes to break upon centrifugation, rendering the test unacceptable.

Continued

PROCEDURE 42-2—cont'd

10. Secure the cover to the centrifuge to avoid tube breakage and start the centrifuge timer for the desired time as indicated by the manufacturer's or your instructor's specifications.

11. Listen for the timer to go off. Allow the centrifuge to come to a complete stop before opening it.

12. Inspect the tubes, making sure they are intact and not broken.

13. Read the results. Depending on the type of microhematocrit centrifuge, the cover may have the reading grid on it or you may have to use a handheld hematocrit reader grid.

14. Dispose of both capillary tubes in a biohazard waste container.

15. Record the results in the patient's chart.

Date	
10/26/08: 2:32 p.m.	*Performed microhematocrit: 43% ------ S. Gonzales, CMA*

16. Disinfect the centrifuge if indicated. A dirty or contaminated centrifuge can cause unnecessary exposure to biohazardous material.

17. Dispose of the gloves and wash or sanitize your hands.

Front office–Back office connection

Understanding Hematological Abbreviations

There are many times when someone from the clinical laboratory will call the office to give a CBC result. Some of the terminology used when giving that report may be different or abbreviated from what is actually written on a report form. Although the clinical medical assistant may be more familiar with such terminology because she is using it every day in the POL, it is also important for the administrative medical assistant to recognize standard hematological abbreviations so that she can understand certain tests or test results. Here are some common hematology abbreviations used in the POL:

• *baso*—basophil

• *diff*—differential count

• *eos*—eosinophil

• *lymph*—lymphocyte

• *mono*—monocyte

• *plt*—platelet

• *seg* or *poly*—neutrophil

Other Hematology Department Tests

For hematology tests that may not be performed in a POL, the medical assistant may be involved in processing blood specimens for such testing or reading the final laboratory results received by the office. The medical assistant should familiarize herself with the most common hematology tests in order to facilitate better patient care. In addition to the

CBC and H&H, two other tests related to hematology include:

• *erythrocyte sedimentation rate (ESR),* which determines the rate of red blood cell sedimentation and is usually ordered as a screening test to determine nonspecific inflammation

• *reticulocyte count* (also called *retic count*), which evaluates the ability of the bone marrow to produce and release red blood cells into the bloodstream and, if abnormally increased, could indicate such conditions as hemolytic anemia or a problem with the bone marrow.

Diseases Associated with Hematology Tests

The medical assistant will see patients with many different diseases and conditions. Understanding these conditions will allow the medical assistant to better relate the tests used to diagnose and treat such conditions. Here are some common diseases diagnosed using hematology tests:

• *anemia,* which is characterized by a decrease in the number of red blood cells or in the amount of hemoglobin in the circulating blood and includes sickle cell anemia and iron deficiency anemia

• *leukemia,* which is a marked increase in the number of abnormal or immature white blood cells in the bone marrow and the circulating blood and can be classified by the type of white blood cell affected, such as chronic lymphocytic leukemia (CLL), which affects the patient's lymphocytes, and chronic myelogenous leukemia (CML), which affects the monocyte blood cell (See *Managing a patient's treatment.*)

• *polycythemia,* which is a rare disorder of unknown cause that involves an excess of red blood cells in the circulating blood and causes the blood to have a viscous consistency

- *leukocytosis*, which is an abnormal increase in white blood cells and is usually caused by a bacterial infection or dehydration
- *leukopenia*, which is an abnormal decrease in the number of white blood cells and can be caused by some medications, failure of the bone marrow to produce enough white blood cells, or chemotherapy
- *thrombocytopenia*, which is an abnormal decrease in the amount of circulating platelets characterized by bruising or frequent nosebleeds and can be caused by a decrease in platelet production by the bone marrow or increased platelet destruction from unknown factors.

Tests and Procedures Associated with Coagulation

The coagulation laboratory is usually a section of the hematology department, but in larger laboratories, coagulation may be a separate department. The coagulation section evaluates the overall process of hemostasis (the process of forming a blood clot), including the function of platelets, blood vessels, coagulation factors, and anticoagulant therapy, such as heparin and warfarin (Coumadin).

The process of hemostasis involves several steps. First, collagen released by an injured blood vessel causes circulating platelets to bind with the collagen and then adhere to the site of injury. The platelets form what is known as a *platelet plug*. Also circulating in the blood are substances known as *plasma proteins*. These plasma proteins are coagulation factors that become activated upon injury to a blood vessel. The coagulation factors go through a complex series of reactions called *pathways*. One of the last steps in these pathways consists of a fibrin clot that combines with the platelet plug to stabilize and strengthen the injured blood

vessel. The final stage in the process is **fibrinolysis**, when the fibrin clot eventually breaks down after the blood vessel has healed.

Many offices have begun using recently developed CLIA-waived prothrombin instruments in their POLs. (See Figure 42-6.) Patients on warfarin (Coumadin) therapy must undergo frequent blood tests to ensure that the anticoagulation therapy is effective. Now that the medical assistant can perform these tests in the POL, the physician can receive patient results immediately and thus make decisions regarding the effectiveness of the patient's therapy without delay. (See *Procedure 42-3: Measuring prothrombin time using a CLIA-waived analyzer,* page 900.)

Other Coagulation Department Tests

Even though some additional coagulation tests may not be performed in a POL, a medical assistant may be involved with processing blood specimens for such testing or reading the final laboratory results received by the office. The medical assistant should familiarize herself with the most

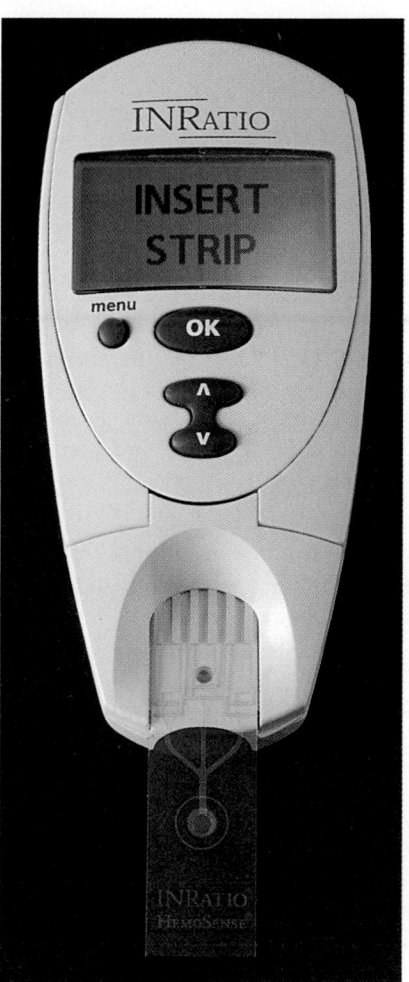

FIG 42-6 CLIA-waived prothrombin time analyzer.

Front office–Back office connection

Managing a Patient's Treatment

A patient diagnosed with leukemia may need to undergo various procedures, treatments, and laboratory tests. The administrative medical assistant may have to coordinate such appointments for the patient. The medical assistant should keep handy a list of the various facilities to which the patient may be referred. In addition, she should familiarize herself with what these procedures, treatments, and tests may entail so she can answer questions the patient may have regarding the amount of time a certain procedure may take or any specialized patient preparation.

■ **PROCEDURE 42-3**

Measuring prothrombin time using a CLIA-waived analyzer

Task
Measure prothrombin time using a CLIA-waived analyzer.

Conditions
- Prothrombin time analyzer
- Test strips
- Lancet
- Alcohol preparation
- Gauze
- Biohazard waste container
- Gloves

Standards
In the time specified and within the scoring parameters determined by the instructor, the student will successfully measure prothrombin time using a CLIA-waived analyzer.

Performance Standards
1. Wash or sanitize your hands and put on gloves and any other personal protective equipment (PPE) as designated by your facility.
2. Assemble the supplies.
3. Greet and identify your patient and introduce yourself. Explain the procedure.
4. Turn the meter on.

5. Insert the test strip into the meter and check the code. The test strip code must match the meter code to ensure accurate results.
6. Perform a capillary puncture on the patient.
7. Apply a large hanging drop of blood to the test strip when prompted by the meter. A sample that is too small will cause erroneous results.
8. Wait for results to appear on the display.
9. Read the results.
10. Record the results correctly in the patient's chart.

Date	
05/26/08; 9:45 a.m.	INR 1.00. --------------------------------- S. Gonzales, CMA

11. Dispose of the cuvette in the biohazard waste container.
12. Disinfect the equipment if indicated. A dirty or contaminated machine may cause erroneous results.
13. Dispose of the gloves and wash or sanitize your hands.

---

common coagulation tests in order to facilitate better patient care. Here are some commonly ordered coagulation tests:

- **prothrombin time (PT)**, which determines how long it takes for blood to clot and is used to screen for bleeding abnormalities, evaluate the entire coagulation process, and monitor warfarin (Coumadin) therapy. (See *Therapeutic ranges for oral anticoagulant therapy*.)
- *International Normalized Ratio (INR)*, which provides uniform prothrombin time results for physicians in all parts of the country, as recommended by the World Health Organization
- *activated partial thromboplastin time (APTT or PTT)*, which evaluates the intrinsic system of the coagulation cascades, monitors heparin therapy, and, if prolonged, may indicate disseminated intravascular coagulation (DIC), hemophilia, or cirrhosis
- *bleeding time (BT)*, which evaluates the function of platelets and, if increased, may indicate decreased level of platelets or decreased platelet function
- *thrombin time (TT)*, which determines if adequate fibrinogen is present for normal coagulation and, if prolonged, may indicate the presence of fibrin degradation products (FDPs) or an increased level of heparin

- *fibrin degradation product (FDP)*, which measure the body's clot dissolving system and, if increased, may indicate disseminated intravascular coagulation (DIC), primary fibrinolysis, or pulmonary embolus.
- *D-dimer*, which measures abnormal clotting and fibrinolysis and, if increased, may indicate deep vein thrombosis, pulmonary embolism, DIC, or myocardial infarction
- *fibrinogen*, which determines the amount of fibrinogen in plasma and indicates the body's clotting ability and clotting activity in the body.

Diseases Associated with Coagulation
Diseases associated with coagulation include:

- *disseminated intravascular coagulation (DIC)*, a severe blood disorder caused by certain cancers, septicemia, blood transfusion reaction, and such complications of pregnancy as eclampsia and abruptio placenta and in which a person's blood coagulates throughout the body, possibly resulting in blood clots, severe bleeding, or death
- *thrombophilic disorder*, an inherited disease in which a person is at risk of developing or has developed thrombosis or blood clots that can occur in veins and arteries and cause strokes and heart attacks

Therapeutic ranges for oral anticoagulant therapy

The following table shows normal International Normalized Ratio (INR) ranges according to various conditions.

Condition	INR
Treatment of venous thrombosis	2.0 to 3.0
Treatment of pulmonary embolism	2.0 to 3.0
Prevention of thrombosis in patients with:	
• atrial fibrillation	2.0 to 3.0
• myocardial infarction	2.0 to 3.0
• mechanical prosthetic heart valve	2.5 to 3.5
• recurrent systemic embolism	2.5 to 3.5

- *hemophilia,* a rare hereditary blood disease usually affecting males more than females in which blood does not clot normally and is characterized by excessive bleeding due to the decrease or lack of a certain blood substance that is responsible for the clotting of blood, known as a *clotting factor.* (Hemophilia is differentiated into two types based on the deficiency of a specific factor. Type A is known as *classic hemophilia;* type B is known as *Christmas disease.*)

Chapter Summary

- Hematology is the study of formed elements in the blood.
- Hematological tests a medical assistant may perform include: CBC, Hgb, HCT, and ESR.
- Coagulation is the study of the clotting process.
- Coagulation tests a medical assistant may perform include the CLIA-waived PT test.
- Diseases associated with hematology include: anemia, leukemia, polycythemia, leukocytosis, leucopenia, and thrombocytopenia
- Diseases associated with coagulation include: disseminated intravascular coagulation and hemophilia.

Team Work Exercises

1. Divide into groups of two to three students. Your instructor will assign each group a different type of white blood cell. Each group should provide the following information on their assigned cell:
   a. colored drawing or image (approximately 8" × 10" or bigger) of the cell with its correct anatomy
   b. function of the cell type
   c. normal range for the cell type
   d. diseases or conditions associated with an increase and a decrease of this cell type.
2. The coagulation process is complicated and follows what is known as a cascade or pathway. Your instructor will divide the class into two groups. One group will research the intrinsic pathway of coagulation and the other group will research the extrinsic pathway. After each group has done its research, it will develop a visual representation of its cascade and present it to the class. Discussion of how the two pathways relate to the entire coagulation process should take place as a full class discussion.

Case Studies

1. Mr. Bomba is on warfarin therapy because of atrial fibrillation and he goes to your POL for his regular prothrombin time with INR test. Blood was drawn and submitted for processing, and the result came back with prothrombin time of 9.5 and INR of 0.8. What is the interpretation of these results? After alerting Dr. Mahoney of Mr. Bomba's results, he asks you to interview the patient. What question(s) are you going to ask of Mr. Bomba?
2. Edna Lorenkiewicz has just been diagnosed with polycythemia vera and, as she leaves the office, she seems distraught. Although you have heard of the disease, you do not know much about it but want to educate yourself for the next time Edna comes to the office. What type of information will you find on this disease?

Resources

- American Society for Clinical Pathology: *www.ascp.org/*
- American Society of Hematology: *www.hematology.org/*
- Hematology atlas: *www.hematologyatlas.com/principalpage.htm*
- Public resource for clinical laboratory testing: *www.labtestsonline.org/*
- Sacher, R.A., and McPherson, R.A.: *Widmann's Clinical Interpretation of Laboratory Tests,* 11th ed. Philadelphia: F.A. Davis, 2000.
- Strasinger, S.K., and Di Lorenzo, M.S.: *The Phlebotomy Workbook,* 2nd ed. Philadelphia: F.A. Davis, 2003.

Clinical Chemistry and Serological Procedures

Learning Objectives

Upon completion of this chapter, the student will be able to:

- define the key terms in the glossary
- explain the basic principles of a blood chemistry test
- state the proper collection, handling, and processing of specimens
- state the proper instruction for patient preparation for a fasting blood glucose specimen
- state the process of quality control and maintenance of a basic chemistry analyzer
- state the restrictions that must be followed by the patient undergoing a glucose tolerance test
- understand and explain the desirable ranges for some chemistry panels
- perform blood chemistry tests using an automated chemistry analyzer
- explain the antigen–antibodies reaction in relation to blood typing
- explain the principles of ABO and Rh typing
- understand the basic principles of serological methodologies
- perform basic serological procedures and accurately interpret results.

CAAHEP Competencies

Diagnostic Testing
  CLIA-Waived Tests
    Perform chemistry testing
    Perform immunology testing
Operational Functions
  Use Methods of Quality Control

ABHES Competencies

Clinical Duties
  Use quality control
  Collect and process specimens
  Perform chemistry testing
  Perform immunology testing

Procedures

  Performing a blood glucose test and patient education for a glucose monitoring system
  Performing cholesterol or lipid panel testing
  Performing a CLIA-waived mono test

Chapter Outline

Key Terms

agglutination
Type of antibody–antigen reaction in which a solid antigen clumps with a soluble antibody

analyte
Measurable chemical substance

antibody
Protein produced by B lymphocytes in response to the presence of an antigen

antigen
Substance that, when introduced into the body, elicits an immune response

atherosclerosis
Thickening and hardening of the walls of the arteries; also called *arteriosclerosis*

methodology
System of principles and procedures used in scientific testing

microsample
Very small amount of a specimen

panel
Group of blood tests that evaluates the function of a particular body system; also called *profile*

photometric reflectance
Measurement of the amount of light reflected by a specimen

Testing in the POL

Advances in automated chemistry analyzers, the utilization of microsample testing, and the development of specific, rapid, antibody testing have made it possible to perform some basic chemistry and serology tests in the physician's office laboratory (POL). Medical assistants should know how to properly handle, maintain, and operate the instruments in the POL as well as perform quality control testing on these instruments. In addition, medical assistants should be aware of the normal ranges for various chemistry analytes and serological results in order to alert the physician to an abnormal or critical laboratory result. (See *Know the format.*)

Clinical Chemistry

Clinical chemistry is the most automated area of the clinical laboratory. Testing involves the quantitative measurement of a chemical substance, or **analyte**, in the circulating blood and other body fluids. Common measurable blood constituents include glucose, hormones, drugs, and antibodies. The instruments are designed to perform single or multiple tests from a **microsample** (very small amount) of serum or plasma.

The menu of tests available in the POL may not be as varied as in a hospital or reference laboratory. Even so, the medical assistant must have an understanding of all types of chemistry tests that might be ordered for a patient. This knowledge will help the medical assistant better assist the patient and the physician. (See *Common blood chemistry tests.*)

Chemistry Analyzers
The types of chemistry analyzers used in the clinical laboratory have been adapted for the POL. However, they share

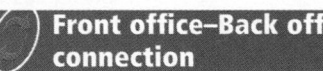
Front office–Back office connection

Know the Format
Many hospital and reference laboratories provide the physician's office with direct access to laboratory reports via faxes, printers, and, most recently, secure electronic transfer. The administrative medical assistant may be responsible for collecting and reviewing the reports prior to alerting the physician. The administrative medical assistant should familiarize herself with each laboratory's report format, knowing how results are arranged and identifying when a report has a critical or out-of-range (abnormal) value so that she can notify the physician immediately and facilitate proper patient care.

Common blood chemistry tests

The following table provides a list of common blood chemistry tests and their normal ranges.

Test	Normal Range
General Chemistry	
albumin	3.5 to 5.0 g/dl
alkaline phosphatase	31 to 97 units/L
alanine aminotransferase (ALT)*	10 to 40 units/L
aspartate aminotransferase (AST)†	10 to 37 units/L
ammonia	10 to 65 micromoles/L
amylase	25 to 125 units/L
bilirubin, total	0.1 to 1.0 mg/dl
blood urea nitrogen (BUN)	6 to 19 mg/dl
calcium (Ca)	8.4 to 10.2 mg/dl
cholesterol	< 200 mg/dl§
cortisol	6 to 23 mcg/dl
creatinine	0.5 to 1.4 mg/dl
creatine kinase (CK)	
• male	38 to 174 units/L
• Female	96 to 140 units/L
CK-MB	< 4.0 ng/ml
gamma-glutamyl transferase (GGT)	5 to 85 units/L
glucose (FBS)	70 to 110 mg/dl
glycosylated hemoglobin (Hgb A1C)	3.0% to 6.1%
iron (Fe)	35 to 150 µg/dl
lactate dehydrogenase (LD)‡	91 to 180 units/L
lipase	7 to 58 units/L
lithium	0.6 to 1.2 mmol/L

Test	Normal Range
General Chemistry	
magnesium	1.6 to 2.6 mg/dl
phosphorus	2.7 to 4.5 mg/dl
prostate-specific antigen (PSA)	0 to 4.0 ng/ml
total protein	6.0 to 8.3 g/dl
troponin I	< 1.0 ng/ml
uric acid	2.6 to 7.2 mg/dl
Electrolytes	
carbon dioxide (CO_2)	22.0 to 30.0 mmol/L
chloride (Cl–)	101 to 110 mmol/L
potassium (K+)	3.5 to 5.0 mmol/L
sodium (Na+)	135 to 145 mmol/L
Thyroid Panel	
thyroglobulin	0 to 56 mg/ml
thyroid stimulating hormone (TSH)	0.34 to 5.6 million International Units/ml
thyroxine (T_4)	6.1 to 12.2 ug/dl
triiodothyronine (T_3) uptake	32% to 48.4%

* Formerly known as *serum glutamic-pyruvic transaminase (SGPT)*.
† Formerly known as *serum glutamic-oxaloacetic transaminase (SGOT)*.
‡ Formerly known as *LDH*.
§Cholesterol results vary with age, gender, and testing facility.

the same **methodology**, or system of principles and procedures, used in scientific testing. Blood chemistry analyzers use photometric reflectance (measurement of the amount of light reflected by a specimen) or photometric absorbance (measurement of the amount of light absorbed by a specimen) for quantitative measurements of analytes in the blood. Many of these analyzers are waived by the Clinical Laboratory Improvement Amendment (CLIA).

The medical assistant should familiarize herself with all laboratory equipment and instruments before using them, including the chemistry analyzer. Before operating an analyzer, the medical assistant should read the instrument's operating manual provided by the manufacturer completely. Information found in the operating manual includes specimen collection and type, step-by-step operating instructions, quality control measures, troubleshooting information, and preventive maintenance measures. Some manufacturers provide customer support or a maintenance agreement if the analyzer malfunctions. The medical assistant may be able to call customer support and a technician may be able to run through a series of steps over the phone to fix the problem with the instrument.

Specimen Types

Depending on the chemistry analyzer and the analyte being tested in the medical office, proper specimen collection should be strictly followed in order to obtain the most accurate results. Some chemistry analyzers measure serum, plasma, and whole blood samples; others measure only serum or plasma. Occasionally, the POL cannot evaluate a specimen and must refer it to a reference laboratory. Such a referral might be necessary because the result was inconclusive or the specimen could not be tested on a POL instrument. In such cases, the medical assistant should refer to the manual provided to collect, store, and transport the appropriate specimen.

Common POL Chemistry Tests

Chemistry tests commonly performed in a POL include blood glucose and lipids testing.

Blood Glucose Testing

When carbohydrates are digested, simple sugars, such as glucose, are generated. The glucose travels from the bloodstream to provide energy to the body's cells and tissues. The body produces two hormones that aid in the regulation of blood glucose levels: insulin and glucagon. Glucagon converts the stored form of glucose (glycogen) into glucose when blood glucose levels become low. In contrast, the pancreas releases insulin to facilitate the transport of glucose from the bloodstream to the tissues and cells, thus lowering blood glucose levels.

Blood glucose is one of the most common tests performed in the chemistry department of the laboratory. It is used to detect abnormalities in carbohydrate metabolism. Several collection procedures are used to measure blood glucose, such as fasting blood glucose , 2-hour postprandial blood glucose (2° pp), and glucose tolerance tests (GTT), including a 3-hour GTT to diagnose diabetes mellitus and a 6-hour GTT to diagnose hypoglycemia.

Fasting Blood Glucose

Blood glucose is best measured when the patient has been fasting. The medical assistant should advise the patient undergoing a fasting blood glucose (FBG) test, formerly called *fasting blood sugar (FBS)test*, to refrain from eating or drinking anything (except water) for 12 hours before the test. Although the normal range for fasting blood glucose is 70 to 110 mg/dl, the range can vary depending on the specimen, methodology, and laboratory. If a patient's FBG is elevated and the patient has complied with pretesting instructions, the physician may order additional testing, such as a 2-hour postprandial test or a glucose tolerance test.

2-hour Postprandial

The 2-hour postprandial (2° pp) glucose test is used as a screening test for diabetes mellitus. The test measures the amount of blood glucose in the bloodstream 2 hours after a patient has ingested a meal. Ideally, blood glucose levels should return to fasting levels within 2 hours after a meal. The normal range for a 2° pp is less than 140 mg/dl. Results of 140 mg/dl or higher may indicate that the patient has diabetes mellitus. Sometimes a physician will order the 2° pp with the patient ingesting a controlled amount of glucose by drinking 100 g of Glucola. It is the medical assistant's responsibility to instruct the patient on the manner in which

the test will be performed. If the patient is to eat a meal and then report to the laboratory 2 hours later, the medical assistant should instruct the patient to eat at least 100 g of carbohydrates and arrive at the laboratory at the appropriate time. (See *100-gram meal.*)

Glucose Tolerance Test

If a patient's 2-hour postprandial results are inconclusive or above normal, the physician may order a 3-hour glucose tolerance test (GTT). The GTT assists in the diagnosis of diabetes mellitus. The test measures the body's ability to metabolize glucose using insulin in response to a glucose load. Ideally, after 3 hours, the patient's blood glucose levels should return to the normal fasting range.

A physician may order a 6-hour GTT if he suspects the patient has hypoglycemia. A hypoglycemic patient's fasting blood sugar dips below the normal 70 to 110 mg/dl. (Because some institutions may consider a range below 70 mg/dl as normal, the medical assistant should take care to check with the testing facility regarding its range of normal values.) The procedure is the same as the 3-hour GTT except the test lasts

---

📖 Patient Education

100-Gram Meal

Here are some examples of meals with 100 g of carbohydrates.

Breakfast
- 30 g of cereal
- 1 banana
- 200 ml of milk
- 500 ml of orange juice

OR

- 4 slices of toast
- 1 piece of fruit
- 6 to 8 oz of yogurt (that does not contain a sugar substitute)

Lunch
- 1 large baked potato
- 200 ml of fruit juice or milk
- 400 mg of rice or pasta

OR

- 300 g of homemade fruit salad
- 6 to 8 oz of yogurt (that does not contain a sugar substitute)
- 500 ml of fruit juice

for 6 hours in order to observe a below-normal fasting blood sugar.

Patient preparation is essential for a successful GTT. The medical assistant may be responsible for scheduling the test for the patient and should understand how the test is administered as well as the proper patient preparation in order to instruct the patient correctly. (See *Instructions for GTT*.) On the day of the test, the medical assistant must gather the equipment necessary to conduct a GTT, including the urine specimen containers, the glucose solution the patient will drink, the proper venipuncture tubes (usually gray-stoppered or SST tubes), a timer, and stickers to indicate specimen one, two, and three. (See Figure 43-1.)

Glucose Monitors

Medical assistants can provide better patient care if they use glucose monitors in the medical office. The benefits of testing in the office include ease, speed, and convenience for the patient. In addition, the physician is provided with immediate results that will aid in assessment and treatment of the patient.

There are many glucose monitoring systems available to patients and the POL. The latest monitors require fewer specimens, provide faster results, and can even generate a computer printout. The patient is able to monitor and document her levels and provide her physician with a history of her blood glucose results. Not only is the monitoring convenient but it also provides the patient with an immediate indication of her blood glucose level, which will allow her to know how much insulin she has to take. Several glucose monitoring systems, such as One Touch Ultra (Lifescan), are CLIA-approved and easy to use. (See Figure 43-2.)

In addition to testing the patient's blood glucose when she comes to the office, the medical assistant may be responsible for providing instructions to the patient on the use and maintenance of her personal glucose machine. (See *Procedure 43-1: Performing a blood glucose test and patient education*

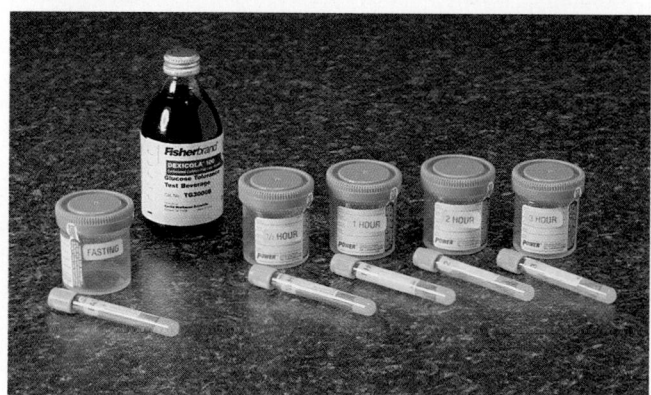

FIG 43-1 Supplies for glucose tolerance test.

> ### Patient Education
>
> #### Instructions for GTT
>
> When preparing a patient for a 3-hour glucose tolerance test (GTT), be sure to include these instructions:
>
> - The test is usually ordered for the early morning, such as 7 a.m.
> - The procedure takes approximately 4 hours. Make sure to arrive on time for the test so that the phlebotomist will have the opportunity to prepare for and begin the test before the laboratory becomes busy.
> - Fast for 12 hours.
> - Consume a high-carbohydrate diet 3 days prior to the examination, as ordered.
> - A fasting blood glucose test and a urine glucose test will be done before you ingest the glucose.
> - You must ingest a measured amount of liquid glucose within 5 minutes.
> - You will need to provide multiple blood and urine samples at specific times during the test. Time intervals include: 30 minutes, 1 hour, 2 hours, and 3 hours.
> - Bring a book to read or something else to keep busy during the examination because you may not be able to leave the laboratory.
> - You cannot eat or drink during the testing (although you may be encouraged to drink some water in order to provide the required urine samples).
> - You may experience minor symptoms, such as lightheadedness, dizziness, and nausea, during the examination.
> - It is important to follow instructions exactly, because the test may have to be repeated if you do not comply.

for a glucose monitoring system, page 908.) A patient who is newly diagnosed with diabetes may experience various emotions, including denial and anxiety. By explaining the purpose and process of using a glucose monitoring instrument, the medical assistant can help allay the patient's fears and empower the patient to take control of her treatment. (See *Glucose monitoring tips,* page 909.) The medical assistant may also want to discuss with the patient the implications of failing to follow the physician's advice or not complying with proper glucose monitoring.

The medical assistant should stress to the patient that, in addition to the daily glucose monitoring he performs, the physician may still require an FBG or a glycosylated hemoglobin test. Long-term blood glucose regulation, and thus

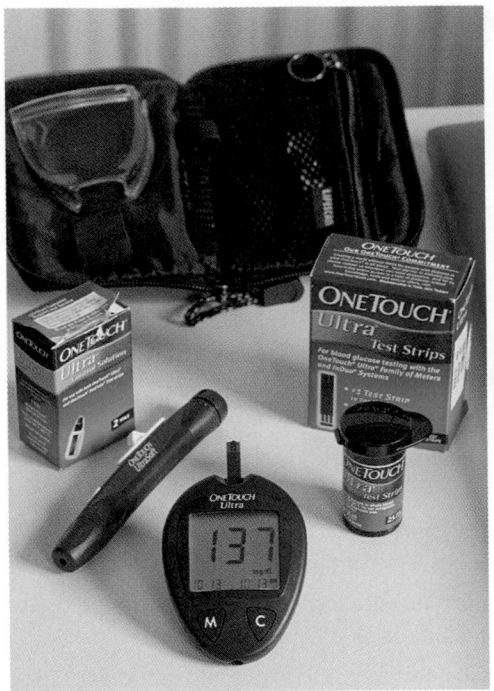

FIG 43-2 One Touch Ultra glucose monitoring system.

effectiveness of treatment and patient compliance, can be objectively assessed by determining a patient's glycosylated hemoglobin (Hgb A1c) levels. If a patient with diabetes mellitus has carefully regulated his blood glucose levels over a period of 5 or 6 weeks, his HgbA1c levels will be normal or just slightly above normal. If the patient has had uncontrolled levels during the same time period, his HgbA1c level will be elevated. For a patient who is not regulating his insulin properly, the physician may suggest an insulin pump. The medical assistant should understand how an insulin pump operates and provide patient teaching on its use. (See *Insulin pump,* page 910.)

Lipids

Lipids are fats or fatlike substances that are insoluble in water. They include fatty acids, waxes, and sterols. Lipids provide an alternative source of energy and, therefore, are essential to the body. Blood lipids that are responsible for cardiovascular disease are classified as *lipoproteins.* Lipoproteins are fats that are attached to proteins. Examples of blood lipids include cholesterol and triglycerides. Analysis of these levels in the bloodstream can provide information on a patient's risk of atherosclerosis and cardiovascular disease.

■ PROCEDURE 43-1

Performing a blood glucose test and patient education for a glucose monitoring system

Task
Properly perform a capillary puncture and glucose test and instruct the patient in the care and use of a glucose monitoring system.

Conditions
- Glucose monitoring system
- Gloves
- Alcohol wipe
- Gauze
- Lancet
- Adhesive bandage
- Test strips
- Glucose control
- Biohazard disposable container

Standards
In the time specified and within the scoring parameters determined by the instructor, the student will successfully perform a capillary puncture and glucose testing and instruct the patient in the care and use of a glucose monitoring system.

Performance Standards
1. Wash or sanitize your hands and assemble the supplies.
2. Put on gloves.
3. Identify the patient and explain the procedure.
4. Perform quality control measures, including:
   a. Turn the meter on.
   b. Check the code number on the display with the code number on the test strip package, making sure they match or inaccurate results may occur.
   c. Insert the test strip when prompted.
   d. When APPLY SAMPLE appears, apply one drop of quality control reagent.
   e. Read the meter for results.
   f. Check the results against the proper control range, as set by the manufacturer. Quality control results must be in the proper range before patient testing can occur.
   g. Repeat the process if necessary using additional control reagents, such as high or low values.

PROCEDURE 43-1—cont'd

h. Record the results. If you do not document quality control results, there is no proof that you performed them. Notify the instructor if controls are out of range. If quality control results are out of range, you must take corrective action before conducting patient testing.

5. Instruct the patient on how to operate the glucose monitoring system, Topics should include:

    a. Turning on the monitor

    b. Display area

    c. Proper code reading

    d. Proper testing strips

    e. Proper cleaning and care.

6. Perform patient testing, including:

    a. Press the ON–OFF button.

    b. Insert the test strip.

    c. Prepare the patient for capillary puncture.

    d. Perform the puncture and wipe away the first drop of blood to ensure that the testing drop does not include tissue fluid, which may alter the results. Then apply one drop of blood to the test strip without touching the test strip or smearing the blood to avoid altering test results.

    e. Bandage the patient's finger.

    f. Read the results after hearing the beep.

    g. Correctly record the results in the patient's chart because proper documentation is key to patient care.

    h. Discuss with the patient the physician's orders and any necessary follow-up visits to ensure patient compliance and follow-up.

    i. Remove the test strip and discard all biohazard material in the appropriate container.

Date	
05/26/08: 9:45 a.m.	*Provided patient with proper care and operation of glucose monitoring system. Performed FBG. FBG: 86 mg/dl. ——————————————————————— S. Gonzales, CMA*

Patient Education

Glucose Monitoring Tips

Here are some tips for the medical assistant to follow when educating patients about glucose monitoring. The medical assistant should:

- have the patient bring in his own monitor, along with the test strips and operating instructions, if possible

- read the operating manual before testing if she is unfamiliar with the patient's monitor

- show the patient how to turn on the monitor

- explain how the test strip code must correlate with the code in the monitor and, if the code is different, show the patient how to change the code

- explain to the patient the importance of running a high, low, and normal control prior to testing his own blood

- show the patient how to use the automatic puncture device

- show the various acceptable puncture sites

- have the patient perform his own puncture and apply the sample to the test strip

- have the patient read and record his results

- tell the patient that, if he is on insulin, he may also need to record the time of his meals, keep a diary of food eaten, the times and dosages of insulin, and any exercise undertaken

- show the patient how to use the memory function to retrieve past results

- have the patient read troubleshooting and maintenance procedures as described in the operating manual

- allow the patient time for questions.

Cholesterol

Cholesterol is the main lipid associated with atherosclerotic vascular disease. **Atherosclerosis** is the general term used to describe thickening and hardening of the walls of the arteries. It is synthesized in the liver and a normal constituent of bile. Cholesterol is also important in metabolism and responsible for the production of steroid hormones. Cholesterol testing is an important tool in helping to identify patients who are at risk for heart disease and is just one component of the lipid panel. A *panel*, sometimes called a *profile*, is a group of blood tests that evaluates the function of

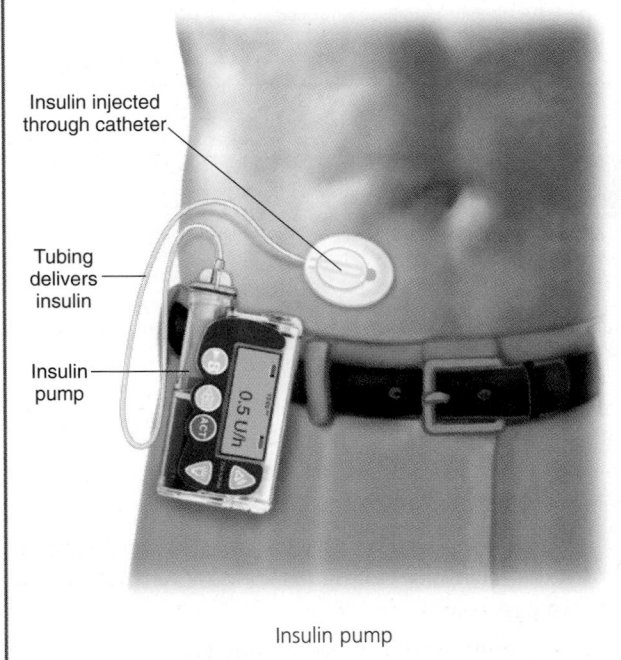
a particular body system. The lipid panel evaluates the health of a patient's arteries.

HDL and LDL Cholesterol

There are two types of lipoproteins that contain cholesterol:

• low-density lipoprotein (LDL)
• high-density lipoprotein (HDL).

HDL, commonly called the "good" cholesterol, removes excess cholesterol from cells and carries it to the liver for excretion. A high HDL cholesterol level shows a reduced risk of heart disease, whereas a low level of HDL cholesterol (less than 35 mg/dl) is a risk factor for coronary artery disease (CAD).

LDL is referred to as the "bad" cholesterol because, in excessive amounts, it can cause plaque to build up in arterial walls. The ingestion of saturated and trans fats can cause LDL levels to increase. A third type of lipoprotein, called *very-low-density lipoprotein (VLDL),* is composed mostly of cholesterol with little protein. VLDL is also known as "bad" cholesterol because, like LDL, it deposits cholesterol on the walls of arteries. Increased levels of VLDL are associated with atherosclerosis and CAD.

Lipid Panel

One of the most commonly performed chemistry tests in the POL is the lipid panel. It is very easy to perform, uses a small amount of blood, and provides the physician with an immediate indication of the patient's coronary artery health.

The lipid panel includes tests of:

• total cholesterol (TC)
• HDL
• LDL
• VLDL
• triglycerides
• TC-to-HDL ratio. (See *Normal ranges for the lipid panel.*)

A commonly used chemistry analyzer in the POL is the Cholestech LDX. (See Figure 43-3.) The Cholestech can provide cholesterol results or perform an entire lipid panel. Newer versions of the analyzer can also perform blood glucose testing. In the POL, the medical assistant may be responsible for the proper maintenance, quality control, and operation of the analyzer. (See *Procedure 43-2: Performing cholesterol or lipid panel testing.*)

Normal ranges for the lipid panel

The table lists the tests included in a lipid panel and the normal ranges for each.

Test	Normal Range
Total cholesterol	< 200 mg/dl
High-density lipoprotein (HDL)	35 to 60 mg/dl
Low-density lipoprotein (LDL)	< 130 mg/dl
Very low-density lipoprotein (VLDL)	20 to 40 mg/dl
Triglycerides	35 to 160 mg/dl

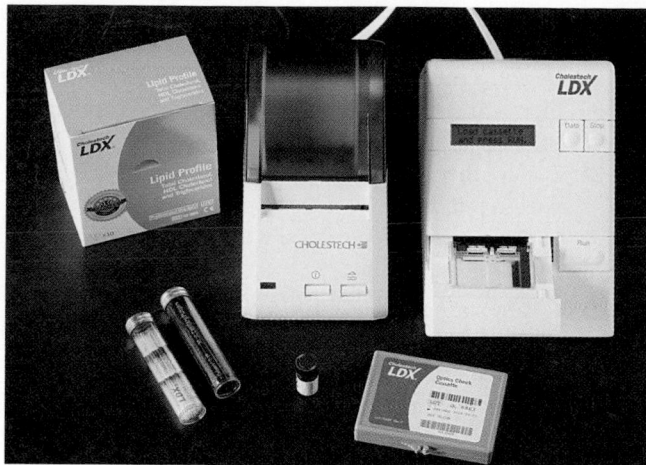

FIG 43-3 Cholestech LDX instrument.

Interpretation of CAD risk

Several factors affect coronary artery disease (CAD), including hypertension, smoking, diabetes, severe obesity, and premature CAD. However, determining CAD risk is done by comparing the total cholesterol (TC) level to the high-density lipoprotein (HDL) level, or the *TC-to-HDL ratio*. The table shows the TC-to-HDL ratio for men and women.

Risk	Ratio	
	Men	*Women*
Half the average risk	3.4	3.3
Average risk	5.0	4.4
Two times the average risk	9.6	7.1
Three times the average risk	23.4	11.0

Patient Preparation

Some physicians prefer the patient to be in a fasting state for any testing. Although total cholesterol and HDL cholesterol determination are not affected significantly by food consumption, triglyceride levels are affected. Therefore, if a physician orders a lipid panel, the medical assistant should instruct the patient to fast.

Interpretation of Results

Cholesterol values vary with gender, age, and the testing facility. Cholesterol levels under 200 mg/dl for adult and elderly patients are desirable. Levels between 200 mg/dl and 239 mg/dl are considered borderline high, and levels of 240 mg/dl and above are high. HDL levels above 60 mg/dl are considered optimal and levels below 35 mg/dl constitute a risk factor for CAD. (See *Interpretation of CAD risk.*)

Other Chemistry Department Tests

Although there are many chemistry tests that may not be performed in a POL, a medical assistant may be involved with processing blood specimens for such testing or reading the final laboratory results received by the office. The medical assistant should familiarize herself with the most common chemistry tests and panels in order to facilitate better patient care. Some of these tests include:

- *renal panel,* which assesses kidney function and includes tests for albumin, calcium, carbon dioxide (CO_2), chloride, creatinine, glucose, phosphorous, potassium, sodium, and blood urea nitrogen (BUN)
- *electrolyte panel,* which assesses acid–base balance and, possibly, hydration status and includes tests for sodium, potassium, CO_2, and chloride

---

PROCEDURE 43-2

Performing cholesterol or lipid panel testing

Task

Perform cholesterol or lipid panel testing using a CLIA-waived instrument.

Conditions

- Cholesterol instrument
- Gloves
- Alcohol wipe
- Gauze
- Lancet
- Capillary tubes and other supplies as required by manufacturer

- Adhesive bandage
- Test strips
- Control reagents
- Calibration cassette
- Biohazard disposable container

Standards

In the time specified and within the scoring parameters determined by the instructor, the student will successfully perform cholesterol or lipid panel testing.

Continued

PROCEDURE 43-2—cont'd

Performance Standards

1. Wash or sanitize your hands and assemble supplies.
2. Put on gloves.
3. Identify the patient to ensure accurate results and explain the procedure.
4. Perform quality control measures, including:
   a. Turn the instrument on, and watch as it performs a self-test.
   b. Remove the cassette from the pouch without touching the black bar or magnetic strip because touching the magnetic strip may interfere with test results. Place the cassette on a flat surface.
   c. Apply a quality control reagent to the well of the cassette. Place the cassette in the drawer and press the RUN button.
   d. Read the results after you hear the beep.
   e. Check the results against the control range, as set by the manufacturer. Quality control results must be in the proper range before any patient testing can occur.
   f. Repeat the process if necessary using additional control reagents, such as high or low values.
   g. Record the results because if quality control results are not documented, there is no proof that they were ever performed. Notify the instructor if a control is out of range. If quality control results are out of range, corrective action must take place prior to any patient testing.
5. Perform patient testing steps, including:
   a. Prepare the patient for capillary puncture.
   b. Remove the cassette from the pouch without touching the black bar or magnetic strip. Place the cassette on a flat surface.

   c. Perform the puncture, wipe away the first drop of blood, and then collect the blood in the capillary tube.
   d. Apply the sample to the well of the cassette within 5 minutes of collection because blood may coagulate after 5 minutes, which could cause erroneous test results.
   e. Place the cassette in the drawer and press the RUN button.
   f. Bandage the patient's finger.
   g. Read the results after hearing the beep.
   h. Record the results in the patient's chart because proper documentation is key to patient care.

Date	
12/20/08: 8:45 a.m.	*Capillary blood tested via Cholestech. Results: 256 mg/dl. Physician referred patient for further laboratory studies.* -- *S. Gonzales, CMA*

   i. Talk to the patient about the physician's orders and follow-up. Communication with the patient is vital to patient compliance and follow-up.
   j. Remove the test strip and discard all biohazard material appropriately.
   k. Remove the results and wash your hands.

- *basic metabolic panel*, which assesses electrolytes, glucose, and kidney function and includes tests for calcium, CO_2, chloride, creatinine, glucose, potassium, sodium, and BUN
- *comprehensive metabolic panel*, which assesses various body systems and organs and includes tests for albumin, total bilirubin, calcium, bicarbonate, chloride, creatinine, glucose, alkaline phosphatase, potassium, total protein, sodium, BUN, alanine aminotransferase (ALT), and aspartate aminotransferase (AST)
- *hepatic panel*, which assesses liver function and includes tests for ALT, AST, lactate dehydrogenase (LD), gamma-glutamyl transferase (GGT), bilirubin, and alkaline phosphatase

- *thyroid panel*, which assesses thyroid function and includes tests for triiodothyronine (T_3), thyroxine (T_4), thyroid stimulating hormone (TSH), and thyroglobulin
- *cardiac panel*, which aids in the diagnosis of myocardial infarction and includes tests for creatine kinase (CK), CK-MB, and troponin.

Diseases Associated with Chemistry Tests

The medical assistant will see patients with many different diseases and conditions. Understanding these conditions will allow the medical assistant to better relate the tests used to diagnose and treat such conditions. Here are some common diseases that are diagnosed using chemistry tests:

- *diabetes mellitus,* which is a chronic disorder of carbohydrate metabolism in which there is an inadequate production or use of insulin and demonstrates such symptoms as excessive thirst, excessive urine production, dizziness, loss of coordination, and sweet-smelling breath
- *hypoglycemia,* which is an abnormal decrease in blood glucose levels and demonstrates such symptoms as lightheadedness, dizziness, fatigue, and fainting
- *hyperlipedemia,* which is an excessive amount of fat in the blood, giving the serum a milky appearance but otherwise is usually asymptomatic
- *hyperthyroidism,* which is characterized by increased triiodothyronine (T_3) and thyroxine (T_4) levels with a possibly normal, increased, or decreased thyroid stimulating hormone (TSH) level and demonstrates such symptoms as palpitations, heat intolerance, nervousness, insomnia, fatigue, weight loss, and hair loss
- *hypothyroidism,* which is characterized by decreased T_3 and T_4 levels with usually increased TSH levels and demonstrates such symptoms as fatigue, weakness, hair loss, dry skin, constipation, intolerance to cold, and irritability.

Serology

Serology is defined as the study of the serum of the blood. Serology testing deals with the study of antigen and antibody reactions. **Antigens** are substances that are perceived by the body as foreign and are capable of stimulating the production of antibodies. **Antibodies** are formed from B lymphocytes as a response to the foreign substance (antigen) invading the body. An antigen–antibody reaction is formed when the protective antibody seeks out, attacks, and combines with the antigen to destroy it. The medical assistant needs a basic knowledge of the antibody–antigen reaction to understand the serological methodologies of many tests performed in the POL.

Antibody–Antigen Reactions

An antigen–antibody reaction can be simulated in the laboratory and thus aid in the diagnosis of certain diseases and conditions. The various methods used in testing include agglutination and enzyme-linked immunosorbent assay. (See Figure 43-4.)

Agglutination

The **agglutination** method of testing consists of an antibody–antigen reaction in which a solid antigen clumps with a soluble antibody. The most common type of agglutination testing consists of mixing a patient's serum with a

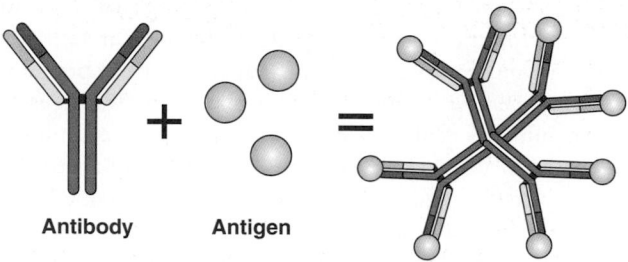

Antibody **Antigen**

Antibody-antigen complex

FIG 43-4 Antibody-antigen reaction.

known antigen coated with latex particles. If the suspected antibody is present in the patient's serum, it will react with the antigen-coated latex and, upon mixing, will cause a visual clumping reaction. Conversely, if an antigen is suspected in a patient's serum, then the specimen would be tested against a known latex-coated antibody. Certain test kits for mononucleosis and rheumatoid arthritis utilize the agglutination method. The advantages of agglutination tests are that they can be performed quickly, are easy to read, and usually contain a positive and negative control for quality control purposes. (See Figure 43-5.)

ELISA

Many CLIA-waived test kits incorporate the enzyme-linked immunosorbent assay (ELISA) method of antibody

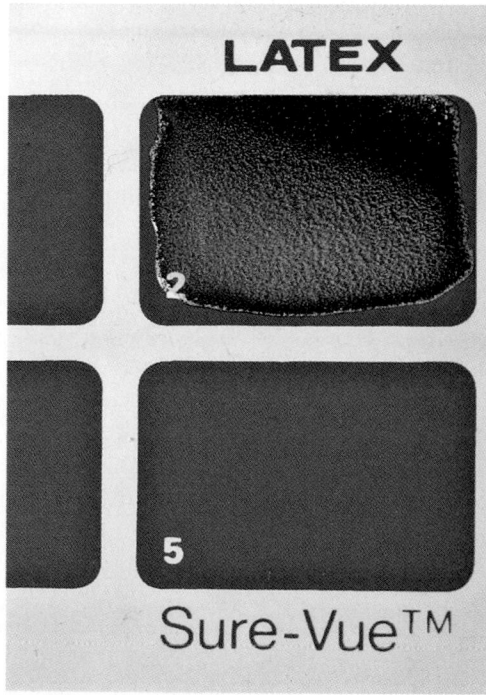

FIG 43-5 Agglutination reaction.

or antigen detection. A manufacturer develops a test kit to identify a specific analyte in a patient's blood—an antibody or an antigen. For example, a kit that tests for the presence of the *Streptococcus* antigen in a throat specimen would use a known antibody to the *Streptococcus* organism. The antibody couples with an enzyme as a result of the manufacturing process or during the course of the test. The enzyme helps accelerate the antibody–antigen reaction. When the antibody, enzyme, and patient specimen containing the *Streptococcus* antigen combine and react, the reaction that is created causes a color change in the testing well. The HIV test and the rapid *Streptococcus* test both incorporate the ELISA method. (See Figure 43-6.)

Blood Groups and Typing

There are four principal blood types, or *groups*, that a person can possess: A, B, AB, or O. A person's blood type is based on the antigen that is present on the surface of her red blood cells (RBCs). In addition, that person has a noncorresponding antibody in her serum. (See *Blood type, antigens, and antibodie*.) Knowing a patient's blood type is the first step when that patient needs a blood transfusion. Administering the wrong type of blood could cause a life-threatening reaction. (See Figure 43-7.)

Another antigen, known as *Rh factor*, may also be present on a person's RBCs. People whose red blood cells contain Rh factor are known as Rh-positive (Rh+). Conversely, if people do not have the Rh factor antigen, they are considered Rh-negative (Rh−). Although it is important for a

Blood type, antigens, and antibodies

The following chart lists the ABO blood types with their associated antigens on the red blood cells and antibodies circulating in the serum.

Blood Type	Antigen	Antibody
A	A	B
B	B	A
AB	A and B	None
O	None	A and B

person to know her ABO type, it is equally important, especially for a woman, to know her Rh type as well. (See *Rh incompatibility*.)

Medical assistants do not typically perform blood typing in the POL. However, it is important for medical assistants to understand the procedure and how it works. A simple blood typing procedure involves a capillary puncture to obtain a few drops of blood. The examiner mixes one drop of blood with a commercially prepared anti-serum A and another drop with anti-serum B. Then the examiner observes both mixtures for agglutination. If a patient's blood agglutinates with anti-serum A and not with anti-serum B, the patient's blood type is A. Conversely, if the patient's blood agglutinates with anti-serum B and not with anti-serum A, then her blood type is B. A patient whose blood does not agglutinate with either anti-sera has blood type O. To determine a person's Rh status, a drop of the person's blood is mixed with the known anti-serum D (the name given to the commercially prepared Rh anti-serum). If the patient's blood agglutinates with anti-serum D, then the person is considered Rh+. For example, if a person's blood agglutinates with the anti-serum A and anti-serum D, that person's blood type is A+.

While simple blood typing is common in the POL, a hospital laboratory would conduct a more complex procedure. Traditionally, hospital laboratories use serum for blood typing and screening procedures. However, use of plasma has become more common. Medical assistants who may work as hospital phlebotomists should become familiar with the facility's blood bank specimen collection policies and procedures.

Common POL Serological Tests

There are a variety of serological tests that can be performed in the POL. Most are CLIA-waived and can be performed by the medical assistant. Some serological tests, such as syphilis

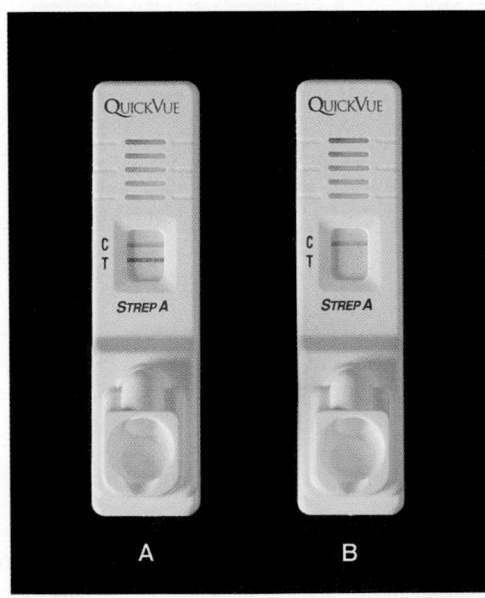

FIG 43-6 QuickVue In-Line *Strep* test using the ELISA serological method. (A) Positive. (B) Negative.

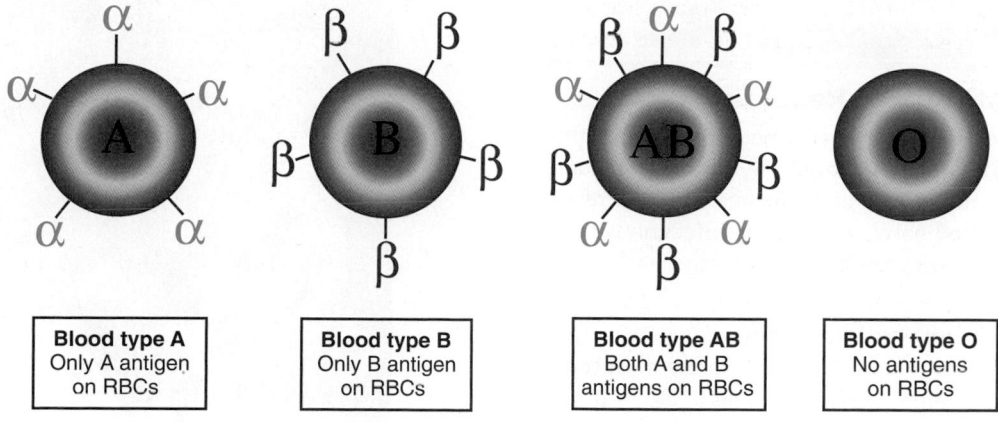

Blood type A
Only A antigen
on RBCs

Blood type B
Only B antigen
on RBCs

Blood type AB
Both A and B
antigens on RBCs

Blood type O
No antigens
on RBCs

FIG 43-7 Red blood cell antigens.

Rh incompatibility

If a pregnant woman's blood type is Rh-negative and the baby she is carrying happens to be Rh-positive, then the condition of Rh incompatibility could occur. In Rh incompatibility, when the baby's blood mixes with the mother's blood during delivery, the mother's body recognizes the Rh protein as a foreign substance and begins producing antibodies (protein molecules in the immune system that recognize and, later, work to destroy foreign substances) against the Rh proteins introduced into her blood. These antibodies that the mother produces are not harmful to her; however, they may be harmful to her fetus during a subsequent pregnancy.

If, during the next pregnancy, the mother is carrying an Rh-positive baby, her Rh antibodies will attack the Rh antigen that is on the baby's red blood cells (RBCs). The baby's RBCs will undergo lysis (destruction), a disorder called *hemolytic disease of the newborn (HDN)*.

A physician can prevent HDN by testing a pregnant woman's blood for type and Rh factor. If the woman is Rh-negative, the physician can administer a series of two Rh immune-globulin (RhoGAM) shots to the woman at 28 weeks' gestation and then again within 72 hours after giving birth. The RhoGAM prevents the mother's antibodies from attacking the baby's RBCs if the baby is Rh-positive. A woman who has experienced a miscarriage, abortion, or blood transfusion may also receive RhoGAM because those events put the woman at risk for having been exposed to the Rh-positive antigens from a fetus or blood transfusion.

testing, should not be performed in the physician's office. However, the medical assistant should understand the test and its results. (See *Syphilis testing and reporting*, page 916.)

Mononucleosis Testing

Mononucleosis (typically referred to as *mono*) is an acute infectious disease commonly seen in children and young adults. It is caused by the Epstein-Barr virus (EBV) and causes such symptoms as a sore throat, fatigue, lymphadenopathy, and splenomegaly. A physician who suspects that a patient has mononucleosis will order a test for mononucleosis, called a *mono test*, as well as other clinical tests, including a complete blood count (CBC) and liver enzymes. (See Figure 43-8.) Most mononucleosis tests do not specifically look for EBV, but instead test for heterophile antibodies, which are sometimes present when a patient is acutely infected with EBV. (See *Procedure 43-3: Performing a CLIA-waived mono test*, page 916.)

Rheumatoid Factor

Rheumatoid arthritis (RA) is a chronic inflammatory disease that usually affects the connective tissue or joints of the body. Symptoms of rheumatoid arthritis include joint stiffness and pain, swelling, and difficulty moving. Patients with RA develop an antibody called *rheumatoid factor*. Rheumatoid factor can be detected in a patient's serum during serological testing. (See Figure 43-9.)

HIV Testing

Human immunodeficiency virus (HIV) causes acquired immune deficiency syndrome (AIDS). Early HIV detection helps the physician choose the best course of treatment to delay the rate at which HIV weakens the immune system. Some early symptoms of HIV infection include fatigue,

Front office–Back office connection

Syphilis Testing and Reporting

Syphilis is a sexually transmitted disease caused by the bacterium *Treponema pallidum.* Symptoms include headache, fever, fatigue, and a chancre at the site of infection. If detected early enough, the infection can be successfully treated with antibiotics.

Syphilis testing

The Venereal Disease Research Laboratory (VDRL) test and the rapid plasma reagin (RPR) test are the most common serological screening tests for syphilis. If either test is positive, then the microhemagglutination–*Treponema pallidum* (MHA-TP) test is performed to confirm the diagnosis of syphilis.

Reporting results and confidentiality

Regardless of where screening tests are performed, the medical assistant must keep positive results confidential. When an office receives positive results for certain tests, such as human immunodeficiency virus or syphilis, the medical office must send a report to the local and state Departments of Public Health. It may be the responsibility of the administrative medical assistant to notice such results and to collaborate with the clinical medical assistant in order to complete and submit the required form to the proper agency. It is a good idea to have the phone numbers for the local and state Department of Public Health at hand for easy reference.

Usually, the physician will want to meet with the patient to review the results and gather information on the patient's sexual history and other pertinent information in order to complete the required forms. When the medical assistant calls the patient to come in for an appointment, she must make sure not to leave any information regarding the results of the tests on the patient's answering machine.

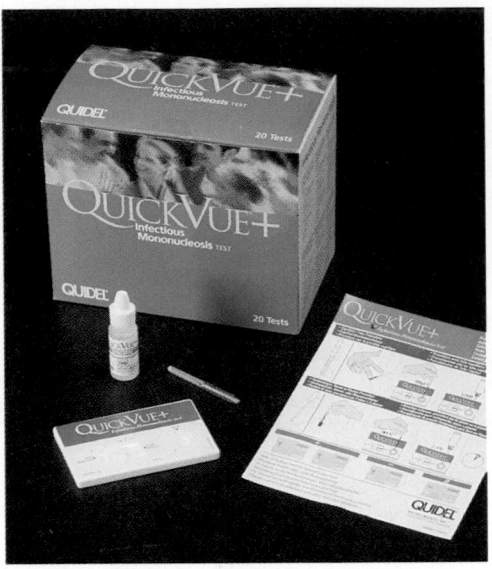

FIG 43-8 QuickVue+ mono test kit.

weight loss, fever, malaise, and lymphadenopathy. The ELISA method is widely used by clinical laboratories for initial testing for HIV infection. If the test indicates HIV antibodies are present in a patient's serum, the Western blot assay test confirms those results. HIV tests that actually detect the presence of the virus and not the antibody are becoming more common and provide earlier detection of infection. Although typical POLs do not perform the more advanced tests, CLIA-waived HIV tests are available for use in the POL and test for the presence of HIV antibodies in blood or oral specimens. (See Figure 43-10.)

PROCEDURE 43-3

Performing a CLIA-waived mono test

Task
Perform a CLIA-waived mono test.

Conditions
- CLIA-waived mono test kit
- Gloves
- Lancet
- Alcohol wipe
- Gauze
- Adhesive bandage
- Biohazard waste container

Standards
In the time specified and within the scoring parameters determined by the instructor, the student will successfully perform a mono test using a capillary blood specimen.

PROCEDURE 43-3—cont'd

Performance Standards

1. Assemble supplies and prepare the testing cassette (commonly referred to as a *reaction unit*). Refer to the manufacturer's test procedure directions to familiarize yourself with the proper procedure.

2. Run quality control (QC) according to the manufacturer's specifications before testing the patient specimen. Record the results on the proper QC chart. Quality control results must be within limits and properly documented or the patient specimen cannot be tested.

3. Greet and identify your patient. Introduce yourself and explain the procedure to prevent errors and ease patient anxiety.

4. Wash or sanitize your hands and apply gloves to ensure infection control.

5. Collect capillary blood from the patient's ring or middle finger using the collection capillary tube supplied by the manufacturer.

6. Dispense the patient's blood sample to the ADD well of the testing cassette.

7. According to the manufacturer's instructions, add the proper number of drops of developer to the ADD well to avoid adding the incorrect amount and rendering the results invalid.

8. Wait 5 minutes (or the amount of time specified by instructions). Underestimating or overestimating the reaction time can render the patient results invalid.

9. Read the test results in the TEST COMPLETE or RESULTS window. Refer to the manufacturer's instructions about reading the results.

10. Properly dispose of all supplies and wash your hands to ensure infection control.

11. Chart the procedure to ensure the accuracy of the medical record.

Date	
06/11/08: 9:35 a.m.	Mono Test performed, results: negative ——————————— ———————————————— S. Gonzales, CMA

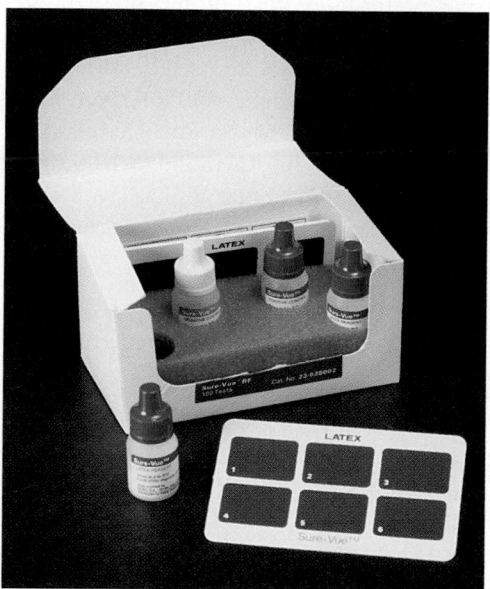

FIG 43-9 Typical CLIA-waived test kit for rheumatoid factor.

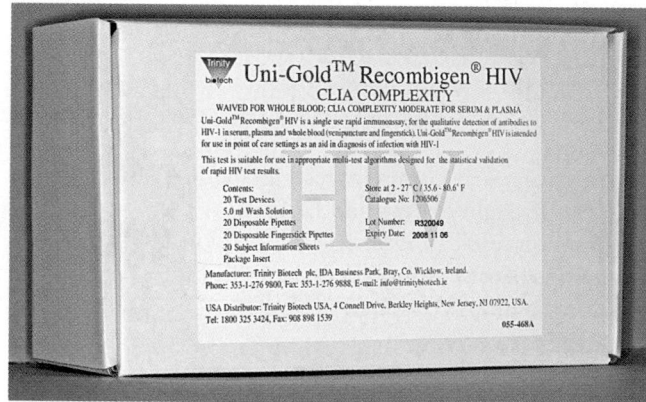

FIG 43-10 CLIA-waived HIV test kit.

Chapter Summary

- The clinical chemistry department in a hospital or reference laboratory is highly automated and performs a large inventory of tests.
- Most chemistry tests require a serum specimen, but some POL testing uses plasma.
- Medical assistants must be aware of normal ranges for each chemistry test result.
- The most common chemistry tests performed in a POL include glucose, cholesterol, and lipid panel.
- Medical assistants often provide patient education and instructions for proper blood glucose monitoring.
- Increased lipids are a common factor in cardiovascular disease.
- Panels associated with the chemistry department include:

  - renal panel
  - electrolyte panel
  - basic and comprehensive metabolic panels
  - hepatic panel
  - thyroid panel
  - cardiac panel.

- Some diseases associated with chemistry tests include:

  - diabetes mellitus
  - hypoglycemia
  - hyperlipidemia
  - hyperthyroidism
  - hypothyroidism.

- *Serology* is the study of serum.
- Antibodies and antigens are key components in serology testing.
- The two most common testing methodologies in the POL are agglutination and ELISA.
- Common serological tests performed in the POL include mononucleosis testing, rheumatoid factor testing, syphilis testing, and HIV testing.

Team Work Exercises

1. Divide into groups of 2 to 3 students. Your instructor will provide each group with one of the following blood glucose tests:
   a. FBG
   b. 1-hour postprandial
   c. 2-hour postprandial
   d. 3-hour postprandial
   e. 5-hour postprandial

Each team will research its assigned test and provide the following information in report format:
   a. reason for test
   b. patient education and preparation
   c. supplies required for testing
   d. normal and abnormal test results.
The instructor may have each group discuss its results with the rest of the class.

2. This chapter discusses the two most common serological testing methods used in the POL. There are various other testing methods used in the clinical laboratory:
   a. agglutination
   b. ELISA
   c. Western blot
   d. complement fixation
   e. agar gel immunodiffusion test.
Divide into groups of 2 to 3 students and research the serological method assigned to you by your instructor and provide the following information to the class:
   a. description of the method
   b. difficulty of performance (including length of time, elaborate equipment, and training)
   c. uses of the method (such as specific condition or disease identified with this method).

Case Studies

1. Stephanie performs a lipid profile on Mr. Dean. As required, the patient fasted for 12 hours. Mr. Dean's results are: total cholesterol, 185; triglycerides, 210; LDL, 80; HDL, 60. How would you interpret Mr. Dean's results? Are they normal or abnormal? Explain.
2. Dr. Burgess examines Jill Raymond, a 16-year-old high school student. She notes that Jill has swollen glands in her neck and splenomegaly. Which tests would you expect Dr. Burgess to order for Jill?

Resources

- Brassington, C., and Goretti, C.: *MA Notes: Medical Assistant's Pocket Guide.* Philadelphia: F.A. Davis, 2006.
- Sacher, R.A., and McPherson, R.A.: *Widmann's Clinical Interpretation of Laboratory Tests,* 11th ed. Philadelphia: F.A. Davis, 2000.
- American Society for Clinical Pathology: *www.ascp.org*
- Laboratory Corporation of America: *www.labcorp.com*
- Overview of CLIA: *www.cms.hhs.gov/clia*
- Public resource for clinical laboratory testing: *www.labtestsonline.org*

Urinalysis

Learning Objectives

Upon completion of this chapter, the student will be able to:

- define the key terms in the glossary
- understand the basic structures of the urinary system
- describe the importance of urinalysis
- explain the importance of medical terms related to the urinary system
- explain the importance of the different methods of urine collection
- explain and educate the patient in the proper method of urine collection
- identify the various tests that are included in the physical and chemical examination of urine
- explain the basis for urine pregnancy testing
- recognize the various structures or elements that may be found in normal and abnormal urine under the microscope.

CAAHEP Competencies

Clinical Competencies

Specimen Collection
Instruct patients in the collection of a clean-catch, midstream urine specimen

Diagnostic Testing
CLIA-waived tests
Perform urinalysis

General Competencies

Operational Functions
Use methods of quality control

ABHES Competencies

Clinical Duties
Use quality control
Instruct patients in the collection of a clean-catch midstream urine specimen
Perform urinalysis
Collect and process specimens

Procedures

Instructing the patient on collecting a clean-catch, midstream urine specimen
Performing a urinalysis
Performing a urine pregnancy test

Chapter Outline

Urinalysis in the POL

Urinalysis is the testing of a urine specimen. It is one of the most common tests performed in the physician's office laboratory (POL). Urinalysis can tell a lot about the patient's metabolism and overall health as well as diagnose conditions of the urinary system.

The medical assistant must know the structures and functions of the urinary system as well as proper collection, storage, and testing procedures in order to provide quality urine specimens. As with many procedures, proper patient education is an essential component in urinalysis to ensure accurate results.

Urinary System Overview

The urinary system regulates fluid, electrolyte, and acid-base balance and removes unwanted waste products. (See *Urinary system structures and functions*.) The structures of the urinary system include the kidneys, ureters, urinary bladder, and urethra. (For a more in-depth explanation of the anatomy and physiology of the urinary system, see Chapter 31, "Urology and the Male Reproductive System," page 567.)

Characteristics of Urine

Urine is a liquid excreted by the kidneys, stored in the bladder, and expelled by the urethra. It is mainly composed of 95% water. The other 5% is made up of organic and inorganic waste products. The organic substances include ammonia, urea, uric acid, creatine, and creatinine. Inorganic waste products include calcium, phosphorus, and magnesium. Urine is considered a sterile fluid when it is in the body and remains sterile if collected via a catheter or aspiration. When urine is discharged during normal urination, it may become contaminated from microorganisms inside or outside the urethra.

The typical healthy adult will produce approximately 1000 to 1500 ml of urine per day. However, various factors can affect urine production or output:

- **anuria**, the absence of urine production, can be caused by uremia, nephritis, or obstruction
- **dysuria**, the condition of difficult or painful urination, can be caused by cystitis, urinary tract infection (UTI), urethritis, or enlarged prostate
- **nocturia**, the condition of excessive urination during the night
- **oliguria**, a decrease in the amount of urine formation, can be caused by decreased fluid intake, vomiting, diarrhea, and dehydration

Urinary system structures and functions

This table lists the components of the urinary system along with a description and the functions for each.

Structure	Description	Function
Kidneys	Paired, kidney-bean shaped organs located in the back of the peritoneal cavity	• Filter waste materials from the blood • Regulate water, electrolyte, and acid-base content of the blood • Excrete urine
Ureters	Consist of two narrow tubes located behind the peritoneum	• Carry urine from the kidneys to the urinary bladder
Urinary bladder	Muscular, membranous organ that rests on the anterior part of the pelvic floor	• Receptacle for urine • Receives urine from the kidneys via the ureters and discharges urine from the body through the urethra
Urethra	Tube that extends from the bladder to the exterior of the body	• Discharges urine from the bladder to outside the body

- *polyuria*, an increase in the amount of urine formation and excretion, can be caused by diabetes mellitus, diabetes insipidus, increased fluid intake, and diuretics, such as caffeine and digoxin.

Collecting a Urine Specimen

The medical assistant should be sure to obtain a urine specimen properly so that it is the true representation of the patient's metabolic state. When collecting a specimen, the medical assistant should consider certain aspects, including the time and method of collection and the patient's medication and diet.

Urine Specimen Types

The medical assistant may collect many types of urine specimens from a patient. The type of specimen collected will depend on the test ordered:

- *Random* urine testing yields the most common type of specimen collected in the medical office. This test is used for routine urinalysis screening. It is not recommended for urine culture.
- *First morning* urine testing yields the most concentrated type of specimen and is best for pregnancy testing and routine urinalysis because it increases the chances of the detection of abnormal results.
- *Clean-catch, midstream (CCMS)* urine testing, also known as *clean voided midstream* testing, yields a common type of

specimen for urine culture and detection of UTIs via routine urinalysis. The medical assistant should ensure strict adherence to the proper collection procedure to reduce false-positive results.

- *24-hour* urine testing is used for quantitative chemical analysis. A special collection container is required and the medical assistant may need to add a preservative to the container prior to specimen collection.
- *Catheterized* testing yields the best specimen for urine culture. It may also be used for cytological testing. The medical assistant must follow aseptic technique to ensure the integrity of the specimen. (See Figure 44-1.)
- *Suprapubic aspirate* testing involves collecting aspirate from the urinary bladder by introducing a syringe directly into the bladder to withdraw urine. This test is sometimes performed on pediatric patients. This tests yields a sterile specimen for urine culture.

Collection Procedure

The clinical medical assistant is usually responsible for providing urine specimen collection instructions to the patient as well as handling and processing the specimen. (See *Urine specimens in the front office*, page 922.) When collecting a urine specimen in the office, the following guidelines should be followed. The medical assistant should:

- Make sure that specimen is correctly labeled with the patient's name, collection date and time, and the type of specimen collected, being sure to place the label on the

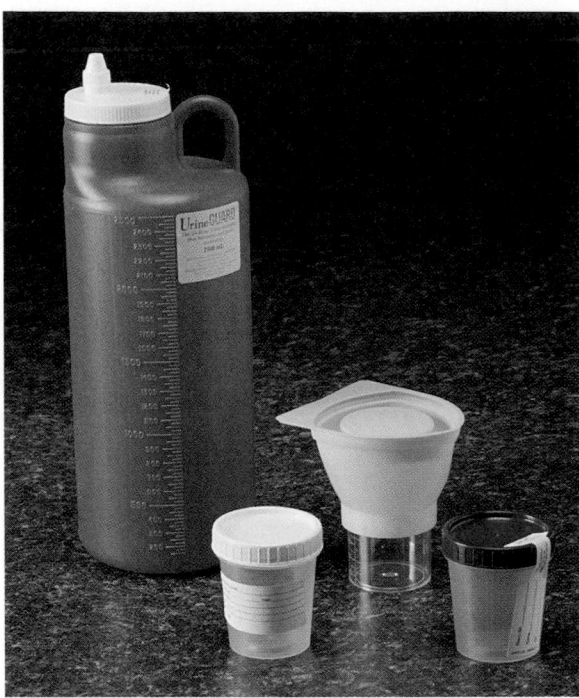

FIG 44-1 Urine collection containers.

container itself and not the lid, because the lid might become separated from the specimen.

- Make sure that the volume is sufficient for the type of test ordered. Usually, 25 to 50 ml is adequate for routine testing.
- Always use the proper urine container as provided by the medical office or hospital laboratory. Specimens collected in household jars are unsterile and not acceptable for testing.
- Provide verbal and written instructions for specimen collection. (See *Urine specimen collection*, and *Procedure 44-1: Instructing the patient on collecting a clean-catch midstream urine specimen*.)
- Be sure to test specimens within 30 to 60 minutes of collection. If a delay in testing might occur, the specimen can be refrigerated for up to 4 hours. Urine that has been sitting at room temperature can go through various physical and chemical changes, altering the results for that specimen.
- Make sure the specimen is gently stirred prior to testing specimens that may have been sitting still or refrigerated. In such specimens, solutes may have settled to the bottom. Gentle stirring evenly distributes the solutes. (For information on pediatric urine collection, see Chapter 33, "Pediatrics," page 641.)

Front office–Back office connection

Urine Specimens in the Front Office

Checking a specimen to make sure it is acceptable is normally the task of a clinical medical assistant. However, there may be times when an administrative medical assistant or other front office staff receive a urine specimen from a patient. When this happens, the administrative medical assistant must inspect the specimen before the patient leaves the office. Items to check include:

- proper container
- proper labeling
- when the specimen was collected
- all information noted on the requisition form.

If the administrative medical assistant notes inconsistencies, she may want to ask the patient to collect another specimen, preferably in the office.

Patient Education

Urine Specimen Collection

For some patients, especially children and adolescents, collecting a urine specimen may be a new experience. Such patients may be apprehensive about the procedure. The medical assistant should provide clear instructions on collection as well as show the collection container and supplies and explain their usage. Other topics to discuss include:

- how much specimen is needed
- telling a child that his parent can help him
- preservative in the collection container for a patient collecting a 24-hour specimen, which might be hazardous or irritating to the skin
- avoiding touching the inside of the container and lid because doing so may contaminate the specimen

Increase compliance

For increased collection compliance, the medical assistant should post collection instructions for collecting a clean-catch, midstream urine specimen in the bathroom used by patients. Also, she should provide written as well as verbal instructions on proper specimen collection and storage to the patient collecting a 24-hour specimen.

PROCEDURE 44-1

Instructing the patient on collecting a clean-catch, midstream urine specimen

Task

Instruct a patient on how to collect a clean-catch, midstream urine specimen.

Conditions

- Sterile screw-cap container
- Computer-generated patient label
- Antiseptic towelettes (2)

Standards

In the time specified and within the scoring parameters determined by the instructor, the student will successfully instruct a patient on how to collect a clean-catch, midstream urine specimen.

Performance Standards

1. Wash or sanitize your hands and assemble the equipment.
2. Greet the patient, introduce yourself, and explain the proper collection procedure.

For female patients

3. For female patients, instruct the patient to:
   a. Wash her hands and then open the lid of the cup and place the lid on the counter facing up. If the lid is placed facing down on the counter, it could become contaminated and cause a false-positive result.
   b. Lower her underwear and expose the urinary meatus by spreading the labia apart with the nondominant hand.
   c. Take one of the towelettes and clean one side of the urinary meatus from the front to the back on one side. Repeat the same procedure with the other towelette on the opposite side of the meatus. If the kit contains a third towelette, clean from front to back down the middle. Proper cleaning of the skin area will avoid contamination of the specimen by microorganisms on the skin.
   d. Continue to keep the labia spread apart and begin voiding a small amount of urine into the toilet for 1 or 2 seconds to clear the urethra of contaminants and ensure accurate results.
   e. Position the collection container into the stream of urine without stopping the flow. Stopping the flow

could cause bacteria and other contaminants to be washed into the specimen.
   f. After filling the container adequately (30 to 50 ml), void the remaining urine into the toilet.
   g. Wipe the area and wash her hands.
   h. Securely cap the specimen container and place it in the specified area. (The area in the physician's office laboratory or hospital laboratory designated for specimens.) Placing specimens in the proper collection area ensures prompt specimen testing and results reporting.

For male patients

4. For male patients, instruct the patient to:
   a. Wash his hands and then open the lid of the cup and place the lid on the counter facing up. If the lid is placed facing down on the counter, it could become contaminated and cause a false-positive result.
   b. Lower his underwear and, if uncircumcised, retract the foreskin and hold it back during the entire procedure to avoid contaminating the specimen with microorganisms present on the foreskin, which can cause erroneous results.
   c. Clean the area around the penile opening (glans penis) by starting at the tip of the penis and cleaning downward using a separate towelette for each side.
   d. Void a small amount of urine into the toilet. Excreting a small amount of urine before collection clears the urethra of contaminants and thus ensures accurate results.
   e. Collect the next amount of urine by voiding into the sterile container, being careful not to touch the inside of the container with the hand or penis.
   f. After filling the container adequately, void the last amount of urine into the toilet.
   g. Dry the area and wash his hands.
   h. Securely cap the specimen container and place it in the specified area. Placing specimens in the proper collection area ensures prompt specimen testing and results reporting.

Preparation for Urinalysis

Before conducting a urinalysis, the medical assistant must make sure that she is familiar with the equipment, including the reagent strip and urine analyzer, and quality control measures involved in the procedure.

Reagent Strip

There are several commercial testing strips commonly used in the POL, including Bayer Multistix 10SG and Roche Chemstrip 10SG. (See Figure 44-2.) The test strip contains individual color pads that correlate with a urine component, such as glucose or blood. After the medical assistant dips the test strip in the urine, she compares the individual color pads to a color chart and records each result on a urinalysis reporting form. (See Figure 44-3.) The strips can also be read automatically on a urine analyzer, where the results would be printed out by the analyzer. Some results are recorded as an actual amount or value and would be considered quantitative. For example, a urobilinogen result of 0.2 mg/dl is considered normal. Other results may be qualitative and interpreted by using results such as *positive* or *negative*.

Although testing urine using a reagent strip is quick and easy, the medical assistant should be aware of the following guidelines:

- Carefully read and follow the manufacturer's instruction provided in the reagent strip package.

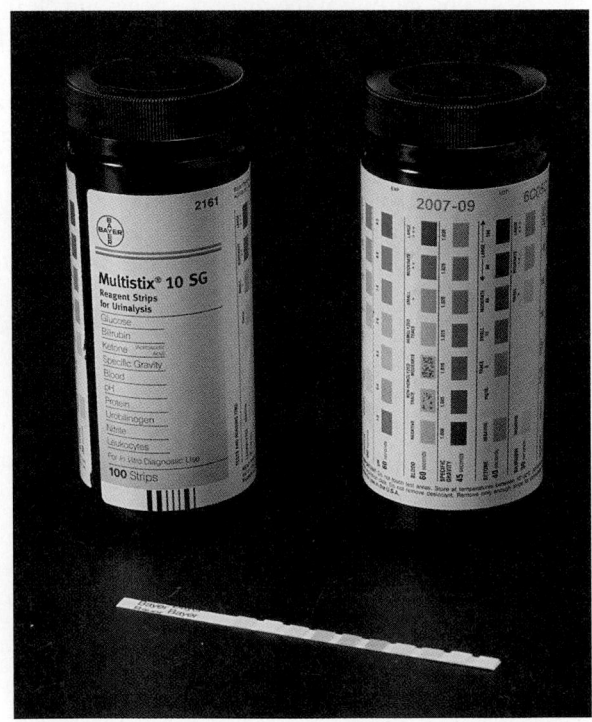

FIG 44-2 Urinalysis reagent strip and container with color chart.

Patient name: *Maggie Benjamin* MR#: 036218
Date of collection: 06/21/08
Time of collection: 8:13 a.m.
Initials: *mag. CMA*

Test	Results
Color	dark yellow
Clarity	clear
Specific gravity	1.020
pH	6.0
Protein	neg
Glucose	neg
Ketones	neg
Bilirubin	neg
Blood	trace
Urobilinogen	0.2
Nitrite	neg
Leukocytes	neg
MICROSCOPIC	
Epithelial cells	2-5/lpf
wbc	None
rbc	0-5/hpf
Casts	None
Crystals	None
Bacteria	None
Mucus	None
Miscellaneous	

FIG 44-3 Completed urinalysis report.

- Always check the expiration date and do not use strips that are outdated.
- Do not use test strips if a color change has occurred to the reagent pads.
- Store reagent strips in a cool, dark area with the cover always on the container. Do not refrigerate the strips.

Urine Analyzer

Many POLs read the urine reagent strip using a urine analyzer, such as the Clinitek analyzer manufactured by Bayer Corporation. (See Figure 44-4.) The benefits of using the analyzer include:

- computer printout of the results (color and clarity included) with abnormal values flagged
- ability to process results for a greater number of urine tests in a shorter amount of time
- decreased exposure of the medical assistant to the urine specimen, compared with reading the results manually.

If, at any time, the medical assistant questions the results obtained by the urine analyzer, she should confirm the

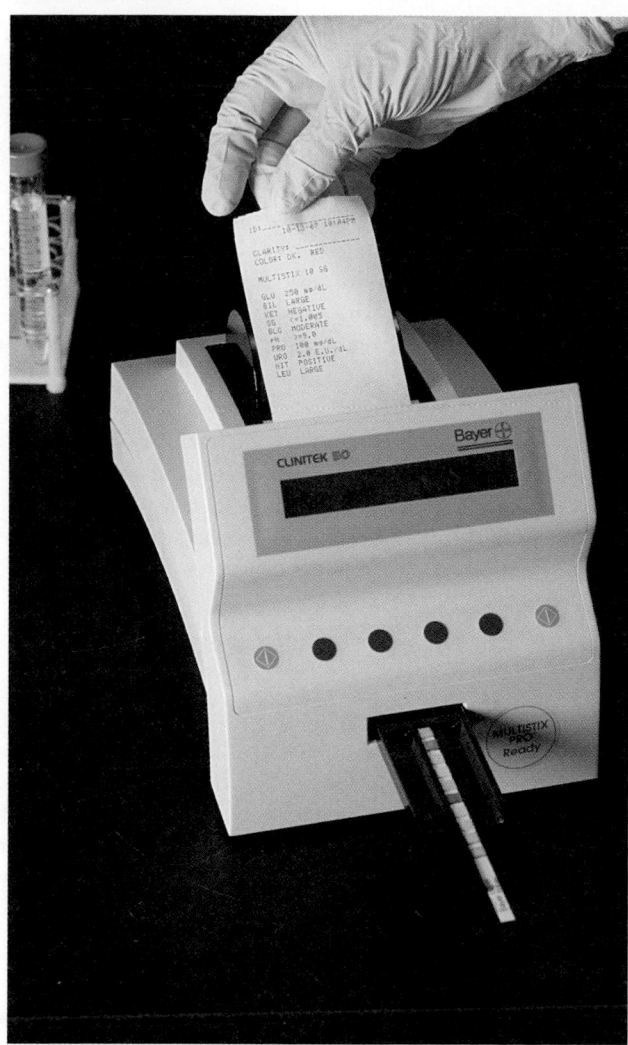

FIG 44-4 Bayer Clinitek urine analyzer with printed results.

results by performing a manual (visual) chemical reagent test using a new test strip.

Quality Control

Regardless of which method the medical assistant uses to read a urine reagent strip, she must perform quality control to ensure accurate results. Performing quality control not only certifies that the reagent strips are acceptable for use but also tests the procedure and technique of testing personnel. As with any quality control procedures, quality control should be run prior to any patient testing and results must be documented properly and according to the manufacturer's and laboratory protocol.

Most manufacturers that supply reagent test strips also provide quality control reagents and supplies as well as instructions for testing, control ranges, results reporting, troubleshooting, and corrective action procedures.

Urinalysis Components

Although relatively simple, urinalysis consists of three components:

- physical
- chemical
- microscopic.

Under regulations set by the Clinical Laboratory Improvement Amendment (CLIA) of 1988, the medical assistant is qualified to perform only physical and chemical analysis; the physician or other CLIA-sanctioned professional must perform and record the microscopic evaluation.

Evaluating the Physical Components of Urine

The physical examination of urine evaluates the specimen's color, clarity, odor, and specific gravity. The medical assistant should make sure that the urine is collected in a clear container or should transfer the specimen into a clear glass or plastic container so that color and clarity can be determined.

Color

Urochrome is a pigment responsible for giving urine its varying shades of yellow color. The normal color of urine can vary from pale yellow or straw-colored to amber. Urine that is colorless or pale is diluted, while urine that is dark yellow is concentrated. The first urine voided in the morning tends to be a darker yellow because it is more concentrated, which means that it contains a greater amount of substances compared to the volume of water. The more water or fluid a person takes in, the greater the volume of water, which would dilute the urine and cause its color to be lighter.

Urine that has a color other than yellow may indicate an underlying disorder, including:

- orange or brownish color—possible liver disease, such as hepatitis
- red or reddish—a UTI, trauma, or a renal disorder
- milky—possibly fat globules in the urine or a UTI.

Certain foods, vitamins, and drugs cause urine to change color as well. (See *Urine color changes,* page 926.)

Clarity

The clarity, or *transparency,* of urine is one aspect of the evaluation of its appearance. Fresh urine is usually clear or transparent but it may become cloudy when refrigerated or left standing at room temperature. Such substances as mucus, bacteria, and cells can contribute to the cloudy appearance of urine. When assessing the

Urine color changes

Certain foods, vitamins, or medications a patient ingests could cause his urine to be a different color. Generally, if the color change is caused by something the patient normally ingests, it is not considered an indication of a pathological condition. The following lists include foods, vitamins, and medications that can cause a urine color change.

Foods
- Carrots—orange
- Beets—red-tinged
- Blackberries—red-tinged

Vitamins
- Vitamin C—bright yellow or orange
- B vitamins—bright yellow or orange

Medications
- Antibiotics, such as sulfamethoxazole (Bactrim) and nitrofurantion (Furadantin)—yellowish-brown
- Rifampin (Rifadin) or phenazopyridine (Pyridium)—reddish-orange

clarity of urine, the medical assistant should use such terms as *clear, cloudy, slightly cloudy,* or **turbid**, which means "thick" or "opaque."

Odor

A fresh urine specimen normally has a slight aromatic odor; however, upon standing, urine develops an ammonia odor. This odor is caused by the breakdown of urea by bacteria that may be present in the specimen. A sweet or fruity odor may be an indication of the presence of ketones, which are found in urine of patients with uncontrolled diabetes. Foul-smelling urine may be a symptom of a UTI, while a mousy, or musky, smell from an infant's urine may indicate phenylketonuria. Certain foods can also change the odor of urine. For example, asparagus can cause a strange or musty odor, and saffron or sandalwood oil may create a spicy odor. Although urine can have varying degrees of odor, the odor is not generally recorded when performing a urinalysis unless something abnormal is noted.

Specific Gravity

Specific gravity is the weight of a substance compared with an equal amount of water. The specific gravity of

urine measures the concentration of dissolved substances in urine and is an indication of how well the kidneys are functioning. The specific gravity of water is 1.000, whereas the normal range for urine is 1.005 to 1.030. Urine that is too concentrated will have a higher specific gravity, and urine that is diluted will have a lower specific gravity. A person's specific gravity may change throughout the day, depending on that person's fluid intake and output. Specific gravity is highest upon the first morning voiding, because the urine has concentrated during the night. Conditions that may affect a specific gravity result include dehydration, heart disease, renal disease, and diabetes mellitus.

Specific gravity can be measured manually, using a refractometer, or chemically, using a reagent testing strip. Because most urine reagent strips have a specific gravity test component, most POLs use this method rather than the refractometer method.

Evaluating the Chemical Components of Urine

Urine may contain various chemical substances that, when detected, could indicate a range of pathological conditions, such as renal disorders, UTIs, and diabetes. Urine may also contain various hormones and metabolites that, if detected, can help determine pregnancy or detect drug use. Routine urinalysis chemical tests include pH for alkalinity or acidity, glucose, protein, ketones, blood, bilirubin, urobilinogen, nitrite, and leukocytes.

pH

Alkalinity or acidity of urine is represented by pH. The pH scale ranges from 0.0 to 14.0, with a pH of 7.0 being neutral. An acidic measurement ranges from 0.0 to 6.0, and an alkaline measurement ranges from 8.0 to 14.0. Although normal urine pH can range from 4.5 to 8.0, freshly voided urine tends to be more acidic than alkaline and generally has a pH result around 6.0. If urine is not tested when received and sits at room temperature, it will become alkaline and its pH will become elevated. Results of pH testing vary due to changes in a person's diet or condition. An acid pH may indicate acidosis, diabetes mellitus, or starvation; an alkaline pH may indicate a UTI.

Glucose

The presence of glucose in the urine is not a normal condition. Normally, the kidneys will filter and then reabsorb glucose back into the bloodstream. However, if glucose levels in the bloodstream increase, glucose will reach its renal threshold. **Renal threshold** is the concentration at which substances in the blood not normally excreted by the kidneys begin to appear in the urine. The renal threshold for glucose is 160 to 180 mg/dl. If blood glucose levels exceed the renal threshold, **glucosuria**, a condition where glucose spills back into the urine, will result.

The main cause of glucosuria is diabetes mellitus but it can also result from pancreatic insufficiency, disorders of the endocrine glands, and excessive carbohydrate intake. Urine glucose results may be reported as *negative, trace, 1+, 2+, 3+,* and *4+*. However, some reagent strip charts provide quantitative results measuring 100 mg/dl to 2 g/dl.

Protein

The presence of a large amount of protein in the urine is called **proteinuria**. Protein results are graded as *negative, trace, 1+, 2+, 3+,* or *4+*. A temporary increase in urine protein may be caused by fever, stress, or strenuous exercise. Chronic proteinuria may be due to renal failure or other renal conditions.

Ketones

Ketones are the by-products of excessive fat metabolism and are oxidized by the muscles as a source of energy. **Ketonuria** is the presence of ketone bodies in the urine and can result from a starvation or high-fat diet, pregnancy, or uncontrolled diabetes mellitus. Ketone results are recorded as *negative, trace, small, moderate,* or *large* or as *negative, 1+, 2+,* or *3+*.

Bilirubin

Bilirubin is formed as a result of the breakdown of hemoglobin. It is carried to the liver via the bloodstream, where it is then excreted as bile. Urine that contains high levels of bilirubin may be yellow-orange to dark brown in color. High levels of bilirubin in the urine can indicate liver damage or obstruction, hepatitis, or cirrhosis. Bilirubin results may be recorded quantitatively as *negative, small, moderate,* or *large* or qualitatively as *negative, 1+, 2+,* or *3+*.

Urobilinogen

As bilirubin passes through the intestines, it is converted to urobilinogen by bacterial enzymes and then excreted through the feces. Small amounts of urobilinogen in the urine are normal; however, increased amounts may indicate a biliary obstruction, cirrhosis, heart failure, or excessive red blood cell destruction. Urobilinogen results may be from 0.2 mg/dl (normal) to 8 mg/dl.

Blood

Hematuria is the condition in which blood is found in the urine. Blood is not normally present in urine except as a contaminant during menstruation. The medical assistant should always document if the patient has her menses during urine collection. The presence of hemoglobin in the

urine without red blood cells (RBCs), called *hemoglobinuria,* is a rare condition that can be caused by a transfusion reaction, hemolytic anemia, arsenic poisoning, or malaria. Blood results are graded as *negative, trace, small, moderate,* or *large* or as *negative, trace, 1+, 2+,* or *3+*. Reasons for blood in the urine include trauma to the kidneys, UTI, and kidney stones.

Nitrite

Nitrate (NO_3) is a compound of nitrogen and oxygen found in many food items in a person's diet. It is normally precipitated out in urine. Some pathogenic bacteria possess the ability to convert nitrate to nitrite. Nitrite in the urine suggests the presence of these pathogenic bacteria and indicates a possible UTI. Because not all bacteria that can cause a UTI produce nitrite, leukocyte test results must also be taken into consideration when considering an infection. Nitrites are reported as *negative* or *positive*. A positive nitrite test should be followed by a urine culture and identification of the organism.

Leukocytes

The presence of leukocytes, or white blood cells (WBCs), in urine usually indicates a UTI and should be compared with a nitrite test. Leukocyte results are graded as *negative, trace, small, moderate,* or *large*. Microscopic evaluation of the specimen should confirm the reagent strip results with a visual confirmation of leukocytes.

Evaluating the Microscopic Components of Urine

Physicians or other qualified personnel examine the microscopic components of urine to evaluate the sediment, or solid material, found in urine. (See *Common microscopic components in urine,* page 928 to 932.) This method is also used to confirm the results of the physical and chemical urine evaluation. Although the medical assistant can prepare a urine specimen for microscopic evaluation, according to CLIA, a physician or other qualified health care profession must read and record the results. Upon completing the physical and chemical aspects of urinalysis, the medical assistant should centrifuge the urine, pour off the excess fluid, and prepare the sediment for microscopic examination.

The examiner may look at the sediment with or without the aid of a stain, based on her preference. The examiner will first observe the specimen under a low power field and scan it for casts. Then she may view it under a high power field to look for the presence of RBCs, WBCs, epithelial cells, crystals, bacteria, and other substances. (See *Procedure 44-2: Performing a urinalysis,* page 932.)

Urine Pregnancy Testing

There are various rapid methods of determining pregnancy. All of them rely on detection of the human chorionic gonadotropin (HCG) hormone, which is secreted by the developing fertilized egg. HCG levels are detectable in the urine or blood as soon as 1 to 5 days after conception. HCG levels continue to rise during the beginning of the first trimester, with levels peaking at about 8 weeks.

There are many CLIA-waived pregnancy test kits on the market. Most of them are based on the same immunologic principle (immunoassay) and perform a qualitative detection

Common microscopic components in urine

The following table lists common components found in urine using microscopic examination along with a description of each.*

Component	Description
Red blood cell (RBC) 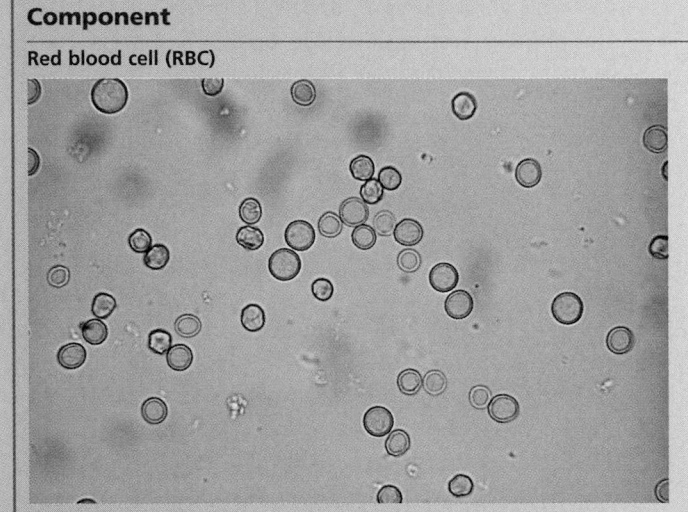 (From Strasinger/Di Lorenzo. *Urinalysis and Body Fluids*, 4th ed. FA Davis, Philadelphia, 2001, p 77, with permission.)	• Round, colorless, biconcave disc that is highly refractile in unstained urine • Not normally seen in urine sediment, but may be present during menstruation • If present, commonly reported as *0 to 2, 2 to 5, 5 to 10, 10 to 20, >50, >100,* or *too numerous to count (TNTC)* per high power field (hpf)
White blood cell (WBC) 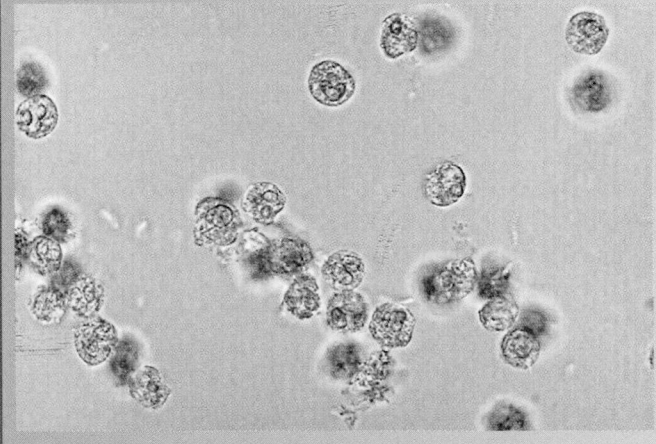 (From Strasinger/Di Lorenzo. *Urinalysis and Body Fluids*, 4th ed. FA Davis, Philadelphia, 2001, p 79, with permission.)	• Slightly larger than RBCs and possibly granular or containing a multilobed nucleus • Possibly indicating a urinary tract infection (UTI), prostatitis, or urethritis in amounts greater than 5 to 10/hpf • If present, commonly reported as *0 to 5, 5 to 10, 10 to 20,* up to *TNTC* per hpf

Common microscopic components in urine—cont'd

Component	Description
Epithelial cells	• Larger than WBCs

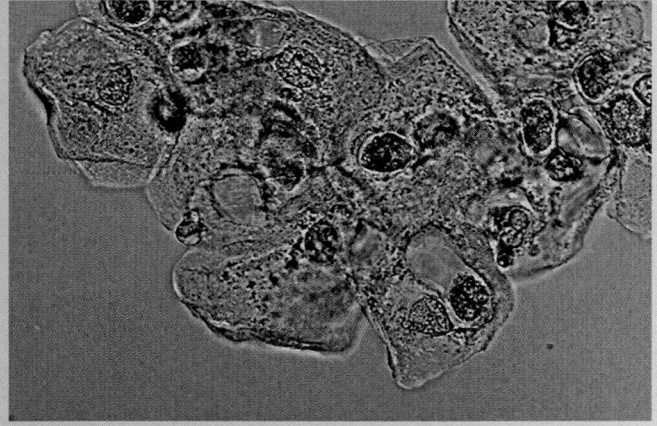

(From Strasinger/Di Lorenzo. *Urinalysis and Body Fluids*, 4th ed. FA Davis, Philadelphia, 2001, p 81, with permission.)

Description (Epithelial cells)

- Larger than WBCs
- Three different types: squamous, renal tubular, and transitional
- Possibly seen in urine; presence of transitional and renal epithelial cells considered normal
- If present, commonly reported as *rare, few, moderate,* or *many* per hpf or low power field (lpf), depending on physician office laboratory (POL) protocol.

Casts

(From Strasinger/Di Lorenzo. *Urinalysis and Body Fluids*, 4th ed. FA Davis, Philadelphia, 2001, p 87, with permission.)

Description (Casts)

- Usually clear and rectangular in shape but possibly containing blood cells
- Formed in the lumen of the tubules of the nephron
- Mainly consisting of protein but, when forming, possibly include urinary substances, such as RBCs and WBCs
- Various kinds, classified by what they contain, including the most common type, the hyaline cast, but also RBC, WBC, waxy, and granular
- Usually indicative of a pathological condition
- If present, commonly reported as *0 to 2, 2 to 5, 5 to 10,* up to *TNTC* per lpf
- If present, formal identification of cast type made at high power field

Continued

Common microscopic components in urine—cont'd

Component	Description
Crystals	• Can be many different shapes that refract light and appear shiny or colored (as in a prism) on microscopic evaluation • Formed when there are changes in urine pH, temperature, or concentration • Usually classified based on urine pH and include calcium oxalate, tyrosine, amorphous urates, triple phosphate, uric acid, and calcium carbonate • Possibly caused by certain foods, medications, or disorders • If present, commonly reported as *rare, few, moderate,* or *many* per hpf

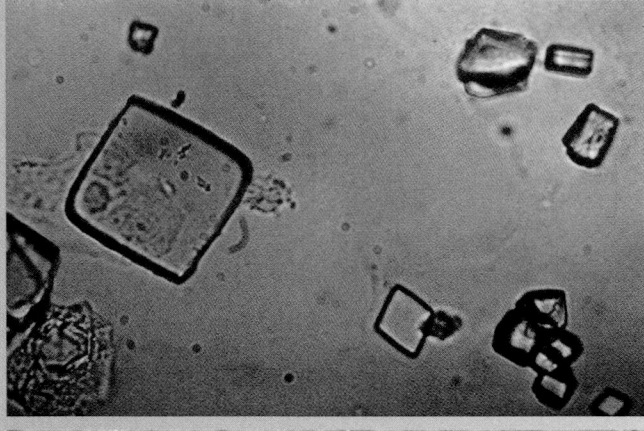

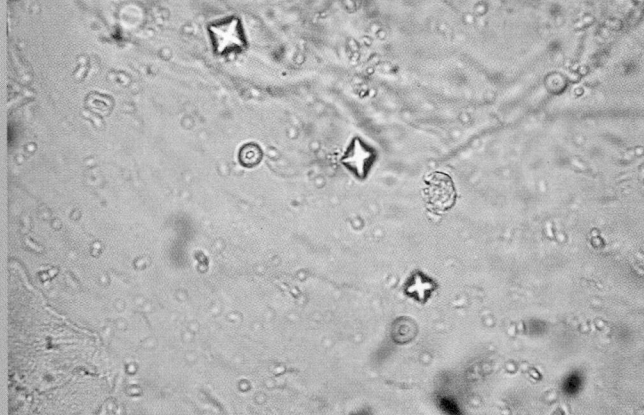

(From Strasinger/Di Lorenzo. *Urinalysis and Body Fluids*, 4th ed. FA Davis, Philadelphia, 2001, p 96-97, with permission.)

Component	Description
Bacteria	• Tiny round or rod-shaped structures • Possibly indicating a UTI in large amounts • If present, commonly reported as *rare, few, moderate,* or *many* per hpf

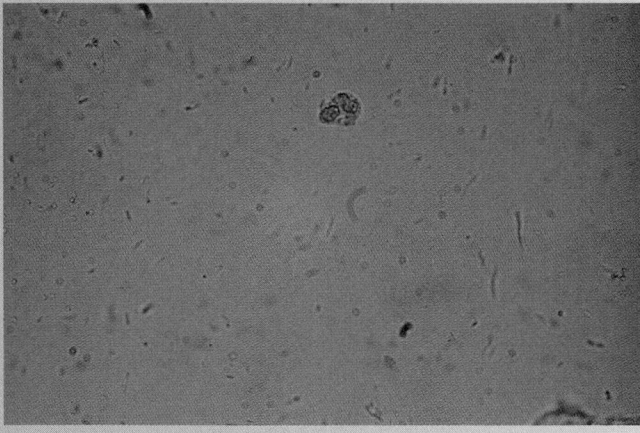

(From Strasinger/Di Lorenzo. *Urinalysis and Body Fluids*, 4th ed. FA Davis, Philadelphia, 2001, p 85, with permission.)

Common microscopic components in urine—cont'd

Component	Description

Yeast

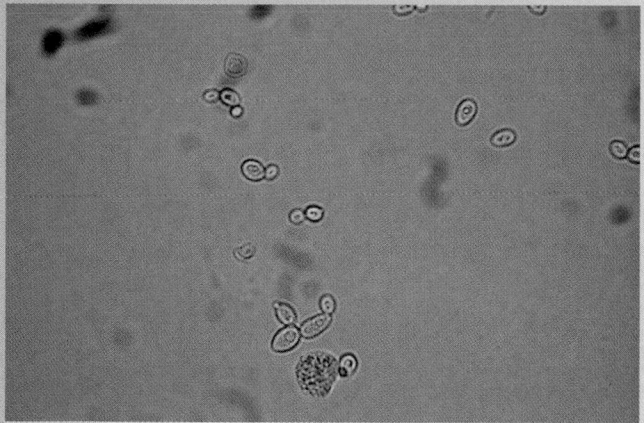

(From Strasinger/Di Lorenzo. *Urinalysis and Body Fluids*, 4th ed. FA Davis, Philadelphia, 2001, p 77, with permission.)

- Single-celled or budding oval structure that is larger than bacteria
- Grouped under "miscellaneous" on the laboratory report form
- If present, commonly reported as *rare, few, moderate,* or *many* per hpf

Trichomonas vaginalis

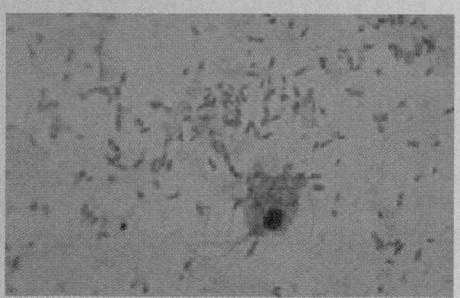

(From Strasinger/Di Lorenzo. *Urinalysis and Body Fluids*, 4th ed. FA Davis, Philadelphia, 2001, p 64, with permission.)

- Parasite that causes trichomonas infection
- Grouped under "miscellaneous" on the laboratory report form
- If present, commonly reported as *rare, few, moderate,* or *many* per hpf

Sperm cells

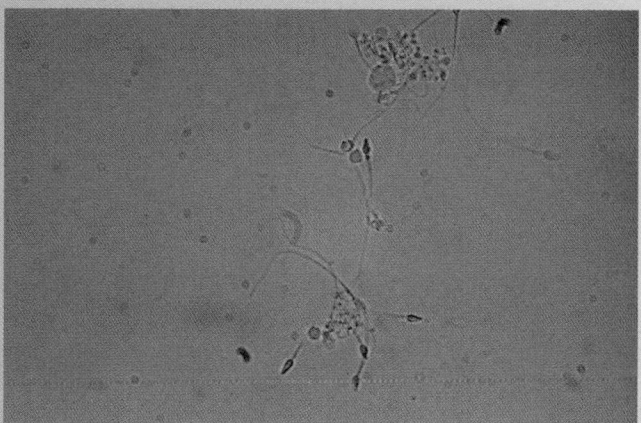

(From Strasinger/Di Lorenzo. *Urinalysis and Body Fluids*, 4th ed. FA Davis, Philadelphia, 2001, p 85, with permission.)

- Possibly seen in urine sediment
- Grouped under "miscellaneous" on the laboratory report form
- If present, commonly reported as *few, moderate,* or *many* per hpf

Continued

Common microscopic components in urine—cont'd

Component	Description
Mucus threads 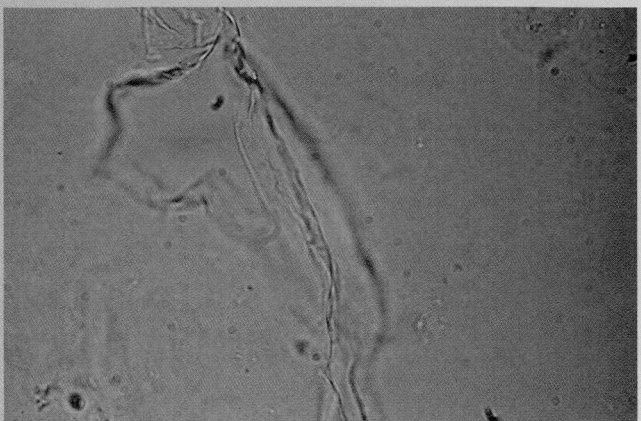 (From Strasinger/Di Lorenzo. *Urinalysis and Body Fluids*, 4th ed. FA Davis, Philadelphia, 2001, p 86, with permission.)	• Possibly seen in urine sediment • Grouped under "miscellaneous" on the laboratory report form • If present, commonly reported as *few, moderate,* or *many* per hpf

* Please note: Normal values and reporting ranges for urine sediment constituents are not clearly defined. Use suggested reporting ranges as a guide and always refer to your physician's office laboratory reporting protocol.

PROCEDURE 44-2

Performing a urinalysis

Task
Perform and document a urinalysis.

Conditions
- Sterile specimen cup
- Computer-generated label
- Urine reagent strips or Cliniteck automatic urine analyzer
- Clean glass microscope slide
- Clean glass microscope coverslip
- Microscope
- Blank urine report form or the patient's chart
- Paper towel
- Disposable examination gloves
- Plastic centrifuge tube
- Gown or laboratory coat with a zipper or button closure
- Biohazard waste container

Standards
In the time specified and within the scoring parameters determined by the instructor, the student will successfully perform and document a urinalysis.

Performance Standards

1. Assemble the supplies. Accurately complete the label and affix it to the specimen cup (not to the lid). Efficiency during procedures is greater with advance preparation. Applying the label to the cup ensures that the specimen will remain accurately labeled and not confused with other specimens in the laboratory after the lid has been removed.
2. Greet and identify your patient. Introduce yourself and explain the procedure for collecting a clean-catch, midstream urine specimen to prevent errors and ease patient anxiety.
3. Wash or sanitize your hands and apply gloves to ensure infection control.
4. Obtain the urine specimen from the patient.
5. Observe the specimen for physical characteristics, such as color, clarity, and odor.
6. Record your observations on the blank urine report form or in the patient's chart.

PROCEDURE 44-2—cont'd

7. Pour the specimen into a conical centrifuge tube. Testing with a reagent strip is easier to perform in a centrifuge tube than in a specimen container.
8. Test the urine using a chemical reagent strip, making sure all test pads have been exposed to the urine.
9. Tap the side of the strip gently on a paper towel to remove excess urine.
10. After waiting for the required time, according to the manufacturer's guidelines, read each reagent pad and record the results on the urine report form or in the patient's chart.
11. Centrifuge the tube for 5 minutes at 1500 rpm.
12. Pour off the fluid and tap the bottom of the tube to mix the remaining contents.
13. Place a drop of sediment on a glass slide and cover with a coverslip.
14. Place the slide on the microscope stage.

15. Notify the physician that the slide is ready for evaluation and provide the urine report form or the patient's chart so the physician can document the results. According to CLIA regulations, only physicians or other trained health care professionals are qualified to read a urine microscopic slide.
16. Dispose of the biological materials in appropriate containers.
17. Remove your gloves and wash your hands.
18. Record the procedure in the patient's chart.

Date	
06/11/08: 9:35 a.m.	Urine specimen collected and urinalysis performed. ---------- --- S. Gonzales, CMA

---

of HCG. (See Figure 44-5.) All of these kits have the benefits of procedural ease, specificity, and rapid results. (See *Confidentiality and pregnancy results*.) Some kits now allow for serum as well as urine testing and most include an internal control, in addition to containing positive and negative control reagents. The medical assistant should follow the manufacturer's instructions for testing, specimen requirements, and storage. As with performing any laboratory testing, the medical assistant should check the kit for expiration date and degradation or contamination of reagents. (See *Procedure 44-3: Performing a urine pregnancy test,* page 934.)

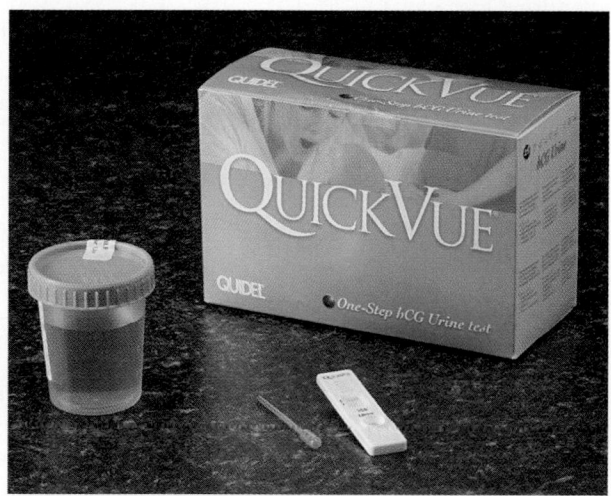

FIG 44-5 QuickVue urine pregnancy test kit.

Front office–Back office connection

Confidentiality and Pregnancy Results

In some medical offices, reporting test results is the responsibility of the clinical medical assistant. However, the administrative medical assistant should be familiar with the procedure as well as the confidentiality issues involved. The medical assistant must take care when reporting pregnancy test results and should never leave the results on the patient's answering machine. Conversely, if a patient calls looking for her pregnancy test results, the administrative medical assistant must take care to make sure she is giving the results to the correct patient. She should follow all office policies and procedures for such calls.

Chapter Summary

- The urinary system includes the kidneys, ureters, urinary bladder, and urethra.
- Urine is mainly composed of 95% water. The other 5% is made up of organic and inorganic waste products.
- Various types of urine specimens include random, first-morning, clean-catch midstream, catheterized, suprapubic, and 24-hour.
- A complete urinalysis consists of physical, chemical, and microscopic evaluation.

PROCEDURE 44-3

Performing a urine pregnancy test

Task

Perform a urine pregnancy test according to the manufacturer's instructions.

Conditions

- Disposable examination gloves
- Patient urine specimen
- Urine pregnancy test kit
- Biohazard waste container

Standards

In the time specified and within the scoring parameters determined by the instructor, the student will successfully perform a urine pregnancy test according to the manufacturer's instructions.

Performance Standards

1. Wash or sanitize your hands to ensure infection control and gather the supplies.
2. Obtain a testing cassette or stick, reagents, and a urine specimen.

3. Following the manufacturer's instructions, perform and document the necessary quality control measures. Quality control ensures that the test kit is working properly.
4. Following the manufacturer's instructions, apply urine to the testing cassette or stick.
5. Wait the appropriate time interval to ensure the accuracy of results.
6. Apply other reagents if specified by the manufacturer.
7. Read the results.
8. Remove your gloves and wash your hands to ensure infection control.
9. Document the procedure to ensure the accuracy of the medical record.

Date	
02/07/08: 11:15 a.m.	*Urine pregnancy test results: negative.* ------------------------ -- *S. Gonzales, CMA*

- The physical components of urine include color, clarity, odor, and specific gravity.
- Chemical components of urine include pH, glucose, protein, ketones, bilirubin, urobilinogen, blood, nitrite, and leukocytes.
- The microscopic portion of the urinalysis must be performed by a physician or CLIA-approved health care professional.
- Urine pregnancy testing is a CLIA-waived test performed in the POL.

Team Work Exercises

1. Separate into groups of 2 to 3 students. Your instructor will assign one of the following components of urinalysis collection and testing:
   a. collection for female
   b. collection for male
   c. physical component of testing
   d. chemical component of testing
   e. microscopic component of testing.
   Each group should gather information on its component and work together to develop a presentation that includes a demonstration to the rest of the class.
2. Separate into groups of 2 to 3 students. Your instructor will assign each group a different condition or disease of the urinary system for the group to research. The group should design a poster that explains the condition or

disease and relates the testing performed in the urinalysis department to the diagnosis or monitoring of that condition or disease.

Case Studies

1. Mrs. Robidoux has come to the office with a complaint of flank pain. She has brought in a urine specimen (first-morning) for a possible urinalysis and culture. The urine was in a glass fruit jar and she claims that she boiled the container. What would you say to Mrs. Robidoux about the urine specimen?
2. Linda Piniela has just given Robin, CMA, a freshly voided urine specimen. Robin performed a urine dipstick and the specimen was positive for blood. What questions should Robin ask Linda?

Resources

- King Strasinger, S., and Schaub DiLorenzo, M.: *The Phlebotomy Workbook*, 2nd ed. Philadelphia: F.A. Davis, 2003.
- CLIA categorization of laboratory tests: *www.cms.hhs.gov/CLIA/10_Categorization_of_Tests.asp*
- Information on urinalysis: *labtestsonline.org/understanding/analytes/urinalysis/test.html*
- Information and current issues and procedures on urinalysis: *www.labcorp.com* and *www.ascp.org*

Microbiology

Learning Objectives

Upon completion of this chapter, the student will be able to:

- define the key terms in the glossary
- discuss the major scientists who have contributed to the field of microbiology
- describe the importance of normal flora
- explain the different groups of microorganisms capable of causing human disease
- discuss the different types of microbiological specimens and proper specimen collection techniques
- describe the procedure for culturing a microbiological specimen
- describe the types of microbiological tests performed in a physician's office laboratory (POL)
- discuss the procedure involved in rapid streptococcal testing
- describe antimicrobial susceptibility testing.

CAAHEP Competencies

Clinical Competencies
  Specimen Collection
    Obtain specimens for microbiological testing
  Diagnostic Testing
    CLIA-waived tests
      Perform microbiology testing

ABHES Competencies

Clinical Duties
  Obtain throat specimen for microbiological testing
  Perform wound collection procedure for microbiological testing
  Perform microbiology testing

Procedures

  Collecting a throat specimen for microbiological testing
  Collecting a wound specimen for culture
  Collecting a sputum specimen for culture
  Performing a rapid streptococcal test
  Processing a throat culture

Chapter Outline

History of Microbiology

Microbiology is the study of microorganisms. **Microorganisms** are living organisms that cannot be seen by the naked eye and can only be viewed through the use of a microscope. Clinical microbiology focuses on identifying the pathogens that cause disease in humans.

One of the most important events early in the field of microbiology was the invention of the microscope by Anton van Leeuwenhoek in 1673. Van Leeuwenhoek's microscope, albeit crude, enabled him to view various samples, such as rainwater and scrapings from his teeth, to observe live microorganisms. He was the first to view such organisms, and he described the various shapes he viewed in letters to scientific groups, such as the Royal Society of England. Since van Leeuwenhoek's invention and subsequent discoveries, the field of microbiology has grown considerably. (See *Microbiology contributors.*)

Infection and Disease

An **infectious disease** is one in which a microorganism is transmitted directly or indirectly between individuals, causing infection. The direct link between infection and disease is well proven. Medical assistants should understand the sources of infection as well as the ways in which infectious diseases can spread. Sources of human infection include other humans, animals, and, sometimes, the soil. When a pathogen enters the body, it attempts to invade the tissues so it can grow and multiply. The body then responds to the invasion by producing antibodies and white blood cells that together try to fight off the infection. If the pathogen is successful in evading the body's response, then an infection occurs, and the person becomes sick.

Many infectious diseases are **contagious**, which means that the disease-causing pathogen can spread from one individual to another through different transmission routes. Various routes of transmission include contact, airborne, or droplet. Contact transmission can occur through direct contact with an infected person, such as touching or kissing, or indirect contact, such as touching a door knob that an infected person just touched after he sneezed into his hand. Airborne and droplet transmission spread infectious particles through such activities as coughing and sneezing. (See *Proper specimen storage.*)

Normal Flora

Not all microorganisms are **pathogenic**, or cause disease. Some organisms normally live in the body and can be

Microbiology contributors

The accompanying table provides a brief history of contributions to the field of microbiology.

Year	Scientist	Contribution
1673	Anton Van Leeuwenhoek	• Unofficially known as the "Father of Microbiology" • Creator of the first microscope • First person to observe and describe live microorganisms
1798	Edward Jenner	• Invented the first vaccine (for smallpox) • Successfully vaccinated against smallpox by injecting the cowpox virus into a healthy boy to vaccinate him against the deadly smallpox virus
1864	Louis Pasteur	• Invented the process of pasteurization, a method of sterilizing liquids
1867	Joseph Lister	• Practiced aseptic surgery by using phenol to kill bacteria on surgical instruments and wounds
1876	Robert Koch	• Developed *Koch's Postulates,* a series of experimental steps to prove that a disease is caused by a certain microorganism • Discovered *Bacillus anthracis,* the causative organism for anthrax
1884	Hans Christian Gram	• Developed the *Gram stain,* a method of staining bacteria in order to further classify them
1910	Paul Ehrlich	• Discovered a chemical means to kill a pathogen inside a host without harming the host and coined the phrase "magic bullet" to describe it • Discovered chemotherapeutic agent salvarsan
1928	Alexander Fleming	• Discovered antibiotic penicillin

Front office–Back office connection

Proper Specimen Storage

Although the clinical medical assistant will usually be responsible for collecting and handling clinical specimens, there may be times when the administrative medical assistant will receive patient specimens that cannot be processed immediately and must be stored in a refrigerator. The medical assistant must ensure that she places the specimens in the refrigerator that is designated solely for patient specimens. Conversely, she should never place her personal food items in a refrigerator designated for specimens. All medical office staff should adhere strictly to this major safety guideline to avoid contaminating food and infecting employees.

beneficial to the body. **Normal flora,** also known as *indigenous flora,* are harmless microorganisms that normally reside in many different parts of the body but do not cause disease. They are permanent residents of certain body sites, especially the skin, nasopharynx, gastrointestinal tract, and vaginal tract. Although normal flora extensively populate many areas of the body, the internal organs are usually sterile. Normal flora mainly consists of **bacteria,** which are one-celled microorganisms that sometimes produce disease in humans. Examples of bacteria that are considered normal flora include *Staphylococcus epidermidis, Streptococcus mitis,* and *Lactobacillus* species. Such areas as the central nervous system, blood, lower bronchi and alveoli, liver, spleen, kidneys, and bladder are essentially free of all organisms.

Although normal flora does not usually cause disease, if these bacteria are introduced into another body site, infection could occur. For instance, normal gastrointestinal tract bacteria such as *Escherichia coli* can cause a urinary tract infection if it is introduced into the urinary tract.

Types of Microorganisms

Although not all microorganisms are pathogenic, the pathogenic forms are of most importance when studying clinical microbiology. There are vast numbers of different microorganisms; however, most of them can be classified into a few main types:

- bacteria
- viruses and prions
- fungi
- protozoa and parasitic worms. (See *Common pathogenic microorganisms.*)

Common pathogenic microorganisms

The following table lists the various types of microorganisms and the common human infections they may cause.

Microorganism	Associated Conditions
Bacteria	
Bacillus anthracis	Anthrax
Borrelia burgdorferi	Lyme disease
Chlamydia trachomatis	Genitourinary infection, neonatal sepsis
Clostridium difficile	Pseudomembranous colitis
Escherichia coli	Urinary tract infection, gastrointestinal infection, bacteremia
Helicobacter pylori	Peptic ulcer
Klebsiella pneumoniae	Pneumonia, urinary tract infection, bacteremia
Haemophilus influenzae	Otitis media, pneumonia, conjunctivitis, bacteremia, meningitis
Mycoplasma pneumoniae	Pneumonia
Neisseria meningitidis	Meningitis, bacteremia
Neisseria gonorrhoeae	Gonorrhea, neonatal conjunctivitis
Pseudomonas aeruginosa	Nosocomial infections, pneumonia, urinary tract infection
Salmonella species	Food-borne illness, bacteremia
Staphylococcus aureus	Wound infection, bacteremia, food-borne illness, impetigo, boils, carbuncles, pneumonia
Streptococcus agalactiae (Beta *Streptococcus* group B)	Neonatal sepsis, wound infections
Streptococcus pneumoniae	Otitis media, pneumonia, sinusitis, bronchitis, bacteremia
Streptococcus pyogenes (Beta *Streptococcus* group A)	Streptococcal throat infection, impetigo, wound infections, scarlet fever, rheumatic fever
Fungi	
Aspergillus niger	Pneumonia
Candida albicans	Thrush, genitourinary infection
Cryptococcus neoformans	Meningitis
Viruses	
Adenovirus	Common cold
Avian influenza	Infectious bronchitis
Ebola	Hemorrhagic fever
Human herpesvirus 1	Genitourinary infections and skin infections
Human immunodeficiency virus	Acquired immune deficiency syndrome
Rubella	German measles
Varicella-zoster	Chickenpox

Common pathogenic microorganisms—cont'd

Microorganism	Associated Conditions
Protozoa	
Cryptosporidium	Gastrointestinal infection
Entamoeba histolytica	Gastrointestinal infection
Giardia lamblia	Gastrointestinal infection
Plasmodium species	Malaria
Trichomonas vaginalis	Genitourinary infection
Parasitic Worms	
Ascaris lumbricoides	Gastrointestinal infection
Enterobius vermicularis	Pinworm

Bacteria

Bacteria are microscopic unicellular organisms that do not have a nuclear membrane enclosing their genetic material. Such a simple cell is called a *prokaryote* (prenucleus). Bacteria are classified into three basic groups based on their shape:

- cocci
- bacilli
- spiral bacteria.

Bacteria can be further classified based on their characteristics upon a Gram staining. The Gram stain, discovered by Hans Christian Gram, is a simple method to further classify bacteria into two groups: gram-positive and gram-negative. For a Gram stain, the examiner must prepare a **smear**, which is a bacterial growth sample spread onto a microscope slide. After the slide has dried and the examiner has ensured that the smear is attached, or *fixed*, to the slide using heat or alcohol, the slide is ready for staining. (See *Gram staining*, page 940.) The examiner can determine the Gram classification based on the color (purple or pink) that the organism stains as well as the bacteria's shape by viewing the smear under a microscope. Because it is a quick, relatively simple test, the Gram stain can aid the physician in quickly determining the proper treatment for a patient. Most bacteria are easily treated with antibiotics such as penicillin, ciprofloxacin (Cipro), or azithromycin (Zithromax), and the selection of an antibiotic is partially based on the bacteria's Gram stain reaction. (See Figure 45-1.)

Cocci

Cocci are round or spherical bacteria that, depending on their pattern of growth or arrangement, can be further categorized as:

- *diplococci*, which are arranged in pairs and include *Streptococcus pneumonia* (common cause of otitis media, bacteremia, and pneumonia, especially in children) and *Neisseria gonorrhoeae* (a common sexually transmitted disease)
- *tetrads*, which are arranged in double pairs that appear to look like a square and include *Micrococcus luteus* that, although considered normal respiratory flora in humans, has been known to cause infection in immunocompromised patients
- *streptococci*, which are arranged in chains and include *Streptococcus pyogenes* (cause of streptococcal throat infection, or *strep throat*, and scarlet fever as well as the emerging disease necrotizing fasciitis)
- *staphylococci*, which are arranged in clusters sometimes known as *grapelike clusters* and include *Staphylococcus aureus*, commonly known as *Staph aureus* (common cause of skin infections and toxic shock syndrome). (See Figure 45-2.)

Bacilli

Bacilli are rod-shaped bacteria that are commonly found in the soil and air. Like cocci, bacilli can have different arrangements. However, unlike the cocci in which a specific bacterium always arranges itself in only one way, most bacilli bacteria—with the exception of coccobacilli—do not adhere strictly to one arrangement type. For example, most of the bacteria found in the gastrointestinal tract, such as *Escherichia coli* and *Enterobacter*, can be in any arrangement of bacilli except for coccobacilli. Bacilli arrange themselves as:

- *single bacilli*, which are arranged as single, separate rods
- *diplobacilli*, which are arranged in pairs
- *streptobacilli*, which are arranged in chains
- *coccobacilli*, which are rods with rounded ends and include *Bordetella pertussis* (cause of whooping cough) and *Haemophilus influenzae* (cause of bacteremia and pneumonia). (See Figure 45-3.)

Gram staining

Although most medical assistants will not be performing Gram stains in the medical office, it is necessary to understand the theory and practice of Gram staining as it applies to identification of pathogenic bacteria. Bacteria can be classified into two different categories based on their staining. *Gram-positive* bacteria stain a dark purple, and *gram-negative* bacteria stain a pink color. After smearing a few colonies of bacteria on a sterile glass microscope slide, an examiner will follow these steps to stain the slide:

1. Flood the slide with crystal violet stain and let it sit for 1 minute.

2. Rinse the slide with running tap water or sterile water.

3. Flood the slide with iodine and let it sit for 2 minutes.

4. Rinse the slide with water.

5. Flood the slide with acetone and let it sit for 5 seconds.

6. Rinse the slide with water.

7. Flood the stain with safranin red stain and let it sit for 30 seconds.

8. Rinse with water.

9. Let the stained slide air-dry and read it under a microscope.

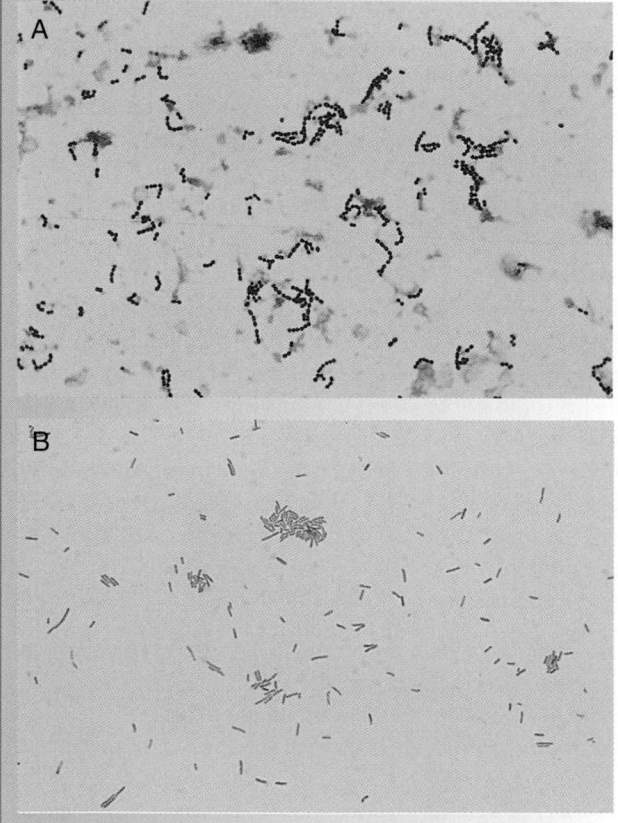

Gram Stain Slides. (A) Gram-Positive Bacteria. (B) Gram-Negative Bacteria. (From Bartlet. *Diagnostic Bacteriology*. FA Davis, Philadelphia, 2000, color plate #2 & #5, with permission)

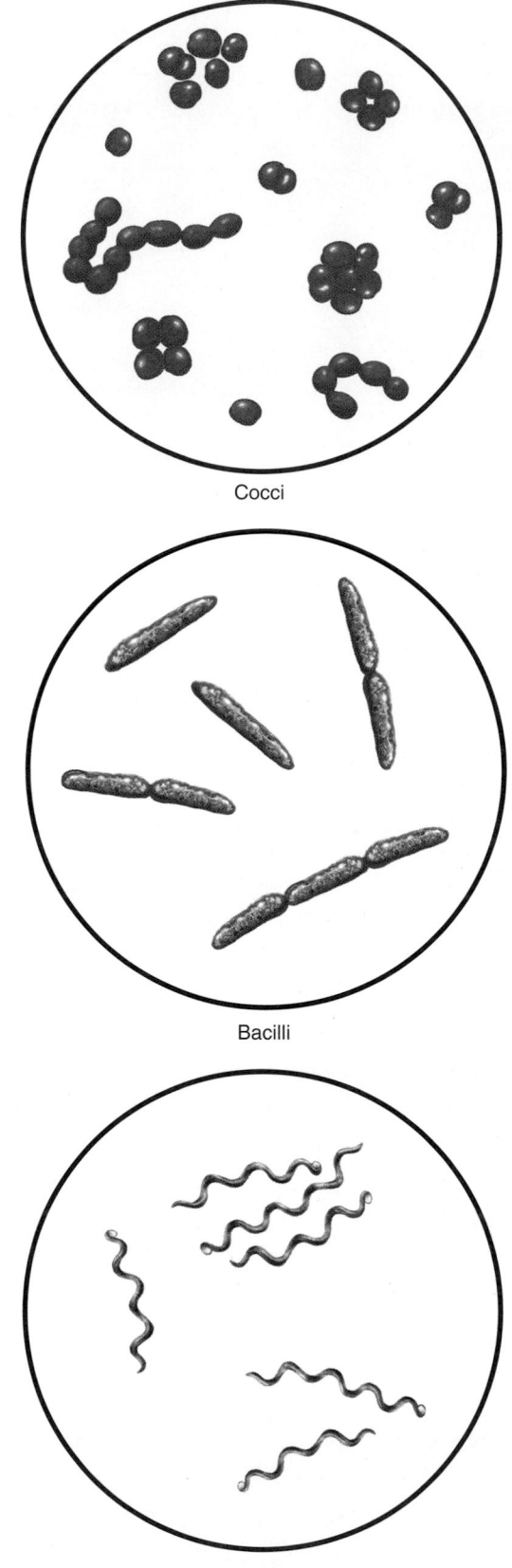

Cocci

Bacilli

Spiral bacteria

FIG 45-1 Classification of bacteria based on shape.

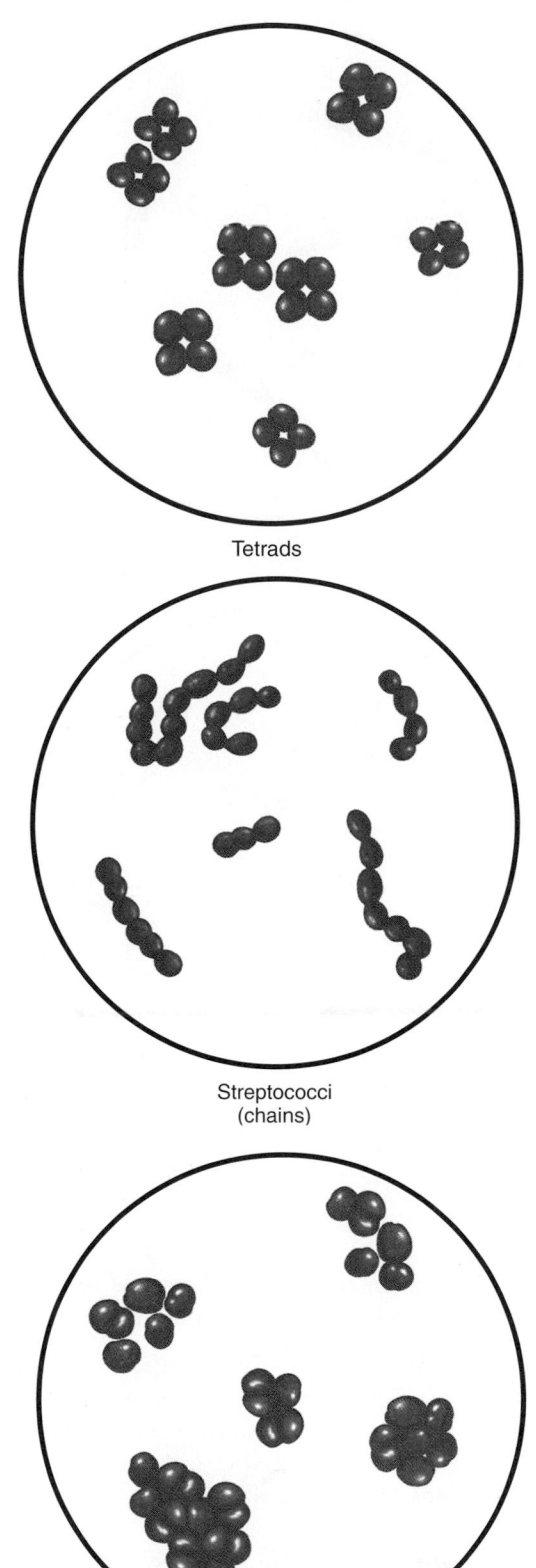

Tetrads

Streptococci
(chains)

Staphylococci
(clusters)

FIG 45-2 Cocci

Spiral

Unlike bacilli and cocci, spiral bacteria are classified as rods having a curved or spiral shape. They can be further classified as:

- *spirilla*, which appear as curved rods and include *Vibrio cholera* (cause of cholera)
- *spirochetes*, which appear as helical, or corkscrew-shaped, and include *Borrelia burgdorferi* and *Treponema pallidum*. (See Figure 45-4.)

Viruses and Prions

Viruses are pathogens, consisting of a nucleic acid surrounded by a protein coat, that can grow and reproduce only after infecting a host cell. They are extremely small microorganisms and require the use of an electron microscope to view them. Structurally, viruses come in various shapes and sizes. They are considered nonliving because they cannot exist on their own, but require a living cell to reproduce. For example, a virus enters a host cell, takes over that cell, and uses the cell's nutrients to multiply. Once the virus has multiplied within the cell, the cell will then burst, thus releasing more virus into the body. (See Figure 45-5.) Viruses possess DNA or RNA and they are insensitive to antibiotics. Unlike bacteria, viruses are not easily classified, but they are distinguished by their size and shape and whether they contain RNA or DNA. Viral shapes also differ from bacterial shapes, with viruses considered more three dimensional, such as helical, icosahedral, and spherical. (See Figure 45-6.) Virus taxonomy is slightly different from that of bacteria and quite complicated. They are grouped as families and their names do not include a genus or species name (although their detailed classification can include subfamilies and genus groupings). Instead, viruses are usually named after the infection they cause or the family in which they are classified. For example, the virus that causes rubella (German measles) is known as the *rubella virus* and is classified under the Togaviridae family of viruses.

Like other pathogenic microorganisms, viruses have the ability to spread from host to host. Infectious diseases caused by viruses include smallpox, chickenpox, rubeola (measles), rubella (German measles), mumps, rabies, herpes simplex, herpes zoster, yellow fever, and hepatitis. Viral infections cannot be treated with antibiotics. There are a few antiviral medications, such as ribavirin (Rebetol) to treat patients with respiratory syncytial virus, acyclovir (Zovirax) for various viral infections, and zanamivir (Relenza) and oseltamivir (Tamiflu) for the influenza virus.

A **prion**, also classified as nonliving, is even less complex than a virus because it consists of only a protein. A prion is a proteinaceous infectious particle that, when transmitted to a human, can cause a spongiform encephalopathy. Creutzfeldt-Jakob disease and kuru are two untreatable and fatal human diseases caused by a prion.

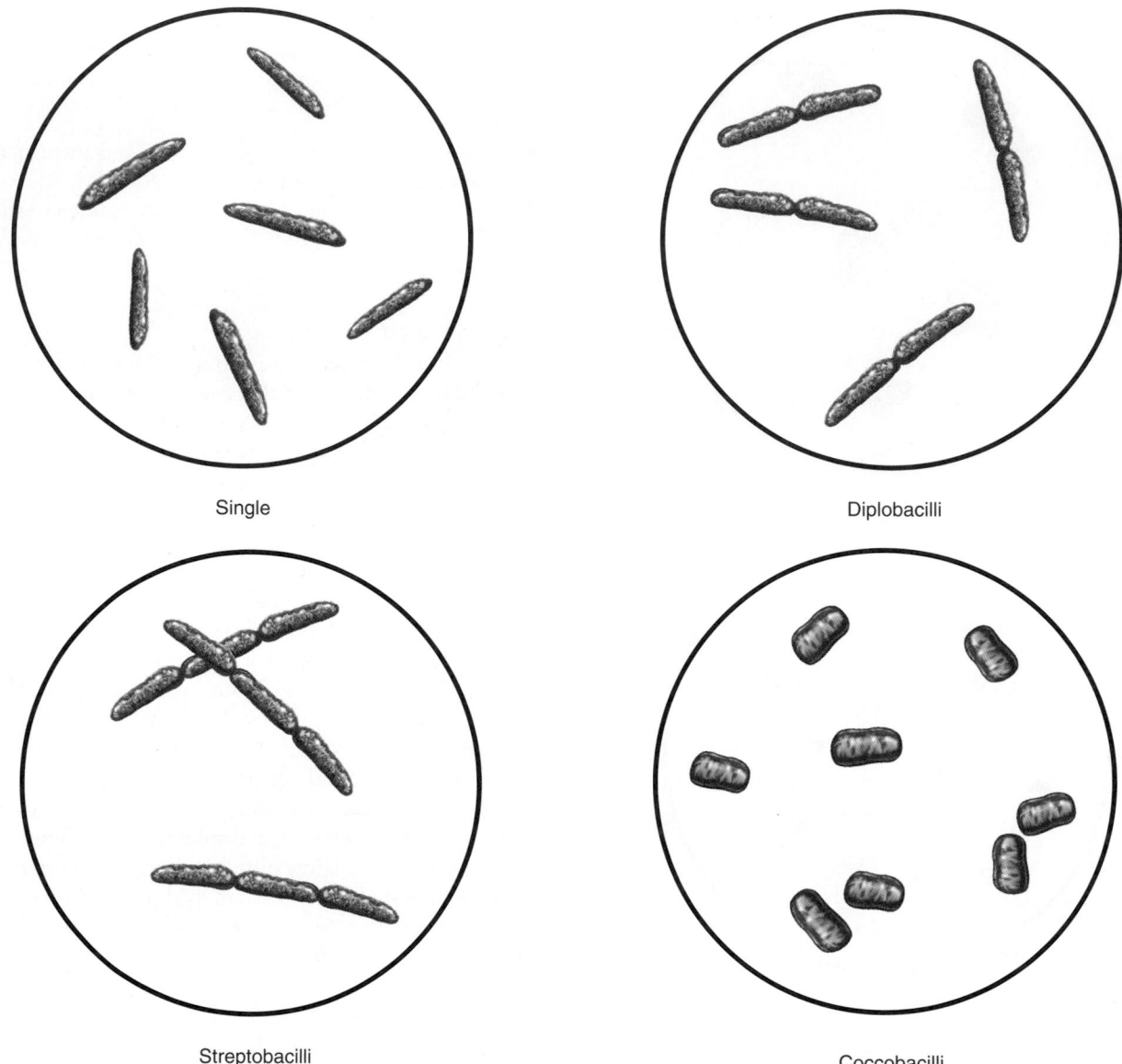

Single

Diplobacilli

Streptobacilli

Coccobacilli

FIG 45-3 Bacilli.

Fungus

A **fungus** is an eukaryotic organism, which means it possesses a true nucleus with a nuclear membrane. There are unicellular types of fungi, such as yeasts, and more complex multicellular types, such as molds and mushrooms. Fungi play an important role in the environment by decomposing plant and animal wastes. Additionally, some fungi are still used as a source of antibiotics. Human fungal infections can be caused by:

- yeasts, such as *Candida albicans* (cause of such local infections as thrush or vulvovaginal infection) and *Cryptococcus neoformans* (cause of serious systemic infections, such as meningitis, especially in patients with suppressed immune systems)

- molds, such as the black mold *Aspergillus niger* (possible cause of lung and ear infections in humans).

As with viral infections, fungal infections cannot be treated with antibiotics. Some antifungal medications, such as amphotericin (Amphocin), miconazole (Lotrimin), and fluconazole (Diflucan), are used to treat systemic and local fungal infections. (See Figure 45-7.)

Protozoa and Parasitic Worms

Protozoa are eukaryotic unicellular microscopic organisms that inhabit soil and water. The majority of protozoa do not cause infection and many of them play an important role in ecology by preying on unicellular microorganisms such as

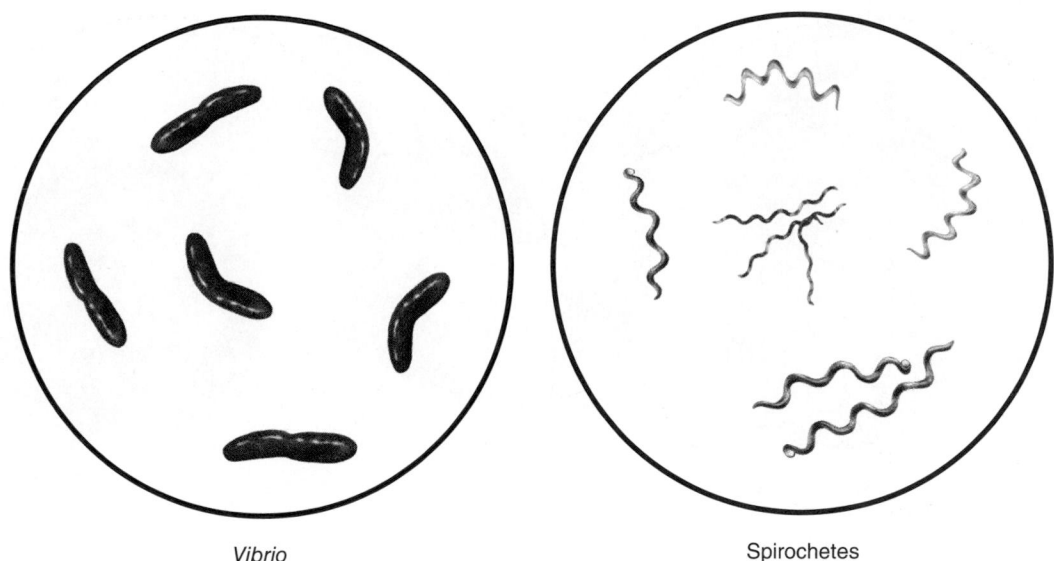

Vibrio

Spirochetes

FIG 45-4 Spiral bacteria.

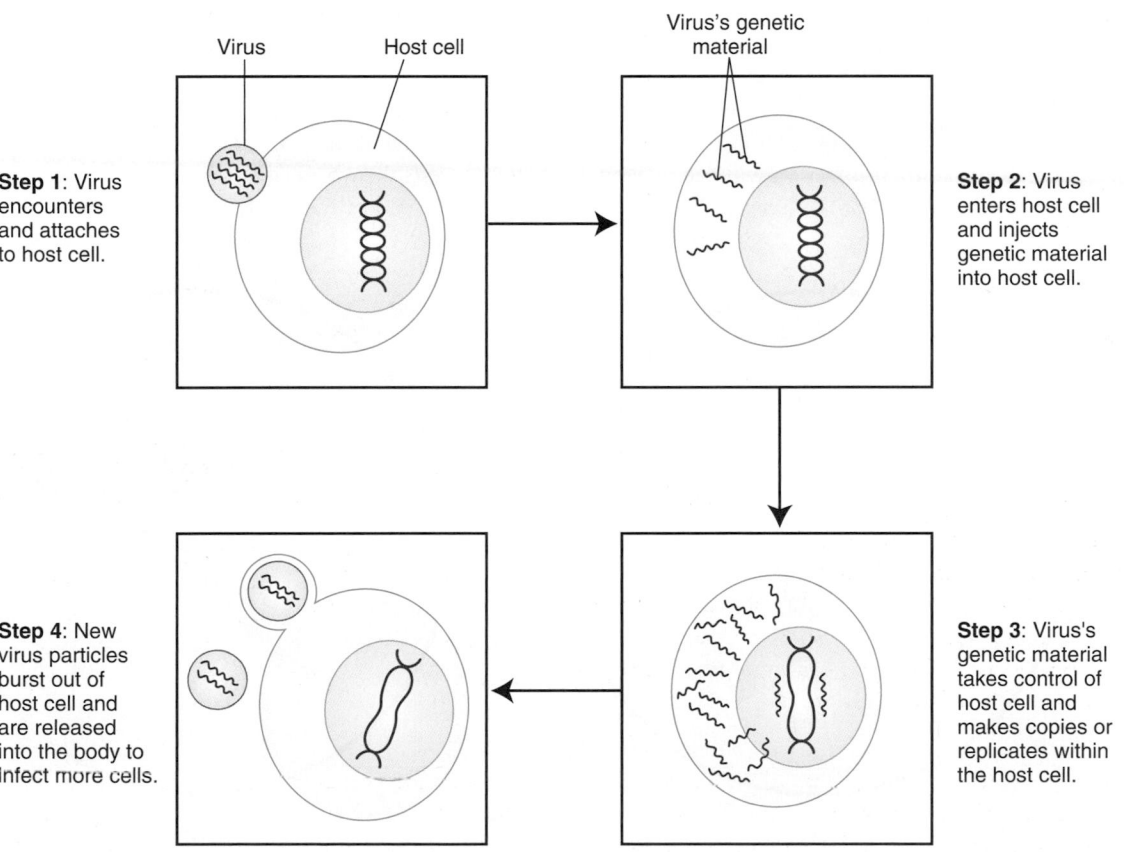

Virus Host cell

Virus's genetic material

Step 1: Virus encounters and attaches to host cell.

Step 2: Virus enters host cell and injects genetic material into host cell.

Step 4: New virus particles burst out of host cell and are released into the body to infect more cells.

Step 3: Virus's genetic material takes control of host cell and makes copies or replicates within the host cell.

FIG 45-5 Life cycle of a virus.

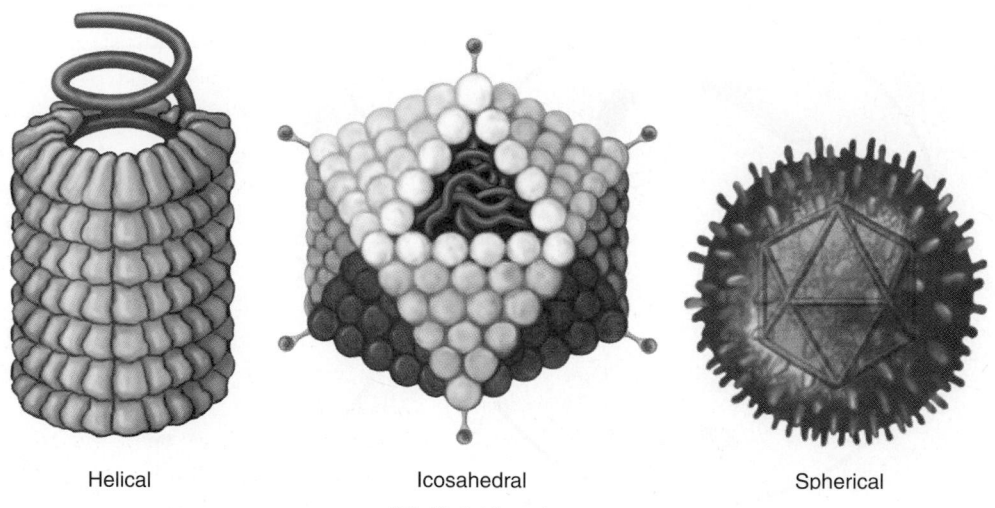

Helical   Icosahedral   Spherical

FIG 45-6 Virus shapes.

bacteria, breaking down organic material, and serving as a food source for other animals. Some protozoa are parasitic, which means they require another living organism in order to live and reproduce.

Human infections caused by protozoa are serious and can sometimes be difficult to diagnose because, unlike bacteria that simply divide to reproduce, protozoa have a life cycle that includes a trophozoite stage and a cyst stage. The trophozoite stage is considered the growth phase while the cyst stage is the dormant stage. During this dormant stage, the protozoa is protected from various environmental factors that may kill it. If a cyst is ingested by a human, the protozoa's life cycle begins and human infection will occur. Medically important protozoa include *Giardia lamblia, Trichomonas*

vaginalis, Pneumocystis carinii, Cryptosporidium, and *Plasmodium.* Various treatments for protozoal infections include metronidazole (Flagyl), tinidazole (Tindamax), and chloroquine (Aralen). (See Figure 45-8.)

A parasitic worm is a **parasite**, or a pathogen that requires another living organism to survive. These worms are not microscopic. However, they are commonly discussed with protozoa because many parasitic worm infections involve the ingestion of soil or water that may be contaminated with microscopic worm eggs. Most parasitic worms infect a human's intestinal tract; however, some can migrate to other body systems, such as the lungs and liver. If a person accidentally ingests the worm eggs, the eggs will hatch in the person's intestines and release a worm. Diagnosis is determined by

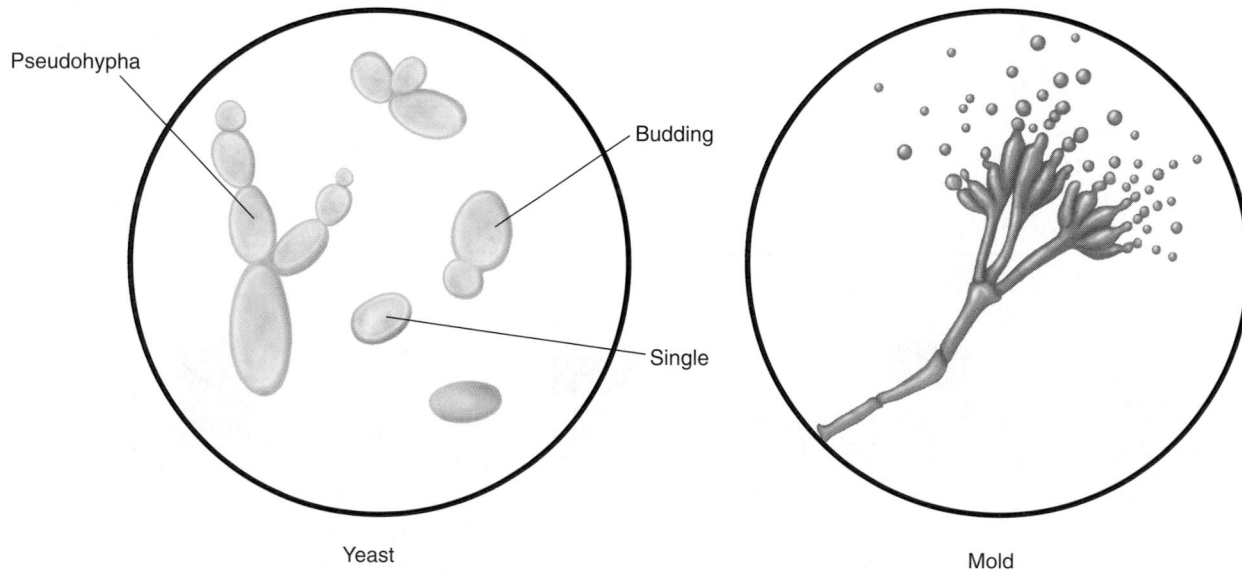

Pseudohypha

Budding

Single

Yeast   Mold

FIG 45-7 Fungi.

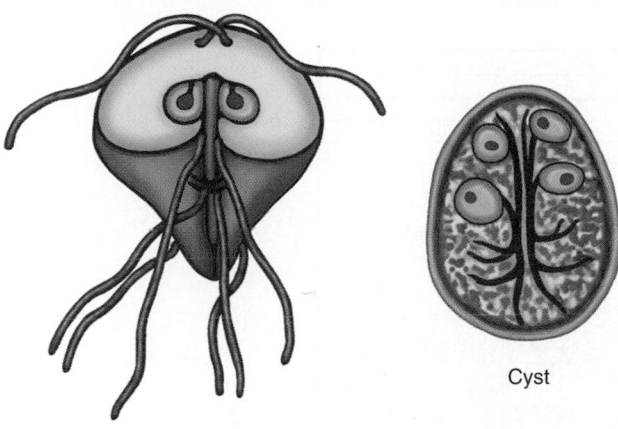

Trophozoite

Cyst

FIG 45-8 *Giardia lamblia.*

visual examination of parasite eggs in the feces or the capture of the actual worm. Commonly seen parasitic worm infections include *Enterobius vermicularis*, otherwise known as pinworm, and *Ascaris lumbricoides*. (See Figure 45-9.) Treatment of parasitic worm infections includes the use of medications such as albendazole (Albenza), mebendazole (Vermox), and niclosamide (Niclocide).

Microbiological Testing

Although many different types of microorganisms cause human infection and disease, only a few general tests are used to detect them, including:

- culture and sensitivity (C&S) test
- Gram stain
- fungal culture

- viral culture
- acid-fast bacillus (AFB) stain
- potassium hydroxide (KOH) stain
- ova and parasite (O&P) determination.

The specificity of the testing is not in the type of test, but, instead, in the body site or specimen type collected for testing. The most common test in the microbiology department is called a *culture and sensitivity* (C&S) test. In order to ensure accurate, specific results from a C&S test, the medical assistant must indicate the site from which the specimen was collected. For example, if the patient comes in with a rash on his lower right arm that looks infected, the physician will order a C&S test of the rash. The medical assistant should collect the specimen from the arm, check off *culture and sensitivity* on the requisition slip, and write in the site area *infected rash from lower right arm*. The site of the specimen tells the microbiologist exactly how to process the specimen in order to cultivate the suspected pathogen. In addition to the C&S test, another commonly ordered test is a Gram stain. Although a Gram stain helps identify bacteria that have already grown in a culture, it also helps the microbiologist observe potential bacteria directly from the patient's specimen. (See Figure 45-10.)

Bacterial Culture

A bacterial **culture** is the most common test performed by a typical hospital microbiology laboratory. A physician can request a viral or fungal culture of a patient sample; however, these requests require highly specialized processing and testing. If a physician suspects a person has a protozoal or parasitic gastrointestinal infection, she should order an ova and parasite (O&P) examination of the patient's feces. Because the method of testing and the procedure for specimen collection may be different from collecting the typical specimen for a bacterial culture order, the medical assistant should contact

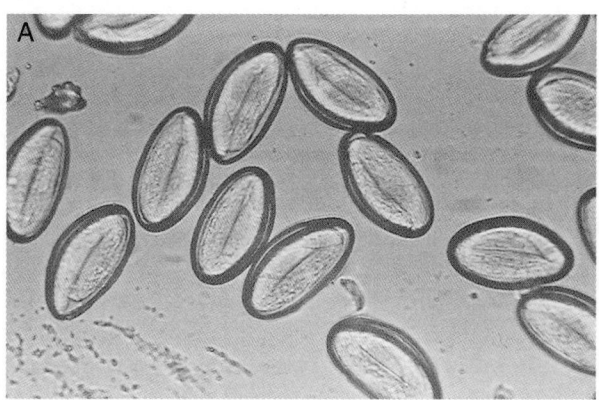

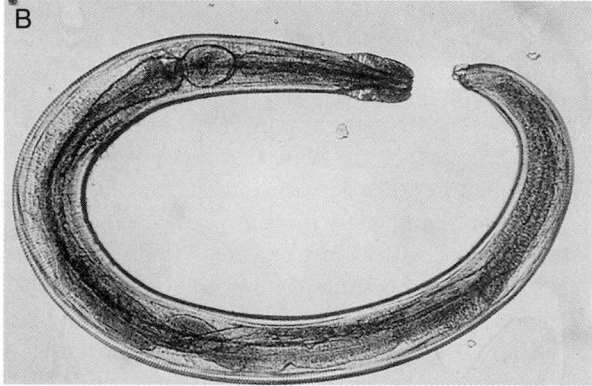

FIG 45-9 *Enterobius vermicularis.* (A) Egg stage. (From Leventhal/Cheadle: Medical Parasitology, 5th ed. FA Davis, Philadelphia, 2002, color plate #1, with permission.) (B) Worm stage. (From Leventhal/Cheadle: Medical Parasitology, 5th ed. FA Davis, Philadelphia, 2002, color plate #5E, with permission.)

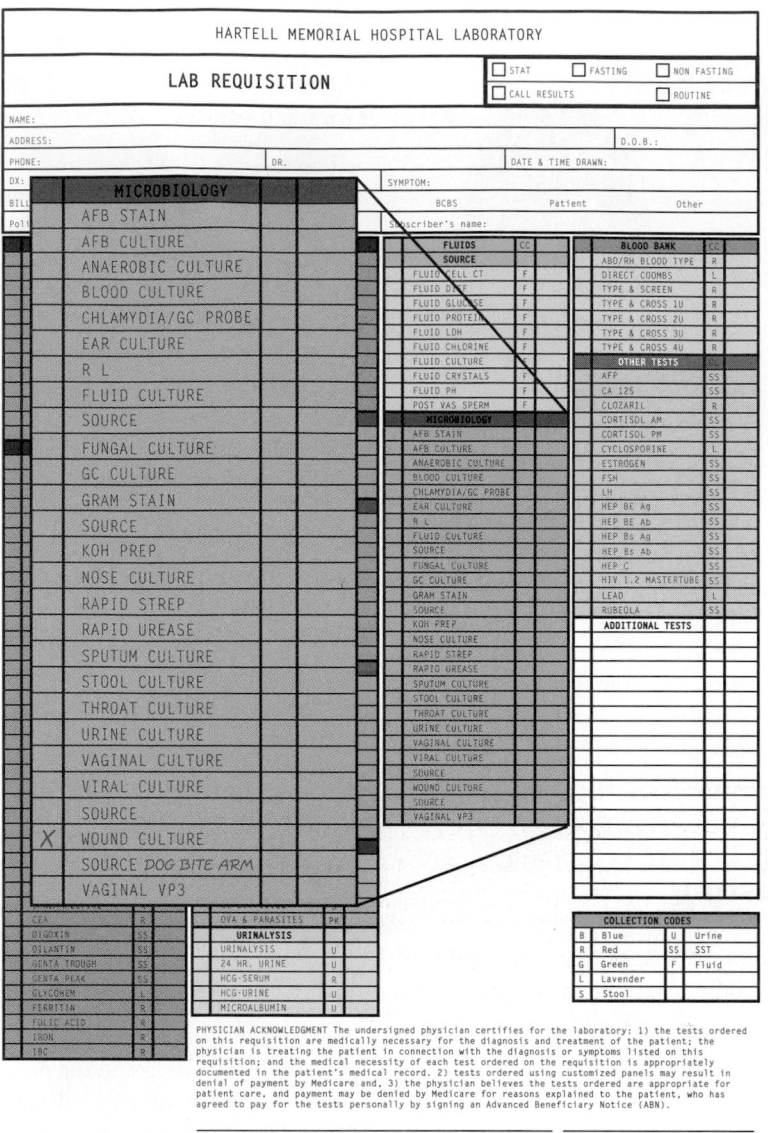

HARTELL MEMORIAL HOSPITAL LABORATORY

LAB REQUISITION

☐ STAT ☐ FASTING ☐ NON FASTING
☐ CALL RESULTS ☐ ROUTINE

NAME:
ADDRESS: D.O.B.:
PHONE: DR.   DATE & TIME DRAWN:
DX: SYMPTOM:
BILL   BCBS   Patient   Other
Poli   Subscriber's name:

MICROBIOLOGY

MICROBIOLOGY		
AFB STAIN		
AFB CULTURE		
ANAEROBIC CULTURE		
BLOOD CULTURE		
CHLAMYDIA/GC PROBE		
EAR CULTURE		
R L		
FLUID CULTURE		
SOURCE		
FUNGAL CULTURE		
GC CULTURE		
GRAM STAIN		
SOURCE		
KOH PREP		
NOSE CULTURE		
RAPID STREP		
RAPID UREASE		
SPUTUM CULTURE		
STOOL CULTURE		
THROAT CULTURE		
URINE CULTURE		
VAGINAL CULTURE		
VIRAL CULTURE		
SOURCE		
X WOUND CULTURE		
SOURCE *DOG BITE ARM*		
VAGINAL VP3		

FLUIDS	CC
SOURCE	
FLUID CELL CT	F
FLUID DIFF	F
FLUID GLUCOSE	F
FLUID PROTEIN	F
FLUID LDH	F
FLUID CHLORINE	F
FLUID CULTURE	
FLUID CRYSTALS	F
FLUID PH	F
POST VAS SPERM	F

MICROBIOLOGY	
AFB STAIN	
AFB CULTURE	
ANAEROBIC CULTURE	
BLOOD CULTURE	
CHLAMYDIA/GC PROBE	
EAR CULTURE	
R L	
FLUID CULTURE	
SOURCE	
FUNGAL CULTURE	
GC CULTURE	
GRAM STAIN	
SOURCE	
KOH PREP	
NOSE CULTURE	
RAPID STREP	
RAPID UREASE	
SPUTUM CULTURE	
STOOL CULTURE	
THROAT CULTURE	
URINE CULTURE	
VAGINAL CULTURE	
VIRAL CULTURE	
SOURCE	
WOUND CULTURE	
SOURCE	
VAGINAL VP3	

BLOOD BANK	CC
ABO/RH BLOOD TYPE	R
DIRECT COOMBS	L
TYPE & SCREEN	R
TYPE & CROSS 1U	R
TYPE & CROSS 2U	R
TYPE & CROSS 3U	R
TYPE & CROSS 4U	R

OTHER TESTS	
AFP	SS
CA 125	SS
CLOZARIL	R
CORTISOL AM	SS
CORTISOL PM	SS
CYCLOSPORINE	L
ESTROGEN	SS
FSH	SS
LH	SS
HEP BE Ag	SS
HEP BE Ab	SS
HEP Bs Ag	SS
HEP Bs Ab	SS
HEP C	SS
HIV 1.2 MASTERTUBE	SS
LEAD	L
RUBEOLA	SS

ADDITIONAL TESTS	

CEA	R
DIGOXIN	SS
DILANTIN	SS
GENTA TROUGH	SS
GENTA PEAK	SS
GLYCOHEM	L
FERRITIN	R
FOLIC ACID	R
IRON	R
IBC	R

OVA & PARASITES	PK

URINALYSIS	
URINALYSIS	U
24 HR. URINE	U
HCG-SERUM	R
HCG-URINE	U
MICROALBUMIN	U

COLLECTION CODES				
B	Blue	U	Urine	
R	Red	SS	SST	
G	Green	F	Fluid	
L	Lavender			
S	Stool			

PHYSICIAN ACKNOWLEDGMENT The undersigned physician certifies for the laboratory: 1) the tests ordered on this requisition are medically necessary for the diagnosis and treatment of the patient; the physician is treating the patient in connection with the diagnosis or symptoms listed on this requisition; and the medical necessity of each test ordered on the requisition is appropriately documented in the patient's medical record. 2) tests ordered using customized panels may result in denial of payment by Medicare and, 3) the physician believes the tests ordered are appropriate for patient care, and payment may be denied by Medicare for reasons explained to the patient, who has agreed to pay for the tests personally by signing an Advanced Beneficiary Notice (ABN).

SIGNATURE   DATE

FIG 45-10 Laboratory requisition slip with microbiological tests.

the clinical laboratory for the proper collection procedure for a viral or fungal culture request or O&P determination.

There are a few ways that the testing performed in the microbiology department of the clinical laboratory differs from tests performed in other departments, such as hematology and chemistry. First, while most testing in hematology and chemistry departments involves blood samples, the majority of microbiological testing involves body substances other than blood. Second, specimen processing is more involved in microbiological testing. Most hematological or chemistry testing is done by putting the blood sample in an autoanalyzer; microbiological specimens require specialized cultures that involve placing the specimen on various culture media and then putting them in a temperature-controlled environment for 24 to 72 hours. The culture medium's main ingredient is agar, a gel-like substance. Thus, the medium is commonly known as an *agar plate*. It also contains various substances that the bacteria need in order to grow (if present in the patient sample). Some of the common growth substances used in manufacturing commercially prepared culture media include glucose, sucrose, maltose, and sheep's blood. (See Figure 45-11.) The laboratory maintains the required temperature-controlled environment by using an incubator. Because most pathogenic bacteria grow best at body temperature (37°C), the incubator is usually set to 37°C. (See Figure 45-12.)

Finally, the laboratory tests typical blood samples when they arrive and usually generates a final report within a few interprets the bacterial growth, identifies the type or types of bacteria present, and generates a laboratory report indicating the name of the pathogen and the quantity present in the sample. (See Figure 45-13.)

Antimicrobial Susceptibility Testing

Susceptibility is the degree to which a microorganism's growth can be inhibited by an **antimicrobial agent**, which is any chemical substance (such as an antibiotic) that has the ability to kill or stop the growth of a microorganism. A pathogenic bacteria that is reported as being susceptible to ciprofloxacin (Cipro), for example, indicates that this drug will kill or inhibit the growth of the bacteria and may be used to treat the patient's infection. **Resistance** refers to a microorganism's ability to withstand the effects of an antimicrobial agent. Thus, a drug to which bacteria are reported as *resistant* should not be used to treat a patient's infection because the test demonstrates that the drug does not kill or inhibit the growth of the bacteria.

When a culture enables the microbiologist to identify a pathogenic bacteria in a patient specimen, the microbiologist will most likely perform an antimicrobial susceptibility test. This test determines the correct antimicrobial agent to use to kill the pathogen. An antibiotic is a type of antimicrobial agent. There are two types of antimicrobial susceptibility testing in the microbiological laboratory: the disk-diffusion method and minimum inhibitory concentration (MIC) method.

The *disk-diffusion method* is an older, more manual method that involves diluting the pathogenic bacteria and spreading the sample onto the surface of a Mueller-Hinton

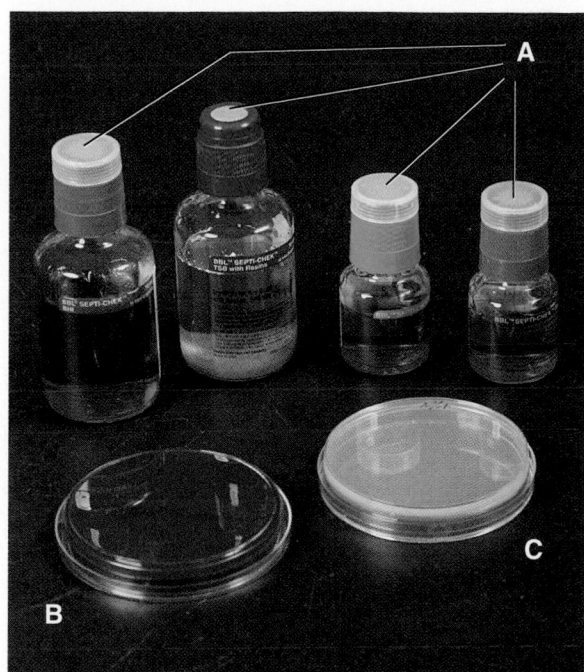

FIG 45-11 Culture media used in the microbiology laboratory. (A) Blood culture bottles. (B) Blood agar plate. (C) Nutrient agar plate.

hours. However, the laboratory may wait up to 72 hours to generate a final patient report on a microbiological specimen because of the bacteria's **incubation period**, or the time the bacteria need to multiply and grow. If bacteria are present in the patient sample, colonies of bacteria will become visible on the culture media. The microbiologist then identifies and

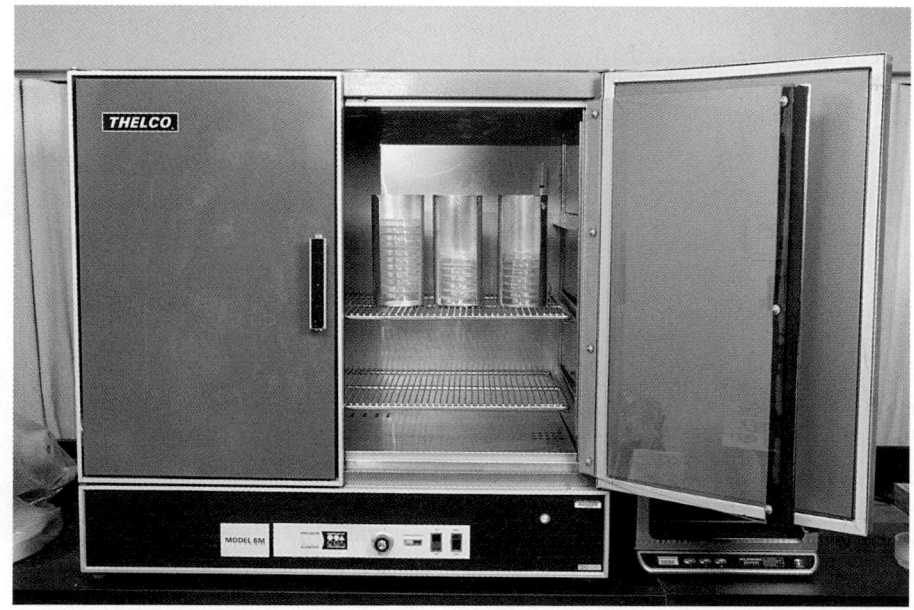

FIG 45-12 Typical microbiological incubator in which the agar plates are placed.

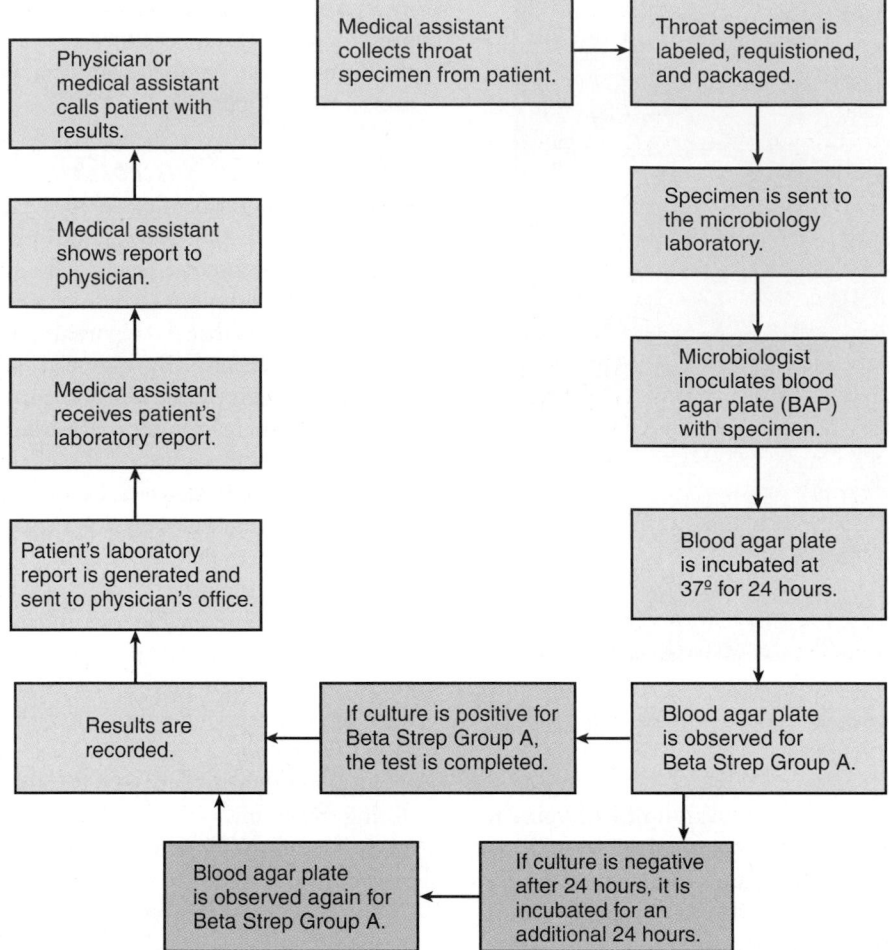

FIG 45-13 Life cycle of a throat culture.

agar medium. Then, individual paper discs that are impregnated with a known concentration of an antibiotic are placed on the agar plate. Usually five to ten antibiotics are tested against one known pathogenic bacteria. The microbiologist sets the agar plate in the incubator for 18 to 24 hours and then observes the plate to see if a zone of inhibition appears around any of the antibiotic discs. (See Figure 45-14.) The microbiologist then measures each zone and lists the susceptibility of the pathogen to each antibiotic qualitatively as *sensitive, moderately susceptible,* or *resistant,* based on guidelines developed by the National Committee for Clinical Laboratory Standards (NCCLS).

The MIC is a more advanced and, usually, automated method of determining an antimicrobial agent's usefulness against certain bacteria. However, the MIC tests only for antibiotics and not other antimicrobial agents. Thus, it is useful when testing for susceptibility to bacteria but not viruses and other pathogens. Instead of using an agar medium for testing, the MIC involves the use of a plastic,

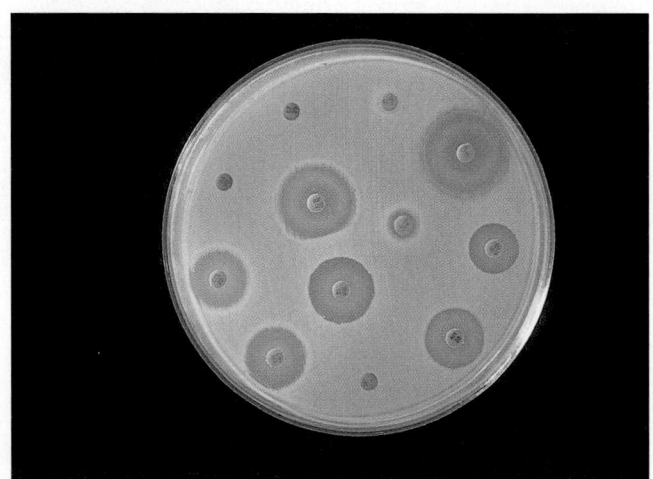

FIG 45-14 Disk-diffusion method for antimicrobial susceptibility testing. (From Bartlet. *Diagnostic Bacteriology*. FA Davis, Philadelphia, 2000, color plate #54, with permission)

square panel with rows of wells. Each well has a predetermined dilution of antibiotic as provided by the manufacturer and is labeled with the antibiotic name and the dilution. The microbiologist introduces the pathogenic bacteria suspended in sterile saline solution into each well, incubates the panel for 24 to 48 hours, and then looks at each well to see if there is growth, determined by a cloudiness within the well. A well that is clear is considered *no-growth*, which means that the pathogen is susceptible to the effects of the antibiotic in that well. The no-growth well with the lowest dilution of an antibiotic is considered the *minimum inhibitory concentration (MIC)*, or the lowest level of antibiotic that will be effective against the pathogen. The microbiologist reports the MIC dilution number for each antibiotic tested.

Although the pathogen may be isolated prior to MIC testing, it may not be identified. Thus, sometimes MIC testing involves identification of the pathogen in the patient sample. In such a case, the microbiologist will use a special panel from the manufacturer, called an *ID-MIC panel*, that will also include wells in an *identification section*. The identification section is a series of wells that contain different chemicals that may change color, depending on the type of bacteria tested. The microbiologist will analyze the various color change patterns in the wells and identify the pathogen. (See Figure 45-15.)

Regardless of the method, the microbiologist generates a report that will indicate to the physician the best antimicrobial agents to use to treat the patient's infection. (See Figure 45-16.) The physician will read the entire susceptibility report and make a decision based on the patient's condition and his medical history of tolerance or allergy to antimicrobial agents, if any. The report will usually identify the pathogen as *susceptible, moderately susceptible,* or *resistant*. Some bacteria are highly resistant to most antimicrobial agents and, thus, create a dilemma for physicians when

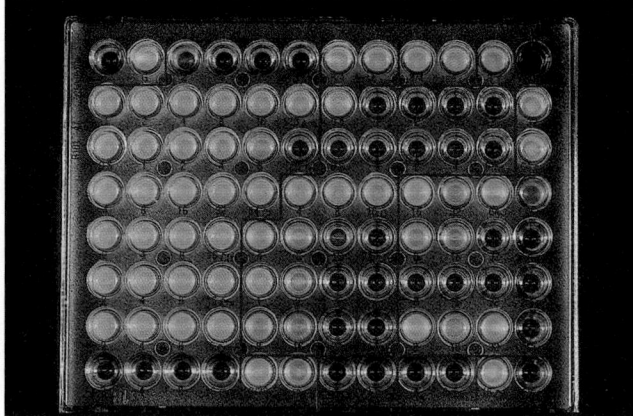

FIG 45-15 MIC test for antimicrobial susceptibility on bacteria. (From Bartlet. *Diagnostic Bacteriology*. FA Davis, Philadelphia, 2000, color plate #71, with permission)

prescribing a drug to treat infections caused by those bacteria. (See *MRSA*, page 950.)

Microbiology Procedures

Proper specimen collection procedures are the first step in accurate patient specimen testing. Most POLs have a specimen collection procedure manual that explains the correct procedure. To ensure proper collection, the medical assistant should be sure to select the proper site, use the proper collection swab and container, provide a complete requisition slip, and, finally, package and transport the specimen appropriately. When the laboratory receives the specimen, the microbiologist will determine the adequacy of the specimen. If she finds it to be inadequate for any reason, she will reject it. (See *Specimen rejection*, page 951.)

Specimen Collection for Microbiological Analysis

Microbiological testing can analyze almost any body tissue, fluid, or secretion. Specimens routinely collected using a sterile culture swab include:

- eye drainage, usually to detect bacteria that cause conjunctivitis
- ear drainage, possibly to confirm serous otitis media or fungal infection
- throat specimen, typically to detect beta *Streptococcus* group A (See *Procedure 45-1: Collecting a throat specimen for microbiological testing*, page 951.)
- urogenital specimen, typically to detect a sexually transmitted disease (STD)
- rectal specimen, sometimes collected from babies to detect a food-borne illness
- wound drainage, such as drainage from a rash, an infected surgical incision, and an animal bite, to detect various kinds of bacteria. (See *Procedure 45-2: Collecting a wound specimen for culture*, page 952.)

Specimens routinely collected using a sterile container include:

- urine, to detect infections of the urinary tract, bladder, or kidneys
- blood, to detect any bacteria that have entered the bloodstream and caused bacteremia
- sputum, to confirm pneumonia (See *Procedure 45-3: Collecting a sputum specimen for culture*, pages 952 and 953.)
- feces, to confirm food-borne illness (See *Stool specimen collection*, page 953.)
- body fluids, such as ascites, peritoneal fluid, and synovial fluid, to detect any pathogen that may have infected these normally sterile body fluids.

```
══════════════════ PATIENT LABORATORY REPORT ══════════════════
```

HARTELL MEMORIAL HOSPITAL LABORATORY

Name: Seth Banas   Sex: M   Date ordered: 08/30/2008
M/R#: 032608   Date collected: 08/30/2008
D.O.B.: 05/02/63   45   Time collected: 0
Physician: Greer, R.   Date tested: 08/30/2008
Location: Outpatient   Time tester: 21:41
                                                  Accession Number: 0007413225

CULTURE WOUND
SOURCE: Abdominal wound
GRAM STAIN:
    10–20 WBC
    few gram-negative rods

<<<<<<<<<<24 HOUR PRELIMINARY REPORT>>>>>>>>>>

ORGANISM #1: Many growth gram negative rods

<<<<<<<<<<48 HOUR FINAL REPORT>>>>>>>>>>

COLONY COUNT: Many
ORGANISM: Enterobacter aerogenes

drug	MIC	Interpretation
ampicillin	>16	R
ampicillin/sulbactam	16/18	I
cefazolin	>16	R
cepotetan	≤8	S
ceftriaxone	≤8	S
cefuroxime	>16	R
ciprofloxacin	≤1	S
gentamicin	≤1	S
nitrofurantoin	–	–
TMP/SMX	2/38	S
levofloxacin	≤1	S
pipercillin/tazobact	16/4	S

S = Susceptible   MS = Moderately Susceptible   I = Intermediate   R = Resistant

FIG 45-16 Antimicrobial susceptibility report.

MRSA

Some strains of *Staphylococcus aureus* are resistant to most forms of penicillin, such as methicillin and nafcillin. These strains are commonly known as *methicillin-resistant Staphylococcus aureus (MRSA)*. When the microbiology laboratory identifies a strain of *S. aureus* as resistant to methicillin, it is most likely resistant to all other antibiotics. Patients identified as infected with this highly resistant strain of bacteria have an increased chance of mortality because there may be no other antibiotic to treat the infection.

As is with other types of specimens, the medical assistant must take care when collecting and processing a microbiological specimen to avoid contaminating the specimen or exposing herself to a pathogenic microorganism. The medical assistant should observe standard precautions at all times:

- Wear appropriate personal protective devices, such as gloves, gowns, and a mask.
- Upon collection, properly label the specimen with the patient's name, the date and time of the culture, and the specific site of the specimen.
- Put the specimen in a biohazard transport bag.
- Wash her hands after specimen collection.

Specimen rejection

Clinical laboratory personnel will always assess a patient specimen submitted to the laboratory for microbiological testing before processing the specimen. If the laboratory determines that a specimen is unacceptable for processing, the microbiologist will usually call the medical office to tell them to collect another specimen as well as send a written report about the reason for specimen rejection. Some common reasons for rejection include:

- unlabeled or improperly labeled specimen
- delayed transport
- improper container (nonsterile)
- oropharyngeal contaminated sputum
- unsuitable specimen (such as a request for an anaerobic culture on a specimen collected on an aerobic swab)
- quantity not sufficient (QNS).

In addition to these precautions, the medical assistant should remember that proper timing is essential in many ways to successful collection and analysis of microbiological specimens. For example, the laboratory will decide if it needs optional specimens based on the infectious process being tested and the laboratory's ability to process the specimens in the required time frame. In addition, the first early morning sputum and urine specimens are optimal for recovery of pathogens. Although specimens collected at other times are acceptable, the medical assistant should consider the best method for achieving the desired result. Finally, the physician determines blood culture timing. The standard order for blood culture collection is three cultures within a 24-hour period. (See *Completing a microbiological requisition slip*, page 953.)

Microbiological Testing Performed in the POL

The most common microbiological tests performed in the physician's office laboratory (POL) is the rapid streptococcal test. The second most common test in the POL is a complete throat culture. Both tests detect the presence of the

---

PROCEDURE 45-1

Collecting a throat specimen for microbiological testing

Task
Collect a throat specimen for culture or rapid *Strep* testing.

Conditions
- Disposable examination gloves
- Tongue depressor
- Sterile culture swab
- Label
- Laboratory requisition slip
- Biohazard specimen transport bag
- Biohazard waste container

Standards
In the time specified and within the scoring parameters determined by the instructor, the student will successfully collect a throat specimen for culture or rapid *Strep* testing.

Performance Standards
1. Greet and identify your patient. Introduce yourself and explain the procedure to prevent errors and ease patient anxiety.
2. Wash or sanitize your hands to ensure infection control and gather supplies.
3. Position the patient in an upright, sitting position and adjust the light if necessary to maximize the viewing of and access to the patient's oropharynx.
4. Put on the gloves and mask per standard precautions. Instruct the patient to open his mouth widely.
5. Remove the swab from the tube. While depressing the patient's tongue with a tongue depressor, swab the back of the patient's throat and tonsils, taking care to thoroughly swab areas that appear inflamed or covered in exudate. Also take care to avoid touching the patient's tongue or teeth to ensure accuracy of results.
6. Place the swab back in the tube and crush the transport media ampule to moisten and preserve the specimen.
7. Dispose of the tongue blade in the waste container to ensure infection control. Apply the label to the culture tube and attach the completed requisition slip per laboratory policy to ensure timely processing of the specimen.
8. Remove the gloves and mask and wash your hands to ensure infection control. Document the procedure to ensure accuracy of the medical record.

Date	
06/11/08: 9:35 a.m.	Sputum specimen collected and sent to lab for culture. ———————————————————— S. Gonzalez, CMA

PROCEDURE 45-2

Collecting a wound specimen for culture

Task
Collect a wound specimen for culture.

Conditions
- Sterile culture swab
- Label
- Laboratory requisition slip
- Biohazard specimen transport bag
- Disposable examination gloves
- Gown or laboratory coat with a zipper or button closure
- Biohazard waste container

Standards
In the time specified and within the scoring parameters determined by the instructor, the student will successfully collect a wound specimen for culture.

Performance Standards
1. Assemble the supplies. Advance preparation facilitates efficiency during the procedure.
2. Greet and identify your patient. Introduce yourself and explain the procedure to prevent errors and ease patient anxiety.
3. Wash or sanitize your hands to ensure infection control.
4. Clean and decontaminate the surrounding skin area to avoid contaminating the specimen with normal skin flora.

5. Swab the infected area, being sure to swab any purulent discharge. Purulent discharge contains pathogenic organisms.
6. Properly insert the swab into the collection tube and activate the transport medium by squeezing the bottom of the tube to moisten and preserve the specimen.
7. To ensure timely processing of the test, label the culture swab with the patient's name, the date and time, and the specific site of the specimen and place it in the proper biohazard transport bag.
8. Complete the laboratory requisition slip and attach it to the specimen bag, according to facility policy. Send the specimen to the laboratory in a timely manner. A lost or missing requisition slip will delay specimen processing, which may compromise the accuracy of test results.
9. Properly dispose of all supplies and wash your hands to ensure infection control.
10. Document the procedure to ensure the accuracy of the medical record.

Date	
02/07/08; 11:15 a.m.	*Throat specimen collected and sent to lab for culture.* ―――― ――――――――――――――――――― *S. Gonzalez, CMA*

PROCEDURE 45-3

Collecting a sputum specimen for culture

Task
Collect a sputum specimen for culture.

Conditions
- Sterile specimen cup
- Label
- Laboratory requisition slip
- Approved specimen container bag
- Disposable examination gloves
- Face shield or mask and goggles
- Gown or laboratory coat with a zipper or button closure
- Biohazard waste container
- Cup of water

Standards
In the time specified and within the scoring parameters determined by the instructor, the student will successfully collect a sputum specimen for culture.

Performance Standards
1. Assemble the supplies. Advance preparation facilitates efficiency during the procedure. Complete the label and affix it to the specimen cup (not to the lid) to ensure that the specimen will remain labeled and will not get confused with other specimens in the laboratory after the lid is removed.
2. Greet and identify your patient. Introduce yourself and explain the procedure to prevent errors and ease patient anxiety.
3. Wash or sanitize your hands and apply the face shield or mask and goggles to ensure infection control.
4. Hand a glass of water to the patient and ask her to rinse her mouth to remove food particles from her mouth.
5. Instruct the patient to take two deep breaths, cough deeply, and spit the sputum into the cup. Deep

PROCEDURE 45-3—cont'd

coughing is needed to bring secretions up from the lungs. Saliva from the mouth will not provide an adequate specimen.

6. Make sure that no one touches the inner surfaces of the cup or lid to ensure that external microorganisms do not enter the cup to compromise the results, and apply the lid and secure it snugly to ensure that the specimen does not leak out. Place the specimen cup into the specimen bag and seal it.

7. Affix the requisition slip to the specimen bag, according to facility policy, and send it to the laboratory in a timely manner. A lost or missing requisition slip will

delay specimen processing, which may compromise the accuracy of test results.

8. Properly dispose of all supplies and wash your hands to ensure infection control. Document the procedure to ensure accuracy of the medical record.

Date	
06/12/08: 9:10 a.m.	Infected surgical wound. Specimen collected for culture and sent to lab. ------------------------- S. Gonzalez, CMA

---

bacteria beta *Streptococcus* group A, also known as *Streptococcus pyogenes*, in throat specimens. *Streptococcus* group A is the causative agent for streptococcal throat infection, commonly called *Strep throat* or *streptococcal pharyngitis*.

Rapid Streptococcal Test

Early diagnosis and treatment of streptococcal throat infection is important because the pathogen can develop into a more severe systemic infection, such as scarlet fever or rheumatic fever. Most commercially prepared streptococcal test kits are CLIA-waived, are easy to perform, and provide results in 5 minutes. The medical assistant should familiarize herself with the quality control steps required for the kit as well as the proper procedure for performing the test. (See *Procedure 45-4: Performing a rapid streptococcal test*, page 954 and 955.)

Throat Culture Test

Although most commercial rapid streptococcal test kits are extremely sensitive for the pathogen that causes streptococcal throat infection, these kits may sometimes give a false-negative result. For this reason, manufacturer's instructions may instruct the physician to order a throat culture if the patient's clinical assessment warrants the test. For this

 Patient Education

Stool Specimen Collection

A patient may be confused about how to collect a stool specimen for analysis and may feel uncomfortable discussing it. However, the medical assistant must explain the procedure clearly so that the patient can collect the specimen properly. The medical assistant should include these steps:

1. Using the plastic wrap, loosely line the outside of the toilet seat so that it will catch the specimen.

2. Do not collect the specimen from the toilet bowl because it may be contaminated with urine.

3. Use the plastic wrap to handle the stool and carefully slide the required amount of the specimen from the wrap into the container.

4. When collecting a specimen from an infant's diaper, line the diaper with plastic wrap as well. Because an infant's stool is commonly loose in consistency, it may be absorbed into the diaper's fibers; a specimen that contains diaper fibers would be unacceptable. Use the plastic wrap to handle the stool and carefully slide the specimen into the sterile container supplied by the office.

 Front office–Back office connection

Completing a Microbiological Requisition Slip

Usually, the clinical medical assistant is responsible for completing a laboratory requisition slip for microbiological testing. However, in a small office or on a busy day, the administrative medical assistant may be required to fill out the slip. Although the slip may not list the exact specimen type, it should always include an area where the medical assistant can indicate the specimen type. For instance, for a specimen collected from a wound caused by a dog bite, the medical assistant should indicate the cause of the wound instead of simply writing *wound on arm*. Such information is essential for the laboratory technologist, because wounds caused by a dog or cat bite may be infected with rare bacteria that a technologist may not normally attempt to detect when testing a specimen.

PROCEDURE 45-4

Performing a rapid streptococcal test

Task
Perform a rapid streptococcal test.

Conditions
- Commercial rapid streptococcal test kit
- Disposable examination gloves
- Gown or laboratory coat with a zipper or button closure
- Biohazard waste container

Standards
In the time specified and within the scoring parameters determined by the instructor, the student will successfully perform a rapid streptococcal test.

Performance Standards
1. Assemble the supplies and prepare the test kit. Advance preparation facilitates efficiency during the procedure. Run quality control procedures before testing the patient specimen. Quality control results must be within limits or the patient specimen cannot be tested.
2. Greet and identify your patient. Introduce yourself and explain the procedure to prevent errors and ease patient anxiety.
3. Wash or sanitize your hands and put on the gloves to ensure infection control.
4. Properly collect a throat specimen, taking care to avoid touching the patient's tongue or teeth with the swab because doing so will contaminate the specimen.
5. To ensure the accuracy of results, follow the manufacturer's directions and place the required number of reagent drops into the plastic testing tube.
6. Place the throat specimen swab into the swab chamber of the test cassette.

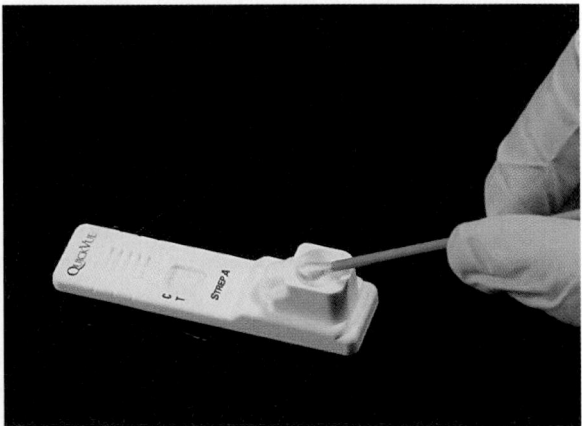

Placing the throat swab into the test cassette

7. Add the extraction solution to the chamber. Fluid should fill the chamber to the rim (approximately 10 drops). When the fluid has been added, watch for the liquid to move across the results window, which indicates that you performed the test properly.

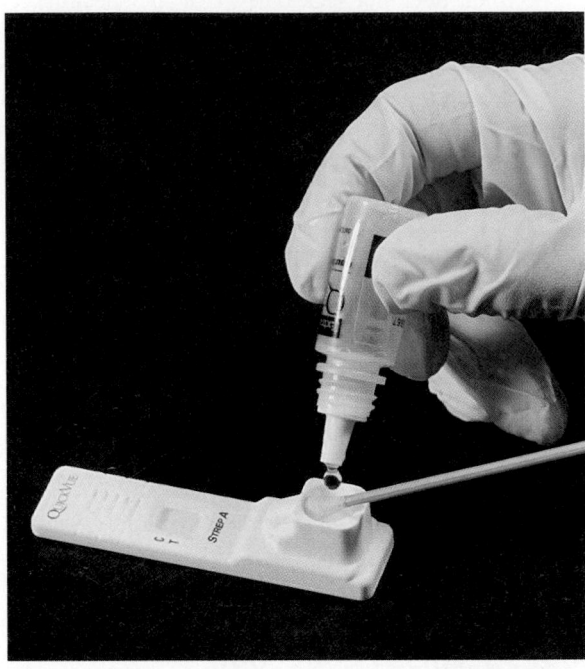

Putting the required amount of drops in the test cassette

8. Begin timing after adding the solution.
9. After 5 minutes, read the results using the manufacturer's result chart.

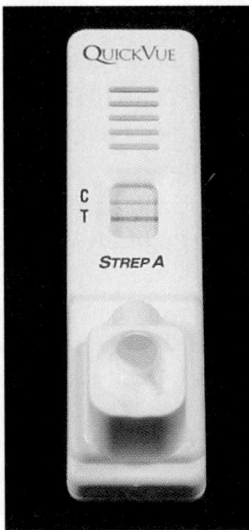

Positive result for beta *Streptococcus* group A

PROCEDURE 45-4—cont'd

10. Dispose of the throat swab and all testing supplies in a biohazard waste container to ensure infection control. Document the results in the patient's chart to ensure accuracy of the medical record.

Date	
06/13/08:	*Rapid strep test performed. Result: positive.* -----------------
10:30 a.m.	-- *S. Gonzalez, CMA*

---

reason, some medical offices prefer to perform the actual throat culture instead of conducting a rapid streptococcal test. Results of a throat culture will not be available for 24 to 48 hours—considerably longer than a rapid streptococcal test result. However, because a throat culture is a simple procedure that can be done in the POL, preliminary results may be available within 24 hours.

In addition to collection of a throat specimen, the medical assistant must also be familiar with the processing and testing of the actual culture procedure. (See *Procedure 45-5: Processing a throat culture.*)

PROCEDURE 45-5

Processing a throat culture

Task
Process a throat culture.

Conditions
- Sterile culture swab
- Tongue depressor
- Sheep blood agar media plate
- Sterile disposable inoculation plastic loop
- Bacitracin disc
- 37°C incubator
- Approved specimen container bag
- Disposable examination gloves
- Gown or laboratory coat with a zipper or button closure
- Biohazard waste container

Standards
In the time specified and within the scoring parameters determined by the instructor, the student will successfully process a throat culture.

Performance Standards
1. Assemble the supplies. Advance preparation facilitates efficiency during the procedure.
2. Greet and identify your patient. Introduce yourself and explain the procedure to prevent errors and ease patient anxiety.
3. Wash or sanitize your hands and put on the gloves to ensure infection control.
4. Properly collect the throat specimen, taking care to avoid touching the patient" tongue or teeth because doing so will contaminate the specimen.
5. Roll the swab onto the top quarter of the blood agar plate to reserve room on the plate to make subsequent

streaks and enable an accurate reading of the results. This streak is known as the *primary streak.*

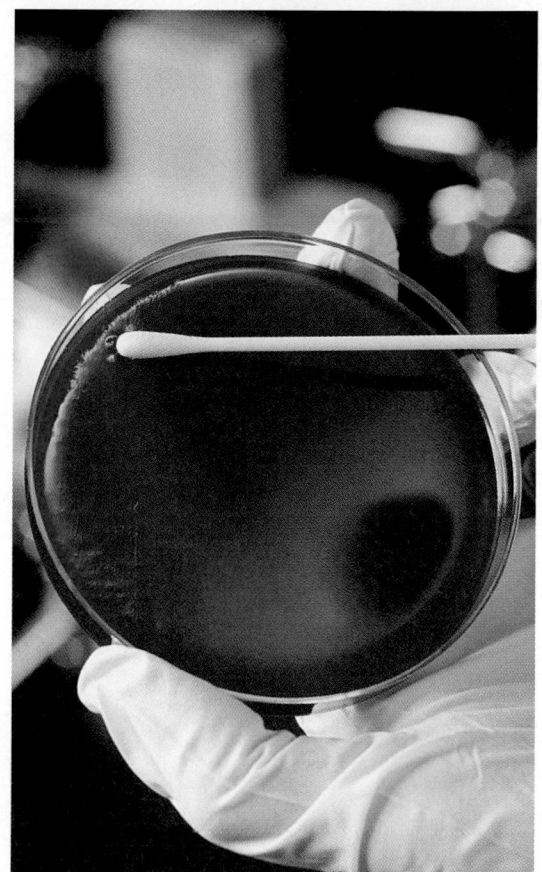

Rolling the throat swab onto the top quarter of the blood agar plate

Continued

PROCEDURE 45-5—cont'd

6. Using a sterile disposable plastic inoculation loop, spread the specimen from the primary streak into a secondary and tertiary streak to dilute the specimen and make it easier to read the results.

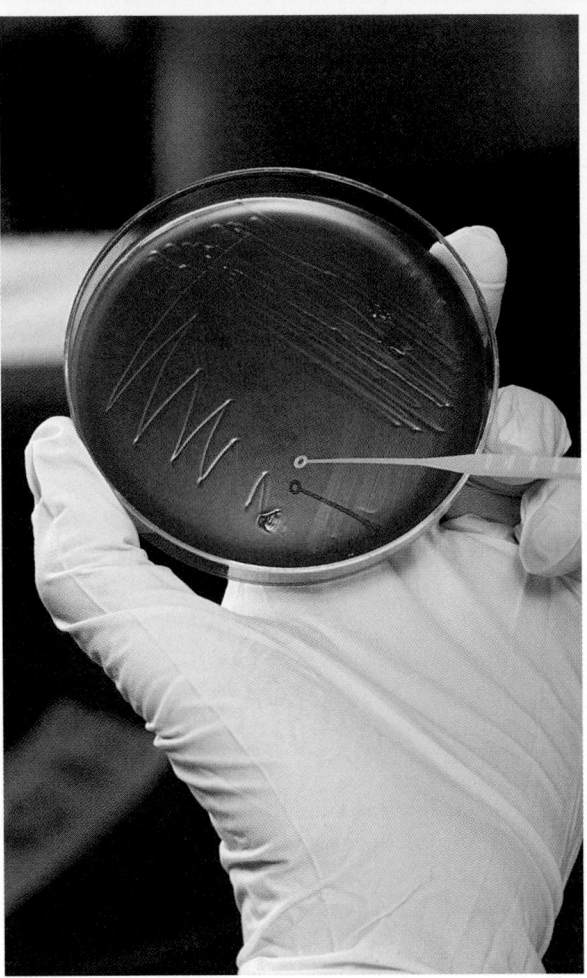

Making a third streak using the same disposable loop

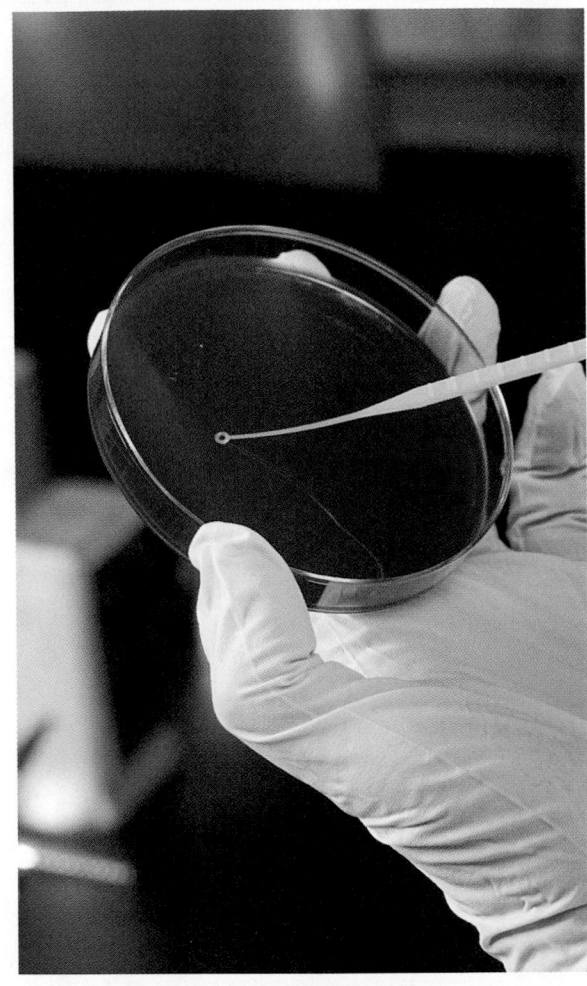

Streaking the primary streak into a secondary streak using a sterile disposable plastic loop

7. Place the bacitracin disc on the primary streak of the sheep blood agar plate.

PROCEDURE 45-5—cont'd

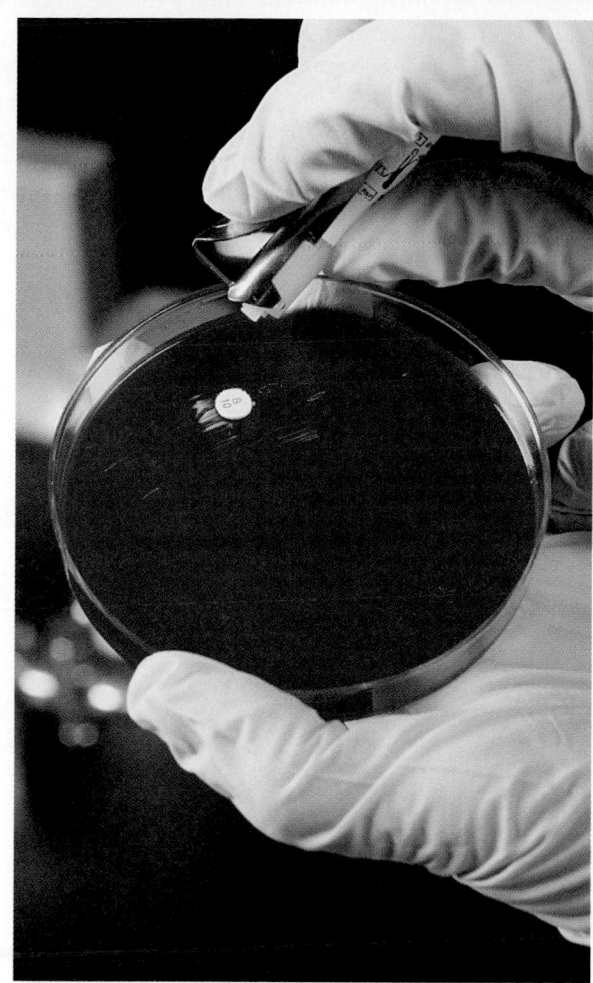

Applying the bacitracin disk to the primary streak

8. Incubate the sheep blood agar plate in the 37°C incubator for 18 to 24 hours to facilitate growth of the pathogen, if present. Do not incubate the specimen for more than 24 hours because overincubation could cause overgrowth of normal flora and may cause erroneous results.

9. After 18 to 24 hours, remove the sheep blood agar plate from the incubator and read the results. If beta *Streptococcus* group A is present, there will be a zone of inhibition around the bacitracin disc.

10. Properly dispose of all supplies and wash your hands to ensure infection control. Document the procedure in the patient's chart to ensure accuracy of the medical record.

Date	
06/27/08: 1:25 p.m.	Throat culture taken and processed. Culture will be read tomorrow and patient will be notified of results. ------------ --- S. Gonzalez, CMA

Chapter Summary

- Microbiology is the study of microorganisms. Although there are thousands of microorganisms in the world, only about 5% are pathogenic to humans.
- The scientists Van Leeuwenhoek, Jenner, Ehrlich, Pasteur, Koch, Lister, Gram, and Fleming made great contributions to the field of microbiology.
- Not all microorganisms are pathogenic. Some bacteria are considered normal flora because they reside in the body and do not cause harm and can be beneficial to the body.
- Bacteria are prokaryotic microorganisms that are classified according to their shape and Gram stain characteristics.
- There are three basic shapes of bacteria: cocci, bacilli, and spiral.
- Viruses are nonliving parasites that cause disease. They require a host to live and replicate.
- Prions are protein particles that, when introduced into the body, can cause an incurable condition.
- Fungi are eukaryotic microorganisms that can be unicellular or multicellular.
- Fungi are classified as yeasts or molds.
- Protozoa are eukaryotic microorganisms that inhabit soil and water.
- Many protozoa cause gastrointestinal infections.
- Parasitic worms start out as microscopic eggs but grow to be a macroscopic animal.
- The majority of testing performed in the microbiology department consists of such bacterial cultures as throat culture, sputum culture, and wound culture.
- Viral and fungal cultures require special collection and testing techniques.

- After a microbiologist isolates and identifies a pathogenic bacteria, she will perform an antimicrobial susceptibility test to help the physician determine which antibiotic will treat the specific infection.
- The rapid streptococcal test is the most commonly performed microbiological test in the POL.
- The throat culture test can also be performed in a POL but requires more specialized supplies, equipment, and interpretation than a rapid strep test.

Team Work Exercises

1. Divide into groups of 2 to 3 students. Your instructor will assign each group a different microbiological infection for your group to research. Please provide the following information in your report:
   a. name of the infection
   b. causative agent for the infection
   c. how the infection is diagnosed
   d. how the infection is treated.
2. Divide into groups of 2 to 3 students. Your instructor will assign a local medical office for your group to contact. Ask your assigned office about which method it is using to test for streptococcal throat infection (rapid streptococcal test kit, throat culture, or sending the specimen out to a reference laboratory). Ask the office the reason for its testing choice. Then compare your results with the class.

Case Studies

1. You just performed a rapid streptococcal test on Alyssa Gadois, a 4-year-old girl who did not hold still while you were taking the throat specimen. The quality control was in range, and her test result was negative. What is your next course of action?
2. Dr. Yang has just finished examining Gary Quinn's abdominal surgical wound. She has asked you to take a culture of the wound. Describe what you would do.

Resources

- American Society for Microbiology: *www.asm.org*
- Centers for Disease Control and Prevention: *www.cdc.gov*
- Clinical Laboratory Standards Institute: *www.nccls.org*
- Tortora, G.J., et al.: *Microbiology: An Introduction*, 9th ed. Menlo Park, CA.: Benjamin Cummings, 2007.

Bioemergency Response and Preparedness

Key Terms

bioterrorism
Intentional or threatened use of biological agents or toxins to produce death, disease, or fear in an individual or a population

bioterrorism agent
Any substance, such as a bacteria, virus, or other germ that is released during a bioterrorism attack

covert event
Unannounced event that involves the release of an agent or toxin without any advanced warning

epidemic
The occurrence of a disease or health-related event in which many individuals within an area or population are affected at the same time

influenza
Highly infectious acute respiratory infection that is characterized by a sudden onset of fever, chills, body aches, and cough

overt event
Attack that is announced prior to or after the release of the bioterrorism agent

pandemic
Occurrence of a disease that has reached epidemic proportions in many different parts of the world at the same time

pandemic flu
Virulent human flu that causes a global outbreak, or pandemic, of serious illness

Emergency Preparedness

Two of the largest threats to public health in the United States include a bioterrorism attack and an influenza pandemic. **Bioterrorism** is the intentional or threatened use of biological agents or toxins to produce death, disease, or fear in an individual or a population for political, religious, or personal reasons. A **pandemic** is the occurrence of a disease that has reached epidemic proportions in many different parts of the world at the same time. After the events of September 11, 2001, U.S. local, state, and federal governments began developing procedures and protocols in the event that either of these threats occurs. This proactive preparedness has in turn spurred preparedness planning by health care facilities, local school systems, colleges and universities, businesses, and individuals. Preparedness activities include planning responses to an attack or outbreak, monitoring an outbreak, determining methods of communicating with the public and emergency responders, and establishing diagnosis and treatment plans as well as evacuation plans.

Bioterrorism

The threat of a bioterrorism attack has been in the forefront of U.S. national security planning since the attacks on September 11. However, bioterrorism attacks are not something new to this era. In fact, they have occurred throughout history and as far back as 600 B.C.E., when the Assyrians poisoned the wells of their enemies with rye ergot. During American colonial times, colonists supplied a Native American tribe with blankets infected with smallpox, eventually wiping out the tribe.

Bioterrorism attacks can be classified as *overt* or *covert* events. An **overt event** is an attack that is announced prior to or after the release of the bioterrorism agent by the individual or group responsible. Such an announcement might name the agent that has been released as well as the location. An overt event may be a hoax; however, an emergency response must occur until the threat can be disproved. A **covert event** is an unannounced event that involves the release of an agent or toxin without advanced warning. If a covert event occurs, medical office staff may observe an increase in the number of patients with the same symptoms from unknown causes or an infection that is not normally seen in that area. Regardless of the nature of the potential attack, a rapid response and notification of the proper authorities is essential to the successful management of the attack.

Agents Used in Bioterrorism

A **bioterrorism agent** is any substance, such as a bacteria, virus, or other germ, that may be released during a bioterrorism attack. Agents involved in an attack may be biological or chemical. If an incident were to occur in a community, medical office personnel such as medical assistants, nurses, and physicians would most likely be the first heath care professionals to see patients who may have been exposed to such agents. Health care professionals must take some important steps if they suspect a patient has been exposed to a bioterrorism agent. The first step is to have knowledge of various bioterrorism agents and the infectious diseases they cause. Second, once a health care professional suspects that a patient has been exposed to a bioterrorism agent, she should limit exposure to the patient. She should isolate the patient from other patients and protect herself and other health care professionals by ensuring that they are wearing the proper personal protective equipment (PPE). (For a review of proper standard precautions as well as a list of PPE, please refer to Chapter 19, "Infection Control and Medical and Surgical Asepsis," page 285.)

Categories of Bioterrorism Agents

The Centers for Disease Control and Prevention (CDC) has separated bioterrorism agents into three categories based on the ease with which each can spread disease and the severity of that disease. The categories range from A to C, with category A considered the highest risk and category C an emerging threat for disease. (See *Bioterrorism agents*.) Individuals can suffer exposure to most of these agents through inhalation, ingestion, or physical contact.

Bioterrorism agents

The following table lists three categories of bioterrorism agents, as defined by the Centers for Disease Control and Prevention (CDC), along with the major characteristics of those agents and some examples of each.

Category	Characteristics	Example
Category A—highest risk to public health and national security	• Potential for mass casualty • Easily disseminated if aerosolized • Easily spread from person to person • Could cause high death rates • Causes high level of panic • Requires special action for public health preparedness	• *Bacillus anthracis*—causative agent of anthrax • *Clostridium botulinum*—causative agent of botulism • *Yersinia pestis*—causative agent of the plague • *Francisella tularensis*—causative agent of tularemia • *Variola major virus*—causative agent of smallpox
Category B—second highest risk to public and national security	• Moderately easy to spread • Results in moderate illness rates and low death rates • Requires specific enhancements of CDC's laboratory capacity and enhanced disease monitoring	• *Brucella species*—causative agent of brucellosis • *Coxiella burnetii*—causative agent of Q fever • *Salmonella species*—causative agent of salmonellosis • *Escherichia coli* O157:H7—causative agent of hemolytic uremic syndrome and food poisoning
Category C—third highest risk to public and national security	• Emerging pathogens • Easily available • Easily produced and spread • Potential for high illness and death rates	• *Mycobacterium tuberculosis*—causative agent of tuberculosis (TB) • Nipah virus • *Hantavirus*—causative agent of hemorrhagic fever or pneumonia

Laboratory Response Network

The key to identifying a possible threat to public health is the development of a network consisting of national, governmental, private reference, state public health, and local hospital laboratories. In 1999, the CDC, along with the Association of Public Health Laboratories (APHL), the Federal Bureau of Investigation (FBI), the Department of Defense (DOD), and each state's public health laboratories established a collaborative, voluntary system of laboratories called the *Laboratory Response Network (LRN) for Bioterrorism.* Staff at the laboratories in this network are trained in identifying and handling not only bioterrorism attacks but any other threat to public health, such as emerging infectious diseases and a possible pandemic caused by a known or unidentified microorganism.

The goals of the LRN are early detection and disease prevention. The role of clinical laboratories in early detection and disease prevention is critical to preventing or limiting the effects of a bioterrorism attack or a pandemic. These laboratories would be the first to isolate or identify microorganisms from such an event. They must develop the capability to rule out suspected microorganisms in a given specimen or send isolated microorganisms to another laboratory for identification. Development of a fully capable LRN is based on strengthening existing local, state, and federal public health laboratories and improving relationships among all laboratories in the network. The LRN organizes laboratories based on their diagnostic capabilities and safety facilities into a three-tiered network, including:

- federal laboratories
- reference laboratories
- hospital clinical laboratories.

Federal Laboratory

A federal laboratory is one that receives funding as well as direction from the federal government. These laboratories are able to perform specialized identification procedures and contain the highest level of biosafety isolation equipment to handle highly infectious agents. Laboratories such as the CDC, U.S. Army Medical Research Institute for Infectious Diseases (USAMRIID), and the Naval Medical Research Center (NMRC) are examples of federal laboratories. Most federal laboratories have the highest biosafety level designation from the CDC. (See *Laboratory biosafety levels.*)

Laboratory biosafety levels

The Centers for Disease Control and Prevention (CDC) developed biosafety levels to ensure the safe handling of materials in biological laboratories. A laboratory's biosafety level is determined based on several criteria, the most important of which is the agents isolated or tested in that laboratory. The more potentially dangerous an agent is, the higher the biosafety level classification for that laboratory. Other criteria address the type of personnel who can perform the testing, specialized training for laboratory personnel, facility management, decontamination practices, medical surveillance, safety equipment, and security procedures.

Biosafety Level 1

- Handle agents not known to consistently cause disease in most people and present minimal potential hazard to laboratory personnel, including *Escherichia coli, Bacillus subtilis,* and *Chlamydia* species
- No special facility or containment requirements
- Use of basic PPE

Biosafety Level 2

- Handle agents that pose a moderate hazard to laboratory personnel and the environment, including *Streptococcus pneumonia, Staphylococcus aureus,* and the rhinoviruses

- Specialized training in handling pathogenic agents for laboratory personnel
- Restricted access to laboratory
- Biosafety cabinets used when handling agents
- Medical surveillance provided and appropriate immunizations offered to laboratory personnel

Biosafety Level 3

- Handle agents that may cause serious or potentially lethal disease via inhalation exposure and may be exotic in nature, including *Mycobacterium tuberculosis, Rickettsia rickettsii,* West Nile virus, human immunodeficiency virus, and hepatitis B and C viruses

- Special training, handling, and environmental control requirements
  - Laboratory personnel with demonstrated proficiency in specialized procedures
  - Specialized clothing for laboratory personnel, such as scrub suits and coveralls, that must be put on prior to entering the laboratory
  - Self-closing laboratory doors with locks and sealed windows

Laboratory biosafety levels—cont'd

Biosafety Level 4

- Handle dangerous and exotic agents that pose a high risk of life-threatening disease and may have an unknown risk of transmission, including *Ebola* virus, Marburg virus, and hemorrhagic fever virus
- Special training, handling, and environmental control requirements
  - Special decontamination procedures followed by laboratory personnel

- Positive pressure protective suits worn by laboratory personnel, as necessary
- Strict clothing removal and changing procedures
- Strict medical surveillance and support of laboratory personnel
- Strictly controlled access to the laboratory
- For example, laboratories at the CDC and U.S. Army Medical Research Institute for Infectious Diseases

Reference Laboratory

A reference laboratory is able to perform some specialized biological agent identification procedures and may have a lower level of biosafety than federal laboratories. When a reference laboratory isolates a potential bioterrorism agent, proper procedure may include sending the isolate to a federal laboratory, such as the CDC, for additional specialized testing. Reference laboratories may be public health, private, or international (outside the United States) clinical laboratories as well as veterinary laboratories and laboratories that perform environmental testing, such as water and soil testing.

Hospital Clinical Laboratories

A hospital clinical laboratory may be the first facility to obtain a patient specimen that could contain a potential bioterrorism agent. Such a laboratory may be unable to rule out a potential bioterrorism agent and would need the assistance of a more specialized laboratory for further identification. Clinical laboratories include those in hospitals and larger clinics.

Bioterrorism Response and the Medical Assistant

A medical assistant can play a key role in the initial response to a suspected bioterrorism attack. Actions a medical assistant might take include initiating communication protocols as well as conducting specimen collection and transport. For example, if a physician suspects that her patient may have been exposed to a bioterrorism agent, she may ask the medical assistant to call the local hospital and health department to report the findings and transcribe and deliver instructions provided by the hospital or health department. The medical assistant must make sure that these essential contact numbers are easily accessible. In addition, the medical assistant may be required to collect a body specimen for testing.

Specimen procurement may include specialized collection, packaging, and transporting to a laboratory such as the CDC or state public health laboratory. The medical assistant must be sure to follow the exact directions for collection and processing of the specimen to ensure the integrity of the specimen and protection from the suspected bioterrorism agent. (See *Bioterrorism specimen collection and submission.*)

Bioterrorism specimen collection and submission

The medical assistant may collect many types of specimens to test for a suspected bioterrorism agent, including blood, stool, sputum, enema fluid, food samples, nasal swabs, bronchial or tracheal washings, biopsies, scabs, or vesicular fluid. The medical assistant should follow these guidelines when collecting and submitting a specimen that is suspected of containing a bioterrorism agent:

- Always note the specimen site and volume collected. Use the correct requisition form, specimen container, test kit, and shipping requirements for safe transport of the specimen.
- Submit good-quality specimens for analysis.
- Properly label all specimens for identification.
- Include a complete requisition form with all the necessary and pertinent patient health history and information with each specimen submitted.
- Do not attach the specimen to the requisition form or wrap the requisition form around the specimen.
- In serological testing, collect the specimen at the appropriate times and note in the form the time it was collected.
- Follow instructions for proper temperature control.

Continued

Bioterrorism specimen collection and submission—cont'd

- Transport or ship the specimen to the laboratory as soon as possible

- Make sure the correct laboratory name is printed on the return address label.

- Many state laboratories and departments of public health will supply collection and transport containers to medical offices. Make sure the medical office has plenty of these containers on hand.

- Follow proper state and federal biological hazardous material transportation guidelines if you are mailing the specimen.

- If you have a question about how to collect or process a specimen, call the laboratory *before* collecting it to get the exact directions.

Pandemic Influenza

Three **pandemic influenza** outbreaks have occurred in the 20th century. The most severe, the Spanish influenza pandemic, occurred in 1918 and caused around 500,000 deaths in the United States and 40 million deaths worldwide. Other pandemics include the 1957 Asian flu and the 1968 Hong Kong flu pandemics. (See *Epidemic or pandemic?*)

Scientists worldwide think the world is on the brink of another pandemic. Many scientists and health officials believe an **influenza** (flu) pandemic may occur in the near future and that a new virus such as avian flu or an old virus such as the Hong Kong flu will begin infecting people and then spread worldwide. (See *WHO pandemic phases*.)

An influenza pandemic can occur when a new virus subtype emerges that has not previously circulated in humans. Because people have never been exposed to this new subtype, their bodies have not produced the antibodies to fight off the virus in their system. Currently, the avian H5N1 virus has mostly affected birds, but there have been documented cases in which the virus has infected other

Epidemic or pandemic?

An *epidemic* occurs when more individuals than normally expected are infected with a disease. Usually, an epidemic is contained within a certain area or region.

A *pandemic* is an epidemic involving an infectious disease that has spread from region to region and the people infected are from many geographical areas.

animals, such as pigs, as well as confirmed cases of human infection by avian H5N1 in various Asian countries.

Pandemic Response Plan

Because the medical office may be the first to experience an increase in patients suspected of having the flu, the office should have a plan in place that includes steps for preparing for a pandemic before it happens as well as a response plan if a pandemic occurs. It is also important for the office to inform patients about preparing for disaster or a pandemic. (See *Preparing for pandemic*.) Following are some ideas for preparing for a pandemic before it happens:

WHO pandemic phases

The following table lists six pandemic phases defined by the World Health Organization (WHO) along with characteristics of each.

Phase	Characteristics
Phase 1	• Interpandemic phase • No new human influenza virus subtypes • Subtype that can infect humans may be present in animals
Phase 2	• Interpandemic phase • No new human influenza virus subtypes, but existing virus subtype in animals poses a significant risk to humans
Phase 3	• Pandemic alert • Human infection with a new subtype but no human-to-human spread
Phase 4	• Pandemic alert • Small clusters with limited human-to-human transmission • Virus not well adapted to humans
Phase 5	• Pandemic alert • Larger clusters of human-to-human spread • Virus better adapted to humans (substantial pandemic risk)
Phase 6	• Pandemic period • Increased and sustained transmission in general population

- Keep important information handy, such as phone numbers for local hospitals, pharmacies, and state and local public health departments.
- Practice and promote good hygiene techniques, such as frequent hand washing and proper disinfection of surfaces.
- Promote yearly influenza vaccinations to your patients. Make sure the office has an ample supply of influenza vaccine.
- Be alert to symptoms of the flu, such as fever, muscle pain, cough, and runny nose. These symptoms are similar to seasonal flu but may be more severe.
- Stay informed of the latest updates. Go to *http://www.pandemicflu.gov* for the most current information.

It is estimated that if an influenza pandemic occurs, approximately 25% of the population may become infected. In the event that a pandemic occurs, the medical office should also have a plan in place for communicating with patients, potentially closing the office, addressing payroll practices, and handling other financial responsibilities such as vendor payment and billing. (See *Pandemic plan*.)

Patient Education

Preparing for Pandemic

Many local, state, and federal public health agencies have developed guides for individuals and families on how to plan for a pandemic influenza outbreak. The medical office staff should obtain the information these agencies have and distribute it to patients. It is important to display or distribute the information in a way that does not cause the patient to panic. Some suggestions for patients include:

- Keep a list of important phone numbers handy, such as the numbers for the local police and fire departments, nearest hospital, and pharmacy, as well as the numbers of relatives and neighbors.

- Keep some items handy, such as flashlights, batteries, candles, matches, a battery-powered radio, wood, bottled water, canned foods and juices, a manual can opener, a first-aid kit, pet food (if applicable), bleach, and hand sanitizer.

- Remember to keep a list of medications for each member of the family, including the full name of the medication, the dosage, and instructions for administering it.

Front office–Back office connection

Pandemic Plan

It is essential for a medical office to establish a plan for responding to a pandemic well before the event occurs. The plan should include how to deal with patients and how to run the day-to-day operations of the medical office. Essentially, medical staff from the front and back office should come together to create a plan for such an emergency. To avoid straining already crowded appointment schedules, many offices choose to conduct such planning during a working lunch so that everyone can be involved.

Making a Plan

To start planning, staff members should explain their daily responsibilities to help assign tasks and responsibilities during an emergency. For example, the administrative medical assistant may be responsible for backing up the billing system and the clinical medical assistant may back up the other computer applications. With a little planning and training, only one of these medical assistants may be responsible for backing up both systems in the event of an emergency so that the other person can be assigned another task. Likewise, an administrative medical assistant may normally call patients to remind them of their next day's appointment, while the clinical medical assistant may call patients with laboratory results. When making an emergency plan, both of these persons may share the responsibility of calling patients to alert them to the closing of the office.

Chapter Summary

- Bioterrorism is a real threat and the medical office should have an emergency plan already in place in the event of such an occurrence.
- Various microorganisms such as *Bacillus anthracis*, *Yersinia pestis*, and *Clostridium botulinum* are biological agents that can be used in a biological attack.
- The medical assistant should know how to communicate with local, state, and federal public health and safety agencies in the event of a bioterrorism threat.
- The medical assistant should know how to properly collect, package, and transport specimens that may contain a possible biological agent.
- Health officials think it is a matter of time before the United States will be involved in a pandemic influenza outbreak.

- Medical offices should have a pandemic response plan in place as well as educational material for their patients.

Team Work Exercises

1. In groups of 2 to 3 students, develop a fact sheet on pandemic influenza as well as a checklist or plan for patients on how to prepare for such an incident.
2. Working in groups of 2 to 3 students, research the various microorganisms that can be classified as bioterrorism agents. Provide the following information on each agent:
   a. type of microorganism
   b. pathogenicity and virulence
   c. mode of transmission for infection
   d. symptoms of human infection
   e. treatment.

Case Studies

1. Your seventh grader's principal has asked you to speak to the middle school students about what influenza is, how it is spread, and the ways to prevent it. What type of information will you access and present? What will you take into consideration when speaking to this age group?

2. During her many office visits, Mrs. Szlozek frequently tells you about her granddaughter, who works for the CDC. She states that her granddaughter mentioned she is doing surveillance studies of Rift Valley fever. You are intrigued by this because you have never heard of this disease. How would you go about finding more information on this disease? What regions have experienced outbreaks of Rift Valley fever?

Resources

- Association of Public Health Laboratories: *www.aphl.org*
- Centers for Disease Control and Prevention (CDC): *www.cdc.gov*
- CDC emergency preparedness and response guidelines: *www.bt.cdc.gov*
- CDC National Laboratory Training Network: *www.nltn.org*
- Examples of state health department checklists for specimen transport: *www.state.ma.us/dph/bls*
- U.S. government avian and pandemic flu information: *www.pandemicflu.gov/index.html*

Office Emergencies

Learning Objectives

Upon completion of this chapter, the student will be able to:

- define the key terms in the glossary
- describe steps medical office personnel can take to prepare for emergencies
- list the typical contents of a crash cartz
- differentiate between a standard defibrillator and an AED
- explain the concept of triage
- list and describe the ABCs of basic emergency care
- list the information that needs to be gathered in a medical emergency
- describe typical presenting symptoms and emergency treatment for various emergencies seen in the medical office.

CAAHEP Competencies

General Competencies
Patient Instruction
Instruct individuals according to their needs

ABHES Competencies

Clinical Duties
Recognize emergencies
Perform first aid and CPR
Instruction
Teach patients methods of health promotion and disease prevention

Chapter Outline

Emergency Preparedness
Emergency Planning
Common Emergency Equipment
Triage

Responding to Common Office Emergencies
Common Signs and Symptoms in Office Emergencies
Dyspnea
Chest Pain
Altered Consciousness
Acute Abdominal Pain
Common Office Emergencies
Hemorrhage
Poisoning
Environmxental Injuries
Musculoskeletal Injury
Eye Injury
Chapter Summary
Team Work Exercises
Case Studies
Resources

Key Terms

automated external defibrillator
Small automated device used to deliver an electrical shock to a patient suffering from a life-threatening cardiac arrhythmia

crash cart
Wheeled supply cabinet in which emergency equipment and supplies are kept

debrief
Discussion of events, thoughts, and feelings among persons who have experienced an important or stressful event

defibrillator
Specialized device used to deliver an electrical shock to a patient suffering from a life-threatening cardiac arrhythmia

mock code
Practice drill for responding to a medical emergency

protocol
Expected behavior during a given situation

recorder
Person designated to document a medical emergency

team captain
Person designated to coordinate activities of all team members during a medical emergency

triage
Process of sorting patients and setting priorities for their treatment

Emergency Preparedness

Everyone who works in a medical office should be trained and prepared to respond to emergencies. Such preparation includes establishing a written plan of response in case of fire, disaster, workplace violence, or medical emergency. Fortunately, most emergencies in the medical office are minor and include such events as a patient arriving unexpectedly with a nosebleed or fractured arm. However, emergencies of all types can and do occur in the medical office. Therefore, the professional medical office team must always be ready for any emergency, small or large.

All health care facilities must make an effort to create an environment that is safe for patients and staff alike. Workplace safety programs provide instruction in cardiopulmonary resuscitation (CPR), standard precautions, proper body mechanics, and other safety issues. New employees undergo safety training upon hire and are required to update their knowledge and regularly demonstrate competence (usually annually) on specific skills, such as CPR.

The appropriate response to an emergency depends on the nature of the emergency, the patient population being served, and the proximity of other medical facilities. The physician or most highly trained clinician in the office should be summoned for immediate help. If the office has staff trained in advanced cardiac life support (ACLS) and the needed equipment is on hand, the staff can provide ACLS measures at the office. In the case of life-threatening emergencies, the staff should institute basic cardiac life support (BCLS) measures while summoning emergency medical service (EMS) personnel. EMS staff are experienced experts in evaluation, treatment, and transport of persons experiencing a medical emergency. (See *ABCs of first-aid.*)

Emergency Planning

The medical assistant must understand the basics about responding to an emergency. (See *General emergency guidelines,* page 970.) In addition to the basics, however, the medical assistant and each member of the medical office staff must understand how to respond to specific emergencies. To ensure an effective, smooth response to medical emergencies, everyone in the medical office must respond according to a **protocol**, which is a predetermined plan about how to respond. Such treatment protocols, agreed upon in advance, help ensure that all members of the medical team understand their roles so they can work together cohesively. Such a protocol might include supplies and equipment needed, the roles for each staff member, and the step-by-step procedure for responding to that particular emergency.

All members of the health care team should know where the emergency equipment is located and obtain proper

ABCs of first-aid

All health care providers, regardless of their credentials or role in the health care team, must understand the basics of first-aid. These basics are designated as the ABCs, for *airway, breathing, and circulation,* the three highest priorities, in order of importance, when assisting a person in an emergency.

Airway

Establishing the presence of an adequate airway is the top priority in first-aid. If the patient cannot get oxygen, other interventions are futile. To open the patient's airway, the rescuer uses the head tilt–chin lift maneuver or the jaw-thrust maneuver for patients with potential cervical spine injuries.

Breathing

To determine a patient's breathing, the rescuer should look, listen, and feel. She should lean low over the patient's face and *look* to see if his chest is rising, *listen* for breath sounds, and see if she can *feel* his breath on the side of her face. If not, she must reposition the patient's head again to open the airway. She should then begin rescue breaths if necessary.

Circulation

Circulation is necessary to deliver oxygenated blood to the brain and other parts of the body. The rescuer should check the patient's circulation by evaluating the carotid pulse in the unconscious patient or radial pulse in the conscious patient. If the patient is pulseless, the rescuer should place her hands, one on top of the other, on the lower half of the patient's sternum and begin chest compressions.

The rescuer should continue these basic cardiac life support (BCLS) measures until more advanced help arrives. She should alternate 15 chest compressions with two breaths (for adults) and recheck for a pulse every few minutes.

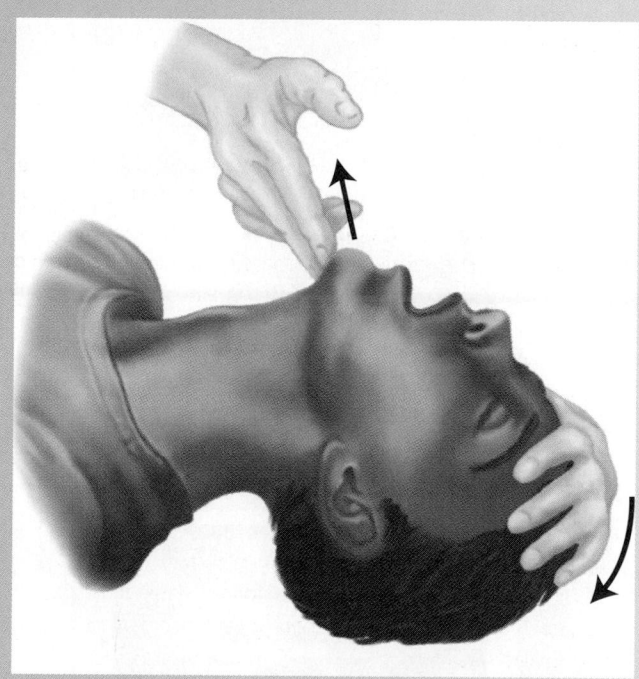

Head-tilt–chin-lift maneuver

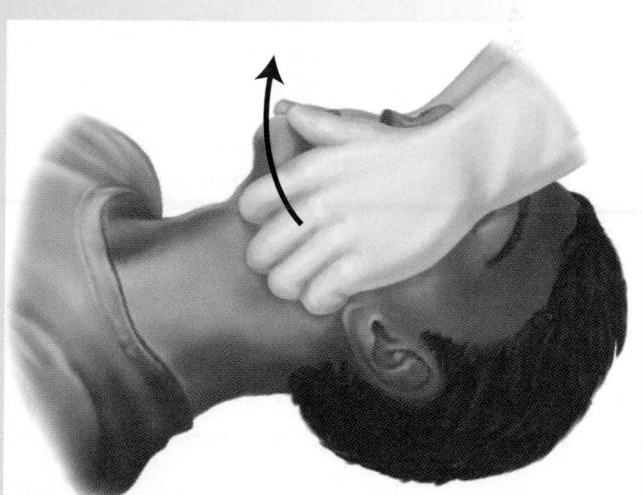

Jaw-thrust maneuver

training in its use. In some cases, a **team captain** is designated to guide members of the team throughout the emergency. The team captain may be the physician; however, in many cases a charge nurse or another staff member will serve as the captain in order to leave the physician free to focus on immediate patient care.

Many facilities routinely run **mock codes**, which are drills that allow all members of the health care team to practice and develop their skills in responding to medical emergencies. Such drills rehearse the staff's response to bomb scares, fires, infant or child abduction, a threat of violence and, most commonly, a patient experiencing cardiac or respiratory failure. These drills are referred to as *codes* because most facilities have a special code system that assigns each type of emergency its own code. When an emergency occurs, a staff member announces the code, usually through an intercom *cart,* which is specifically used for emergencies. (See Figure 47-1.) Specific equipment stored on the cart varies, depending on the patient population seen by the office.

One item almost always present on a crash cart is a **defibrillator**. This specialized device is used to deliver an electrical shock to a patient suffering from a life-threatening cardiac arrhythmia, such as ventricular fibrillation and ventricular tachycardia. During such arrhythmias, some or all heart muscle fibers contract in a disorganized fashion. Delivery of an electrical shock causes all cardiac muscle fibers to contract in unison, which sometimes stimulates the heart to convert back to normal sinus rhythm. Because some risk is associated with operating this device, all staff members who use it must be properly trained. (See *Common crash cart supplies and equipment.*)

General emergency guidelines

General guidelines apply to any emergency in the medical office, including:

- Follow standard precautions and wear personal protective equipment (PPE) to prevent the transmission of disease through blood or body secretions.
- Follow airway, breathing, and circulation (ABCs) to prioritize actions.
- Act in a manner consistent with the standard of care.
- Perform tasks only within your scope of practice.
- Summon help early. It is better to summon more help than is needed than to fail to call for adequate help in a timely manner.
- Never leave an unstable patient alone.
- Document the event carefully, including the action taken by medical office staff and the patient's response.

system, to alert all staff so they can respond according to the specific protocol for that type of emergency.

After each mock code, members of the team should **debrief**, which is a discussion of the event among all team members to determine what worked during the event and what did not, so that appropriate changes can be made in the response plan. Such debriefing should also take place after an actual emergency as well.

An important, but sometimes overlooked, part of emergency preparedness is the designation of a team member to document the emergency, called a *recorder* in some care settings. This person should assume her role from the beginning of the emergency so she can accurately record the events in a chronological fashion. Otherwise, reconstructing events after the fact will be difficult, especially in a complex medical emergency.

In addition to protocols, availability of critical supplies and properly working equipment are essential in an emergency. Therefore, medical staff must be sure to maintain inventory of needed supplies and medications and restock following each emergency event. In addition, staff must carefully maintain and routinely check emergency equipment so that it is always ready.

Common Emergency Equipment

Not all medical offices keep emergency equipment on hand; however, many do. If an office does stock emergency equipment and medication, the physician and other staff members must be familiar with its use. Many supplies are stored in a portable, wheeled supply cabinet, called a *crash cart* or *code*

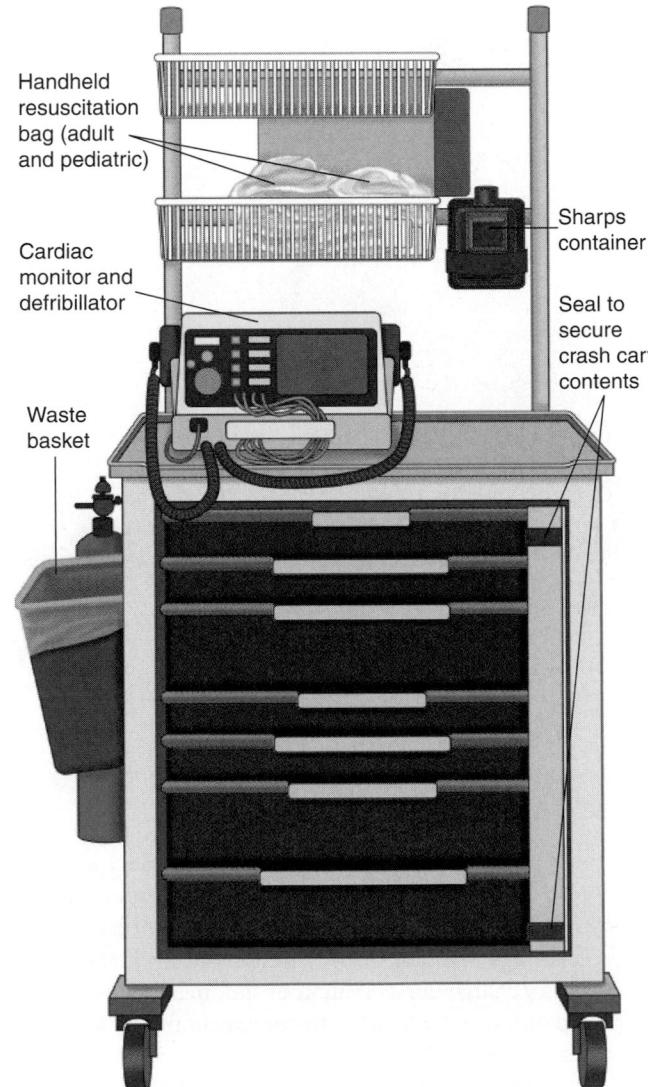

Handheld resuscitation bag (adult and pediatric)

Cardiac monitor and defibrillator

Waste basket

Sharps container

Seal to secure crash cart contents

FIG 47-1 Typical crash cart.

Common crash cart supplies and equipment

The specific items kept in a crash cart vary with the office specialty and patient population seen. Here are some of the most common types of equipment, supplies, and medications kept in a crash cart for emergencies.

Emergency Equipment
- Personal protective equipment, including:
  - gowns
  - masks
  - goggles
  - examination gloves
- Portable oxygen delivery equipment, including:
  - oxygen tanks
  - oxygen tubing
  - various types of oxygen masks
  - handheld resuscitation bags
  - airways (oral and nasal)
  - endotracheal tubes
  - laryngoscopes
- Blood pressure cuffs
- Suction equipment
- Defibrillator or automated external defibrillator (AED)
- Stethoscope

Emergency Supplies
- Adhesive tape
- Assorted dressings and bandages
- Alcohol wipes
- Constriction band
- Cotton swabs
- Antibiotic ointment
- Sterile and nonsterile gloves
- Flashlight or penlight
- Hot and cold packs (instant)
- IV catheters
- Assorted IV fluids

- IV tubing
- Bandage scissors
- Biohazard sharps container
- Assorted syringes
- Assorted needles

Emergency Medication
- Activated charcoal
- Antihistamines
- Aspirin
- Atropine
- Dextrose
- Diphenhydramine
- Dopamine
- Epinephrine
- Furosemide
- Glucagon
- Insulin
- Ipecac syrup
- Digoxin
- Lidocaine
- Nitroglycerine
- Pancuronium
- Sodium bicarbonate
- Sterile water
- Sterile saline
- Xylocaine
- Controlled substances (must be kept in a locked compartment), including:
  - morphine
  - diazepam
  - midazolam
  - lorazepam

Recently, development of simpler devices known as **automated external defibrillators** (AEDs) make operation of this type of emergency equipment much easier. In addition, the AED's manufacturers have programmed them to give automatic, step-by-step instructions for their use. They are smaller and more portable than the original defibrillators. Because of these technological advances, AEDs are now present in many places in addition to medical offices, including fitness centers, airplanes, college campuses, ski resorts, and even shopping malls. As a result, persons suffering from cardiac arrest receive help more quickly and the survival rate for this population is increasing.

Triage

The term **triage** is derived from the French word *trier*, which means "to sort." In the medical setting, triage involves making a quick determination about the nature of the patient's emergency, the type of immediate care needed, and the most appropriate response. If more than one patient is involved, triage may also involve determining which patient should be treated first. In many settings, a registered nurse performs triage; however, other staff members may perform this task, depending on their qualifications. In some cases, medical assistants must perform triage. Most offices have written guidelines in place that guide the process. Even so, no guidelines are as valuable as experience and practice. Therefore, the person assigned triage duties should be an experienced health care provider.

A significant number of the phone calls received by the medical office involve potentially urgent or even emergency situations. In such cases, the administrative medical assistant sometimes transfers the call to a nurse or clinical medical assistant. However, she should never put a caller with a medical emergency on hold. Therefore, anyone who answers telephones in the medical office must know how to handle such calls. (For more information on telephone triage, see Chapter 11, page 121.)

Responding to Common Office Emergencies

When a medical emergency occurs, the patient's exact diagnosis may be unclear at first. The patient may simply display a collection of signs and symptoms, such as dyspnea or chest pain. Thus, the medical assistant's response to such an emergency should be to evaluate the signs and symptoms, rather than attempt to determine a diagnosis. In other situations, the cause of the patient's condition may be clear, as in a laceration to the hand. Thus, the medical assistant must be aware of common signs and symptoms of emergencies as well as the potential causes.

Common Signs and Symptoms in Office Emergencies

Office emergencies commonly involve such signs and symptoms as dyspnea, chest pain, altered consciousness, and acute abdominal pain.

Dyspnea

Any time a patient complains of dyspnea (difficulty breathing), a potential emergency exists. The medical assistant should make a quick evaluation to determine the severity of the dyspnea and institute appropriate interventions. When possible, the medical assistant should attempt to identify the underlying cause, which is useful in formulating a treatment plan. However, the medical assistant should not ask a patient in extreme distress to answer questions that would delay treatment. There are many potential causes of dyspnea and

the severity may range from temporary loss of breath to total airway obstruction or respiratory failure. (See *Common causes of dyspnea*.) When in doubt regarding severity, the medical assistant should summon a nurse or physician to perform a quick assessment of the patient and provide help. Appropriate intervention depends on the nature and severity of the problem and ranges from assisting the patient to a chair where he can catch his breath to calling EMS and beginning rescue breathing.

In order to determine the severity of the patient's dyspnea, the medical assistant must quickly obtain the patient's vital signs, including his oxygen saturation level. Such information helps determine the severity of the emergency and provides important baseline data for later comparison. The medical assistant can also look for other clues to determine severity. Paying close attention to these clues will help the medical assistant determine an appropriate response. Such clues include:

- skin appearance
- character of respirations
- respiratory rate
- use of accessory muscles
- breath sounds
- mental or emotional state.

Skin Appearance

In mild dyspnea, skin appears pink or pale (in light-skinned people) with possible diaphoresis (sweating). In moderate dyspnea, the skin appears dusky with circumoral cyanosis (blue tint around the mouth) and diaphoresis. In severe dyspnea or apnea (absence of breathing), the skin appears cyanotic (bluish tint) and is moist and clammy.

Character of Respirations

In a patient with mild dyspnea, respiratory effort and depth is regular or the depth of respirations is slightly deeper than normal. In moderate dyspnea, respirations may be labored and deep or, if breathing is painful, shallow and rapid. In severe dyspnea or apnea, respirations are labored, deeper, or more shallow than normal, and irregular in pattern.

Respiratory Rate

A patient with mild dyspnea will have a normal respiratory rate or slight tachypnea (rapid breathing). In moderate dyspnea, respiratory rate is moderately tachypneic. A patient with severe dyspnea or apnea has severe tachypnea or severe bradypnea (slow breathing).

Use of Accessory Muscles

A patient with dyspnea commonly uses his accessory muscles to breathe. These muscles include the intercostal and supraclavicular muscles. In mild dyspnea, use of these muscles is mild. In moderate dyspnea, the use of accessory muscles becomes more pronounced. Slight nasal flaring may also be present. In severe dyspnea, nasal flaring and the patient's use of accessory muscles become even more apparent. He also will insist on sitting upright in order to make full use of his diaphragm and commonly displays a wide-eyed, panicked expression.

Breath Sounds

In mild dyspnea, the patient's breath sounds are clear with minimal noise. The medical assistant may hear mild crackles, rhonchi, or wheezing with a stethoscope. In moderate dyspnea, the medical assistant should be able to hear wheezes or other signs of congestion without a stethoscope and moderate crackles, rhonchi, or wheezing with a stethoscope. In

severe dyspnea or apnea, the medical assistant may hear extreme wheezing, crackles, rhonchi, stridor, and other abnormal sounds, or breath sounds may be abnormally quiet, signaling respiratory failure.

Mental or Emotional State

In mild dyspnea, the patient may seem alert and slightly anxious. In moderate dyspnea, the patient may be alert, anxious, or even frightened. In severe dyspnea or apnea, the patient may be extremely anxious; however, his level of consciousness rapidly declines as fatigue and lethargy from oxygen deprivation set in.

Common causes of dyspnea

The following table lists some of the most common causes of dyspnea, along with typical signs and symptoms, and emergency management measures.

Cause	Signs and Symptoms	Emergency Management
Complete foreign body airway obstruction (choking) *ICD-9-CM code: 934.9 (complete or partial obstruction)*	• Universal choking sign by person with his hands at his throat and his eyes wide and frightened • Absent breath sounds • Rapid development of cyanosis and loss of consciousness	• Call for immediate assistance from the physician or nurse and follow these steps: 1. Ask the victim, "Are you choking?" If the person nods yes or is unable to speak, cough, or breathe, administer the Heimlich (abdominal thrust*) maneuver until it is effective or the person loses consciousness. 2. Check the mouth of an unconscious person for a foreign body. 3. Open the person's airway and attempt to deliver rescue breaths. 4. Continue these steps until they are effective or other help arrives.
Partial foreign body airway obstruction *ICD-9-CM code: 934.9 (complete or partial)*	• Universal choking sign by person with his hands at his throat and his eyes wide and frightened • Abnormal breath sounds with possible whistling or stridorous sound • With severe obstruction, cyanosis and possible loss of consciousness as efforts to breathe become less effective	• Allow the person to cough as long as coughing is forceful and breathing is adequate. • If the person's efforts become weak and ineffective, begin the Heimlich (abdominal thrust*) maneuver. • Summon emergency medical services (EMS).
Asthma attack *ICD-9-CM code: 493.90*	• Mild to severe wheezing • Dyspnea • Possible coughing	• Assist the patient to use an inhaler if he has one. • Administer medications such as a nebulizer per a physician's order. • Apply oxygen if ordered.
Anaphylaxis *ICD-9-CM code: 995.0 (unspecified cause; use additional codes for cause and E code for external cause)*	• Stridorous breath sounds as the airway closes • Wheezing • Anxiety and other signs of severe dyspnea • Possibly blotchy skin with hives • Possibly rapidly decreasing blood pressure	• Administer medications per a physician's order, which may include epinephrine, prednisone, and antihistamines. • Apply oxygen per order.

Continued

Common causes of dyspnea—cont'd

Cause	Signs and Symptoms	Emergency Management
Pneumonia *ICD-9-CM code: 486 (organism unspecified)*	• Chest discomfort with breathing • Productive cough with yellow or green sputum • General ill appearance • Mild to moderate dyspnea	• Pneumonia is not an emergency. • Administer antibiotics per a physician's order. • Administer oxygen per order.
Chronic obstructive pulmonary disease (COPD) exacerbation *ICD-9-CM code: 492.9 (emphysema)*	• Mild to severe dyspnea • Wheezing • Prolonged expiratory phase • Other signs of dyspnea, depending on severity	• Administer oxygen and medications per a physician's order.

Pneumothorax
ICD-9-CM code: 512.8
	• Depending on severity, possibly includes:
	  • dyspnea
	  • sharp chest pain with inspiration
	  • cyanosis
	  • decreased oxygen saturation
	  • tachycardia
	  • hypotension
	  • tachypnea
	  • anxiety
	  • decreased or absent breath sounds on affected side
		• Administer oxygen.
		• Place an occlusive dressing over the injury site taped on three sides (if injury is present).
		• Position the patient for comfort and optimal lung expansion (usually in semi-Fowler position).
		• Prepare to assist with possible chest tube insertion.

Myocardial infarction (MI) or heart failure *ICD-9-CM code: 410.9 (MI, unspecified site), 428.0 (heart failure)*	• Dyspnea as primary symptom (in patients suffering from a silent MI or from heart failure)	• Administer oxygen, morphine, nitroglycerine, aspirin, thrombolytic agents, and, if needed, anti-arrhythmic agents per a physician's order. • Instruct the person to rest in a position of comfort to reduce the heart's oxygen demands. • Provide BCLS or advanced cardiac life support (ACLS) as needed.

* Use chest compressions for pregnant patients.

Chest Pain

The medical assistant must always take seriously any complaint of chest pain because it could indicate a myocardial infarction (MI). (See *Common causes of chest pain*.) During an MI, the heart is starved for oxygen. Therefore, the medical assistant must take immediate action to decrease the heart's workload and maximize oxygen supply. The medical assistant should immediately notify the physician and then assist the patient to an examination room by wheelchair and position him in a manner that maximizes comfort and breathing. Most offices have a protocol for such situations that includes removing clothing above the waist, obtaining a stat ECG, and administering oxygen. If the office has an emergency code cart, a medical assistant or other staff member should bring it into the room. The medical assistant or other staff member should do a quick review of the patient's medications and ask him what medications he has taken that day. (See *Working as a team*.)

Altered Consciousness

ICD-9-CM code: 780.09 (alteration of consciousness excluding coma)

There are many causes of a sudden alteration in consciousness. Common causes include seizures, conditions related to diabetes management, and head injury as well as stroke, cardiac arrhythmias, and cardiac arrest; however, the cause is usually unclear at first. (See *Medical alert*, page 977.) Regardless of the cause, when a patient suddenly loses consciousness in the medical office, the medical assistant must immediately summon help and check the patient's ABCs. When a

Front office–back office connection

Working as a team

There are few emergencies more serious than the patient with a possible myocardial infarction (MI). Therefore, all members of the office team should be alerted so they can make themselves available to help as needed. Having a written protocol and practicing mock codes will help everyone perform their jobs more efficiently. Some considerations might include designating the following assignments to the following team members:

- Administrative medical assistant: make phone calls and enter orders into the computer system for stat blood draws and lab tests, emergency cardiology consultations, and contacting EMS for hospital transport and contacting a family member for the patient.

- Second administrative medical assistant, receptionist, or office manager: attend to other patients who are checking in and if necessary reschedule their appointments.

- Team captain (needed in the event of a code): coordinate the activities of everyone involved in direct patient care.

- Clinical medial assistant: assist in patient care as directed by the physician.

- Nurse (if present): may also serve as team captain, aid in direct patient care including starting the IV and administering IV medications.

Common causes of chest pain

The accompanying table lists some of the most common causes of chest pain along with the typical signs and symptoms and emergency management measures.

Cause	Signs and Symptoms	Typical Emergency Management
Myocardial infarction (MI) *ICD-9-CM code: 410.9* *(unspecified site)*	• Sensation of pain, discomfort, squeezing, or heaviness in the chest, jaw, left arm, or left shoulder that is unrelieved by nitroglycerine, oxygen, or rest • Dyspnea • Diaphoresis • Nausea • In female patients, any of the above symptoms or back pain, syncope, gastric symptoms, heart palpitations	• Monitor airway, breathing, and circulation (ABCs). • Administer oxygen, morphine, nitroglycerine, aspirin, thrombolytic agents and, if needed, antiarrhythmic agents as ordered by the physician. • Provide the patient with a restful environment, encourage him to rest, and move the patient in a wheelchair, rather than letting him walk. • Provide basic cardiac life support (BCLS) or advanced cardiac life support (ACLS) measures as needed.
Angina *ICD-9-CM code: 413.9*	• As in MI, sensation of pain, discomfort, squeezing, or heaviness in the chest, jaw, left arm, or left shoulder, except that symptoms are relieved by nitroglycerine, oxygen, or rest • Dyspnea • Diaphoresis • Nausea • In female patients, any of the above symptoms or back pain, syncope, gastric symptoms, heart palpitations	• Administer nitroglycerine and oxygen. • Provide the patient with a restful environment and encourage rest.

Continued

Common causes of chest pain—cont'd

Cause	Signs and Symptoms	Typical Emergency Management
Gastroesophageal reflux disease (GERD) *ICD-9-CM code: 530.81*	• Belching with heartburn triggered by large meals, spicy foods, alcohol, and eating before bedtime • Worsening of symptoms about 1 hour after meals	• GERD is not an emergency. • Tests may rule out cardiac causes. • Treatment includes GI evaluation and medications to reduce stomach acid production.
Pericarditis *ICD-9-CM code: 420.91 (unspecified; if applicable, code underlying cause first)*	• Chest pain that is worse with inspiration • Fever • Malaise • Dyspnea • Chills	• Pericarditis is not an emergency. • Tests may rule out other cardiac causes. • Treatment includes anti-inflammatory medication and, possibly, antibiotics.
Cholecystitis *ICD-9-CM code: 575.12 (acute and chronic)*	• Colicky epigastric pain that radiates into the right upper quadrant (RUQ), right shoulder, and back • Nausea and vomiting • Fever • Jaundice and pruritus • Tachycardia • Light stools and dark urine	• Cholecystitis is not an emergency, although pain may be severe. • Tests may rule out cardiac causes. • Patients may be hospitalized for cholecystectomy or lithotripsy.
Costochondritis *ICD-9-CM code: 733.6*	• Chest pain over the sternum that may radiate into the shoulders and arms and is worse with a deep breath • Tenderness on and around the sternum to palpation	• Costochondritis is not an emergency and is usually identified by a brief physical examination. • Tests may rule out a cardiac cause. • Treatment includes nonsteroidal anti-inflammatory drugs (NSAIDs) and ice (or cold) application.
Pulmonary embolism *ICD-9-CM code: 415.1*	• Chest pain with inspiration • Cough • Low-grade fever • Dyspnea • Tachypnea • Occasional hemoptysis • Cyanosis • Shock	• Monitor ABCs. • Administer oxygen and ventilatory support as needed and ordered by a physician. • Measures to rule out a cardiac cause may include ECG and cardiac enzyme studies.
Spontaneous pneumothorax *ICD-9-CM code: 512.8*	• Sudden, sharp, pleuritic chest pain • Mild to moderate dyspnea • Decreased breath sounds on affected side • Decreased oxygen saturation • Tachycardia • Tachypnea • Anxiety	• Administer oxygen as directed by a physician. • Position the patient for comfort and optimal lung expansion. • The physician may order chest x-ray to confirm diagnosis. • Prepare to assist with possible chest tube or Heimlich valve placement. • Patient may be transported to the hospital for further care.
Panic attack *ICD-9-CM code: 300.01*	• Sudden onset of chest palpitations, tachycardia, diaphoresis, trembling, dyspnea, chest pain, nausea, paresthesias, dizziness, chills or hot flashes • Feelings of anxiety or impending doom	• Panic attack is not an emergency. • Tests may rule out cardiac and GI causes. • Treatment may include reassurance and anti-anxiety medications.

person loses consciousness and falls, he may suffer an injury from the fall itself. Therefore, the medical assistant should keep the patient still until a nurse or physician can evaluate him, even if she must keep him on the floor for a few minutes. Well-intentioned staff members can cause further injury to a patient by moving him prematurely. If the physician or nurse suspects a spinal injury, the medical assistant should summon EMS to properly immobilize and move the patient.

Causes of a slower change in consciousness include hyperglycemia, hypoglycemia, drug toxicities, dementia, and other neurological disorders. Although these conditions can be quite serious or even life-threatening, the changes generally occur gradually, which enables evaluation, diagnosis, and initiation of treatment before the situation becomes an emergency.

Generalized Seizure
ICD-9-CM code: 345.90 (epilepsy, unspecified)
Many triggers may cause loss of consciousness from a generalized seizure. While a seizure may signal a serious condition, it is not usually life-threatening on its own unless prolonged. The medical assistant should not attempt to restrain the patient experiencing a tonic-clonic seizure (also called *grand mal seizure*) but should keep him as safe as possible by removing nearby objects that might inflict injury if struck and placing something soft under his head. She should not place or force anything into his mouth, because in doing so she risks injuring the patient and herself. A general misconception regarding seizures is that the patient could swallow his tongue, which is, in fact, not possible. However, the medical assistant can help protect the patient's airway by placing him on his side and can increase his comfort by loosening his tie or other tight clothing. She should also note the duration of the seizure and type of activity. After the seizure, the medical assistant should reorient and reassure the patient, obtain a set of vital signs, allow the patient to rest, and provide other care as directed by the physician. She should not offer the patient anything to eat or drink until he is fully awake.

Syncope
ICD-9-CM code: 780.2 (blackout, fainting, or code according to identified cause)
When a patient experiences syncope (fainting) and quickly regains consciousness, she is sometimes embarrassed by the attention that ensues. However, it is still important that the physician evaluate her before the medical staff allows her to leave. The physician must investigate two potential problems. First, there may be an underlying disorder that triggered the syncopal episode. Second, the patient may have suffered injury when she fainted and fell.

Patient Education

Medical Alert

Many patients have chronic conditions that can result in life-threatening emergencies, such as those with severe allergies and diabetes. Because altered consciousness may occur as a result of many of these conditions, the medical assistant should encourage these patients to wear a medical alert bracelet or necklace. Doing so can provide essential information to a health care provider in the event that the patient is unable to provide the information himself. Data may include:

- nature of the condition, such as allergy and diabetes
- person's name
- code status
- emergency contact number.

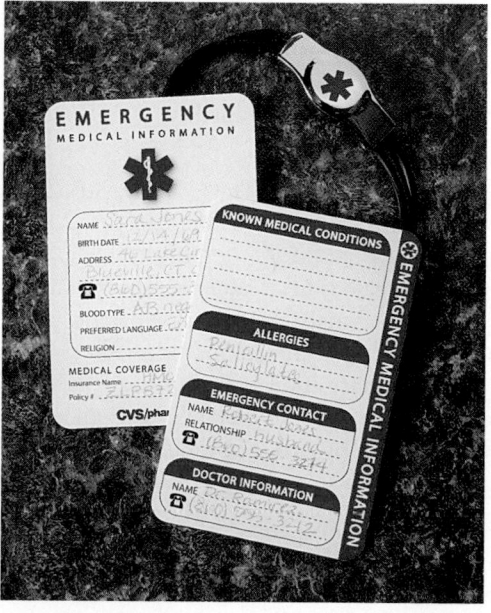

Diabetic Emergencies

ICD-9-CM code: 250.90 (diabetes mellitus, coding digits added according to clinical manifestations, diabetes type, and specific pathology)

A patient with diabetes can experience altered consciousness when his blood glucose level rises to dangerously high levels (hyperglycemia) or drops to dangerously low levels (hypoglycemia). A person with hyperglycemia demonstrates a gradual change over a period of hours or days. Typical symptoms include fatigue, dry skin, tacky (semi-dry) mucous membranes, and lethargy that progresses to stupor and then coma. Respirations become increasingly deep and rapid and the patient has a fruity breath odor, which is sometimes mistaken for alcohol breath. The medical assistant can help by keeping the patient safe, performing glucometer testing, and assisting the physician with evaluation and treatment as directed. She may also need to arrange for transfer of the patient to the hospital for careful management, including administration of IV fluids and insulin.

The patient with hypoglycemia demonstrates a more sudden change in consciousness (minutes to hours) with hunger, irritability, confusion, combativeness, weakness, tremulousness, headache, dizziness, sweating, seizures, coma, and death. The medical assistant can help by keeping the patient safe, performing glucometer testing, and assisting the physician with evaluation and treatment as directed. If the patient is alert enough to safely swallow, the medical assistant may administer some form of oral sugar, such as fruit juice, per office protocol. If he is unable to safely swallow, the nurse or physician must start an IV for administration of IV dextrose.

Hypoglycemia has the potential to progress more quickly than hyperglycemia and can rapidly result in death. Therefore, when the cause of altered consciousness is unknown in a patient with diabetes, the medical staff should treat the situation as an emergency, as if he has hypoglycemia, until an accurate diagnosis is determined.

Head Injury

ICD-9-CM code: 852 (subarachnoid, subdural, and extradural hemorrhage caused by injury), 852.4 (epidural hematoma), 852.2 (subdural hematoma)

A patient with a serious head injury is usually transported to the hospital immediately. However, a patient with a less severe head injury is common in the medical office. The medical assistant must always treat any patient with a head injury seriously and quickly escort him to an examination room. While beginning care, she should help gather specific data, including:

- description of the mechanism of injury
- presence or absence of neck or spinal pain
- whether the patient lost consciousness and, if so, for how long

- time the event occurred
- whether the event was witnessed and, if so, whether the witness is available to answer questions.

The medical assistant should also obtain baseline vital signs, monitor him for changes in consciousness, and assist the physician with patient care as directed. If there is any question of spinal cord injury, she must help immobilize the patient immediately until the physician can obtain and review x-rays.

Acute Abdominal Pain

Acute abdominal pain has many potential causes, some of which may be life-threatening. In addition, some causes of abdominal pain may not originate in the abdomen. Occasionally, disorders that originate in the pelvic region, , such as urinary tract infection (UTI) and ectopic pregnancy, or vascular disorders, such as a dissecting (tearing) aortic aneurysm, cause pain that may be felt in the abdomen or back. (See *Common causes of abdominal pain*.)

When a patient complains of acute abdominal pain, the cause is seldom immediately clear. Therefore, the medical assistant must take all such cases seriously and provide care according to office protocol, including informing the physician so that she can begin prompt evaluation and treatment. Because of the possibility of emergency surgery, the medical assistant must determine when the patient last had anything to eat or drink and not allow the patient to take anything by mouth without the physician's approval. She must obtain baseline vital signs immediately as well.

Common Office Emergencies

Common emergencies encountered in a medical office include hemorrhage, poisoning, environmental injuries, musculoskeletal injuries, and eye injuries.

Hemorrhage

Numerous types of injuries result in hemorrhage (bleeding), which may be minor or life-threatening. After checking airway, breathing, and circulation, the medical assistant must take measures to control bleeding. Two of the most common conditions that involve hemorrhage in the medical office are laceration and epistaxis.

Laceration

ICD-9-CM code: 879.8 (site unspecified)

A common office emergency involves a patient entering the medical office with a blood-soaked towel wrapped around his lacerated hand. A laceration is a cut or tear in the flesh that may bleed slightly or may hemorrhage profusely. The medical assistant should put on examination gloves before greeting the patient and should escort him to an examination room and help him lie down. If bleeding is severe, the medical assistant should apply direct pressure with an

Common causes of abdominal pain

The accompanying table lists some common causes of abdominal pain along with signs and symptoms and emergency management measures.

Cause	Signs and Symptoms	Emergency Management
Appendicitis *ICD-9-CM code: 540*	• Classic symptoms of nausea, vomiting, and severe periumbilical pain that eventually localizes to the RLQ (in less than 50% of patients) • RLQ rebound tenderness to palpation possible • Fever • Diarrhea or constipation	• Keep the patient on nothing-by-mouth (NPO) status. • Help arrange for appendectomy if directed. • Administer antibiotics to prevent or resolve infection if ordered.
Bowel obstruction *ICD-9-CM code: 560.9*	• More severe symptoms with complete obstruction than with partial obstruction • Nausea and vomiting • Abdominal pain • Abdominal distention • Inability to pass gas or stool	• Keep the patient on NPO status and assist with care as directed. • The patient will require hospitalization for further care and possible surgery.
Cholecystitis *ICD-9-CM code: 575.12* *(acute and chronic)*	• Colicky epigastric pain that radiates into the right upper quadrant, right shoulder, and back • Nausea and vomiting • Fever • Jaundice • Tachycardia • Light stools and dark urine • Pruritus	• Cholecystitis is not an emergency, although pain may be severe. • Tests rule out cardiac causes. • The patient may be hospitalized for cholecystectomy or lithotripsy.
Crohn disease (also called *regional enteritis*) *ICD-9-CM code: 555.9*	• Chronic diarrhea • Fever • Weight loss, anorexia • Fatigue • Abdominal pain • Cramping that may localize to right lower quadrant (RLQ)	• Crohn disease is not usually an emergency. However, surgery may be necessary in cases of perforation or to remove the involved portion of the colon. • Administer fluid replacement, anticholinergics, and opioid analgesics to control pain and reduce bowel motility; antimicrobials for infection; and corticosteroids to reduce inflammation per the physician's order.
Diverticulitis *ICD-9-CM code: 562.11* *(without hemorrhage), 562.13* *(with hemorrhage)*	• Fever • Nausea • Blood-streaked stools • Left lower quadrant abdominal pain	• Diverticulitis is not normally an emergency. However, surgery may be necessary in cases of bowel perforation. • Administer antibiotics to treat infection and analgesics for pain per the physician's order.
Gastroenteritis *ICD-9-CM code: 558.9*	• Varies with the cause • Watery diarrhea • Abdominal cramps • Anorexia • Nausea and vomiting • Headache • Fever • Weakness	• Gastroenteritis is rarely an emergency. • Administer fluid and electrolyte replacement, antiemetics, and antibiotics per the physician's order. • Provide a restful environment and encourage the patient to rest.

Continued

Common causes of abdominal pain—cont'd

Cause	Signs and Symptoms	Emergency Management
Peptic ulcer disease *ICD-9-CM code: 531.90 (gastric), 532.90 (duodenal), 533.90 (peptic)*	• Indigestion • Heartburn • Epigastric pain • Uncomfortable fullness • Nausea and vomiting • Peak of symptoms about 2 hours after eating	• PUD is usually not an emergency. • Tests may rule out cardiac causes. • Treatment includes GI evaluation, anti-ulcer medications, and, possibly, antibiotics.
Ulcerative colitis *ICD-9-CM code: 556.9*	• Episodic flare-ups with as many as 10 to 20 episodes of bloody, mucoid diarrhea per day • Pain • Cramps • Urgency to defecate • Weight loss • Fever • Malaise	• Ulcerative colitis is not usually an emergency. However, surgery may be necessary in cases of severe hemorrhage or perforation. • Administer anticholinergic and antidiarrhea medications per the physician's order to reduce bowel motility, corticosteroids to reduce inflammation, and analgesics for pain.

adequate amount of absorbent dressing material and remain with the patient while another staff member summons the physician. (See *Tourniquets*.) She should measure vital signs as quickly as possible to establish baseline information because hemorrhage can quickly result in tachycardia, hypotension, and shock. In such a case, the medical assistant or other staff member should summon EMS to transport the patient to the hospital. The physician or a nurse may also begin intravenous (IV) fluid administration in order to stabilize the patient for transport.

Patient Education

Tourniquets

Tourniquet use is no longer an approved care measure for bleeding, because a tightly applied tourniquet cuts off circulation to the distal extremity. Resulting tissue death may require amputation of the extremity. Instead, the medical assistant should teach patients to control hemorrhage by taking one of these measures:

• applying direct pressure with an absorbent dressing

• applying direct pressure to the nearest pulse point

• applying a constricting band tight enough to reduce, but not completely stop, bleeding, which still allows some circulation to distal tissue.

For less severe lacerations, the physician may choose to administer a local anesthetic to the wound so the medical assistant can clean it. Most commonly, the medical assistant will use sterile saline solution or warm water and antibacterial soap. If the patient has not had a tetanus vaccination in more than 10 years, the physician will usually order a booster. The physician will also typically close minor lacerations with a butterfly closure, adhesive strips, or a tissue adhesive. (See *Tissue adhesive: Why use it?*) The medical assistant may help the physician close more severe lacerations with sutures.

Epistaxis
ICD-9-CM code: 784.7

Epistaxis (nosebleed) is caused by erosion or rupture of small vessels within the nasal mucosa. In most cases, epistaxis is minor; however, it can be severe in the case of an arterial bleed. Causes of epistaxis are numerous and include trauma, irritation from nasal sprays, abuse of drugs inhaled nasally, and bleeding disorders. Contributors include hypertension and the use of antiplatelet medications, such as aspirin, or anticoagulant medications, such as warfarin. To treat epistaxis, the medical assistant should immediately escort the patient to an examination room and position him sitting up and leaning forward while applying direct pinching pressure high on the nostrils. Unless the patient is feeling faint, the medical assistant should not have him lie down because doing so will cause drainage of blood down to the patient's stomach, which will likely result in nausea and

Tissue adhesive: Why use it?

In some cases, minor lacerations can be sealed with a liquid tissue adhesive, such as Dermabond, rather than sutures. There are several advantages to using tissue adhesive, including:

- It is brushed on and bonds in less than 3 minutes.
- It comes off naturally as the wound heals.
- It forms a strong, flexible seal that protects the wound while it heals.
- It acts like glue to hold skin edges together.
- Bandages are usually not required.
- Getting the wound wet is not a problem.
- Needles are not necessary, so children (and some adults) experience less anxiety.

vomiting. If epistaxis is severe, the physician may perform electrocautery to cauterize the bleeding vessel. The physician may also refer the patient to an otolaryngologist for follow-up care.

Poisoning

ICD-9-CM code: varies depending on agent and pathology (add E code to indicate accidental poisoning, E850 to E858; suicidal intent, E950 to E952.9; homicidal intent, E962 to E962.9; or undetermined intent, E980 to E982.9)

Poisoning most commonly occurs from oral ingestion of a substance, such as a drug, household cleaner, plant, or vitamin. Other causes of poisoning include injection (accidental administration of medication or overdose of illicit drugs), absorption (through skin exposure to chemicals), and inhalation (as with carbon monoxide poisoning). Symptoms of poisoning vary depending on the offending agent and may include nausea, vomiting, abdominal cramps, changes in skin color, seizures, diaphoresis, dizziness, tearing, drooling, drowsiness, and decreased level of consciousness. Burns or stains may also appear on the patient's hands, mouth, or clothing.

When providing care for a patient with possible poisoning, the medical assistant must attend to the ABCs and provide care as directed by the physician. She should also help gather data to aid the physician in determining an appropriate treatment plan, including:

- patient name, age, and weight
- substance the patient ingested or was exposed to
- time the poisoning occurred
- quantity ingested or injected

- whether the patient vomited
- any first-aid measures attempted
- whether the patient has dyspnea.

If the patient calls before coming to the medical office, the medical assistant should instruct the caller to bring the poison container (if known) and, if possible, the emesis if the patient vomited. The best treatment for poisoning is prevention, so the medical assistant should always take the opportunity to educate patients about ways to prevent poisoning. (See *Preventing poisoning.*)

Environmental Injuries

Occasionally, patients enter the medical office with environmental injuries, such as burns, animal bites, or insect stings. Less common environmental injuries seen in this setting include heat stroke, hypothermia, and others. (See *Less common environmental injuries,* page 982.) After attending to ABCs, the medical assistant must gather information about the mechanism of injury, which helps guide the physician in appropriate treatment.

Patient Education

Preventing Poisoning

Most accidental cases of poisoning occur in young children (under age 6). Thus, the medical assistant should instruct parents of young children to take the following measures to try to prevent accidental poisoning:

- Keep toxic substances, such as pesticides and cleaning supplies, locked up and out of reach of children.
- Keep toxic substances in their original containers and replace them if the labels become illegible.
- Prior to using pesticides (indoors or outdoors), remove children and their toys from the area.
- Never leave pesticides, cleaning solutions, or other potentially toxic substances unattended when children are around.
- Keep a current bottle of syrup of ipecac in your medicine cabinet or first-aid kit.
- Keep all medications and vitamins locked up and out of reach of children.
- Never coax children to take medication or vitamins by telling them that it is candy.
- Keep the telephone number of your state Poison Control Center by your telephone. All numbers are available (24 hours, 7 days per week) by calling the National Poison Control Center at 1-800-222-1222.

Less common environmental injuries

The following table lists some environmental injuries that are less commonly treated in an office setting, along with their signs and symptoms and emergency management measures.

Cause	Signs and Symptoms	Emergency Management
Heat exhaustion ICD-9-CM code: 992.5 (unspecified effects)	• Diaphoresis, pallor • Muscle cramps, fatigue, weakness • Dizziness, headache, fainting • Nausea, vomiting • Tachycardia, orthostatic hypotension • Elevated body temperature (up to 105°F)	• Administer cooling measures, including a cool shower or sponge bath, moving the patient to a cool environment, and rehydration with cool nonalcoholic beverages. • Allow the patient to rest. • Monitor the patient's temperature.
Heat stroke ICD-9-CM code: 992.0 (unspecified effects)	• High body temperature (above 105°F); hot, flushed, dry skin • Headache, confusion, agitation, anxiety, delirium, paresthesias, seizures, coma • Tachycardia, hypertension • Tachypnea, dyspnea • Loss of coordination	• Administer cooling measures, including removing excess clothing, applying cool or tepid water to the skin (but avoiding immersion in icy water), and placing covered ice packs in the arm pits and groin. • Administer IV fluids. • Arrange transport of the patient to the hospital. • Monitor the patient's temperature.
Hypothermia ICD-9-CM code: 991.6	• Body temperature less than 95°F (mild), less than 89°F (moderate), or less than 79°F (severe); shivering, cold, pale skin • Lethargy, fatigue, loss of coordination • Confusion, slurred speech, progressive unresponsiveness, eventual coma	• Warming measures, including moving the patient to a warm environment, removing wet clothes, applying dry clothing and blankets, and administering warm fluids by mouth if the patient is able to swallow safely. • Administer warm oxygen and warm IV fluids if ordered.
Frostbite ICD-9-CM code: 991.3 (unspecified sites)	• Very cold or frozen tissue on exposed body parts, such as the ears, cheeks, and nose, and extremities, such as fingers and toes • Skin that appears white (in light-skinned people) or ashen (in dark-skinned people) and feels little pain until it thaws • Tissue that is stiff and has a waxy appearance (in deep frostbite)	• Warming measures that include placing the patient in a warm environment and warming affected body parts in warm water (less than 105°F). (Rewarming deep frostbite should take place in the hospital setting.) • Monitor the patient's vital signs. • *Never* rub the body part because doing so will cause further injury. • Administer opiate analgesics for severe pain as rewarming occurs, as ordered by the physician.

Animal Bite

ICD-9-CM code: 879.8 (uncomplicated, open wound)
An animal bite normally leaves marks and may involve skin puncture, laceration or tearing, pain, bleeding, and bruising of surrounding tissue. The medical assistant should clean the wound as directed by the physician with sterile saline solution, antibacterial solution, or warm water and soap. She should apply antibiotic ointment and a dressing as directed or assist the physician with surgical repair if needed. The physician will order a tetanus booster if needed. The medical assistant should question the patient or accompanying family or friends in order to attempt to identify the animal involved and whether rabies should be a concern.

Snake Bite

ICD-9-CM code: 989.5 (venomous snakes, lizards and spiders)
Snake bites may be nonvenomous or venomous. Nonvenomous bites leave fang marks in the skin, local tissue pain, discoloration, burning, edema, and inflammation. Venomous snake bite symptoms vary with the type of snake and include the same local symptoms as in nonvenomous bites, plus blurred vision, convulsions, diarrhea, dizziness, diaphoresis, syncope, fever, thirst, loss of coordination, nausea, vomiting, tachycardia, and weakness. The medical assistant should calm and reassure the patient and keep the affected body part below heart level. She should assist the patient to rest in

a position of comfort and remove jewelry on the affected body part. She should also monitor the patient's vital signs and try to identify the type of snake, if possible, without putting anyone in danger by trying to capture the snake for identification purposes. She should clean the bite with warm water and soap or antibacterial solution and apply antibacterial ointment and dressing per the physician's order. She may also order antivenin if needed by calling a regional Poison Control Center (in the United States, the University of Arizona Poison and Drug Information Center at 1-520-626-6016, which is available 24 hours a day.)

Insect Sting

ICD-9-CM code: 919.4 (nonvenomous insect bite)

An insect sting or bite causes a sharp stinging sensation, redness, itching, and localized edema. A systemic allergic reaction may cause generalized edema, rash, itching, and, possibly, respiratory compromise (anaphylaxis). The medical assistant should determine if the stinger is still present in the skin and, if so, remove it by scraping across it with a plastic card. She should then clean the site with water and soap and apply a cold pack, anesthetic spray, or dry dressing as directed by the physician. She should continually observe for signs of allergic reaction. She may administer antihistamines, corticosteroids, and epinephrine as ordered by the physician for moderate to severe reactions and anaphylaxis.

Burns

First-degree burn—ICD-9-CM code: 940.1 to 949.1 (4th digit indicates degree; 5th digit indicates BSA)
Second-degree burn—ICD-9-CM code: 940.2 to 949.2 (4th digit indicates degree; 5th digit indicates BSA)
Third-degree burn—ICD-9-CM code: 940.3 to 949.3 (4th digit indicates degree; 5th digit indicates BSA)

Burns are classified according to severity as *first-degree*, *second-degree*, or *third-degree*. Part of evaluating the patient with burns includes an estimation of the percentage of the person's body surface area (BSA) affected. A commonly used tool for this process is a chart, called the Rule of Nines, which divides the body up into sections that are 9% of total BSA. (See Figure 47-2.) By referring to this chart, the medical assistant can make a quick, fairly accurate estimation. This data is essential in determining the person's condition and making appropriate treatment decisions.

First-Degree

First-degree burns, also called *superficial burns,* involve only the epidermis. (See Figure 47-3.) They are generally considered minor injuries. When a patient experiences a first-degree burn, his skin becomes red, blanches to pressure, is moderately painful to the touch, and is dry with no blisters. Permanent tissue damage is rare and may consist of minor changes in skin color. Sunburn is an example of a first-

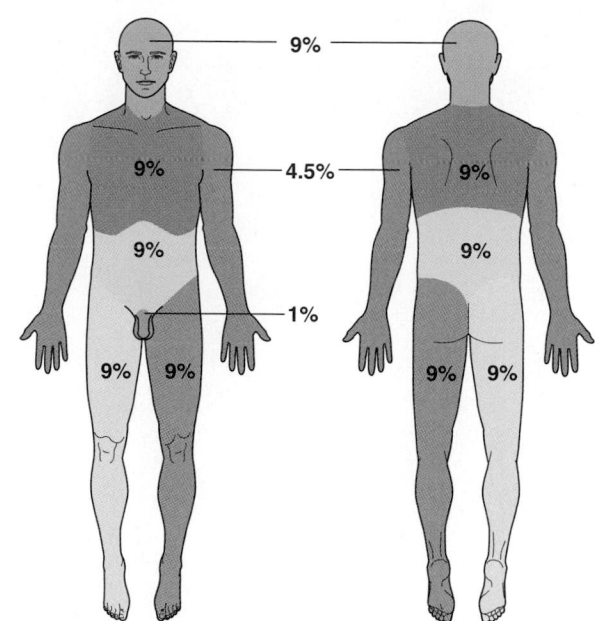

FIG 47-2 Rule of Nines.

degree burn. First-degree burns usually heal without further treatment and do not require treatment from a physician.

Second-Degree

Second-degree burns, also called *partial-thickness burns,* involve the epidermis and part of the dermis. The patient experiences intense pain and his skin appears red, edematous, and wet, shiny, or blistered. Second-degree burns usually result from exposure to flames, scalding liquids, steam, or direct contact with a very hot object. A patient with second-degree burns should be seen by the physician immediately. A patient with extensive second-degree burns should be treated in an emergency room and will most likely require hospitalization. A physician in a medical office can usually treat a patient with second-degree burns covering less than 10% of her BSA. At the direction of the physician, the medical assistant can clean the wound and apply silver sulfadiazine cream or another antibiotic ointment and a nonadherent dressing. The physician may also prescribe analgesics for pain and antibiotics to prevent infection. The medical assistant can also instruct the patient on other ways to avoid infection. (See *Preventing infection in burn wounds,* page 985.)

At the direction of the physician, the medical assistant can help treat second-degree burns that cover a small part of the body (2" to 3" in diameter) by cooling the burn with cold water or cold compresses. However, she should never apply ice directly to the site because doing so can cause frostbite. The medical assistant should cover loosely with a sterile bandage any areas where the skin is blistered or broken. The

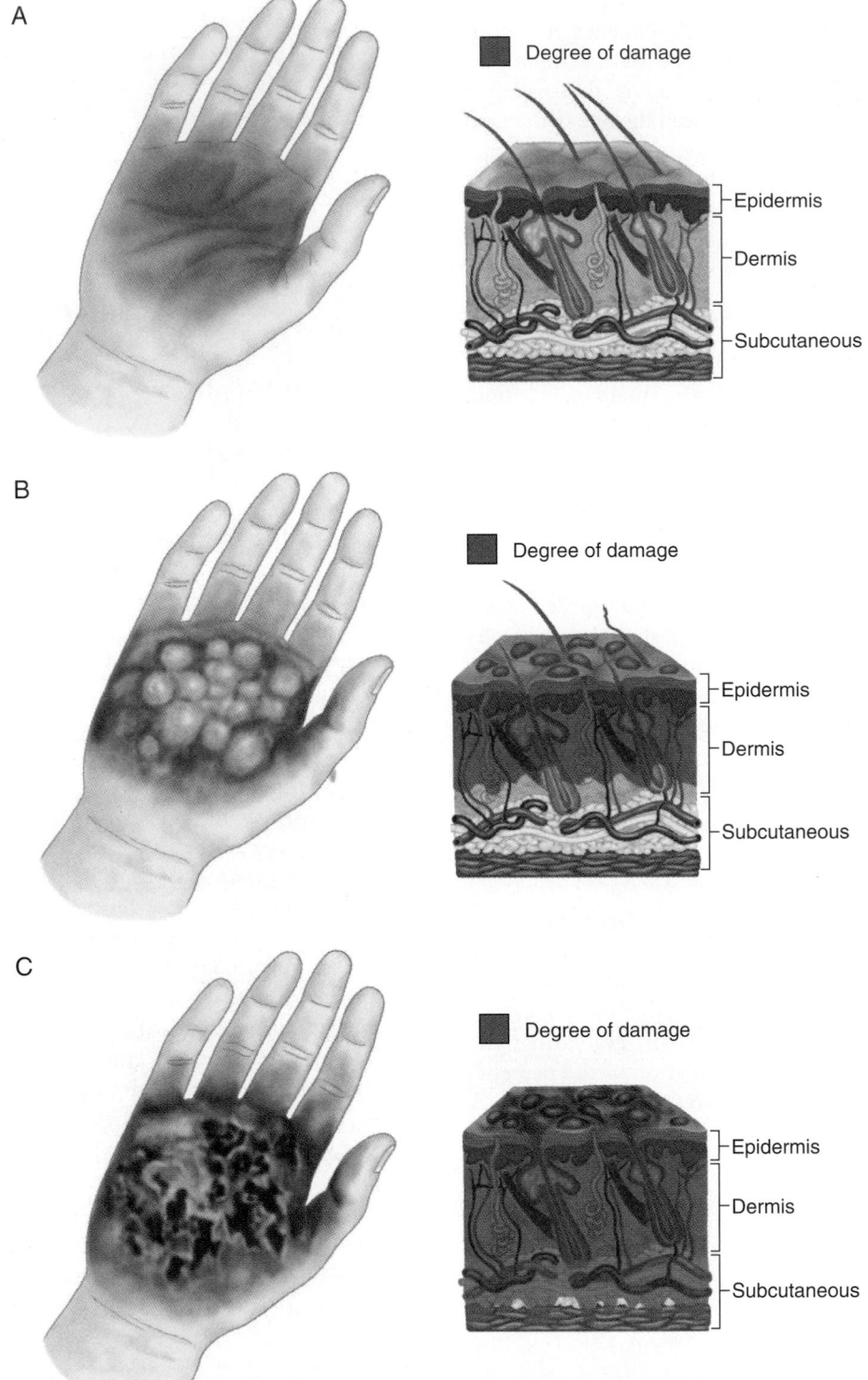

FIG 47-3 Classification of burns. (A) First-degree. (B) Second-degree. (C) Third-degree.

physician may order analgesics such as ibuprofen or acetaminophen to alleviate mild to moderate pain and opiate analgesics for severe pain. The medical assistant should administer such medications as ordered.

Second-degree burns covering a larger area of the body or located on the hands, the feet, a major joint, the face, the buttocks, or the groin may require special treatment because of a greater risk of complications. The medical assistant should be sure to consult with the physician for special instructions on treating such burns.

Third-Degree

Third-degree burns, also called *full-thickness burns,* destroy the epidermis, dermis, and subcutaneous layers of the skin. Fatty tissue, muscle, bone, and tendon may be involved as well, although some experts further classify burns with such involvement as *fourth-degree burns.* These burns may appear black and charred, brown, yellow, or even white. They are also dry and leathery. The patient feels no pain from third-degree burns because the nerves are destroyed. However, he may have first- and second-degree burns in the surrounding area that may be very painful. Typical causes of third-degree burns include scalding liquids, contact with flames, chemicals, extended contact with a hot object, or electrical burns.

Patients with third-degree burns should receive treatment in a hospital, preferably one with a burn unit because of the risk of profound dehydration, shock, infection, septicemia, and other life-threatening complications.

Treatment of patients with third-degree burns includes IV fluid and electrolyte replacement, wound debridement, antibiotics, analgesics, a diet high in protein and calories, and extensive rehabilitation. These patients may also be candidates for skin grafting and reconstructive surgery.

Musculoskeletal Injury

Musculoskeletal injuries are common in a medical office. While they may be less serious than some conditions, many are considered emergencies that require immediate attention. The medical assistant should assist the patient into a position of greatest comfort and quickly evaluate circulation distal to the injured site. This is especially important if a fracture may be present because such an injury can impair circulation. If she is unable to confirm circulation, the medical assistant must contact the physician immediately, because the patient's limb may be in peril. Common musculoskeletal injuries include fracture, sprain, and muscle strain.

Fractures and Sprains

Fractures—ICD-9-CM code: 800 to 829 (coded according to site, type, and other factors)
Sprains—ICD-9-CM code: 840 to 848 (coded according to site, type, and other factors)

Fractures and sprains are among the most common forms of musculoskeletal injuries seen in the medical office. A *fracture* is a break or crack in a bone. A sprain is trauma to a joint that causes a brief, partial dislocation, resulting in tearing of the ligaments that stabilize the joint. In either case, the patient may also have suffered injury to surrounding tissue, including blood vessels, nerves, muscles, and tendons. Thus, the patient commonly complains of pain, edema (swelling), ecchymosis (bruising), and decreased function. Symptoms of sprain include pain, weakness, decreased function, and, possibly, numbness. Bruising is usually not apparent. Fractures and sprains are almost always caused by some form of trauma or repetitive motion. Osteoporosis is also a major risk factor for fractures in elderly patients.

With most types of fracture or sprain, the patient's condition is typically unclear at first. Thus, most medical office protocols include sending the patient for an immediate x-ray before seeing the physician to help determine whether the injured body part is fractured or sprained. However, the physician should immediately examine a patient with an obvious compound (open) fracture, in which the bone is protruding from the skin. Such a fracture can cause severe pain, hemorrhage, numbness, and circulation impairment and has a high risk of infection. Such patients will also need x-rays but should be quickly examined by the physician first because the injury may constitute a surgical emergency.

While the patient is waiting for x-rays or treatment, the medical assistant should help him into the position of greatest comfort and offer a way to stabilize his injured body part, such as with a pillow. The medical assistant can also apply ice packs or instant cold packs as approved by the physician to reduce swelling and pain. Basic care measures for a sprain or uncomplicated fracture help minimize edema formation, which helps minimize discomfort. To treat a sprain or uncomplicated fracture, the medical assistant can apply a splint and an elastic bandage or air splint, per the physician's order. Before and after applying a splint or dressing to an injured extremity, the medical assistant should always make sure there is adequate circulation to the injured tissue by checking circulation, motion, and sensation and document her findings. (See *Safety alert: CMS.*) She can also continue cold therapy and help the patient elevate the injured body part above heart level. (See *RICE.*) In addition, the physician may prescribe NSAIDs, opiates, and muscle relaxants to alleviate pain and reduce muscle spasms.

Muscle Strain
ICD-9-CM code: 840 to 848 (code specific site)
A muscle strain injury involves overstretching and tearing of muscles and tendons. Symptoms include pain, decreased function, and weakness. Mild cases of muscle strain resolve with rest. Treatment for moderate to severe muscle strain

includes the *RICE* approach, analgesics for pain, and muscle relaxants to reduce muscle spasm. Physical therapy may also help to ease discomfort and restore function.

Eye Injury
ICD-9-CM code: 930.9 (foreign body)
The medical assistant should quickly place a patient with an eye injury or a foreign body in the eye in an examination room and gently apply patches to both eyes to minimize movement while she awaits examination by the physician. The medical assistant should instruct the patient to refrain from rubbing her eyes because doing so could cause further injury.

Treatment for a foreign body in the eye usually includes irrigation with sterile saline solution. If the patient is in pain from inflammation, the medical assistant can instill anesthetic drops as directed by the physician. The physician may prescribe antibiotic drops or ointment if infection is present or if the patient is at risk for infection. Other care may include application of cold compresses and administration of NSAIDs to alleviate inflammation and pain. The medical assistant can help the physician with examination and treatment as needed.

Safety alert: CMS

To remember to check circulation before and after applying a splint or dressing to an injured extremity, the medical assistant should remember *CMS:*

• **Circulation**—Check pulses or capillary refill.

• **Motion**—Ask the patient to wiggle his fingers or toes.

• **Sensation**—Ask the patient to close his eyes and verify when you touch his fingers or toes.

RICE

To remember basic care measures for the patient with a sprain or uncomplicated fracture, the medical assistant can use the acronym *RICE:*

• **Rest** (splint application)

• **Ice** (application of a cold pack)

• **Compression** (air splint or elastic bandage)

• **Elevation** of injured part above the heart.

Chapter Summary

• Everyone who works in a medical office should be trained and prepared to respond to emergencies. Such preparation includes establishing a written plan of response in case of fire, disaster, workplace violence, or medical emergency.

• All health care facilities must make an effort to create an environment that is safe for patients and staff alike. Workplace safety programs provide instruction in cardiopulmonary resuscitation (CPR), standard precautions, proper body mechanics, and other safety issues.

• Medical staff must be sure to maintain inventory of needed supplies and medications and restock following each emergency event. In addition, staff must carefully maintain and routinely check emergency equipment so that it is always ready.

• Many facilities routinely run mock codes, which are rehearsals for responding to specific emergencies, so that all members of the health care team can practice and develop their skills in responding to medical emergencies.

• An important, but sometimes overlooked part of emergency preparedness is the designation of a team member to document the emergency, called a *recorder* in some care settings.

• Not all medical offices keep emergency equipment on hand, but many do. If an office does stock emergency equipment and medication, staff should be familiar with its use.

- A defibrillator is a specialized device used to deliver an electrical shock to a patient suffering from a life-threatening cardiac arrhythmia to convert the heart back to normal sinus rhythm. An AED is a smaller, more portable version of a defibrillator.

- Triage is the process of making a quick determination about the nature of the patient's emergency, the type of immediate care needed, and the most appropriate response. If more than one patient is involved, triage may also involve determining which patient should be treated first.

- When a medical emergency occurs, the patient's exact diagnosis may be unclear at first. The patient may simply display a collection of signs and symptoms.

- A common emergency is the patient with dyspnea. The medical assistant can look for clues to identify the severity of the patient's distress and determine an appropriate response. Such clues include skin color, character of respirations, respiratory rate, use of accessory muscles, breath sounds, and the patient's mental or emotional state. Common causes of dyspnea include choking, asthma attacks, anaphylaxis, pneumonia, COPD exacerbation, chemical or smoke inhalation, pneumothorax, and MI or heart failure.

- The medical assistant must always take seriously any complaint of chest pain. Common causes of chest pain include MI, angina, GERD, cholecystitis, costochondritis, pulmonary embolism, spontaneous pneumothorax, and panic attack.

- Numerous types of injuries result in hemorrhage (bleeding), which may be minor or life-threatening. After checking airway, breathing, and circulation, the medical assistant must take measures to control bleeding. A laceration is a cut or tear in the flesh that may bleed slightly or may hemorrhage profusely. Epistaxis (nosebleed) is caused by erosion or rupture of small vessels within the nasal mucosa. Common causes include seizures, conditions related to diabetes management, and head injury as well as stroke, cardiac arrhythmias, and cardiac arrest; however, the cause is usually unclear at first.

- Causes of a slower change in consciousness include hyperglycemia, hypoglycemia, drug toxicities, dementia, and other neurological disorders. Although these conditions can be quite serious or even life-threatening, the changes generally occur gradually, which enables evaluation, diagnosis, and initiation of treatment before the situation becomes an emergency.

- Poisoning most commonly occurs from oral ingestion of a substance. Other causes include injection, absorption, and inhalation.

- Occasionally patients enter the medical office with environmental injuries such as animal bites, insect stings, or burns. Less common injuries seen in this setting include heat exhaustion, heat stroke, and hypothermia. After attending to ABCs, the medical assistant must gather information about the mechanism of injury to help ensure appropriate treatment.

- Burns are classified according to severity as first-degree, second-degree, and third-degree burns. First-degree burns usually heal without further treatment and do not require treatment from a physician. The physician should see patients with second- and third-degree burns immediately. Those with extensive second- and third-degree burns should be treated in an emergency room and will most likely require hospitalization.

- Acute abdominal pain has many potential causes, some of which may be life-threatening. When a patient complains of acute abdominal pain, the cause is seldom immediately clear. Therefore, the medical assistant must take all such cases seriously and provide care according to office protocol, including informing the physician so that she can begin prompt evaluation and treatment. Common causes of abdominal pain include peptic ulcer disease, gastroenteritis, ulcerative colitis, diverticulitis, Crohn disease, cholecystitis, and appendicitis.

- Fractures and sprains are among the most common forms of musculoskeletal injuries seen in the medical office.

- A sprain is trauma to a joint that causes a brief, partial dislocation, resulting in tearing of the ligaments that stabilize the joint.

- A muscle strain injury involves overstretching and tearing of muscles and tendons.

- The medical assistant should quickly place a patient with an eye injury or a foreign body in the eye in an examination room and gently apply patches to both eyes to minimize movement while she awaits examination by the physician. Treatment for a foreign body in the eye usually includes irrigation with sterile saline solution.

Team Work Exercises

1. Divide into teams and select one of the following assignments. Report your findings to the rest of the class in a manner specified by your instructor.
   a. Contact a medical office in your town and ask them to describe:
      - what protocols they have in place for responding to medical emergencies, such as the patient with chest pain
      - what types of patients they usually take immediately into examination rooms, rather than having them wait in the reception area
      - whether they have an emergency cart (crash cart) and what type of equipment and supplies it contains
      - whether they have a special code system for alerting staff to emergencies, such as a medical emergency,

fire, bomb threat, and so on, and if so, what are some examples.

b. Create a protocol for dealing with a patient who walks into your office with chest pain. Role-play a scenario for the rest of class in which you demonstrate the protocol that you created.

c. Create a protocol for dealing with a patient who walks into your office with a severe nosebleed. Role-play a scenario for the rest of class in which you demonstrate the protocol that you created.

d. Create a protocol for dealing with a patient in your office experiencing severe dyspnea. Role-play a scenario for the rest of class in which you demonstrate the protocol that you created.

e. Create a protocol for dealing with a patient who has a tonic-clonic seizure in the reception room. Role-play a scenario for the rest of class in which you demonstrate the protocol that you created.

2. Divide into teams of three to five students each. Develop a triage plan for the order in which the following patients would be cared for (assuming they could only be seen one at a time). Present your list of patients in the order in which they would be cared for to the rest of the class and explain your rationale for the order. (Two teams will have the same list in order to compare how the teams triaged their patients.)

a. Teams 1 and 2
- 19-year-old female with severe RLQ pelvic pain and vaginal spotting
- 65-year-old man with moderate dyspnea and left shoulder pain
- 35-year-old man with first- and second-degree burns over his face, right arm, and chest
- 12-year-old boy with a bite on his right leg from a snake, which may have been a rattlesnake
- 51-year-old man with severe abdominal pain and a distended belly
- 25-year-old man with a potentially fractured right forearm
- 19-year-old woman with severe wheezing and history or asthma

b. Teams 3 and 4
- 45-year-old woman with LLQ pain
- 72-year-old woman with second- and potentially third-degree burns on her arms from hot cooking oil
- 18-month-old lethargic infant who is hot, fussy, and diaphoretic and was left in the car in 90°F heat while the mother was in a store for 45 minutes
- 47-year-old man who walks in with his hand wrapped in a blood-soaked towel
- 17-year-old with glass fragment in his eye
- 20-year-old with swollen right eye from a bee sting

- 38-year-old woman with nausea and pain in her RUQ and right shoulder

c. Teams 5 and 6
- 66-year-old with COPD and moderate dyspnea
- 55-year-old with pneumonia, fever, chills, and moderate dyspnea
- 67-year-old with severe pain in the abdomen that radiates to his back
- 17-year-old with an obvious compound leg fracture who was brought in by friends after a skateboard accident
- 32-year-old woman with pelvic and low back pain, frequency, and dysuria
- 40-year-old man with chronic heartburn, which is worse today
- 27-year-old woman who fainted at the grocery store but is now alert and oriented

Case Studies

1. Albert Gomez is a medical assistant working in an urgent care clinic. He notices that a patient waiting in the reception area who brought her 9-year-old granddaughter in with a sore throat is having chest pain and dyspnea. As he walks across the room to talk with her, an elderly couple enters the reception area. The elderly woman, who appears upset, calls out "I think my husband is having a heart attack!"

a. Describe a way in which Albert can respond to this situation so that the needs of both patients are met.

b. There is currently only one unoccupied examination room and one crash cart with a defibrillator available. Where should each of these patients be cared for? How should the staff allocate the use of the defibrillator?

c. Describe how the administrative and clinical medical assistants can work together to facilitate efficient care for these patients.

d. Describe strategies the staff might employ to tend to the needs of the six other patients waiting in the reception area and the five patients currently in examination rooms.

2. Claudia Benevides is a medical assistant working in a family medicine practice. Describe how she ought to respond to the following patients who arrive at the office without prior notice:

a. A concerned mother brings her 10-year-old son, who was stung by a bee on his right forearm 30 minutes ago. It is red and swollen to about the size of a golf ball. He has no other symptoms.

b. A 32-year-old woman states that she had blood-streaked stool this morning and thinks she might also have a fever.

c. A 68-year-old woman arrives with her husband, who is experiencing a sudden onset of confusion, difficulty speaking, and right-sided weakness.

d. A woman arrives with her 14-year-old daughter, who has grease burns on her right leg and foot from a spill that occurred 20 minutes ago.

e. A worried mother arrives with her 22-year-old son, who has a severe nosebleed that won't stop.

Resources

- BCLS and ACLS certification courses from the American Heart Association: *www.americanheart.org /presenter.jhtml?identifier=3011795*

- Emergency preparedness guidelines from the American Red Cross: *www.redcross.org/services/prepare/0,1082,0_239_, 00.html*

- Frequently asked questions about poisoning: *www .poisonprevention.org/faq.htm*

- Guidelines for patients on burn prevention: *www .healthline.com/sw/wl-what-you-need-to-know-about -burn-prevention*

- Guideline for treating patients with animal bites: *www.nlm.nih.gov/medlineplus/ency/article/000034.htm*

Radiology and Diagnostic Imaging

Objectives

Upon completion of this chapter, the student will be able to:

- define and use the terms in the glossary
- list the four views for chest x-ray, describing the patient positioning for each
- discuss patient positioning for back, neck, and extremity x-ray and how to comfort the patient in pain
- explain the patient preparation necessary for mammography
- explain the difference between film-screen radiography and fluoroscopy
- explain the function of contrast media and special considerations of their use with patients
- describe how ultrasound waves create images of soft tissue and internal organs.

CAAHEP Competencies

Clinical Competencies
Patient Care
Perform telephone and in-person screening
Prepare and maintain examination and treatment areas
Prepare patients for and assist with routine and specialty examinations
Screen and follow up test results

General Competencies
Professional Communications

Recognize and respond to verbal communications
Recognize and respond to nonverbal communications

Legal Concepts
Identify and respond to issues of confidentiality

Patient Instruction
Instruct individuals according to their needs

ABHES Competencies

Professionalism
Maintain confidentiality at all times
Conduct work within scope of education, training, and ability

Communication
Adapt what is said to the recipient's level of comprehension
Serve as a liaison between the physician and others
Recognize and respond to verbal and nonverbal communication
Adaptation for individualized needs
Application of electronic technology

Clinical Duties
Prepare patients for procedures
Prepare and maintain examination and treatment area
Prepare patient for and assist physician with routine and specialty examinations and treatments and minor office surgeries

Legal Concepts
Determine needs for documentation and reporting
Document accurately

Procedures

Assist x-ray technician with patient positioning as needed
Schedule patients for diagnostic testing

Chapter Outline

Key Terms

angiogram
Diagnostic radiograph of the blood vessels using a contrast medium

cholecystogram
Radiograph of the gallbladder

claustrophobia
Fear of closed spaces

computed tomography
Computerized procedure that views the target organ or body area from different angles in a three-dimensional view

contrast medium
Radiopaque substance that enhances an image

digital radiographic imaging
Radiography using computer imaging instead of conventional film or screen imaging

dosimeter
Device that monitors the quantity of x-ray exposure to health care workers

fluoroscopy
Radiographic imaging that can be viewed as a moving picture

intravenous pyelogram
Radiographic view of the kidneys using contrast medium injected intravenously

ionization
Process of gaining or losing an electron from an atom

lower gastrointestinal series
Radiographic examination of the lower intestinal tract during and after introduction of barium, which acts as the contrast medium

magnetic resonance imaging
Procedure in which a strong magnetic field and radio waves are used to produce images to view body structures

mammography
Radiographic imaging of the breast to screen for breast cancer

nuclear medicine
Techniques that use radioactive material for the diagnosis and treatment of patients

open MRI
Imaging table with more open space than a traditional MRI tube

positron emission tomography
Procedure in which the brain is viewed using positron-emitting radionuclides

radiograph
Image produced on radiosensitive film by x-rays passed through an object

radiography
Process of producing an image for diagnosis using a radiographic modality

radiology
Branch of medicine concerned with radioactive substances, including x-rays or other sources of ionizing radiation used to assist in diagnosis and treatment

radiolucent
Penetrable by x-rays

radiopaque
Impenetrable to x-rays or other forms of radiation

tomography
Radiographic technique that selects a level in the body and blurs out structures above and below that plane, leaving a clear image of the selected anatomy

tracer
Radioactive isotope that can identify a specific portion of a molecule to follow its course

transducer
Device that moves over the skin to record sound waves

ultrasound
Use of high-frequency sound waves to produce an image of an organ or tissue

upper gastrointestinal series
Radiographic examination of the esophagus, stomach, and upper small intestine during and after the introduction of barium as a contrast medium; also called *upper GI series* or *barium swallow*

x-ray film
Special photographic film that blackens on exposure to light

x-ray tube
Vacuum tube that creates electromagnetic radiation with a wavelength between 0.1 and 100 angstrom units

Radiography and the Medical Assistant

Radiography is a diagnostic technique that uses radiation to produce an image of the body. The branch of medicine concerned with radioactive substances, including x-rays or other sources of ionizing radiation, sound, or radiofrequencies, for diagnosis and treatment is referred to as *radiology*. Radiograph procedures can include x-ray, ultrasound, magnetic resonance imaging (MRI), computed tomography (CT) scan, mammogram, and radionuclide imaging.

In a radiography setting, the medical assistant's main duties include instructing the patient before, during, and after the procedure and assisting with positioning the patient, as directed. The patient's health care provider (such as an MD or APRN) will typically order the procedure, a radiologic technologist (or *radiographer*), will perform the procedure, and the patient's health care provider or a radiologist will interpret, or *read,* the image, or **radiograph**. (See *Radiography roles.*)

The health care provider is responsible for explaining the images to the patient. The medical assistant can assist the provider by placing the images on the view box during a patient visit and filing the radiology report in the patient's medical record. View boxes are lighted and often mounted on the wall of the treatment room or office. The image is placed in front of the light and the light shining through the image allows the physician to view it. The medical assistant should check the name on the image before putting it on the view box. If the patient asks the medical assistant about the findings, the medical assistant should not offer an interpretation. She should instead tell the patient that the physician or nurse will explain findings when she arrives.

In addition to understanding the techniques, procedures, and patient care associated with radiology, the medical assistant must have a good understanding of terminology related to radiology and diagnostic imaging. (See *Radiography terminology,* page 994.)

Radiography roles

In radiography, a radiologic technologist performs radiography procedures as ordered by the patient's health care provider, who may interpret the results or may consult with a radiologist.

Radiologic technologist

A radiologic technologist, or *radiographer,* performs imaging procedures ordered by physicians or other health care providers. To become a radiologic technologist, a person must graduate from a 2- or 4-year program and then pass a national examination administered by the American Registry of Radiologic Technologies. If the person passes the examination, he can use the title *Registered Radiologic Technologist* (RRT).

Radiologist

The patient's health care provider should interpret, or *read,* the radiography results. If the procedure is performed outside of the medical practice, such as at a hospital or imaging center, a radiologist (a medical doctor who specializes in x-rays) will interpret the images and send a report of his findings along with the images to the health care provider. The provider must then read the radiologist's report and view the images herself.

X-Ray

X-rays were discovered by German physicist Wilhelm Konrad Roentgen in 1895. X-rays are a type of light wave within the electromagnetic spectrum. A special **x-ray tube** is a vacuum tube that causes **ionization** (gain or loss of an electron from an atom) of the x-rays, creating electromagnetic radiation with a wavelength between 0.1 and 100 angstrom units. This ionization causes fluorescence of certain substances, which in turn creates the x-ray picture. The process revolutionized diagnosis of disease because, for the first time, physicians could "see" inside a patient's body without cutting it open.

X-ray imaging, typically referred to simply as *x-ray,* is the most common radiographic technique. In the procedure, a patient is positioned between an x-ray tube and **x-ray film,** a special photographic film that blackens on exposure to light. The x-ray machine then directs electromagnetic radiation through the patient's body from the tube onto the x-ray film. As the radiation passes through the patient's body, structures that are **radiopaque** (impenetrable by electromagnetic radiation) prevent the radiation from reaching the film. The radiation passes easily through structures that are **radiolucent** (penetrable by electromagnetic radiation). (See Figure 48-1.)

Because radiopaque structures are impenetrable to electromagnetic radiation, they will appear white on the x-ray film because the x-ray beam could not penetrate them. Bone is the densest tissue in the body and will appear white on the x-ray film. Other radiopaque structures include teeth, surgical metal implants, and calcified structures of the body. Because radiolucent structures allow x-ray radiation to pass through the patient's body to the x-ray film, they appear darker on the film. Such soft tissues of the body as muscle, fascia, and fat are radiolucent. Thus, the resulting image, called an *x-ray* or *radiograph,* shows definition of bony structures and absence of soft tissues. (See Figure 48-2.)

Radiography terminology

The medical assistant should be familiar with the terminology used in the x-ray department or in the physician's office. Here are some of the most common terms she will encounter in such a setting:

- *anteroposterior* (AP)—x-ray view in which the patient is positioned facing the x-ray tube or lying supine
- *prone*—x-ray view in which the patient is positioned lying prone (face down)
- *supine*—x-ray view in which the patient is positioned lying supine (on back)
- *posteroanterior* (PA)—x-ray view in which the patient is positioned facing the x-ray film or lying prone
- *oblique*—x-ray taken at a 45-degree angle
- *lateral*—x-ray taken from the side view (right or left)
- *weightbearing*—indication on an x-ray order that the

patient must bear weight for the view (typically used for the foot, knee, and back)

- *plain film*—term used for an x-ray image to differentiate it from other types of images
- *bucky*—moving grid device in which the cassette loaded with radiographic film is placed
- *cassette*—holder in which the technician places the radiographic film in the darkroom to protect it from exposure to light until exposure to x-rays.

Word Elements

In addition to radiology terms, the medical assistant should be familiar with some of the most common word elements associated with radiology. The following table lists common combining forms, prefixes, and suffixes related to radiology.

Word Element	Meaning	Example	Meaning
Combining Forms			
actin/o	ray; some form of radiation	actinotherapy (ăk-tĭn-ō-THĔR-ă-pē)	treatment of a disease with rays of light
anter/o	anterior, front, before	anteroinferior (ăn-tĕr-ō-ĭn-FĒ-rē-or)	in front and below
fluor/o	luminous; fluorescence	fluorochrome (FLOO-ŏr-krōm)	coloring agent that adds fluorescent glow to an object
later/o	side	bilateral (bī-LĂT-ĕr-ăl)	pertaining to or affecting two sides
mamm/o	breast	mammoplasty (MĂM-ō-plăs-tē)	reconstructive surgery of the breast
oste/o	bone	osteodynia (ŏs-tē-ō-DĬN-ē-ă)	pain in bone
poster/o	posterior, behind, toward the back	posteromedial (pŏs-tĕr-ō-MĒ-dē-ăl)	toward the back and middle
pyel/o	pelvis	pyelotomy (pī-ĕ-LŎT-ō-mē)	incision of the renal pelvis
radi/o	radiant energy; a radioactive substance	radiobiology (rā-dē-ō-bī-ŎL-ō-jē)	branch of biology that deals with ionizing radiation and the effects on living tissues
Prefixes			
cine-	movement	cinematics (sĭn-ĕ-MĂT-ĭks)	science of movement
contra-	against	contraindication (kŏn-tră-ĭn-dĭ-KĀ-shŭn)	any reason that makes treatment with a drug unsafe
trans-	across; over; beyond; through	translucent (trăns-LŪ-sĕnt)	permitting the passage of some light through an object
ultra-	beyond; excess	ultrasound (ŬL-tră-sownd)	inaudible sound frequency used to create images
Suffixes			
-graph	instrument used to make a drawing or record	radiograph (RĀ-dē-ō-grăf)	image produced on radiosensitive film by x-rays passed through an object
-scope	instrument for viewing or examining	fluoroscope (FLOO-or-ō-skōp)	instrument that produces moving images
-scopy	examination	fluoroscopy (floo-or-ŎS-kō-pē)	examination that produces moving images

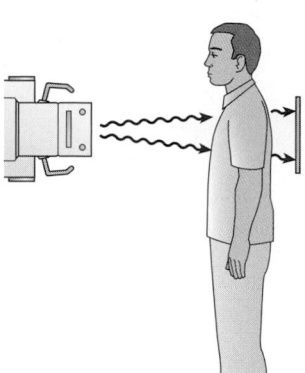

FIG 48-1 X-ray technique.

X-Ray Film

X-ray, or radiographic, film is manufactured to be sensitive to energy from the x-ray machine. It is coated with a photosensitive fluid on both sides, which makes it easy to load film into cassettes. Film must be stored in a clean, cool, dry area. Humidity will fog the film, causing poor x-ray quality. Film has an expiration date, so the medical assistant who loads film into cassettes should check the date on the film. Boxes of film should be stored with the expiration date visible, with the closest date in the front to be used first. Film and cassettes come in standard sizes:

- 8″ × 10″ (20 × 25 cm)
- 9″ × 9″ (23 × 23 cm)
- 10″ × 12″ (25 × 30 cm)
- 11″ × 14″ (28 × 35 cm)
- 7″ × 17″ (18 × 43 cm)
- 14″ × 14″ (36 × 36 cm)
- 14″ × 17″ (36 × 43 cm).

X-Ray Views

X-ray views are named for the direction of the beam in relation to the body part that the beam of radiation passes through. There are five major x-ray views:

- posteroanterior
- anteroposterior
- right lateral
- left lateral
- oblique.

Thus, a patient that is positioned for a chest x-ray (CXR) with his back toward the x-ray tube would produce a posteroanterior (PA) chest film. If the patient then turns around to face the x-ray tube, the x-ray produced would be an anteroposterior (AP) view. Placing the patient at a 90-degree angle for a chest film produces a right lateral (LAT) or left lateral chest view. When the patient is positioned at a 45-degree angle, the x-ray produces an oblique view. X-ray views of extremities have the same terminology; thus, an anteroposterior knee film would show the front of the knee. (See Figure 48-3.)

Patient Preparation for X-ray

Before the x-ray procedure, the medical assistant should explain the procedure to the patient. If appropriate, she should ask the patient if she is pregnant because exposing a fetus to x-rays can damage its growth and development. Thus, health care providers rarely order x-rays for a pregnant

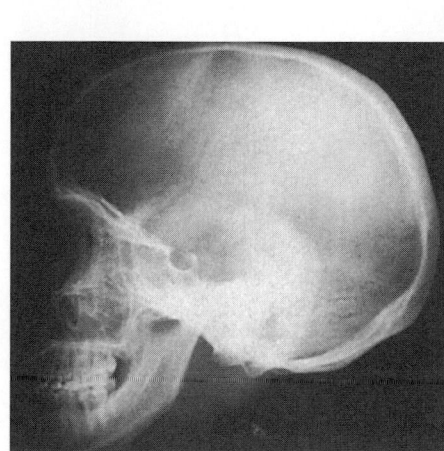

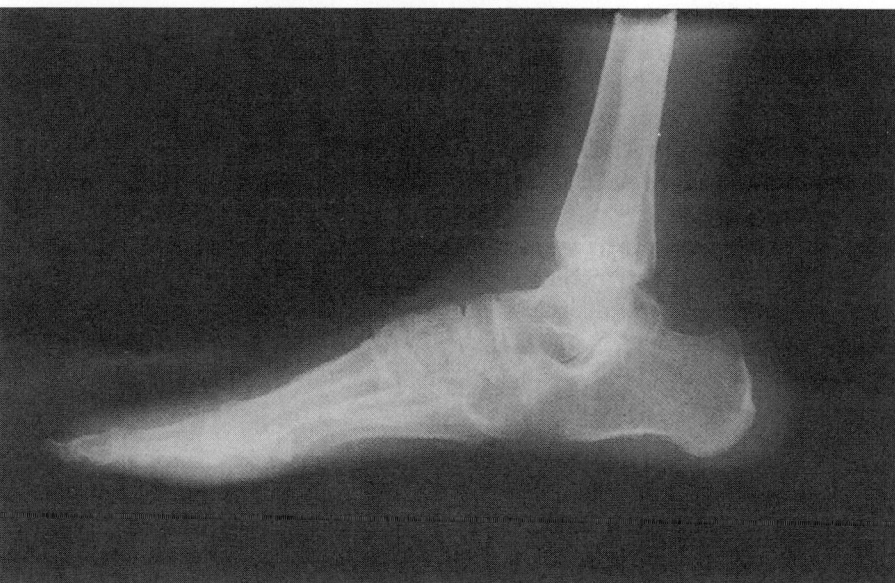

FIG 48-2 Plain film x-rays.

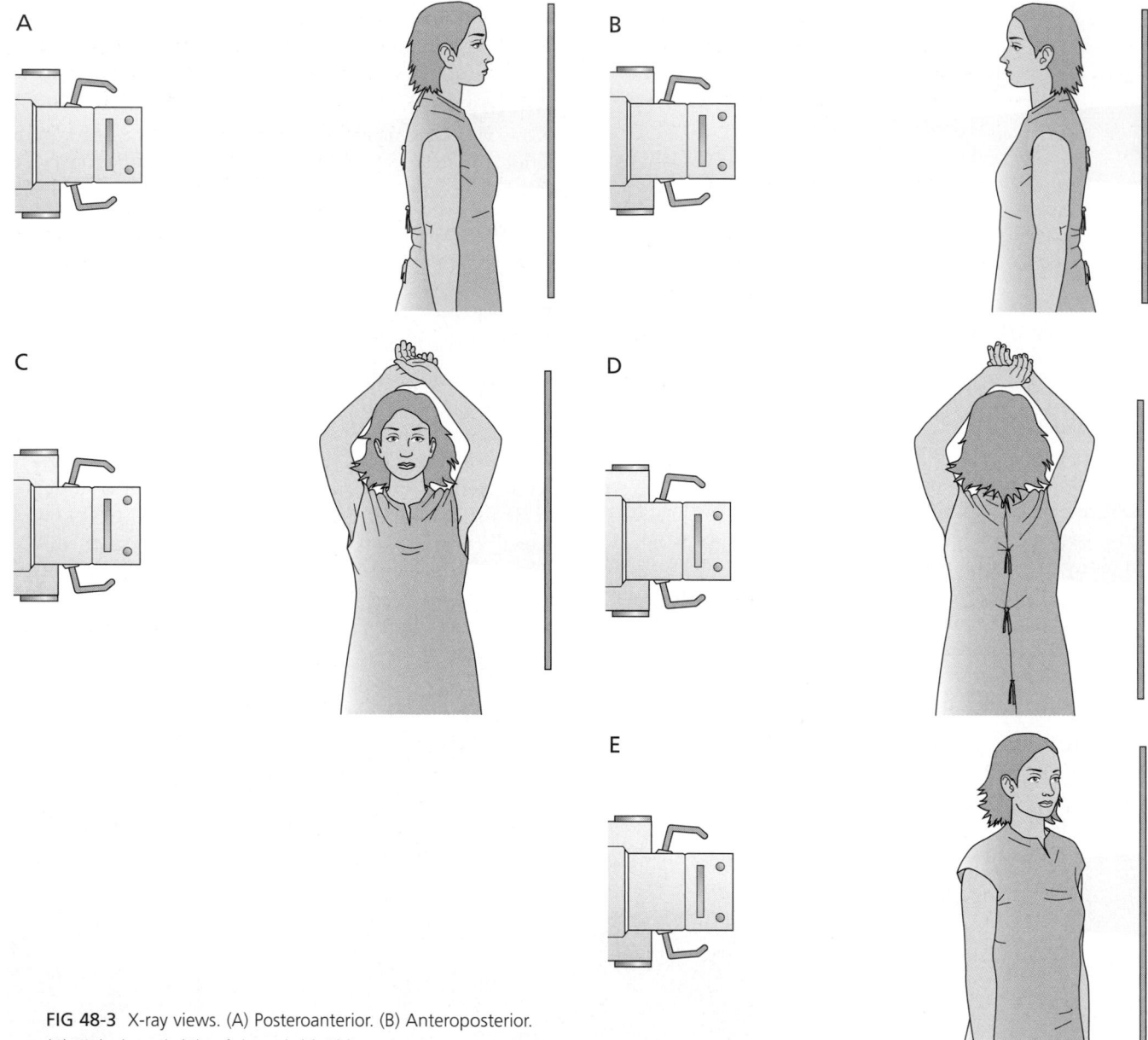

FIG 48-3 X-ray views. (A) Posteroanterior. (B) Anteroposterior. (C) Right lateral. (D) Left lateral. (E) Oblique.

woman. In the case of an emergency, it may be acceptable to x-ray a pregnant woman's extremity.

The medical assistant should instruct the patient to remove all jewelry and female patients to remove underwire bras; these objects are radiopaque, so they will appear on the x-ray image and limit the view of the patient's body. When the patient is ready, the medical assistant should position the patient appropriately for the x-ray. For weightbearing x-ray studies of the chest or back, the medical assistant should position the patient standing. These same areas are viewable via x-ray with the patient lying down on an x-ray table

(nonweightbearing). The medical assistant should always mark the x-rays as weightbearing or nonweightbearing.

There are four major areas that undergo x-ray. The medical assistant may be asked to assist the radiologic technologist in positioning a patient for x-ray or comforting an injured patient, so she must be familiar with these areas and the appropriate patient positioning and instruction for each:

- *chest x-ray*—The medical assistant should ask the patient to stand or lie down (as directed), remain still, and take a deep breath and hold it until directed to release it.

- *lower back*—The medical assistant should ask the patient to stand or lie down (as directed) and remain still (no need to take a deep breath).
- *cervical spine*—The medical assistant should ask the patient to stand. She should then place the x-ray tube at the patient's head and neck level, check the order for open- or closed-mouth x-ray, and direct the patient to open or close his mouth, as appropriate.
- *extremities*—The medical assistant should ask the patient to sit or lie on the x-ray table and then place the x-ray film under the affected body part. (See Figure 48-4.) She

should drape a lead apron across the patient's shoulders and lap to protect his reproductive organs from ionizing radiation. (See *Gonad shields,* page 998.) Because extremity x-rays diagnose injury, she should be careful moving the affected area. Directing the patient to move the extremity on their own (if possible) is commonly the least traumatic for the patient. She should allow the patient to move slowly without rushing him and ask him to remain still during the x-ray. (See *Procedure 48-1: Preparing a patient for and assisting with x-ray examination,* page 999.)

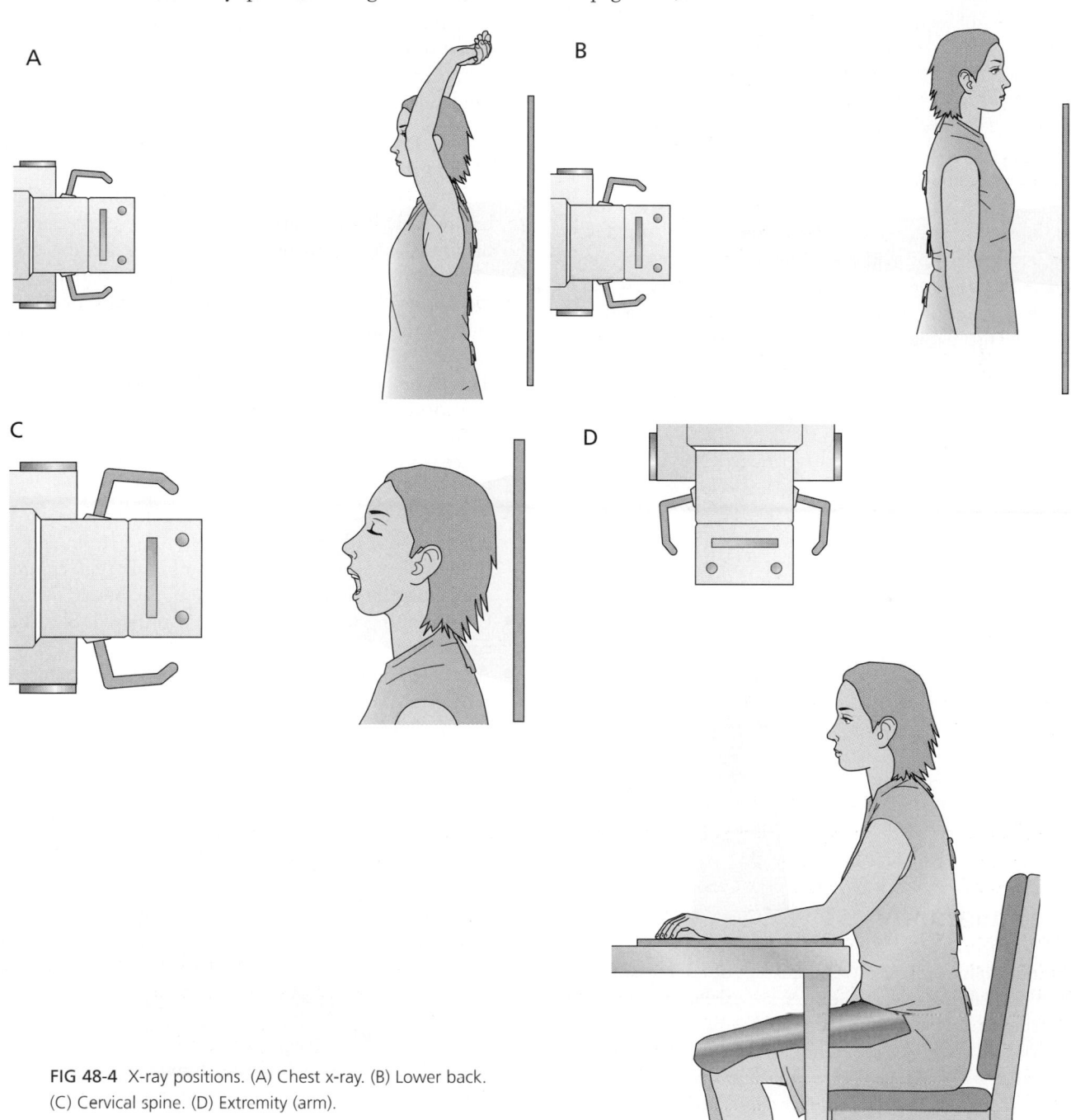

FIG 48-4 X-ray positions. (A) Chest x-ray. (B) Lower back. (C) Cervical spine. (D) Extremity (arm).

Gonad shields

Exposure of reproductive organs to radiation can cause cellular damage that can lead to sterility. The medical assistant and radiologic technologist should always shield patients who are at reproductive age (or younger) from exposure using a gonad shield. The medical assistant can explain the need for the gonad shield to her patient and place the shield appropriately before the procedure. The shield consists of at least 0.5 mm of lead and will not interfere with the x-ray. The medical assistant can strap the shield around the patient for x-rays in the standing position or drape it over his lap for seated x-rays (such as of the arm, shoulder, or head.) For pelvic x-rays, done with the patient lying supine (face up), the medical assistant should place the shield directly over the patient's reproductive organs to allow an accurate image of the pelvis while protecting reproductive organs from radiation. For male patients, the medical assistant should place the upper margin of the shield 1″ below the symphysis pubis. For females, she should place the lower margin of the shield on the upper margin of the symphysis pubis. No matter the position, proper placement of the shield is vital to ensure that reproductive organs are protected from damage by ionizing radiation.

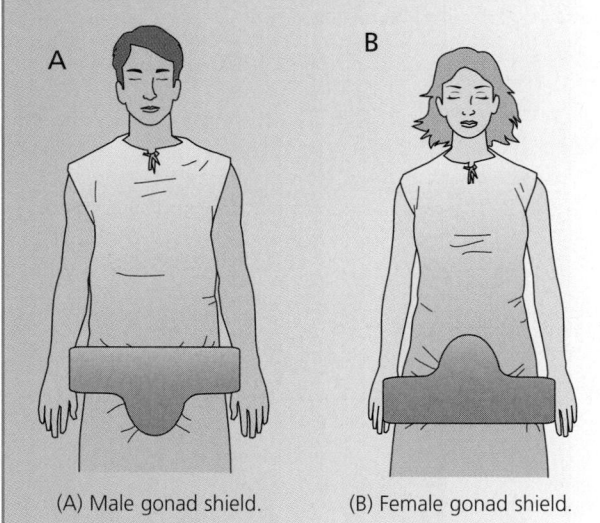

(A) Male gonad shield.   (B) Female gonad shield.

Mammography

Mammography is the x-ray examination of the breast to detect abnormalities, such as cancer or calcium deposits. It is considered one of the most effective methods for early detection of breast cancer along with regular breast self-examinations. Women should receive their first mammogram at age 40 and have follow-up mammograms yearly or as directed by the physician. Males may also undergo a mammogram if abnormalities are detected in male breast tissue.

To undergo a mammogram, the patient must stand facing the mammogram machine. The radiologic technologist or medical assistant will then position the patient's breast on a flat plate on the machine. The machine applies pressure from the top and bottom of the breast and laterally from each side, compressing the breast. When the breast is compressed, the machine will take x-ray images of it. (See Figure 48-5.)

Patient Preparation for Mammography

Before the patient schedules a mammogram, the medical assistant should give her verbal and written instructions. She should address any questions the patient has before the examination. Instructions for the patient include:

- Avoid caffeine for several days before the test to reduce swelling and soreness that caffeine may exacerbate.
- If possible, do not schedule the examination immediately before or during the patient's menstrual cycle because the breasts are commonly tender at that time and the examination may be more uncomfortable for the patient.
- Do not use lotions, powders, antiperspirants, or deodorants on the morning of the test because they may interfere with the image quality.
- The patient will be standing for approximately 15 minutes for the procedure. If standing for this amount of time would be difficult, notify the mammography department to see if accommodations could be made before the examination.
- The machine will compress each breast superiorly to inferiorly and medially to laterally (top to bottom and side to side). There may be some discomfort, but full compression allows for an accurate picture of the breast.
- Only clothing from the waist up is removed. Slacks and comfortable shoes are recommended.
- After the examination, take an analgesic as directed by the physician if soreness or pain are present.

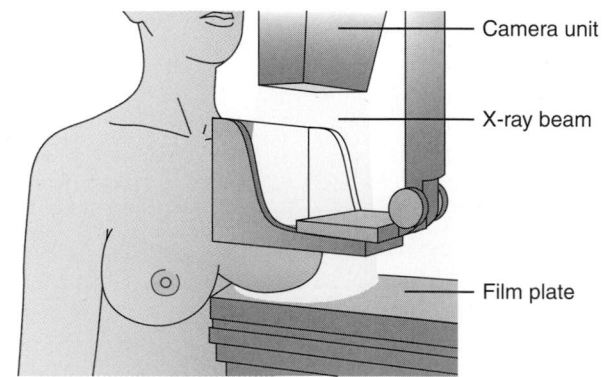

Camera unit

X-ray beam

Film plate

FIG 48-5 Mammography.

PROCEDURE 48-1

Preparing a patient for and assisting with x-ray examination

Task

Prepare and position a patient for x-ray examination, label and store the x-ray, and document the procedure.

Conditions

- Physician's order for x-ray examination
- Patient identification card to imprint x-ray
- X-ray machine and cassette with film loaded
- Lead shield
- Patient's medical record
- X-ray processor, darkroom

Standards

In the time specified and within the scoring parameters determined by the instructor, the student will successfully prepare and position the patient for x-ray examination by the radiologic technologist, label and store the x-ray, and document the procedure.

Performance Standards

1. Greet and identify the patient and explain the examination procedure to reassure the patient and calm his fears about the procedure.
2. Check the x-ray examination order to ensure that the correct procedure is performed.
3. Explain the procedure to the patient and obtain consent verbally or in written form, per office policy.
4. Ask a childbearing-age woman if she may be pregnant. If she is or might be, discontinue the procedure because x-rays can cause injury to a developing fetus.
5. Place the x-ray cassette in the machine.
6. Ask the patient to remove clothing and jewelry, as needed for the procedure, to avoid causing obstruction and ensure the quality of the image.
7. Check to make sure that the patient has removed all metal objects from the area to be examined to avoid

the need for a second x-ray and limit the patient's exposure to radiation.

8. Assist the radiologic technologist with these steps, as requested:
   a. Position the patient against the x-ray film cassette. Proper positioning is required to obtain a clear view.
   b. Align the x-ray tube and cassette at the correct distance and set controls to deliver the appropriate x-ray quantity.
   c. Ask the patient to hold her breath, if necessary, to prevent the diaphragm from moving, which will cause blurring of the image.
9. While the x-ray machine is in use, leave the room with the radiologic technologist and stand behind the lead shield to limit exposure to radiation as much as possible.
10. Ask the patient to relax while the x-ray develops because the patient must wait in case the x-ray quality is poor and another image is required.
11. After the radiologic technologist develops the x-ray and confirms that he does not need to repeat the procedure, ask the patient to dress.
12. Obtain the x-rays from the radiologic technologist and ensure that the films are properly named and dated to avoid misdiagnosis or having to repeat the procedure.
13. Create a labeled x-ray envelope and place the x-rays in it.
14. Document the procedure in the patient's medical record to ensure a complete, accurate medical record.

Date	
05/28/08: 9:45 a.m.	AP/Lat chest x-ray. ----------------------- S. Gonzales, CMA

Fluoroscopy

Unlike an x-ray that produces a still picture, **fluoroscopy** is a type of x-ray procedure that produces a moving picture. The radiologist views the fluoroscopy during the procedure and records it for the physician to review at a later time. This technique contributes valuable information on the functioning of organs, in addition to the structure. Most fluoroscopic examinations require a **contrast medium**, which is a type of substance that makes normally radiolucent structures radiopaque. Normally, such soft tissues as the esophagus, stomach, and small intestines would be radiolucent and, thus,

appear black when viewed on x-ray film. (See Figure 48-6.) Contrast media can be administered orally, through injection, or with an enema. When the patient swallows a contrast medium such as barium, the radiopaque substance outlines the organs, enabling the physician to view the organs. When the physician injects a contrast medium such as iodine into a vein, she can see vascular structures in the kidney. (See *Common diagnostic tests requiring contrast media*, page 1001.)

Patient Preparation

Patient preparation for diagnostic testing with contrast medium requires specific instructions. These instructions

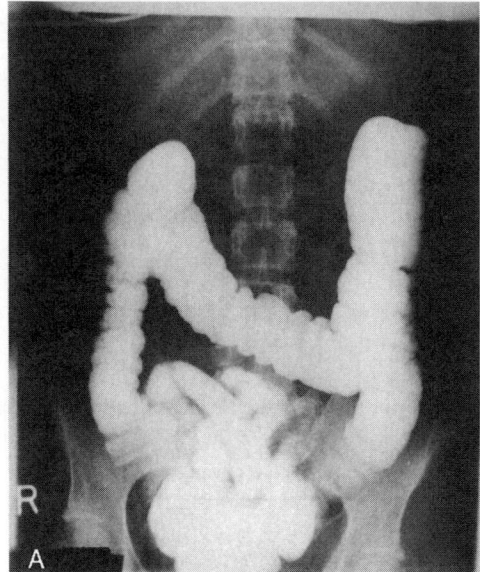
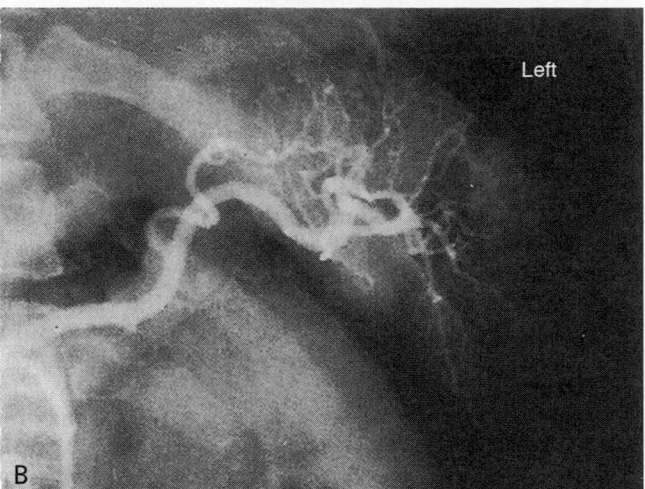

FIG 48-6 Fluoroscopy. (A) Barium in intestines. (From Williams & Hopper. *Understanding Medical Surgical Nursing*, 3rd ed. FA Davis, Philadelphia, 2007, page 650, with permission.) (B) Angiogram with iodine in veins and arteries. (From Tortorici & Apfel. *Advanced Radiographic and Angiographic Procedures*. FA Davis, Philadelphia, 1995, page 236, with permission.)

should always be given in writing and sometimes require a prescription for pretest medication. When scheduling testing, the medical assistant should explain to the patient the importance of following pretest instructions. She should emphasize that if the patient cannot follow the instructions, the test may not be performed. She must also discuss allergies to iodine or shellfish with the patient. If the patient is allergic to iodine, alternative testing is indicated.

Computer Imaging

Computer imaging, or **digital radiographic imaging**, uses x-ray technology but offers an alternative to using x-ray film. Film can expire; become exposed to light, ruining its ability to create images; or arrive from the manufacturer in damaged condition. If the medical assistant or radiologic technologist does not realize that the film is not in good condition, the patient must undergo the discomfort and inconvenience of more testing and will be exposed to more radiation. Because computer imaging does not rely on film, it provides clearer, error-free images. The computer creates the image while the patient is undergoing the test. The interpreter of the image (physician or technologist) can see the image while performing the test, ensuring that no repeat images will be necessary. Computer imaging

techniques include ultrasound, magnetic resonance imaging, computed tomography, and nuclear medicine.

Ultrasound

Ultrasound uses high-frequency sound waves to create an image of soft tissue and internal organs. It is a noninvasive procedure and, because no ionizing radiation is used, it is considered safe to use to view a fetus. The machine consists of a computer screen to view the images, a keyboard to label and save images, a printer to save images for further review, and a **transducer**, which is a device that focuses sound waves into the body. Sound waves enter the body as the transducer passes over the skin. (See Figure 48-7.) The sound waves emitted from the transducer bounce off the deep tissues and differences in the tissue densities create the image. Ultrasound is painless and the patient will only feel the cool conducting gel that is applied to the skin.

Patient Preparation

Patient preparation for ultrasound procedures is limited. Common ultrasound tests include abdominal ultrasound, pelvic ultrasound, and fetal ultrasound.

Abdominal

Abdominal ultrasound is used to view the liver, gallbladder, kidneys, pancreas, spleen, and aorta. Patient preparation

Common diagnostic tests requiring contrast media

The following table lists common diagnostic tests that use a contrast medium, along with the type of medium used, the test's purpose, specific patient preparation considerations, and a description of the procedure.

Test and Purpose	Contrast Medium	Patient Preparation	Procedure Description
Upper GI series Radiographic examination of the esophagus, stomach, and upper small intestines (duodenum) with contrast medium to detect obstruction	Barium sulfate	• Light evening meal • Nothing by mouth (NPO) after midnight	• Patient removes all clothing and wears a gown. • Medical assistant or technologist positions the patient with his back against the film. • Patient drinks barium during examination.
Lower GI series Radiographic examination of the colon with contrast medium to detect polyps, inflammation, diverticula, and other abnormalities	Barium sulfate	• Low-residue diet for 2 days • No dairy products • Use of special bowel preparation kit to evacuate bowel contents • Light evening meal and NPO after midnight • Enema and rectal suppositories the morning of the examination	• Patient removes all clothing and puts on gown with opening in the back. • Medical assistant or technologist positions the patient in Sims position. • Physician inserts barium sulfate as an enema. • Medical assistant helps patient with frequent side-to-side turning to allow barium to move through the intestines.
Intravenous pyelogram (IVP) Radiograph of the urinary tract during excretion of radiopaque material to examine the renal pelvis, ureters, and bladder to detect cysts, tumors, stones, or strictures and provide information about structure and function	Iodine	• Light evening meal • Laxative taken the night before • NPO after midnight • Before the test, drink fluids, empty bladder before procedure	• Nurse or physician injects dye through intravenous (IV) catheter. • As the kidneys excrete the dye, multiple radiographs record excretion of the material.
Cholecystogram Radiograph of the gallbladder to record movement of bile through the gallbladder	Iodine	• Low-fat evening meal • Oral medication the evening before • NPO after medication	• Technologist performs a series of x-ray films. • Patient consumes fatty meal to stimulate gallbladder after initial films. • Technologist performs subsequent series of x-rays.
Angiogram Radiographic record of the size, shape, and location of the heart and blood vessels to detect tumors and obstructions as well as lung, heart, and other organ problems	Iodine	• NPO after midnight	• Nurse or physician administers a sedative. • Nurse or physician injects dye into a vein using an IV catheter. • Technologist takes series of x-ray films.

guidelines include nothing by mouth (NPO) after midnight before the day of the test.

Pelvic

Pelvic ultrasound is used to view various structures in the pelvis. The approach used may be transvaginal or transrectal. Patient preparation guidelines include no dietary restrictions. However, the test must be performed while the patient's bladder is full. Thus, the patient must drink four to six 8-oz glasses of fluid 1 hour before the examination.

Fetal

Fetal ultrasound is used to view the developing fetus to approximate gestational age, determine the sex of the fetus, measure head circumference, and assess the position of the placenta. It can also detect abnormalities of the fetus or

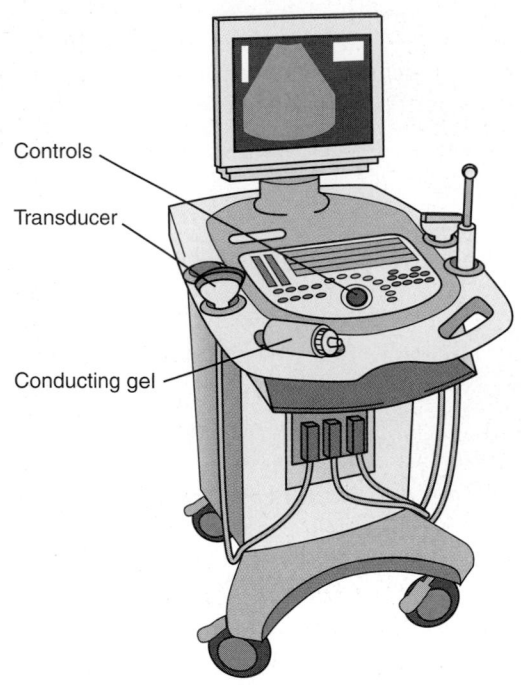

Controls

Transducer

Conducting gel

FIG 48-7 Ultrasound machine and equipment.

placenta. There are no special patient preparation guidelines for fetal ultrasound.

Magnetic Resonance Imaging

Magnetic resonance imaging (MRI) uses a strong magnetic field and radio waves to view anatomical structures. MRI scans create a three-dimensional image of the body that can show blood clots, nerve damage, torn ligaments and tendons, and other soft tissue abnormalities that x-ray technology cannot differentiate. MRI scans are noninvasive and patient preparation is limited to pretest questions.

Patient Preparation

Dietary restrictions are not necessary for MRI scans. In addition, patients can continue their prescription medications without restriction. The medical assistant must ask the patient these questions before the scan:

- *Do you have any medical devices with metal, such as pacemakers, surgical rods or pins, or dental bridges?* The medical assistant must be sure to explain to the patient that the strong magnetic field of the MRI can pull loose metal fragments out of the patient's body, causing injury. She should also explain that permanent metal objects in the body will blur the picture. Objects that contain metal that can be removed for the scan include hearing aids, glasses, hair clips, and dentures. Because clothing could contain metal, the medical assistant should tell the patient that he must remove all clothing and wear the gown provided. She should also tell the patient not to wear eye shadow,

transdermal patches, or aluminum-based antiperspirants, as they all contain metal.

- *Does your occupation involve small particles of metal?* The medical assistant should explain that welders, plumbers, and ironworkers may be exposed to particulate metal on the job. These patients may require ophthalmic x-rays before the examination to rule out metal fragments in the eyes to avoid injury during the examination.
- *Could you be pregnant?* The medical assistant should ask this question of all female patients of childbearing age. MRI scans are contraindicated during pregnancy because the effects of a strong magnetic field on a developing fetus are not well documented.
- *Will you be able to lie still for at least 30 minutes?* The medical assistant should explain that movement will blur the image. MRI scans may not be feasible for patients with lower back pain or other conditions that induce pain when maintaining the same position for an extended time period.
- *Do you suffer from claustrophobia (fear of enclosed spaces)?* The medical assistant should explain to the patient that the MRI scanner is a tubelike structure in which the patient must remain still for an extended period. A patient who may feel anxious can receive a mild sedative before the scan for comfort.

During the examination, the patient must lie supine (on her back) with her arms at her sides. The medical assistant can place a small pillow behind the patient's knees if necessary for comfort. When the patient is comfortably positioned on the bed, the technologist slides the bed into the magnetic tube. The scan takes 30 to 45 minutes, depending on the body areas to be scanned. The patient will hear a humming or thumping sound. The medical assistant can provide earplugs to lessen the noise.

For obese or severely claustrophobic patients, an **open MRI** scanner may provide some relief from anxiety or difficulty. The scanner produces the same images but the imaging table is wider and the sound less noticeable. Children who may be fearful of the noise and closed-in feeling of the MRI scanner can also benefit from the open MRI. (See Figure 48-8.)

Computed Tomography

Computed tomography (CT), or *computerized axial tomography* (CAT), is a technology that produces cross-sectional views of the body, or *slices,* along varying axes (hence, the word *axial*). The machine is able to focus on the structures of the body in one specific plane to create each image. The computer uses these two-dimensional images to create a three-dimensional image, which can rotate in many directions to provide many views of the body. Unlike an ultrasound, which uses sound waves, or an MRI, which uses a strong magnetic field, **tomography uses** x-ray. The CT scanner x-ray tube focuses a narrow x-ray beam across a layer

A

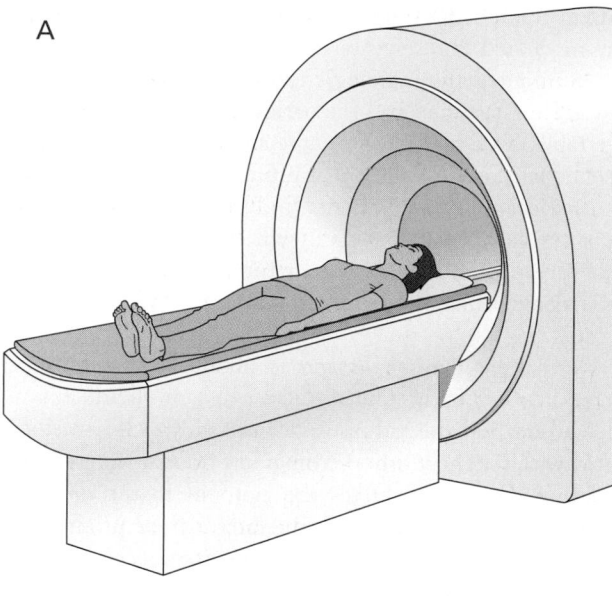

B

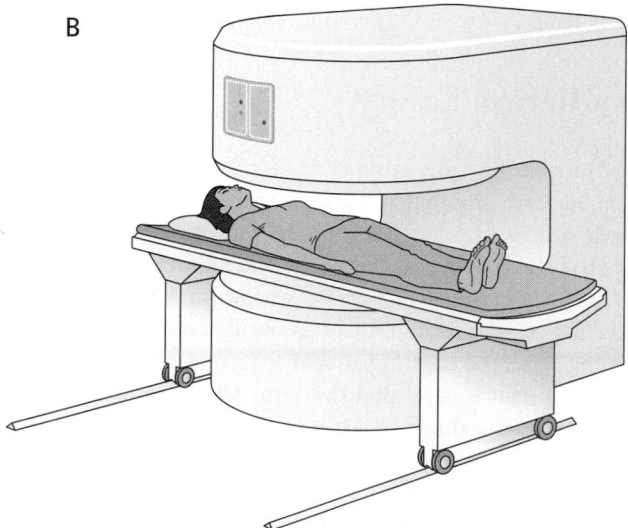

FIG 48-8 MRI scanners. (A) Regular scanner. (B) Open MRI scanner.

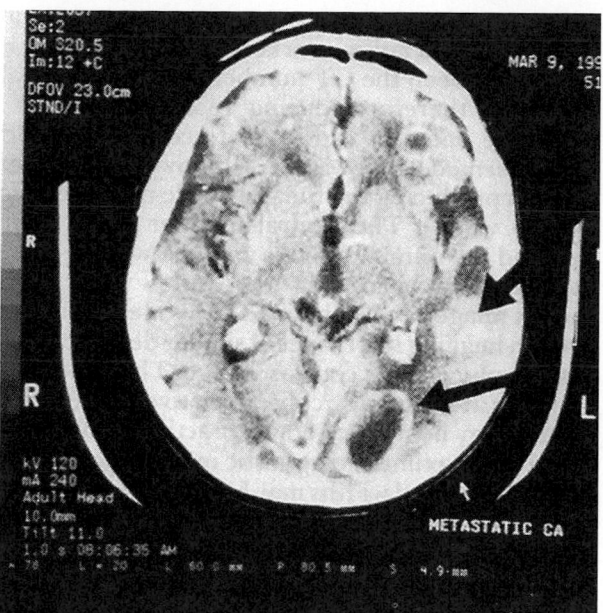

FIG 48-9 CT scan of the head. (From Tortorici & Apfel. *Advanced Radiographic and Angiographic Procedures*. FA Davis, Philadelphia, 1995, page 312, with permission.)

of the body. The computer analyzes the absorption of x-ray energy by body structures (according to their density) and produces an image.

CT scan may involve the use of a contrast medium introduced into an intravenous (IV) line. The nurse or physician injects the dye directly into the vein so the technologist can follow the path of the dye on the scan. (See Figure 48-9.)

Nuclear Medicine

Nuclear medicine includes techniques that use radioactive material for diagnosis and treatment. Nuclear medicine used to treat diseases such as cancer is called *radiation therapy*. **Positron emission tomography** (PET) scanning is a nuclear medicine technique used for diagnosis.

Radiation Therapy

Radiation therapy delivers a specific dose of radiation to a specific area of the body to destroy cancer cells. Radiation alters the cells' structure so that they can no longer reproduce. Healthy cells are affected by radiation but can repair themselves after damage. Although healthy and cancerous cells are affected by radiation, the aim is to kill more cancer cells than healthy body cells. There are two forms of radiation therapy: external and internal.

External Radiation Therapy

In external radiation therapy, the technologist administers calculated doses of radiation from a machine positioned at a specific distance from a tumor. The tumor must be well-defined before radiation therapy begins. A CT scan or ultrasound determines the exact location and size of the tumor. The technologist then marks the patient with a small, permanent tattoo so the radiation continually hits the tumor directly and limits damage to healthy tissue. A patient receives external radiation treatments over a period of weeks or months. The physician carefully monitors the patient's course of treatment and her response through reports from the radiologic technologist and physical examination of the patient.

Internal Radiation Therapy

Internal radiation therapy involves implanting containers of radioactive material near a tumor. Such substances as cesium-137 and cobalt-60 are sealed in gold containers, or *seeds,* and implanted in or near the site of the tumor. The patient can also take radioactive iodine-131, phosphorus-32, or gold-198 by mouth or IV.

Patient Preparation

Patients treated with external or internal radiation therapy may experience adverse effects related to the radiation. The medical assistant can help her patient by providing strategies for reducing symptoms. Common symptoms include anorexia (loss of appetite), nausea, vomiting, and diarrhea. The medical assistant can encourage the patient to eat cool, soft foods in small portions. Because a patient will typically undergo one to two radiation treatments per week, the medical assistant should encourage her to eat on the days that she does not receive radiation in an effort to build strength for the next dose. The medical assistant should instruct the patient to plan time for sleeping and relaxing after treatment. She should also emphasize that the patient should ask a friend or family member to drive her home after the treatment.

Positron Emission Tomography

Positron emission tomography (PET) uses a **tracer**, which is a radioactive isotope that identifies cancer cells and follows their course through the body. The nurse or physician injects tracer material into the patient's vein, and the cancer cells or other cells (such as brain cells) take up the tracer. The tracer, the radioactive sugar isotope fluorodeoxyglucose, attaches to the cancer cells and sends a signal to the PET scanner. The scanner converts the signal into an image on the screen that depicts the exact size and location of the cancer cells. The computer produces images in colors that indicate the degree of metabolism (activity) or blood flow.

Unlike CT and MRI scans, a PET scan can show the functioning of organs. Other tracers, such as carbon-14, calcium-42, and iodine-131 (not sugar tracers), may also be chemically designed to attach to cells of the brain or heart (healthy cells) to create a picture of the functions of that organ. Patients with iodine allergies must receive a carbon or calcium tracer. PET scanning can be a useful tool in assessing potential benefits of coronary bypass surgery because it shows not only obstructed blood flow but also where blood is able to flow. The functional picture obtained with PET scanning enables the physician to safely divert blood flow in a bypass procedure. It can also help in diagnosis of Alzheimer disease, Parkinson disease, and other neurological disorders by enabling a physician to view the cells of the brain and observe areas of decreased activity, an indication of such pathologies.

Patient Preparation

The medical assistant must instruct the patient to fast for 6 hours before a PET scan. She should also explain to the patient that during the procedure, he will be seated in a reclining chair and receive an IV injection of sugar tracer. After 45 minutes, the radiologic technologist takes the patient to the PET scanner, and the patient lies down on the scanner table. The medical assistant should advise the patient that he will need to remain still on the scanner for up to 2 hours. Because many patients find the test difficult, physicians typically prescribe it only when information from the scan is vital, such as to determine tumor size, activity, and location or vascular abnormalities that other testing may not identify.

The patient may be concerned about a radioisotope injected into his body. The medical assistant should reassure the patient that the radioisotopes used in nuclear medicine decay within a short time—from a few hours to a few days—and that the body excretes the isotopes in the urine and feces. She should explain that the radioisotope produces less radioactivity than most x-ray examinations or even a cross-country airplane flight.

Radiation Safety

Because health care workers can be exposed to particles of ionizing radiation when working with x-ray machines, they must follow safety procedures to prevent exposure. Some safety measures are instituted by the facility in which they work. For example, walls of x-ray rooms are lined with lead, limiting exposure through the walls and into adjacent rooms. Also, the control panel of the x-ray machine is placed behind a lead wall so that the x-ray technician is protected while exposing the film. Other safety measures are the responsibility of the health care worker. For example, all health care workers who work in an area with potential exposure to radiation must wear a personal monitor called a *dosimeter*, commonly called a *film badge*. The dosimeter measures the quantity of radiation to which the person is exposed. The person must wear the dosimeter on the outside of her anterior surface, usually on her laboratory coat, between the chest and waist level. If the person wears a lead apron to assist the patient during an x-ray procedure, she must wear the dosimeter on the outside of the apron. She must wear the badge at work at all times and cannot share it with other employees. The facility will send the dosimeters for evaluation of radiation exposure weekly, monthly, or quarterly, depending on the quantity of x-rays taken at the facility and the facility's policy. Employees receive an annual report of their occupational exposure. (See Figure 48-10.)

Although the dosimeter monitors radiation exposure, health care workers can take measures to limit exposure to radiation. During x-ray examinations, the medical assistant or radiologic technologist should stand behind the lead

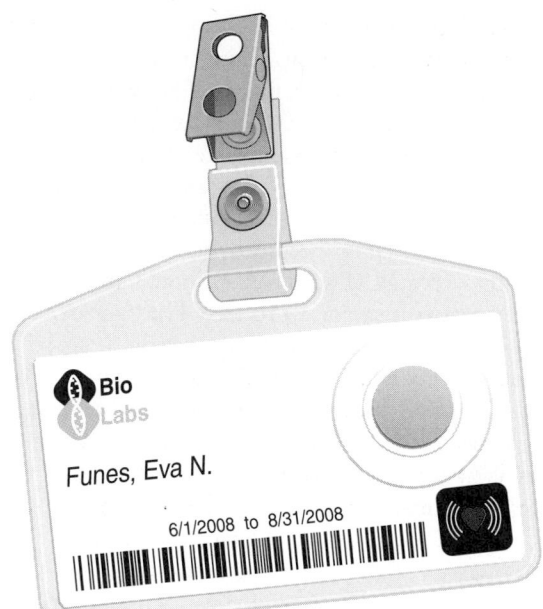

FIG 48-10 Dosimeter.

barrier so that she is not exposed to radiation. Although exposure to radiation during pregnancy can result in birth defects, the pregnant medical assistant or radiologic technologist can avoid exposure by following safety procedures and can work safely through a pregnancy if she desires to do so.

Scheduling Diagnostic Imaging Procedures

The medical assistant commonly schedules diagnostic imaging procedures. Because patient pretest instructions are required for many tests, the medical assistant must explain the pretesting requirements and answer questions that arise at the time of scheduling. The medical assistant should give the patient written pretest instructions, an appointment card with the date and time of the test, and directions to the hospital department or imaging center. Some offices require medical assistants to call patients to remind them of the scheduled testing 24 hours before the appointment. (See *Procedure 48-2: Scheduling a patient for diagnostic examinations.*)

PROCEDURE 48-2

Scheduling a patient for diagnostic examinations

Task
Schedule a patient for diagnostic examinations.

Conditions
- Physician's order for specialty examination
- Written instructions
- Appointment card
- Patient's medical record

Standards
In the time specified and within the scoring parameters determined by the instructor, the student will successfully explain pretesting instructions to the patient and schedule the procedure with an outside provider.

Performance Standards
1. Review the physician's order for testing to prevent mistakes in scheduling testing.
2. Give the patient written instructions for pretest preparation to avoid noncompliance that would require cancellation of the test.
3. Explain the pretest preparation verbally to the patient to allow the patient to ask questions at the visit.
4. Call the provider of the examination to be scheduled (hospital or radiology group) and ask to make an appointment for the examination.

5. Tell the patient the available dates and times for the examination and ask the patient to choose a date and time.
6. Confirm the date, time, and type of examination on the phone with the scheduling personnel to ensure that you and the scheduling personnel hear each other correctly and you give the proper date and time to the patient.
7. Give the patient an appointment card with the date and time of the examination. Provide driving directions to the examination site as needed to ensure that the patient has the correct appointment location, date, and time.
8. Record the scheduled examination in the patient's medical record.

Date	
05/27/08; 11:00 a.m.	Scheduled MRI of left knee for 05/30/08 at 4:30 p.m. at Lincoln Memorial Hospital Radiology, written pretest instructions provided. ———————— C. Chapin, CMA

Chapter Summary

- Radiographic procedures provide important diagnostic information.
- The medical assistant can assist the radiologic technologist in proper patient placement for radiologic procedures.
- Having an understanding of the various types of diagnostic imaging procedures such as x-ray, mammography, ultrasound, and MRI, CT, and PET scanning enables the medical assistant to properly prepare and educate patients.
- Because valid test results rely on proper patient preparation, the medical assistant must communicate pretest preparations to patients and answer questions as they arise.
- The medical assistant can schedule diagnostic and therapeutic hospital radiologic procedures and alert hospital staff to any special needs of her patient.
- Awareness of safety precautions and adherence to safety procedures will allow the medical assistant to perform duties safely.

Team Work Exercises

1. Divide into groups of four to six students. Each group must create a poster or computer presentation on one of these technologies:
   a. CT scan
   b. MRI scan
   c. PET scan
   d. fluoroscopy.
   Each group should be sure to include how the machine works, what patient preparation is required for the examination, whether the technology is used for diagnosis, treatment, or both, and what contraindications or special concerns there might be with its use.
2. Divide into groups of three to five students. Each group must create patient preparation instructions for these examinations:
   a. upper GI series
   b. lower GI series
   c. MRI scan
   d. ultrasound (fetal)
   e. ultrasound (abdominal)
   f. mammogram.

Case Studies

1. Gary Edwards tells the medical assistant that he suffers from claustrophobia and is unsure if he will be able to lie still for the MRI that Dr. Greer has prescribed for his knee. The medical assistant realizes that Gary does not understand that his entire body does not go into the scanner. How should the scheduling medical assistant help Gary? If Gary becomes panicked at the mere thought of the MRI scan, what should the scheduling medical assistant say or do to allay Gary's fears? Should she involve Dr. Greer in the conversation. If so, why?
2. Robert Jenkins is a 78-year-old patient with Parkinson disease who fell and has a large bruise on his left knee. Dr. Rodriguez has ordered an x-ray for Mr. Jenkins's knee. What can the medical assistant do to assist the radiologic technologist in x-raying Mr. Jenkins?

Resources

- American Society of Radiologic Technologists: *www.asrt.org*
- How x-rays are made: *www.colorado.edu/physics/2000/xray/making_xrays.html*
- Labeled normal x-rays: *www.accessexcellence.org/RC/VL/xrays/*
- NASA explains x-rays in medicine and space: *www.science.hq.nasa.gov/kids/imagers/ems/xrays.html*
- Radiology information for patients: *www.radiologyinfo.org/index.cfm?bhcp=1*
- X-ray information: *www.nlm.nih.gov/medlineplus/xrays.html*

Externship and Career Strategies

Key Terms

certification continuation program
Program of documenting ongoing professional activities whereby RMAs may earn continued certification

chronological resume
Resume that lists work experience and education in chronological order, with most recent first

cover letter
Letter that accompanies a resume to highlight the applicant's qualifications and requests a job interview

externship
Scheduled, on-the-job experience that helps a student bridge the gap between the classroom and workplace

functional resume
Resume that emphasizes specific skill sets and describes the most valuable experiences and abilities of the applicant

human resources department
Office or department that advertises job vacancies, accepts applications, arranges interviews, and manages documentation of employee benefits

informational interview
Interview conducted to gain information about an organization to determine whether a person is interested in applying for work there

networking
Exchange of information related to a person's profession with coworkers, friends, and acquaintances

performance evaluation
Assessment of an employee's performance conducted at the end of a probationary period and annually thereafter

preceptor
Experienced medical assistant or other health care provider who agrees to work closely with a student in the medical office

program coordinator
Medical assistant program staff member who arranges externship placement and monitors progress

proofread
Check of a written document for accuracy in spelling, punctuation, grammar, word choice, and sentence structure

resume
Document that summarizes a job applicant's experiences, qualifications, and education

short-timer's syndrome
Tendency of an employee to demonstrate a reduction in the quality of, quantity of, and interest in work after giving notice of the intent to leave the position

skill set
Group of related work abilities

targeted resume
Document that identifies the position desired and summarizes specific experiences and abilities that are relevant to the job for which the person is applying

white space
Blank space in a document to create a more organized, less cluttered presentation

Bridging the Gap

Externship, sometimes called an *internship* or *practicum*, is a scheduled work experience that helps medical assisting students bridge the gap between classroom and workplace. It involves the placement of medical assisting students in medical offices, where they learn by observation and hands-on experience. The externship is an opportunity for the medical assisting student to apply her newly obtained skills and knowledge in a real-world setting, while still benefiting from instruction and supervision from more experienced health care providers. (See *Procedure 49-1: Applying skills for final competency assessment.*)

The **program coordinator** arranges the externship, placing students in medical offices with preceptors. **Preceptors** are experienced medical assistants or other health care providers who agree to work closely with students in the medical office to help them transition from the role of student to the role of professional medical assistant. Program coordinators make occasional site visits to evaluate the student's progress and communicate with preceptors. Programs accredited by the AAMA require students to participate in 160 hours of an unpaid externship experience.

Key Benefits of an Externship

Participation in an externship provides several key benefits to the medical assisting student. She receives real-world experience in her chosen profession, which increases her competence and confidence. Also, an externship can help her identify possible areas for future employment. In addition, she can attain a much higher level of competence than she would if her entire training were restricted to campus classroom and laboratory settings.

Employers also benefit from the externship. They are able to contribute to a student's learning and help students become the kind of employees they would like to hire. In addition, they have a firsthand opportunity to observe the student's work behaviors, interpersonal skills, and attitudes before hiring them for a long-term position. Employers who are impressed by a student's attitude, work ethic, professionalism, and eagerness to learn commonly offer the externship student a position before she graduates.

Externship Placement

The program coordinator carefully selects externship sites to create the best possible experience for students. Ideal placement allows a student to get experience in clinical, administrative, and general areas with staff who are interested in

PROCEDURE 49-1

Applying skills for final competency assessment

Task
Apply various skills learned throughout the clinical medical assisting course to a patient mock scenario.

Conditions
- Patient's medical record
- Supplies and equipment as needed for the given scenario

Standards
In the time specified and within the scoring parameters determined by the instructor, the student will successfully apply various skills learned throughout the clinical medical assisting course to a patient mock scenario.

Performance Standards
1. Greet and identify the patient.
2. Review the patient's medical record.
3. Obtain and document the patient's health history and chief complaint.
4. Demonstrate professional, therapeutic communication skills throughout the scenario.
5. Recognize and respond to verbal and nonverbal communications.
6. Identify and respond to issues of confidentiality and perform within legal and ethical boundaries.
7. Wash your hands. Follow standard precautions throughout the procedure.
8. Perform vital signs measurement and document appropriately.
9. Measure height and weight and document appropriately.
10. Put on appropriate PPEs for the procedure.
11. Prepare the patient for the procedure.
12. Perform the specialized procedure and quality control if applicable, according to the given scenario.
13. Dispose of biohazardous materials.
14. Provide patient education, including instruction on health maintenance and disease prevention. Instruct the patient according to his needs.
15. Document the procedure and teaching in the patient's medical record.

---

supporting their learning. Some of the best externship placements are with staff who realize that the externship student they work with today may well become their work colleague tomorrow. The externship gives such staff members the opportunity to help train students to become the type of future team members they would like to work with.

In some cases, students are offered positions before graduation. Although this may be an exciting development for the student, it can confuse the issue of paid work hours versus unpaid externship hours. Programs accredited by the American Association of Medical Assistants (AAMA) require the externship to be an unpaid experience. Therefore, the medical office that wishes to hire the externship student before the externship is complete must make an arrangement for the student to spend additional *unpaid* time on the job.

Although there may be some advantages for students who get their externship hours in a familiar setting, there are disadvantages as well. The top priority for students is *learning,* which allows them the luxury of asking questions and observing and participating in procedures purely for learning's sake. The top priority for an employee is to meet the needs of employer and patients, which may mean sacrificing the student's opportunity to observe interesting procedures and ask questions. When students try to get externship hours in the place they normally work, these two priorities may come into conflict.

Making a Good Impression

Medical office staff members must observe a student throughout the externship and note student behaviors regarding attendance, punctuality, attitude, flexibility, willingness to learn, work ethic, and professionalism. Students who display good work habits are quickly hired, commonly before they graduate. Even if the externship site is not currently hiring, students should try to make the best impression possible because they may want to list their externship experience on their resume.

Students who work hard and seek opportunities to learn and help others quickly earn the trust and respect of the office staff. Receiving correction and constructive feedback does not come easily for many people. However, students who receive such feedback in a positive, professional manner and modify their performance accordingly will earn high praise from preceptors. During their time in the externship rotation, students are expected to demonstrate an increasing ability to work independently. At the same time, they must be aware of their limitations and always be willing to ask for advice or guidance when unsure of themselves.

A key ability of the professional medical assistant is to maintain an awareness of and respect for professional boundaries. Therefore, students should never attempt to develop a romantic relationship with patients or coworkers. They should not ask the physician for prescriptions to treat themselves or family members and should never use office drug samples unless specifically given permission to do so by the physician. Even entering the drug storage area alone or without permission should be avoided.

The Job Search

The medical assistant has a reputation as one of the health care industry's most versatile members. For this reason, medical assistants are in high demand and some graduating students may find it easy to obtain their first job. On the other hand, job markets change over time and demand for medical assistants may fluctuate, so students should never assume that they will obtain their dream job as soon as they graduate. Therefore, all students should know how to conduct an effective job search.

Many people learn about job opportunities through **networking**, which is the exchange of information about job opportunities with coworkers, friends, and acquaintances. Students should begin networking early in their training and continue throughout their careers. The medical assistant can obtain all kinds of information through networking, including information about financial aid, job openings, and educational opportunities.

By graduation, many students have identified some of the places they would like to work. Direct contact with these facilities can be an effective method of searching for a job. If a student is unsure where she would like to work, she must conduct some research. She can learn a lot about an organization by visiting its website or reading brochures or the annual report distributed by the organization. Other methods include communicating with friends or acquaintances who work there and setting up an **informational interview**. Rather than applying for a job, the student uses such an interview to learn more about the organization to determine if she would like to work there. The student should dress and behave professionally, because making a good impression may lead to a future job. However, she should not ask for a position at the time of the interview. (See *Tips for the informational interview*.)

Other traditional methods of conducting a job search include searching newspaper classified advertisements and working with employment agencies. Such agencies charge a fee for their services to the employer or the applicant. In a tight job market, using such services may be well worth the fee if it means the difference between landing a good job or remaining unemployed.

Applying for a Position

When a medical assistant decides to apply for a position, she should submit her resume in person, along with a cover letter that requests an appointment for a job interview. Although the applicant may be in the office just long

---

Tips for the informational interview

The medical assisting student should keep these tips and guidelines in mind when conducting an informational interview.

General Tips
- Arrive on time.
- Dress professionally.
- Make eye contact.
- Use a firm handshake.
- Do *not* ask for a job.
- Send a thank-you note.

Topics to Ask About
- company mission statement
- size of the organization (such as number of employees, physicians, nurses, and medical assistants)
- typical ratio of medical assistants to physicians
- qualities the organization looks for in employees.

---

enough to hand her resume and cover letter to the receptionist, she must take care to make a positive, professional impression. Good hygiene and professional attire are an absolute must. Making a positive impression will virtually guarantee that the resume and cover letter will be read by a person with hiring authority. A bad impression may make the receptionist or other staff member toss the resume and cover letter in the nearest garbage can.

In small offices, the applicant may meet directly with the office manager or even the physician. In larger facilities, she will be directed to the **human resources department** (also called the *personnel office*), which advertises job vacancies, accepts and reviews all applications, and arranges initial interviews as well as manages documentation of employee benefits.

The Resume

A **resume** is a document that lists contact information, such as address, phone number, and e-mail address, and summarizes the applicant's experiences, qualifications, and education. The resume's purpose is to help the applicant obtain a job interview. Therefore, the applicant should resist the temptation to put too much information in the resume. In most cases, the resume should be just one page long. A resume that appears organized and uncluttered with strategic use of **white space**, or blank space, is more likely to be read.

The applicant should always resist the temptation to include untrue information in her resume in an attempt to make a good impression. Such practices reflect dishonesty and a lack of integrity and create unrealistic expectations on the part of an employer. In addition, lying on a resume is grounds for termination if discovered after the organization hires the applicant. Finding creative ways to highlight and emphasize true experiences and qualifications, regardless of how limited they may be, is the best course of action when compiling a resume. With time, experience, and effort, the medical assistant will accumulate plenty of impressive information to include. When the applicant creates the resume, she should always keep a computerized and hard copy for future modification and use.

In addition to the resume, the applicant should keep a list of references ready in case the hiring office requests them. They should be neatly typed in a style similar to the resume and on the same type of paper. The applicant may also wish to include a comment on the resume that she will provide references "upon request." However, she should not use valuable space on the resume for this information.

Resume Types

There are many types and styles of resume. The applicant may purchase software to help her design her resume or find examples and services on the Internet. The applicant should never copy another resume entirely. Instead, she should create one that is unique and specific to her own experiences and qualifications. The three most common types of resume are the chronological resume, the functional resume, and the targeted resume.

Chronological Resume

A **chronological resume** summarizes the applicant's qualifications and experiences in chronological order, with the most recent information listed first. It includes information on two key areas: education and work experience. The applicant should list first whichever information she thinks is her greatest strength. For example, new graduates with little or no relevant work experience should list education first. Because this same applicant may have limited work experience of any kind, she can highlight community activities and professional affiliations as well. (See Figure 49-1.) As the medical assistant accumulates more relevant professional experience, she can modify her resume to reflect such experience and condense the sections on community activities and professional affiliations. The medical assistant with many years of experience should list her work experience first.

Functional Resume

A **functional resume** does not follow a chronological pattern but emphasizes specific **skill sets** (groups of related work abilities) and describes the most valuable experiences and abilities of the applicant. (See Figure 49-2.) This type of resume may be best for the job applicant who has been out

of the job market for several years or has a history of many short-term jobs.

Targeted Resume

A **targeted resume** identifies the position desired and summarizes the applicant's specific experiences and abilities that are relevant to the job. (See Figure 49-3.) This type of resume is ideal for applicants who know exactly what position they want.

The Cover Letter

The purpose of a **cover letter** is to highlight the applicant's best qualifications and to request a job interview. Cover letters should be professional in appearance and should sell the applicant without being too grandiose (that is, exaggerated with the intention of impressing someone). The applicant should carefully **proofread** the letter, checking for accuracy in spelling, punctuation, grammar, word choice, and sentence structure, to make sure the letter is free of errors. In addition, she should tailor the cover letter to the resume it accompanies and the specific job the applicant is applying for. The cover letter should be addressed respectfully to the appropriate person. If this information is unknown, a phone call is appropriate to ask to whom she should address a letter of application. The applicant should never send a photocopied, generic resume and cover letter, which usually make a poor impression.

Inexperienced job applicants commonly find that one of the most challenging aspects of writing cover letters is determining how to "sell" themselves without appearing conceited. As a result, they tend to be overly modest and create cover letters that are too vague or reflect a lack of confidence. Thus, it is essential for the applicant to demonstrate self-confidence and assertiveness in her resume and cover letter, as well as to explain how her best qualities would benefit the employer, in order to obtain an interview. (See Figure 49-4.)

The Interview

After the applicant has submitted a resume and cover letter, the organization may invite her to come for a job interview. The applicant's goal in an interview should be to convince the prospective employer that she would make a valuable contribution to the organization. She must do this in a way that demonstrates a positive, professional demeanor, without appearing overly confident or aggressive. The applicant's behavior can also cause her to lose a job opportunity. The inability to secure a position is usually related to behaviors or mannerisms demonstrated during the interview process, of which the applicant may be unaware. Some applicants never understand the reason why they do not obtain the job they are hoping for. (See *Interviewing tips*, page 1016.)

Depending on the type and size of the organization, the applicant may interview with the human resources manager,

Nicole Daniels
305 Apple Lane
Fruitdale, CT 06101

Home: (860) 123-3827
Cell: (861) 453-2345
E-mail: ndan@fruit.com

Education

2008 Certificate, Fruitdale Community College, Fruitdale, CT
Major: Medical Assisting

2005 Diploma, Fruitdale High School, Fruitdale, CT

Work Experience

6/06 – 6/08   Food server, Julio's Ristorante Italiano, Fruitdale, CT
                 Duties: waited tables, filled in for hostess and busser,
                 inventoried and ordered supplies, assisted with scheduling

8/04 – 5/06   Barista, Coffee Cupboard, Fruitdale, CT
                 Duties: made assorted coffee drinks, cashiered, weekend opener

Professional Affiliations

• American Assocation of Medical Assistants
• Connecticut Society of Medical Assistants
• Douglas County Chapter of Medical Assistants

Community Activities

• American Cancer Society volunteer
• Fruitdale Community Theater
• Fruitdale Middle School Volunteer Reading Tutor

References: Furnished upon request

FIG 49-1 Sample chronological resume.

the office manager, the physician, or all of them. One person or a committee may conduct the interview. The interview process is commonly a stressful experience for an applicant. However, she can reduce her stress by preparing carefully, including identifying where the interview will take place. If the location is unknown, the applicant may want to drive to the facility the day before to avoid getting lost on the day of the interview. In addition, preparing clothing ahead of time and practicing answering typical interview questions will help the applicant feel prepared and more confident. (See *Common interview questions,* page 1017.)

After the Interview

After an interview, the applicant should always send a thank-you note to the person who conducted the interview. Doing so displays courtesy and professionalism and makes an added positive impression. In addition, it reminds the employer of the applicant's sincere interest in the job. However, the applicant should take care to ensure that the note is written neatly and free of spelling or grammatical errors. Depending on when the employer stated a decision would be made, it is generally considered appropriate to call a week later to inquire whether the position has been filled. If it has not, the applicant should politely relate her continued interest in the position. Continued inquiries should not be made more than once or twice per week. The person in charge of hiring may perceive an applicant who calls more frequently as too aggressive and annoying. Conversely, that person may perceive an applicant who does not call at all as too passive or lacking sincere interest in the job.

Karen Stephens
233 Apple Road
Fruitdale, CT 06101

Home: (860) 123-3344
Cell: (861) 453-6798
E-mail: bdbud@fruit.com

OBJECTIVE
To obtain a position as an administrative Medical Assistant

EDUCATION
2008 Certificate, Fruitdale Community College, Fruitdale, CT
Major: Medical Assisting

STRENGTHS AND ABILITIES
▶ Professional communication skills with clients in person and on the
  telephone
▶ Detail-oriented and organized
▶ Strong multi-tasking skills
▶ Double-entry bookkeeping
▶ Typing: 65 wpm

RELEVANT EXPERIENCE
▶ 2008   Medical Assisting Externship (160 hrs), Eastside Medical Clinic
                    Duties: prepared patients for examinations and procedures,
                    medication administration, phlebotomy, EKGs, medical asepsis,
                    WAIVE testing, data entry, reception, appointment scheduling,
                    filing, coding, inventoried and ordered supplies
▶ 2006 – present   Receptionist, Fruitdale Family Dental Clinic
▶ 2000 – 2006   Homemaker
▶ 1995 – 2000   Stephens Chiropractic Center, Secretary/Bookkeeper

COMMUNITY ACTIVITIES
▶ American Red Cross volunteer
▶ Eastside Daycare Cooperative President
▶ Eastside Community Church Secretary

AFFILIATIONS
▶ Fruitdale Business and Professional Women's Organization
▶ Crested County Chapter of Medical Assistants
▶ Connecticut Society of Medical Assistants

FIG 49-2 Sample functional resume.

Career Advancement

Most employers will place a new employee on a probationary period for up to the first 90 days after beginning a new job. A performance that does not meet employer expectations may result in termination during this time. This time is also an opportunity for the employee and staff to become acquainted. An employee has only one chance to make a first impression, so the newly hired medical assistant should take care to be punctual, arriving a few minutes early, and never try to leave early. She should avoid taking time off for any reason other than significant illness or extreme emergency. Even legitimate absences will make a poor impression if they occur too frequently. A new employee should focus her energy on learning the routine and rhythm of the office, adapting to the various personalities of staff members, and learning the details of the new job. An employee who brings extensive experience to her new job may be tempted to make suggestions about different, more efficient ways of carrying out day-to-day duties. However, she should wait to make such suggestions until after she has earned the trust and respect of other staff members and gains an understanding of the rationale for current practices.

The keys to keeping a new job and advancing in a career revolve around maintaining a professional attitude. (For more information, see Chapter 3, "Professionalism," page 19.) In addition, the professional medical assistant can demonstrate a strong work ethic with her punctuality, consistent

Brenda Williams

2321 Grant Road
Fruitdale, CT
(860) 123-8976
bwill@anyserve.com

Objective: Full-time Medical Assistant position in a primary care practice

Summary: Seven years' experience in emergency and primary health care

Skills and Abilities
Administrative Skills
- Reception and appointment scheduling
- ICD-9-CM and CPT coding

Clinical Skills
- First-aid and CPR
- Phlebotomy
- Electrocardiography
- Medication administration
- Preparation and assistance with sterile procedures

General Skills
- Strong work ethic
- Effective written and verbal communication ability
- Detail-oriented, yet good at multitasking
- Fluent in Spanish

Achievements
- Helped organize new local chapter of AAMA
- Organized and managed children's booth at local health fair
- Taught first-aid course to seventh-grade students at summer camp
- Earned CPR and CMA credential

Education
2008 – present	Fruitdale Community College, Fruitdale, CT
	Major: Nursing
2003	Certificate, Fruitdale Community College, Fruitdale, CT
	Major: Medical Assisting
2001	Certificate, Fruitdale Community College, Fruitdale, CT
	Major: Emergency Medical Technician

Employment History
2006 – 2008	Fruitdale Family Medicine, Fruitdale, CT
	Clinical Medical Assistant
2003 – 2006	Hartell Memorial Hospital, Blueville, CT
	Administrative Medical Assistant
2001 – 2003	Gibbons Ambulance Service, Fruitdale, CT
	Emergency Medical Technician

References: Furnished upon request

FIG 49-3 Sample targeted resume.

attendance, good organizational skills, willingness to stay late if needed, thoroughness, accuracy, and general willingness to help others. A positive, solution-focused attitude and avoiding gossip or other negative behaviors will earn the medical assistant the respect and trust of coworkers. Effectively handling responsibility and tactful, professional communication skills are keys to career advancement.

Performance Evaluation

A medical assistant will typically undergo a **performance evaluation** at the end of the probationary period and each year thereafter. This process involves evaluation of the medical assistant by the manager and, possibly, the medical assistant's peers as well as herself. Although many people feel uncomfortable under such close scrutiny, the medical assistant should welcome it as an opportunity to identify

October 13, 2008

Brenda Williams
2321 Grant Road
Fruitdale, CT

Marcie Cross, Office Manager
1400 Peach Avenue
Fruitdale, CT 06101

Dear Ms. Cross,

I am interested in a position as a medical assistant for your family practice office. I have worked as a medical assistant for the past five years and very much enjoy helping people with their health care needs.

I am currently enrolled in the nursing program at FCC and am excited about a continuing career as a health care professional. I believe my varied experience and skills will enable me to be a versatile, valuable member of your health care team. As you can see from my enclosed resume, I have experience in clinical and administrative medical assisting. I would be happy to work in whatever capacity you may need. However, I would especially enjoy working in both areas if possible, as doing so will enable me to continue to develop and maintain my knowledge and skills in both areas.

Please call me at (860) 123-8976 so that we may schedule an interview and further discuss your needs and my qualifications. I can be contacted during the week after 3:00 p.m. and on weekends. I also have voicemail and respond to all messages promptly. I look forward to hearing from you.

Sincerely,

Brenda Williams

Brenda Williams, CMA (AAMA)

enclosure: resume

FIG 49-4 Sample cover letter.

strengths as well as areas of desired growth. One result of such evaluations should be a plan for professional development to guide future growth and learning. These evaluations are also an opportunity for the medical assistant to share with her manager specific goals for career development.

Employers do not approve of "job-hopping," a practice in which a person moves from position to position without staying in one position for an appropriate length of time. However, after a respectable length of time on the job, a medical assistant may wish to change jobs for personal reasons or for career advancement. Whatever the reason, the medical assistant should leave her current position on a positive, professional note. She should give a minimum of 2 weeks' notice and take care to keep her work effort at a high level through the last minute on the job. The medical assistant will leave a bad impression if she develops **short-timer's syndrome**, the tendency of an employee to reduce the quality, quantity, and interest in work after giving notice of the intent to leave.

Interviewing tips

Here are some key do's and don'ts to help the medical assistant make the best possible impression during a job interview and to avoid unwittingly making a poor impression.

Do's

- Complete and turn in a neat application form.
- Make frequent direct eye contact.
- Appear alert, yet relaxed.
- Remember to smile.
- Keep makeup minimal and conservative.
- Wear minimal jewelry, such as a watch, wedding band, and one pair of stud-type earrings.
- Wear professional dress, such as a suit and closed-toe shoes.
- Be prepared with identified personal goals (that are also in the best interest of the organization).
- Use a firm, brief handshake.
- Be early.
- Prepare questions to ask at the end of the interview.
- Have a plan for self-improvement and professional growth.
- Demonstrate interest in the organization.
- Save money-related questions for later.
- Speak clearly, using good diction and proper grammar.
- Use good hygiene (body, hair, mouth and teeth, nails).
- Keep nails short and smooth with clear, neutral polish or no polish.
- Have a small note pad or planner and pen to take notes.

Don'ts

- Fidget, bite nails, or use other nervous mannerisms
- Keep hands tightly clasped
- Smoke before or during the interview
- Chew gum
- Overdo makeup
- Wear too much jewelry (multiple earrings, dangly earrings, bracelets, necklaces, and so forth)
- Forget to shower or bathe (including hair)
- Let hair hang limp or loose over shoulders or face
- Appear sleepy or bored
- Emphasize or ask about money
- Use poor grammar, pronunciation, or diction
- Talk disrespectfully of past employers
- Keep eyes on the floor
- Use a handshake that is limp or too lengthy
- Arrive late
- Act like a know-it-all
- Make excuses for poor past performance
- Act in an indecisive manner
- Turn in a sloppy application form
- Ask for a temporary position unless it is advertised as such
- Discuss personal life or personal problems
- Wear long or acrylic nails in bold colors
- Say or do anything that might convey intolerance, prejudice, sexism, and so forth
- Act too aggressive
- Wear perfume or cologne
- Take anyone else with you.

Because the medical assistant will want to add the position to her resume and allow the prospective employer to contact her former supervisor for a job reference, she will want to be sure to carry out her duties well to the end of her employment. A positive recommendation from a previous employer can open the door to a new, desirable position.

Credentialing

There are two credentials for medical assistants: the Certified Medical Assistant (CMA) and the Registered Medical Assistant (RMA). These credentials are not legally required for employment as a medical assistant. However, employers seek out medical assistants with these credentials because they understand that these individuals have demonstrated a specific level of competence in educational knowledge as well as in clinical and administrative skills.

Certified Medical Assistant

A medical assistant earns the Certified Medical Assistant (CMA) credential by passing an examination offered by the American Association of Medical Assistants (AAMA). To be eligible for the examination, the person must have

Common interview questions

This table lists some common job interview questions with examples and tips for how the applicant might respond.

Type of Question	Example	Response
The interviewer wants to know what motivates the applicant and whether she will stick around for the long term.	• What are your long-range goals? • Where do you see yourself in 5 years? • Why did you choose a career as a medical assistant?	The applicant should identify reasons that will be of interest to the employer (such as an interest in health care, a desire to help others, a desire to "make a difference," and enjoyment of challenging, stimulating work environments). She should *not* mention money.
The interviewer wants to see if the applicant feels confident and competent and wants to know how the organization will benefit by bringing her on board.	• Why should we hire you? • How will you contribute to this organization? • What are your greatest strengths?	The applicant should share what she will contribute to the organization in a confident manner that is not boastful.
Interviewer wants to know if the applicant has enough humility and insight to identify her own flaws.	• What are your greatest weaknesses?	The applicant should be careful to avoid the potential trap in this type of question. Rather than discussing her flaws at length, which might give a negative impression, she should briefly mention goals she has identified for personal improvement or professional growth and then describe her current plan to achieve these goals.
The interviewer wants to know how the applicant responds to authority.	• Describe an experience in which you had a major conflict with a manager and describe how you handled it. • Describe a time when you felt you were unfairly criticized by your boss. How did you respond?	The applicant should be careful to avoid the potential trap in this type of question. She should avoid speaking in a disrespectful or disparaging manner about previous managers, as the prospective employer might wonder if she has difficulty working cooperatively with persons of authority. Rather she should share an example of a time when she used a positive, professional approach to resolve an issue in a manner that achieved a win-win result for everyone.
Interviewer wants to know how the applicant deals with conflict and whether she uses effective communication and problem-solving skills.	• Describe an experience in which you had a conflict with a coworker. How did you deal with it?	The applicant should share an example of a time when she was able to professionally resolve a conflict with a coworker or at least found a way to work professionally together, despite what may have been a personality conflict.
Interviewer wants to know if the applicant is a team player.	• Describe a previous situation in which you worked as part of a team. What was your role and how did you contribute?	The applicant's answer should stress her willingness to work cooperatively for the good of the team, the patients, and the employer—not to achieve personal goals to the detriment of others.
Interviewer wants to know how the applicant responds to stress.	• Describe a time when you had too much work to get done with pressing deadlines. How did you cope with this?	The applicant should be careful to avoid the potential trap in this type of question. She must avoid complaining about previous work experiences, which conveys to the employer that she might be an employee who complains and harbors resentment. Rather, she should describe a situation in which she rose to the challenge and found creative, cooperative ways to achieve work goals.

graduated from a program of medical assisting accredited by the Commission on Accreditation of Allied Health Education Programs (CAAHEP) or by the Accreditation Bureau of Health Education Schools (ABHES). Students who wish to take the AAMA certification examination can sit for the examination within a three-month period after applying for the examination. Upon successful completion of the examination, the medical assistant earns the privilege of using the credential *CMA* after her name on her name badge and on all official documents. She must recertify her credentials every 5 years by undergoing continuing education or reexamination.

Registered Medical Assistant

A medical assistant earns the Registered Medical Assistant (RMA) credential by passing an examination offered by the American Medical Technologists (AMT), a national certifying organization for laboratory professionals. There are three ways that a medical assistant can qualify for the examination: She must graduate from an ABHES-accredited medical assisting program or an organization approved by the U.S. Department of Education; she must graduate from a formal medical services program of the U.S. Armed Forces; or she must have been employed in the profession of medical assisting for at least 5 years. RMA examinations are offered every week at testing center locations throughout the United States. Upon successful completion of the examination, the medical assistant earns the privilege of using the title *RMA* after her name on her name badge and on all official documents.

Preparing for the Credentialing Examination

The medical assistant can employ a number of strategies when preparing for the credentialing examination. The AAMA will send each medical assistant a copy of the Curriculum Content Outline along with the application form for the CMA examination. The medical assistant can obtain a similar outline and application for the RMA examination on the AMT website. The medical assistant should review this outline carefully when creating her study plan, paying special attention to any areas in which she feels deficient. The content for the CMA and RMA examinations is similar. (See *Credentialing examination content*.)

Credentialing examination content

The Certified Medical Assistant (CMA) and the Registered Medical Assistant (RMA) credentialing examinations are similar. Here are basic outlines of the content for each.

CMA Examination

The CMA examination includes 100 questions in each of three areas: general, administrative, and clinical.

General
- medical terminology
- anatomy and physiology
- psychology
- professionalism
- communication
- medicolegal guidelines and requirements.

Administrative
- data entry
- equipment
- computer concepts
- records management
- screening and processing mail
- scheduling and monitoring appointments
- resource information and community services
- maintaining the office environment

- office policies and procedures
- practice finances.

Clinical
- principles of infection control
- treatment area
- patient preparation and assisting the physician
- patient history interview
- collecting and processing specimens; diagnostic testing
- preparing and administering medications
- emergencies
- first aid
- nutrition.

RMA Examination

The RMA certification examination includes 200 to 210 multiple-choice questions that require the test-taker to recall facts, interpret graphic illustrations, analyze and apply data pertaining to case studies, and perform general problem solving. The examination covers three areas: general (41% of the examination), administrative (24%), and clinical (35%).

General
- anatomy and physiology
- medical terminology

Credentialing examination content—cont'd

- medical law
- medical ethics
- human relations
- patient education.

Administrative
- insurance
- financial and bookkeeping
- medical receptionist/secretarial/clerical.

Clinical
- asepsis
- sterilization

- instruments
- vital signs and mensurations
- physical examinations
- clinical pharmacology
- minor surgery
- therapeutic modalities
- laboratory procedures
- electrocardiography
- first aid.

In order to get the greatest value from her time and effort, the medical assistant should adapt study strategies to her learning style. (For more information on learning styles, see Chapter 1, page 3.) For example, a social learner may wish to organize a study group that meets regularly to discuss specific topics. Such a group can help the medical assistant process information and clarify her understanding of concepts. However, the temptation to socialize can distract members from their main purpose, so adhering to the agenda should be a top priority. To review subject matter that may be included in either examination, the medical assistant may wish to review current publications and text books that include clinical and administrative content as well as anatomy and physiology, medical terminology, and laboratory procedures. In addition, the medical assistant can take several measures on the day of the examination to help her remain relaxed and focused for the examination. (See *Tips for examination day*.)

Recertification

CMAs must recertify their credentials every 5 years by one of two methods:

- retaking the certification examination
- earning continuing education units (CEUs) by attending appropriate educational offerings.

Some CMAs retake the examination, but most CMAs prefer to recertify through continuing education. A CMA must accumulate a total of 60 CEUs in 5 years, 30 of which must be AAMA-approved CEUs. The other 30 may be from other programs and events. It is the responsibility of the medical assistant to determine whether the programs are appropriate for continuing education.

The AMT recently announced a **certification continuation program (CCP)**, which is a program that documents ongoing professional activities that can earn an RMA

Tips for examination day

Here are some tips for the medical assistant to follow before and during the examination to help her relax and remain focused.

Before the Examination
Before the examination, the medical assistant should:

- refrain from traveling or lodging with anyone whose behavior increases her own feelings of anxiety
- get an adequate amount of sleep the night before and avoid studying or other late-night activities
- physically locate the testing center the day before and stay nearby so that she has a short drive the next morning

- plan relaxing activities the night before, such as a nice meal, pleasant music, and perhaps a movie
- eat a nutritious breakfast, including complex carbohydrates and protein—even if she does not usually eat breakfast—so her blood sugar does not fluctuate widely and her energy level remains constant
- consider drinking a small caffeinated beverage to boost mental alertness (However, she should avoid excessive amounts of caffeine as this will make her feel anxious and edgy. Caffeine also has a diuretic effect, so too much may result in the frequent need to empty her bladder.)

Tips for examination day—cont'd

- use anxiety reduction exercises
- trust in herself and use positive self-talk to boost her feelings of confidence and competence.

During the Examination
During the examination, the medical assistant should:

- try to sit near the front of the room or in a corner so that the activities of others are less visible and, thus, less distracting
- ask permission to wear ear plugs if room noise distracts her
- perform an "information dump" if the test administrator permits writing on the examination or a blank piece of paper by writing memorized facts on paper—for example, formulas, laboratory values, and normal vital signs for various age groups

- cover up all areas of a written examination below the test question she is reading until she has read it twice, then uncover each potential answer one at a time and read it twice before moving on
- read all options even if she thinks she has already identified the correct one and then go back and read the question one more time before selecting her answer to avoid missing key words and important clues so that she is more likely to select the correct answer
- avoid overanalyzing the questions and, instead, select the best answer from the choices available, based on the data at hand, and then move on
- trust her first inclination and avoid going back to change her answer unless she has an extremely good reason for doing so, because she is more likely to change a correct response to an incorrect one than vice versa.

---

continued certification. This program applies to members certified or reinstated since January 2006. The AMT does not require those certified before that date to participate in the CCP, but strongly urges them to do so.

The RMA may earn points toward continuing certification through a variety of activities, including continuous employment, continuing education, employer evaluations, instructional presentations, and authoring written works. Proof of compliance is required every 3 years.

Chapter Summary

- Externship is a scheduled work experience that helps the medical assisting student bridge the gap between the classroom and workplace. A program coordinator arranges the externship and places the student in a medical office with a preceptor, who works closely with her. Externship provides the medical assistant with opportunities to learn by observation and hands-on experience.
- The program coordinator carefully selects externship sites to create the best possible experience for the student. Ideal placement allows a student to get experience in clinical, administrative, and general areas with staff who are interested in supporting her learning.
- The medical assisting student who works hard and seeks opportunities to learn and help others will quickly earn the trust and respect of the office staff and may even receive a job offer at her externship site.

- Because job markets change over time and demand for medical assistants may fluctuate, a medical assisting student should never assume that she will obtain her dream job right after graduation. Therefore, she must know how to conduct an effective job search.
- Job-search strategies include networking, looking online, searching the newspaper classified advertisements, and working with employment agencies. The most effective strategy is making personal contact with a prospective employer by visiting in person with a professional resume and cover letter.
- The job applicant should be prepared to interview with the office manager, a physician, or someone in the human resources office.
- A resume is a document that lists contact information, such as address, phone number, and e-mail address, and summarizes the applicant's experiences, qualifications, and education. The purpose of a resume is to obtain an interview for the applicant.
- An applicant should resist the temptation to embellish her resume by including untrue information. Such practices reflect dishonesty and a lack of integrity and create unrealistic expectations from employers.
- There are many types of resume, including the chronological resume, functional resume, and targeted resume. An applicant should design a personalized resume that best highlights her strengths and minimizes her weaknesses.
- A cover letter highlights the applicant's best qualifications and requests a job interview.
- The applicant's goal in an interview should be to convince the prospective employer that she would make a valuable

contribution to the organization. She must do this in a way that demonstrates a positive, professional demeanor, without appearing overly confident or aggressive.

- The applicant should always send a thank-you note to the person who conducted the interview. Doing so displays courtesy and professionalism and makes an added positive impression. In addition, it reminds the employer of the applicant's sincere interest in the job.
- Most employers will place a new employee on a probationary period for up to the first 90 days of the job. A performance that does not meet employer expectations may result in termination during this time. Therefore, the newly hired medical assistant must take care to make a good impression.
- Employers do not approve of job-hopping, a practice in which a person moves from position to position without staying in one position for an appropriate length of time. However, after a respectable length of time on the job, a medical assistant may wish to change jobs for personal reasons or for career advancement. Whatever the reason, the medical assistant should leave her current position on a positive, professional note, because a previous employer can open the door to a new, desirable position.
- There are two credentials for medical assistants: the Certified Medical Assistant (CMA) and the Registered Medical Assistant (RMA). These credentials are not legally required for employment as a medical assistant. However, employers seek out medical assistants with these credentials because they understand that these individuals have demonstrated a specific level of competence in educational knowledge as well as in clinical and administrative skills.
- Medical assistants earn the certified medical assistant (CMA) credential by passing an examination offered by the American Association of Medical Assistants (AAMA). Medical assistants earn the registered medical assistant (RMA) credential by passing an examination offered by the American Medical Technologists (AMT), a national certifying organization for laboratory professionals.
- The medical assistant can employ a number of strategies to prepare for the credentialing examination, including obtaining copies of the examination content outlines from the certifying organizations and carefully reviewing the content. She should pay close attention to any areas in which she feels deficient.
- CMAs must recertify their credentials every 5 years by retaking the certification examination or earning continuing education units. RMAs can take part in the certification continuation program (CCP), which allows recertification activities every 3 years.

Team Work Exercises

1. Divide into small groups of four to six students. Randomly assign two students to the role of interviewers. The other students must be job applicants. The interviewers must meet alone and identify a list of 5 to 10 interview questions they would like to ask. The interviewers (together) will then interview each applicant, asking exactly the same questions of each. The interviewers may take notes. When the interviewers have interviewed all applicants, they may take only 10 minutes to decide whom they wish to hire. When they have made a decision, they must provide feedback to the entire group about whom they decided to hire and why. They should give each applicant feedback about her strengths and positive qualities as well as any weakness identified. If time allows, students can reverse the roles and repeat the process.

2. Organize a "Career Day" for your program. This event can be imaginary or actual, depending on the instructor. Divide into teams and select the following assignments:

   a. Team 1 must organize a "Graduate Panel" for Career Day by identifying working medical assistants in the community and inviting them to be part of a guest panel. Activities might include asking guest panel members to introduce themselves and talk about the jobs they have held since graduation, how they landed their current job, what they like most about being a medical assistant, what they like least, and any advice they have to offer. After each member of the panel has spoken for a few minutes, provide time for questions and answers.

   b. Team 2 must organize an "Employer Panel" for Career Day by identifying health care employers in the community who hire medical assistants and inviting them to be part of a guest panel. Activities might include asking guest panel members to introduce themselves and talk about their current job and what qualities they look for when interviewing and hiring medical assistants. After each member of the panel has spoken for a few minutes, provide time for questions and answers.

   c. Team 3 must design a "mock interview" for Career Day. Job applicants can be members of the team or other volunteers whom the team recruits. Let the applicants interview as a group so that no one individual is put on the spot. Give them permission to demonstrate some interviewing "don'ts" as well as "do's" so that it can be a fun, informative event. Designate who the interviewers are and provide them with a list of questions. During the interview, each member of the applicant panel will have an opportunity to answer the question. Provide members of the audience with some type of score sheet on which they can make notes and possibly score each applicant on her answers and behaviors. At the conclusion, the audience may vote on whom they would hire.

   d. Team 4 must organize a resume review session in which members of the class may bring drafts of their resumes and cover letters for review. Reviewers might be medical assistant program instructors, English professors, or other on-campus and health care employers. This session should be a nonthreatening opportunity for students to get honest, helpful feedback on resume preparation.

e. Team 5 must organize a "Dress for Success" session, including advice about how to dress for the job interview and possibly even a fashion show. Be sure to address business fashion do's and don'ts. Include information about community resources that can help the new medical assistant obtain professional attire. For example, the YWCA commonly maintains a clothing bank with free business attire for homeless or low-income women who need clothing for interviews or new jobs.

Case Studies

1. Marci is a medical assisting student in her fourth and final quarter. She and one of her classmates, Lisa, have been placed in a family practice office to complete their externship hours. Marci has arrived a few minutes late on several occasions and has called in sick twice. She does everything she is asked but rarely volunteers to do anything extra. She usually seems eager to leave at the end of the day to go home or to go to her "real" job. Out of concern one day, Lisa commented on some of these behaviors. Marci responded by saying "It's not like this is a real job. When I'm hired and paid to be a medical assistant, then I'll do great work." What comments might Marci's preceptor have about her level of professionalism? How might Marci's performance impact her future efforts to get a job as a medical assistant? What feedback and suggestions might the externship coordinator have for Marci?

2. Gary is a medical assisting student who will be graduating soon. He is interested in applying for work as a CMA at a local medical center and would very much like to work in the urgent care clinic. Gary's work history includes 3 years in construction, followed by 9 months of unemployment, then 2 years as a handyman doing yard cleanup and maintenance. He was then hired at the local aluminum plant, where he worked for 5 years before he lost that job due to downsizing. After 1 year on unemployment, he decided to go back to school to become a medical assistant. Gary must prepare a resume and cover letter. What type of resume would best suit Gary's needs and why? What skills and abilities in his former jobs will be useful in his career as a medical assistant? Draft a cover letter for Gary to accompany his resume.

Resources

- Job searches, resumes, interviewing
  - Career and job-search information: *www.ajb.org*
  - Extensive information on searching for a job, resume preparation, and so forth: *www.monster.com*
  - Information about different types of interview questions: *www.jobinterviewquestions.org*
  - YWCA clothing services: *www.ywca.org*
- Medical assisting and examination review and preparation
  - Elsevier, Inc.: *www.us.elsevierhealth.com/specialty.jsp?lid=3&sid=441*
  - F.A. Davis Company: *www.fadavis.com/prof_aisle/profdetail.cfm?catid=28&disccode=HP 1915*
  - Lippincott Williams & Wilkins: *www.lww.com/browsemediaspec/Book/0,0,129,00.html*
  - Thomson Delmar Learning: *http://www.healthcare.delmar.cengage.com/Medical_Assisting/*
- Credentialing
  - An application form and other information regarding the CMA credentialing examination, continuing education, and recertification: *www.aama-ntl.org*
  - An application and further information about the RMA credentialing examination and the AMT's CCP: *www.amt1.com*

Glossary

A

Abandonment Failure to make arrangements for a patient's continued medical care

Abduction Motion away from the midline of the body

Ablation Therapeutic destruction of a part, pathway, or function using surgery, chemicals, electrocautery, or radiofrequency

Abortion Spontaneous or induced termination of pregnancy before the fetus reaches a viable age

Absorption Process of transferring nutrients from the digestive tract into the bloodstream; passage of a drug into the body's bloodstream through the digestive system, mucous membranes, or skin

Acceptance Stage of grief and loss when a person acknowledges the reality and permanence of life changes

Accessibility Degree of a person's ability to gain entrance to a facility when using a wheelchair or other assistive device

Accession record Record of numbers assigned to each new patient medical record

Accommodation Ability of the eye to see objects in the distance and then adjust to focus on a close object

Accountable Willingness to account for or be responsible for one's own actions

Accounts payable Amount of money a practice owes to outside vendors, rent or mortgage, supplies, salaries, and so forth

Accounts receivable Amount of money owed to a practice for patient services performed

Accounts receivable ratio Comparison of the amount of money charged to a practice and the amount collected by the practice

Accredit To certify as meeting specific standards set by regional or national organizations

Acronym Word created from the first letters of a series of words

Action Ability of a drug to act on body processes at the cellular level

Active files Medical files of patients who are currently seen in the office

Active listening Nonverbal communication method used to indicate that the listener has heard the message and concerns of the patient

Acute care Setting in which short-term health care is delivered to patients who are experiencing sudden illness or injury

Additive Substance, such as an anticoagulant or preservative, that may be added to an evacuated blood collection tube

Adduction Motion toward the midline of the body

Adenomyosis Benign invasive growth of endometrial tissue into the myometrium

Adenosine triphosphate Usable energy of cells

Administer To give a medication to a patient as directed by a physician

Administrative medical assistant Person who works in a medical office primarily in the front office areas performing clerical, reception, or medical records duties

Adolescent Person from approximately age 12 to age 18

Adverse effect Nontherapeutic result of drug administration that may also be unpleasant or harmful

Affect Emotional state or mood

Affective domain Thought processes involving emotions, values, and attitudes

Against medical advice Designation for a patient who leaves the hospital despite his doctor's recommendation to remain

Age of majority Legal status of adulthood as recognized by the state

Ageism Form of prejudice and discrimination against individuals because of their age

Agenda Items of business to be addressed at a staff meeting

Agent Representative of a facility, hospital, or doctor's office who represents the supervising physician in word and action

Agglutination Type of antibody–antigen reaction in which a solid antigen clumps with a soluble antibody

Aggressive Quality of striving to meet one's own needs while disregarding the rights and needs of others

Aging accounts Method used to identify how long an account has been overdue

Alimentary canal Route of digestion that includes all structures from the mouth to the anus, excluding the accessory organs of digestion; also known as the *digestive tract* or *gastrointestinal tract*

Allergen Substance that produces a hypersensitivity reaction

Allergy Immune response to a medication that results in inflammation and organ dysfunction

Alphabetical filing Organizing system based on the alphabet, usually using the patient's last name

Ambiguity State of uncertainty or vagueness

Ambulation Action of walking

Ambulatory care Facility, such as a medical clinic, that provides medical care to nonresidential patients, who arrive and leave on the same day

Analgesic Medication that relieves pain

Analyte Measurable chemical substance

Analyzer Automated instrument used to test blood and other body fluids for various substances

Anaphylaxis Severe allergic reaction

Anatomical laboratory Section of the laboratory that includes histology and cytology

Anemia Condition marked by a decrease in the number of red blood cells or the amount of hemoglobin

Anesthesia Absence of sensation

Anger Stage of grief and loss when a person experiences feelings of rage

Angiogram Diagnostic radiograph of the blood vessels using a contrast medium

Angioplasty Endovascular procedure that reopens narrowed blood vessels

Antecubital space Space inside the arm at the bend of the elbow that is the best site for routine venipuncture

Antibody Immunoglobulin produced by white blood cells in response to a specific antigen

Anticoagulant Substance that inhibits blood clotting

Antigen Marker that identifies a cell as being part of the body (self) or not part of the body (nonself); substance that, when introduced into the body, elicits an immune response

Antimicrobial agent Any chemical substance that has the ability to kill or stop the growth of microorganisms

Antipyretic Medication that lowers fever

Antitussive Medication that suppresses the cough reflex

Anuria Absence of urine production

Apical pulse Pulse felt or heard over the apex of the heart

Apnea Temporary absence of breathing

Aponeurosis Flat, fibrous sheet of connective tissue that attaches muscle to bone or other tissues

Apothecary System of weights and measures based on the yard

Appointment matrix Grid or schedule (computerized or manual) that shows the times available for scheduling patients and the days and hours the practice is open (excluding lunches and breaks)

Approximation Bringing wound edges together closely and evenly

Archives Storage place for records that are no longer in use but are kept for legal purposes

Articulate To verbally express oneself clearly and easily

Articulation Juncture between two or more bones; also called a *joint*

Artifact Signal interference on an ECG caused by patient movement, faulty equipment, or other factors

Asepsis State of cleanliness that is free from disease-causing microorganisms or the practice of maintaining such an environment

Aspiration Unintentional inhalation of any substance other than air

Assault Threat or perceived threat to do bodily harm to another person

Assertive Quality of advocating for one's own rights while respecting the rights of others

Assets Property owned by a business, such as equipment, supplies, and accounts receivable

Assisted living Residential facilities with minimal health care, common dining and social activities, and usually transportation assistance

Associate practice Sole proprietors who share resources, such as office space, equipment, and employees

Astigmatism Abnormality of the eye in which the refraction of a ray of light is spread over a diffuse area rather than sharply focused on the retina

Atherosclerosis Thickening and hardening of the walls of the arteries; also called *arteriosclerosis*

Atopic Type of allergic reaction for which there is a genetic predisposition

Atrophy Decrease in mass of a muscle or organ; also called *wasting*

Audiometer Instrument used to measure hearing

Aura Subjective sensation that occurs prior to and signals the onset of a migraine headache or a seizure

Auscultation Method of listening to body sounds with a stethoscope

Auscultatory gap Disappearance of tapping sounds during phase II of a blood pressure measurement

Authorization Written permission to disclose protected health information (PHI) when a consent form does not apply or another exception is evident

Automated external defibrillator Small, automated device used to deliver an electrical shock to a patient suffering from a life-threatening cardiac arrhythmia

Automated method Laboratory test performed on an automated instrument or machine

Autonomy Right to self-determination

B

Bacilli Rod-shaped bacteria

Bacteria One-celled organism, some of which are capable of producing disease

Balance sheet Statement of financial condition that contains itemized assets, liabilities, and owner's equity

Bandage Nonsterile material applied over the top of dressings to secure them

Bargaining Stage of grief and loss when a person makes irrational attempts to negotiate for unlikely or impossible changes

Bartholin glands Two small glands located at the opening of the vagina

Battery Intentional act of touching another person in a socially unacceptable manner without her consent

Beneficence Duty to provide good or benefit

Beneficiary Recipient of insurance coverage

Benefit year 12-month period starting with the date of initial insurance coverage

Bias Unfair or incorrect belief that stems from prejudice and inhibits impartial judgment or action

Bilingual Capable of conversing in two languages

Bioethics Study of the ethical implications of discoveries and advances in modern medicine and health care

Biopsy Procedure in which a representative sample of tissue is obtained for microscopic examination

Bioterrorism Intentional or threatened use of biological agents or toxins to produce death, disease, or fear in an individual or a population

Bioterrorism agent Any substance, such as a bacteria, virus, or other germ released during a bioterrorism attack

Birthday rule Insurance regulation that uses the subscribers' dates of birth to determine primary and secondary coverage for dependents

Blastocyte Group of cells in early gestation that will form an embryo

Blood pressure Tension exerted by blood against the arterial walls during ventricular contraction and relaxation

Body mechanics Conscious coordination of the nervous and musculoskeletal systems to preserve and protect posture, balance, and body alignment while bending, lifting, and performing activities of daily living

Bolus Mass of masticated (chewed) food

Bone Individual unit of osseous tissue that is part of the framework of the body

Boundary Physical or psychological space that indicates the limit of appropriate versus inappropriate behavior

Bradykinesia Extreme slowness in movement

Bradypnea Abnormally slow breathing

Brainstorming Process in which individuals in a group offer ideas to solve a specified problem

Breach of contract Failure to comply with an established agreement as specified in a written contract

Bronchoscopy Examination of the bronchi through a specialized instrument called a *bronchoscope*

Brudzinski sign Patient response in which neck flexion causes flexion of the hips when the patient is lying in a supine position

Buccal Route of administration that involves placement of a drug between the cheek and gum

Buffy coat Middle layer of a whole blood tube that has been allowed to settle or has been centrifuged and contains leukocytes and platelets

Burnout Decreased physical, emotional, or mental energy caused by ongoing intensive demands without sufficient physical or emotional rest

Business associate Person who, on behalf of the covered entity, performs or assists in the performance of a function or activity involving the use of individually identifiable health information (IIHI)

Business associate contract Document that describes the obligation of an outside entity that uses PHI to protect the privacy of the PHI as an extension of the physician's office (also called *data use agreement*)

Business letter Formal document sent by mail that contains information related to business, rather than personal, affairs

C

Caduceus Ancient symbol of the Greek god Hermes that consists of a staff with two serpents entwined around it, surmounted by two wings, and used today by some medical groups to symbolize medical care

Call forwarding Technology that enables a telephone call to reach a specific person, department, or desk

Calorie Unit by which food energy is measured

Capillary puncture Process of performing a skin puncture to obtain blood

Capitation System of payment in which physicians are paid a flat rate per patient

Capsule Special container made of gelatin sized to contain a single dose of an oral medication

Carbohydrate Compound containing carbon, hydrogen, and oxygen atoms

Cardiac cycle One complete contraction and relaxation cycle of the heart

Cardiac sphincter Circular muscle at the top of the stomach that allows food from the esophagus to enter the stomach

Cardioversion Restoration of normal sinus rhythm by chemical or electrical means

Cash flow Amount of available cash that a business maintains to cover expenses

Catabolism Body process that converts large structures into smaller ones

Cataract Opacity (clouding) of the lens of the eye

Catch-up time Time in the schedule that is not booked with appointments to let doctors and staff catch up on paperwork, return phone calls, or catch up with appointments if patient visits take longer than anticipated

Central nervous system Nerve tissue that comprises the brain and spinal cord

Cerebral concussion Brief loss of consciousness or brief episode of disorientation or confusion following a head injury

Cerebral contusion Injury involving bruising of brain tissue

Certification Issuance of a certificate by a professional organization to an individual who has met a specified standard of education or training and has, therefore, earned the right to exercise certain skills

Certification continuation program Program of documenting ongoing professional activities whereby registered medical assistants (RMAs) may earn continued certification

Cerumen Yellow or brown waxy substance produced in the ceruminous glands of the ear

Channel Mode of conveying a message, including vision, hearing, and touch

Chemical peel Destruction of superficial layers of the skin using a chemical application in order to remove scars, tattoos, or abnormal pigmentation

Chest physiotherapy Type of therapy that includes percussion (clapping) over the thorax or vibration and positioning to facilitate loosening and removal of respiratory secretions

Child Person from age 1 to around age 12

Cholecystogram Radiograph of the gallbladder

Cholesterol Multiringed, waxy lipid found in all body cells

Chronological resumé Resumé that lists work experience and education in chronological order, with the most recent first

Chyme Mixture of partially digested food and saliva

Circumcision Surgical removal of the prepuce

Circumduction Circular motion of a body part

Circumoral cyanosis Blue coloring around the mouth due to inadequate oxygenation

Civil law Branch of private law that deals with accidental, rather than intentional, injury to a person or personal property

Claustrophobia Fear of closed spaces

Clinical diagnosis Diagnosis based on actual observations, diagnostic results, and symptoms

Clinical medical assistant Person who works in a medical office primarily in the back office areas assisting the physician with patient care, procedures, and diagnostic testing

Cloning Creation of cells, tissue, or an embryo without the fertilization of an egg

Closed question Question that can be answered with one word

Closed records Medical records of patients who no longer seek treatment in the office

Cluster booking Scheduling technique that involves consecutive booking of patients who have similar problems or are undergoing similar procedures

Cocci Round or spherical bacteria that can arrange themselves in chains, clusters, or tetrads

Cognitive domain Thought processes that involve the intellect and include thinking on several levels

Coitus Sexual intercourse

Collection agency Business that recovers bad debts for a percentage of the debt or a fixed fee

Collection ratio Comparison of outstanding debt amount and amount collected

Color coding Alphabetical filing system that adds colored stickers to the open end of a file to facilitate visual maintenance of files

Color deficiency Genetic or acquired abnormality in color perception

Colposcope Instrument used to examine the tissues of the vagina and cervix

Colposcopy Examination of vaginal and cervical tissues by means of a colposcope

Combining form Word element created by joining a word root with a combining vowel

Combining vowel Vowel placed between word parts to link them together and make the term easier to pronounce

Communication Process of sending and receiving information between two or more individuals

Compensation Psychological response in which a person offsets feelings of inadequacy in one aspect of that person's life by achievement in another aspect

Compliance Patient's adherence to the plan of care as instructed by the health care provider

Computed tomography Computerized procedure that views the target organ or body area from different angles in a three-dimensional view

Conception Time at which an ovum is fertilized

Confidentiality Principle of keeping personal medical and financial information private and avoiding divulgence of such information to any unapproved party

Congruent Consistent or matching

Conjunctivitis Inflammation of the conjunctiva caused by bacteria or a virus

Consecutive filing Filing system that uses sequential numbers to order medical records

Consent To agree or give permission

Constructive criticism Method of instruction that focuses on actions that can improve an employee's job performance, rather than focusing on the negative aspects of the person's performance

Contagious Easily spread from one person to another

Continuing education units Credits awarded for the attendance of classes, workshops, or seminars

Contrecoup Rapid acceleration-deceleration injury of the brain that bruises the front and back of the brain

Contracture Movement that shortens or tightens a muscle

Contraindication Condition under which a drug should never be used

Contrast medium Radiopaque substance that enhances an image

Coordination of benefits Insurance carrier's explanation of how it will pay benefits if a patient has more than one insurance plan

Copayment Patient's share of the cost of an office visit

Core temperature Temperature within the body's deep internal structures

Corneal abrasion Injury to the translucent anterior structure of the eye

Corporation Organization that is granted legal status with rights, privileges, and liabilities separate from those of its members

Corpuscallosotomy Surgical procedure in which the central part of the brain is partially divided in two

Corticosteroids Medications that suppress the immune response and decrease inflammation

Cost ratio Comparison of total expenses to number of procedures

Courteous Behavior that is polite, considerate, and helpful

Cover letter Letter that accompanies a resume to highlight the applicant's qualifications and request a job interview

Covert event Unannounced event that involves the release of an agent or toxin without any advanced warning

Crackles Abnormal crackly lung sound heard with a stethoscope

Crash cart Wheeled supply cabinet that contains emergency equipment and supplies

Criminal law Branch of public law that deals with the rights and responsibilities of the government to maintain public order

Cross-reference Guide placed where a medical record could be misfiled to indicate the correct location of the file

Cryosurgery Technique that destroys tissue by subjecting it to very cold temperatures; also called *cryotherapy*

Cryotherapy Removal of heat from a body part to decrease cellular metabolism and swelling

Culture Growth of microorganisms in a laboratory-prepared medium

Cumulative medication action Action of repeated doses of a medication that are not immediately eliminated from the body

***Current Procedural Terminology*, 4th ed.** Coding manual used to identify the procedures performed by physicians and their staff; also called *CPT-4*

Cycle billing Method of billing that divides patients into groups that are mailed billing statements at various times throughout the month

Cystoscopy Visual examination of the bladder

D

Damages Monetary award paid by the physician to the patient as directed by the court

Debrief Discussion of events, thoughts, and feelings among persons who have experienced an important or stressful event

Decoding Process by which the receiver of a message extracts its meaning

Defamation Providing false information (written or spoken) that causes harm to the reputation of another

Defecation Passage of feces from the bowels

Defense mechanism Unhealthy coping strategy that a person may employ when feeling emotionally threatened in some way

Defibrillator Specialized device used to deliver an electrical shock to a patient suffering from a life-threatening cardiac arrhythmia

Deglutition Swallowing

Dehydration Condition in which body water output exceeds water input

De-identified information Health information data set from which all personal identifiers are removed

Delegation Act of assigning tasks to another person who then legally acts as the assigner's representative

Demographics Personal information used to identify a patient

Denial Psychological response by which a person refuses to acknowledge the validity or reality of something that is obvious to others; stage of grief and loss when a person refuses to accept the reality of a situation

Deontology Ethical philosophy concerned with duties and rights

Dependable Characteristic of being reliable and trustworthy

Depolarization Electrical change in cells in which the inside becomes positive in relation to the outside

Deposition Formal method of gathering information in which a person testifies to the actions of herself and coworkers

Dermabrasion Procedure in which outer layers of the skin are removed by abrasion with a wire brush or other device

Dermaplaning Procedure in which a dermatome is used to skim off surface layers of the skin to remove scars, tattoos, and fine wrinkles

Dermatome Band or region of skin supplied by a single sensory nerve; instrument used to cut thin slices of skin

Diascopy Procedure in which a glass plate is held against the skin to observe changes related to pressure application

Diastole Period of cardiac muscle relaxation when blood is filling the chambers of the heart and blood pressure is lowest

Diastolic pressure Blood pressure between heart contractions

Dictation Creation of a tape or computer voice file to be transcribed

Digestion Chemical and physical breakdown of food in the gastrointestinal tract

Digital radiographic imaging Radiography using computer imaging instead of conventional film or screen imaging

Dilation Increase in size

Directional term Term used to indicate specific areas on the body

Directive statement Statement that guides the listener in discussing topics as directed

Disability Deficiency, especially physical, that prevents or restricts normal performance

Disclosure Process of releasing, transferring, providing access to, or divulging information in any manner to a second party

Disease Any condition characterized by subjective complaints, a specific history, clinical signs or symptoms, and laboratory or radiographic findings

Disinfection Application of a substance to materials and surfaces to destroy pathogens

Dispense To prepare or deliver medicines

Displacement Psychological response by which a person expresses anger or another emotion at a person or object that is not the cause of those feelings

Dissection Separation and delineation of animal or human tissues for study

Distribution Transport of a drug to body fluids, tissues, and cells

Distributive justice Principle regarding the fair distribution of scarce resources

Diurnal rhythm Normal daily cyclic fluctuation in body temperature

Dorsal recumbent position Position in which the patient is lying flat with knees bent and feet on the examination table

Dosage Physician's indication of how much and how often a patient should take a drug

Dose Amount of a drug a patient takes each time

Dosimeter Device that monitors the quantity of x-ray exposure to health care workers

Double booking Scheduling technique in which several patients are scheduled for the same appointment time and are attended to at the same time in different rooms

Dressing Material placed in or on a wound

Drug Any substance that, when taken into a living organism, may modify one or more of its functions

Drug class Grouping of drugs by their therapeutic effect, the body system affected, or their action

Durable power of attorney Written legal designation of a person to make medical decisions on behalf of another person

Dyspnea Labored or difficult breathing

Dysuria Painful or difficult urination

E

Effacement Thinning of the cervix during labor

Efficacy Ability of a medication to produce a desired effect

Electrocardiogram Record or tracing of electrical activity of the heart

Electrocardiograph Instrument used to record an electrocardiogram

Electrocardiography Process of recording the electrical activity of the heart

Electrodesiccation Destructive drying of cells by applying electrical energy

Electrosurgery Use of high-frequency electric current to cut, remove, or destroy tissue; also called *electrocautery*

Emancipated minor Person under the age of majority who has been declared by a court to be independent and responsible for his own debts

Embolic Caused by a moving mass in a blood vessel (embolus)

Empathy Understanding of the emotions and thoughts of another

Emulsification Process of making an emulsion, allowing fat and water to mix

Endocrinologist Medical doctor who specializes in the diagnosis and treatment of endocrine diseases and disorders

Endocrinology Study of the structures and functions of the endocrine system

Endometrium Mucous membrane that lines the uterus

Endoscopy Use of a specialized scope to visually examine a structure

Enema Introduction of a solution into the rectum to stimulate bowel activity

Enteric-coated Drug formulation in which tablets or capsules are coated with a compound that does not dissolve until exposed to the fluids of the small intestine

Enunciation Act of pronouncing words distinctly

Environment Setting in which a communication experience occurs

Epiglottis Uppermost cartilage of the larynx

Episiotomy Incision made into the perineum to facilitate delivery of a baby

Equilibrium State of balance, which is controlled by structures of the inner ear

Ergonomics Science of equipment or workplace design that aims to minimize operator fatigue

Erythema Redness of the skin

Erythrocyte Red blood cell responsible for carrying oxygen to all cells and tissues in the body

Established patient Patient who has previously received care at the office

Ether Organic compound once used for anesthesia; also called *diethyl ether*

Ethics Study of human behavior and moral choices based on a set of principles; rules or standards governing professional conduct

Etiquette Rules for socially acceptable behavior

Evacuated tube Plastic tube that contains a vacuum, which draws blood from the vein into the tube through a dual needle system

Eversion Movement of a body part outward

Excretion Process of eliminating waste products of digestion

Exhalation Act of breathing out; also called *expiration*

Exophthalmos Symptom of protruding eyeballs, usually caused by a severe form of hyperthyroidism called *Graves disease*

Expectorant Medication that liquefies and loosens respiratory secretions to aid in expelling them

Expert witness Person who is called to testify in court due to her status as an expert on a given subject or in a specialty

Expiration Act of exhaling

Extension Movement that straightens a body part

External marketing Methods of informing people who have not been patients of the practice about the practice and its services

External respiration Movement of air into and out of the lungs

Externship Scheduled, on-the-job experience that helps a student bridge the gap between the classroom and workplace

F

Fascia Sheet of fibrous connective tissue that covers, separates, or supports muscle

Fasciculation Visible involuntary muscle twitching

Fasting Practice of denying the body all food or nutrition, usually for a specified period of time before laboratory tests or surgical procedures

Fatty acid Long, unbranched fat used by the body to manufacture various lipoproteins

Febrile Fever causing

Fee for service Payment method based on each item billed to the insurance company

Feedback Message returned by a receiver as a response to the sender's message

Felony Serious crime against the public that is punishable by serving time in prison

Fetus Term used to describe a developing human in utero from 9 weeks' gestation (after the embryonic stage) until birth

Fibrillation Spontaneous muscle contraction or quivering

Fidelity Concept of loyalty or faithfulness

Film-screen radiography Radiography using special photographic film that blackens in response to the light from intensifying screens

Filtrate Mixture of water, electrolytes, urea, and other small molecules first filtered in the glomerulus

Financial accounting Process of tracking monetary expenditures and income for outside entities, such as the federal government

Fixed costs Expenses that do not depend on the number of patients being seen in a practice

Flexible Adaptable to change; able to bend without breaking

Flexion Movement that bends a body part

Float Ability to fulfill a temporary assignment to work in a different area from the one in which an individual usually works

Fluent Ability to speak and write well in a given language

Fluoroscopy Radiographic imaging that can be viewed as a moving picture

Fomite Any object that adheres to and transmits infectious material (such as a comb, countertop, or drinking glass)

Forced vital capacity Test that measures the amount of air that can be maximally exhaled after a maximum inspiration and the time required for that expiration

Fowler position Position in which the patient sits with his head as close to 90 degrees as possible and his legs resting outstretched on the examination table

Fraud Intentional misrepresentation of a situation for financial gain

Frequency Need for frequent urination

Functional resumé Resumé that emphasizes specific skill sets and describes the most valuable experiences and abilities of the applicant

Fundus Area of the uterus above the openings to the fallopian tubes

Fungi Kingdom of organisms that includes yeasts, molds, and mushrooms and is usually not pathogenic to humans

G

Gait Manner of walking

Gastroenterologist Physician who diagnoses and treats disorders of the gastrointestinal tract

Gastroenterology Study of the gastrointestinal tract

Genome Complete set of chromosomes and, thus, the complete genetic information present in a cell

Gestation Time from conception to birth

Glaucoma Disorder that involves increased intraocular pressure, resulting in atrophy of the optic nerve and, possibly, blindness

Glucagon Hormone that cleaves bonds in glycogen to release glucose

Glucometer Instrument used to measure glucose levels in the blood

Glucose Monosaccharide used by the brain and tissues for fuel

Glucosuria Presence of glucose in the urine

Glycemic index Scale that lists the amount of time it takes for a food to raise blood glucose levels

Goiter Enlarged thyroid gland

Goniometry Process of measuring joint movements and angles

Gravidity Total number of pregnancies

Gross negligence Intentional failure to provide care or the commission of an act by an individual with reckless disregard for consequences that endanger a patient

Group practice Medical group with three or more licensed, full-time physicians

Growth hormone Hormone secreted by the pituitary gland to stimulate growth of bones and tissues; also called *somatotropin*

Gustation Sense of taste

H

Health care operations Business activities of the practice, including employee training, marketing, fundraising, licensing, and quality assessments

Hematocrit Volume of packed red blood cells

Hematology Study of blood and blood-forming tissues

Hematoma Discoloration of the area around a puncture site caused by an accumulation of blood around the site; also called *bruise*

Hematopoiesis Production and development of blood cells

Hematuria Presence of blood in the urine

Hemiplegia Paralysis of one side of the body

Hemoconcentration Accumulation of blood caused by leaving the tourniquet on the venipuncture arm longer than one minute, causing an increase in red blood cells and a decrease in plasma volume

Hemodialysis Artificial means of removing urea, wastes, toxins, and excess fluid from the blood

Hemoglobin Iron-containing protein found in red blood cells that is responsible for transporting oxygen to cells and carbon dioxide to the lungs

Hemolysis Destruction or breakdown of red blood cells, causing a red tinge in serum

Hemoptysis Coughing up blood

Hemostasis Blood clotting process

Hippocratic Oath Oath of medical ethics created by Hippocrates

Histologist Specialist in the study of cells and microscopic tissues

Home care Health care assistance for a person living in his own home

Home health care agency Private company that employs nursing

assistants and nurses who make home visits to provide patients with limited nursing services

Homeostasis State of equilibrium in the body

Hormone Chemical substance released from a gland or organ

Hospice Program that provides special end-of-life care for the terminally ill

Hospital privileges Permission granted by a hospital that allows a physician to see patients and practice medicine within that hospital

Household System of volume measurement using the teaspoon and tablespoon

Human resources department Office or department that advertises job vacancies, accepts applications, arranges interviews, and manages documentation of employee benefits

Humor Term created by Claudius Galen that refers to any fluid or semifluid substance in the body

Hyperextension Position of maximum extension, or extending a body part beyond its normal limits

Hyperglycemia Abnormally high blood glucose level

Hyperopia Error of refraction in which affected individuals can see distant objects clearly but cannot see near objects; also called *farsightedness*

Hypersecretion Increased amount or excessive secretion

Hyperthyroidism Condition of having excessive levels of thyroid hormone in the body

Hypertrophy Excessive growth of tissue

Hyperventilation Increased ventilation resulting in a higher blood pH

Hypoglycemia Abnormally low blood glucose levels

Hypoglycemic Drug that lowers blood glucose levels

Hyposecretion Decreased secretion

Hypothyroidism Condition of inadequate levels of thyroid hormone in the body

Hypoxia Deficient level of oxygen

Hypoxic drive Backup system of respiration that stimulates breathing in a patient who is retaining carbon dioxide

I

Implied consent Acceptance of treatment expressed through a patient's actions, such as rolling up his sleeve for blood pressure measurement

Inactive records Records of patients who have not been seen for an extended period of time (usually 1 to 6 years) but who may return for care

Incentive spirometer Handheld device used by the patient to inhale a maximal breath to keep lungs expanded and functional

Income statement Report of itemized monthly expenses and profits

Incubation Interval between exposure to infection and the appearance of the first symptoms; period of time it takes for a microbiological culture to grow and multiply before actual bacterial colonies are visible on the medium

Indication Approved use of a drug, as approved by the Food and Drug Administration

Individually identifiable health information Medical information contained in a patient's record that could be used to identify the patient

Infant Child between ages 1 month and 1 year

Infectious disease Any disease caused by a microorganism that may be directly or indirectly transmitted between individuals, causing infection

Influenza Highly infectious acute respiratory infection that is characterized by a sudden onset of fever, chills, body aches, and cough

Informational interview Interview conducted to gain information about an organization to determine whether a person is interested in applying to work there

Informed consent Document that a patient signs, which is a written agreement for treatment

Inhalation Act of breathing in; also called *inspiration*

In-home care Care provided in the home by spouses, family, close friends, or paid, live-in caregivers

Insoluble fiber Indigestible food components that do not dissolve in water

Inspection Process of gathering information about the patient through observation

Inspiration Act of inhaling; also called *inhalation*

Insulin Hormone that binds to glucose allowing its transport from the bloodstream to the tissues

Interaction Effect in the body as the result of a combination of a drug with food or another drug

Internal marketing Method used to stimulate business with existing patients through mailings and other means

Interpersonal variables Factors that impact a receiver's interpretation of a message

Intradermal Route of administration that involves injection of a drug just under the epidermis

Intramuscular Route of administration that involves injection of a drug into the muscle

Intravenous Route of administration that involves injection of a drug into a vein

Intravenous pyelogram Radiographic view of the kidneys using contrast medium injected intravenously

Inversion Movement of a body part inward

Ionization Process of gaining or losing an electron from an atom

J

Jack-knife position Position in which the patient sits on a special examination table in a semisitting position with the thighs flexed to 90 degrees

Jargon Abbreviations or technical, specialized language used by professionals that is generally confusing to other people

Job description Written description of the qualifications and duties of a position

Justice Concept of fairness or equity

K

Kernig sign Reflexive hamstring contraction and pain when attempting to extend the leg after flexing the hip

Ketonuria Presence of ketones in the urine

Knee-chest position Position in which the patient sits on her knees with her chest and face and arms resting forward and her buttocks in the air

Korotkoff sounds Sounds heard when auscultating the blood pressure

L

Lactation Process by which a mother's body produces milk for her newborn infant

Lancet Capillary puncture device that usually contains a retractable blade

Laser resurfacing Use of short pulses of light to treat some skin conditions

Laser surgery Treatment of tissue by means of colored light beams

Layperson Nonmedical person

Learning domains Modes of learning conducted by different parts of the brain

Learning objectives Goals or outcomes to be achieved in the learning process

Learning style Manner in which a person most effectively learns

Leukocyte White blood cell responsible for fighting off infection and producing antibodies

Leukocytosis Abnormal increase in circulatory white blood cells

Leukopenia Abnormal decrease in circulatory white blood cells

Liability Money owed to a creditor

Libel Dishonoring or defaming a person through written documents

Licensure Designation signifying that a person has met standards and requirements of her profession and is legally able to offer specific services for monetary reimbursement

Ligament Band or sheet of fibrous tissue that connects two or more bones or cartilage

Ligation Application of a band, thread, or wire to tie a blood vessel or other structure in order to constrict or fasten it

Lipid Family of compounds that are insoluble in water, including fatty acids, triglycerides, phospholipids, and sterols; also called *fat*

Lithotomy position Position in which the patient reclines face up, with legs apart and feet in stirrups

Lithotripsy Treatment that uses shock or sound waves to crush stones in the kidneys or urinary tract

Litigation In medicine, a legal action that determines the rights and remedies a patient can pursue in the event of suspected medical malpractice

Living will Written directions to a physician that instruct the physician about whether or not to maintain life-support systems in the event of a patient's terminal illness

Lobectomy Surgical removal of a lobe of a lung

Local effect Impact of a medication that is specific only to a certain part of the body

Locus of control Person's belief about the degree of control that he has over events in his life

Lower gastrointestinal series Radiographic examination of the lower intestinal tract during and after introduction of barium, which acts as the contrast medium

Lumen Space within a vessel or other tubelike structure

Lymph Clear, colorless, alkaline fluid found within lymph vessels made up of water, protein, salts, urea, fats, and white blood cells

Lymphadenopathy Swollen, tender cervical lymph nodes

M

Macrophage Type of white blood cell that destroys cellular debris and foreign invaders within tissues and organs

Magnetic resonance imaging Procedure in which a strong magnetic field and radio waves are used to produce images to view body structures

Malfeasance Unlawful act that causes harm

Malnutrition Condition caused by insufficient intake of nutrients

Malpractice Action by a health care professional that injures a patient and fails to meet reasonable standards of professional care

Mammary glands Milk-producing glands in a female

Mammography Radiographic imaging of the breast to screen for breast cancer

Managerial accounting Process of tracking monetary expenditures and income for a practice's managers or physician owners

Manipulation Application of touch to assess joint symmetry and passive range of motion, or the therapeutic application of force to increase mobility and realign dislocated joints

Mantoux test Test to identify tuberculosis exposure

Manual method Test method in which the steps of testing are done by hand instead of by an automated instrument

Marketing Process of letting customers or potential customers know of a product or service

Mastication Process of chewing food

Medical asepsis Practice that frees a specific environment from microorganisms that might cause disease

Medical jargon Terminology and abbreviations used in medicine that are not readily understood by laypersons

Melanocyte Melanin-forming skin cell

Menarche Age of first menstruation or onset of menstruation

Ménière disease Syndrome characterized by recurring episodes of hearing loss, tinnitus, and vertigo that can progressively lead to deafness

Meniscus Curved upper surface of a liquid in a container

Menopause Permanent cessation of menstruation, usually occurring between ages 38 and 58

Menstruation Female cycle of producing and expelling the unfertilized ovum

Mensuration Measurements of body parts, including height, length, and circumference

Message Content of a communication, including verbal, nonverbal, and symbolic language

Metabolism All physical and chemical changes within the body that build and break down substances; change to a medication by the body, which converts it to an inactive water-soluble compound for excretion

Metered dose inhaler Handheld device used to inhale medication into the lungs

Methodology System of principles and procedures used in scientific testing

Metric System of weights and measures based on the meter

Microdermabrasion Gentle abrasion of the skin to reduce fine lines, age spots, and acne scars and stimulate growth of new skin cells and collagen

Microorganism Living organism too small to be seen with the naked eye

Microsample Very small amount of a specimen

Microsurgery Any procedure completed with the use of a special operating microscope

Micturition reflex Bladder reflex that creates the urge to urinate

Middle digit filing Numeric system that uses the middle digits of an identification number as the primary indexing unit

Mineral Inorganic element

Mnemonic Technique used to enhance memory, such as creating a word from the first letters of a series of words

Mock code Practice drill for responding to a medical emergency

Modality Method of applying a therapy, usually a physical device

Modified wave Scheduling technique in which two or three patients are scheduled at the beginning of each hour and then one patient is scheduled every 10 to 20 minutes into the hour

Modifier Two-digit number added to the end of a procedure code that changes and further defines the procedure

Monthly billing Method of billing in which all patients are mailed billing statements on the same date, usually the first of the month

Morals Judgment regarding the value of certain behaviors based on personal belief

Motor nerves Nerves involved in movement

Multilingual Proficient in several languages

Muscle Tissue made up of contractile fibers that produce movement

Muscle testing Process of evaluating muscle strength and range of motion

Myelin Layer of phospholipids and protein that forms the myelin sheath of neurons and acts as electrical insulation

Myofascia Tissue consisting of muscle and underlying fascia

Myopia Error of refraction in which light rays are focused in front of the retina, enabling the person to see distinctly for only a short distance; also called *nearsightedness*

N

Nasal cannula Oxygen tubing designed to deliver oxygen into a patient's nose

Nebulizer Device that produces a fine spray or mist to deliver medication to the air passages and lungs

Negative feedback system Control system in which an increase or decrease in a substance stimulates an opposite response by a hormone

Negligence Unintentional failure of a health care professional to meet his responsibilities to a patient, resulting in injury to the patient

Neonate Newborn baby to age 28 days

Networking Exchange of information related to a person's profession with coworkers, friends, and acquaintances

Neuritic plaque Accumulation of bundled fibers surrounding normal and damaged nerve cells in the brain

Neurofibrillary tangles Tangles of neurofibrils that make up part of the nerve cell body

Neuron Nerve cell

Neurotransmitter Chemical that plays an important role in nerve impulse transmission

New patient Patient who has not previously received care at the office

Nocturia Excessive urination during the night

Noncompliance Failure of a patient to follow his physician's treatment plan

Nonconsecutive filing Numeric system that does not use consecutive ordering for medical records

Nonfeasance Failure of a health care professional or organization to perform a task or deliver a service, resulting in harm or injury to a patient

Nonmaleficence Duty to do no harm

Normal flora Organisms found on and in a person's body that do not cause disease and are sometimes beneficial

Normal range Range of values in which a test result should fall for most healthy individuals

Norms Unwritten rules of socially acceptable behavior

No-show Patient who has a scheduled appointment but fails to appear

Notice of Privacy Practices Document that describes the use of protected health information for carrying out treatment, payment, or health care operations

Nuchal rigidity Condition that involves pain and stiffness of the neck and a resulting reluctance to flex the head forward

Nuclear medicine Techniques that use radioactive material for the diagnosis and treatment of patients

Numeric filing System that assigns an identification number to each patient file

Nursing center Facility in which custodial and nursing care are provided to individuals who need assistance with activities of daily living; also called a *skilled nursing facility* or *nursing home*

Nutrient Chemical substance obtained from food and used in the body to provide energy, build structural materials, support growth and maintenance, or repair body tissues

O

Olfaction Sense of smell

Oliguria Deficiency of urine production

Open hours Block of time in which patients are seen by the physician on a first-come, first-served basis

Open MRI Imaging table with more open space than a traditional MRI tube

Open-ended question Question that requires more than a one-word answer

Ophthalmoscope Handheld instrument used to view the internal structures of the eye, including the retina, optic nerve, and blood vessels

Opiate Class of analgesic drugs that depress the central nervous system; also called *narcotic*

Oral route Route of administration of a medication through the mouth and into the GI tract

Otitis Inflammation of the ear

Otoscope Handheld instrument used to visualize the internal structures of the ear, ear canal, and eardrum

Out guide Marker used to indicate that a medical record has been taken from the filing system

Ovaries Glands that produces ova, the cells from the female necessary for procreation

Overnutrition Condition caused by excess intake of nutrients

Overt event Attack that is announced prior to or after the release of the bioterrorism agent

Over-the-counter Type of drug that can be obtained without a prescription

Owner's equity Amount that business assets exceed business liabilities; also called *net worth*

P

Palpation Examination of the patient's body by touching it with the hands and pads of the fingers

Palpitation Sensation of rapid or irregular beating of the heart sometimes described as a thudding or fluttering sensation

Palliative care Medical care aimed at alleviating disease symptoms, rather than providing a cure

Pandemic Occurrence of a disease that has reached epidemic proportions in many different parts of the world at the same time

Pandemic flu Virulent human flu that causes a global outbreak, or pandemic, of serious illness

Panel Group of blood tests that evaluate the function of a particular body system; also called *profile*

Papanicolaou test Test used to detect cancer of cervical cells

Parasite Pathogen requiring another living organism in order to survive

Paresthesia Abnormal sensation

Partnership Creation of a legal agreement between two or more licensed physicians that specifies the rights, obligations, and responsibilities of each

Passive Quality of submitting or yielding without offering resistance

Passive-aggressive Manipulative behavior that appears initially passive but seeks to control by retaliation in the form of procrastination, stubbornness, and "forgetfulness"

Pasteurization Process of heating a fluid to a moderate temperature to destroy bacteria without changing the chemical composition of the fluid

Patch test Skin test in which a low concentration of a presumed allergen is applied to the skin beneath an occlusive dressing to see if a reaction occurs

Paternalism Practice of providing for people without giving them rights or responsibilities

Pathogen Disease-producing microorganism

Pathogenic Causing disease

Pathological term Term that refers to a disease or disorder of the body

Peak flow meter Handheld device used to measure an individual's lung capacity

Pediatrician Specialist in the treatment of children's diseases

Pediatrics Medical science relating to the care of children

'Percussion Tapping on the body surface with the fingers or a small hammer and noting the sound elicited to determine the position, size, or density of underlying structures

Performance evaluation Assessment of an employee's performance conducted at the end of a probationary period and annually thereafter

Perfusion Circulation of blood, nutrients, and oxygen through tissues and organs

Perineum Area between the vaginal opening and anus

Peripheral Away from the trunk of the body; in the extremities

Peripheral nervous system Portion of the nervous system outside the central nervous system that conveys sensory and motor impulses

Peristalsis Wavelike muscular contractions that move food down the esophagus

Peritoneal dialysis Dialysis in which the lining of the peritoneal cavity is used as the dialyzing membrane

Perjury Act of lying in court, despite taking an oath to tell the truth

pH scale Scale used to measure acidity or alkalinity of a substance

Phagocytosis Process in which specialized white blood cells (phagocytes) engulf and destroy microorganisms, foreign antigens, and cellular debris

Pharmacodynamics Study of the body's biochemical and physiological response to drugs

Pharmacokinetics Study of the action of drugs as they move through the body, including absorption, distribution, metabolism, and excretion

Pharmacology Study of drugs and their origin, nature, properties, and effects on living organisms

Pharmacotherapeutics Study of the use and effect of drugs in the treatment and prevention of disease

Phlebotomy Process of collecting blood for analysis

Photometric reflectance Measurement of the amount of light reflected by a specimen

Physician's office laboratory Laboratory within the medical office

Placenta Uterine structure that is connected to the fetus by the umbilical cord and from which the fetus obtains nourishment and oxygen

Plaintiff   Person bringing charges in court

Plasma   Liquid portion of blood that contains clotting factors

Pleural membranes   Double membranes that cover the lungs and line the thoracic cavity

Pneumonectomy   Surgical removal of an entire lung

Point of maximal impulse   Point on the chest wall at which cardiac contractions are best seen or felt

Policies and procedures manual   Handbook that provides detailed information about regulations regarding tasks and how to perform the tasks

Policyholder   Person who purchases an insurance policy

Polycythemia   Abnormal increase in the amount of red blood cells

Polydipsia   Increased thirst

Polyphagia   Increased appetite

Polypharmacy   High-risk situation in which a patient is taking multiple medications, thus increasing the risk of adverse effects

Polyuria   Increase in the amount of urine formation and excretion

Positron emission tomography   Procedure in which the brain is viewed using positron-emitting radionuclides

Postmenopausal   Period occurring after permanent cessation of menstruation

Postpartum   Time from birth up to 6 weeks

Postural vital signs   Vital signs performed to test for orthostatic hypotension

Practice-based   Scheduling technique that designates special days for common treatments based on time limits and staff and equipment availability

Preceptor   Experienced medical assistant or other health care provider who agrees to work closely with a student in the medical office

Preferred provider organization   Managed care plan that contracts with physicians to furnish services to its members

Prefix   Word element placed at the beginning of a word that modifies the word's meaning

Premium   Money paid to an insurer to obtain insurance

Prenatal   Time of gestation before birth

Presbyopia   Permanent loss of accommodation of the crystalline lens that occurs in people over age 40

Prescribe   To indicate a drug to be administered

Pressure point   Point at which an artery may be compressed to decrease blood flow in the event of hemorrhage

Prion   Proteinaceous infectious particle that can cause a spongiform encephalopathy

Privacy standard   Policies and procedures in a facility that determine who has access to protected health information

Problem-oriented medical record   System of documentation that includes the database, problem list, plan, and progress notes

Prodromal   Interval between earliest symptoms and appearance of a rash or fever

Productivity   Extent of a person's ability to perform a job function

Proficiency testing   Tests on unknown specimens provided by an external monitoring agency, such as the state health department and the College of American Pathologists, to meet quality control requirements

Program coordinator   Medical assistant program staff member who arranges externship placement and monitors progress

Projection   Psychological response in which a person accuses others of that person's own feelings, attitudes, or behaviors

Prolactin   Hormone that stimulates breast development and production of milk

Pronation   Movement of the arm so the palm is down or movement of the foot outward and up

Pronunciation   Generally accepted sound of a spoken word

Proofread   Check of a written document for accuracy in spelling, punctuation, grammar, word choice, and sentence structure

Protected health information   Information from a patient's record that contains details that could be used to identify the patient

Protein   Dietary source of amino acids used to build various body tissues, hormones, and antibodies

Proteinuria   Presence of protein in the urine

Prothrombin time   Blood test that determines how long it takes for blood to clot and monitors warfarin (Coumadin) therapy

Protocol   Expected behavior during a given situation

Protozoa   Unicellular, animal-like organism mainly found in soil that is capable of producing disease

Proxemics   Study of how much personal space people prefer and how it relates to culture and environment

Pruritus   Feeling of itchiness

Psychomotor domain   Processes that involve physical activity and the senses (sight, sound, touch, smell, and taste)

Pulmonary function test   Measurement of air flow and lung volumes; also called *spirometry*

Pulmonologist   Physician who specializes in the diagnosis and treatment of respiratory disorders

Pulmonology   Field of medicine that studies and treats respiratory disorders

Pulse deficit   Difference between the apical pulse and radial pulse

Pulse pressure   Difference between systolic and diastolic pressures

Purge   Permanent removal of medical records that are no longer in use

Purulent   Consisting of or containing pus

Q

Qualitative result   Laboratory result that is descriptive, rather than providing a numerical value

Quality control   Methods used to monitor the accuracy of laboratory results

Quantitative result   Laboratory result that includes a numerical value

R

Radioallergosorbent test   Blood test for allergy that measures small quantities of immunoglobulin E in blood

Radiograph   Image produced on radiosensitive film by x-rays passed through an object

Radiography   Process of producing an image for diagnosis using a radiographic modality

Radiology   Branch of medicine concerned with radioactive substances, including x-rays or other sources of ionizing radiation used to assist in diagnosis and treatment

Radiolucent   Penetrable by x-rays

Radiopaque   Impenetrable to x-rays or other forms of radiation

Range of motion   Outer limit of joint movement

Rapport   Empathetic relationship

Rationalization   Psychological response in which a person makes excuses to justify inappropriate behaviors

Reactive   Responding without considering the situation at hand

Reagent   Substance used in a chemical reaction

Receiver   Person who receives a message and decodes it

Recorder   Person designated to document a medical emergency

Redirecting   Guiding the patient back to relevant subject matter

Reduction   Manual manipulation of a bone to return it to its normal position

Reference laboratory   Independent laboratory used by physician office and hospital laboratories to perform specialized testing

Referent   Stimulation or motivation to communicate

Referral   Request by a physician to have another physician examine a patient

Reflecting   Validating the patient's feelings and concerns

Registration   Process of collecting patient demographic and insurance information when the patient begins care

Regression   Psychological response in which a person reverts to behaviors associated with earlier (younger) developmental stages

Renal colic   Pain that radiates from the flank into the abdomen or groin area

Renal threshold   Concentration at which substances in the blood not normally excreted by the kidneys begin to appear in the urine

Repetitive motion injury   Physical injury caused by a specific repeated motion

Repression   Psychological response in which a person eliminates from conscious thought traumatic experiences or certain impulses that the person believes are unacceptable

Requisition slip   Form used to order laboratory tests

Reservoir host   Organism that provides a hospitable environment in which pathogens can grow

res ipsa loquitur   Latin phrase, which means "the thing speaks for itself" and is used in legal situations when negligence is clearly evident

Resident   Physician who obtains further medical training after internship, usually as a member of the house staff of a hospital

Resistance   Microorganism's ability to withstand the effects of an antimicrobial agent

Resolution   Stage of grief and loss when a person expresses emotions more freely and begins to identify changes in life caused by the loss

Respectful   Behavior that treats a person or object with honor or esteem

respondeat superior   Latin phrase, which means "let the master answer" and is a legal doctrine that places responsibility on a physician for the actions of her employee

Restating   Rewording a statement to check for accuracy

Restitution   Monetary compensation for loss or injury

Resumé   Document that summarizes a job applicant's experiences, qualifications, and education

Rickettsia   Genus of bacteria that are intracellular parasites

Risk management   Proactive management that seeks to reduce potential risks of a lawsuit before it occurs

Roentgenography   Practice of using radiation technology to examine the bones and other dense structures of a patient's body; also called *radiology* and *x-ray*

Rhonchi   Coarse gurgling sound heard on auscultation that is caused by secretions in the air passages

Rotation   Movement that turns a body part around its axis

Route of administration   Way in which medication is introduced into the body

Routine test   Laboratory test ordered as part of a regular office visit

Rugae   Folds on the internal surface of the stomach

S

Saliva   Oral secretions that moisten food for tasting, chewing, and swallowing

Sanitize   Remove microorganisms from reusable equipment and surfaces by using chemicals, heat, or ionizing radiation

Scope of practice   Legal description of professional responsibilities and duties that may be performed by a licensed or certified individual

Scratch test   Test in which a dilution of a potential allergen is placed in a lightly scratched area of the skin

Security standard   Policy that protects the confidentiality, integrity, and availability of protected health information

Self-care   Activity that supports and nurtures an individual's physical, mental, spiritual, or emotional health and well-being

Self-efficacy   Person's perception of how capable and confident he feels about being able to make a specified change or accomplish a goal

Semi-Fowler position   Position in which the patient reclines at 45 degrees with legs outstretched

Sender   Person who delivers a message

Sensory nerves   Nerves that convey sensory information

Serum   Liquid portion of blood that does not contain clotting factors

Short timer's syndrome   Tendency of an employee to demonstrate a reduction in

the quality and quantity of and interest in work after giving notice of the intent to leave the position

Silence   Communication strategy that allows the patient time to process information and formulate a response

Sims position   Position in which the patient lies on his side with the upper arm forward on the table, lower leg flexed slightly, and upper leg flexed sharply

Sinusitis   Inflammation of the sinuses, which can be caused by a virus, bacteria, or an allergy

Skill set   Group of related work abilities

Skin turgor   Resistance of the skin to deformation when grasped between the fingers that is used to assess the state of hydration

Slander   Dishonoring or defaming a person through verbal attacks

Slang   Unconventional word or phrase used in place of a conventional word that is commonly clinical or complex in some way

Sleep apnea   Temporary cessation of breathing during sleep

Smear   Bacterial growth sample that is spread onto a microscope slide for staining purposes

Sole proprietor   Physician in a solo practice

Soluble fiber   Indigestible food component that dissolves in water to form a gel

Source-oriented medical record   System of documentation that includes a note for each patient visit, arranged in reverse chronological order

Specific gravity   Weight of a substance compared with an equal amount of water

Specimen   Blood, other body fluid, or body tissue submitted for laboratory analysis

Sphygmomanometer   Blood pressure cuff

Spinal fusion   Surgical immobilization of adjacent vertebrae

Spores   Bacterial or fungal cells that are resistant to temperature extremes

Staff of Asclepius   Ancient symbol of the Greek god Asclepius that consists of a staff with a single serpent entwined around it and used today as a symbol of medical care

Statute   Law

Statute of limitations   Law that sets a time limit within which a person can bring a lawsuit

Stent   Device that holds tissue in place and maintains an opening

Sterile technique   Method that involves performing invasive procedures in a manner that protects patients from pathogens

Sterile toss   Technique for placing sterile items on the sterile field without contaminating either one

Stream   Most common scheduling technique in which patients are seen in a steady stream at set appointment times of 15-, 30-, 45-, or 60-minute intervals

Subacute care   Health care setting in which temporary care is provided with the goal of helping the patient to regain strength, mobility, and function in order to return home or to an assisted-living setting

Subcutaneous   Route of administration that involves injection of a drug into the fatty layer under the skin

Sublingual   Route of administration that involves placement of a drug under the tongue

Subpoena   Legal document that notifies a person that he is required to appear in court or be available for deposition

subpoena ducas tecum   Latin phrase that means "bring with you under penalty of punishment" and is a legal document that requires a person to appear in court with specified documents, such as patient records

Suffix   Word element placed at the end of a word that modifies the word's meaning

Summarizing   Clarifying the patient's key issues

Summary of care   Written description of assessment, services (procedures), and outcomes of care provided to a patient

Superbill   Document used in a medical office to indicate the services provided by a physician to a patient during an office visit

Supination   Movement of the arm so the palm is up or movement of the foot inward and up

Supine position   Position in which the patient is lying flat, face up toward the ceiling

Surgical asepsis   Destruction of all pathogenic organisms before they enter the body

Susceptibility   Degree to which a microorganism's growth can be inhibited by an antimicrobial agent

Suspension   Solid particles mixed in a liquid but not dissolved

Suture   Material used to sew wound edges together or the act of sewing wound edges together

Swage   To fuse a suture to a needle

Symptomatic   Having symptoms, such as fever, sore throat, nausea, and vomiting

Syrup   Concentrated solution of sugar and water to which medicine is added and taken orally

Systemic circulation   Circulation throughout the entire body

Systemic effect   Impact of a medication throughout the body

Systole   Period during contraction of chambers of the heart when blood pressure is the highest

Systolic pressure   Tension exerted against arterial walls during ventricular contraction and represented by the top number in a blood pressure reading

T

Tablet   Small, disklike mass of medicine in compressed powder form taken orally

Tachycardia   Abnormally rapid heart rate

Tachypnea   Abnormally rapid breathing

Tactful   Displaying sensitivity and courtesy in behavior and comments to avoid offending others

Targeted resumé   Document that identifies the position desired and summarizes specific experiences and abilities that are relevant to the job for which the person is applying

Teaching hospital   Hospital that is affiliated with a medical school where residents provide much of the physician-related care under the supervision of licensed physicians

Team captain   Person designated to coordinate activities of all team members during a medical emergency

Teleological philosophies   Philosophies that focus on consequences or the end, more than on actions or the means, in determining value

Tendon   Band of dense fibrous tissue that attaches muscle to bone

Teratogenic effect   Adverse effect of a drug on a developing embryo or fetus

Terminal digit filing   System that uses the last digits of an identification number as the primary indexing unit

Termination policy   Written policy that mandates termination of an employee who fails to comply with internal privacy policies and procedures

Therapeutic effect   Desired response in the body from a prescribed drug

Thermotherapy   Therapeutic application of heat used to treat various muscle injuries

Thoracentesis   Surgical puncture of the chest wall into the pleural space to obtain a fluid specimen for testing

Thrombocytes   Platelets responsible for clot formation

Thrombocytopenia   Abnormal decrease in platelets

Thrombotic   Caused by a blood clot

Tickler file   Reminder file used to prompt such activities as supply orders and equipment inspection

Tinnitus   Ringing in the ears

Tolerance   Need for increased dose of a drug to produce the same effect

Tomography   Radiographic technique that selects a level in the body and blurs out structures above and below that plane, leaving a clear image of the selected anatomy

Tort   Wrongful act committed by a person that causes harm to another person or property

Tourniquet   Device used to aid vein protrusion

Toxic   Poisonous or harmful

Toxicology   Division of medical and biological science concerned with toxic substances

Tracer   Radioactive isotope that can identify a specific portion of a molecule to follow its course

Transaction   Exchange of information between two parties to carry out financial or administrative activities related to health care

Transaction code sets   Standardized codes used to represent health care concepts and procedures for health-care-related financial and administrative procedures

Transcription   Creation of a written document from dictated tapes or computer voice files

Transducer   Device that moves over the skin to record sound waves

Transection   Cutting

Trendelenburg position   Position in which the patient lies with her head approximately 30 degrees lower than her outstretched legs and feet

Triage   Process of screening patients to determine which need immediate medical treatment and in what order each patient must be seen, and which patients must go to the emergency room or if they can be worked into the physician's schedule for the day

Troponin   Protein that is released into the blood by damaged heart muscle and, therefore, a highly sensitive and specific indicator of recent myocardial infarction

Turbid   Thick or opaque

U

Ultrasonography   Use of high-frequency sound waves to produce an image of an organ or tissue

Ultrasound   Application of high-frequency sound waves to warm tissues, increasing tissue extensibility and improving local blood flow

Undernutrition Condition caused by insufficient intake of calories and, sometimes, nutrients

Unit Each part of a patient's name or identification number used in a filing system

Upcode Illegal practice of using a procedure code that yields higher reimbursement than the procedure that is actually performed

Upper gastrointestinal series Radiographic examination of the esophagus, stomach, and upper small intestine during and after the introduction of barium as a contrast medium; also called *upper GI series* or *barium swallow*

Urgency Sudden, nearly uncontrollable need to urinate

Urinalysis Laboratory analysis of urine

Urinary catheterization Procedure that involves insertion of a sterile drainage tube into the bladder to drain or withdraw urine

Urine culture Growth and study of microorganisms isolated from a urine specimen

Utilitarianism Ethical philosophy concerned with achieving the greatest good for the greatest number of people

Utilization review Determination by a managed care organization of the medical necessity of a procedure or service

Uvula Soft tissue hanging from the upper mouth that prevents food from entering the nasal cavity

V

Vaccine Preparation used to improve immunity to a particular disease

Variable costs Expenses that increase with an increase in the number of patients seen

Vasectomy Procedure that involves removal of a segment of the vas deferens to achieve male sterilization

Vasoconstriction Decrease in diameter of blood vessels, which decreases blood flow and raises blood pressure

Vasodilation Dilation or enlargement of blood vessels, especially small arteries and arterioles

Vector Carrier, usually an insect, that transmits a disease from an infected person to a noninfected person

Venipuncture Process of puncturing a vein with a needle to obtain blood

Venous Pertaining to the veins or the blood in the veins

Veracity Quality of truthfulness

Verification Process of confirming insurance benefits with the patient's insurance carrier

Vicarious liability Liability of an employer for the wrongdoing of an employee while on the job

Villi Projections of the small intestines that absorb water and nutrients

Virus Pathogen that can grow and reproduce only after infecting a host cell

Visual acuity Ability to see at different distances

Vitamin Organic molecule that contains carbon and several different elements needed by the body to support chemical reactions

Voice mail System that enables a caller to leave a recorded message for the recipient

W

Wave Scheduling technique in which patients are scheduled in the first half-hour of each hour

Wedge resection Surgical removal of a small part of a lung

Wheeze Somewhat musical sound heard in the lungs, usually with a stethoscope, that is caused by partial airway obstruction

White space Blank space on a document to create a more organized, less cluttered presentation

Whole blood Blood composed of formed elements (cells) and plasma

Word root Main stem of a word that conveys the word's meaning

Workflow Physical space that facilitates accomplishment of work-related duties

Write-off Difference in the amount charged for a service and the amount contractually allowed by an insurance company

X, Y

X-ray film Special photographic film that blackens on exposure to light

X-ray tube Vacuum tube that creates electromagnetic radiation with a wavelength between 0.1 and 100 angstrom units

Z

Z-track injection Intramuscular injection technique where the skin is pulled to one side to prevent medication from leaking into the subcutaneous tissues

Zygote Fertilized ovum

Abbreviations

This appendix includes two lists of abbreviations. The first includes commonly used abbreviations and the second lists discontinued abbreviations. Even so, the medical assistant should always check her facility's policy on the appropriate use of abbreviations.

Commonly Used Abbreviations

The table below lists abbreviations commonly used in the medical office and other health care settings along with their spelled-out terms.

A

a	before
ABGs	arterial blood gases
ac, AC	before meals
AC	air conduction
ACL	anterior cruciate ligament
ACTH	adrenocorticotropic hormone
AD	Alzheimer disease
ad lib	as desired
ADD	attention deficit disorder
ADH	antidiuretic hormone
ADHD	attention deficit hyperactivity disorder
ADL	activities of daily living
AGA	appropriate for gestational age
AIDS	acquired immune deficiency syndrome
AK	above the knee
ALS	amyotrophic lateral sclerosis
ALT	alanine aminotransferase
AMD, ARMD	age-related macular degeneration
APGAR	activity, pulse, grimace, appearance, respiration
aq	water
ARDS	acute respiratory distress syndrome
ARF	acute renal failure
AS	ankylosing spondylitis
ASHD	arteriosclerotic heart disease
AST	aspartate aminotransferase

B

BaE, BE	barium enema
BC	bone conduction
BG	blood glucose
bid	twice a day
BK	below the knee
BM	bowel movement
BMG	bone mineral density
BOM	bilateral otitis media
BP	blood pressure
BPH	benign prostatic hypertrophy
BS	blood sugar
BSA	body surface area
BUN	blood urea nitrogen
Bx	biopsy

C

C&S	culture and sensitivity
C	Celsius
c̄	with
c/o	complaint of
Ca	calcium
Ca, CA	cancer
CABG	coronary artery bypass graft
CAD	coronary artery disease
cap	capsule
CBC	complete blood count
CK	conductive keratoplasty, creatine kinase
CKD	chronic kidney disease
Cl	chloride
cm	centimeter
CNS	central nervous system
CO_2	carbon dioxide
COPD	chronic obstructive pulmonary disease
CPAP	continuous positive airway pressure
CPR	cardiopulmonary resuscitation
CRF	chronic renal failure
C-section	cesarean section
CSF	cerebrospinal fluid
CT	computed tomography
CVA	cerebrovascular accident (stroke)

D

D&C	dilatation and curettage
DDH	developmental dysplasia of the hip
decub.	decubitus (ulcer)
disc	discontinue
DJD	degenerative joint disease
DM	diabetes mellitus
DNR	do not resuscitate
DPT	diphtheria, pertussis, and tetanus
DRE	digital rectal examination
DTR	deep tendon reflexes
DVT	deep vein thrombosis
Dx	diagnosis

E

EAC	external auditory canal
EC	enteric coated

ED	erectile dysfunction; emergency department	IV	intravenous
EEG	electroencephalography	IVC	intravenous cholangiogram
EMG	electromyogram	IVF	in vitro fertilization
ENT	ears, nose, and throat	IVP	intravenous pyelogram
EOM	extraocular movement	IVPB	intravenous piggy back
ERCP	endoscopic retrograde cholangiopancreatography		
ESR	erythrocyte sedimentation rate	**J, K**	
ESRD	end-stage renal disease	JRA	juvenile rheumatoid arthritis
		K	potassium
F		kg, Kg	kilogram
		KUB	kidney, ureter, bladder
FBG	fasting blood glucose		
FBS	fasting blood sugar	**L**	
Fe	iron		
FH	family history	L	liter
fl, fld	fluid	LA	left atrium
fsbs	finger stick blood sugar	LASIK	laser-assisted keratomileusis
FSH	follicle-stimulating hormone	LD	lactate dehydrogenase
		LDL	low-density lipoprotein
G		LFT	liver function test
		LH	leuteinizing hormone
g, G, Gm	gram	LLE	left lower extremity
GERD	gastroesophageal reflux disease	LMP	last menstrual period
GFR	glomerular filtration rate	LP	lumbar puncture
GGT	gamma-glutamyl transferase	LTC	long-term care
GH	growth hormone	LTK	laser thermal keratoplasty
GI	gastrointestinal	LUE	left upper extremity
gr	grain	LV	left ventricle
gtt	drop	lytes	electrolytes
GYN	gynecology		
		M	
H			
		mcg	microgram
H&H	hemoglobin and hematocrit	MD	muscular dystrophy; medical doctor
h, hr	hour	mEq	milliequivalent
HCT	hematocrit	Mg	magnesium
HDL	high-density lipoprotein	mg	milligram
HEENT	head, eyes, ears, nose, and throat	ml, mL	milliliter
Hep B	hepatitis B vaccination	mm	millimeter
Hgb	hemoglobin	MMR	measles, mumps, and rubella
Hgb A1C	glycosylated hemoglobin	MRI	magnetic resonance imaging
HiB	*Haemophilus influenzae* type B vaccine	MS	multiple sclerosis
HIV	human immunodeficiency virus	MVA	motor vehicle accident
HPV	human papillomavirus		
HSV-1	herpes simplex virus type 1	**N**	
HSV-2	herpes simplex virus type 2		
HTN	hypertension	N&V	nausea and vomiting
Hx	history	Na	sodium
		NaCl	sodium chloride
I		NG	nasogastric
		NIDDM	non-insulin-dependent diabetes mellitus
I&D	incision and drainage	NIHL	noise-induced hearing loss
IBD	inflammatory bowel disease	noc, noct, n	night
IBS	irritable bowel syndrome	NPC	nonproductive cough
ICP	intracranial pressure	NPO, npo	nothing by mouth (*nil per os*)
ID	intradermal	NSAID	nonsteroidal anti-inflammatory drug
IDDM	insulin dependent diabetes mellitus		
IM	intramuscular	**O**	
INR	International Normalized Ratio		
IOL	intraocular lens	O₂	oxygen
IOP	intraocular pressure	OA	osteoarthritis
IPV	inactivated poliovirus vaccine	OB-GYN	obstetrics and gynecology
IUD	intrauterine device	OC	oral contraceptive

ORIF	open reduction and internal fixation
OT	occupational therapy
OTC	over-the-counter
oz	ounce

P

P	pulse
p̄	after
PAC	premature atrial contraction
Pap test	Papanicolaou test
pc	after meals
PCP	*Pneumocystis* pneumonia
PCV	pneumococcal conjugate vaccine
PDA	patent ductus arteriosis
PE	physical examination
PE tube	pressure-equalizing tube
Peds	pediatric
PERRLA	pupils equal, round, and reactive to light and accommodation
pH	parts hydrogen
PID	pelvic inflammatory disease
PKD	polycystic kidney disease
Plt	platelets
PM, pm	afternoon
PMH	prior medical history
PND	paroxysmal nocturnal dyspnea; postnasal drip; postnasal drainage
PNS	peripheral nervous system
PO, po	by mouth, orally (*per os*)
PR	per rectum
PRN, prn	whenever necessary (*pro re nata*)
PSA	prostatic-specific antigen
PT	prothrombin time; physical therapy
PTCA	percutaneous transluminal coronary angioplasty
PTH	parathormone, parathyroid hormone
PTT	partial thromboplastin time
PUD	peptic ulcer disease
PVC	premature ventricular contraction

Q

q	every
q2h	every 2 hours
q3h	every 3 hours
qam	every morning
qh	every hour
qhs	every day at bed time (or each evening)
qid	four times a day
QNS	quantity not sufficient
QS, qs	quantity sufficient

R

R	respiration; rectal
RA	right atrium; rheumatoid arthritis
RAST	radioallergosorbent test
RBC	red blood cell
RK	radial keratotomy
RLE	right lower extremity
ROM	range of motion
ROP	retinopathy of prematurity

RP	retrograde pyelogram; retinitis pigmentosa
RR	respiratory rate
RUE	right upper extremity
RV	right ventricle
Rx	prescription

S

s̄	without
SARS	sudden acute respiratory syndrome
SBO	small bowel obstruction
SubQ, subcu, or subq	subcutaneous
sed rate	erythrocyte sedimentation rate
SIDS	sudden infant death syndrome
SL	sublingual
SLE	systemic lupus erythematosus
SOB	shortness of breath
sol	solution
SOM	serous otitis media
SR	sustained release
stat	immediately
STD	sexually transmitted disease
STI	sexually transmitted infection
supp	suppository
Sx	symptom
syr	syrup

T

T	temperature
T, Tbsp, Tbs	tablespoon
t, tsp, Tsp	teaspoon
T&A	tonsillectomy and adenoidectomy
T3	triiodothyronine
T4	thyroxine
tab	tablet
TAH	total abdominal hysterectomy
TAH-BSO	total abdominal hysterectomy with bilateral salpingo-oophorectomy
TB	tuberculosis
TC	total cholesterol
TENS	transcutaneous electrical nerve stimulation
TIA	transient ischemic attack
tid	three times a day
tinct, tr	tincture
TM	tympanic membrane
TMJ	temporomandibular joint
TO	telephone order
TPR	temperature, pulse, respiration
TSE	testicular self-examination
TSH	thyroid stimulating hormone
TURP	transurethral resection of the prostate
Tx	treatment

U

UA	urinalysis
ung	ointment
URI	upper respiratory infection
US	ultrasound
UTI	urinary tract infection

V

VA	visual acuity
vag	vaginal
VC	vital capacity
VF	visual field
VLDL	very-low-density lipoprotein
VO	verbal order

W, X, Y, Z

WBC	white blood cell
WNL	within normal limits

Discontinued Abbreviations

The abbreviations below, although commonly used in the past, have been identified as the cause of many errors and much confusion. Thus, the medical assistant should refrain from using these abbreviations. Even so, many of these abbreviations will appear in medical records; thus, medical assistants should know the abbreviated and spelled-out forms for each.

AD	right ear (*auris dextra*)
AS	left ear (*auris sinistra*)
AU	both ears (*auris utraque*)
cc	cubic centimeter
DC, dc	discharge (confused with discontinue)
hs, HS	bedtime
OD	right eye (*oculus dexter*), overdose
OS, os	left eye (*oculus sinister*)

OU	both eyes together (*oculus uterque*)
IU	International Unit
μg	microgram
qd	every day
qod	every other day
SC, SQ	subcutaneous
U	unit

Index of Competencies

Below are lists of competencies as determined by the Commission on Accreditation of Allied Health Education Programs (CAAHEP) and Accrediting Bureau of Health Education Schools (ABHES). Each list includes the individual competency and every chapter in which it appears. The CAAHEP list also includes a column to indicate those competencies that require a work product.

CAAHEP Competencies

Competency	Work Product	Chapter
Administrative Competencies		
Perform Clerical Functions		
Schedule and manage appointments	• Appointment schedule • Appointment schedule showing changes, such as rescheduling and no-shows	11, 12
Schedule inpatient and outpatient admissions and procedures	• Completed referral forms for each of the four components	12
Organize a patient's medical record	None required	7, 14
File medical records	None required	14
Perform Bookkeeping Procedures		
Prepare a bank deposit	• Completed bank deposit slip	18
Post entries on a day sheet	• Completed day sheet	18
Perform accounts receivable procedures	• Completed day sheet	17, 18
Perform billing and collection procedures	• Completed billing form • Documentation of collection activity	17, 18
Post adjustments	• Completed day sheet or ledger including adjustments	18
Process a credit balance	• Completed day sheet or ledger including credit balance	18
Process refunds	• Completed day sheet or ledger including refund or indication of refund issued	18
Post nonsufficient fund (NSF) checks	• Completed day sheet or ledger including NSF check	18
Post collection agency payments	• Completed day sheet or ledger including collection agency payment	18
Process Insurance Claims		
Apply managed care policies and procedures	None required	7, 16
Apply third party guidelines	None required	7, 16
Perform procedural coding	• Completed CMS 1500	16
Perform diagnostic coding	• Completed CMS 1500	25, 28, 29, 16
Complete insurance claim forms	• Completed CMS 1500	16
Clinical Competencies		
Fundamental Principles		
Perform hand washing	None required	19
Wrap items for autoclaving	None required	19
Perform sterilization techniques	None required	19
Dispose of biohazardous materials	None required	19, 30, 38, 40, 41, 46
Practice standard precautions	None required	19, 22, 30, 40, 41, 46

Continued

Competency	Work Product	Chapter
Clinical Competencies		
Specimen Collection		
Perform venipuncture	None required	41
Perform capillary puncture	None required	41
Obtain specimens for microbiological testing	None required	40, 45, 46
Instruct patients in the collection of a clean-catch, midstream urine specimen	None required	44
Instruct patients in the collection of a fecal specimen	None required	30
Diagnostic Testing		
Perform electrocardiography	• ECG tracing to accompany the checklist as evidence of the achievement	27
Perform respiratory testing	• Results of the testing attached with the checklist or recorded on the checklist	28
CLIA-Waived Tests		25, 32, 40, 42, 43, 44, 45,
• Perform urinalysis	• Reporting of the results of the urinalysis with or on the checklist	40, 44
• Perform hematology testing	• Reporting of the results of the hematology test with or on the checklist	40, 42
• Perform chemistry testing	• Reporting of the results of the chemistry test with or on the checklist	40, 43
• Perform immunology testing	• Reporting of the results of the immunology test with or on the checklist	25, 40, 43
• Perform microbiology testing	• Reporting of the results of the microbiology test with or on the checklist	40, 45
Patient Care		
Perform telephone and in-person screening	• Chart notes referring to the screening process between the medical assistant and the "patient"	12, 48
Obtain vital signs	• Charting examples on a "medical record" or the checklist that demonstrates the student has recorded her results	21, 33
Obtain and record patient history	• A patient history form completed by the student	20
Prepare and maintain examination and treatment areas	None required	22, 27, 30, 32, 33, 48
Prepare patients for and assist with routine and specialty examinations	None required	22, 25, 26, 27, 28, 29, 30, 31, 32, 33, 36, 48
Prepare patients for and assist with procedures, treatments, and minor office surgeries	None required	22, 24, 25, 26, 28, 29, 30, 31, 33, 35
Apply pharmacology principles to prepare and administer oral and parenteral (excluding IV) medications	• Documentation of the administration of the oral and parenteral medications in the "chart" or on the checklist	36, 38, 39
Maintain medication and immunization records	• Documentation in a patient's "chart" or on a medication log showing both medications and immunizations (could be separate logs for different patients)	33, 39
Screen and follow up test results	• Documentation of calling or writing the patient to follow up on the test results	40, 48
General Competencies*		
Professional Communications		
Respond to and initiate written communications	• Sample of the written communication used to document the achievement of this competency (for example, a letter or memorandum)	13, 23
Recognize and respond to verbal communication	None required	12, 15, 20, 23, 34
Recognize and respond to nonverbal communications	None required	3, 5, 6, 9, 10, 11, 34, 48, 49

Competency	Work Product	Chapter
*General Competencies**		
Professional Communications		
Demonstrate telephone techniques	None required	11, 12
Legal Concepts		
Identify and respond to issues of confidentiality	None required	6, 7, 8, 11, 10, 13, 15, 34, 48
Perform within legal and ethical boundaries	None required	6, 7, 8, 11, 13, 15, 39
Establish and maintain the medical record	None required	6, 7, 13, 20, 32
Document appropriately	• Sample of documentation associated with the procedure used to document achievement of this competency (For example, if "Obtain vital signs" was the basis for achievement of this competency, then the sheet used to record vitals signs should be attached.)	6, 7, 11, 20, 22, 26, 32, 38, 39, 40, 41
Demonstrate knowledge of federal and state health care legislation and regulations	None required	6, 7, 38, 39,
Patient Instruction		
Explain general office policies	None required	10, 11, 17
Instruct individuals according to their needs	None required	1, 9, 10, 11, 23, 25, 26, 27, 28, 29, 30, 32, 34, 35, 36, 37, 38, 39, 47, 48
Provide instruction for health maintenance and disease prevention	None required	9, 10, 19, 22, 23, 25, 27, 28, 29, 31, 32, 34, 35, 37
Identify community resources	None required	4, 10, 32, 34, 37
Operational Functions		
Perform an inventory of supplies and equipment	• Completed inventory sheet showing status of supplies • Completed inventory sheet showing status of equipment	15
Perform routine maintenance of administrative and clinical equipment	• Sample of routine maintenance log for the administrative equipment used to document achievement of this competency • Sample of routine maintenance log for the clinical equipment used to document achievement of this competency	15, 40
Utilize computer software to maintain office systems	• Printed sample from the computer software used to document achievement of this competency (for example, a letter for word processing, an insurance form or report for medical office software, sent e-mail message for e-mail software, and a printout of a website page for research)	15, 12, 16, 18
Use methods of quality control	• Sample of quality control log for the test performed to document achievement of this competency	40, 42, 43, 44

*Documentation of achievement of General Competencies may include materials other than checklists.

ABHES Competencies

Competency	Chapter
Professionalism	
Project a positive attitude	3, 10, 15, 49
Maintain confidentiality at all times	7, 8, 10, 34, 48
Be a "team player"	3, 15
Be cognizant of ethical boundaries	7, 8, 10, 49
Exhibit initiative	3, 15, 49

Continued

Competency	Chapter
Professionalism	
Adapt to change	3
Evidence a responsible attitude	3, 8, 10, 15, 39
Be courteous and diplomatic	3, 5, 8, 10, 20
Conduct work within scope of education, training, and ability	6, 7, 39, 48
Communication	
Be attentive, listen, and learn	5, 10, 11, 15, 20
Be impartial and show empathy when dealing with patients	5, 7, 10, 32
Adapt what is said to the recipient's level of comprehension	7, 10, 11, 20, 32, 34, 38, 39, 48
Serve as a liaison between the physician and others	4, 11, 32, 38, 39, 48
Use proper telephone techniques	11, 12
Interview effectively	12, 15, 20
Use appropriate medical terminology	10, 12, 23, 25, 26, 30
Receive, organize, prioritize, and transmit information expediently	11, 13, 20
Recognize and respond to verbal and nonverbal communication (and recognition and response to verbal and nonverbal communication)	3, 5, 10, 12, 20, 30, 41, 48, 49
Use correct grammar, spelling, and formatting techniques in written works	10, 13, 49
Principles of verbal and nonverbal communication	5, 10, 20
Adaptation for individualized needs	9, 20, 34, 48
Application of electronic technology	13, 48
Fundamental writing skills	6, 13
Professional components	3
Allied health professions and credentialing	3
Administrative Duties	
Perform basic secretarial skills	13
Prepare and maintain medical records	20
Schedule and monitor appointments	11, 12
Apply computer concepts for office procedures	12, 18
Locate resources and information for patients and employers	7, 13, 34
Manage physician's professional schedule and travel	15
Schedule inpatient and outpatient admissions	12
File medical records	14
Prepare a bank statement and deposit record	18
Reconcile a bank statement	18
Post entries on a day sheet	18
Perform billing and collection procedures	17, 18
Prepare a check	18
Establish and maintain a petty cash fund	18
Post adjustments	18
Process credit balance	18
Process refunds	18
Post NSF funds	18
Post collection agency payments	18
Apply managed care policies and procedures	16
Obtain managed care referrals and precertification	16
Perform diagnostic coding	16, 25, 26, 29
Complete insurance claim forms	16
Use physician fee schedule	16
Clinical Duties	
Interview and record patient history	20, 31, 32, 33
Prepare patients for procedures	22, 25, 26, 27, 28, 29, 30, 31, 32, 33, 35, 36, 48
Apply principles of aseptic technique and infection control	19, 24, 32, 36, 39, 41
Take vital signs	21, 32, 33
Recognize emergencies	47
Perform first aid and CPR	47
Prepare and maintain examination and treatment areas	30, 32, 33, 35, 36, 48

Competency	Chapter
Clinical Duties	
Prepare patient for and assist physician with routine and specialty examinations and treatments and minor office surgeries	22, 24, 25, 26, 27, 28, 29, 30, 31, 32, 35, 36, 48
Use quality control	40, 41, 42, 43, 44
Collect and process specimens	25, 26, 31, 32, 40, 41, 42, 43, 44, 46
Perform selected CLIA-waived tests that assist with diagnosis and treatment	32, 40
Screen and follow up patient test results	40, 41
Prepare and administer oral and parenteral medications as directed by the physician	39
Maintain medication and immunization records	33
Wrap items for autoclaving	19
Perform sterilization techniques	19
Dispose of biohazardous materials	30, 32, 39, 41, 42, 43, 44, 45
Practice standard precautions	32, 39, 41, 42, 43, 44, 45
Perform venipuncture	41
Perform capillary puncture	33, 41
Obtain throat specimen for microbiological testing	33, 45
Perform wound collection procedure for microbiological testing	45
Instruct patients in the collection of a clean-catch, midstream urine specimen	44
Instruct patient in the collection of fecal specimen	30
Perform urinalysis	33, 44
Perform hematology testing	41, 42
Perform chemistry testing	43
Perform immunology testing	25, 43
Perform microbiology testing	45
Perform electrocardiograms	27
Perform respiratory testing	28
Perform telephone and in-person screening	11
Legal Concepts	
Determine needs for documentation and reporting	6, 7, 32, 48
Document accurately	6, 7, 20, 30, 32, 35, 48
Use appropriate guidelines when releasing records or information	6, 9, 14
Follow established policy in initiating or terminating medical treatment	6, 9, 13
Dispose of controlled substances in compliance with government regulations	38, 39
Maintain licenses and accreditation	6
Monitor legislation related to current health care issues and practices	6, 38
Perform risk management procedures	6
Office Management	
Maintain physical plant	15
Operate and maintain facilities and equipment safely	15
Inventory equipment and supplies	15
Evaluate and recommend equipment and supplies for practice	15
Maintain liability coverage	15
Exercise efficient time management	15
Instruction	
Orient patients to office policies and procedures	17
Instruct patients with special needs	1, 9, 32, 34, 35, 36, 37
Teach patients methods of health promotion and disease prevention	1, 9, 25, 26, 27, 29, 32, 34, 35, 36, 37, 38, 47
Orient and train personnel	15
Financial Management	
Use manual and computerized bookkeeping systems	18
Implement current procedural terminology and ICD-9-CM coding	16
Analyze and use current third-party guidelines for reimbursement	16
Manage accounts payable and receivable	18
Maintain records for accounting and banking purposes	18
Process employee payroll	18

Commonly Prescribed Drugs

This table includes a list of many of the most commonly prescribed medications in the United States. They are alphabetized according to the generic names with some of the common trade names listed in the second column. Because of the extent of trade name drugs for some generic forms, the list of trade names is not comprehensive in every case.

Generic name	Trade name(s)
acetaminophen	Tylenol, APAP, Abenol, Acephen, Panadol
acyclovir	Zovirax, Acycloguanosine
albuterol	Proventil, Ventolin, Salbutamol, Volmax
alendronate	Fosamax
allopurinol	Zyloprim, Aloprim, Lopurin
alprazolam	Xanax, Niravam
amiodarone	Cordarone, Pacerone
amitriptyline	Elavil, Endep
amlodipine	Norvasc
amlodipine and atorvastatin*	Caduet*
amlodipine and benazepril*	Lotrel*
amoxicillin	Amoxil, Trimox, Wymox
amoxicillin clavulanate	Augmentin
amphetamine	Adderall, Racemic Amphetamine, Sulfate
ampicillin	Principen, Polycillin, Totacillin, Marcillin, Omnipen
aripiprazole	Abilify
aspirin	Bayer, ASA, Acuprin, Artria, Ecotrin, Empirin
atenolol	Tenormin
atomoxetine	Strattera
atorvastin	Lipitor
atropine	Atropen, Sal-Tropine
azithromycin	Zithromax, Zmax
baclofen	Lioresal
bupropion	Wellbutrin, Budeprion SR, Zyban
bupropion hydrochloride	Budeprion, Wellbutrin, Zyban
buspirone	BuSpar
butalbital, acetaminophen, and caffeine*	Fioricet*, Dolmar*, Medigesic*
butalbital sodium	Butisol, Barbased, Butalan, Sarisol No2
calcium carbonate	Caltrate 600, Chooz, Os-Cal 500, Titralac, Tums
calcium chloride, calcium gluceptate, or calcium gluconate	Kalcinate
candesartan cilexetil	Atacand
captopril	Capoten
carbamazepine	Tegretol, Atretol, Carbatrol, Epitol, Equetro, Teril
carbidopa-levodopa	Sinemet, Atamet, Parcopa
carisoprodol	Soma, Rela, Vanadom
carvedilol	Coreg
cefdinir	Omnicef
celecoxib	Celebrex
cephalexin	Cefanex, Keflex, Keftab, Ceporex, Novolexin-A
cetirizine	Zyrtec
ciprofloxacin	Cipro, Proquin
citalopram	Celexa
clarithromycin	Biaxin
clindamycin	Cleocin

*combination product

Continued

Generic name	Trade name(s)
clonazepam	Klonopin
clonidine	Catapres, Duraclon, Dixaril
clopidogrel	Plavix
codeine	Codeine
colchicine	Colchicine
conjugated estrogen	Premarin, Congest
cyclobenzaprine	Cycloflex, Flexeril
desloratidine	Cymbalta
dexamethasone	Decadron, Dexon, Hexadrol, Mymethasone
diazepam	Valium, Diastat, Valrelease
diclofenac	Cataflam, Volatren, Solaraze
dicyclomine	Bentyl, Antispas, Byclomine, Dibent, Nospaz
digoxin	Lanoxicaps, Lanoxin
diltiazem	Cardizem, Dilacor XR, Tiazac, Tiamate
diphenhydramine	Benadryl, Benylin, Compoz, Diphon
divalproex sodium (valproic acid)	Depakote, Depacon, Depakene, Zalkote
donepezil hydrochloride	Aricept
dopamine	Intropin, Dopastat
doxazosin	Cardura
doxepin	Doxepin, Sinequan
doxycycline	Adoxa, Doxy, Monodox, Vibramycin, Vibra-Tabs, Vivox
duloxetine	Cymbalta
enalapril	Vasotec
enoxaparin	Lovenox
erythromycin	E-Mycin, Ery-Tab, Erythrocin
escitalopram oxalate	Lexapro
esomeprazole	Nexium
estradiol	Estrace, Estraderm, Alora, Climara
eszopiclone	Lunesta
etanercept	Enbrel
ethinyl estradiol and drospirenone*	Yasmin*, Yaz28*
ethinyl estradiol and norelgestromin	Ortho Evra
etodolac	Lodine
exenatide	Byetta
ezetimibe	Zetia
ezetimibe and simvastatin*	Vytorin*
famotidine	Mylanta AR, Pepcid
fenofibrate	Tricor, Antara, Lofibra, Triglide
fentanyl	Actiq, Sublimaze, Duragesic (transdermal), Oralet
fexofenadine	Allegra
finasteride	Proscar, Propexia
flucanazole	Diflucan
fluoxetine	Prozac, Sarafem
fluticasone	Flovent, Butivate, Flonase, Cutivate
furosemide	Lasix
gabapentin	Neurontin, Gabarone
glimepiride	Amaryl
glipizide	Glucotrol
glyburide	DiaBeta, Glynase, Micronase
haloperidol	Haldol
heparin	Lipo-Hepin, Liquaemin Sodium
hydralazine	Apresoline
hydrochlorothiazide	Esidrix, HCTC, Hydro-Chlor, HydroDIURIL
hydrocodone bitartrate	Hycodan, Robidone
hydrocodone bitartrate and acetaminophen	Vicodin, Norco, Zydone, Lortab
hydrocortisone	Cortef, Cortifoam, Hydrocortone, SoluCortef
hydromorphone	Dilaudid , Hydrostat
hydroxyzine	Atarax, Hyzine-50, Vistacon, Visteril
ibandronate sodium	Boniva

*combination product

Generic name	Trade name(s)
ibuprofen	Advil, Excedrin IB, Motrin, Nuprin
indomethacin	Indocin
insulins:	
Rapid Acting: lispro	Humalog
Short Acting: regular	Humulin R, Novolin R
Intermediate Acting: isophane suspension (NPH)	Humulin N, Novolin N,
Long Acting: glargine	Lantus
Mixtures: isophane suspension and regular*	Humulin 70/30*, Novolin 70/30*
ipratropium	Atrovent
irbesartan	Avapro
isosorbide dinitrate	Iso-Bid, Isorbid, Isordil, Sorbitrate, Imdur, Monoket
ketorolac	Toradol
lamotrigine	Lamictal
lansoprazole	Prevacid
leuprolide	Lupron, Eligard, Viadur
levetiracetam	Keppra
levofloxacin	Levaquin, Iquiz, Quixin
levothyroxine	Levoxyl, Levo-T, Levothyroid, Synthroid
lidocaine	Xylocaine, Anestacon, Dilocaine, Lidoderm
lisinopril	Prinivil, Zestril
lithium	Eskalith, Lithonate, Lithotabs
loratadine	Claritin, Dimetapp, Tavist ND
lorazepam	Ativan
losartan	Cozaar
losartan potassium and hydrochlorothiazide*	Hyzaar*
lovastatin	Mevacor, Altoprev, Mevinolin
magnesium hydroxide	Phillips' Magnesia Tablets, Phillips' Milk of Magnesia, MOM
meclizine	Antivert, Antrizine, Bonine, Meni-D, Vergon
medroxyprogesterone	Provera, Amen, Curretab, Cycrin, Depr-Provera
meloxicam	Mobic
memantine	Namenda
meperidine	Demerol, Pethidine
metaxalone	Skelaxin
metformin	Fortamet, Glucophage, Glumetza, Riomet
methadone	Dolophine, Methadose
methocarbamol	Carbacot, Robaxin
methotrexate	Rheumatrex, Amethopterin, Trexall
methylphenidate	Ritalin, Concerta, Daytrana, Methylin, Methidate
methylprednisolone	Medrol, A-Methapred, Solu-Medrol, Duralone
metoclopramide	Metoclopramide Octamide, Reglan Sensamide IV
metoprolol	Lopressor, Toprol-XL
metronidazole	Flagyl, Protostat, Metizol
midazolam	Versed
mirtazapine	Remeron
modafinil	Provigil
mometasone	Nasonex, Asthmanex Twisthaler, Elocon
montelukast	Singulair
morphine	Duramorph, Roxanol, MS-Contin
moxifloxacin Hcl	Avelox, Vigamox
nabumetone	Relafen
naproxen	Naprosyn, Aleve, Anaprox, Midol ER
niacin	Niaspan, Nia-Bid, Niac, Niacor
nifedipine	Adalat, Procardia
nitrofurantoin	Macrobid, Furadantin, Macrodantin
nystatin	Mycostatin, Nilstat, Nystex, OV Statin
olanzapine	Zyprexa
olmesartan medoxomil	Benicar
omeprazole	Prilosec, Zegerid
ondansetron	Zofran
oseltamivir	Tamiflu

*combination product

Continued

Generic name	Trade name(s)
oxcarbazepine	Trileptal
oxybutynin	Ditropan, Oxytrol
oxycodone	Roxicodone, Endocodone, Oxycontin, M-Oxy
oxycodone and acetaminophen	Percocet, Endocet, Roxicet, Tylox
pantoprazole	Protonix
paroxetine	Paxil, Asimia
penicillins (many variations)	Pentids, Bicillin, Permapen, Wycillin, Veetids, Penacillin VK
phentermine	Adipex-P, Fstin, ObeNix-30, Zantryl
phenylephrine, phenylpropanolamine, and guaifenesin*	Entex
phenytoin	Dilantin
pioglitazone hydrochloride	Actos
piroxicam	Feldene
potassium	K-Lyte, K-Dur, Micro-K, SlowK
pravastatin	Pravachol
prednisolone	Delta-Cortef, Key-Pred, Predalone, Prelone
prednisone	Deltasone, Meticorten, Orasone, Panasol
pregabalin	Lyrica
prochlorperazine	Compazine, Ultrazine, Chlorpazine
promethazine	Phenergan, Phenadoz
promethazine	Phenergan, Phenadoz
propoxyphene	Darvon, Darvon-N, Dolene
propoxyphene and acetaminophen*	Darvocet*
propranolol	Inderal, InnoPran XL
propranolol	Inderal, InnoPran LX
pseudoephedrine	Halofed, Sudafed, Triaminic AM Decongestant Formula
quetiapine	Seroquel
quinapril	Accupril
quinine	Quinamm, Quiphile
rabeprazole	Aciphex
raloxifene	Evista
ramelteon	Rozerem
ramipril	Altace
ranitidine	Zantac
risedronate	Actonel
risperidone	Risperdal
ropinirole	Requip
rosiglitazone maleate	Avandia
rosuvastatin	Crestor
sertraline	Zoloft
sildenafil	Viagra, Revatio
simvastatin	Zocor
spironolactone	Aldactone
sumatriptan	Imitrex
tadalafil	Cialis
tamsulosin	Flomax
tegaserod mesylate	Zelnorm
temazepam	Restoril, Razepam
terazosin	Hytrin
terbinafine	Lamisil
tetracycline	Panmycin, Robitet, Sumycin, Teline, Tetracap, Tetracyn
thyroid	Amour, Thyrar
tiotroppium	Spiriva
tizanidine	Zanaflex
tolterodine	Detrol
topiramate	Topamax
tramadol	Ultram, Zydol
tramadol and acetaminophen*	Ultracet*
trazodone	Desyrel
triamcinolone	Amcort, Aristocort, Azmacort, Kenacort, Kenalog
triamterene	Dyrenium

*combination product

Generic name	Trade name(s)
trimethoprim and sulfamethoxazole	Bactrim, Septra, Cotrim, Co-Rimoxazole
valacyclovir	Valtrex
valsartan	Diovan
vancomycin	Lyphocin, Vancocin, Vancoled
vardenafil	Levitra
venlafaxine	Effexor
verapamil	Calan, Covera-HS, Isoptin, Verelan PM
warfarin	Coumadin, Panwarfarin
ziprasidone	Geodon
zolpidem	Ambien

*combination product

Certification Examination Content Outlines

This appendix provides detailed information about the content students can expect on the medical assistant certification examinations. Students may use this as a study guide along with other examination preparation materials when preparing to take the certified medical assistant (CMA) or registered medical assistant (RMA) examination. However, because examination content is revised annually, students should check with the certifying organization for updates after 2009.

CMA (AAMA)
Certification-Recertification Examination

I. A–F General

A. Medical Terminology

  1. Word building and definitions
    a. Basic structure
      1. roots or stems
      2. prefixes
      3. suffixes
      4. abbreviations
    b. Surgical procedures
    c. Diagnostic procedures
    d. Medical specialties

  2. Uses of terminology
    a. Spelling
    b. Selection and use (e.g., data entry, reports, records, documents, patient education, correspondence, medicolegal documentation, letters, memos, messages, facsimiles)
    c. Reference sources

B. Anatomy and Physiology

  1. Body as a whole, including multiple systems
    a. Structural units
    b. Anatomical divisions
    c. Positions and directions
    d. Body planes
    e. Common diseases and pathology

  2. Systems, including structure, function, related conditions and diseases, and their interrelationships
    a. Integumentary
    b. Musculoskeletal
    c. Nervous
    d. Cardiovascular, hematopoietic, and lymphatic
    e. Respiratory
    f. Digestive
    g. Urinary
    h. Reproductive
    i. Endocrine
    j. Sensory

C. Psychology

  1. Basic principles
    a. Understanding human behavior
      1. Behavioral theories
      2. Death and dying

  2. Developmental stages of the life cycle
    a. Developmental theories used to explain behavior and development
    b. Human growth and development

  3. Defense mechanisms
    a. Recognition
    b. Management

D. Professionalism

  1. Displaying professional attitude
    a. Supporting professional organization
    b. Accepting responsibility for own action

  2. Job readiness and seeking employment
    a. Resumé and cover letter
    b. Methods of job searching
    c. Interviewing as a job candidate

  3. Working as a team member to achieve goals
    a. Member responsibility
    b. Promoting competent patient care
    c. Utilizing principles of group dynamics

E. Communication

  1. Adapting communication according to an individual's needs
    a. Blind
    b. Deaf
    c. Elderly
    d. Children
    e. Seriously ill
    f. Mentally impaired
    g. Illiterate
    h. Non-English-speaking
    i. Anxious
    j. Angry/distraught
    k. Culturally different

2. Recognizing and responding to verbal and nonverbal communication
   a. Body language
   b. Listening skills
   c. Eye contact
   d. Barriers to communication
   e. Identifying needs of others

3. Professional communication and behavior
   a. Professional situations
      1. Tact
      2. Diplomacy
      3. Courtesy
      4. Responsibility/integrity
   b. Therapeutic relationships
      1. Impartial behavior
      2. Empathy/sympathy
      3. Understanding emotional behavior

4. Patient interviewing techniques
   a. Types of questions
      1. Exploratory
      2. Open-ended
      3. Direct
   b. Evaluating effectiveness
      1. Observation
      2. Active listening
      3. Feedback
   c. Legal restrictions

5. Receiving, organizing, prioritizing, and transmitting information
   a. Modalities for incoming and outgoing data (e.g., mail, fax telephone, computer)
   b. Prioritizing incoming and outgoing data (e.g. importance, urgency, recipient availability)

6. Telephone techniques
   a. Incoming calls management criteria
      1. Screening
      2. Maintaining confidentiality
      3. Gathering data
      4. Multiple-line competency
      5. Transferring appropriate calls
      6. Identifying caller, office, and self
      7. Taking messages
      8. Ending calls
   b. Monitoring special calls
      1. Problem calls (e.g., unidentified caller, angry patient, family member)
      2. Emergency calls

7. Fundamental writing skills
   a. Sentence structure
   b. Grammar
   c. Punctuation

F. Medicolegal Guidelines and Requirements

1. Licenses
   a. Medical practice acts
   b. Revocations/suspension of license
      1. Criminal/unprofessional conduct
      2. Professional/personal incapacity

2. Legislation
   a. Advanced directives

b. Anatomical gifts
c. Reportable incidences
   1. Public health statutes (e.g., communicable diseases, vital statistics, substance abuse/chemical dependency, abuse against persons)
   2. Wounds of violence
d. Occupational Safety and Health Act (OSHA)
e. Food and Drug Administration (FDA)
f. Clinical Laboratory Improvement Act (CLIA '88)
g. Americans with Disabilities Act (ADA)
h. Health Insurance Portability and Accountability Act (HIPPA)

3. Documentation/reporting
   a. Sources of information
   b. Drug Enforcement Administration (DEA)
   c. Internal Revenue Service (e.g., personnel forms)
   d. Employment laws
   e. Personal injury occurrences
   f. Workers' compensation
   g. Medical records
      1. Patient activity
      2. Patient care
      3. Patient confidentiality
      4. Ownership
   h. Personnel records
      1. Performance evaluation
      2. Privacy

4. Releasing medical information
   a. Consent
      1. Patient written authorization
      2. Federal codes
         (1) Right to privacy
         (2) Drug and alcohol rehabilitation records
         (3) Public health and welfare disclosures
         (4) HIV-related issues
         (5) Subpoena duces tecum
      3. Rescinding authorization for release

5. Physician-patient relationship
   a. Contract
      1. Legal obligations
      2. Consequences for noncompliance
   b. Responsibility and rights
      1. Patient
      2. Physician
      3. Medical assistant
   c. Guidelines for third-party agreements
   d. Professional liability
      1. Current standard of care
      2. Current legal standards
      3. Informed consent
   e. Arbitration agreements
   f. Affirmation defenses
      1. Statue of limitations
      2. Comparative/contributory negligence
      3. Assumption of risk
   g. Termination of medical care
      1. Establishing policy
      2. Elements for withdrawal
      3. Patient notification and documentation
   h. Medicolegal terms and doctrines

6. Maintaining confidentiality
   a. Agent of the physician
      1. Patient rights
      2. Releasing patient information
   b. Intentional tort
      1. Invasion of privacy
      2. Slander and libel

7. Performing within ethical boundaries
   a. Ethical standards
      1. AAMA Code of Ethics
      2. AMA Code of Ethics
   b. Patient rights
   c. Current issues in medical bioethics

II. G–Q Administrative

G. Data Entry

1. Keyboard fundamentals and functions
   a. Alpha, numeric, and symbol keys
   b. Tabulation

2. Formats
   a. Letters
   b. Memos
   c. Reports
   d. Envelopes
   e. Chart notes

3. Proofreading
   a. Proofreader's marks
   b. Making corrections from rough draft

H. Equipment

1. Equipment operations
   a. Calculator
   b. Photocopier
   c. Computer
   d. Fax machine
   e. Telephone services and features
   f. Scanners

2. Maintenance and repairs
   a. Contents of instruction manual
   b. Routine maintenance
      1. Agreements
      2. Warranty
      3. Repair service

3. Protection and Safety

I. Computer Concepts

1. Computer components
   a. Terminology
   b. Central processing unit (CPU), monitor, keyboard
   c. Printer
   d. Disk drive
   e. Storage devices (e.g., hard drives, magnetic tapes, CD-ROMs, flash drives)
   f. Operating systems
   g. Basic commands

2. Computer applications
   a. Word processing
   b. Database (e.g., menu, fields, records, files)
   c. Spreadsheets, graphics
   d. Electronic mail
   e. Networks
   f. Security/password
   g. Medical management software
      1. Patient data
      2. Report generation

3. Internet services

J. Records Management

1. Needs, purposes, and terminology of filing systems
   a. Basic filing systems
      1. Alphabetic
      2. Numeric/terminal digit
      3. Subject
   b. Special filing systems
      1. Color-code
      2. Tickler file
      3. Electronic data processing files (EDP
      4. Cross-reference/master file

2. Filing guidelines
   a. Storing
   b. Protecting/safekeeping
   c. Transferring

3. Medical records (paper/electronic)
   a. Organization of patient's medical record
   b. Types
      1. Problem oriented
      2. Source oriented
   c. Collecting information
   d. Making corrections
   e. Retaining and purging
      1. Statue of limitations

K. Screening and Processing Mail

1. U.S. Postal Service
   a. Classifications
   b. Types of mail services

2. Postal machine/meter

3. Processing incoming mail

4. Preparing outgoing mail
   a. Labels
   b. Optical Character Reader (OCR) guidelines

L. Scheduling and Monitoring Appointments

1. Utilizing appointment schedules/types
   a. Stream
   b. Wave/Modified wave
   c. Open booking
   d. Categorization

2. Appointment guidelines
   a. Appointment schedule matrix
   b. Legal aspects
   c. New/established patient
   d. Patient needs/preference
   e. Physician preference/habits
   f. Facilities/equipment requirements

3. Appointment protocol
   a. Follow-up visits
     1. Routine
     2. Urgent
   b. Emergency/acutely ill
   c. Physician referrals
   d. Cancellations/no-shows
   e. Physician delay/unavailability
   f. Outside services (e.g., lab, x-ray, surgery)
   g. Reminders/recalls
     1. Appointment cards
     2. Phone calls

M. Resource Information and Community Services

1. Patient advocate
   a. Services available
   b. Appropriate referrals
   c. Follow-up

N. Intentionally left blank (currently there are no items for this category)

O. Maintaining the Office Environment

1. Physical environment
   a. Arrangement of furniture, equipment, and supplies
   b. Facilities and equipment
     1. Maintenance and repair
     2. Safety regulations
       (1) Occupational Safety and Health Act (OSHA)
       (2) Centers for Disease Control and Prevention (CDC) guidelines
       (3) Americans with Disabilities Act (ADA)
       (4) Fire regulations
       (5) Security systems

2. Equipment and supply inventory
   a. Inventory control
   b. Purchasing

3. Maintaining liability coverage
   a. Types of coverage
   b. Recordkeeping

4. Time management
   a. Establishing priorities
   b. Managing routine duties

P. Office Policies and Procedures

1. Patient information booklet

2. Personnel manual

3. Policy and procedures manuals/protocols

Q. Practice Finances

1. Bookkeeping principles
   a. Daily reports, charges slips, receipts, ledgers, etc.
     1. Charges, payments, and adjustments
     2. Identifying and correcting errors
   b. Petty cash

2. Coding systems
   a. Types
     1. Current Procedural Terminology (CPT)
     2. International Classification of Diseases, Clinical Modifications (ICD-CM) (current schedule)

3. Healthcare Financing Common Procedural Coding System (HCPCS Level II)
   b. Relationship between procedures and diagnosis codes

3. Third-party billing
   a. Types
     1. Capitated plans
     2. Commercial carriers
     3. Government plans
       (1) Medicare
       (2) Medicaid
       (3) Tricare
       (4) CHAMPVA
     4. Prepaid HMO, PPO, POS
     5. Worker's compensation
   b. Processing claims
     1. Manual and electronic preparation of claims
     2. Tracing claims
     3. Sequence of filing (e.g., primary versus secondary)
     4. Reconciling payments/rejections
     5. Inquiry and appeal process
   c. Applying managed care policies and procedures
     1. Referrals
     2. Precertification
   d. Fee schedules
     1. Methods for establishing fees
       (1) Relative Value Studies
       (2) Resource-Based Relative Value Scale (RBRVS)
       (3) Diagnosis Related Groups (DRGs)
     2. Contracted fees

4. Accounting and banking procedures
   a. Accounts receivable
     1. Billing procedures
       (1) Itemization
       (2) Billing cycles
     2. Aging/collection procedures
       (1) Collection agencies
       (2) Consumer protection acts
   b. Accounts payable
     1. Ordering goods and services
     2. Monitoring invoices
     3. Tracking merchandise
   c. Banking procedures
     1. Processing accounts receivable
     2. Preparing bank deposit

5. Employee payroll
   a. Calculating wages
   b. Payroll forms

III. R–Z Clinical

R. Principles of Infection Control

1. Principles of asepsis

2. Aseptic technique
   a. Medical asepsis
     1. Handwashing
     2. Sanitization
     3. Chemical disinfection
   b. Surgical asepsis
     1. Scrubbing
     2. Gowning
     3. Gloving

4. Surgical assisting
5. Preparing equipment
6. Preparing items for autoclave
7. Performing sterilization techniques

3. Disposal of biohazardous material

4. Standard precautions

S. Treatment Area

1. Principles of equipment operation
   a. Autoclave/sterilizer
   b. Cast equipment/materials
   c. Electrocardiograph
   d. Examination tables
   e. Microscope
   f. Ophthalmoscope/otoscope/stethoscope
   g. Oxygen
   h. Physical therapy modalities
   i. Endoscopes
   j. Scales
   k. Sphygmomanometers
   l. Spirometer
   m. Thermometers
   n. Nebulizers
   o. Mobility assistive devices
   p. Oximeter

2. Restocking supplies

3. Preparing/maintaining treatment areas

4. Safety precautions

T. Patient Preparation and Assisting the Physician

1. Vital signs
   a. Performing
   b. Recording

2. Examinations
   a. Types
   b. Body positions
   c. Body mechanics

3. Procedures
   a. Instruments, supplies, and equipment
   b. Explanation and instructions

4. Providing education for health maintenance and disease prevention

U. Patient History Interview

1. Components of patient history
   a. Personal data
   b. Chief complaint
   c. Past, present, family, and social history
   d. Review of systems

2. Documentation guidelines

V. Collecting and Processing Specimens; Diagnostic Testing

1. Methods of collection
   a. Blood
      1. Vein
      2. Capillary
   b. Urine

c. Stool
d. Sputum
e. Cultures
   1. Throat
   2. Vaginal
   3. Wounds
   4. Urine
   5. Blood

2. Processing specimens
   a. Centers for Disease Control and Prevention (CDC) guidelines
   b. Proper labeling
   c. Contamination
   d. Specimen preservation
   e. Recordkeeping

3. Quality control

4. Performing selected tests
   a. Urinalysis
      1. Physical
      2. Chemical
      3. Microscopic
   b. Hematology
      1. Hematocrit
      2. Hemoglobin
      3. Erythrocyte sedimentation rate
      4. Automated cell counts
         (1) Red blood cell (RBC)
         (2) White blood cell (WBC)
         (3) Platelet
      5. Coagulation testing
   c. Blood chemistry
      1. Glucose
      2. Kidney function tests
      3. Liver function tests
      4. Lipid profile
      5. Hemoglobin A1c
   d. Immunology
      1. Mono test
      2. *Strep* test
      3. C-reactive protein (CRP)
      4. Pregnancy testing
   e. Microbiology
      1. Theory/terminology
         (1) Bacteria
            i. Gram's staining
         (2) Virus
         (3) Fungus
         (4) Parasites
         (5) Protozoa
   f. Tuberculosis testing
   g. Guaiac testing

5. Electrocardiography (EKG/ECG)

6. Vision testing

7. Hearing testing

8. Respiratory testing
   a. Pulmonary function
   b. Spirometry
   c. Pulse oximetry
   d. Nebulizer treatment

9. Medical imaging
   a. Safety principles
   b. Patient preparation
   c. Patient instruction

W. Preparing and Administering Medications

1. Pharmacology
   a. Classes of drugs
   b. Drug forms
   c. Drug actions/uses
   d. Side effects/adverse reactions
   e. Emergency use
   f. Substance abuse

2. Preparing and administering oral and parenteral medications
   a. Calculation of dosage
   b. Routes of administration
   c. Types of injections
   d. Injection sites

3. Prescriptions
   a. Safekeeping
   b. Medication recordkeeping
   c. Controlled substance guidelines

4. Immunizations
   a. Childhood
   b. Adult vaccines
   c. Storage
   d. Recordkeeping

5. Principles of IV therapy
   a. Terminology
   b. Theory (excludes administration of IV medications)

X. Emergencies

1. Preplanned action
   a. Policies and procedures
   b. Legal implications and action documentation
   c. Equipment
      1. Crash cart
      2. Automated external defibrillator

2. Assessment and triage

3. Emergency preparedness

Y. First Aid

1. Identifying and responding to
   a. Bleeding/pressure points
   b. Burns

c. Cardiac and respiratory arrest/CPR
d. Choking/Heimlich maneuver
e. Diabetic coma/insulin shock
f. Fractures
g. Poisoning
h. Seizures
i. Shock
j. Stroke
k. Syncope
l. Wounds

Z. Nutrition

1. Basic principles
   a. Dietary guidelines
   b. Food nutrients (e.g., vitamins, minerals)

2. Special needs
   a. Diets
   b. Restrictions

Registered Medical Assistant Examination

General Medical Assisting Knowledge—41%*

- Anatomy and physiology
- Medical terminology
- Medical law
- Medical ethics
- Human relations
- Patient education

Administrative Medical Assisting—24%*

- Insurance
- Financial and bookkeeping
- Medical receptionist/secretarial/clerical

Clinical Medical Assisting—35%*

- Asepsis
- Sterilization
- Instruments
- Vital signs and mensurations
- Physical examinations
- Clinical pharmacology
- Minor surgery
- Therapeutic modalities
- Laboratory procedures
- Electrocardiography
- First aid

---

* Approximate percentages of questions in content areas

Index